AVOIDING COMMON ERRORS IN THE EMERGENCY

This book is due for return on or before the last date shown below.

- 7 APR 2015

1 5 MAY 2019

D1380369

Acquisitions Editor: Frances DeStefano
Product Manager: Julia Seto
Production Manager: Alicia Jackson
Senior Manufacturing Manager: Benjamin Rivera
Senior Marketing Manager: Angela Panetta
Design Coordinator: Holly McLaughlin
Production Service: SPi Technologies

© 2010 by **LIPPINCOTT WILLIAMS & WILKINS**, a **WOLTERS KLUWER** business
Two Commerce Square
2001 Market Street
Philadelphia, PA 19103 USA

Printed in China

Library of Congress Cataloging-in-Publication Data
Avoiding common errors in the emergency department / editors, Amal Mattu ... [et al.].
    p. ; cm. — (Errors series)
  Includes bibliographical references.
  ISBN 978-1-60547-227-0
 1. Emergency medicine. 2. Medical errors. I. Mattu, Amal. II. Series: Errors series.
  [DNLM: 1. Critical Care—methods. 2. Emergency Service, Hospital. 3. Medical Errors—prevention & control. WX 215 A9605 2011]
  RC86.7.A96   2011
  616.02'5—dc22

                                                                            2010004704

Care has been taken to confirm the accuracy of the information presented and to describe generally accepted practices. However, the authors, editors, and publisher are not responsible for errors or omissions or for any consequences from application of the information in this book and make no warranty, expressed or implied, with respect to the currency, completeness, or accuracy of the contents of the publication. Application of the information in a particular situation remains the professional responsibility of the practitioner.

The authors, editors, and publisher have exerted every effort to ensure that drug selection and dosage set forth in this text are in accordance with current recommendations and practice at the time of publication. However, in view of ongoing research, changes in government regulations, and the constant flow of information relating to drug therapy and drug reactions, the reader is urged to check the package insert for each drug for any change in indications and dosage and for added warnings and precautions. This is particularly important when the recommended agent is a new or infrequently employed drug.

Some drugs and medical devices presented in the publication have Food and Drug Administration (FDA) clearance for limited use in restricted research settings. It is the responsibility of the health care provider to ascertain the FDA status of each drug or device planned for use in their clinical practice.

To purchase additional copies of this book, call our customer service department at (800) 638-3030 or fax orders to (301) 223-2320. International customers should call (301) 223-2300.

Visit Lippincott Williams & Wilkins on the Internet: at LWW.com. Lippincott Williams & Wilkins customer service representatives are available from 8:30 am to 6 pm, EST.

CCS1010

DISCLAIMER

The editors and authors of this textbook strongly believe that the complex practice of medicine, the vagaries of human diseases, the unpredictability of pathologic conditions, and the functions, dysfunctions, and responses of the human body cannot be defined, explained, or rigidly categorized by any written document. *It is neither the purpose nor the intent of our textbook to serve as a final authoritative source on any medical condition, treatment plan, or clinical intervention, nor should our textbooks be used to rigorously define a rigid standard of care that should be practiced by all clinicians.*

Every medical encounter must be individualized, and every patient must be approached on a case-by-case basis. At any given moment in time, a physician's actions and interventions should be guided by real-time, unique circumstances, the current clinical and historical milieu, available resources, his or her individual experience, and, most importantly, clinical judgment.

Every attempt has been made to ensure the accuracy of management recommendations and medication dosages. However, the reader is urged to consult other resources for confirmation of recommendations and medication dosages.

The editors are pleased to accept comments, corrections, and suggestions. Please send them to insidesurgery@gmail.com

There is no question that emergency medicine is a high-risk specialty. Emergency physicians and other acute care providers are tasked with caring for patients they do not know in a time-pressured and crowded environment. Complicating matters further is the fact that the majority of patients in the emergency department have non–life-threatening conditions, so providers may be easily lulled into a false sense of security that the patient in front of them has a benign condition. The great challenge in emergency medicine is to sort through the morass of benign conditions and properly diagnose and treat the deadly ones. Emergency care providers face many other challenges: delivering care efficiently, communicating with patients effectively, and discharging patients with instructions that ensure a safe transition to further care. Errors in this fast-paced setting are inevitable.

To help providers minimize errors, we have focused on those that occur most frequently, those with the greatest potential to cause harm to our patients, and those that pose significant medicolegal risk to providers. Errors and pitfalls are organized by organ system. In addition, sections that focus on nonclinical aspects of emergency medicine practice such as proper documentation, communication with consultants, and interactions with lawyers are also included. It is our expectation that the sections will be read not in a single sitting but in short sessions over the course of weeks or months. For that reason, some redundancy has been built into the text in order to emphasize key points.

We would like to thank the authors and associate editors for the significant time and effort that they have devoted to making their chapters informative, cutting-edge, and practical. We also thank the Errors Series Editor Dr. Lisa Marcucci for giving us this opportunity to make what we believe is an important educational contribution to our specialty and the staff at Lippincott Williams & Wilkins for their support of this work. Finally, on behalf of all of the authors and editors, we would like to thank our patients, our colleagues, and our families for providing the inspiration to carry on our work.

It is our sincere hope that the reader finds this text practical and usable and that our focus on these common errors produces a tangible improvement in patient care. Our best wishes to you and your patients!

AMAL MATTU, MD
ARJUN S. CHANMUGAM, MD, MBA
STUART P. SWADRON, MD, FRCPC
CARRIE D. TIBBLES, MD
DALE P. WOOLRIDGE, MD, PHD

ACKNOWLEDGMENTS

I would like to thank my wife, Sejal, for her constant support and encouragement. I thank my children, Nikhil, Eleena, and Kamran, for always reminding me of my proper priorities in life. I thank the faculty, residents, and students at the University of Maryland School of Medicine for providing me the inspiration for the work I do every day. Finally, thanks are also due to Dr. Lisa Marcucci and Lippincott Williams & Wilkins for giving us this opportunity to contribute to our specialty.

—Amal Mattu, MD

This book is dedicated to Karen, my beloved wife; to Sydney, William, and Nathan who have made me appreciate the really important things in life; to my parents who fostered a spirit of growth; and to the residents and students of emergency medicine who help us all to remember the joy of learning and who reinforce a commitment to one of the greatest specialties.

—Arjun S. Chanmugam, MD, MBA

I would like to thank my wife, Joyce, and the residents, students, faculty, and patients at the Los Angeles County/University of Southern California Medical Center for their constant support and inspiration.

—Stuart P. Swadron, MD, FRCPC

To God, Michael and the boys, and my family and friends, for providing me with joy and inspiration. To the past and current Beth Israel Deaconess Medical Center emergency medicine residents from whom I have learned so much.

—Carrie D. Tibbles, MD

My ability to contribute to this project derives directly from those who support me in my day-to-day life. So, this is for them: my wife, Michelle, my daughter, Anna, and son, Garrett. I would be remiss without also thanking the University of Arizona's combined emergency medicine and pediatric residents who make every day a day of learning.

—Dale P. Woolridge, MD, PhD

ASSOCIATE EDITORS

CRAIG T. CARTER, DO
Assistant Professor
Medical Director, Pediatric Emergency Medicine
Department of Emergency Medicine and
    Pediatrics
University of Kentucky College of Medicine
Lexington, Kentucky

BRIAN D. CLOTHIER, MD, MS
Emergency Physician
Department of Emergency Medicine
Salem Hospital
Salem, Oregon

SERIC CUSICK, MD
Assistant Professor and Director
Ultrasound Fellowship Program
Department of Emergency Medicine
Sacramento, California

**JORGE A. FERNANDEZ, MD,
FAAEM, FACEP**
Assistant Professor
Department of Emergency Medicine
Keck School of Medicine
University of Southern California
Medical Student Clerkship Director
Department of Emergency Medicine
Los Angeles County/University of Southern
    California Medical Center
Los Angeles, California

**ALBERT FIORELLO, MD, RDMS,
FAAEM, FACEP**
Assistant Professor, Clinical Emergency Medicine
Associate Residency Director
Director, Emergency Medicine Ultrasound
Department of Emergency Medicine
University of Arizona
Attending Physician
Department of Emergency Medicine
University Medical Center
Tucson, Arizona

SEAN M. FOX, MD
Adjunct Clinical Instructor
Department of Emergency Medicine
University of North Carolina School of Medicine
Chapel Hill, North Carolina
Faculty in Pediatric & Adult Emergency Medicine
Department of Emergency Medicine
Carolinas Medical Center
Charlotte, North Carolina

ELLIOTT R. HAUT, MD, FACS
Assistant Professor
Department of Surgery and Anesthesiology
    and Critical Care Medicine
The Johns Hopkins University School of
    Medicine
Director, Trauma/Acute Care Surgery Fellowship
The Johns Hopkins Hospital
Baltimore, Maryland

TARLAN HEDAYATI, MD
Assistant Professor
Department of Emergency Medicine
Rush Medical College
Attending Physician
Department of Emergency Medicine
John Stroger Hospital of Cook County
Chicago, Illinois

JULIANNA JUNG, MD, FACEP
Assistant Professor
Department of Emergency Medicine
Johns Hopkins University School of Medicine
Attending Physician
Department of Emergency Medicine
Johns Hopkins Hospital
Baltimore, Maryland

CHRISTINE A. KLETTI, MD
Assistant Program Director
Hennepin County Medical Center
Department of Emergency Medicine
Minneapolis, Minnesota

CONTRIBUTORS

DIEGO ABDELNUR, MD
Attending Staff Physician
Department of Emergency Medicine
Long Beach Memorial Medical Center
Long Beach, California

JASON D. ADLER, MD
Resident Physician
Department of Emergency Medicine
University of Maryland Medical Center
Baltimore, Maryland

RICHARD AMINI, MD
Resident
Department of Emergency Medicine
University Medical Center
Tucson, Arizona

JONATHAN S. ANDERSON, MD
Resident Physician
Beth Israel Deaconess Medical Center
Harvard Affiliated Emergency Medicine Residency
Boston, Massachusetts

ROBERT S. ANDERSON, JR, MD
Chief Resident
Department of Emergency Medicine and
  Internal Medicine
University of Maryland School of Medicine
Baltimore, Maryland

NATHANIEL ARNONE, MD
Resident Physician
Department of Emergency Medicine
University of Arizona
Tucson, Arizona

JENNIFER M. BAHR, MD
Emergency Physician and EMS Medical Director
Department of Emergency Medicine
Divine Savior Healthcare
Portage, Wisconsin

JENNIFER BAINE, MD
Resident Physician
Stanford University Hospital
Stanford, California

AMIRA BASS, MD
Resident Physician
Stanford University Hospital
Stanford, California

SALAH BAYDOUN, MD
St Luke's-Roosevelt Hospital
New York City, New York

JONATHAN C. BERGER, MD
Surgery Resident
Department of Surgery
Johns Hopkins Univeristy School of Medicine
Surgery Resident
Department of Surgery
Johns Hopkins Hospital
Baltimore, Maryland

RUSSELL BERGER, MD
Resident Physician
Harvard Affiliated Emergency Medicine Residency
Beth Israel Deaconess Medical Center
Boston, Massachusetts

EDWARD S. BESSMAN, MD, MBA
Assistant Professor
Department of Emergency Medicine
The Johns Hopkins University
Chairman
Department of Emergency Medicine
Johns Hopkins Bayview Medical Center
Baltimore, Maryland

COLLEEN BIRMINGHAM, MD
Resident
Department of Emergency Medicine
Beth Israel Deaconess Medical Center
Boston, Massachusetts

ATANU BISWAS, MD, MSc
Resident
Department of Surgery
University of Arizona
Resident
Department of Surgery
University Medical Center
Tucson, Arizona

SHARON BORD, MD

Instructor
Department of Emergency Medicine
Johns Hopkins University
Instructor
Department of Emergency Medicine
Johns Hopkins Bayview Medical Center
Baltimore, Maryland

EDUARDO BORQUEZ, MD

Assistant Professor
Department of Emergency Medicine
Keck School of Medicine
University of Southern California
Assistant Residency Program Director
Department of Emergency Medicine
Los Angeles County/University of Southern
  California Medical Center
Los Angeles, California

HANS BRADSHAW, MD

Chief Resident
Department of Pediatrics and Emergency
  Medicine
University of Arizona
Tucson, Arizona

BENJAMIN BRASLOW, MD

Assistant Professor
Department of Surgery
University of Pennsylvania Medical School
Division of Traumatology/Surgical Critical Care
  & Emergency General Surgery
Hospital of The University of Pennsylvania
Philadelphia, Pennsylvania

RANDOLPH N. BROWN, MD

Emergency Medicine Resident
Department of Emergency Medicine
Johns Hopkins Hospital
Baltimore, Maryland

TERRENCE W. BROWN, MD, JD, MS

Attending Physician
Department of Emergency Medicine
Emergency Professional Services, P.C.
Banner Good Samaritan Medical Center
Phoenix, Arizona

CHARLES A. BRUEN, MD

Resident Physician
Department of Emergency Medicine
Hennepin County Medical Center
Minneapolis, Minnesota

BRYAN BUCHANAN, MD

Resident
Emergency Department
Christus Spohn Memorial/Texas A&M
  University
Corpus Christi, Texas

JOHN W. BURGER, MD

Chief Resident
Department of Emergency Medicine
Johns Hopkins School of Medicine
Chief Resident
Department of Emergency Medicine
Johns Hopkins Hospital
Baltimore, Maryland

LAURA BURKE, MD

Resident Physician
Harvard Affiliated Emergency Medicine
  Residency
Beth Israel Deaconess Medical Center
Boston, Massachusetts

J. BRACKEN BURNS, JR, DO

Assistant Professor
Department of Surgery Division of Acute Care
  Surgery
University of Florida College of
  Medicine—Jacksonville
Medical Director of Flight Services
Associate Program Director of General Surgery
  Residency
Department of Surgery Division of Acute Care
  Surgery
University of Florida Health Science Center
  Jacksonville
Jacksonville, Florida

XZABIA CALISTE, MD

Trauma Research Fellow
Department of Surgery, Trauma Services
Washington Hospital Center
Washington, District of Columbia

EMILIE J. B. CALVELLO, MD, MPH

Clinical Instructor
Department of Emergency Medicine
Johns Hopkins Hospital
Baltimore, Maryland
Staff Physician
Department of Emergency Medicine
Howard County General Hospital
Columbia, Maryland

DARRYL V. CALVO, MD
Resident Physician
Department of Emergency Medicine
Hennepin County Medical Center
Minneapolis, Minnesota

EMILY A. CARPENTER ROSE, MD
Assistant Professor
Department of Emergency Medicine
Keck School of Medicine
University of Southern California
Attending Staff
Department of Emergency Medicine
Los Angeles County/University of Southern
   California Medical Center
Los Angeles, California

STEPHANIE M. CASTRILLO, MD
Pediatric Resident
Department of Pediatrics
University of Arizona
Pediatric Resident
Department of Pediatrics
University Medical Center
Tucson, Arizona

ESTHER I. CHANG, MD
Resident
Wilmer Eye Institute
Baltimore, Maryland

RICHARD J. CHANG, MD
Resident Physician
Department of Emergency Medicine
Hennepin County Medical Center
Minneapolis, Minnesota

YIAN (MICHAEL) CHENG, MD
Resident Clinical Instructor
Department of Emergency Medicine
Keck School of Medicine
University of Southern California
Chief Resident
Department of Emergency Medicine
Los Angeles County/University of Southern
   California Medical Center
Los Angeles, California

TIMOTHY P. CHIZMAR, MD
Senior Resident
Department of Emergency Medicine
University of Maryland School
   of Medicine
Senior Resident
Department of Emergency Medicine
University of Maryland Medical Center
Baltimore, Maryland

SARAH CHRISTIAN-KOPP, MD
Emergency Medicine Resident
Department of Emergency Medicine
Maricopa Medical Center
Phoenix, Arizona

CONRAD J. CLEMENS, MD, MPH
Associate Professor of Clinical Pediatrics
Department of Pediatrics
University of Arizona
Director, Pediatric Residency Program
Department of Pediatrics
University Medical Center
Tucson, Arizona

KRISTIN COCHRAN, MD
Resident Physician
Beth Israel Deaconess Medical Center
Harvard Affiliated Emergency Medicine
   Residency
Boston, Massachusetts

JON B. COLE, MD
Medical Toxicology Fellow
Department of Emergency Medicine
Regions Hospital
St Paul, Minnesota

ANGELA P. CORNELIUS, MD
Resident Physician
Christus Spohn Emergency Medicine Program
Department of Emergency Medicine
Texas A&M University
Resident Physician
Department of Emergency Medicine
Christus Spohn Memorial Hospital
Corpus Christi, Texas

JAMES E. CORWIN, MD
Assistant Clinical Faculty
Department of Emergency Medicine
Johns Hopkins University School of Medicine
Urgent Care Division Director
Department of Emergency Medicine
The Johns Hopkins Hospital
Baltimore, Maryland

MELISSA W. COSTELLO, MD, FACEP
Associate Professor
Department of Emergency Medicine
University of South Alabama
Mobile, Alabama

STEPHEN A. CRANDALL, MD
Good Samaritan Regional Medical Center
Corvalis, Oregon

JUSTIN A. DAVIS, MD, MPH
Associate Physician
Subchief for Emergency Ultrasound Services
Kaiser Oakland Medical Center
Oakland, California

TROY DEAN, MD
Resident Physician
University of California Davis Medical Center
Sacramento, California

MATTHIEU DE CLERCK, MD
Resident Clinical Instructor
Department of Emergency Medicine
Keck School of Medicine
University of Southern California
Chief Resident
Department of Emergency Medicine
Los Angeles County/University of Southern
   California Medical Center
Los Angeles, California

JAMES DE LA TORRE, MD, MMM
Clinical Instructor
Department of Emergency Medicine
USC-Los Angeles County
Los Angeles, California
Associate Director of Emergency Services
Department of Emergency Medicine
West Hills Hospital/Medical Center
West Hills, California

**LAWRENCE A. DELUCA, JR,
EDD, MD**
Instructor
Department of Clinical Emergency Medicine
University of Arizona
UPH at University Medical Center and
   University Physicians Hospitals
Tucson, Arizona

**GERARD DEMERS, DO, DHSC,
MPH**
Academic Chief Resident
Emergency Medicine Department
Naval Medical Center of San Diego
San Diego, California

SAMIT DESAI, MD
Resident
Department of Emergency Medicine
Johns Hopkins Hospital
Baltimore, Maryland

SHOMA DESAI, MD
Assistant Professor
Department of Emergency Medicine
Keck School of Medicine

University of Southern California
Quality Improvement Director
Department of Emergency Medicine
Los Angeles County/University of Southern
   California Medical Center
Los Angeles, California

**STEPHEN DOCHERTY, DO,
FAAEM, FACEP**
Assistant Professor
Department of Emergency Medicine
Keck School of Medicine
University of Southern California
Director
Center for Life Support Training and Research
Department of Emergency Medicine
Los Angeles County/University of Southern
   California Medical Center
Los Angeles, California

JOSEPH J. DUBOSE, MD, FACS
Clinical Assistant Professor of Surgery
University of Maryland Medical System
R Adams Cowley Shock Trauma Center
Baltimore, Maryland

ANDREA DUGAS, MD
Resident Physician
Harvard Affiliated Emergency Medicine
   Residency
Beth Israel Deaconess Medical Center
Boston, Massachusetts

STEPHEN J. DUNLOP, MD
Assistant Professor
Department of Emergency Medicine
University of Minnesota
Fellow in International Emergency Medicine
Department of Emergency Medicine
Hennepin County Medical Center
Minneapolis, Minnesota

**ANITA W. EISENHART, DO,
FACOEP, FACEP**
Assistant Program Director
Emergency Medicine Residency
Pediatric Emergency Department
Arizona Childrens Hospital
Maricopa Medical Center
Phoenix, Arizona

MICHAEL L. EPTER, DO, FAAEM
Assistant Professor
Department of Emergency Medicine
University of Nevada School of Medicine
Program Director
Department of Emergency Medicine
University Medical Center
Las Vegas, Nevada

DAVID FARMAN, MD
Attending Physician
Department of Emergency Medicine
Hendricks Regional Health
Danville, Indiana

ADAM G. FIELD, MD
Staff Physician
Department of Emergency Medicine
Naval Medical Center of San Diego
San Diego, California

ERINE OI MING FONG, MD
Resident Physician
Department of Emergency Medicine
Hennepin County Medical Center
Minneapolis, Minnesota

NICOLAS P. FORGET, MD, DTMH
Clinical Instructor
Department of Emergency Medicine
Keck School of Medicine
University of Southern California
Merkin Fellow of International Emergency
    Medicine
Department of Emergency Medicine
Los Angeles County/University of Southern
    California Medical Center
Los Angeles, California

LISA FORT, MD
St Luke's-Roosevelt Hospital
New York City, New York

**HEIDI L. FRANKEL, MD, FACS,
FCCM**
Chief
Department of Trauma, Acute Care and Critical
    Care Surgery
Penn State Milton S. Hershey Medical Center
Hershey, Pennsylvania

ADAM D. FRIEDLANDER, MD
Departments of Emergency Medicine and
    Pediatrics
University of Maryland School of Medicine
Baltimore, Maryland

**DREW L. FULLER, MD, MPH,
FACEP**
Instructor
Department of Emergency Medicine
Johns Hopkins Medical Institute
Director, Patient Safety
Department of Emergency Medicine
Johns Hopkins Bayview Medical Center
Baltimore, Maryland

JASON GAJARSA, MD
Fellow
Division of Cardiology
Harbor-UCLA Medical Center
Torrance, California

CHARLIE GALANIS, MD
Chief Resident
Department of Surgery
Johns Hopkins University
Chief Resident
Department of Surgery
The Johns Hopkins Hospital
Baltimore, Maryland

GREG GARDNER, MD
Department of Emergency Medicine
University of Arizona
Department of Emergency Medicine
University Medical Center
Tucson, Arizona

FIONA M. GARLICH, MD
Resident Physician
Department of Emergency Medicine
Hennepin County Medical Center
Minneapolis, Minnesota

**JACQUELINE GARONZIK-WANG,
MD**
Surgery Resident
Department of Surgery
Johns Hopkins Hospital
Baltimore, Maryland

ARTI GEHANI, MD
Resident Clinical Instructor
Department of Emergency Medicine
Keck School of Medicine
University of Southern California
Senior Resident Physician
Department of Emergency Medicine
Los Angeles County/University of Southern
    California Medical Center
Los Angeles, California

JEFFREY T. GERTON, MD, MBA
Department of Emergency Medicine
Upper Chesapeake Medical Center
Bel Air, Maryland

ALBERT L. GEST, DO
Assistant Professor
Department of Emergency Medicine
Corpus Christi Emergency Medicine Residency
Assistant Professor
Christus-Spohn Hospital–Corpus Christi,
    Memorial
Corpus Christi, Texas

LALEH GHARAHBAGHIAN, MD
Associate Director
Department of Emergency Ultrasound
Stanford University Medical Center
Stanford, California

ALISA GIBSON, MD, DMD
Resident
Department of Emergency Medicine
University of Maryland
Baltimore, Maryland

COLLEEN ANNA GIBSON, MD
Senior Resident
Department of Emergency Medicine
University of Maryland Medical Center
Baltimore, Maryland

CHARLES G. GILLESPIE, MD
Resident Physician
Department of Emergency Medicine
University of Arizona
Tuczon, Arizona

EVAN S. GLAZER, MD, MPH
Resident
Department of Surgery
The University of Arizona
Resident
Department of Surgery
University Medical Center
Tucson, Arizona

KEVIN GREER, MD
Resident
Department of Emergency Medicine
Harvard Medical School
Resident Physician
Harvard Affiliated Emergency Medicine Residency
Beth Israel Deaconess Medical Center
Boston, Massachusetts

SARAH E. GREER, MD, MPH
Instructor
Department of Surgery
Dartmouth Medical School
Hanover, New Hampshire
Resident
Department of Surgery
Dartmouth Hitchcock Medical Center
Lebanon, New Hampshire

MICHAEL D. GROSSMAN, MD, FACS
Associate Professor
Department of Clinical Surgery
Division of Trauma and Surgical Critical Care
University of Pennsylvania
Philadelphia, Pennsylvania
Chief, Division of Trauma, Emergency Surgery
    and Surgical Critical Care
St Luke Hospital
Bethlehem, Pennsylvania

KHAWAR M. GUL, MD
Fellow
Division of Cardiology
Harbor-UCLA Medical Center
Torrance, California

JOHN GULLETT, MD
Assistant Professor
Department of Emergency Medicine
SUNY Downstate Medical Center/Kings
    County Hospital
Brooklyn, New York

RAJAN GUPTA, MD, FACS, FCCP
Associate Professor
Department of Surgery
Dartmouth Medical School
Hanover, New Hampshire
Attending Staff
Department of Surgery
Dartmouth Hitchcock Medical Center
Lebanon, New Hampshire

ADIL HAIDER, MD, MPH
Assistant Professor
Department of Surgery and Anesthesiology and
    Critical Care Medicine
The Johns Hopkins University School of
    Medicine
Assistant Professor Surgery & Health Policy
    and Management
The Johns Hopkins Hospital
Baltimore, Maryland

DIANA A. HANS, DO
Chief Resident
Department of Emergency Medicine
Maricopa Medical Center
Phoenix, Arizona

LISA M. HAYDEN, MD
Resident Physician
Department of Emergency Medicine
Hennepin County Medical Center
Minneapolis, Minnesota

ASHLEIGH HEGEDUS, MD
Resident Physician
Beth Israel Deaconess Medical Center
Harvard Affiliated Emergency Medicine Residency
Boston, Massachusetts

ERIC J. HEMMINGER, MD
Fellow
Division of Cardiology
Harbor–UCLA Medical Center
Torrance, California

JESSICA HERNANDEZ, MD
Resident
Department of Emergency Medicine
St Luke's-Roosevelt Hospital
Columbia College of Physicians & Surgeons
New York

CHANDLER H. HILL, MD
Emergency Physician
Department of Emergency Medicine
Mercy Hospital
Coon Rapids, Minnesota

KATHERINE M. HILLER, MD, FACEP
Assistant Professor
Department of Emergency Medicine
University of Arizona
Assistant Professor
Department of Emergency Medicine
University Medical Center
Tucson, Arizona

EVELINE A. HITTI, MD
Instructor of Clinical Medicine
Department of Emergency Medicine
American University of Beirut
  Medical Center
New York City, New York

BEATRICE HOFFMANN, MD, PHD, RDMS
Assistant Professor
Department of Emergency Ultrasound
Department of Emergency Medicine
Johns Hopkins University
Fellowship Director
Department of Emergency Medicine
Johns Hopkins Medical Institutions
Baltimore, Maryland

STEPHEN G. HOLTZCLAW, MD, FACEP
Instructor
Department of Emergency Medicine
Johns Hopkins
Baltimore, Maryland
President and Chief Medical Officer
Team Health Southeast
Fort Lauderdale, Florida

JOHN E. JESUS, MD
Resident Physician
Harvard Affiliated Emergency Medicine
  Residency
Beth Israel Deaconess Medical Center
Boston, Massachusetts

NATHANIEL R. JOHNSON, MD, PHD
Resident
Pediatrics
Department of Emergency Medicine
University of Arizona
Tucson, Arizona

SONIA Y. JOHNSON, MD
Resident Clinical Instructor
Department of Emergency Medicine
Keck School of Medicine
University of Southern California
Senior Resident Physician
Department of Emergency Medicine
Los Angeles County/University of Southern
  California Medical Center
Los Angeles, California

CLAYTON P. JOSEPHY, MD
Department of Emergency Medicine
University of Arizona
Tucson, Arizona

SAI-HUNG JOSHUA HUI, MD
Assistant Clinical Professor
Department of Emergency Medicine
David Geffen School of Medicine at UCLA
Los Angeles, California
Director of Simulation
Department of Emergency Medicine
Olive View–UCLA Medical Center
Sylmar, California

MISHA KASSEL, MD
Resident Physician
Stanford University Hospital
Stanford, California

ERIC D. KATZ, MD, FAAEM, FACEP
Associate Professor—Clinical
Department of Emergency Medicine
University of Arizona College of
  Medicine—Phoenix
Vice-chair for Education and Program Director
Department of Emergency Medicine
Maricopa Medical Center
Phoenix, Arizona

CLINTON D. KEMP, MD
Resident
Department of Surgery
The Johns Hopkins University School of
    Medicine
Resident
Department of Surgery
The Johns Hopkins Hospital
Baltimore, Maryland

MAURA KENNEDY, MD
Resident Physician
Beth Israel Deaconess Medical Center
Harvard Affiliated Emergency Medicine Residency
Boston, Massachusetts

ANDREW J. KERWIN, MD
Associate Professor
Department of Surgery
Division Chief, Acute Care Surgery
University of Florida College of
    Medicine—Jacksonville
Trauma Medical Director
Shands Jacksonville
Jacksonville, Florida

KATHERINE W. KHALIFEH, MD
Surgical Resident
Department of Surgery
Johns Hopkins Hospital
Baltimore, Maryland

FAHAD KHAN, MD
St Luke's-Roosevelt Hospital
New York City, New York

POOJA KHANDELWAL, MD
Resident
Department of Pediatrics
University of Arizona College of Medicine
Tucson, Arizona

SAMIUR R. KHANDKER, MD
Resident Physician
Department of Emergency Medicine
Johns Hopkins University School of Medicine
Baltimore, Maryland

ALICIA N. KIENINGER, MD
Assistant Professor
Department of Surgery
Washington University
Associate Program Director, General Surgery
    Residency Program
Barnes_Jewish Hospital
St Louis, Missouri

JONATHAN KIRSCHNER, MD
St Luke's-Roosevelt Hospital
New York City, New York

DOHWA KIM, MD
Assistant Professor
Section Head, Geriatric Medicine
Department of Internal Medicine
Keck School of Medicine
University of Southern California
Program Director, Geriatric Fellowship Program
Los Angeles County/University of Southern
    California Medical Center
Los Angeles, California

JESSE H. KIM, MD
Clinical Instructor
Department of Medicine
University of Washington
Seattle, Washington
Attending Physician
Emergency Department
St Francis Hospital
Federal Way, Washington

EDWARD KIMLIN, MD
Resident Physician
Harvard Affiliated Emergency Medicine Residency
Beth Israel Deaconess Medical Center
Boston, Massachusetts

THOMAS D. KIRSCH, MD, MPH
Associate Professor
Department of Emergency Medicine
Johns Hopkins School of Medicine
Director of Faculty Practice
Department of Emergency Medicine
Johns Hopkins Hospital
Baltimore, Maryland

ALEXANDER A. KLEINMANN, MD
Senior Resident
Department of Emergency Medicine
Thomas Jefferson University Hospital
Philadelphia, Pennsylvania

COLLEEN C. KNIFFIN, MD
Resident Physician
Department of Emergency Medicine
Hennepin County Medical Center
Minneapolis, Minnesota

MONICA KUMAR, MD
Resident Clinical Instructor
Department of Emergency Medicine
Keck School of Medicine

University of Southern California
Senior Resident Physician
Department of Emergency Medicine
Los Angeles County/University of Southern
   California Medical Center
Los Angeles, California

ZULEIKA LADHA, MD
Attending Physician
Department of Emergency Medicine
Long Island College Hospital
Brooklyn, New York

ALDEN LANDRY, MD
Resident Physician
Harvard Affiliated Emergency Medicine Residency
Beth Israel Deaconess Medical Center
Boston, Massachusetts

SARAH J. LANNUM, MD
Attending Physician
Department of Emergency Medicine
Kaiser Permanente
Walnut Creek, California

JONATHAN LARSON, MD
Metropolitan Methodist Hospital
San Antonia, Texas

TINA M. LATIMER, MD, MPH
Medical Education Fellow
Department of Emergency Medicine
The Johns Hopkins University School of
   Medicine
Instructor
Department of Emergency Medicine
The Johns Hopkins Hospital
Baltimore, Maryland

JENNIFER LAW, MD
Resident Physician
University of California Davis Medical Center
Sacramento, California

**BENJAMIN J. LAWNER, DO,
EMT-P**
Clinical Instructor and Attending Physician
Department of Emergency Medicine
University of Maryland School of Medicine
Baltimore, Maryland

BRYAN S. LEE, MD, JD
Resident
Wilmer Eye Institute
Johns Hopkins University
Resident
Wilmer Eye Institute
Johns Hopkins Hospital
Baltimore, Maryland

JAE LEE, MD
Attending Emergency Physician
Florida

JARONE LEE, MD, MPH
Chief Resident
Department of Emergency Medicine
Columbia University
Chief Resident
Department of Emergency Medicine
St Luke's Roosevelt Hospital Center
New York City, New York

BEN A. LEESON, MD, FACEP
Assistant Professor
Emergency Department
Christus Spohn Memorial/Texas A&M University
Corpus Christi, Texas

KIMBERLY A. B. LEESON, MD
Assistant Professor
Department of Emergency Medicine
Texas A & M Christus Spohn Emergency
   Medicine Residency
Emergency Physician
Department of Emergency Medicine
Christus Spohn Memorial
Corpus Christi, Texas

MATTHEW J. LEVY, DO, MSc
Instructor
Department of Emergency Medicine
Johns Hopkins University School of Medicine
Baltimore, Maryland
Attending Physician
Department of Emergency Medicine
Howard County General Hospital
Columbia, Maryland

ZHANNA LIVSHITS, MD
Fellow, Medical Toxicology
Department of Emergency Medicine
New York University School of Medicine
New York City Poison Control Center
Fellow, Medical Toxicology
Department of Emergency Medicine
Bellevue Hospital Center
New York

**STEPHEN YUAN-TUNG
LIANG, MD**
Fellow
Division of Infectious Diseases/Department of
   Medicine
Washington University School of Medicine/
   Barnes-Jewish Hospital
Saint Louis, Missouri

BRIAN LIN, MD
Kaiser Permanente
San Francisco, California

BONNIE E. LONZE, MD, PHD
Resident
Department of Surgery
The Johns Hopkins University School of Medicine
Resident
Department of Surgery
The Johns Hopkins Hospital
Baltimore, Maryland

LE N. LU, MD
Fellow
Division of Emergency Medicine
University of California, San Diego
Fellow
Division of Pediatric Emergency Medicine
Rady Children's Hospital
San Diego, California

YING WEI LUM, MD
Fellow
Division of Vascular Surgery,
Department of Surgery
The Johns Hopkins University School of Medicine
Baltimore, Maryland

CHRISTOPHER MAJOR, MD, FAAEM
Clinical Instructor
Department of Emergency Medicine
Keck School of Medicine
University of Southern California
Fellow
Department of Emergency Medicine
Los Angeles County/University of Southern
    California Medical Center
Los Angeles, California

MICHAEL P. MALLIN, MD
Cheif Resident
Department of Surgery, Division of Emergency
    Medicine
University of Utah
Salt Lake City, Utah

WILLIAM K. MALLON, MD, FAAEM, FACEP
Associate Professor
Department of Emergency Medicine
Keck School of Medicine
University of Southern California
Director
Department of Emergency Medicine
Los Angeles County/University of Southern
    California Medical Center
Los Angeles, California

CRAIG A. MANGUM, MD
Associate Professor
Department of Surgery
Duke University Medical Center
Durham, North Carolina

CHRISTINA MANNINO, DO
Resident
Department of Emergency Medicine
Columbia College of Physicians
    and Surgeons
Resident
Department of Emergency Medicine
St Luke's-Roosevelt Hospital
New York

ROBERT R. MARSHALL, JR, MBA
Clinical Administrator
Department of Emergency Medicine
Johns Hopkins Bayview Medical Center
Baltimore, Maryland

MARY LOUISE MARTIN, MD
Staff Emergency Physician
Department of Emergency Medicine
Our Lady of the Lake Regional Medical Center
Baton Rouge, Louisiana

MINA MASRI, DO
Assistant Professor
Department of Emergency Medicine
Keck School of Medicine
University of Southern California
Attending Staff Physician
Department of Emergency Medicine
Los Angeles County/University of Southern
    California Medical Center
Los Angeles, California

JAMES M. MATERN, MD, MPH
Attending Physician
Department of Emergency Medicine
The Hospital of Central Connecticut
New Britain, Connecticut

KAZUHIDE MATSUSHIMA, MD
Fellow
Division of Trauma, Acute Care & Critical Care
    Surgery
Penn State Milton S. Hershey
    Medical Center
Hershey, Pennsylvania

ANGELA MCKELLAR, MD
Resident Physician
Department of Emergency Medicine
University of Arizona
Tucson, Arizona

MICHAEL MCLAUGHLIN, MD
Department of Emergency Medicine
Santa Clara Valley Medical Center
San Jose, California

KAMAL MEDLEJ, MD
Resident
Department of Emergency Medicine
Columbia University, College of Physicians and
    Surgeons
Resident
Department of Emergency Medicine
St Luke's-Roosevelt Hospital Center
New York

ROBERT A. MEGUID, MD, MPH
Chief Resident
Department of Surgery
Johns Hopkins University School of Medicine
Chief Resident
Department of Surgery
The Johns Hopkins Hospital
Baltimore, Maryland

JEREMY D. MEIER, MD
Chief Resident
Otolaryngology—Head and Neck Surgery
University of California, Davis
Chief Resident
Otolaryngology—Head and Neck Surgery
UC Davis Medical Center
Sacramento, California

SAMUEL N. MELTON, MD
Attending Staff Physician
Department of Emergency Medicine
Community Hospital of the Monterey Peninsula
Monterey, California

CHRISTIAN MENARD, PHD, MD
Senior Resident
Department of Emergency Medicine
St Luke's-Roosevelt Hospital
Columbia College of Physicians & Surgeons
New York City, New York

SARAH L. MILLER, MD
Resident
Combined Emergency Medicine and Pediatrics
    Program
Department of Emergency Medicine/Pediatrics
University of Maryland
Baltimore, Maryland

KELLY M. MILKUS, MD
Emergency Physician
Department of Emergency Medicine
North Memorial Medical Center
Robbinsdale, Minnesota

JAMES M. MONTOYA, MD
University of California Davis
    Medical Center
Sacramento, California

JOHANNA C. MOORE, MD
Resident Physician
Department of Emergency Medicine
Hennepin County Medical Center
Minneapolis, Minnesota

MELINDA J. MORTON, MD
Resident Physician
Department of Emergency Medicine
Johns Hopkins University School
    of Medicine
Resident Physician
Department of Emergency Medicine
Johns Hopkins Hospital
Baltimore, Maryland

JARROD MOSIER, MD
Chief Resident
Department of Emergency Medicine
University of Arizona
Tucson, Arizona

JOSHUA MOSKOVITZ, MD, MPH
Resident
Department of Emergency Medicine
University of Maryland
Baltimore, Maryland

ANDRE' J. MOULEDOUX, JR, MD
Emergency Physician
Department of Emergency Medicine
Terrebonne Medical Center
Houma, Louisiana

DEBRAJ MUKHERJEE, MD, MPH
Resident
Department of Neurosurgery
Cedars-Sinai Medical Center
Los Angeles, California

KOUSTAV MUKHERJEE, MD
Attending Physician
Department of Emergency Medicine
Bronx Lebanon Hospital Center
Bronx, New York

GERHARD S. MUNDINGER, MD
Resident
Division of Plastic, Reconstructive, Aesthetic, and
    Maxillofacial Surgery
Johns Hopkins Hospital
Baltimore, Maryland

STEVEN NAZARIO, MD
Volunteer Faculty
Assistant Professor
Department of Emergency Medicine
University of Central Florida College of Medicine
Associate Residency Director
Department of Emergency Medicine
Florida Hospital
Orlando, Florida

PAULA M. NEIRA, RN, JD, CEN
Nurse Educator
Department of Emergency Medicine
The Johns Hopkins Hospital
Baltimore, Maryland

JAMES A. NELSON, MD, FACEP
Assistant Professor
Department of Emergency Medicine
University of California
San Diego, California
Medical Director
Emergency Department
Pioneers Memorial Hospital
Brawley, California

MÁRIA NÉMETHY, MD
Senior Resident
Department of Emergency Medicine
St Luke's-Roosevelt Hospital
Columbia College of Physicians & Surgeons
New York City, New York

VLADIMIR K. NEYCHEV, MD, PhD
Resident
Department of Surgery
Johns Hopkins Hospital
Baltimore, Maryland

TAY NGUYEN, MD
Resident Physician
Department of Emergency Medicine
Texas A&M University
Corpus Christi, Texas

MICHAEL E. NOTTIDGE, MD, MPH
Attending Physician
Department of Emergency Medicine
St Mary's Hospital
Waterbury, Connecticut

KATHLEEN O'BRIEN, MD
Resident Physician
Department of Emergency Medicine
University of Arizona
Tucson, Arizona

FRANCIS J. O'CONNELL, MD
Resident Physician
Beth Israel Deaconess Medical Center
Harvard Affiliated Emergency Medicine Residency
Boston, Massachusetts

KELLY OLINO, MD
Resident
Department of Surgery
The Johns Hopkins School of Medicine
Housestaff
Department of Surgery
The Johns Hopkins Hospital
Baltimore, Maryland

JEREMY OLSEN, MD
Staff Physician
Department of Emergency Medicine
Christus St Vincent Hospital
Santa Fe, New Mexico

BABAK JOHN ORANDI, MD, MSc
General Surgery Resident
Johns Hopkins University
General Surgery Resident
The Johns Hopkins Hospital
Baltimore, Maryland

BENJAMIN S. OROZCO, MD
Resident Physician
Department of Emergency Medicine
Hennepin County Medical Center
Minneapolis, Minnesota

EMILY B. J. OSBORN, MD
Physician
Department of Emergency Medicine
Inova Fairfax Hospital
Falls Church, Virginia

MASARU RUSTY OSHITA, MD
Kaiser Permanente
South Sacramento, California

MATTHEW P. OSTROM, MD
Fellow
Division of Cardiology
Harbor-UCLA Medical Center
Torrance, California

EMMANOUIL PAPPOU, MD
Assistant Resident
Department of Surgery
The Johns Hopkins University School of Medicine
Assistant Resident
Department of Surgery
The Johns Hopkins Hospital
Baltimore, Maryland

VIRGINIA S. PARK, MD
General Surgery Resident
Department of Surgery
Washington Hospital Center
Washington, District of Columbia

TYLER R. PEARCE, MD
Resident
Department of Emergency Medicine and Pediatrics
Indiana University School of Medicine
Resident
Department of Emergency Medicine and Pediatrics
Methodist Hospital
Indianapolis, Indiana

TONY PEDUTO, MD
Resident Clinical Instructor
Department of Emergency Medicine
Keck School of Medicine
University of Southern California
Chief Resident
Department of Emergency Medicine
Los Angeles County/University of Southern
    California Medical Center
Los Angeles, California

JAMES PENG, MD
Kaiser Permanente Sacramento Medical Center
Sacramento, California

CATHERINE E. PESCE, MD
Resident Physician
Department of Surgery
The Johns Hopkins University School of Medicine
Resident Physician
The Johns Hopkins Hospital
Baltimore, Maryland

SUSAN MARIE PETERSON, MD
Emergency Medicine Resident
Johns Hopkins University School of Medicine
Baltimore, Maryland

KIMBALL POON, MD
Fellow
Division of Cardiology
Harbor-UCLA Medical Center
Torrance, California

MARC E. PORTNER, MD
Adjunct Assistant Professor of Surgery
The University of Pennsylvania School of Medicine
Associate Director, Trauma and Critical Care
    Fellowship
Trauma and Surgical Critical Care
St Luke's Hospital and Health Network
Bethlehem, Pennsylvania

JACOB POULSEN, MD
Resident
Department of Emergency Medicine
University of Arizona
Tucson, Arizona

SHANNON B. PUTMAN, MD
Assistant Professor and Staff Physician
Department of Emergency Medicine
Johns Hopkins Hospital
Baltimore, Maryland

JEFFREY S. RABRICH, DO
Medical Director
Department of Emergency Medicine
St Luke's–Roosevelt Hospital Center
New York City, New York

AMRITHA RAGHUNATHAN, MD
Resident Physician
Stanford University Hospital
Stanford, California

PRAKASH RAMSINGHANI, MD
Resident
Department of Emergency Medicine
St Luke's–Roosevelt Hospital Center
New York

RALPH J. RIVIELLO, MD, MS, FACEP
Associate Professor
Department of Emergency Medicine
Drexel University College of Medicine
Attending Physician
Department of Emergency Medicine
Hahnemann University Hospital
Philadelphia, Pennsylvania

DILLON ROACH, MD
Resident
Department of Emergency Medicine
University of Kentucky
Chandler Medical Center
Lexington, Kentucky
Staff Physician
Department of Emergency Medicine
Integris Baptist Hospital
Oklahoma City, Oklahoma

LINDSAY ROBERTS, MD
Resident
Department of Emergency Medicine
Harvard Medical School
Resident Physician

Harvard Affiliated Emergency Medicine
Residency
Beth Israel Deaconess Medical Center
Boston, Massachusetts

JENNIE K. ROBIN, MD
Resident Physician
Stanford University Hospital
Stanford, California

CHRISTINA L. ROLAND, MD
Resident
Department of General Surgery
UT Southwestern
Dallas, Texas

CHAD E. ROLINE, MD
Resident Physician
Department of Emergency Medicine
Hennepin County Medical Center
Minneapolis, Minnesota

MICHAEL ROSSELLI, MD, MPH
Sports Medicine Fellow
Department of Emergency Medicine
New York University
New York City, New York
Sports Medicine Fellow
Department of Emergency Medicine
North Shore University Hospital—Manhasset
Manhasset, New York

JENNIFER K. ROSSI, MD
Resident Physician
Stanford University Hospital
Stanford, California

WILLIAM F. RUTHERFORD, MD
Assistant Clinical Professor
Department of Emergency Medicine
Indiana University School of Medicine
Medical Director
Emergency Department
Indiana University Medical Center
Indianapolis, Indiana

MARY SADEGHI, MD
Resident Clinical Instructor
Department of Emergency Medicine
Keck School of Medicine
University of Southern California
Senior Resident Physician
Department of Emergency Medicine
Los Angeles County/University of Southern
California Medical Center
Los Angeles, California

ROXANNA SADRI, MD
Resident Clinical Instructor
Department of Emergency Medicine
Keck School of Medicine
University of Southern California
Senior Resident Physician
Department of Emergency Medicine
Los Angeles County/University of Southern
California Medical Center
Los Angeles, California

HOUMAN SAEDI, MD
Surgical Critical Care/Trauma Fellow
Department of Surgery
University of California,
San Diego Medical Center
San Diego, California

MUSTAPHA SAHEED, MD
Clinical Instructor
Department of Emergency Medicine
Johns Hopkins University
Assistant Chief of Service
Johns Hopkins Hospital
Baltimore, Maryland

ESTEBAN SCHABELMAN, MD, MBA
Attending Physician
Department of Emergency Medicine
University of Pittsburgh Medical Center
Passavant Hospital
Pittsburgh, Pennsylvania

ELISSA SCHECHTER-PERKINS, MD, MPH
Assistant Professor
Department of Emergency Medicine
Boston University School of Medicine
Attending Physician
Department of Emergency Medicine
Boston Medical Center
Boston, Massachusetts

MIREN A. SCHINCO, MD, FACS
Associate Professor of Surgery
University of Florida
Medical Director, Surgical
Intensive Care
Program Director, Surgical Critical Care
Fellowship
Department of Surgery
Shands, Jacksonville
Jacksonville, Florida

DIANA C. SCHNEIDER, MD
Assistant Professor
Departments of Family and Internal Medicine
Keck School of Medicine
University of Southern California
Medical Director, Adult Protection Team
Los Angeles County/University of Southern
   California Medical Center
Los Angeles, California

ERIKA DEE SCHROEDER, MD, MPH
Resident
Division of Emergency Medicine
University of Utah
Salt Lake City, Utah

HOLLY SCHRUPP-BERG, MD
Resident Physician
Beth Israel Deaconess Medical Center
Harvard Affiliated Emergency Medicine Residency
Boston, Massachusetts

CHRISTOPHER M. SCIORTINO, MD, PhD
Administrative Chief Resident
Department of Surgery
The Johns Hopkins Hospital
Baltimore, Maryland

NATHANIEL L. SCOTT, MD
Resident Physician
Department of Emergency Medicine
Hennepin County Medical Center
Minneapolis, Minnesota

SONYA C. SECCURRO, MD, MS
Chief Resident
Department of Emergency Medicine
St Luke's-Roosevelt Hospital
Columbia College of Physicians & Surgeons
New York City, New York

OSCAR K. SERRANO, MD
Surgery Resident
Department of Surgery
Johns Hopkins Hospital
Baltimore, Maryland

ATMAN P. SHAH, MD, FACC, FSCAI
Assistant Professor
Department of Medicine
University of Chicago
Interventional Cardiologist
Department of Medicine
University of Chicago
Chicago, Illinois

SAJID HUSSAIN SHAH, MD
Surgical Resident
Division of Plastic, Reconstructive, and
   Maxillofacial Surgery
Johns Hopkins Hospital
Baltimore, Maryland

CYRUS SHAHPAR, MD, MPH
Chief Resident
Department of Emergency Medicine
Johns Hopkins University School
   of Medicine
Baltimore, Maryland

MELISSA L. SHERMAN, MD
Resident Physician
Department of Emergency Medicine
Hennepin County Medical Center
Minneapolis, Minnesota

MARTINE SILVER, MD
Resident
Department of Emergency Medicine
St Luke's-Roosevelt Hospital
New York

MICHAEL A. SILVERMAN, MD
Instructor of Emergency Medicine
Department of Emergency Medicine
The Johns Hopkins University School of
   Medicine
Chairman
Department of Emergency Medicine
Harbor Hospital
Baltimore, Maryland

MORGAN SKURKY-THOMAS, MD
Resident
Department of Emergency Medicine
Beth Israel Deaconess Medical Center
Boston, Massachusetts

ROBERT J. SOBEHART, MD
Associate Professor
Department of Military & Emergency
   Medicine
Uniformed Services University of the Health
   Sciences
Bethesda, Maryland
Staff Emergency Physician
Emergency Department
Naval Medical Center
San Diego, California

JENNIFER TAITZ SOIFER, MD
Clinical Instructor in Medicine
Department of Emergency Medicine

Columbia University College of Physicians and Surgeons
Assistant Attending Physician
Department of Emergency Medicine
New York-Presbyterian Columbia University Medical Center
New York City, New York

SARAH K. SOMMERKAMP, MD
Resident Physician
Department of Emergency Medicine
University of Maryland Medical Center
Baltimore, Maryland

COLIN STACK, MD
Resident
Department of Emergency Medicine
Resident Physician
Beth Israel Deaconess Medical Center
Boston, Massachusetts

KENT STEVENS, MD, MPH
Assistant Professor
Department of Surgery and Anesthesiology and Critical Care Medicine
The Johns Hopkins University School of Medicine
Assistant Professor, Division of Acute Care Surgery & Adult Trauma
Department of Surgery
The Johns Hopkins Hospital
Baltimore, Maryland

ASHLEY R. STOKER, MD
Resident Physician
Department of Emergency Medicine
University of Kentucky
Resident Physician
Department of Emergency Medicine
University of Kentucky Chandler Medical Center
Lexington, Kentucky

ANDREW STOLBACH, MD
Assistant Professor
Department of Emergency Medicine
Johns Hopkins University
Attending Physician
Department of Emergency Medicine
Johns Hopkins Hospital
Baltimore, Maryland

LORI ANN STOLZ, MD
Resident
Department of Emergency Medicine
University of Arizona College of Medicine
University Medical Center
Tucson, Arizona

DAVID STORY, MD
Duke University Hospital
Durham, North Carolina

JAMES H. STREET III, MD
Attending Surgeon
Department of Surgery, Trauma Services
Washington Hospital Center
Washington, District of Columbia

ZACHARY STURGES, MD
Associate Professor
Department of Surgery, Division of Emergency Medicine
University of Utah
Salt Lake City, Utah

LIZA TAN, MB, BCH, BAO
Resident
Department of General Surgery
Johns Hopkins Hospital
Baltimore, Maryland

PEDRO G. R. TEIXEIRA, MD
Resident Physician
Department of Surgery
University of Southern California
Keck School of Medicine
Los Angeles, California

BRYAN C. THIBODEAU, MD
Attending Physician
Department of Internal Medicine, Division of Emergency Medicine
Medical City Hospital, Dallas
Dallas, Texas

JANSEN M. TIONGSON, MD
Primary Care Sports Medicine Fellow
Department of Orthopedic Surgery
Harvard Medical School
Children's Hospital
Boston, Massachusetts

RIZWAN N. TOKHI, MD
Assistant Clinical Professor
Department of Emergency Medicine
University Medical Center—Las Vegas
Las Vegas, Nevada

CHRISTINE T. TRANKIEM, MD, FACS
Attending Surgeon
Trauma, Emergency General Surgery & Surgical Critical Care
Department of Surgery
Washington Hospital Center
Washington, District of Columbia

GARY M. VILKE, MD
Professor of Clinical Medicine
Department of Emergency Medicine
University of California
Chief of Staff
Department of Emergency Medicine
University of California, San Diego Medical Center
San Diego, California

FRANK E. VILLAUME IV, MD
Staff Physician
Department of Emergency Medicine
Camp Pendleton Naval Hospital
Camp Pendleton, California

EMILY E. VOGEL, MD
Resident Physician
Department of Emergency Medicine
Hennepin County Medical Center
Minneapolis, Minnesota

HEIDI F. WALZ, MD
Resident Physician
Department of Emergency Medicine
Hennepin County Medical Center
Minneapolis, Minnesota

SEAN WANG, MD
St Luke's-Roosevelt Hospital
New York City, New York

ANNA L. WATERBROOK, MD
Assistant Professor
Department of Emergency Medicine
University of Arizona
Tucson, Arizona

CHERI N. M. WEAVER, MD
Clinical Fellow
Department of Medicine
Harvard Medical School
Emergency Medicine Resident
Department of Emergency Medicine
Beth Israel Deaconess Medical Center
Boston, Massachusetts

JONATHAN CRAIG WENDELL, MD
Resident Physician
Department of Emergency Medicine
University of Maryland
Baltimore, Maryland

BJORN C. WESTGARD, MD, MA
Staff Physician
Department of Emergency Medicine
Regions Hospital
St Paul, Minnesota

WARREN WIECHMANN, MD
University of California
Medical Center
Irvine, California

ERIN E. WILKES, MD
Resident Clinical Instructor
Department of Emergency Medicine
Keck School of Medicine
University of Southern California
Senior Resident Physician
Department of Emergency Medicine
Los Angeles County/University of Southern California Medical Center
Los Angeles, California

DAVID T. WILLIAMS, MD, FAAEM
Assistant Professor
Department of Emergency Medicine
Keck School of Medicine
University of Southern California
Attending Staff Physician
Department of Emergency Medicine
Los Angeles County/University of Southern California Medical Center
Los Angeles, California

JEFFERSON G. WILLIAMS, MD, MPH
Resident
Department of Emergency Medicine
Harvard Medical School
Resident
Department of Emergency Medicine
Beth Israel Deaconess Medical Center
Boston, Massachusetts

GEORGE C. WILLIS, MD
Faculty Development Fellow, Clinical Instructor
Department of Emergency Medicine
University of Maryland School of Medicine
Attending Physician
Department of Emergency Medicine
Mercy Medical Center
Baltimore, Maryland

J. MICHAEL WILSON, MD, MPH
Senior Emergency Medicine Resident
Department of Surgery, Emergency Medicine Division
University of Utah
Salt Lake City, Utah

MICHAEL P. WILSON, MD, PHD
Fellow
Department of Emergency Medicine
University of California
San Diego, California

WESLEY S. WOO, MD
Clinical Instructor
Geriatric Medicine & Palliative Medicine
Kaiser Permanente, Los Angeles Medical Center
Staff Physician
Continuing Care Services
Kaiser Permanente, Los Angeles Medical Center
Los Angeles, California

CHAD DAVID WRIGHT, MD
Staff
Department of Emergency Medicine
University of Kentucky
Department of Emergency Medicine
Physician
Department of Emergency Medicine
University of Kentucky Good Samaritan Hospital
Lexington, Kentucky

JIM YEN, MD
Resident Clinical Instructor
Department of Emergency Medicine

Keck School of Medicine
University of Southern California
Chief Resident
Department of Emergency Medicine
Los Angeles County/University of Southern
 California Medical Center
Los Angeles, California

BRENNA K. YURSIK, MD, MPH
Department of Emergency Medicine
Maricopa Medical Center
Phoenix, Arizona

AMY MAY ZHENG, MD, MPHIL
Assistant Clinical Professor
Department of Medicine
University of California, San Diego
Staff Physician
Medicine Service
Veteran's Affairs San Diego Healthcare
 System
San Diego, California

CONTENTS

SECTION VI CLINICAL PRACTICE

SECTION VII EMERGENCY MEDICAL SYSTEMS

SECTION VIII EARS, NOSE, THROAT

Section IX Environmental

Section X Geriatrics

SECTION XI HEMATOLOGY/ONCOLOGY

SECTION XII INFECTIOUS DISEASE

SECTION XIII LEGAL ISSUES

Section XVII Neurological

Section XVIII Obstetrical/Gynecological

SECTION XIX PEDIATRIC

SECTION XXI PSYCHIATRIC

SECTION XXII PULMONARY

SECTION XXIII RESUSCITATION

SECTION XXIV TOXICOLOGY

SECTION XXVIII WOUND CARE

ABDOMINAL/GASTROINTESTINAL

1

OBTAIN THE APPROPRIATE IMAGING TEST WHEN EVALUATING ABDOMINAL PAIN

JAMES H. STREET III, MD AND XZABIA CALISTE, MD

Acute abdominal pain is one of the most common presenting symptoms in emergency departments (EDs) worldwide. Utilizing the correct imaging modality can affect patient outcome, prevent delay, and influence the type and onset of treatment. The purpose of this chapter is to compare imaging modalities available to the emergency medicine physician in the evaluation of common etiologies of abdominal pain in patients who present to the ED.

Two of the most frequent modalities utilized in the ED in the evaluation of abdominal pain are the abdominal radiograph and CT, and oftentimes, the initial screening is via radiograph. This, however, is not the optimal initial modality for many abdominal pathologies, and its routine use as a screen is discouraged except under certain circumstances. Abdominal radiograph is an unsatisfactory primary tool because it has a low sensitivity for elucidating the common causes of abdominal pain with the exception of depicting a foreign body. The sensitivity and specificity for delineating a foreign body are 90% and 100%, respectively, with an accuracy of 100%. Nonetheless, the abdominal radiograph should be employed as a tool in specific clinical settings. For patients in whom there is a suspicion of free air secondary to small bowel obstruction (SBO) or perforated peptic ulcer, abdominal x-ray is the first imaging modality of choice. For patients in whom there is a high clinical suspicion of intra-abdominal disease, abdominal CT is the recommended primary imaging test, with the exception of biliary disease. CT has a higher sensitivity for bowel obstruction, urolithiasis, appendicitis, pancreatitis, pyelonephritis, and diverticulitis as compared to abdominal radiograph.

ACUTE ABDOMEN

Acute abdomen is a condition in which a patient will present with sudden, severe abdominal pain usually of <24-h duration. There are a multitude of etiologies, many of which may need urgent surgical intervention. Some of the pathologies include acute appendicitis, cholecystitis, pancreatitis, intestinal ischemia, diverticulitis, and bowel perforation. A rapid diagnosis of the acute abdomen is imperative to decrease morbidity and mortality. The helical CT scan with intravenous and oral contrast is the diagnostic imaging of choice because it is reliable and highly accurate.

SMALL BOWEL OBSTRUCTION

Patients presenting to the ED with the triad of symptoms, namely, nausea/vomiting, obstipation, and abdominal pain, are likely to be diagnosed with an SBO. In the ED, the abdominal series is most often the initial imaging test used in the evaluation of an SBO. It is most readily available and is inexpensive. However, recently in the literature, CT scan is advocated as the initial imaging modality for SBO as it has been proven to be the more sensitive and specific test to diagnose this pathology, and the abdominal series has been noted to have a low diagnostic yield (*Table 1.1*). It is of particular use in patients who present with confusing or vague symptoms. The abdominal series is limited in its diagnostic abilities and in identifying a cause of SBO. Nonetheless, in a select group of patients with a high-grade SBO and/or suspected perforation, it is pertinent to perform an abdominal series first. Allowing some patients to ingest contrast and subsequently undergo CT hours later can place them at risk of aspiration.

    CT scan is advocated when the diagnosis is indeterminate and when x-ray findings are equivocal. The CT scan can determine the level, cause, and type of obstruction: closed loop versus simple. Therefore, CT scan is a highly useful imaging modality for SBOs; however, if suspicions are present for a high-grade SBO, it would be remiss not to perform an abdominal series initially.

ACUTE CHOLECYSTITIS

When assessing acute right upper quadrant pain and when acute cholecystitis is suspected, the initial/screening imaging utilized should be ultrasound (US) rather than CT. The initial use of CT scan can lead to under diagnosis or misdiagnosis. The sensitivity (Se), specificity, positive predictive value (PPV), and negative predictive value (NPV) of US versus CT are seen in *Table 1.2*. These

TABLE 1.1	STATISTICS OF ABDOMINAL X-RAY VERSUS CT IN THE EVALUATION OF SBO	
	ABDOMINAL X-RAY (%)	**CT (%)**
Sensitivity	49	75
Specificity	98	99
Accuracy	96	98

TABLE 1.2	STATISTICS OF US VERSUS CT IN THE EVALUATION OF ACUTE BILIARY DISEASE	
	US (%)	CT (%)
Sensitivity	83	39
Specificity	95	93
PPV	75	50
NPV	97	89

statistics indicate that US alone is enough to screen for acute biliary disease. The lower Se/PPV/NPV of CT demonstrates that it is unnecessary to use when ruling acute biliary disease in or out. There is no need for follow-up CT after diagnosis by US. US can grasp more findings than CT, and CT does not change the clinical treatment in patients. CT is recommended in the analysis of patients presenting with confusing symptoms or when a wider differential diagnosis is considered.

SUMMARY
The three most accessible imaging modalities available to the emergency medicine physician when delineating abdominal pain are the x-ray, CT, and US. The use of x-rays should be employed when a foreign body or free air is suspected secondary to etiologies such as perforated peptic ulcer or SBO. US is best utilized in the evaluation of acute cholecystitis, and CT scan is optimal for a variety of intra-abdominal diseases: pancreatitis, appendicitis, pyelonephritis, and diverticulitis, to name a few. Overall, utilization of the correct mode of imaging can and will positively affect patient outcome.

SUGGESTED READINGS
Ahn SH, Mayo-Smith W, Murphy B, et al. Acute nontraumatic abdominal pain in adult patients: Abdominal radiography compared with CT evaluation. *Radiology*. 2002;225:159–164.

Bono M. Gastrointestinal imaging. In: Tintinalli JE, Kelen GD, Stapczynski JS, eds. *Emergency Medicine: A Comprehensive Study Guide*. 6th ed. McGraw Hill, 2004.

Harvey RT, Miller WT Jr. Acute biliary disease: Initial CT and follow-up US versus initial US and follow-up CT. *Radiology*. 1999;213(3):831–836.

Mindelzun R, Jeffrey R. Unenhanced helical CT for evaluating acute abdominal pain: A little more cost, a lot more information. *Radiology*. 1997;205:43–45.

Torreggiani WC, Harris AC, Lyburn ID, et al. Computed tomography of acute small bowel obstruction: Pictorial essay. *Can Assoc Radiol J*. 2003;54(2):93–99.

Urban BA, Fishman EL. Targeted helical CT of the acute abdomen: Appendicitis, diverticulitis, and small bowel obstruction. *Semin Ultrasound CT MR*. 2000;21(1):20–39.

Vicario S, Price T. Intestinal obstruction. In: Tintinalli JE, Kelen GD, Stapczynski JS, eds. *Emergency Medicine: A Comprehensive Study Guide*. 6th ed. McGraw Hill, 2004.

DO NOT MISS A SIGMOID VOLVULUS

JASON D. ADLER, MD

The elderly patient who presents to the emergency department complaining of abdominal pain, distention, or constipation may, in fact, have a benign course of constipation. Unfortunately, the assumption that this is the case without a thorough workup can lead to disastrous consequences. An ileus or a small bowel obstruction (SBO) is frequently considered in the differential, and the experienced clinician may think about an obstructing mass and large bowel obstruction (LBO). But sigmoid volvulus (SV), despite being the third leading cause of LBO, is rarely considered. This is perhaps the most unique cause of LBO, because the rotated bowel creates a closed-loop obstruction, entrapping the mesentery causing decreased blood flow, ischemia, perforation, and gangrene of the affected segment. Failure to consider this potentially fatal diagnosis is the most important pitfall in managing elderly patients with constipation.

Your index of suspicion should vary according to the patient's age and background. In developing countries, SV is more common among middle-aged patients, while developed countries have a higher occurrence in elderly patients. In the United States, a third of cases are seen in institutionalized patients, often with a history of chronic constipation. These patients can be poor historians with difficult-to-interpret exams, further illustrating the need for a high index of suspicion.

The classic triad of SV, that is, abdominal pain, distention, and constipation, occurs in patients less than a third of the time. More likely, patients will present with distention and pain, occurring in 93% and 75% of patients with SV, respectively. Interestingly, the number of patients who presented with constipation was equal to the number presented with diarrhea in one study. Never let the absence of constipation or presence of diarrhea deter you from considering the diagnosis of SV! Another pearl is to inquire about a history of similar symptoms in the past, as nearly half of all cases involve recurrent attacks.

The history in these patients is often misleading. Similarly, the physical exam and laboratory evaluation seldom illuminate the diagnosis. Certainly, there are findings that are consistent with the diagnosis. The abdomen may be massively distended and tympanic with asymmetry favoring the upper quadrants. Bowel sounds can be increased or decreased. A lack of stool in the rectal vault is suggestive of volvulus. Patients may have electrolyte abnormalities and azotemia secondary to third spacing. All of these findings are very sensitive but not nearly specific enough to diagnose the condition.

When your history and physical exam let you down, you should take a picture! Imaging is important in the diagnosis of SV. Plain abdominal radiographs can be useful and are diagnostic in nearly 80% of SV cases. A "bent inner tube," with its point directed toward the right upper quadrant, can implicate the condition (*Fig. 2.1*). Unfortunately, a normal plain x-ray does not rule out the entity. A CT scan is more sensitive and can further describe the site of obstruction and demonstrate ischemia. If your physical exam is abnormal, then a plain film is warranted as it can expedite care; otherwise, CT scans have largely supplanted it.

Once suspected, emergent surgical consultation should be obtained as death can occur within 24 h of presentation. SV has an overall mortality rate of 20% and nearly 53% after the development of gangrene. Think of it, find it, and then treat it. Initial treatment should consist of supportive care with aggressive hydration and correction of electrolyte disturbances. Patients who are actively vomiting may benefit from a nasogastric tube for symptomatic relief, but this has little utility in deflating a dilated colon. Immediate surgical involvement is essential. A patient who is illappearing, febrile, hypotensive, and tachycardic should raise a

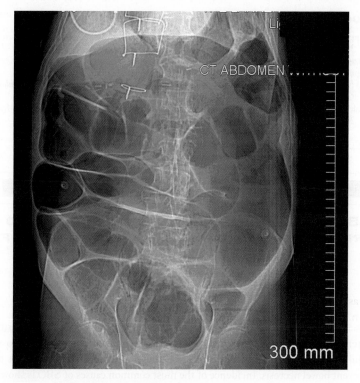

FIGURE 2.1. Plain abdominal radiograph.

suspicion for perforation or ischemia. Start antibiotics with Gram-negative and anaerobic coverage early, and prepare the patient for the OR.

SV is a rare and potentially lethal condition that presents many diagnostic challenges for the emergency physician. You can avoid the first pitfall by maintaining a high index of suspicion for the condition. A thorough history is paramount looking for sudden onset and recurrent history of abdominal distention and pain. As with other causes of abdominal pain, those patient populations that are at greatest risk, such as the elderly and institutionalized, are often unable to provide a reliable history, making the diagnosis more difficult. Do not rely on the classic triad to diagnose SV, and never allow the absence of constipation to alleviate your concern for SV. A plain abdominal radiograph can be diagnostic 80% of the time. This is helpful, but you should have a low threshold to order a CT scan in any patient you are considering to have an SV. Once suspected, immediate surgical consultation should be initiated and IV antibiotics started. SV can progress rapidly and have disastrous consequences. Thinking of it early and often will help avoid a major pitfall in emergency medicine care.

SUGGESTED READINGS

Cappell MS, Batke M. Mechanical obstruction of the small bowel and colon. *Med Clin N Am*. 2008;92:575–597.
Frizelle FA, Wolff BG. Colonic volvulus. *Adv Surg*. 1996;29:131–139.
Gibney EJ. Volvulus of the sigmoid colon. *Surg Gynecol Obstet*. 1991;173:243–255.
Lal SK, Morgenstern R, Vinjirayer EP, et al. Sigmoid volvulus an update. *Gastrointest Endosc Clin N Am*. 2006;16:175–187.
Tiah L, Goh SH. Sigmoid vollulus: Diagnostic twists and turns. *Eur J Emerg Med*. 2006;13(2):84–87.

3

BE AGGRESSIVE WITH INTRAVENOUS FLUID RESUSCITATION IN ACUTE MANAGEMENT OF SMALL BOWEL OBSTRUCTION

ROBERT A. MEGUID, MD, MPH

Small bowel obstruction (SBO) is a surgical emergency, demanding priority attention and urgent focused investigations aimed at confirming the diagnosis while simultaneously initiating corrective fluid and acid-base management to prevent bowel necrosis. Incidence of the most common causes of SBO is shown in *Table 3.1*.

| TABLE 3.1 | MOST COMMON CAUSES OF SBO |
CAUSE OF SBO	FREQUENCY (%)
Postoperative adhesions	75
Hernia	15
Tumor	5
Other: appendicitis or Meckel diverticulitis with abscess, intussusception, volvulus, gallstone ileus, Crohn disease, bezoar, foreign body, helminthic diseases	5

The suspicion of SBO is made from a careful history and a physical examination, including a rectal exam and is confirmed by a judicious use of appropriate radiographic studies. A careful history is invaluable and frequently suggests the diagnosis. Different age groups present with a more probable diagnosis, while a history of bleeding problems, allergies, and medications as well as a past medical history of surgery provides valuable information focusing the direction of further management, examination, and investigation. Constellation of pathenomonic complaints includes fever, nausea and vomiting, anorexia, crampy abdominal pain (frequently periumbilical), abdominal distension, and the cessation of flatus and bowel movements. Not all elements of the constellation need to be present. The degree and severity of findings depends on the duration of their symptoms. A reasonably high suspicion of SBO should trigger a surgical consultation. A history of laparoscopic surgery should not decrease suspicion for SBO, as no decrease in SBO has been observed even as the use of laparoscopy has increased. Tumor is the cause of SBO in half of patients having no past medical history of abdominal or pelvic surgery or a hernia on examination.

Physical examination should assess fever, hydration status, degree of abdominal distension and tenderness, presence of peritonitis, hernias, and the characteristics of stool as determined by rectal exam, including the presence of occult or gross blood. External hernias causing SBO include ventral/incisional, umbilical, inguinal, and femoral hernias. The presence of fever, peritonitis, incarcerated hernias, or rectal blood mandates a surgical consultation, because surgery may be necessary to prevent deterioration of a patient's fluid and acid-base condition and to prevent perforation or bowel necrosis. In the mean time, workup and treatment should continue on an urgent basis as outlined below.

Evaluation in the emergency room should include the measurement of serum electrolytes and a complete blood count. The former is key to determining the degree of metabolic derangement (metabolic acidosis), dehydration, and renal status and may be crucial to the type and volume of fluid replacement, particularly in patients with prolonged SBO, vomiting, or strangulated bowel. An elevated or depressed white cell count or the presence of hemoconcentration provides useful additional information to guide therapeutic management; however, normal leukocyte and hematocyte counts do not exclude SBO. Given that the patient with an SBO will be admitted to the hospital and surgery may be necessary, additional laboratory investigations should include coagulation studies, blood type and screening, urinalysis, and an EKG.

Supine and erect x-ray views of the abdominal are obtained to evaluate the presence of air-fluid levels in the small or large bowel, a possible transition point, intestinal emphysema or edema, pneumobilia, foreign bodies, or the suggestion of a mass effect of intussusception or volvulus. Also indicated is an erect chest x-ray to determine signs of aspiration, or subdiaphragmatic free air signifying GI tract perforation. Should these studies prove inconclusive, a CT scan of the abdomen and pelvis with oral and intravenous contrast medium is obtained. This may reveal a transition point, the degree of obstruction, and often the cause of obstruction, including the complications from SBO (pneumoperitoneum, ischemic bowel, and abscess). This information alters the urgency of patient management and preparation for operation. CT scans should not be delayed in patients who will not tolerate oral contrast due to vomiting, where a CT scan with intravenous contrast may still elucidate diagnosis. Ultrasound may be used in lieu of CT scans in a pregnant patient.

Concurrent with evaluation of possible SBO, patients should be aggressively volume resuscitated via intravenous access (two 18-gauge cannulae). Given that vomiting results in upper GI fluid losses, infusion of D_5 ½NS with 20 mEq/L of potassium chloride should be performed unless the patient has renal insufficiency. A urinary catheter should be placed to monitor volume status (goal urine output 0.5 mL/kg/h). Gastric decompression should be initiated with the placement of a nasogastric (NG) tube into the stomach, on low, continuous suction with frequent attendance to prevent clogging, and the placement confirmed with chest and abdominal x-rays. In addition to providing retrograde decompression of the GI tract, NG tube decompression helps to decrease the risk of vomiting and aspiration. Electrolytes should be repleted, again being cognizant of impaired renal function. Regarding pain control, masking of symptoms by analgesics remains debatable. However, it is undeniable that patients should not be kept in pain to facilitate the examination.

In summary, once diagnosis of SBO is made, NG tube decompression should be initiated, and the patient should be aggressively resuscitated by intravenous fluids and repletion assessed via urine output measurement with a urinary catheter and electrolyte assessment. This should be done expeditiously, and initiated prior to consultation and continued in consultation with the surgery team.

SUGGESTED READINGS

Cappell MS, Batke M. Mechanical obstruction of the small bowel and colon. *Med Clin North Am.* 2008;92(3):575–597, viii.

Cope Z. *Early Diagnosis of the Acute Abdomen.* 21st ed. London, UK: Oxford University Press; 2005.

Diaz JJ Jr, Bokhari F, Mowery NT, et al. Guidelines for management of small bowel obstruction. *J Trauma.* 2008;64(6):1651–1664.

McCloy C, Brown TC, Bolton JS, et al. The etiology of intestinal obstruction in patients without prior laparotomy or hernia. *Am Surg.* 1998;64(1):19–22; discussion 3.

4

DO NOT MISS THE DEADLY CAUSES OF PAINLESS JAUNDICE IN THE EMERGENCY SETTINGS

VLADIMIR K. NEYCHEV, MD, PhD

Icterus or jaundice is yellowish staining of the skin, sclera, and mucous membranes due to increased levels of serum bilirubin. In most patients, jaundice is apparent when hyperbilirubinemia reaches levels 2.5 to 3 mg/dL or greater. Jaundiced patients often present to the ED with related symptoms including abdominal pain, fever, or vomiting; however, ED physicians may face cases in which jaundice is found incidentally and the patient does not have abdominal pain or discomfort.

Although the majority of patients with painless jaundice present in the ED with a more indolent course, jaundice can reflect a serious hematologic or hepatobiliary dysfunction such as massive hemolysis or fulminant hepatic failure. Expedient diagnosis and appropriate therapy can be lifesaving in these settings. Therefore, a systematic approach is warranted to clarify the cause quickly so that treatment can begin as soon as possible.

The differential diagnosis of painless jaundice can be challenging to even the most experienced emergency physician. It includes a wide variety of conditions that can be caused by defects in any of the three phases of bilirubin metabolism: prehepatic, intrahepatic, and posthepatic. Although painless jaundice is the typical presentation of pancreatic cancer, this correlation is not universally applicable, and several other clinical and diagnostic features must be kept in mind while managing jaundiced patient in the ED. Patients should be asked of the use of medications (toxic hepatitis), drug and alcohol use (hepatitis B, C; alcohol liver disease), family history (G6PD deficiency, Gilbert syndrome), and social (HIV) and travel histories (hepatitis A, malaria).

One of the errors that can be made when working up painless jaundice is not thinking about acetaminophen toxicity, since missing that diagnosis and not implementing treatment can be disastrous. This can be due to an intentional overdose or an accidental overdose due to taking supratherapeutic doses of acetaminophen-containing medications. It is noticeable that acetaminophen overdose results in more calls to poison control centers in the United States than the overdose of any other pharmacological substance, accounting for more than 100,000 calls, 56,000 emergency room visits, 2,600 hospitalizations, and 458 deaths due to acute liver failure per year. Although hepatotoxicity and jaundice usually develop gradually, liver toxicity may be evident in 12 h after the ingestion, depending on the dose of the acetaminophen ingested. N-acetyl-L-cysteine (NAC) therapy should be initiated immediately regardless of the time of ingestions, although NAC has been shown to be most beneficial when given in the first 8 h. Likewise, although activated charcoal therapy has been shown to be most beneficial if it is initiated within 2 h of acetaminophen ingestion, activated charcoal administration should be started immediately regardless of the time of ingestions, because it is beneficial to the clinical outcome. Perform gastric lavage if decontamination can be started within 60 min of ingestion. Estimate the risk of toxicity based on the serum concentration of acetaminophen at a given number of hours after ingestion. Admit the patient for close observation, and call poison center consultation. Patients with a pH < 7.30, renal insufficiency, a rise in prothrombin time, and hepatic encephalopathy have poor prognosis with a mortality rate of 95% without transplant.

In conclusion, if you incorrectly diagnose and manage a patient with painless jaundice, there can be disastrous consequences. The bottom line is that painless jaundice should be approached as a potential medical emergency until proven otherwise. Patients with hemodynamically stable, new-onset jaundice, with no evidence of liver failure or acute biliary obstruction, can be discharged with close follow-up; otherwise, admission with appropriate consultation is warranted.

SUGGESTED READINGS

Buckley NA, Whyte IM, O'Connell DL, et al. Activated charcoal reduces the need for N-acetylcysteine treatment after acetaminophen (paracetamol) overdose. *J Toxicol Clin Toxicol.* 1999;37:753–757.

Lee WM. Acetaminophen and the U.S. Acute Liver Failure Study Group: Lowering the risks of hepatic failure. *Hepatology.* 2004;40:6–9.

Rumack BH, Matthew H. Acetaminophen poisoning and toxicity. *Pediatrics.* 1975;55:871–876.

Stedman's Medical Dictionary. 28th ed. Philadelphia: Lippincott Williams & Wilkins; 2006.

Vale JA, Kulig K, et al.; American Academy of Clinical Toxicology. Position paper: Gastric lavage. *J Toxicol Clin Toxicol.* 2004;42:933–943.

5

ADMINISTER MEDICATIONS TO PATIENTS WITH LIVER FAILURE WITH GREAT CARE

ROBERT S. ANDERSON, JR, MD

According to Greek mythology, Prometheus angered Zeus and was thus chained naked to a pillar in the Caucasian mountains. For years, a vulture tore at his liver, yet with each sunrise, the liver was whole again. Showing insight into human pathophysiology, the ancient Greeks correctly identified the liver's amazing regenerative capacity. In fact, the liver can regenerate itself almost completely with only one eighth of the original tissue. Indeed, the human liver has large functional reserve and does not easily fail. Therefore, the prevalence of acute liver failure is relatively rare and has been estimated at 5.5 cases per million population or approximately 1,600 cases annually in the United States. Nevertheless, it should not be ignored during care of acutely ill patients.

The assessment of liver dysfunction, however, is hampered by the lack of a single test to measure liver function. Furthermore, for added confusion, the literature is replete with case studies of hepatic injury from a variety of drugs and herbal supplements from which it is difficult to draw clinical conclusions.

What is clear, however, is that alcohol, acetaminophen, and viral hepatitis have carried on in the tradition of the mythical vulture and are occasionally more successful. Of these, the primary cause of acute hepatic failure in the United States is drug-induced injury from acetaminophen. Even therapeutic doses of acetaminophen taken by regular alcohol drinkers may lead to acute hepatic failure.

Often, the emergency physician (EP) is tasked with caring for sick cirrhotic patients who, because of their condition, have a 10% mortality rate if admitted to the hospital. While the liver disease places the patient at risk for a variety of complications (i.e., spontaneous bacterial peritonitis), the EP must exercise great care and thought with the selection of therapeutic drugs and their delivery in order to not further adversely affect the patient's condition. Pirmohamed presents a succinct summary with recommendations in his 2002 paper "Prescribing in Liver Disease." Paraphrased here are the major medication risks with patients who have liver failure:

Risk of increased bioavailability: highly extracted drugs (see *Table 5.1*) and phenytoin.
Risk of bleeding: warfarin.
Risk of excess sodium and water retention: corticosteroids and NSAIDS.
Risk of hypokalemia: corticosteroids and diuretics.

TABLE 5.1	**DRUGS THAT NEED TO HAVE THEIR INITIAL PO DOSE REDUCED**

COMMON AND/OR ED USAGE

Morphine

Isosorbide dinitrate

Nitroglycerine

Imipramine

Sertraline

Venlafaxine

Promethazine

Lovastatin

Sumatriptan

Chlorpromazine

Quetiapine

Labetolol

Metoprolol

Propranolol

Nicardipine

Verapamil

Buspirone

Clomethiazole

Midazolam

Sildenafil

Risk of precipitating hepatic encephalopathy: sedatives/hypnotics, lithium, loop diuretics, and opiates.

Risk of adverse drug reaction:

- ACE-I: hypotension
- Aminoglycosides: nephrotoxicity
- Cimetidine: confusion
- NSAIDS: GI bleeding, nephrotoxicity
- Oral hypoglycemics: hypoglycemia
- Quinolone antibiotics: CNS toxicity

For a handful of drugs that undergo high hepatic extraction, a basic understanding of hepatic extraction is necessary to allow the EP to make logical decisions about the initial oral dose. In healthy subjects, drugs that have a high hepatic extraction will have low bioavailability. Such drugs are dosed in healthy subjects with the understanding that most of the drugs will be rendered unavailable after first-pass metabolism by the liver. In those with liver dysfunction, it follows logically that hepatic compromise leads to an increase in the bioavailability of these drugs that could be detrimental.

With this in mind, the drugs listed in *Table 5.1* need to have their initial PO dose reduced.

This concept of hepatic extraction holds only for the **initial PO dose** of these drugs and is not related to initial IV dosing (since the hepatic "first-pass effect" is not relevant with IV dosing). With a few exceptions, initial IV dosing does not need to be adjusted (see below). Subsequent maintenance dosing, whether PO or parental, does require adjustment based on the assessment of hepatic blood flow, and this is often difficult to do. Fortunately, unless your ED has a real, significant problem with patient boarding, the maintenance dosing will not be your problem.

In an effort to do no harm, it is imperative that the previously mentioned medications be used cautiously, yet there are three groups that deserve further attention. **Morphine, benzodiazepines,** and **NSAIDs** have notoriously dangerous pharmacodynamic effects. Morphine, IV or PO, should be used with caution because it has unpredictable effects in cirrhotic patients due to higher bioavailability and impaired elimination. Benzodiazepines are interesting, in that, cirrhotics are extremely sensitive to diazapam and midazolam yet more tolerant of oxazepam and lorazepam, since the latter drugs undergo phase II reactions (conjugation metabolism), which are less affected by cirrhosis. NSAIDs must be respected as well. NSAIDs negate the vasodilator effects of prostaglandins that the kidneys need for sufficient filtration pressure, and they have been known to precipitate renal failure in patients with hepatic disease. This also reminds us that many of these patients with liver disease have concurrent renal disease and require renal adjustment of their medications using calculated glomerular filtration rate (GFR) rather than serum creatinine.

As is the case with most emergency medicines, the EP is charged with large responsibility in light of little clinical information in often chronically ill patients. Liver failure patients highlight this dilemma and put the spotlight on care provided in the ED. While it may be true that a vulture has been tearing a liver away for decades, the bird will be largely forgotten if the physician makes a life-threatening medication error.

SUGGESTED READINGS

Bower WA, Johns M, Margolis HS, et al. Population-based surveillance for acute liver failure. *Am J Gastroenterol.* 2007;102:2459–2463.

Crotty B, Watson KJ, Desmond PV, et al. Hepatic extraction of morphine is impaired in cirrhosis. *Eur J Clin Pharmacol.* 1989;36:501–506.

Delcò F, Tchambaz L, Schlienger R, et al. Dose adjustment in patients with liver disease. *Drug Saf.* 2005;28(6):529–545.

Guyton A, Hal J. *Textbook of Medical Physiology*. Philadelphia: W.B. Saunders Company; 1996:37.

Hasselstrom J, Ericksson S, Persson A, et al. The metabolism and bioavailability of morphine in patients with severe liver cirrhosis. *Br J Clin Pharmacol.* 1990;29:289–297.

Navarro VJ, Senior JR. Drug-related hepatotoxicity. *N Engl J Med.* 2006;354:731–731.

Pirmohamed M. Prescribing in liver disease. *Medicine.* 2002;35:31–34.

Rodighiero V. Effects of liver disease on pharmacokinetics. *Clin Pharmacokinet.* 1999;37(5):399–431.

Tlawalkar JA, Kamath P. Influence of recent advances in medical management of clinical outcomes of cirrhosis. *Mayo Clin Proc.* 2005;80(11):1501–1508.

William N, Paredes AH, Lewis JH. Drug induced liver injury in 2007. *Curr Opin Gastroenterol.* 2008;24(3):287–297.

6

Do not ignore the possibility of spontaneous bacterial peritonitis in patients with liver disease who "look good"

Timothy P. Chizmar, MD

Spontaneous bacterial peritonitis (SBP) is a well-recognized, severe complication in cirrhotic patients presenting to the emergency department (ED) with ascites. The prevalence of this disease varies widely among study populations, with a range of 10% to 30% in hospitalized patients with ascites, compared to 0% to 3.5% among asymptomatic outpatient clinic populations. The most recent prospective ED-based study found an SBP prevalence of 12% in all patients undergoing paracentesis. Mortality rates from treated SBP range from 20% to 30% in-hospital to nearly 50% at 1 year.

This significant condition is defined as an infection of ascitic fluid with no apparent intra-abdominal source (i.e., abscess, perforated viscus). Most sources postulate that this infection arises from translocation of bacteria from the intestines to the systemic circulation in the context of an impaired immune system, secondary to hepatic disease. The diagnostic evaluation for SBP centers on the analysis of ascitic fluid. Although this analysis remains somewhat controversial, the diagnosis of SBP and its variants is generally agreed upon:

- **SBP:** polymorphonuclear (PMN) count in ascites >250 cells/mm^3 with the growth of pathogenic bacteria from ascites fluid (however high false-negative rate of the culture).

- **Culture-negative neutrocytic ascites (CNNA):** the PMN count is >250 cells/mm³, but there is no culture growth (should be treated as SBP).
- **Bacterascites:** positive culture result, but with a PMN count <250 cells/mm³ (most sources regard this as transient intestinal colonization or skin flora contamination).

While the definitions are important to know, it is important to realize that you could be missing the diagnosis in patients with SBP who "look good." Most patients will NOT display classic signs and symptoms of SBP. Likewise, there is no single clinical characteristic that we can rely upon to effectively rule in or rule out SBP. In fact, clinical impression has a sensitivity of only 76% and specificity of 34% for the detection of SBP. Fever was present in only 50% to 68% of patients, while abdominal pain was noted in only 49% to 60% of patients. Confusion or encephalopathy was seen in 50% to 60% of patients. Rebound tenderness was present in only 10% to 42% of patients.

Because there is no reliable clinical finding that can rule in or rule out the condition, the ED physician must maintain a HIGH index of suspicion for SBP in all patients with ascites. Certainly, during a busy shift, you would prefer to call the medicine team and let them worry about tapping the belly, but you MUST PERFORM a paracentesis in any patient with new-onset ascites or with ascites and associated fever, abdominal pain, peritoneal signs, leukocytosis, unexplained encephalopathy, or worsening liver and renal function.

Once you have come to the realization that you must consider SBP and that the only way to truly investigate the condition is by performing a paracentesis, it is incumbent upon you to make sure the results are as valid as possible. The standard for diagnosis of SBP is a PMN count of >250 cells/mm³ in ascitic fluid, with or without a subsequent positive culture. Interestingly, ascitic cultures yield a pathogenic bacterium in only 40% to 50% of cases. In an effort to maximize your yield and improve patient care, the following are evidence-based considerations to help you clinch an early and accurate SBP diagnosis:

- Use sterile approach, with patient positioned at 30 to 45 degrees. Use a 20- or 22-gauge, 2.5-in. needle.
- Use ultrasound guidance. Left lower quadrant (LLQ) is preferred to the infraumbilical approach (less bleeding and greater depth of ascites).
- Note the clarity of fluid (sensitivity of 98.1%, specificity 22.7% for SBP if hazy, cloudy) and send for cell count.
- Inoculate 10 mL of ascitic fluid directly into aerobic and anaerobic blood culture bottles to increase the yield of cultures to 50% to 80%.
- Use a urine dipstick test on the ascites at bedside, as this can provide rapid diagnosis if leukocyte esterase positive (varies by manufacturer, but generally >stage 2 on the strip). A sensitivity of 89% to 100% with a specificity of 98% to 100%.

Certainly, there are risks to the procedure that need to be discussed but do not talk yourself out of performing the paracentesis because of the possible complications. You should counsel patients and their families concerning the benefits of diagnostic paracentesis and the relatively low rate of risks. These are the facts that should encourage you and patients:

- **Bleeding risk**: 0.2% to 1% even in mild–moderate coagulopathy and thrombocytopenia; risk is increased with renal failure
- **Perforation of bowel or bladder**: <1% (empty bladder, use ultrasound)
- **Infection**: theoretical risk, no statistics available
- **Persistent leak at puncture site**: <1% (using Z-Track technique)
- **Death**: <1.2%

After successfully performing a safe and efficacious procedure, you should initiate broad-spectrum antibiotics immediately in all patients with an ascitic PMN count >250 cells/mm³. Intravenous third-generation cephalosporins are considered first-line treatment at present by some authors, with reported 75% to 90% treatment success; however, recent data show an increasing incidence of SBP caused by Gram-positive and drug-resistant bacteria. In a small prospective validation study, there was treatment failure in 41% of cases treated with cefotaxime. The microbial etiology of SBP is changing, and you should anticipate this and initiate the therapy with broad-spectrum antibiotics. Choosing imipenem or piperacillin-tazobactam, for any patient with an ascitic PMN count >250 cells/mm³, will not only prove that you are well read on the subject but also improve your patients' care.

SUGGESTED READINGS

Angeloni S, Leboffe C, Parente A, et al. Efficacy of current guidelines for the treatment of spontaneous bacterial peritonitis in the clinical practice. *World J Gastroenterol.* 2008;14(17):2757–2762.

Castellote J, Girbau A, Maisterra S, et al. Spontaneous bacterial peritonitis and bacterascites prevalence in asymptomatic cirrhotic outpatients undergoing large-volume paracentesis. *J Gastroenterol Hepatol.* 2008;23(2):256–259 [Epub 2007 Aug 7].

Chinnock B, Hendey GW. Can clear ascitic fluid appearance rule out spontaneous bacterial peritonitis? *Am J Emerg Med.* 2007;25(8):934–937.

Chinnock B, Afarian H, Minnigan H, et al. Physician clinical impression does not rule out spontaneous bacterial peritonitis in patients undergoing emergency department paracentesis. *Ann Emerg Med.* 2008;52(3):268–273 [Epub 2008 Apr 23].

Evans LT, Kim WR, Poterucha JJ, et al. Spontaneous bacterial peritonitis in asymptomatic outpatients with cirrhotic ascites. *Hepatology.* 2003;37(4):897–901.

Koulaouzidis A, Bhat S. Karagiannidis A, et al. Spontaneous bacterial peritonitis. *Postgrad Med J.* 2007;83:379–383; doi:10.1136/pgmj.2006.056168.

McGibbon A, Chen GI, Peltekian KM, et al. An evidence-based manual for abdominal paracentesis. *Dig Dis Sci.* 2007;52(12):3307–3315 [Epub 2007 Mar 28].

Obstein KL, Campbell MS, Reddy KR, et al. Association between model for end-stage liver disease and spontaneous bacterial peritonitis. *Am J Gastroenterol.* 2007;102(12): 2732–2736.

Romney R, Mathurin P, Ganne-Carrié N, et al. Usefulness of routine analysis of ascitic fluid at the time of therapeutic paracentesis in asymptomatic outpatients. *Gastroenterol Clin Biol.* 2005;29(3):275–279.

Thévenot T, Cadranel JF, Nguyen-Khac E, et al. Diagnosis of spontaneous bacterial peritonitis in cirrhotic patients by use of two reagent strips. *Eur J Gastroenterol Hepatol.* 2004;16(6):579–583.

Wong CL, Holroyd-Leduc J, Thorpe KE, et al. Does this patient have bacterial peritonitis or portal hypertension? How do I perform a paracentesis and analyze the results? *JAMA.* 2008;299(10):1166–1176.

7

USE COMPUTED TOMOGRAPHY SCANS TO HELP GUIDE THE CARE OF PATIENTS WITH ACUTE PANCREATITIS

ATANU BISWAS, MD, MSc

When a patient with acute pancreatitis presents in the emergency department, it may be in various stages of inflammatory insult depending on how long the patient's symptoms have been present prior to arriving at the hospital. The inflammatory mediators associated with pancreatitis cause an increase in vascular permeability leading to hemorrhage, edema, and ultimately pancreatic necrosis. When evaluating a patient with acute pancreatitis in the emergency department, quick and accurate diagnosis of pancreatitis, as well as knowing what stage in the course of the disease the patient is in, will aid in the proper management protocol for the patient's pancreatitis. Errors in the management of acute pancreatitis are often the result of inadequate knowledge of the stage of the pancreatitis, causing delayed treatment and interventions.

Ranson criteria were introduced in 1974 and have been widely used as a clinical stratification tool for predicting the severity of acute pancreatitis. With a predictive mortality, sensitivity and specificity of 73% and 77%, respectively, the limitations of Ranson criteria are apparent. First, Ranson criteria are only valid after 48 h from the onset of disease and not valid at any other time of the disease process. This makes the Ranson criteria almost useless in the ED, since we do not have the complete data set many times. The clinician should be aware that the patient with acute pancreatitis may present well after 48 h from the onset of disease causing Ranson criteria to be invalid with regard to prognostic significance. Second, Ranson criteria are assuming that the pancreatitis is caused by gallstones or alcohol. The clinician should be aware that other causes of pancreatitis are possible and that normal lab values with regard to

Ranson criteria may grossly underestimate the severity of the disease. While the acute physiology and chronic health evaluation (APACHE) score has the advantage of assessing the patient at any time during the disease process, it is too cumbersome for routine clinical practice. In light of these pitfalls, what can the clinical practitioner use to accurately determine the severity of the pancreatitis so that he or she can provide and triage the patient with the appropriate care?

Several studies have prospectively studied the prognostic usefulness of the Balthazar Computed Tomography Severity Index (CTSI) compared to Ranson criteria as well as APACHE II & III scoring systems. The Balthazar CTSI has a reported sensitivity and specificity of 87% and 88%, respectively, which has been stated to be superior to other prognostic scores when compared to Ranson criteria (73% and 77%) and APACHE scoring systems (77% and 84%), as it more accurately detects the presence and extent of pancreatic necrosis. The Balthazar CTSI (*Table 7.1*) was introduced in 1990 by Balthazar and Ranson and was found to significantly correlate with acute pancreatitis severity and mortality, length of stay, and need for necrosectomy. The Balthazar CTSI is a 10–point scoring system derived by assessing the degree of pancreatic and peripancreatic inflammation (zero to two points), the presence and number of peripancreatic fluid collections (zero to two points), and the presence and degree of pancreatic parenchymal nonenhancement or necrosis (zero to six points). Patients with grade A–E pancreatitis are assigned zero to four points plus two points for necrosis of up to 30%, four points for necrosis of 30% to 50%, and six points for necrosis of more than 50% (*Table 7.2*). For example, a patient with CT grade D is assigned three points; if, in addition, the patient has more than 50% necrosis, an additional six points are assigned, for a total index score of 9 (*Table 7.2*). In the study by Balthazar and Ranson, there was a statistically significant correlation, with a continuous increasing incidence of morbidity and mortality in patients stratified according to CT severity index groups. Patients who had a severity index of 0 or 1 xhibited a 0% mortality rate and no morbidity, while patients with severity index of 2 had no mortality and a 4% morbidity

TABLE 7.1	BALTHAZAR COMPUTED TOMOGRAPHY SEVERITY INDEX
GRADE	**CT FINDING**
A	Normal pancreas
B	Pancreatic enlargement
C	Pancreatic inflammation and/or peripancreatic fat
D	Single peripancreatic fluid collection
E	Two or more fluid collections and/or retroperitoneal air

TABLE 7.2	BALTHAZAR COMPUTED TOMOGRAPHY SEVERITY INDEX			
		NECROSIS		
CT GRADE	POINTS	PERCENTAGE	ADDITIONAL POINTS	SEVERITY INDEX
A	0	0	0	0
B	1	0	0	1
C	2	<30	2	4
D	3	30–50	4	7
E	4	>50	6	10

rate. By contrast, a severity index of 7 to 10 yielded a 17% mortality rate and a 92% complication rate. In a recent prospective study by Chatzicostas, the Balthazar CTSI has an overall higher positive and negative predictive value. When comparing the performance of the scoring systems in predicting acute pancreatitis severity, the Balthazar score had a positive and negative predictive values of 89% and 83%, respectively (Ranson 65% and 82%, APACHE II 73% and 76%, APACHE III 73% and 69%).

Because of modern technological advances, computed tomography scanning is a widely available modality for diagnostic purposes. In the emergency setting, the clinician can accurately diagnose and predict the outcome of acute pancreatitis using the Balthazar CTSI. This modality will allow the clinician to guide his or her aggressiveness with resuscitation and also contact the appropriate surgical or gastroenterological services for timely intervention.

SUGGESTED READINGS

Balthazar EJ. Acute pancreatitis: Assessment of severity with clinical and CT evaluation. *Radiology*. 2002;223:603–613.

Balthazar EJ, Robinson DL, Megibow AJ, et al. Acute pancreatitis: Value of CT in establishing prognosis. *Radiology*. 1990:174(2):331–336.

Chatzicostas C, Roussomoustakai M, Vardas E, et al. Balthazar computed tomography severity index is superior to ranson criteria and APACHE II and III scoring systems in predicting acute pancreatitis putcome. *J Clin Gastroenterol*. 2003;36(3):253–260.

Leung TK, Lee CM, Lin SY, et al. Balthazar computed tomography severity index is superior to Ranson criteria and APACHE II scoring system in predicting acute pancreatitis outcome. *World J Gastroenterol*. 2005;11(38):6049–6052.

Simchuk EJ, Traverso LW, Nukui Y, et al. Computed tomography severity index is a predictor of outcomes for severe pancreatitis. *Am J Surg*. 2000;179:352–355.

8

WHAT YOU PROBABLY LEARNED ABOUT THE DIAGNOSIS AND TREATMENT OF CHOLANGITIS IS WRONG

GEORGE C. WILLIS, MD

The diagnosis of cholangitis can be elusive, and many emergency physicians continue to misdiagnose cholangitis in patients leading to increased morbidity and mortality. Misdiagnosis leads to the mismanagement of very ill patients and significantly longer hospital stays. Even when the diagnosis is correctly discovered, patients with cholangitis continue to be mismanaged in the emergency department. One in ten cholangitis patients die regardless of any interventions, and these common errors are only worsening the odds! Therefore, a different approach to diagnosing and managing cholangitis patients must be utilized.

For years, physicians have been basing the diagnosis of cholangitis on the presence of Charcot triad and ruling it out if all three components of the triad were not present. Would you rule out myocardial infarction in patients with atypical chest pain with no shortness of breath? Disease processes are notorious for presenting atypically. Therefore, relying on Charcot triad alone is problematic as the incidence of all three symptoms in patients with cholangitis ranges anywhere between 15% and 70%. The diagnosis is more complicated in elderly and septic patients, where often the patient's complaints are nonspecific in nature and the physical exam is clouded by polypharmacy. Cholangitis can present as sepsis in which asymptomatic bacteriuria or lung scarring leads to a presumptive diagnosis of urosepsis or pneumonia obscuring the true intra-abdominal etiology.

So, how does one make the diagnosis? A wide diagnostic net needs to be cast and the use of supplemental information is necessary. In 2007, an international group of hepatobiliary experts came up with an evidence-based set of guidelines for the diagnosis of cholangitis (*Table 8.1*). These guidelines combine components of the history (including Charcot triad) with imaging (CT or ultrasound) and laboratory evidence (elevated white blood cell count and liver function tests). If a patient presents with an incomplete history of Charcot triad, cholangitis should remain in the differential until labs return demonstrating normal liver enzymes and imaging displaying a normal common bile duct. In the elderly or septic patient, there should be a low threshold to acquire imaging, as misdiagnosing either population of patients will often lead your presence being requested at the next morbidity and mortality conference.

Once the diagnosis of cholangitis has been established, what next? Early management consists of volume resuscitation, early antibiotics after acquiring

TABLE 8.1	DIAGNOSTIC CRITERIA FOR ACUTE CHOLANGITIS (TOKYO GUIDELINES)	
A. Clinical context and clinical	1. History of biliary disease manifestations	
	2. Fever and/or chills	
	3. Jaundice	
	4. Abdominal pain (RUQ or upper abdominal)	
B. Laboratory data	5. Evidence of inflammatory response[a]	
	6. Abnormal liver function tests[b]	
C. Imaging findings	7. Biliary dilatation or evidence of an etiology (stricture, stone, stent, etc)	
Suspected diagnosis	Two or more items in A	
Definite diagnosis	(1) Charcot triad (2 + 3 + 4)	
	(2) Two or more items in A + both items in B + C	

[a]Abnormal WBC (white blood cell) count, increased serum CRP (c-reactive protein) level, and other changes indicating inflammation.
[b]Increased serum ALP (alkaline phosphatase), GGT (gamma glutamyl transpeptidase), AST (aspartate transaminase), and ALT (alanine transaminase) levels

blood cultures, and correction of coagulopathies and electrolyte abnormalities. Choice of initial antibiotics is crucial. Utilizing narrowly focused antibiotic regimens often achieves substandard results. Often, the antibiotics will not cover the inciting pathogen, or it will not be secreted adequately in the bile, where the infection began. Therefore, the piperacillin-tazobactam antibiotic regimen is a first-line therapy, as it has been shown to cover the frequent offenders in cholangitis, such as Gram-negative bacteria and anaerobes, and also has been demonstrated to achieve high concentrations in bile. If the patient is penicillin allergic, the combination of ciprofloxacin and metronidazole is a worthy alternative.

Some patients respond well to antibiotic therapy and volume resuscitation, but what about those who fail medical management? These patients require urgent biliary decompression. Your friendly neighborhood surgeon would salivate at the opportunity to put a zipper line down your patient's midline; unfortunately, this would likely end in your patient's untimely demise. Truthfully, depending on who runs the endoscopy suites in your hospital, this is ONE situation where your surgical colleagues' efforts to pawn these patients off onto the medicine service would be in your patient's best interest. Endoscopic retrograde cholangiopancreatography (ERCP) is the preferred method of treatment in cholangitis. ERCP is more therapeutic and associated with fewer complications than surgery. If an endoscopist is not available and there is an interventional radiologist in-house, percutaneous transhepatic drainage can be performed for urgent biliary decompression. If neither is available, depending on how stable the patient is, a ride in the back of an ambulance to a facility with those available in subspecialties would be appropriate. Surgery should be a last resort, after other methodologies have failed, because it has an increased incidence of complications and increased 30-day mortality when compared to the other modalities, particularly in sicker patients.

Diagnosis and treatment of cholangitis can be extremely challenging and frustrating. Relying on the presentation of Charcot triad will often lead to incorrect diagnoses and diagnostic delays. Casting a wide diagnostic net supplemented with lab work and imaging, especially in your older and sicker patients, can often lead to fruitful results in a more rapid time frame, avoiding lengthy patient stays in the hospital and worse outcomes. After making the diagnosis, prompt resuscitation, broad-spectrum antibiotics, and appropriate disposition to the correct service improve patient outcomes. This approach to cholangitis ultimately leads to better patient care.

SUGGESTED READINGS

Bornman PC, van Beljon JI, Krige JEJ. Management of cholangitis. *J Hepatobiliary Pancreat Surg*. 2003;10:406–414.

Mayumi T, Takada T, Kawarada Y, et al. Results of the Tokyo Consensus Meeting Tokyo Guidelines. *J Hepatobiliary Pancreat Surg*. 2007;14(1):114–121.

Qureshi WA. Approach to the patient who has suspected acute bacterial cholangitis. *Gastroenterol Clin N Am*. 2006;35:409–423.

Wada K, Takada T, Kawarada Y, et al. Diagnostic criteria and severity assessment of acute cholangitis: Tokyo Guidelines. *J Hepatobiliary Pancreat Surg*. 2007;14(1):52–58.

9

DO NOT OVERRELY ON ULTRASOUND FINDINGS IN PATIENTS WITH RIGHT UPPER QUADRANT PAIN

ALBERT FIORELLO, MD, RDMS, FAAEM, FACEP

Abdominal pain is one of the most common presenting complaints to the emergency department, and in many patients, their pain is primarily right upper quadrant (RUQ) or epigastric pain. It is estimated that 35% of women and 20% of men will develop gallstones by the time they are 75 years old. Because of the prevalence of gallstones, symptomatic cholelithiasis and acute cholecystitis must be high on your differential for a patient with upper abdominal pain. Although missing the diagnosis of symptomatic cholelithiasis can be problematic, missing the diagnosis of acute cholecystitis can lead to significant morbidity and mortality. Unfortunately, no single clinical finding or laboratory test can reliably establish or exclude the diagnosis of acute cholecystitis, even though there are still a few old surgeons out there who still believe that you cannot have acute cholecysitis without a fever and an elevated white count. Trowbridge et al. inferred that using only clinical and laboratory data, physicians arrived at a posttest probability for acute cholecystitis of about 60%. This certainly is not a strong enough evidence to send a patient to the OR or home. Therefore, we must rely on imaging to further assess for the presence of acute cholecystitis.

Ultrasound has become the first imaging choice in the evaluation for acute cholecystitis. A meta-analysis of the diagnostic accuracy of ultrasound in acute cholecystitis revealed a sensitivity of 94% and a specificity of 78%. Adjusting for possible verification bias, the sensitivity decreased to 88%. Several studies have demonstrated that emergency physicians can be trained to accurately perform bedside ultrasound evaluation for acute cholecystitis. Although this test has become very accessible to most emergency physicians and has good test characteristics, we must still be cautious interpreting the results in certain cases.

Like all ultrasound exams, RUQ ultrasound is an operator-dependent exam. Patient factors also play into the diagnostic accuracy of the exam. Gallstones can be missed on exam. Acalculous cholecystitis is most commonly seen in the setting of very ill patients. Because of this, you may be tempted to try to explain a somewhat thickened gallbladder wall, when no gallstones are seen, in an otherwise well patient, with a diagnosis other than acute cholecystitis, such as liver disease, congestive heart failure, or hypoalbuminemia. In actuality, you may have missed the stone. This is especially true if the stone is lodged in the neck of the gallbladder and the neck was not completely imaged. One study of 31 patients with gallbladder wall thickness >4 mm, a tender gallbladder on exam, and no stones seen on the first ultrasound showed that 14/21 of those who had follow-up studies had stones that were missed on the first exam! So, if your clinical picture looks like acute cholecystitis and you have a thick wall on ultrasound, it is likely cholecystitis.

Another pitfall is stopping with an ultrasound where the gallbladder was not visualized or only partially visualized. This could be due to air in the gallbladder wall from emphysematous cholecystitis. Ultrasound does not penetrate nicely through air; therefore, objects distal to the air are not well visualized. If you see a bright area where you would expect the wall of the gallbladder to be with poorly visualized structures beyond that, think emphysematous cholecystitis. Emphysematous cholecystitis is disastrous to miss, so order a contrasted CT of the abdomen and pelvis to evaluate for this uncommon but deadly entity.

And lastly, just finding gallstones alone does not mean that symptomatic cholelithiasis is the source of the patient's symptoms. This scenario happens all too frequently. A patient is seen for abdominal pain, gallstones are found on ultrasound without evidence of cholecystitis, and the patient is sent home with the diagnosis of symptomatic cholelithiasis only to return soon after with obvious acute cholecystitis or another cause for his symptoms. Remember that biliary colic from gallstones should be self-limited. The pain comes on, most frequently in the RUQ or epigastric area; lasts at most 4 to 6 h; and resolves. If the patient is having pain lasting longer and has gallstones on ultrasound without other ultrasound evidence of acute cholecystitis, think that it may just be early and other ultrasound findings have not developed yet or were not picked up on. You should observe the patient or repeat an ultrasound later. Do not let the radiologist tell you it cannot possibly be acute cholecystitis from her dark little cave—she has not even touched the patient! If the clinical picture fits, think twice about the imaging results. Also, if the clinical picture does not fit for biliary colic but the patient has gallstones, think of other causes for his pain! The gallstones might be an incidental finding (red herring).

Although ultrasound is a great modality in the assessment for acute cholecystitis and now one that we can perform ourselves (at the bedside in the ED), it is, like all other tests in medicine, not perfect. You must understand the test's limitations and interpret the results with caution. Remember that you are a well-trained clinician. If your clinical suspicion for disease is high, no single test should ever make you dismiss your clinical gestalt.

SUGGESTED READINGS

Ekberg O, Weiber S. The clinical importance of a thick-walled, tender gall-bladder without stones on ultrasonography. *Clin Radiol*. 1991;44(1):38–41.

Gaspari RJ, Dickman E, Blehar D. Learning curve of bedside ultrasound of the gallbladder. *J Emerg Med*. 2009;37(1):51–56 [Epub 2008 Apr 25].

Kendall JL, Shimp RJ. Performance and interpretation of focused right upper quadrant ultrasound by emergency physicians. *J Emerg Med*. 2001;21(1):7–13.

Miller AH, Pepe PE, Brockman CR, Delaney KA. ED ultrasound in hepatobiliary disease. *J Emerg Med*. 2006;30(1):69–74.

Rosen CL, Brown DF, Chang Y, et al. Ultrasonography by emergency physicians in patients with suspected cholecystitis. *Am J Emerg Med*. 2001;19(1):32–36.

Shea JA, Berlin JA, Escarce JJ, et al. Revised estimates of diagnostic test sensitivity and specificity in suspected biliary tract disease. *Arch Intern Med*. 1994;154(22):2573–2581.

Trowbridge RL, Rutkowski NK, Shojania KG. Does this patient have acute cholecystitis? *JAMA*. 2003;289(1):80–86.

10

KNOW WHAT TO LOOK FOR WHEN PATIENTS WITH POST-ERCP COMPLICATIONS PRESENT TO THE EMERGENCY DEPARTMENT

BABAK JOHN ORANDI, MD, MSc

Endoscopic retrograde cholangiopancreatography (ERCP), carried out for diagnostic and/or therapeutic purposes, is an effective and commonly performed procedure for patients with pathology of the pancreas and biliary system. Of all endoscopic procedures, ERCP is the one associated with the highest rates of morbidity and mortality, 10% and 1%, respectively, reflecting the more technically challenging nature of the procedure.

A review of the medicolegal literature surrounding ERCP suggests that there are several major reasons for lawsuits. This information is not for the purpose of lawsuit avoidance (although hopefully that is a secondary benefit)but rather to inform physicians what are considered "unforgivable" mistakes in the eyes of patients (and their lawyers) and how to avoid mismanaging these patients. The major reasons for lawsuits are performing the procedure when not indicated (generally not a relevant issue in the emergency department setting for a post-ERCP patient), postprocedural pancreatitis, perforation, and severe bleeding.

Pancreatitis is the most common complication of ERCP and is more likely to occur in younger patients (age < 40). It often occurs in otherwise healthy patients and almost always presents within 24 h. Post-ERCP pancreatitis is NOT simply a transient elevation of serum amylase. Rather, according to the consensus definition of the American Society of GI Endoscopy, it is new or worsened abdominal pain *and* serum amylase three or more times the upper limit of normal 24 h after the procedure and requiring at least 2 days' hospitalization. Generally, the mainstay of treatment is conservative management with aggressive hydration (except in those with cardiopulmonary contraindications to heavy fluid resuscitation), which prevents necrotizing pancreatitis and secondary pancreatic infection, and bowel rest.

In the case of perforation, there is frequently a delay in diagnosis, and the longer the delay, the more likely it is to be fatal. A conservative mortality rate associated with perforation is nearly 10%, with endoscopic sphincterotomy being a major risk factor for this complication. The appropriate management of these patients remains controversial. Some advocate conservative management, including IV antibiotics, IV fluids, analgesia, and making a patient NPO (nothing by mouth), for hemodynamically stable patients. They recommend that indications for surgery include heavy contrast extravasation on an upper GI study, contrast-enhanced CT demonstrating intraperitoneal or retroperitoneal fluid collections, large amounts of subcutaneous emphysema, or when perforation is assumed to be in relation to retained material (i.e., stones, ERCP basket, or wire). Given the unacceptably high mortality rate of 50% for patients who fail conservative treatment, the excessive rate of morbidity, the obscene length of stay for patients failing conservative management (median of 111 days in one study), and the miniscule patient sample sizes of studies advocating conservative management, definitive surgical treatment is currently the preferred method. Quite frankly, based on the currently available data, the stakes are too high with these patients to err on the side of conservative management.

As with perforation, endoscopic sphincterotomy is a major risk factor for severe bleeding after ERCP. Other risk factors for bleeding include the presence of a coagulopathy, anticoagulation within 3 days of the procedure, the presence of acute cholangitis, and papillary stenosis. While many of these bleeds are apparent at the time of endoscopy and are dealt with then, one half of all bleeds are delayed at least a day from the procedure, and some can occur 1 to 2 weeks out from the procedure. For both perforation and hemorrhage, a thorough history is important, particularly for oncology patients and others who are frequently seen by medical professionals. They may forget to volunteer a history of instrumentation occurring as far back as several weeks ago, so be sure to ask! Unlike patients with post-ERCP perforation, bleeding patients can usually be managed with conservative therapy, with very few patients requiring angiographic or surgical intervention.

To summarize, the key complications of ERCP to be aware of are pancreatitis, perforation, and bleeding. While pancreatitis and bleeding can usually be managed conservatively, do not hesitate to obtain a surgical consult for patients with suspected perforation—delays can prove to be fatal. Besides, surgeons are always happy to get consults from the ED, especially at two in the morning.

SUGGESTED READINGS

Andriulli A, Loperfido S, Napolitano G, et al. Incidence rates of post-ERCP complications: A systematic survey of prospective studies. *Am J Gastroenterol.* 2007;102:1781–1788.

Christensen M, Matzen P, Schulze S, et al. Complications of ERCP: A prospective study. *Gastrointest Endosc.* 2004;60:721–731.

Cotton PB. Analysis of 59 ERCP lawsuits; mainly about indications. *Gastrointest Endosc.* 2006;63:378–382.

Cotton PB, Lehman G, Vennes J, et al. Endoscopic sphincterotomy complications and their management: An attempt at consensus. *Gastrointest Endosc.* 1991;37:383–393.

Elder J. Surgical treatment of duodenal ulcer. *Postgrad Med J.* 1988;64(Suppl):54–59.

Freeman ML, DiSario JA, Nelson DB, et al. Risk factors for post-ERCP pancreatitis: A prospective, multicenter study. *Gastrointest Endosc.* 2001;54:425–434.

Rabenstein T, Schneider HT, Hahn EG, et al. 25 years of endoscopic sphincterotomy in Erlangen: Assessment of the experience in 3498 patients. *Endoscopy.* 1998;30:A194.

Reddy N, Wilcox CM, Tamhane A, et al. Protocol-based medical management of post-ERCP pancreatitis. *J Gastroenterol Hepatol*. 2008;22:385–392.

Stapfer M, Selby R, Stain SC, et al. Management of duodenal perforation after endoscopic retrograde cholangiopancreatography and sphincterotomy. *Ann Surg*. 2000;232:191–198.

11

KNOW THE DIFFERENTIAL FOR POSTCHOLECYSTECTOMY PAIN

LIZA TAN, MB, BCH, BAO

Cholecystectomies carried out for cholelithiasis have a very high success rate. However, in a small proportion of patients, persistent symptoms remain. This has been referred to as a wastebasket diagnosis of "postcholecystectomy syndrome."

Symptomatology of this syndrome can be attributed to be from

1) Within the biliary tract, for example, gallbladder or the ducts.
2) Outside of the biliary tract, for example, stomach or esophagus.

The only common denominator is perhaps pain. In the theme of error prevention, let us briefly review the possible pathology that may arise from each.

Following cholecystectomy, symptoms can be broadly attributed to biliary leaks or strictures. Injury to the biliary tree from cholecystectomy has been quoted to be in the low range of 0.2% in open surgery to a higher incidence of 1.5% if carried out laparoscopically. However, when complications do occur, pain results.

Leaks can arise from misplaced or dislodged cystic duct clips. It can also occur as a result of direct injury to the biliary tree. Biliary leaks can be asymptomatic, or it can present with symptoms relating to the inflammatory response evoked by the presence of bile in the peritoneal cavity. This includes a range of symptoms such as nausea, vomiting, abdominal pain, guarding, and ileus. In those with indwelling drains, outputs may be persistently high and will have the characteristic green tinge of bile.

Biliary strictures on the other hand may manifest with aberrant liver enzymes only to full-blown cholangitis with the typical triad of pain, fever/chills, and jaundice.

In the evaluation of the biliary system, the gold standard remains to be cholangiography, more specifically, endoscopic retrograde cholangiopancreatography (ERCP) which has a sensitivity and specificity rate of 100% and 95%, respectively. In approximately 5% to 10% of cases, the procedure itself causes adverse events, for example, acute pancreatitis and duodenal perforation. Therefore, the algorithm we should adopt in the proper examination of the biliary tree is that ultrasound should be first line in conjunction with liver function test. If the common bile duct is not dilated (diameter of the duct is larger than appropriate for that age group) and liver function tests are normal, further ERCP or Magnetic resonance cholangiopancreatography (MRCP) is unnecessary. However, if stones are present, the next logical step is ERCP. In a small group of patients in whom stones are not visualized and the common duct appears dilated on ultrasound, MRCP should be undertaken. MRCP has a sensitivity, specificity, and accuracy of 100%, 88%, and 93%, respectively. Due to the high sensitivity for detecting bile duct abnormalities, MRCP can be used to triage the patient appropriately for ERCP. Although in some cases, MRCP may yield a false-positive result from a spasmodic ampulla of Vater.

When there is a high suspicion of biliary leak versus biliary stricture, a hepatic iminodiacetic acid (HIDA) scan can be useful. Some investigators have recommended this mode of evaluation as a primary screening test in the diagnosis of biliary leak.

Endoscopy and ERCP remain the investigative procedures of first choice in complex postcholecystectomy cases especially when intravenous cholangiography fails to give a complete picture or suggests normality in the face of continuing symptoms or clinical evidence of residual biliary disease.

In a nutshell, the treatment of bile duct injury is to reestablish flow into the gut. In the presence of choledocolithiasis, endoscopic sphincterotomy and stone extraction from the common bile duct may be sufficient. In other cases, where stones are not the underlying cause of the injury, for example, in biliary strictures, stent placement is effective at bridging the defect and act as a splint to prevent further stricture formation. In leaks, stent placement is also indicated. Biliary leaks probably heal by removing physiological pressure gradient through sphincterotomy and tamponading of the leak site. Bergman et al. compared endoscopic versus surgically placed stents, and it was found that surgically placed stents were more likely to develop late strictures. Therefore, surgery is only recommended if endoscopic means fail.

In the group of "other" causes of postcholecystectomy pain, the patient's true underlying pathology was probably left untreated. In other words, the symptoms of nausea, vomiting, indigestion, heartburn, and belching were not due to gallbladder disease. Cholecystectomy was not the answer. In preventing this error, it is important to think outside the box in the evaluation of each patient and have in our heads or on paper what our teachers have tried to teach us—a list of possible and real differentials. I would recommend that patients who are being evaluated for biliary disease should not be considered for an operation unless other etiologies have been ruled out through detailed history, examination, and consideration of differentials followed by the use of targeted and systemic radiological aids.

SUGGESTED READINGS

Al-Rashed RS, Al Mofleh IA, Al Amri SM, et al. Biliary leak: Endoscopic management. *Ann Saudi Med*. 1996;16(2):126–129.

Callery MP, Strasberg SM, Sopher NJ. Complication of laparoscopic general surgery. *Gastrointest Endosc Clin N Am*. 1996;6(2):423–444.

Pannu HK, Fishman EK. Complications of endoscopic retrograde cholangiopancreatography: Spectrum of abnormalities demonstrated with CT. *Radiographics*. 2001;21(6):1441–1453.

Pasmans HL, Go PM, Gouma DJ, et al. Scintigraphic diagnosis of bile leakage after laparoscopic cholecystectomy: A prospective study. *Clin Nucl Med*. 1992;17(9):697–700.

Ryan ME, Geenen JE, Lehman GA, et al. Endoscopic intervention for biliary leaks after laparoscopic cholecystectomy a multicenter review. *Gastrointest Endosc*. 1998;47(3):261–266.

Terhaar OA, Abbas S, Thorton FJ, et al. Imaging patient with "post-cholecystectomy syndrome": An algorithmic approach. *Clin Radiol*. 2005;60(1):78–84.

12

DO NOT BE FOOLED BY ATYPICAL PRESENTATIONS OF ACUTE APPENDICITIS

JEFFREY T. GERTON, MD, MBA

With 250,000 cases per year in the United States, appendicitis is one of the most common surgical emergencies seen in the emergency department (ED). As we were all taught in medical school, appendicitis classically presents with peri-umbilical abdominal pain that migrates to McBurney point and is associated with fever, anorexia, and an elevated white blood count. If only things were as easy as they seemed in medical school! As with most conditions, the "atypical" presentation is more common and the lack of the "classic" presentation is not reliable enough to rule out the entity. Certainly, it is invigorating to diagnose those patients who present as if they read the textbook before coming to the ED, but what separates the seasoned ED physician from the medical student is the ability to recognize and avoid the common errors that are encountered in the management of appendicitis.

One of the most common misconceptions held is that you can exclude the diagnosis of appendicitis with a normal white blood count. While it is true that you can usually see an elevated white blood count, it is only about 80% sensitive. In other words, you would be missing 2 out of every 10 cases of appendicitis, which would be enough to send a malpractice attorney's kids through college. Looking for a left shift in addition to an elevated white blood count can increase your sensitivity, but it still does not exclude the diagnosis. Patients who are presenting early in the course of the disease process will more likely have a normal number of white blood cells. Similarly, children and older patients can have white cell counts that are not alarming. Therefore, first and foremost, you should never rely on a white blood count to rule out appendicitis, despite what any of your surgical consultants say.

In addition to being prone to having normal white cell counts, children are one group that often present in an atypical fashion, making the diagnosis of appendicitis more challenging. One study of children with appendicitis revealed that 50% had no migration of pain to the right lower quadrant (RLQ). Furthermore, 40% did not have anorexia and 52% had no rebound tenderness. Many of these patients had more than one atypical finding. *Forty-two percent of patients with proven appendicitis had six or more atypical characteristics.* This runs contrary to dogmatic teaching on the subject and makes our jobs much more difficult and can make conversations with consultants more "lively." In an effort to reduce unnecessary exposure to radiation, when confronted with a child with a concerning complaint but an equivocal exam, admit the patient for serial abdominal exams by the surgical team. This method is even advocated by some of our surgical colleagues and is advantageous from the patient's perspective but does require a progressively thinking surgical team with proper hospital resources.

Diagnosing appendicitis in women can also be more difficult. One study revealed a significantly higher negative appendectomy rate in women compared to men. Presumably, this is due to the location of the right ovary, leading to a broad overlap of symptoms between appendicitis and gynecologic pain. This can set up the interesting situation of the surgical consultants recommending another consult by the GYN team, despite the patient having a "classic" presentation. Unfortunately, fever and RLQ tenderness can also be attributable to a tuboovarian abscess; therefore, a CT or ultrasound examination can be particularly useful in women.

While children, the elderly, and women commonly present unique diagnostic challenges, so too do patients who present either early or late in the course. Early on, symptoms can be quite vague and nonspecific, including indigestion, flatulence, and just generally not feeling well. At the other extreme, once an appendix has ruptured, patients often get short-term relief of some of their symptoms. The moral of this story is to always keep appendicitis on your differential diagnosis list, and while you are discharging patients with "gastroenteritis," be sure to educate patients and their family about the possibility that their condition still could be appendicitis and that they should return to the ED if the symptoms worsen or their pain migrates.

Treatment of appendicitis is another area in which dogma may not be a reality. There are some mixed data to suggest that with prompt initiation of antibiotics, appendicitis may not truly be a surgical *emergency* and more of a surgical *urgency*. Often surgeons heavily cite this data around 2 AM. Even if this data are valid, medicolegally, it will be awfully hard to defend a ruptured appendix that occurs in your ED. In order to protect yourself, you must fully document your consultations including the time in which they occur and that you have emphasized the seriousness of the diagnosis and the patient's condition. Regardless of when the patient is going to go to the OR, start the intravenous antibiotics as soon as possible in your ED. Once the appendix has ruptured or a periappendiceal abscess has developed, there is evidence suggesting that patients treated with nonoperative management, at least initially, may do better. But it would be better not to use that as a defense strategy in the courtroom.

Overall, the biggest error in diagnosing appendicitis is not considering it or excluding it in patients with atypical findings. Be wary of the pediatric and geriatric populations. Use CT or ultrasound to help define more ambiguous presentations, or do what people did before fancy scans were available: observe the patient with belly pain.

SUGGESTED READINGS

Addiss DG, Shaffer N, Fowler BS, et al. The epidemiology of appendicitis and appendectomy in the United States. *Am J Epidemiol.* 1990;132(5):910–925.

Becker T, Kharbanda A, Bachur R. Atypical clinical features of pediatric appendicitis. *Acad Emerg Med.* 2007;14(2):124–129 [Epub 2006 Dec 27].

Brown CV, Abrishami M, Muller M, et al. Appendiceal abscess: Immediate operation or percutaneous drainage? *Am Surg.* 2003;69(10):829–832.

Cardall T, Glasser J, Guss DA. Clinical value of the total white blood cell count and temperature in the evaluation of patients with suspected appendicitis. *Acad Emerg Med.* 2004;11(10):1021–1027.

Clyde C, Bax T, Merg A, et al. Timing of intervention does not affect outcome in acute appendicitis in a large community practice. *Am J Surg.* 2008;195(5):590–593.

Ditilio MF, Dziura JD, Rabinovici R. Is it safe to delay appendectomy in adults with acute appendicitis? *Ann Surg.* 2006;244(5):656–660.

Oliak D, Yamini D, Udani VM, et al. Nonoperative management of perforated appendicitis without periappendiceal mass. *Am J Surg.* 2000;179(3):177–181.

Oliak D, Yamini D, Udani VM, et al. Initial nonoperative management for periappendiceal abscess. *Dis Colon Rectum.* 2001;44(7):936–941.

Rothrock SG, Pagane J. Acute appendicitis in children: Emergency department diagnosis and management. *Ann Emerg Med.* 2000;36(1):39–51.

Schuler JG, Shortsleeve MJ, Goldenson RS, et al. Is there a role for abdominal computed tomographic scans in appendicitis? *Arch Surg.* 1998;133(4):373–376; discussion 377.

Yamini D, Vargas H, Bongard F, et al. Perforated appendicitis: Is it truly a surgical urgency? *Am Surg.* 1998;64(10):970–975.

Zarba ME, Mazzocchi P, Lepiane P, et al. The role of surgery in the treatment of appendicular abscesses. *Minerva Chir* 1997;52(5):577–581.

13

DO NOT FEAR RADIOGRAPHY IN PREGNANT PATIENTS WITH SUSPECTED APPENDICITIS

JANSEN M. TIONGSON, MD

When evaluating a pregnant female presenting to the emergency department (ED) with appendicitis, perform any medically indicated diagnostic radiography in order not to compromise the health of the mother despite radiation exposure to the fetus.

When a pregnant woman presents to the ED with abdominal pain, you must take certain considerations into account during evaluation as your choice of radiological modality not only affects the patient herself but also affects the growing fetus. Although the American College of Radiology recommends ultrasonography as the safest choice for evaluation due to its lack of nonionizing radiation, you should not fear using computed tomography (CT) when the morbidity/mortality of the mother becomes compromised if a critical diagnosis is missed via ultrasound as utilization of CT can increase your level of certainty and lead to more timely surgical intervention.

The American College of Obstetricians and Gynecologists (ACOG), in 1995, established that an exposure >50 rad (0.5 Gy), regardless of the stage of gestation, puts the embryo at significant risk. However, they also recommended that the threshold exposure for birth defects during the most sensitive stage of development (gestational days 18 to 40) is 20 rad (0.2 Gy). Moreover, the 8th to 15th week of gestation is the most sensitive period for induction of mental retardation. As such, ACOG recommends accurate gestational dating when considering radiation. Regardless of the gestational stage, they have reported that 5 rad (0.05 Gy) has not been associated with increased fetal anomalies or pregnancy loss; as such, use this threshold as the limit for radiation exposure. In reference, a chest x-ray exposes the fetus to 0.02 to 0.07 mrad, while the CT of the abdomen can be up to 3.5 rad.

During pregnancy, peritoneal signs are often absent as the anterior abdominal wall is lifted and stretched, thus preventing any underlying inflammation to be in contact with the parietal peritoneum. Moreover, the abdominal organs are displaced by the expanding uterus, altering the usual nongestational anatomy. The pregnant woman who has suspected appendicitis does not present with the typical signs and symptoms as in the nongestational period. Graded compression ultrasonography is the recommended diagnostic aid in appendicitis in pregnancy, but the size of the gravid abdomen can often limit visualization of the appendix. Ultrasonography has a reported sensitivity and specificity as high as 100% and 96%, respectively, in diagnosing appendicitis. However, Lazarus et al. stated that CT established the diagnosis in 35% of women with abdominal pain and confirmed appendicitis in 30% of women who had negative ultrasound findings. This study established a negative predictive value of 99% for CT accurately diagnosing appendicitis. It is reported that in the setting of a perforated appendicitis, there exists a 20% risk of fetal loss. Therefore, the diagnosis of appendicitis is critical for both maternal and fetal mortality and morbidity, and so, if you have a high clinical suspicion of appendicitis despite a negative ultrasound, a CT scan of the abdomen should highly be considered. As stated above, the level of radiation exposure is still below the recommended ACOG levels.

Magnetic resonance imaging (MRI) has been under discussion as a radiographic modality in diagnosing appendicitis in pregnancy. Although no adverse fetal effects have been documented by the National Radiological Protection Board, its utility has not been fully investigated. MRI is useful in diagnosing appendicitis when ultrasound is inconclusive with a sensitivity and specificity of 100% and 94%, respectively. However, MRI in the evaluation of appendicitis often involves using gadolinium, and in its free form, this contrast can be toxic to the fetus. Overall, although MRI is a good choice for evaluation, many radiologists still overwhelmingly prefer CT in the evaluation of appendicitis in a pregnant patient when ultrasound is inconclusive.

In conclusion, if you have a high clinical suspicion for appendicitis in a pregnant patient, you should first obtain an ultrasound. If the ultrasound is inconclusive and you believe the risk of appendicitis is significant, you should obtain a CT scan of the abdomen as the risk estimate is critical in assessing the risk-benefit ratio for the patient and the growing fetus. So, the next time one of your radiology colleagues will not approve the use of a CT scan in a pregnant patient with a negative ultrasound study and a high clinical suspicion of appendicitis, tell him or her that the literature published by his or her colleagues recommends going forward with the scan. Do not be afraid to order that scan because if it is appendicitis, you potentially saved the patient and her fetus.

SUGGESTED READINGS

Brent RL. Counseling patients exposed to ionizing radiation during pregnancy. *Rev Panman Salud Publica*. 2006;20(2–3):198–204.

Hurwitz LM, Yoshizumi T, Reiman RD, et al. Radiation dose to the fetus from body MDCT during early gestation. *AJR Am J Roentgenol*. 2006;186(3):871–876.

Jaffe TA, Miller CM, Merkle EM. Practice patterns in imaging of the pregnant patient with abdominal pain: A survey of academic centers. *AJR Am J Roentgenol*. 2007;189(5):1128–1134.

Lazarus E, Mayo-Smith WW, Mainiero MB, et al. CT in the evaluation of nontraumatic abdominal pain in pregnant women. *Radiology*. 2007;244(3):784–790.

Lim HK, Bae SH, Seo GS. Diagnosis of acute appendicitis in pregnant women: Value of sonography. *AJR Am J Roentgenol*. 1992;159(3):539–542.

Pedrosa I, Levine D, Evvazzadeh AD, et al. MR imaging evaluation of acute appendicitis in pregnancy. *Radiology*. 2006;238(3):891–899.

Puylaert JB, Rutgers PH, Lalisang RI, et al. A prospective study of ultrasonography in the diagnosis of appendicitis. *N Engl J Med*. 1987;317(11):666–669.

Rosen MP, Sands DZ, Longmaid HE III, et al. Impact of abdominal CT on the management of patients presenting to the emergency department with acute abdominal pain. *AJR Am J Roentgenol*. 2000;174(5):1391–1396.

1 4

ABDOMINAL PAIN IN THE PATIENT WITH INFLAMMATORY BOWEL DISEASE SHOULD NEVER BE CONSIDERED ROUTINE

BEN A. LEESON, MD, FACEP AND KIMBERLY A. B. LEESON, MD

Abdominal pain is a frequent emergency department complaint. Of these, some causes are life threatening while others have a benign course. Patients with possible or known inflammatory bowel disease (IBD) require special considerations in the emergency department.

These patients usually have a history of chronic insidious abdominal pain that is recurrent in nature. This pain is associated with weight loss, anorexia, and mild diarrhea. Acute exacerbations often present with fever, crampy abdominal pain, tenesmus, urgency and frequent painful passage of stools containing mucus, blood, and occasionally pus. To complicate matters, IBD is often managed with immunomodulator drugs that suppress the immune system. These patients may therefore not manifest typical physical findings that are often associated with underlying infections.

It is easy for the emergency physician to fall into the trap of reflexively treating these patients with a "typical" IBD flare. But occasionally, these patients have severe complications or emergency situations that require expertise and prompt action. Some of these problems include toxic colitis, fistulas, abdominal abscesses, primary sclerosing cholangitis (PSC), and pouchitis. Maintaining an awareness of these complications will improve therapy and patient outcomes.

Toxic megacolon is a severe life-threatening emergency that can occur in either Crohn disease or ulcerative colitis. It is always present with toxic colitis: a constellation of at least six bloody bowel movements a day, a hemoglobin of <10.5 g/dL, sedimentation (SED) rate of at least 30, and a heart rate of at least 90 beats/per min. In addition to radiographic evidence of colonic dilatation, at least three of the following must also be present: temperature >38°C, leukocyte count >10,500/mm^3, and a hematocrit of <60% of normal.

The patient must also have at least one of the following signs or symptoms of systemic toxicity: dehydration, altered mental status, electrolyte abnormalities, or hypotension. Toxic megacolon treatment requires aggressive IV fluid resuscitation, broad-spectrum antibiotics aimed at enteric organisms, and bowel rest. Surgery is the best treatment, so be sure to get the surgeon involved early if you suspect this condition. Remember that peritoneal signs equal immediate surgical consult (do not wait for any studies).

Crohn disease can cause fistulas in any part of the bowel, and 50% of patients who had Crohn diease for more than 20 years had evidence of this complication. Enteroenteric, enterovaginal, enterovesicular, and externalizing fistulas may develop. Symptoms range from nonexistent to severe, depending on the location. Barium studies and CT or MRI can aid diagnosis. Treatment involves bowel rest, total parental nutrition (TPN), antiobiotics (ciprofloxacin and metronidazole), and/or surgery.

IBD patients also develop intra-abdominal abscesses. Suspect this condition in Crohn patients who present with abdominal pain, fever, and leukocytosis. An abdominal CT is diagnostic. Treatment involves abscess drainage, broad-spectrum antibiotics, and avoidance of corticosteroids. Surgery consultation should be obtained to determine if the abscess is operative, since some may be drained percutaneously.

PSC is a fibroinflammatory disorder of the bile ducts. It is characterized by strictures and beading of the bile ducts and chronic cholestasis. It is more frequently seen with ulcerative colitis and has a 2:1 male-to-female ratio. Often PSC is asymptomatic, but symptoms can include fatigue, weight loss, intermittent jaundice, right upper quadrant (RUQ) abdominal pain, and pruritis. It is suspected in IBD patients with abnormally elevated alkaline phosphatase levels and otherwise normal liver enzymes. No cure exists for this condition but antipruretics, steroids, immunosuppressives, biliary dilation, and stenting can improve symptoms. Do not forget to assess coagulation function on all patients you suspect may have liver dysfunction.

Some patients with IBD have total colectomies. Of these, some will have ileostomies and others will have an ileoanal pouch. These patients will not only have the usual postabdominal surgery complications (small bowel obstruction, adhesions, etc) but also have some that are unique to IBD and the ileoanal pouch. The normal colon absorbs a significant amount of water on a daily basis. Once it has been removed, patients have an increased risk of dehydration. So, in the emergency department, do not forget to assess hydration status. The ileoanal pouch is an internal reservoir that is created by folding loops of small bowel back on themselves and removing the internal walls. This pouch can become inflamed and when this occurs it is called pouchitis. The exact etiology is unknown. The most common presenting complaint is increased stool frequency which is watery. Admit if severely dehydrated or toxic appearing (unusual with pouchitis alone). Otherwise, emergency department treatment consists of metronidazole for 7 to 10 days. The patient should be instructed to follow up with a GI specialist.

Patients with IBD require special considerations in the emergency department, and medical immunosuppression will often obscure significant pathology. Extraintestinal complications such as PSC, toxic megacolon, bowel perforation, or an intra-abdominal abscess are real concerns. Work them up completely. You might be surprised with what you find.

SUGGESTED READINGS

Gow PJ, Chapman RW. Liver transplant for primary sclerosing cholangitis. *Liver*. 2000;20: 97–103.

Marrero F, Qadeer MA, Lashner BA. Severe complications of inflammatory bowel disease. *Med Clin North Am.* 2008;92(3):671–686.

Marx J, Hockberger R, Walls R., eds. *Rosen's Emergency Medicine, Concepts and Clinical Practice.* 4th ed., Vol II. St. Louis, MO: Mosby; 1996–1997:2032–2035.

Tintinallii JE, Kelen GD, Staphczynski JS, et al., eds. *Tintinalli's Emergency Medicine: A Comprehensive Study Guide.* 6th ed. New York, NY: McGraw Hill; 2003: 530–539, 560–561.

15

GIVE APPROPRIATE DOSAGES OF ANALGESICS TO PATIENTS WITH ABDOMINAL PAIN

ANGELA MCKELLAR, MD

Abdominal pain is a very common complaint evaluated in the emergency department (ED). According to the Center of Disease Control (CDC), there were roughly 112 million visits to EDs in 2005. The same year the reasons most frequently cited by patients for visiting the ED were stomach and abdominal pain at 6.8% or 7,833,000. With so many patients seen each year with this type of pain, it is important to examine the most common errors we make in the management of acute abdominal pain.

One of the biggest mistakes made in the management of abdominal pain is inadequate analgesia. Stalnikowicz et al. have estimated that up to 70% of patients seen in the ED complaining of pain do not receive any pain medications. The main reason for this conservative (and barbaric) strategy was deeply rooted in the concern of minimizing or masking classic physical exam findings and therefore negatively impacting accurate diagnosis and treatment. Many studies have since shown that withholding analgesia is not necessary to perform an adequate abdominal exam and even narcotics do not increase medical errors.

A systematic review by Ranji et al. in 2006 compiled the data from randomized clinical trials where patients with acute abdominal pain were given opiates or placebos in the ED. They were then assessed to see if there was a difference in physical exam findings or diagnostic accuracy. The findings were similar in trials with adults and children, showing an increased risk toward alterations of physical findings on exam after opiate administration, but there was no change in management errors between the two groups. According to these studies, treatment with opiates was found to be more humane and actually may result in a more accurate diagnosis and treatment. Theories for improved outcomes in patients with adequate pain management are most likely to do with the health practitioners' ability to perform a better physical exam when the patients' pain level is reduced. More specific and classic findings may be able to be recognized. Despite this evidence, a recent study by Graber et al. showed that when surveyed, 67% of surgeons still believe that analgesia interferes with diagnostic accuracy, but now you know better.

Treat the pain!! Morphine is often used as first-line therapy for moderate to severe abdominal pain. The initial loading dose suggested for IV morphine is 0.1 mg/kg. This would mean that for the average 70-kg opiate naïve male, an initial loading dose would be 7 mg IV. In practice that is not a typical starting dose used for patients. As everyone does respond to morphine differently, especially depending on their past narcotic exposure, starting lower than the loading dose and titrating up for pain is reasonable for some patients. However, this titration can and should be done over 5 to 10 min increments—not 1 to 2 h, so reassess and redose frequently. There are also many other choices for pain management, and just remember to dose them adequately.

Another consideration that historically has caused emergency physicians to withhold pain management in acute abdominal pain is the potential for the dreaded "sphincter of Oddi spasm" attributed to morphine. While this is a very rare side effect of morphine, it still seems to be a concern for some of our surgical colleagues and can delay definitive treatment. Wu et al. studied sphincter of Oddi spasm in the presence of meperidine and morphine. They found that there was no increase in the signs of motility within the sphincter using meperidine, while morphine showed some signs of motility. Clinically this may not be significant as very few cases of this actually happening have been reported. Chisholm et al. showed in a retrospective study that there was no increase in the sphincter of Oddi spasm in patients who received opiates before cholecystecomy. If the surgeons where you practice frequently delay or change the treatment plan for patients with biliary disease and if morphine has been given (despite the data showing otherwise) then, by all means, consider giving meperidine instead of morphine. It might be easier than convincing them of the evidence to the contrary. Just keep in mind that the duration of action of meperidines is short and there is an increased risk of seizures.

In summary, treat your patients' abdominal pain. There is overwhelming evidence to show that diagnostic ability is not diminished and may be improved, in patients with acute abdominal pain who are treated with opiod analgesics. Although the dreaded "sphincter of Oddi spasm" is unlikely to be of much clinical significance, if your consultants are plagued by this overwhelming fear and you are unable to educate them otherwise, then it may be reasonable to administer meperidine over morphine and live to fight another day!

SUGGESTED READINGS

Centers for Disease Control and Prevention. National Hospital Ambulatory Medical Care Survey: 2005 emergency department summary. Available at: www.cdc.gov/nchs/data/ad/ad386.pdf. Accessed August 13, 2008.

Chisholm RJ, Davis FM, Billings JD, et al. Narcotics and spasm of the sphincter of oddi: A retrospective study of perative cholangiograms. *Anaesthesia*. 1983;37(7):689–691.

Gallagher EJ, Esses D, Lee C, et al. Randomized clinical trial of morphine in acute abdominal pain. *Ann Emerg Med*. 2006;48(2):161–163.

Graber MA, Ely JW, Clarke S, et al. Informed consent and general surgeons' attitudes toward the use of pain medication in the acute abdomen. *Am J Emerg Med*. 1999;17:113–116.

Ranji SR, Goldman LE, Simel DL, et al. Do opiates affect the clinical evaluation of patients with acute abdominal pain? *JAMA*. 2006;296(14):1764–1774. Review.

Stalnikowicz R, Mahamid R, Kaspi S, et al. Undertreatment of acute pain in the emergency department: A challenge. *Int J Qual Health Care*. 2005;17(2):173–176.

Wu SD, Zhang ZH, Jin JZ, et al. Effects of narcotic analgesic drugs on human Oddi's sphincter motility. *World J Gastroenterol*. 2004;10(19):2901–2904.

16

NEVER ASSUME THAT ANY INTRA-ABDOMINAL CONDITION IN AN ELDERLY PATIENT WILL PRESENT "TYPICALLY"

MICHAEL MCLAUGHLIN, MD

Abdominal pain is a common complaint among elderly patients presenting to the Emergency Department (ED). This complaint must be taken very seriously in this population. Compared to younger patients with abdominal pain, elderly patients are more likely to acquire a specific diagnosis, have a delay in definitive diagnosis, and die of their condition. One third will require surgery. Even in admitted patients, failure to correctly diagnose a surgical condition upon initial evaluation leads to an increase in mortality.

The limitations of the history and physical exam must be understood when evaluating elderly patients with abdominal pain. "Textbook" presentations of disease are uncommon. Fever is absent in more than half of elderly patients with an intra-abdominal infection. Examples abound of atypical pain presentations. In one series of geriatric patients with acute cholecystitis, 84% did not have localized right upper quadrant or epigastric pain and 56% were afebrile. Among 96 elderly patients with appendicitis, only 20% presented classically with right lower quadrant pain, vomiting, fever, and an elevated leukocyte count.

Laboratory studies are recommended to guide the diagnostic workup and to evaluate for specific conditions such as renal failure, pancreatitis, biliary obstruction, and urinary tract infection. However, you must be aware of their limitations. Despite what your surgical colleagues would have you believe, a leukocyte count alone cannot be used to exclude serious pathology. It can be normal in 20% and 40% of patients with appendicitis and cholecystitis, respectively. Lactate is a useful marker of mesenteric ischemia. It is elevated in >90% of patients with mesenteric ischemia. It is not specific, however, being elevated in other surgical conditions associated with sepsis. Also, its usefulness in very early bowel ischemia without infarction is unknown. A normal lactate level does not completely rule out severe pathology, but an elevated lactate should alert the physician to a serious problem and the need for aggressive resuscitation.

Most elderly patients with abdominal pain will require imaging in the ED due to the nonspecific nature of their presentations. Routine use of plain radiographs as a screening tool is not recommended. They may detect free intraperitoneal air and obstruction, but computed tomography (CT) is superior in both of these cases. Plain radiographs will miss free intraperitoneal air from a perforated peptic ulcer 40% of the time. Ultrasound is the preferred diagnostic study in patients with biliary tract disease. CT is an exceptionally useful study in this population of stable patients. It is fast, readily available, and highly sensitive for conditions such as abdominal aortic aneurysm (AAA), appendicitis, diverticulitis, perforation, and obstruction. One study showed that CT altered the ED diagnosis of abdominal pain in elderly patients 45% of the time. It also changed the decision to admit 26% of the time, the need for surgery 12% of the time, and the need for antibiotics in 21% of cases. Liberal use of imaging, particularly CT, is recommended in elderly patients with abdominal pain.

Vascular catastrophes such as mesenteric ischemia and ruptured AAA must always be considered in elderly patients with abdominal pain, as they are uniformly fatal if not treated quickly. Ruptured AAA can present with any combination of abdominal pain, back/flank pain, hypotension, or syncope. Atypical presentations are common. In one study, 30% of patients were initially misdiagnosed. Bedside ultrasound by emergency physicians is a useful tool in evaluating for AAA. Mesenteric ischemia is an elusive diagnosis as well. Patients can present with any combination of abdominal pain, gut emptying (vomiting and diarrhea), and underlying cardiovascular disease. Because of the gut emptying, this disease can be mistaken for gastroenteritis. CT angiography stands to replace conventional angiography as the gold standard and is recommended as the first-line study from the ED. It may show bowel wall thickening, mesenteric edema, portal venous gas, or pneumatosis intestinalis. None of these findings alone are specific for mesenteric ischemia, but together they are highly suggestive of the disease.

Lastly, it must be noted that atypical myocardial infarction (MI) can present with isolated gastrointestinal symptoms. Thirty percent of MIs present atypically (lacking chest pain), most often in elderly females. Abdominal pain is a frequent complaint among this group. Thus, liberal use of ECGs and cardiac markers is recommended, particularly in those patients with known cardiac disease.

In summary, elderly patients with abdominal pain are a high-risk group. Serious diseases often present atypically. Be wary of sending an elderly patient with a diagnosis of gastroenteritis or constipation home without doing a thorough workup. Serious disorders, such as mesenteric ischemia and small bowel obstruction, present in a similar fashion. Do not rely upon one lab test, symptom, or physical finding to exclude pathology. Always consider vascular catastrophes and use imaging, particularly CT, liberally when evaluating these patients.

SUGGESTED READINGS

Bugliosi TF, Meloy TD, Vukov LF. Acute abdominal pain in the elderly. *Ann Emerg Med.* 1990;19(12):1383–1386.

Cooper GS, Shlaes DM, Salata RA. Intraabdominal infection: Differences in presentation and outcome between younger patients and the elderly. *Clin Infect Dis.* 1994;19(1):146–148.

de Dombal FT. Acute abdominal pain in the elderly. *J Clin Gastroenterol.* 1994;19(4): 331–335.

Esses D, Birnbaum A, Bijur P, et al. Ability of CT to alter decision making in elderly patients with acute abdominal pain. *Am J Emerg Med.* 2004;22(4):270–272.

Fenyo G. Acute abdominal disease in the elderly: Experience from two series in Stockholm. *Am J Surg.* 1982;143(6):751–754.

Horratas MC, Guyton DP, Wu D. A reappraisal of appendicitis in the elderly. *Am J Surg.* 1990;160:291–293.

Kim AY, Ha HK. Evaluation of suspected mesenteric ischemia: Efficacy of radiologic studies. *Radiol Clin North Am.* 2003;41(2):327–342.

Kuhn M, Bonnin RL, Davey MJ, et al. Emergency department ultrasound scanning for abdominal aortic aneurysm: Accessible, accurate, and advantageous. *Ann Emerg Med.* 2000;36(3):219–223.

Lange H, Jäckel R. Usefulness of plasma lactate concentration in the diagnosis of acute abdominal disease. *Eur J Surg.* 1994;160(6–7):381–384.

Lange H, Toivola A. Warning signals in acute abdominal disorders: Lactate is the best marker of mesenteric ischemia. *Lakartidningen.* 1997;94(20):1893–1896.

Lusiani L, Perrone A, Pesavento R, et al. Prevalence, clinical features, and acute course of atypical myocardial infarction. *Angiology.* 1994;45(1):49–55.

Marston WA, Ahlquist R, Johnson G Jr, et al. Misdiagnosis of ruptured abdominal aortic aneurysms. *J Vasc Surg.* 1992;16(1):17–22.

Martinez JP, Mattu A. Abdominal pain in the elderly. *Emerg Med Clin North Am.* 2006;24(2):371–388.
Parker LJ, Vukov LF, Wollan PC. Emergency department evaluation of geriatric patients with acute cholecystitis. *Acad Emerg Med.* 1997;4(1):51–55.

17

KNOW HOW TO RISK STRATIFY PATIENTS WITH UPPER GASTROINTESTINAL BLEEDING

JOSHUA MOSKOVITZ, MD, MPH

The chief complaint of "vomiting blood" often provokes an adrenaline rush at the thought of a potentially life-threatening condition with a very sick patient. This call to action is muted by the fact that your most dependable triage nurse has not alerted you to this patient, leading you to believe that this is most likely not variceal bleeding. Upper gastrointestinal bleeding (UGIB) can be divided into two types: variceal and nonvariceal bleeding. Variceal bleeding automatically places patients in a high-risk category, as they have higher morbidity and mortality, and necessitates emergent intervention. What then is required for the patient who is not cirrhotic and has a low probability for the presence of varices? Is your gastroenterologist going to be excited to come see this patient or fall back to sleep while talking to you on the phone? Do you need to advocate for admission with emergent or urgent endoscopy? In general, UGIB is associated with a 14% mortality rate in emergency hospital admissions. These patients have a primary bleeding event not related to chronic diseases, but typically related to duodenal ulcers and *Helicobacter pylori* infections. Your goal is to determine whether or not an admission is warranted and if invasive studying will find anything worthy of intervention. GI physicians have developed multiple decision models to determine the probability of finding an active lesion worthy of intervention on endoscopy. While our internal medicine colleagues may like to ponder and pontificate about them during morning rounds, they are important for us to know about so that we can anticipate our consultants' response when we call them in the wee hours of the morning.

Practically speaking though, much of these predictive scoring models require endoscopic findings, so their utility in the ED is undermined. On the other hand, the Blatchford score relies only on clinical and laboratory variables and has also been validated prospectively to risk stratify those patients with acute nonvariceal UGIB at low risk for requiring blood transfusion or endoscopic or

TABLE 17.1	MODIFIED BLATCHFORD RISK SCORE				
VARIABLE	**0**	**1**	**2**	**3**	**6**
Hgb men	≥13.0	12.0–12.9		10.0–11.9	<10.0
Hgb female	≥12.0	10.0–11.9			<10.0
Systolic BP	≥110	100–109	90–99	<90	
HR	<100	≥100			
Melena	No	Yes			
Liver disease	No		Yes		
Cardiac failure	No		Yes		

mBRS ≤1 → Low risk.

surgical management for bleeding control. Unfortunately, this study did not systematically provide scope for all of the low-risk patients to truly determine what their pathology was and, hence, may cause you to label a patient as a low-risk patient who actually has a visible vessel in an ulcer with an adherent clot. The modified Blatchford risk score (mBRS) (*Table 17.1*) was then developed using a retrospective analysis of patients who had had endoscopy and was able to further define those patients at low risk of requiring intervention. (Can you just imagine the fun internal medicine rounds have discussing whether or not patients with an mBRS score ≤1, have a lower risk of rebleeding [5%] and a lower mortality rate [0.5%] than those with an mBRS >1?)

But what is important to the emergency physician? First, you are able to define a low-risk population. Patients have a low risk of rebleeding (5%) and a low mortality rate (0.5%) if they do not have cardiac disease, liver disease, severe hypotension, or severe anemia. The presence of tachycardia, mild hypotension, and mild anemia does not necessarily increase the probability of the endoscopist finding a significant lesion per the mBRS. Your GI specialist will likely emphasize these data, but remember the second point which states that these data were based on a retrospective analysis. As of yet, there has not been a prospective study defining a group that can be safely discharged from the ED on a proton pump inhibitor with close follow-up and early outpatient endoscopy.

The bottom line is that these scoring modalities are confusing and conflicting. A large retrospective study by Adamopoulos refined 17 variables of active bleeding amenable to intervention into four independent predictors (*Table 17.2*). Hemodynamic instability (systolic blood pressure <100 and a heart rate >100) had an OR of 8.7, hemoglobin level <8 had an Odds Ratio (OR) of 8.1, and a WBC > 12 had an OR of 5.2 for detecting bleeds. But by far, the most significant prognostic indicator for active intervention was bloody nasogastric lavage

TABLE 17.2	INDEPENDENT PREDICTORS FOR ACTIVE BLEEDING	
FINDING		**POINTS**
Bloody NGT		6
Hemodynamic instability		4
Hgb < 8		4
WBC > 12		3
Low risk ≤3.		

with an OR of 16.4. If you are going to remember one scoring modality, know that patients presenting only with an increased WBC have not been found to have any active lesions on endoscopy or in need of acute intervention.

The take-home message is that you can consider sending the patient home for outpatient follow-up who does not have risk factors. But if the patient has risk factors, Google a risk scoring modality and tell the house officer, "The patient's modified Blatchford Risk Score places them at a high probability of having a lesion that will require endoscopic visualization and definition. The gastroenterologist is aware, but would prefer that you admit them for the night."

SUGGESTED READINGS

Adamopoulos A, Baibas N, Efstathiou S, et al. Differentiation between patients with acute upper gastrointestinal bleeding who need early urgent upper gastrointestinal endoscopy and those who do not: A prospective study. *Eur J Gastroenterol Hepatol*. 2003;15:381–387.

Chen I, Hung M, Chiu T, et al. Risk scoring systems to predict need for clinical intervention for patients with nonvariceal upper gastrointestinal tract bleeding. *Am J Emerg Med*. 2007;25:774–779.

Cohen M, Sapoznikov B, Niv Y. Primary and secondary non-variceal upper gastrointestinal bleeding. *J Clin Gastroenterol*. 2007;41(9):810–913.

Masaoka T, Suzuki H, Hori S, et al. Blatchford scoring system is a useful scoring system for detecting patients with upper gastrointestinal bleeding who do not need endoscopic intervention. *J Gastroenterol Hepatol*. 2007;22:1404–1408.

Romagnuolo J, Barkun A, Enns R, et al. Simple clinical predictors may obviate urgent dndoscopy in selected patients with nonvariceal upper gastrointestinal tract bleeding. *Arch Int Med*. 2007;167:265–270.

Taupin D. Admission risk markers for upper gastrointestinal bleeding: Can urgent endoscopy be avoided? *J Gastroenterol Hepatol*. 2007;22:1355–1357.

18

MANAGE ACUTE VARICEAL BLEEDING AGGRESSIVELY

JOSHUA MOSKOVITZ, MD, MPH

The management of patients with upper gastrointestinal bleeds (UGIB) presenting in extremis is enough to make any physician have melena. In an effort to preserve your own clothes, make your life easier by classifying the condition in terms of variceal versus nonvariceal. Varices are present 85% of the time in patients with Child-Pugh Class C (severe) cirrhosis, but do not be fooled by the lack of cirrhosis. Primary biliary cirrhosis patients develop varices long before the establishment of cirrhosis. It is simple plumbing; varices develop and subsequently bleed as a result of increased portal pressure due to increased resistance to flow from the fibrous reorganization of the liver's architecture. Variceal hemorrhage is directly proportional to the hepatic venous pressure gradient (HVPG). The control of bleeding varices is therefore aimed at decreasing the HVPG. Inevitably, variceal bleeders require endoscopic banding.

Variceal bleeding frequently is intermittent and resolves spontaneously in 40% to 50% of patients. Rebleeding will occur (in 30% to 40%) in the first 6 weeks, with peak incidence in the first 5 days. Consider the patient who is currently not bleeding as a disaster waiting to happen. Be aggressive!

There are objective criteria that can assist you in risk stratifying your patients. Adverse outcomes have been associated with five initial findings: hematocrit <30%, systolic blood pressure <100 mm Hg, bloody nasogastric lavage, history of cirrhosis or ascites on exam, and history of vomiting red blood. Many of these are intuitive; if your patient is hypotensive with bright red blood in the nasogastric (NG) tube and a hematocrit of 20%, then there is an ominous outcome looming. However, do not overlook the subjective report of hematemesis. Trust your patients! Do not rely on a negative nasogastric lavage or the absence of melena. Hematemesis, whether subjective or objective, has a relative risk of 2.4 and needs to be taken seriously. Furthermore, look for ascites, as patients with a history of cirrhosis or ascites have poor prognosis with a 36% complication rate.

Now that you know that your patient has the potential for a less than optimal outcome, take action to improve his or her chances. You only have to worry about five things: airway protection, volume resuscitation, bleeding tamponade, prevention of organ dysfunction, and minimization of infection. Naturally, you are a master of the As and Bs, but let us focus on the nuances of this patient's circulation.

Volume resuscitation requires prompt but cautious intervention. Overly aggressive saline resuscitation can lead to increased ascites that will further increase the HVPG, further exacerbating bleeding. Do not be shy about plasma expanders; the average patient requires 4 units of packed red blood cells (PRBCs), 3 units of fresh frozen plasma (FFP), and 1½ units of platelets. Aim for a hemoglobin of 8 g/dL and systolic blood pressure to 100 mm Hg, but not higher, as higher HVPGs cause more rebleeding and increased mortality. Obviously, the patient with rapid ongoing bleeding or ischemic heart disease requires a higher hemoglobin level. Control bleeding first with FFP and platelets, but do not waste your patient's money on recombinant factor VIIa, because there is no benefit.

Now is a great time to break out that new handheld computer and your newest drug reference guide! Vasopressin is a potent splanchnic vasoconstrictor that reduces blood flow and decreases the HVPG; however, it has side effects. Give nitrates to decrease some of these untoward effects if the blood pressure can tolerate it. Octreotide also causes splanchnic vasoconstriction, but watch out for tachyphylaxis. Forget about β-blockers; they are only useful to prevent the occurrence of bleeds in outpatients and will complicate your management by blunting the compensatory increase in heart rate.

Interestingly, while vasoconstrictors make intuitive sense, antibiotics also play an important role in patients with variceal bleeds. Cirrhotic patients with UGIB are at increased risk of severe bacterial infections, which lead to early recurrence of hemorrhage and greater mortality. Fifty percent develop spontaneous bacterial peritonitis, 25% urinary tract infections, and 25% pneumonias. Give short-term prophylactic antibiotic therapy whether or not ascites are present. Norfloxacin or ciprofloxacin is the preferred oral medication, but ceftriaxone is the preferred intravenous medication in the severely cirrhotic patient. Forget about lactulose or lactitol; it has no benefit and only angers the nurses.

Unfortunately, despite your efforts, 10% to 20% of patients cannot have their bleeding controlled despite endoscopic or pharmacologic intervention and may need emergent shunt therapy. If your on-call gastroenterologist is on the golf course with nine holes to go, have your interventionalist's and surgeon's numbers readily available. Balloon tamponade is an effective device to control excessive bleeding temporarily; however, it has potentially lethal complications including aspiration, migration, necrosis, and perforation with a mortality rate of 20%. Only use it if your patient will be definitively getting TIPS (Transjugular Intrahepatic Portosystemic Shunt) therapy within 24 h of placement.

With these tips in mind, you should be able to satisfactorily sign this patient out to your colleague, and thanks to the ever-increasing practice of emergency department boarding, receive this patient again during next day morning's sign out.

SUGGESTED READINGS

Abraldes J, Bosch J. The treatment of acute variceal bleeding. *J Clin Gastroenterol.* 2007;41(S3):S312–S327.

Corley D, Stefan A, Wolf M, et al. Early indicators of prognosis in upper gastrointestinal hemorrhage. *Am J Gastroenterol.* 1998;93(3):336–340.

Garcia-Tsao G, Sanyal A, Grace N, et al. Prevention and management of gastroesophageal varices and variceal hemorrhage in cirrhosis. *Hepatology*. 2007;46(3):922–938.

Sorbi D, Gostout C, Peura D, et al. An assessment of the management of acute bleeding varices: A multicenter prospective member-based study. *Am J Gastroenterol*. 2003;98(11): 2424–2434.

19

DO NOT MISS THE DEADLY CAUSES OF RECTAL BLEEDING AND PAIN

TAY NGUYEN, MD AND ALBERT L. GEST, DO

The initial approach to the patient presenting with rectal bleeding in the emergency department (ED) is to determine if the bleeding is life-threatening. Early recognition and early resuscitation are paramount in the management of the hemodynamically unstable patient, for example, the elderly patient status post Abdominal Aortic Aneurysm (AAA) repair or the cirrhotic patient with ongoing bleeding. Signs that the patient may display include tachycardia, hypotension, diaphoresis, altered mental status, pallor, or decreased urinary output (*Table 19.1*, Medical Emergencies). Resuscitation efforts include continuous hemodynamic monitoring, IV fluids, supplemental oxygenation, and availability of blood products. Obtain stat laboratory workup including complete blood count (CBC), complete metabolic panel with blood urea nitrogen (BUN), creatinine, liver function tests (LFTs), coagulation studies, blood type, and cross-match.

More subtle presentations give time to obtain a complete history and physical exam. Obtaining a detailed history assures that the provider does not miss urgent causes of rectal pain and bleeding such as malignancies, perirectal abscesses, and cryptitis (*Table 19.1*, Medical Urgencies). Relevant information includes the amount and frequency of bleeding, timing of pain, rectal trauma, fever, bowel habits, and other systemic complaints. The persistence of pain between bowel movements should alert the provider to a more serious underlying cause of rectal bleeding. Keep in mind that "rectal bleeding" may actually be bleeding from the upper or lower gastrointestinal tracts.

The anorectal examination begins with a thorough external exam looking for hemorrhoids, fissures, fistulas, abscesses, and other cutaneous abnormalities. A digital rectal exam is necessary to further investigate the source of bleeding and to localize any palpable masses or areas of tenderness. A fecal occult blood test should be performed to confirm the presence of blood. Visualization with anoscopy or sigmoidoscopy, if available, may aid the emergency physician in the localization of bleeding.

Abdominal imaging is required in cases where the ability to obtain a history is limited and the physical exam is unreliable. This population includes patients with comorbid conditions such as diabetes, steroid use, immunocompromised, altered mental status, and advanced age. Plain films are useful in patients with diffuse abdominal pain or if foreign bodies are suspected. Contrast CT scans may aid in the diagnosis of malignancies, rectal abscesses, rectal fistulas, and other causes of gastrointestinal bleeding. Sonography has been described in the literature for imaging rectal abscesses and foreign bodies.

Hospital admission for further workup is indicated in patients with uncontrolled pain, intractable vomiting, or abnormal laboratory or imaging results. In addition, surgical consultation should be obtained for patients with perirectal abscess, anorectal fistula, rectal prolapse, acute abdomen, uncontrolled bleeding, and those with foreign bodies requiring surgical removal. In patients who are discharged, documentation must reflect the fact that they are hemodynamically stable with only mild symptoms and that the etiologies of bleeding or pain are benign, such as anal fissures or hemorrhoids. It is also important to document that the patient has reliable and timely follow-up with his or her primary doctor, surgeon, or reevaluation by the ED physician if there is inadequate follow-up.

Medical legal implications stem from failure to diagnose or treat serious causes or complications of rectal bleeding (*Table 19.1*, Medical Legal Pitfalls).

TABLE 19.1	CATEGORIES OF RECTAL BLEEDING	
MEDICAL EMERGENCIES	**MEDICAL URGENCIES**	**MEDICAL LEGAL PITFALLS**
Massive UGI bleed—varices, PUD	Internal and external hemorrhoids	Abnormal vital signs
Aortoenteric fistula (s/p AAA repair)	Fissures (most common in Peds)	Severe and rapid onset
Angiodysplasia	Cryptitis	Brisk bleeding
Coagulopathies	Perianal abscess	Peritoneal signs
Rectal trauma	Food allergy (common in Peds)	Comorbidities
	Infectious diarrhea	Perirectal abscess
	Inflammatory bowel disease	Foreign bodies
	Malignancy	Child abuse
		Inadequate examination or exposure

Abnormal vital signs and brisk bleeding should prompt the ED physician to take immediate actions to stabilize the patient. Patients with severe and rapid onset of bleeding, elderly patients, and those with comorbidities and peritoneal signs warrant more extensive workup and judicious use of imaging. A child abuse workup and social worker consultation should be obtained in pediatric patients presenting with rectal bleeding with evidence of anorectal trauma. Patients presenting with rectal foreign bodies are often embarrassed and may not disclose much information on history. Likewise, body packers are fearful of legal repercussions of being discovered. Foreign bodies may not always be palpable on digital rectal exams, which necessitates a thorough abdominal exam. In prisoners and psychiatric patients with suspected rectal foreign bodies, abdominal films must be obtained before a digital rectal exam, in order to avoid being injured by sharp objects.

SUGGESTED READINGS

Burgess BE, Bouzoukis JK. Anorectal disorders. In: Tintinalli JE, Kelen GD, Stapczynski JS, eds. *Emergency Medicine: Comprehensive Study Guide*. 6th ed. New York, NY: McGraw-Hill; 2004:539–550.

Coates WC. Anorectum. In: Marx JA, Hockberger RS, Walls RM, eds. *Rosen's Emergency Medicine: Concepts and Clinical Practice*. 6th ed. Philadelphia, PA: Mosby; 2006:1507–1524.

Law PJ, Talbot RW, Bartram CI, et al. Anal endosonography in the evaluation of perianal sepsis and fistula in ano. *Br J Surg*. 1989;76(7):752–755.

Munter DW. Foreign bodies, rectum. Available at: http://www.emedicine.com/emerg/topic933.htm. Last updated July 13, 2007.

Segal WN, Greenberg PD, Rochay DC, et al. The outpatient evaluation of hematochezia. *Am J Gastroenterol*. 1998;93:179.

Walker A, Durie PR, Hamilton JR, et al., eds. *Pediatric Gastrointestinal Diseases*. 4th ed. Philadelphia, PA: BC Decker; 2003.

Zeller JA, Masser BA. Rectal complaints. In: Roppolo LP, Davis D, Kelly SP, Rosen P, eds. *Emergency Medicine: Clinical Concepts for Clinical Practice*. Philadelphia, PA: Mosby Elsevier; 2007:560–570.

20

DO NOT OVERESTIMATE THE VALUE OF THE FAST EXAM

PEDRO G. R. TEIXEIRA, MD

Diagnostic imaging remains an essential tool in the management of injured patients. For unstable injured patients, in whom the primary goal is to diagnose and promptly stop the bleeding, imaging is used to identify the sources of hemorrhage. Blood loss is a major cause of early deaths after injury and remains the primary cause of preventable and potentially preventable deaths at mature trauma centers. For hemodynamically stable patients, imaging is also essential for the diagnosis and characterization of specific injuries.

Focused assessment with sonography for trauma (FAST) is a standardized ultrasound examination that aims to identify the presence of free fluid in the pericardium and peritoneal cavity. As an initial diagnostic adjunct, the ultrasound has several advantages: it is noninvasive, repeatable, accessible, portable, rapid, and cost effective. Ultrasound, however, is highly operator dependent and is limited by the presence of subcutaneous emphysema or a large hemothorax, morbid obesity, severe chest wall injury, and a narrow subcostal area.

Physical examination alone is unreliable for the diagnosis of intra-abdominal injuries in patients who have sustained blunt abdominal trauma. In order to safely exclude significant intra-abdominal injuries, a highly sensitive screening diagnostic modality is warranted.

The use of FAST examination in the workup of blunt trauma patients became widespread after the early reports suggesting high sensitivity for the identification of intraperitoneal free fluid. A significant 18% to 26% of trauma patients with intra-abdominal injuries, however, have no detectable hemoperitoneum, and up to 29% of abdominal injuries may be missed by the ultrasound as the only imaging modality. If an associated pelvic fracture is present, the sensitivity of the FAST examination can be as low as 24%.

Most of the studies reporting high sensitivity for FAST lack consistent application of a gold standard to all patients as well as adequate follow-up, which may contribute to an underestimation of the false negative rates. Even groups that report higher sensitivities and advocate the use of FAST as a screening method are cautious in their recommendations, add a period of clinical observation to their protocols, and suggest that a low threshold for obtaining additional testing should be maintained. Blackbourne et al. demonstrated that the addition of a secondary ultrasound examination significantly increased the sensitivity of the FAST examination in stable blunt injured patients.

More recent studies and systematic reviews have highlighted the FAST inability to rule out significant intra-abdominal injuries, suggesting that the FAST has significant limitations as a screening method in the initial evaluation of blunt trauma patients. Compared to CT scan as the gold standard, the FAST examination had a sensitivity of only 42% for intraperitoneal fluid in hemodynamically stable patients. Likewise, Richards et al. found emergent ultrasound to be 60% sensitive for the detection of intraperitoneal fluid. In a comprehensive review, Stengel et al. demonstrated that the ultrasound lacked sensitivity and negative predictive value for the identification of intra-abdominal injuries and therefore, constituted a poor screening method for this patient population, missing 1 in every 10 abdominal injuries. A Cochrane review analyzing the use of ultrasound-based treatment algorithms suggested that the utilizationofultrasoundintheevaluationoftraumapatientshadminimalimpacton management decision.

For the hemodynamically unstable blunt trauma patient, a positive FAST warrants immediate surgical exploration. A negative FAST in this setting, however, is noncontributory, as 32% to 37% of the unstable patients with a negative ultrasound had intra-abdominal injuries. In the setting of hemodynamic instability and negative FAST without other obvious source of bleeding, the addition of a diagnostic peritoneal aspirate (DPA) to the initial assessment of trauma patients can provide useful information. Compared to FAST, DPA was found to be more sensitive (89% vs. 50%) and specific (100% vs. 95%) for the identification of intra-abdominal bleeding.

A poor sensitivity with the FAST is also observed in the setting of penetrating abdominal injuries. In hemodynamically stable patients sustaining penetrating abdominal trauma, the FAST exam identified only 46% to 71% of the patients with intra-abdominal injury.

In summary, as a result of its low sensitivity and negative predictive value for intraperitoneal free fluid and intra-abdominal injuries, a negative FAST in the initial assessment of the trauma patient should not be used as the only diagnostic modality to exclude significant intra-abdominal injuries. Patients with suspected intra-abdominal injury should be clinically observed or should preferentially undergo further investigation, irrespective of the ultrasound findings.

SUGGESTED READINGS

Bakker J, Genders R, Mali W, et al. Sonography as the primary screening method in evaluating blunt abdominal trauma. *J Clin Ultrasound*. 2005;33:155–163.

Ballard RB, Rozycki GS, Newman PG, et al. An algorithm to reduce the incidence of false-negative FAST examinations in patients at high risk for occult injury: Focused assessment for the sonographic examination of the trauma patient. *J Am Coll Surg*. 1999;189:145–150; discussion 150–151.

Blackbourne LH, Soffer D, McKenney M, et al. Secondary ultrasound examination increases the sensitivity of the FAST exam in blunt trauma. *J Trauma*. 2004;57:934–938.

Bode PJ, Edwards MJ, Kruit MC, et al. Sonography in a clinical algorithm for early evaluation of 1671 patients with blunt abdominal trauma. *AJR Am J Roentgenol*. 1999;172:905–911.

Boulanger BR, Kearney PA, Tsuei B, et al. The routine use of sonography in penetrating torso injury is beneficial. *J Trauma*. 2001;51:320–325.

Boulanger BR, McLellan BA, Brenneman FD, et al. Emergent abdominal sonography as a screening test in a new diagnostic algorithm for blunt trauma. *J Trauma*. 1996;40: 867–874.

Brown MA, Casola G, Sirlin CB, et al. Blunt abdominal trauma: Screening us in 2,693 patients. *Radiology*. 2001;218:352–358.

Chiu WC, Cushing BM, Rodriguez A, et al. Abdominal injuries without hemoperitoneum: A potential limitation of focused abdominal sonography for trauma (FAST). *J Trauma*. 1997;42:617–623; discussion 623–625.

Dolich MO, McKenney MG, Varela JE, et al. 2,576 ultrasounds for blunt abdominal trauma. *J Trauma*. 2001;50:108–112.

Farahmand N, Sirlin CB, Brown MA, et al. Hypotensive patients with blunt abdominal trauma: Performance of screening US. *Radiology*. 2005;235:436–443.

Gruen RL, Jurkovich GJ, McIntyre LK, et al. Patterns of errors contributing to trauma mortality: Lessons learned from 2,594 deaths. *Ann Surg*. 2006;244:371–380.

Healey MA, Simons RK, Winchell RJ, et al. A prospective evaluation of abdominal ultrasound in blunt trauma: Is it useful? *J Trauma*. 1996;40:875–883; discussion 883–885.

Holmes JF, Harris D, Battistella FD. Performance of abdominal ultrasonography in blunt trauma patients with out-of-hospital or emergency department hypotension. *Ann Emerg Med*. 2004;43:354–361.

Kirkpatrick AW, Sirois M, Ball CG, et al. The hand-held ultrasound examination for penetrating abdominal trauma. *Am J Surg*. 2004;187:660–665.

Lee BC, Ormsby EL, McGahan JP, et al. The utility of sonography for the triage of blunt abdominal trauma patients to exploratory laparotomy. *AJR Am J Roentgenol*. 2007;188: 415–421.

Lingawi SS, Buckley AR. Focused abdominal US in patients with trauma. *Radiology*. 2000;217:426–429.

Meyer DM, Jessen ME, Grayburn PA. Use of echocardiography to detect occult cardiac injury after penetrating thoracic trauma: A prospective study. *J Trauma*. 1995;39:902–907; discussion 907–909.

Miller MT, Pasquale MD, Bromberg WJ, et al. Not so FAST. *J Trauma*. 2003;54:52–59; discussion 59–60.

Nural MS, Yardan T, Guven H, et al. Diagnostic value of ultrasonography in the evaluation of blunt abdominal trauma. *Diagn Interv Radiol*. 2005;11:41–44.

Richards JR, Schleper NH, Woo BD, et al. Sonographic assessment of blunt abdominal trauma: A 4-year prospective study. *J Clin Ultrasound*. 2002;30:59–67.

Rodriguez A, DuPriest RW Jr, Shatney CH. Recognition of intra-abdominal injury in blunt trauma victims: A prospective study comparing physical examination with peritoneal lavage. *Am J Surg*. 1982;48:457–459.

Rozycki GS, Ballard RB, Feliciano DV, et al. Surgeon-performed ultrasound for the assessment of truncal injuries: Lessons learned from 1540 patients. *Ann Surg*. 1998; 228:557–567.

Rozycki GS, Ochsner MG, Jaffin JH, et al. Prospective evaluation of surgeons' use of ultrasound in the evaluation of trauma patients. *J Trauma*. 1993;34:516–526; discussion 526–527.

Sauaia A, Moore FA, Moore EE, et al. Epidemiology of trauma deaths: A reassessment. *J Trauma*. 1995;38:185–193.

Schurink GW, Bode PJ, van Luijt PA, et al. The value of physical examination in the diagnosis of patients with blunt abdominal trauma: A retrospective study. *Injury*. 1997;28:261–265.

Sirlin CB, Brown MA, Andrade-Barreto OA, et al. Blunt abdominal trauma: Clinical value of negative screening US scans. *Radiology*. 2004;230:661–668.

Soffer D, McKenney MG, Cohn S, et al. A prospective evaluation of ultrasonography for the diagnosis of penetrating torso injury. *J Trauma*. 2004;56:953–957; discussion 957–959.

Stengel D, Bauwens K, Sehouli J, et al. Emergency ultrasound-based algorithms for diagnosing blunt abdominal trauma. *Cochrane Database Syst Rev*. 2005;2:CD004446.

Teixeira PG, Inaba K, Hadjizacharia P, et al. Preventable or potentially preventable mortality at a mature trauma center. *J Trauma*. 2007;63:1338–1346; discussion 1346–1347.

Udobi KF, Rodriguez A, Chiu WC, et al. Role of ultrasonography in penetrating abdominal trauma: A prospective clinical study. *J Trauma*. 2001;50:475–479.

Yoshii H, Sato M, Yamamoto S, et al. Usefulness and limitations of ultrasonography in the initial evaluation of blunt abdominal trauma. *J Trauma*. 1998;45:45–50; discussion 50–51.

21

DO NOT EXPECT THE "TYPICAL" WHEN TRANSPLANT PATIENTS PRESENT WITH ABDOMINAL PAIN

WILLIAM F. RUTHERFORD, MD

It is a dark and stormy night, and you are the lone gun at Elsewhere General when one of the over 29,000 annual solid organ transplant recipients in the United States staggers through your door with severe abdominal pain. (With 1-year graft survival ranging from 78% for a pancreas transplant to >95% for a living donor kidney transplant, you can run—but you cannot hide!). An appropriately quick call to the transplant surgeon is answered by an Odds Ratio (OR) nurse—"he'll call you back as soon as he can." Tag—you are it.

The first pitfall you must avoid is restricting the differential diagnosis, by assuming either that the pain and accompanying symptoms *must* be related to the transplant or conversely that the transplant *cannot* be relevant. Simply having a transplant does not confer any special immunity to the recipient from the usual suspects—just the opposite is true. Transplanted patients also have their own unique set of problems. For example, left lower quadrant pain may be due to constipation, garden variety diverticulitis, immune suppression–facilitated colitis, or an episode of pyelonephritis and/or acute rejection of the transplanted kidney.

Immunosuppression is the leading reason for the transplants to be remarkably successful and yet is responsible for their chief complication—infection. Infection can lead to rejection (e.g., pyelonephritis in the transplanted kidney) and organ dysfunction (e.g., viral hepatitis in the transplanted liver) and is the leading cause of death in the 1st year after transplant.

Transplant recipients are further predisposed to infection. For example, the ureter of the transplanted kidney is both shorter and more acutely angled at the anastamosis than is the native ureter, facilitating pyelonephritis. Despite glucose stability, the microvascular and neuropathic changes in a lifelong diabetic remain, inviting infection from underperfused and insensate tissues. Transplanted organs themselves may harbor infectious agents. The necessary hospitalization unfortunately exposes patients to multiply resistant organisms. The agents of illness run the gamut from the alphabet of viruses through the usual and opportunistic bacterial and fungal agents.

Transplant recipients simply do not follow "the rules." For example, a kidney-pancreas recipient may have a baseline subnormal temperature due to hyperglycemia from a rejected pancreas, uremia from a failed kidney, or steroids.

Celsus' classic signs of inflammation (*rubor, calor, and dolor et tumor*) may just as easily indicate acute rejection as infection. A normal white blood cell count may be rendered diagnostically impotent by immunosuppressives. Regardless of presenting symptoms and signs, *always* strongly consider infection in your differential, as no single complaint or immediate test can firmly establish or exclude it, and missing it can lead to devastating consequences.

Pain in the area of any transplanted organ should immediately raise the specter of rejection, at least one episode of which occurs in 30% to 50% of renal transplant patients. Rejection episodes may be acute or more chronic in nature. Other nonrejection causes of pain include abcess, obstruction of out-flow (e.g., ureteral stone and stricture), vascular stenosis or thrombosis, bowel obstruction, immunosuppressives (azathioprine-induced pancreatitis and tac-rolimus) and peritonitis without defined cause. Colonic perforation can occur with diverticulitis or ischemic or CMV colitis. Constipation from either chronic opiate use or bowel dysmotility secondary to underlying chronic disease also presents as abdominal pain but requires no less vigorous an evaluation—this is a *diagnosis of exclusion*.

Transplant patients "live on the precipice of renal failure" due to the nephrotoxicity of immunosuppressives (e.g., tacrolimus and cyclosporine), the effects of chronic illness (e.g., diabetes and hypertension), as well as the other issues discussed above. Approximately one fifth of liver recipients show some chronic renal insufficiency or failure at 5 years. Do not "push the patient over the cliff"—DO NOT use intravenous contrast without consulting the transplant physician (unless you want him or her to seize). Non-steroidal anti-inflammatory drugs (NSAIDs) (including ketorolac) and other nephrotoxic agents (e.g., aminoglycosides) are similarly *non grata*. You must also adequately replace any significant volume deficit.

The immediate workup reflects both the organ transplanted and the con-stellation of symptoms. Always obtain a complete blood count (CBC), blood urea nitrogen (BUN), creatinine and electrolytes, and amylase, lipase, transaminases, and bilirubin when appropriate. Medication levels (tacrolimus, cyclosporine, and other incidental drugs) should also be obtained. Cultures should include both blood and urine for bacteria and fungus. Get a formal urinalysis instead of a bedside dipstick. CT scans are a valuable diagnostic tool with the obvious caveat regarding intravenous contrast. Ultrasonography of the pancreas or kidney is useful for evaluating vascular integrity (and therefore viability), or obstruction, and for locating fluid collections but can usually await transfer or daylight.

The patient's transplant surgeon, transplant coordinator, or medical sub-specialist should be contacted early in the encounter and especially prior to disposition. Doing so with confidence and appropriate data rather than an air of befuddlement will benefit the patient, the transplant team, and the emergency medicine physician.

Suggested Readings

Chan L, Gaston R, Hariharan S. Evolution of immunosuppression and continued importance of actue rejection in renal transplantation. *Am J Kidney Dis*. 2001;38(Suppl 6):S2.

Fischer SA. Infections complicating solid organ transplantation. *Surg Clin N Am*. 2006;86:1127–1145.

Gautam A. Gastrointestinal complications following transplantation. *Surg Clin N Am*. 2006;86:1195–1206.

Ojo AO, Held PJ, Port FK, et al. Chronic renal failure after transplantation of a non-renal organ. *N Engl J Med*. 2003;349(10):931–940.

Organ Procurement Transplant Network. Available at: www.optn.org. Accessed August 15, 2008.

Tanphaichitr NT, Brennan DC. Infectious complications in renal transplant recipients. *Adv Ren Replace Ther*. 2000;7(2):131–146.

22

ACT QUICKLY WHEN SUSPECTING MESENTERIC ISCHEMIA

ESTEBAN SCHABELMAN, MD, MBA

Diarrhea. Bloody stools. Old people. Fighting with consultants. This is why we went into emergency medicine, right? Sadly, though, this is a typical course of a deadly disease: mesenteric ischemia (MI). If you think you might have a patient with MI, call your surgeons now and then read this chapter. You have plenty of time, and the surgeons (if they have their way) probably will not come down till after the CT scan is finished anyway.

MI has an extremely high mortality rate, between 60% and 80%, *when diagnosed*. One Swedish study showed that actual mortality may be as high as 90%, but it was considered as a diagnosis only one third of the time. Hopefully, you will do better than the Swedes and consider MI as a diagnosis 100% of the time when you see an elderly patient with abdominal pain. The reason that MI is so difficult to diagnose is that it is really four separate diseases, each with a different presentation, but all leading to ultimate bowel infarction. Remembering the four different causes and presentations of MI is the key to its diagnosis.

1) **Arterial emboli** are the most common cause of MI (40% to 50% of cases). Any cardiac problem that can cause a thrombus, such as an infarction or dysrhythmia, can lead to mesenteric emboli. This kind of MI manifests as sudden onset abdominal pain, oftentimes with diarrhea that eventually becomes bloody.

2) **Mesenteric arterial thrombosis** is generally caused by arteriosclerosis. The course of this disease is similar to the classic thought of myocardial infarction progression: anginal symptoms as the arterial lumens become progressively narrow, followed by acute thrombotic occlusion and infarction when blood flow ceases to meet the demands. In this case, anginal symptoms occur with "mesenteric exercise" (eating), and patients complain of chronic weight loss, nausea, and an urgent need to have a bowel movement.

3) **Nonocclusive MI** is seen in about 20% of cases. It is caused by hypoperfusion of the gut, whether through low cardiac output or splanchnic vasoconstriction. Vasopressors and old age are the greatest risk factors. This type of MI generally occurs in very sick patients with other comorbidities and is insidious in onset. It is frequently missed as a diagnosis until bowel infarction occurs. Keep a lookout for any abdominal pain or bloody diarrhea in your septic patients, patients on vasoactive drugs, and chronically ill patients with multiple cardiovascular comorbidities.

4) **Mesenteric venous thrombosis** is the least common cause of MI. Most venous thromboses are caused by an underlying inherited or acquired coagulopathy. Patients typically present 1 or 2 weeks after the onset of nonspecific abdominal pain, diarrhea, and anorexia.

Sadly, there is not really a convenient test that can rule out MI.

Serum lactate is thought to be a useful adjunct in detecting ischemia of all types. However, a single serum lactate measurement is not specific to MI; it is elevated in so many other conditions that its presence in high amounts does not add to the diagnosis of MI (specificity 62%). Serial lactates that are within normal range, however, can add to the clinical picture by decreasing the probability of MI 10-fold.

Abdominal x-rays, much like CT scan, should be used to look for other sources of abdominal pain, like obstruction, not to diagnose MI. Twenty-five percent of patients with MI have normal x-rays, and classic signs such as thumbprinting and bowel loop thickening only occur in 40% of patients.

Unless your emergency department has an angiography suite in it, you are stuck with CT scans like the rest of us. CT scans are a great choice for the diagnosis of MI; they are fast, noninvasive, and available at most hospitals. But remember "mesenteric ischemia" is really four diseases, and contrast CT is best at diagnosing mesenteric venous thrombosis, while CT angiography is best for arterial emboli. CT generally shows secondary signs that "something is wrong," such as bowel wall thickening, dilation, or intramural air. If you see these signs on CT and do not consider MI, you are not going to save the cute little old lady in room 3!

CT is fairly accurate when it does diagnose MI (specificity of ~95%), but it fails to diagnose MI 12% to 23% of the time (sensitivity 77% to 88%) and cannot be a replacement for your clinical suspicion. Angiography is still the gold standard for diagnosis, and while invasive, it can differentiate between the different types of MI and offers the opportunity for therapeutic options that CT scan cannot. If you are highly suspicious of MI, are at a hospital with appropriate facilities, and have some good friends in interventional radiology who owe you a favor, try sending the patient to angiography first.

You have made the diagnosis of MI (or at least you suspect it). Next broad-spectrum antibiotics should be given as early as possible, in conjunction with anticoagulation (if not contraindicated). MI leads to increased translocation of bacteria through the gut and can lead to sepsis and shock which, of course, only worsen the ischemia. Remember that once the patient has peritoneal signs, the gut is not ischemic anymore—it is infarcted! This is a true surgical emergency and you need to get on the phone and get a surgeon down, now, even if the CT scan is not finished yet.

SUGGESTED READINGS

Acosta S, Ogren M, Sternby NH, et al. Incidence of acute thrombo-embolic occlusion of the superior mesenteric artery: A population-based study. *Eur J Vasc Endovasc Surg.* 2004;27(2):145–150.

Herbert GS, Steele SR. Acute and chronic mesenteric ischemia. *Surg Clin N Am.* 2007;87(5):1115–1134.

Lock G. Acute intestinal ischaemia. *Best Pract Res Clin Gastroenterol.* 2001;15:83–98.

Oldenberg WA, Lau LL, Rodenberg TJ, et al. Acute mesenteric ischemia: A clinical review. *Arch Intern Med.* 2004;164(10):1054–1062.

Tintinalli JE, Kelen GD, Stapczynski JS, eds. *Emergency Medicine: A Comprehensive Study Guide.* 6th ed. New York: McGraw Hill; 2004:496–497.

Wilcox MG, Howard TJ, Plaskon LA, et al. Current theories of pathogenesis and treatment of nonocclusive mesenteric ischemia. *Dig Dis Sci.* 1995;40:709–716.

23

MANAGE DISLODGED GASTRIC FEEDING TUBES QUICKLY

KENT STEVENS, MD, MPH

Enteral tube feeds in the critically ill patient have become the norm for meeting nutritional needs. Feeds are usually started early in the hospital course through a nasogastric tube or nasoduodenal tube. More permanent access is secured if the patient requires prolonged enteral feeds because of conditions such as long-term intubation, paralysis, swallowing dysfunction, stoke, and deficient caloric intake. This access is usually obtained by placement of a gastrostomy tube. Gastrostomy tubes were historically placed surgically with either an open or a laparoscopic procedure, but this technique has been replaced by both percutaneous endoscopic gastrostomy (PEG) and percutaneous radiological gastrostomy (PRG) placement. Done at the bedside or in the radiology suite, this access offers a safe, convenient, and effective means for providing nutrition and can be removed nonsurgically when no longer needed. Complications of gastrostomy tube placement include infection, bleeding, gastrocolocutaneous fistula, and tube dislodgement. The latter is most commonly caused by inadvertent dislodgement during patient movement but can also be caused by excessive traction on the tube, causing abdominal wall necrosis and tube migration.

After placement, a gastric feeding tube is held in position by an intraluminal flange or a fluid-filled balloon, which, in combination with an extra-abdominal bolster at the skin level, holds the tube in place and keeps the stomach against the abdominal wall. To keep the stomach from "dropping away" in an open surgical procedure, the stomach wall is plicated to the anterior. Over a period of weeks to months, a track forms between the stomach cavity and the skin. The track formation has been reported to mature within days to months and varies based on factors such as nutritional status, tube manipulation, body habitus, and corticosteroid use.

The evaluation of a dislodged feeding tube should begin with a history—why was the tube placed, when was it placed, by which technique, is it still being used, and are tube feeds tolerated? Patients may present with a dislodged tube that is no longer needed. Physical exam of the site should evaluate for erythema and purulent drainage (although this can be difficult to differentiate from tube feed formulas). A feeding tube may be partially dislodged, unnoticed by the patient or the caregiver, and feeds inadvertently when delivered subcutaneously. This can lead to subsequent infection, abscess formation, and necrotizing soft tissue infection or fasciitis. Radiographic workup may be necessary if there is clinical suspicion for subcutaneous or intra-abdominal fluid collection or tissue necrosis, which may need drainage and/or debridement.

Some feeding tubes may no longer be needed and may not need to be replaced. This decision should be made in consultation with the medical provider managing the nutritional needs of the patient. If the tube is still being used, it needs to be replaced. This should be done in an expedient manner, although sometimes limited by the time elapsed between dislodgement and patient presentation. A mature track in a malnourished patient may remain patent for a number of days or weeks—in the well-nourished patient, closure may occur in a matter of hours. A designated gastric tube can be used for replacement, but other tubes of similar diameter, such as a Foley catheter, suffice for keeping the track open. A larger tube will help maintain full patency of the track, allowing tube exchange if deemed necessary.

When is it safe to replace a dislodged tube and how can proper location be guaranteed? As mentioned above, the timing to track maturation is multifactorial and will vary in each patient. The replacement of the dislodged tube soon after its initial placement should be done cautiously to avoid pushing the stomach away from the anterior abdominal wall. Minimal resistance should be encountered, and the tube should freely rotate 360 degrees after insertion. If any question exists concerning correct positioning, a radiographic study should be conducted either at the bedside or in the radiology suite. Injection of 30 to 60 mL of gastrografin is injected through the replaced tube, and a single abdominal plain film is obtained shortly (seconds) after injection. The contrast should be seen within the gastric lumen, without extravasation into the subcutaneous tissue nor intraabdominally. If extravasation is seen, further evaluation is necessary.

In summary, management of a dislodged feeding tube should include a thorough history—including if the tube is still needed—prompt replacement, and a follow-up study to confirm the location if in question. Emphasis should be placed on prompt replacement—even if the history was unavailable and there was no need for it initially. Delay will result in loss of enteral access, and if still needed, will necessitate an additional invasive procedure.

SUGGESTED READINGS

Fischer JE, Bland KG, eds. *Mastery of Surgery.* 5th ed. Philadelphia: Lippincott Williams & Wilkins; 2007:843–849.
Nicholson FB, Korman MG, Richardson MA. Percutaneous endoscopic gastrostomy: A review of indications, complications and outcome. *J Gastroenterol Hepatol.* 2000;15:21–25.

24

DIAGNOSE AND TREAT HERNIAS IN THE EMERGENCY DEPARTMENT QUICKLY

JAMES H. STREET III, MD AND VIRGINIA S. PARK, MD

A hernia is defined as a protrusion of visceral contents through a defect in the abdominal wall. There are many different types of hernias with the vast majority being inguinal, followed by ventral, femoral, umbilical, and other various rare types. An uncomplicated hernia is one that spontaneously reduces. Once it is unable to be reduced, even manually, it is considered incarcerated. The feared complication of incarceration is strangulation, when the blood supply to the hernia contents is compromised, which can lead to necrosis and gangrene.

Umbilical hernias have been known to naturally progress to incarceration and eventually strangulation. Femoral hernias have been quoted to have a strangulation risk of up to 60%. There is no definitive history yet known about inguinal hernias. When a hernia is encountered in the emergency room, it is usually either an incidental finding on physical exam or the cause of the symptoms that prompted the patient to seek medical attention. Patients commonly present with pain and obstructive symptoms, since hernias are the second most common cause of small bowel obstruction, the most common being adhesions from prior abdominal surgery.

Even if the hernia is asymptomatic and reducible at the time of discovery, therefore not requiring immediate surgical intervention, it would still behoove the emergency physician to obtain a surgical consult. Studies have shown greatly decreased morbidity and mortality when a hernia is repaired electively soon after diagnosis, in contrast to those requiring an emergent operation, regardless of the location. Current literature recommends elective surgical repair for incarcerated hernias. This recommendation is under investigation via a multicenter, randomized trial commissioned by the U.S. government's Agency for Health Research and Quality to view the value of elective versus urgent repair.

If a hernia is in the differential diagnosis after a thorough history and physical exam and the diagnosis is uncertain, an abdominal x-ray is advised. A CT scan is helpful for confirmation, although not usually necessary. Once diagnosed, one should attempt to reduce the hernia. If complicated, the maneuver of taxis in Trendelenburg position is used if a reliable history reveals recent onset. This is accomplished with the fingers of one hand at the neck of the hernia while the other hand applies gentle, intermittent pressure on the apex of the mass. This maneuver done in a rocking motion with both hands allows guidance of the contents back into the abdomen. If the hernia does not reduce after two attempts, the examiner should abort the procedure and an urgent surgical evaluation is warranted. If there is any question of incarceration or strangulation, no attempts should be made to reduce the hernia. This helps minimize the risk of reducing strangulated, ischemic contents back into the abdomen, which may turn a hernia repair into an exploratory laparotomy in search of ischemic bowel.

Other complications of reduction are perforation and reduction en masse, a rare complication where the hernia contents and sac are reduced together back into the abdominal cavity, with the constricting neck still incarcerating/strangulating the hernia within the abdomen.

A delay in presentation and errors in diagnosis of hernias significantly increase the morbidity and mortality in the hernia population. As simple as the diagnosis may seem, a patient with a strangulated groin hernia may be toxic, febrile with leukocytosis, and present with a tense, tender, erythematous mass without bowel sounds that may be misdiagnosed as a groin abscess or thrombosed femoral artery aneurysm.

A difficult-to-diagnose hernia is the obturator hernia, which contributes to high morbidity and mortality of this subset of hernias. Not only are they rare, making up about 0.073% of all hernias, but the presenting symptoms are also nonspecific, usually obstructive, and physical exam may not be informative without a high index of suspicion. Rectal and pelvic exams in females should always be performed. The pathognomonic sign on physical exam is the Howship-Romberg sign that is present in nearly 50% of patients with an obturator hernia. A physical finding consistent with this diagnosis is when medial thigh pain is elicited by extension, adduction, or medial rotation of the ipsilateral hip. Pelvic CT scan imaging with oral and IV contrast is a very sensitive imaging modality for confirmation of the diagnosis.

SUGGESTED READINGS

Davies M, Davies C, Morris-Stiff G, et al. Emergency presentation of abdominal hernias: Outcome and reasons for delay in treatment—A prospective study. *Ann R Coll Surg Engl.* 2007;89:47–50.

Primatesta P, Goldacre MJ. Inguinal hernia repair: Incidence of elective and emergency surgery, readmission and mortality. *Int J Epidemiol.* 1996;25(4):835–839.

Salameh JR. Primary and unusual abdominal wall hernias. *Surg Clin N Am.* 2008;88:45–60.

25

ACUTE DIVERTICULITIS IS COMMON ... SO KNOW THE DISEASE WELL!

JONATHAN CRAIG WENDELL, MD

You can blame our genetics or our diets, but either way diverticular disease is common in Western society. This disease affects 5% to 12% of people under 40 and over 65% at age 85, of which 5% to 15% will develop diverticulitis during their lifetime. Although still a surgical disease, diverticulitis is now initially managed nonoperatively for uncomplicated courses.

Though crampy, left lower quadrant pain with nausea, vomiting, and change in bowel habits is the most common presentation, the emergency physician must be aware of mimicking conditions. Atypical presentations or abnormal locations of disease often occur in young patients (<40 years old). Diverticulitis of the right colon may mimic acute appendicitis, whereas transverse colon involvement may present as peptic ulcer disease, pancreatitis, or cholecystitis. Additionally, signs of peritonitis, urinary symptoms, leg pain, or leg emphysema from retroperitoneal perforation should prompt concern for complicated diverticulitis.

The diagnosis of diverticulitis can be made by history and physical examination alone, especially if the patient has had previous confirmed cases. However, if there is any question regarding the cause of the abdominal pain, get the CT scan. Via CT, we can assess disease severity, rule out mimicking processes, and demonstrate presence of complications (e.g., soft tissue inflammatory masses, phlegmon, abscess). The CT accuracy is enhanced using oral, intravenous, and rectal contrasts. Plain radiographs are not useful! Ultrasound is emerging as a potential diagnostic modality with recent studies showing equal accuracy (84%) as CT; however, further research and training are needed at this time. Routine laboratory tests are not necessary in uncomplicated cases, but these tests should be ordered if the patient looks ill, if you are concerned about mimicking processes, or if you wish to facilitate consultant services (you know the surgeons will want it). Complete blood count (CBC) may show leukocytosis and/or left shift; however, it is important to remind our surgical colleagues that up to 60% of patients have normal white blood cell count. Urinalysis, liver tests, and lipase can be used to exclude other causes of abdominal pain. Serum electrolytes are used to evaluate renal function prior to IV contrast administration. A pregnancy test is mandatory in women of childbearing age to rule out ectopic pregnancy.

The management of diverticulitis depends on severity. Complicated cases (diffuse peritonitis or failure of nonoperative management, immunosuppression, free-air perforation, sepsis, abscess, fistula, possible carcinoma, obstruction, extremes of age, or recurrent episodes) require prompt surgical consultation. These patients should be made NPO and receive broad-spectrum intravenous antibiotics for Gram-negative and anaerobic colonic flora.

The patient presenting with uncomplicated diverticulitis is more difficult to manage. Conservative (e.g., nonoperative) treatment of acute uncomplicated diverticulitis is successful in 70% to 100% of cases. The decision of whether to admit or treat as an outpatient should take into account all aspects of the patient. The treating physician must consider the severity of presentation, ability to tolerate oral intake, presence of comorbid diseases, and available support systems (including ability to follow-up). In general, anyone who is elderly, immunocompromised, or has significant comorbidities, high fever, or significant leukocytosis should be admitted. All admitted patients should be NPO with intravenous hydration, antibiotics, and adequate pain control.

Outpatient management: Antibiotic choice should cover Gram-negative rods and anaerobes (specifically *Escherichia coli* and *Bacteroides fragilis*) and should continue for 7 to 10 days. Common regimens include ciprofloxacin plus metronidazole or amoxicillin-clavulanate. Do not forget pain control, including stool softeners! Patients should start with a light diet of fluids but can advance as tolerated. To prevent recurrent attacks, patients should be placed on a lifelong high-fiber diet. Despite popular belief, there is NO evidence that seeds or nuts exacerbate diverticulitis. It is important that patients receive follow-up, including colonoscopy or contrast enema, to confirm the diagnosis following resolution of acute inflammation and facilitate discussion of possible elective interventions.

Unfortunately, diverticulitis has a recurrence rate of 1.5% per year, meaning that patients with an initial episode at age 65 will have 21% chance of recurrence in their lifetime, whereas a patient younger than 50 years has a 46% chance of recurrence. Additionally, recurrent attacks are less likely to respond to medical management. Elective resection for patients <40 years and those with frequent recurrence is a viable option. All recurrences do not need CT scan, but your threshold should be lower, especially if the patient quickly fails outpatient therapy or appears ill. Let us face it: if the patient is presenting with frequent recurrence, he or she is failing medical management and likely needs surgical intervention.

Bottom line: Each case of suspected diverticulitis should be considered individually. Complicated patients need surgeons, whereas uncomplicated patients can begin with nonoperative therapy. All patients should be treated with pain control, stool softeners, and antibiotics and require close surgical follow-up. Have a low threshold for CT if any concerning symptoms are present. If the stars align, the patient may be treated at home, but close surgical follow-up must be ensured.

SUGGESTED READINGS

Baker J, Mandavia D, Swadron S. Diagnosis of diverticulitis by bedside ultrasound in the emergency department. *J Emerg Med.* 2006;30:327–329.

Cole CD, Wolfson AB. Case series: Diverticulitis in the young. *J Emerg Med.* 2007;33: 363–366.

Komuta K, Yamanaka S, Okada K, et al. Toward therapeutic guidelines for patients with acute right colonic diverticulitis. *Am J Surg.* 2004;187:233–237.

Peppas G, Bliziotis L, Oikonomaki D, et al. Outcomes after medical and surgical treatment of diverticulitis: A systematic review of the available evidence. *J Gastroenterol Hepatol.* 2007;22:1360–1368.

Rafferty J, Shellito P, Hyman N, et al. Practice parameters for sigmoid diverticulitis. *Dis Colon Rectum.* 2006;49:939–944.

Shen SH, Chen JD, Tiu CM, et al. Colonic diverticulitis diagnosed by computed tomography in the ED. *Am J Emerg Med.* 2002;20:551–557.

26

KNOW HOW TO PROPERLY DIAGNOSE A RUPTURED AAA USING ULTRASOUND

CHAD DAVID WRIGHT, MD AND ASHLEY R. STOKER, MD

The ruptured abdominal aortic aneurysm (AAA) is a condition that is rapidly fatal without immediate diagnosis and management. Fleming et al. stated that AAA may be asymptomatic for years; however, resultant rupture in one in three untreated patients occurs and leads to only 10% to 25% of these patients surviving until hospital discharge. It is important when screening in the ED for AAA that we recognize the limitations of ultrasound (US), ensure accurate technique in US imaging, and supplement our findings with a CT.

As usual, there is much variability in the literature of the diagnostic criteria you may use to evaluate an AAA with US. We suggest using the criteria in Singh et al., which defines aneurysm as being present if one or more of the following apply: aortic diameter at the renal level is equal to or >35 mm in either anterior-posterior or transverse plane; infrarenal aortic diameter is ≥5 mm, larger than renal aortic diameter in either plane; or just simply ≥30 mm of localized aortic dilatation, which is easier to remember.

Alund et al. identified male sex and advanced age as important risk factors with a history of smoking being the highest risk associated with AAA. Other risk factors include having a first-degree relative with AAA and atherosclerosis. This study further reports screening men aged 65 to 80 as cost-effective and reduces AAA-related mortality approximately 50%. Identification of risk factors and early screening in high-risk patients can help decrease the incidence of fatalities.

Safe, cost-effective, easily available, and portable US is quickly becoming an accepted AAA screening modality. The only absolute contraindication to US is delaying immediate intervention. Dent et al. found that emergency US has a sensitivity of 96.3%, specificity of 100%, negative predictive value of 98.6%, and positive predictive value of 100% in detecting AAA.

Aortic US examination should be performed with the patient lying supine. A 2.5- to 3.5-MHz transducer should be used with a lower frequency for deeper penetration in obese patients. Begin your examination by visualizing the aorta in the transverse plane. With the marker to patient's right, start at the xiphoid and follow the aorta down to the umbilicus. The vertebral body will appear inferior with the aorta on the right and the inferior vena cava (IVC) on the left. Return the transducer to the xiphoid and rotate 90 degree clockwise for longitudinal views. The IVC will be pictured superior to the pulsatile, less–compressible, and thicker-walled aorta. Despite following these techniques, US is not without its limitations and pitfalls.

Errors with US detection arise from variations in technique, equipment, and anatomy and can vary with each patient. While age is an important risk factor for AAA, it can also lead to decreased accuracy with US. The aorta often becomes tortuous with age, which can make following its course and finding the correct plane for transverse and longitudinal views difficult. False-negative results are infrequent with US, but they do occur. The most common form of AAA rupture is retroperitoneal, resulting in unreliable US findings. Also, contained ruptures can be missed either due to their location or due to possible presentation as a hypoechoic mixed density surrounding the aorta. Obese patients or the presence of bowel gas may limit our US examination. To partially compensate for these factors, you should place the patient in the left lateral decubitus position, allowing repositioning of the bowels and/or pannus or place the transducer in the right axillary line and use the hepatic acoustic window to visualize the coronal plane of the aorta.

There are two common errors made during US imaging, according to Mateer et al. The first is due to sweeping the plane of the beam into the right parasagittal plane, thus resulting in a long-axis view of the IVC. The IVC is thin walled and compressible like the aorta, but careful examination to visualize the celiac trunk and superior mesenteric artery branching off the aorta helps you with proper identification. The other error is due to the cylinder tangent effect occurring when the plane of the transducer beam enters the cylinder of the aorta tangentially during longitudinal view, leading to incorrect AP diameter measurements. Measuring the AP diameter in transverse view diminishes this effect's incidence.

US has consistently been found to elicit smaller AAA diameters than CT scans with Vidakovich et al. reporting this phenomenon most significantly occurring in AAAs measuring >50 mm in diameter. To avoid this pitfall, use a CT scan to more accurately measure and localize a large AAA.

US is a very useful screening tool for you to use in individuals with appropriate risk factors and for whom you have a high clinical suspicion. Lastly, user experience plays a role in the evaluation of AAA with US. Practice any chance you get while in the ED, especially on patients already getting a CT scan of the abdomen. You can then compare your screening US to the CT aortic measurements. Overall, care should be taken to be thorough; avoid known errors using US, and utilize a CT scan as an adjunct study in your evaluation of AAAs.

SUGGESTED READINGS

Ålund K, Mani K, Wanhainen A. Selective screening for adominal aortic aneurysm among patients referred to the vascular laboratory. *Euro Soc Vasc Surg.* 2008;35:669–674.

Dent B, Kendall RJ, Boyle AA, et al. Emergency ultrasound of the abdominal aorta by UK emergency physicians: A prospective cohort study. *Emerg Med J.* 2007;24(8):547–549.

Fleming C, Whitlock EP, Beil TL, et al. Screening for abdominal aortic aneurysm: A best-evidence systematic review for the U.S. Preventive Services Task Force. *Ann Intern Med.* 2005;142(3):203–211.

Mateer J, Ma O. *Emergency Ultrasound.* New York, NY: McGraw-Hill; 2002.

Singh K, Jacobsen BK, Solberg S, et al. The difference between ultrasound and computed tomography (CT) measurements of aortic diameter increases with aortic diameter: Analysis of axial Images of abdominal aortic and common iliac artery diameter in Normal and aneurysmal aortas. The Tromsø Study, 1994–1995. *Eur J Vasc Endovasc Surg.* 2004;28(2):158–167.

Sprouse LR II, Meier GH III, Lesar CJ, et al. Comparison of abdominal aortic aneurysm diameter measurements obtained with ultrasound and computed tomography: Is there a difference? *J Vasc Surg.* 2003;38(3):466–471.

Vidakovic R, Feringa HH, Kuiper RJ, et al. Comparison with computed tomography of two ultrasound devices for diagnosis of abdominal aortic aneurysm. *Am J Cardiol.* 2007;100(12):1786–1791.

27

DOUBLE-CHECK MEDICATION DOSAGES IN RAPID-SEQUENCE INTUBATION

STEPHEN DOCHERTY, DO, FAAEM, FACEP

Knowing how to expertly manage emergency airways in a vast variety of clinical situations is one of the most important roles of the emergency physician (EP). Rapid-sequence intubation (RSI), involving the use of an induction agent followed by a paralytic agent, has revolutionized airway management in the emergency department.

The paralytic agent should not be given before the induction agent in the awake patient. Some individuals believe that because rocuronium and vecuronium have a longer onset of action than succinylcholine, these agents should be administered first. But these drugs cause progressive muscle weakening almost immediately after administration, which can be very unpleasant and frightening. Ensure that patients are sufficiently sedated first.

Instruct the nurse to push the paralytic agent *immediately* after the induction agent. In a patient with respiratory compromise, the induction agent alone can lead to apnea. If a paralytic agent is not given immediately afterwards, optimal intubating conditions will be delayed, and bag-valve-mask ventilation, with its risks of aspiration, will be necessary prior to the actual intubation attempt.

When performing RSI on a patient whose weight is unknown, it is best to overestimate the weight by approximately 20%. Giving a slightly higher dose of induction and paralytic agents is generally safe and assures adequate sedation and paralysis. Underdosing a paralytic agent may result in incomplete muscle relaxation, making airway management unnecessarily difficult. Midazolam, in particular, is frequently underdosed in RSI, resulting in patients who are awake yet paralyzed during intubation. When used as an induction agent, the dose of midazolam is 0.3 mg/kg intravenously.

Be aware of the contraindications to succinylcholine—these include known or likely hyperkalemia, as well as any evolving neuromuscular process. When a patient is brought to the ED with altered mental status and an unknown past medical history, err on the side of safety and use a nondepolarizing agent such as rocuronium.

The evidence in support of premedicating patients for RSI is weak. Premedication agents are used to block unwanted physiologic responses to intubation and include lidocaine, fentanyl, and small priming doses of a paralytic agent. Atropine is given to children to prevent an exaggerated vagal response to intubation. To be effective, premedications must be given at least 3 min prior to the paralytic. Fentanyl, when given at the recommended 3-μg/kg dose, may cause apnea prior to RSI agent administration. This risk is higher if the drug is pushed too rapidly. Fentanyl should be given slowly over about 30 to 60 s. In the geriatric patient, the dose should be reduced to 1 to 2 μg/kg and administered over a 3-min period. Because of the risk of apnea associated with its use, fentanyl should always be the last premedication administered prior to RSI.

Another common pitfall is to leave the patient unsedated after RSI is complete. Most induction agents, when compared with long-acting paralytic agents (e.g., rocuronium, 45 min), have short half-lives (e.g., etomidate, 7 to 14 min). This may result in the patient regaining awareness while still paralyzed. When this occurs in the operating room during general anesthesia, patients have gone on to develop posttraumatic stress disorder. If additional paralytic agents are necessary in the postintubation period, make sure the patient is well sedated and unaware prior to their use.

With the advent of RSI, great advances in our ability to manage the emergency airway have emerged. Avoiding these key pitfalls will make the procedure safer and less traumatic.

SUGGESTED READINGS

Blanda M, Gallo UE. Emergency airway management. *Emerg Med Clin North Am.* 2003;21;1–26.

Laurin EG, Sakles JC, Panachek EA, et al. A comparison of rocuronium, succinylcholine, and vecuronium for rapid sequence induction of anesthesia in adult patients. *Acad Emerg Med.* 2000;7:1362–1369.

Rose DR, Cohen MM. The airway: Problems and predictions in 18,500 patients. *Can J Anesth.* 1994;41:372–383.

Sagarin MJ, Barton ED, Sakles JC, et al. Underdosing of midazolam in emergency endotracheal intubation. *Acad Emer Med.* 2003;10(4):329–338.

28

DO NOT RELY ON THE CLINICAL EXAMINATION ALONE TO CONFIRM CORRECT ENDOTRACHEAL TUBE PLACEMENT

MINA MASRI, DO

The verification of correct endotracheal tube (ETT) placement after intubation is critical in order to prevent hypoxia and gastric insufflation, which may lead to vomiting and aspiration. A common practice after intubation is to auscultate over the epigastrium to ensure early detection in the case of esophageal intubation. The lateral lung fields are then auscultated to ensure equal air entry bilaterally.

Although using clinical examination is helpful, it is imperfect. Air flowing into the esophagus can produce a similar sound quality to that of air flowing through the trachea. Mainstem intubation may lead to absent breath sounds unilaterally, which if not compared to the opposite side may cause the intubator to assume an esophageal intubation. Although experience clearly plays a role in the ability to rely on clinical examination for confirmation of ETT placement, even experienced intubators can be misled. Similarly, the identification of fog in the ETT and the reliance on pulse oximetry have been shown to be fraught with error. Because of these pitfalls, multiple modalities other than clinical examination are used to assess correct ETT placement.

So, what is the best way to confirm tracheal placement of the ETT? The most common and most reliable method is qualitative end-tidal CO_2 (ETCO$_2$) capnometry. Colorimetric ETCO$_2$ detectors that can be affixed to the end of the ETT provide an assessment of expired CO_2 by producing a color change in the presence of exhaled CO_2. The degree of color change roughly correlates with the amount of CO_2 present, from purple (<0.5%) to tan (0.5% to 2%) to yellow (>2%). Thus, a color change from purple (baseline) to yellow indicates the presence of CO_2. Because CO_2 may be present in small amounts in the stomach and esophagus, especially after ingestion of a carbonated beverage, color change should not be relied upon unless it persists beyond six breaths through the ETT.

Quantitative or waveform capnography is even better than colorimetry since it provides an actual waveform with a numerical reading of CO_2. This has been shown to be the most reliable method for correct ETT placement detection, but it has one main limitation: in cardiac arrest patients, where accurate CO_2 levels may be difficult to quantify secondary to decreased gas exchange in the lungs, a lower-than-expected CO_2 reading may result. If the patient is pulseless, adequate CPR should produce enough tissue perfusion to allow for a detectable waveform. If after careful scrutiny no CO_2 waveform is detected, an esophageal intubation should be presumed.

Another device used to confirm ETT placement is the esophageal detector device (EDD). This consists of a suction bulb attached to the end of a syringe. This device is used to distinguish between the collapsibility of the esophagus around the end of the ETT (preventing the bulb from reexpanding) and the rigidity of the trachea (allowing the bulb to reexpand). The EDD, although not widely used in emergency departments, is used by many emergency medical services (EMS) agencies and has been shown to be very effective.

More recent studies have also demonstrated a role for ultrasonography in verifying ET tube placement. This method requires real-time use of an ultrasound probe placed over the neck during intubation. It remains to be seen if this ultrasound application will gain widespread acceptance.

Although all these methods show varying sensitivities and specificities, using at least two modalities for any given intubation will decrease the likelihood of an unrecognized esophageal placement. No method should be used alone, and $ETCO_2$ capnography should be used whenever possible.

SUGGESTED READINGS

Grmec S. Comparison of three different methods to confirm tracheal tube placement in emergency intubation. *Intensive Care Med*. 2002;28(6):701–704.

Li J. Capnography alone is imperfect for endotracheal tube placement confirmation during emergency intubation. *J Emerg Med*. 2001;20(3):223–229.

Ma G, Davis DP, Schmitt J, et al. The sensitivity and specificity of transcricothyroid ultrasonography to confirm endotracheal tube placement in a cadaver model. *J Emerg Med*. 2007;32(4):405–407.

Werner SL, Smith CE, Goldstein JR, et al. Pilot study to evaluate the accuracy of ultrasonography in confirming endotracheal tube placement. *Ann Emerg Med*. 2007;49(1):75–80.

Zaleski L, Abello D, Gold MI. The esophageal detector device. Does it work? *Anesthesiology*. 1993;79(2):244–247.

29

KNOW THE PROPER USE OF A BOUGIE

STEPHEN DOCHERTY, DO, FAAEM, FACEP

There are several modern-day variants of the gum elastic bougie (intubating stylet) in use today. These are commonly around 60 cm in length and 15 French diameter flexible stylets with an approximately 40–degree angle located 3.5 cm from the smooth distal end.

The bougie is extremely useful in managing difficult intubations when the laryngeal inlet cannot be well seen, such as in patients with very anterior laryngeal openings. In addition, when supraglottic or laryngeal edema is present, the bougie will more easily enter the trachea initially than the endotracheal tube (ETT). The ETT can then be inserted over the bougie into the trachea.

When using the bougie, it is important to obtain the best possible laryngeal view with the laryngoscope. Some authors recommend placing a physiologic bend in the distal third of the bougie to help direct it anteriorly and to accentuate vibration/clicking against the tracheal rings. A small amount of water-soluble lubricant can be placed on the bougie prior to use to allow easier advancement of the ETT. During intubation, if the larynx is not visible, attempts to identify the tip of the epiglottis, the tips of the arytenoid cartilages, or any of the other anatomical landmarks will aid in intubation. By gently probing under the tip of the epiglottis, the trachea can be entered with the bougie. Entry into the trachea can be confirmed even without direct visualization of the vocal cords because there will be a readily palpable clicking sensation while holding the bougie.

Failing to recognize esophageal placement of the bougie is a critical error, preventable by a careful understanding of tracheal anatomy. When the trachea is entered, the angled tip of the bougie will vibrate or click on the tracheal rings. These vibrations should be palpable. If there is any doubt about the vibration being present, the bougie can be gently moved back and forth to accentuate this often subtle sensation. Another option for confirmation of tracheal placement of the bougie is to continue to advance it. A bougie correctly placed in the trachea encounts resistance as it comes to the carina or smaller bronchi and is unable to be advanced any further. If no resistance is felt with continued advancement in the absence of vibration of the tip against the tracheal rings, esophageal placement should be suspected.

It is also important to keep the curved tip of the bougie pointing toward the anterior 180 degrees of the trachea during insertion. This is necessary because the tracheal rings (with the exception of the cricoid cartilage) are incomplete, with the posterior aspect of the trachea made up of soft tissue. A posterior-facing bougie tip may not detect vibration against the tracheal rings and is also less likely to successfully navigate the laryngeal opening. It may also theoretically perforate through the back wall of the trachea. Some bougie devices have markings along the length of the tube to indicate in which direction the tip is pointed.

Once the bougie is confirmed to be in the trachea, the ETT is slid over the bougie. It is extremely important that the laryngoscope remain in place while advancing the ETT along the bougie to allow the tube to be placed with minimal resistance from the tongue and other structures. In addition, keeping the laryngoscope in place helps to keep the bougie in a straight line, preventing it from bending and facilitating passage of the ETT. If resistance is felt when advancing the ETT, rotate the ETT 90 degrees counterclockwise so that the bevel faces posteriorly. In some cases, the beveled edge of the ETT may catch on the right arytenoid cartilage or vocal cord. Rotating the ETT counterclockwise 90 degrees allows the bevel to spread the arytenoids so that minimal force is necessary to advance the ETT. Rotating in a clockwise direction will increase the chances of the bevel catching on the arytenoids. Once the ETT is in place, remove the bougie, inflate the cuff, and verify tube placement in the usual manner.

The bougie is one of the simplest and least expensive airway adjuncts. If the few pitfalls above are avoided, it is also one of the most successful.

SUGGESTED READINGS

Hdzovic I, Wilkes AR, Latto IP. To shape or not to shape … Simulated bougie-assisted difficult intubation in a mannequin. *Anaesthesia*. 2003;58(8):792–797.

Jabre P, Combs X, Leroux B, et al. Use of gum elastic bougie for prehospital difficult intubation. *Am J Emerg Med*. 2005;23(4):552–555.

Latto IP, Stacey M, Mecklenburgh J, et al. Survey of the use of the gum elastic bougie in clinical practice. *Anesthesiology*. 2002;57(4):379–384.

Viswanathan S, Campbell C, Wood DG, et al. The Eschmann Tracheal Tube Introducer. (Gum elastic bougie). *Anesthesiol Rev*. 1992;19(6):29–34.

30

BE WARY OF THE ATYPICAL PRESENTATIONS OF ANAPHYLAXIS

WILLIAM K. MALLON, MD, FAAEM, FACEP

Anaphylaxis is an immunoglobulin E (IgE)-mediated process where mast cells degranulate, releasing massive quantities of histamine, thromboxane, and slow-reacting substance-A (SRS-A). These chemical mediators produce a rapidly progressive clinical picture that may include wheezing, urticaria, mucous membrane and airway edema, and hypotension. The process is treatable but still results in fatalities. The most common provocative allergens are penicillins, iodine, nuts, shellfish, eggs, and hymenoptera stings (bees, ants, wasps, hornets). Early recognition and diagnosis are critical to successful treatment and to avoid complications.

While the disease is obvious in classical cases when the history is clear ("I am allergic to X and I was inadvertently exposed") and the findings are obvious (urticaria, wheezing, lip/tongue edema, and altered vital signs), errors in diagnosis still occur because of less obvious but still serious presentations. Examples of less obvious presentations include isolated syncope from hymenoptera stings (particularly those of wasps).

Although anaphylaxis is considered to be an "immediate" form of hypersensitivity (Type I Gel-Coombs), it can take anywhere from minutes to hours to develop depending on the patient, the allergen, and the type of exposure. In some cases, even tiny amounts of allergen can produce dramatic reactions. When the history of exposure to an allergen is lacking or the presentation is atypical, failure to diagnose anaphylaxis is an understandable mistake.

Patients with food allergies sometimes present with gastrointestinal symptoms as their most prominent clinical feature. Common food allergens that cause reactions in children include milk, egg, wheat, soy, peanuts, tree nuts, fish, and shellfish. While the majority of children outgrow their allergies to milk, egg, wheat, and soy, allergies to peanuts, tree nuts, fish, and shellfish are often lifelong. Patients who present with diarrhea and abdominal cramping as their chief complaint may not be identified as patients with anaphylaxis.

TABLE 30.1   DIAGNOSTIC CRITERIA FOR ANAPHYLAXIS

ANAPHYLAXIS IS HIGHLY LIKELY WHEN ANY ONE OF THE FOLLOWING THREE CRITERIA IS FULFILLED:

---

1. Acute onset of an illness (minutes to several hours) with involvement of the skin, mucosal tissue, or both (e.g., generalized hives, pruritus or flushing, swollen lips-tongue-uvula) and at least one of the following

    (a) Respiratory compromise (e.g., dyspnea, wheeze-bronchospasm, stridor, reduced peak flow, hypoxemia)

    (b) Reduced BP or associated symptoms of end-organ dysfunction (e.g., hypotonia, collapse, syncope, incontinence)

   [*Note: no requirement for a history of exposure to an allergen in this definition*]

2. Two or more of the following that occur rapidly after exposure to a likely allergen for that patient (minutes to several hours)

    (a) Involvement of the skin-mucosal tissue

    (b) Respiratory compromise (e.g., dyspnea, wheeze-bronchospasm, stridor, reduced peak flow, hypoxemia)

    (c) Reduced BP or associated symptoms of end-organ dysfunction (e.g., hypotonia, collapse, syncope, incontinence)

    (d) Persistent gastrointestinal symptoms

3. Reduced BP after exposure to known allergen for that patient

    (a) Infants and children: low systolic BP (age specific) or >30% decrease in systolic BP

    (b) Adults: systolic BP <90 mm Hg or >30% decrease from the patient's baseline

Gastrointestinal symptoms are, however, part of the diagnostic criteria. The diagnostic criteria for anaphylaxis are listed in *Table 30.1*.

The primary reason that allergy/anaphylaxis may not be considered in the differential diagnosis is exposure to an unexpected or unknown, unidentified allergen. The correct diagnosis in such cases relies on the emergency physician to employ his or her "detective" skills. The medical literature is full of case reports describing allergic reactions and anaphylaxis to unusual drugs, cutaneous contacts, household items, inhaled allergens, and other environmental components. Examples of these include a case of anaphylaxis from mold in a pancake mix, MDMA (ecstasy), and celery-dependent exercise-induced anaphylaxis.

Inevitably, a failure to diagnose results in a failure to appropriately treat. Treatment for anaphylaxis includes steroids, antihistamines (H_1 and H_2 blockers), and β agonists. Delayed airway management may also be related to a failure to diagnose anaphylaxis. Lastly, early discharge from the ED may result in disease progression, rebound, and re-presentation.

SUGGESTED READINGS

Bennett AT, Collins KA. An unusual case of anaphylaxis: Mold in pancake mix. *Am J Forensic Med Pathol.* 2001;22(3):292–295.

Reisman RE. Unusual reactions to insect stings. *Curr Opin Allergy Clin Immunol.* 2005;5(4): 355–358.

Sampson HA, Munoz-Furlong A, Campbell RL, et al. Second symposium on the definition and management of anaphylaxis: summary report—Second National Institute of Allergy and Infectious Disease/Food Allergy and Anaphylaxis Network Symposium. *J Allergy Clin Immunol.* 2006;117:391–397.

Sauvageau A. Death from a possible anaphylactic reaction to ecstasy. *Clin Toxicol (Phila).* 2008;46(2):156.

Silverstein SR, Frommer DA, Dobozin B, et al. Celery-dependent exercise-induced anaphy-laxis. *J Emerg Med.* 1986;4(3):195–199.

Wang J, Sampson HA. Food anaphylaxis. *Clin Exp Allergy.* 2007;37(5):651–660.

31

BEWARE OF THE BIPHASIC REACTION OF ANAPHYLAXIS

JAN M. SHOENBERGER, MD, FAAEM, FACEP

Anaphylaxis is a potentially fatal, severe systemic allergic reaction. Typically, it has a rapid onset with multiorgan involvement. Anaphylactic reactions most often follow a uniphasic course; however, up to 20% of reactions are biphasic.

The signs and symptoms of anaphylaxis generally have their onset within minutes but occasionally occur as late as 1 h after exposure to the antigen. With proper treatment, resolution of signs and symptoms may occur within hours of treatment. For most patients, no recurrence will occur, but for up to one in five patients, another episode will follow. The initial paper describing this biphasic response described asymptomatic periods between episodes of anaphylaxis of between 1 and 8 h. Since then, there have been several more studies reporting shorter asymptomatic periods (1 to 3 h) as well as reports of reactivity occurring as late as 24 to 38 h after the initial reaction. A more recent study reported the mean time to onset of this "second-phase reactivity" as 10 h.

In terms of severity of the second phase, approximately one third of episodes will be less severe than the initial episode, one third more severe, and one third of similar severity. Although corticosteroids are the primary recom-mended treatment to prevent or minimize the second phase; there have been case reports of patients who received corticosteroids but nonetheless still experienced severe biphasic reactions.

Predicting which patient is at risk for a second-phase reaction is difficult. In one study, patients who had a biphasic pattern of symptoms took longer to achieve resolution of their initial symptoms. In the same study, time to resolution of initial symptoms positively correlated with time to onset of the second phase; that is, the longer it took to achieve resolution of symptoms, the longer the asymptomatic interval if a second-phase reaction occurred. In addition, patients who developed second-phase reactivity received less epinephrine and less corticosteroid therapy (a possible explanation for the longer time to achieve symptom resolution). Another study by Lee et al. looked at pediatric biphasic reactions. They found an association between the delay in administration of epinephrine and the presence of biphasic reactivity. This is consistent with the theory that undertreatment with epinephrine may be associated with a higher incidence of second reactions.

Once symptoms of the initial presentation of anaphylaxis have resolved, when can the patient be safely discharged? Based on the information available, the safest approach would be to observe patients who have experienced a severe, life-threatening reaction for 24 h. Observation units are perfect settings for these patients to be watched. For many emergency departments (EDs), this is not a practical recommendation, and it may be necessary to admit patients with truly life-threatening presentations to a medical ward for observation.

Patients can be safely discharged from the ED under the following circumstances:

- Adequate supervision is available (i.e., the patient is not being discharged to home alone).
- The patient and caregiver are able to access the 911 EMS system should symptoms recur, and the transport time to an ED is not excessive.
- An epinephrine autoinjector (e.g. EpiPen®) is prescribed upon discharge, and the patient is able to demonstrate an understanding of when and how to use it after specific instructions from the treatment team.

Patients should be informed upon discharge of the possibility of a biphasic response so that if it should occur after discharge, both the patient and the family are prepared and aware.

SUGGESTED READINGS

Ellis AK, Day JH. Biphasic anaphylaxis with unusually late onset second phase: A case report. *Can J Allergy Clin Immunol.* 1997;2(3):106–109.

Ellis AK, Day JH. Incidence and characteristics of biphasic anaphylaxis: A prospective evaluation of 103 patients. *Ann All Asthma Immunol.* 2007;98(1):64–69.

Lee JM, Greenes DS. Biphasic anaphylactic reactions in pediatrics. *Pediatrics.* 2000;106(4):762–766.

Sheikh A, Shehata YA, Brown SG, et al. Adrenaline (epinephrine) for the treatment of anaphylaxis with and without shock. *Cochrane Database Syst Rev.* 2008;(4):CD006312.

Stark BJ, Sullivan TJ. Biphasic and protracted anaphylaxis. *J Allergy Clin Immunol.* 1986;78(1):76–83.

32

UNDERSTAND THE PROPER USE OF EPINEPHRINE IN PATIENTS WITH ALLERGIC REACTIONS

JAN M. SHOENBERGER, MD, FAAEM, FACEP

Anaphylaxis is a severe, life-threatening, systemic reaction that affects patients of all ages. It is characterized by multiorgan involvement including skin, respiratory, gastrointestinal, and cardiovascular systems. Epinephrine remains a lifesaving therapy in the treatment of anaphylaxis. The mechanism of action includes stimulation of α receptors, increasing peripheral vascular resistance, thus improving circulation and coronary perfusion, and decreasing angioedema. The stimulation of β_1 receptors has positive inotropic and chronotropic cardiac effects. The stimulation of β_2 receptors results in bronchodilation as well as an increase in intracellular cyclic adenosine monophosphate production in mast cells and basophils, reducing the release of inflammatory mediators.

Inappropriate utilization, both overusage and underusage, of epinephrine is a common pitfall in allergy and anaphylaxis management. In most circumstances involving anaphylaxis, intramuscular administration of epinephrine is the initial treatment of choice. Although subcutaneous epinephrine was widely recommended in the past, intramuscular epinephrine is currently the preferred route of choice. This change is supported by a recent Cochrane Database Review. Epinephrine autoinjector (e.g. EpiPen®) self-administration devices are designed to deliver the drug intramuscularly (IM). The dose of IM epinephrine in infants and children is 0.01 mg/kg of 1:1,000 dilution (maximum dose 0.3 mg). In North America, the recommended dose in adults is 0.3 to 0.5 mL of 1:1,000 dilution (actual dose 0.3 to 0.5 mg). In Europe, recommended doses are higher, 0.5 to 1.0 mg (1:1,000 dilution). If symptoms do not improve, a repeat dose can be given every 5 min.

Intravenous (IV) epinephrine is the next administration route of choice if IM epinephrine has not resulted in resolution of symptoms or the patient presents to the ED with severe symptoms. Some authors suggest that IV epinephrine should only be given in cases of anaphylaxis-associated circulatory collapse or severe anaphylaxis unresponsive to IM administration of the drug. Intravenous epinephrine can be given in a variety of ways. An initial IV bolus dose can be given at one-tenth the strength that would be used in cardiac arrest. In an emergency, the 1:10,000 concentration that is commonly found on adult crash carts can be used in severe anaphylaxis. Instead of the 1 mg dose that would be given in cardiac arrest, increments of 1 cc (0.1 mg) can be administered slowly IV. The IV infusion rate for adults is 1-4 mcg/minute.

In pediatric anaphylaxis, the approach is similar. The intramuscular route should be the initial approach at a dose of 0.01 mg/kg of 1:1,000 solution repeated every 5-20 minutes. If continued shock is present after volume resuscitation, an IV infusion may be necessary. The dose is 0.1-2 mcg/kg/minute.

The decision to give epinephrine, whether IM or IV, must be carefully weighed against the risks. Administering IV epinephrine when it is not indicated can cause nausea, vomiting, chest pain, hypertension, tachycardia, and worsening panic in a patient whose allergic problem is only mild. There have been several case reports of young adults sustaining acute myocardial infarction after receiving epinephrine (both IM and IV). Nonetheless, failure to administer the drug intravenously when indicated may result in undertreatment and ongoing acceleration of the anaphylactic process with possible shock and airway compromise.

Epinephrine should be given as early in the course of the disease as possible. Several studies have demonstrated that there is an association between poor outcome and delayed administration of epinephrine.

Suggested Readings

Hegenbarth MA. American Academy of Pediatrics Committee on Drugs. Preparing for pediatric emergencies: Drugs to consider. *Pediatrics*. 2008;121(2):433–443.

Joint Task Force on Practice Parameters, et al. The diagnosis and management of anaphylaxis: An updated practice parameter. *J Allergy Clin Immunol*. 2005;115(3 Suppl 2):S483–S523.

McLean-Tooke A, Bethune CA, Fay AC, et al. Adrenaline in the treatment of anaphylaxis: What is the evidence? *Br Med J*. 2003;327;1332–1335.

Pumphrey RS. Lessons for management of anaphylaxis from a study of fatal reactions. *Clin Exp Allergy*. 2000;30(8):1144–1150.

Sampson HA, Mendelson L, Rosen JP. Fatal and near-fatal anaphylactic reactions to food in children and adolescents. *N Engl J Med*. 1992;327(6):380–384.

Shaver KJ, Adams C, Weiss SJ. Acute myocardial infarction after administration of low-dose intravenous epinephrine for anaphylaxis. *CJEM*. 2006;8(4):289–294.

Sheikh A, Shehata YA, Brown SG, et al. Adrenaline (epinephrine) for the treatment of anaphylaxis with and without shock. *Cochrane Database Syst Rev*. 2008;4:CD006312.

33

CONSIDER β-BLOCKER POTENTIATION IN PATIENTS WITH ANAPHYLAXIS WHO ARE NOT RESPONDING TO EPINEPHRINE

WILLIAM K. MALLON, MD, FAAEM, FACEP

In anaphylaxis, β-agonists are a critical element of therapy to augment blood pressure via sympathetic nervous system tone and to counteract the effects of mast cell degranulation and release of bioactive amines. β-Blockade can limit the effectiveness of β-agonist therapy by receptor-based competition at the β-receptors. Furthermore, β₁-receptor blockade can exacerbate anaphylactic shock via modulation of adenylate cyclase and increased release of anaphylacto-genic modulators. Lastly, β-blockers can promote unopposed α-adrenergic and vagotonic effects (both undesirable in anaphylaxis).

Since the introduction of β-blockers in the early 1960s, they have become one of the most commonly prescribed classes of drugs in the world and exist in multiple forms, both generic and trademarked. β-Blocker therapy is now extremely common for short- and long-term suppression of dysrhythmias, hypertension, ischemic heart disease, chronic open-angle glaucoma (e.g., timolol ophthalmic drops), situational anxiety (e.g., propranolol for public speaking), migraine headache prophylaxis, thyrotoxicosis, and skeletal muscle tremor, among other conditions. Several combination preparations include a β-blocker (e.g. Tenoretic®, Ziac®). Not only may patients be unaware that they are on a β-blocker, but patients on combination or eye drop preparations also frequently escape the attention of physicians.

Clinically evident "epinephrine-resistant" anaphylaxis should cause the clinician to consider β-blocker–potentiated anaphylaxis. When anaphylaxis fails to respond to usual interventions (epinephrine, corticosteroids, H₁ and H₂ blockers, fluids, and β-agonist inhalers), immediate circumvention of β-blockade is warranted.

Glucagon is a hormone with potent inotropic and chronotropic actions that are only minimally affected by β-blockers. Although data supporting glucagon as therapy for β-blocker–potentiated (epinephrine resistant) anaphylaxis are limited to case reports, a prospective trial with large numbers is unlikely to be done. The pathophysiologic rationale for therapy is good, and an expert opinion from the American Academy of Allergy, Asthma and Immunology consensus group on the diagnosis and management of anaphylaxis recommends considering 1 to 5 mg of glucagon administered intravenously if other treatments are failing. Isoproterenol may also be considered.

In patients who are at increased risk for anaphylaxis (e.g., those with hymenoptera allergy), β-blocker therapy should be discontinued in favor of alternatives if they exist for the condition being treated. Moreover, clinicians referring patients on β-blocker therapy for contrast imaging studies or angiographic procedures should be aware of the role of glucagon in the treatment of anaphylaxis if an allergic or anaphylactoid reaction occurs. Emergency physicians treat anaphylaxis more often than other specialists and are called to "code" situations in the radiology department where anaphylaxis is a relatively common problem. They should be aware of all of the drugs in treatment armamentarium, especially for those severe cases when hypotension fails to respond to usual therapy.

In summary, while a large body of data supporting glucagon therapy in β-blocker–potentiated anaphylaxis are lacking, a growing consensus exists that supports the concept that glucagon may prevent shock and cardiovascular collapse in some cases. Failure to consider glucagon therapy in refractory anaphylaxis or anaphylaxis in a patient known to be on β-blocker therapy is an error that should be avoided.

SUGGESTED READINGS

Javeed N, Javeed H, Javeed S, et al. Refractory anaphylactoid shock potentiated by β-blockers. *Catheter Cardiovasc Diagn*. 1996;39(4):383–384.

Lang DM. Anaphylactoid and anaphylactic reactions: Hazards of β-blockers. *Drug Saf*. 1995;12(5):299–304.

Mclean-Tooke APC, Bethune CA, Fay AC, et al. Adrenaline in the treatment of anaphylaxis: What is the evidence? *Br Med J*. 2003;327:1332–1335.

Momeni M, Brui B, Baele P, et al. Anaphylactic shock in a β-blocked child: Usefulness of isoproterenol. *Paediatr Anaesth*. 2007;17(9):897–899.

Thomas M, Crawford I. Best evidence topic report: Glucagon infusion in refractory anaphylactic shock in patients on β-blockers. *Emerg Med J*. 2005;22(4):272–273.

34

ALWAYS PROVIDE PROPER INSTRUCTIONS, PRESCRIPTIONS, AND FOLLOW-UP WHEN DISCHARGING PATIENTS AFTER ALLERGIC REACTIONS

JAN M. SHOENBERGER, MD, FAAEM, FACEP

Emergency department (ED) clinicians frequently care for patients who have had moderate-to-severe allergic reactions. Once the patent is deemed stable for discharge, the potential exists for future reactions that may be even more severe. Thirty-five to sixty percent of patients with previous severe systemic reactions to hymenoptera stings will have anaphylaxis if stung again. To prevent potentially fatal events, there are several steps that should be taken upon the patient's discharge from the ED. These recommendations come from guidelines of the American Academy of Allergy, Asthma and Immunology and include the prescription of self-injectable epinephrine, education regarding use of the device and indications for use, and referral to an allergy/immunology specialist.

A study published in 2005, looking at ED visits for severe allergic reactions due to insect stings, found that at ED discharge, only 20% to 30% of patients were prescribed an epinephrine self-injection device, and only 15% to 25% were referred to a specialist. This number is surprisingly low considering the future potential for a possibly life-threatening reaction. Prompt administration of epinephrine by patients and/or caretakers is a key component to survival in an out-of-hospital setting, and self-injectable epinephrine devices should be prescribed to all patients at risk.

Education regarding indications for use of the device and how to actually use it is important as well. When needed, these devices must be used quickly and properly to ensure effective delivery of the treatment. The autoinjector device that is currently used in self-injectable epinephrine devices was first designed for use by military personnel in the delivery of lifesaving antidotes such as atropine. It is designed for use in high-stress situations and thus is useful in severe, quickly developing allergic emergencies. The most commonly prescribed autoinjector devices currently available are called EpiPen® and EpiPen Jr.® These are available as single units or in a twin pack. There is also a device called Twinject® that is designed to administer a second follow-up dose of epinephrine using the same device if symptoms worsen or do not resolve.

The EpiPen® device delivers 0.3 mg of a 1:1,000 solution of epinephrine and is designed for use in adults. EpiPen Jr® contains 0.15 mg of a 1:1,000 solution of epinephrine and is designed for use in children. The recommended dose for adults is 0.3 to 0.5 mg of a 1:1,000 solution of epinephrine. European recommendations state that adults may receive higher initial dosages (0.5–1 mg). In children, the recommended dose is 0.01 mg/kg of a 1:1,000 solution up to 0.3 mg. Current recommendations are that infants weighing <10 kg receive the 0.15-mg device or that a conventional syringe/needle be used with the parent or caregiver drawing from an ampule of 1:1,000 epinephrine. However, parents practicing this technique were studied and were found to be relatively incapable of drawing up the correct dose rapidly or accurately.

Education about how to use the EpiPen® is also important. Essentially, it is a three-step process: grasp the device, remove the safety cap, and administer into the lateral thigh. Videos explaining the process are widely available on the Internet on video-sharing sites such as YouTube. The EpiPen® Web site (www.epipen.com) also has detailed instructions with pictures.

Avoidance of anaphylactic triggers will be lifesaving for patients. It is crucial for emergency providers to counsel patients and families about the nature of allergic reactions and how they can be more serious the next time. Medical alert bracelets should also be advised for all ages.

Referral to an allergist/immunologist is advised by the professional society guidelines. The reason for referral is for further education and allergen testing. This is especially important in cases of moderate-to-severe allergic reactions where the trigger is not clear. In the case of many life-threatening allergen reactions, desensitization may be possible through immunologic therapy.

In summary, the discharge instructions (and their documentation) for patients who suffer moderate-to-severe allergic reactions are extremely important. Prescription of a self-injectable epinephrine device and education about its use are key.

SUGGESTED READINGS

Clark S, Long AA, Gaeta TJ, et al. Multicenter study of emergency department visits for insect sting allergies. *J Allergy Clin Immunol*. 2005;116(3):643–649.
Davis JE. Self-injectable epinephrine for allergic emergencies. *J Emerg Med*. 2009;37(1):57–62. [Epub 2008 Feb 1].
Lieberman P, Kemp S, Oppenheimer J, et al. The diagnosis and management of anaphylaxis: An updated practice parameter. *J Allergy Clin Immunol*. 2005;115(Suppl 3):S483–S523.
Simons FER, Chan ES, Gu X, et al. Epinephrine for the out-of-hospital (first-aid) treatment of anaphylaxis in infants: Is the ampule/syringe/needle method practical? *J Allergy Clin Immunol*. 2001;108(6):1040–1044.

35

BE ON THE LOOKOUT FOR DRUG ALLERGIES

WILLIAM K. MALLON, MD, FAAEM, FACEP

Patient safety initiatives and the United States Federal Drug Administration data indicate that medication-related errors continue to be a major problem. Among the many existing adverse drug reactions (ADRs), allergy and anaphylaxis due to erroneously prescribing or administering a drug to a patient with a known allergy is one of the most serious, and deaths continue to occur from this mistake. Of 447 spontaneously reported cases of fatal ADRs, drug allergies accounted for 19%. These are mostly antibiotic related.

Drug name confusion and allergy recognition are clearly two major parts of the problem. Every drug in the United States has (at least) three names: the chemical name, the generic name (nonproprietary), and the brand name (proprietary).

While brand names are about marketing, generic names are supposed to help clinicians recognize drug classes that can be expected to have similar mechanisms of action, side effects, and allergy issues with potential cross-reactivity. Some ADRs are due to the fact that a brand name is better known than a generic name that contains the stem or prefix indicating the drug class (e.g., -coxib for COX-2 inhibitors, or -mab for monoclonal antibodies). The United States Adopted Names council rejects 25% to 30% of proposed drug names due to fears regarding confusion. Such confusion may result in allergy, anaphylaxis, misprescribing, or misadministration.

Additionally, confusion between true drug allergy and drug intolerance is very common. Of patients reporting a penicillin allergy, it has been found that only 2% to 3% are truly allergic, and false reporting of allergy is very common. One classic example of this misreporting is codeine allergy. When reported, it is usually because of drug intolerance (e.g., nausea and vomiting). The same is true for reported allergies to macrolide antibiotics. Differentiation of true allergy from intolerance is often not attempted. This confusion dilutes the importance of allergy reporting because many physicians are skeptical of the likelihood of a true allergy for a given report. The resultant prescribing behaviors of physicians appear to validate this skepticism and reveal a lack of respect or concern regarding anaphylaxis and allergy when allergy is actually present.

There is further confusion regarding the nature of cross-reactivity among drugs of related classes. True cross-reactivity differs from general hypersensitivity. Some investigators have suggested that many cases identified as cross-reactivity are, in fact, hypersensitivity. Clinical manifestations of allergy with both sulfa drugs and penicillins may actually not be due to sensitization or haptenic determinants of the drug but instead reflect a general hypersensitivity of the patient. Nonetheless, true cross-reactivity, as appears to occur between acetyl salicylic acid (ASA) and nonsteroidal anti-inflammatory drugs (NSAIDs), can result in life-threatening reactions.

Having noted the above problems, all of which indicate that drug allergy issues are likely to persist, the question remains as to how to minimize the problem. Good data are emerging showing that computerized physician order entry with a computer-driven system containing a comprehensive allergy warning system including potential cross-reactivity prevents drug allergy ADRs. Allergy notification forms, conspicuous armband identifiers, and nursing/pharmacy protocols are also effective. Physician awareness of a few key drug allergy issues (*Table 35.1*) can help prevent approximately 65% to 75% of hospital-based allergy and anaphylaxis.

ADR-related presentations may represent 10% or more of all emergency department patient presentations, many of which are related to allergies. Hospital and emergency department allergy issues also frequently increase the length of stay, and many of these errors are not disclosed to patients despite hospital policy statements requiring disclosure. Correction of the prescribing errors that produce these visits would have significant health care economic impact.

TABLE 35.1	KEY DRUG ALLERGY ISSUES	
REPORTED ALLERGY	**PRESCRIBED DRUG**	**COMMENT**
Penicillin	Ampicillin/sulbactam (Unasyn) Piperacillin/tazobactam (Zosyn) Imipenem/cilastatin (Primaxin) Ertapenem (Invanz) Doripenem (Doribax) Amoxicillin Amoxillin/clavulanate (Augmentin)	Prescribers should recognize "-syn" or "-penem" as a penicillin
	Cephalosporins (Cephalexin, etc.)	Cross-reactivity between penicillin and cepha-losporin is low
Sulfa	Trimethoprim/ sulfamethoxazole (Bactrim)	A 2003 study showed that although allergy to a sulfonamide antibiotic is indeed a risk factor for a subsequent allergic reaction to a sulfonamide nonantibiotic, a history of penicillin allergy is at least as strong a risk factor.
Antibiotic drugs	Erythromycin/ sulfisoxazole (Pediazole) Dapsone Furosemide (Lasix)	
Nonantibiotic drugs	Acetazolamide (Diamox) Hydrochlorothiazide Metolazone Sulfonylureas Sumatriptan (Imitrex) Sulfasalazine Celecoxib (Celebrex)	
ASA/NSAID	Aspirin Ketorolac (Toradol) Ibuprofen and other NSAIDs	NSAID and ASA allergy can be severe with cross-reactivity well documented
Opiates	Morphine Hydromorphone (Dilaudid) Oxycodone (Oxycontin) Hydrocodone/ acteominophen (Vicodin) Acetaminophen/codeine (Tylenol no. 3)	True anaphylaxis from opiates is actually rare, but side effects and mild rashes (e.g., histamine release with morphine) are common.

SUGGESTED READINGS

DePestel DD, Benninger MS, Danziger L, et al. Cephalosporin use in treatment of patients with penicillin allergies. *J Am Pharm Assoc*. 2008;48(4):530–540.

Hoffman JM, Proulx SM. Medication errors caused by confusion of drug names. *Drug Saf.* 2003;26(7):445–452.

Kelly WN. Can the frequency and risks of fatal adverse drug events be determined? *Pharmacotherapy*. 2001;21(5):521–527.

Strom BL, Schinnar R, Apter AJ, et al. Absence of crossreactivity between sulfonamide antibiotics and sulfonamide nonantibiotics. *NEJM*. 2003;349(17):1628–1635.

36

A "COMPLICATED" PATIENT IS NOT ALWAYS A LEVEL 5

STEPHEN G. HOLTZCLAW, MD, FACEP

The most important goal of emergency medicine is to provide the necessary health care to those who need it, in the most time-efficient and resource-appropriate manner. This can be a challenge and most of the focus of emergency medicine training is on developing the skills to deliver the most important service. However, in order to provide this care, reimbursements for physician involvement must continue at a level that provides fair compensation. Compensation has become intrinsically intertwined with documentation which, in itself, has become an activity that requires attention and continued education in order to remain proficient.

In 1995 and 1997, the Health Care Financing Administration (HCFA), now the Center for Medicare/Medicaid Services (CMS as of 2003), adopted a system of assessing the clinical content of physicians' charts in relation to each patient interaction. This system is known as the evaluation and management (E&M) of physician services. The critical component of this system is not as much as what service is provided, but instead the level of documentation to support that the service was provided. In many ways, the advent of strict reliance on documentation standards to support billing reflects physicians' inability to self-regulate and set standards across the industry. It is not enough to state that you provided a complex service; your documentation of the service must pass scrutiny and adhere to standards that were set, in part, (or in some cases largely) by nonphysicians. Furthermore, the E&M standards of documentation do not always accurately reflect the time and energy devoted to the care of a particular patient. As many emergency physicians have come to realize, a time-consuming patient does not always yield a more favorable E&M code. In short, does managing a complicated patient result in a higher E&M code?

Sadly, the answer is no. The key point here is how the word "complicated" is used. A laceration on the chin of a 2-year-old active male can take upward of 45 min to manage. Putting sutures in this patient can be a time-consuming activity,

TABLE 36.1	**KEY DOCUMENTATION COMPONENTS OF THE PATIENT ENCOUNTER**
History	History of present illness, review of systems, and past/family/social history
Examination	Physical exam appropriate for presenting problem
Medical decision making	Number of management options, complexity of data, and risk of complications

not only because the child will not hold still and may require restraints, but also because the parents need attention as well. They need their questions answered and, in general, require some reassurance about the management and outcome. In general, the patient care that was provided above would not qualify as a Level 5 E&M code. In comparison, an 80-year-old woman who breaks her hip after a trip and fall would have a more straightforward management. She will be admitted and, in general, will have an undemanding workup, requiring minimal physician effort and limited time. Although this case seems uncomplicated, it will likely qualify as a Level 5 (as long as the documentation requirements are met) due to the severity of the presenting problem and the medical decision making involved.

Put another way, complicated, as it pertains to Level 5 charts, has to do with how complex the medical decision making is, and does not reflect the amount of time and effort you spent.

Although it is probable that the E&M codes will be revised in the future, the current E&M codes will likely be around for a while. For emergency medicine, there are five levels of service that were created based upon key documentation components of the patient encounter. These key components are divided into three domains (*Table 36.1*): The first is the history, reflecting the subjective component and historical elements of the health status of the patient. Second is the examination, which reflects the objective qualitative and quantitative measurements that a physician acquires by physical examination of the patient. The third component is the medical decision making, which reflects the cognitive effort that the physician expends in order to justify the treatment. Medical decision making includes review of the data, management options, and consideration of complications.

All of the components must meet or exceed the stated documentation requirements for a particular level of E&M service. The five levels of service and their appropriate past designation are listed in *Table 36.2*.

For each level of service (E&M) code, HCFA/CMS has determined certain details that must be included in the documentation of each patient encounter, to fulfill the key component requirement. If these components are not included or limited in their scope, appropriate billing for the actual complexity of the visit will not take place and a lower level of service will have to be selected. Put

TABLE 36.2	THE FIVE LEVELS OF SERVICE AND THEIR APPROPRIATE PAST DESIGNATION OF E&M OF PHYSICIAN SERVICES	
ASSESSMENT	**LEVEL OF SERVICE**	**E&M CODE**
Brief	1	99281
Limited	2	99282
Intermediate	3	99283
Extended	4	99284
Comprehensive	5	99285

another way, each area is coded separately and the chart is coded to the lowest level of the three areas.

Emergency medicine reimbursements are increasingly more reliant on the documentation provided by the physician. Regardless of how much time and effort you actually spend on a patient, how well you document with particular attention paid to the required three domains will determine the billing. (A certified coder should review all charts for accuracy.) As often cited in the past, the truism holds true today, "not charted, not done," at least in terms of billing.

SUGGESTED READINGS

AMA. Payment Action Kit for Medicare. Available at: http://www.ama-assn.org/ama/pub/physician-resources/solutions-managing-your-practice/coding-billing-insurance/medicare/payment-action-kit-medicare.shtml.

AMA. *CPT 2009 Professional Edition*. Chicago: American Medical Association; 2008.

CRS Report for Congress. *Medicare: Payments to Physicians*. Updated January 17, 2008. Available at: http://aging.senate.gov/crs/medicare15.pdf.

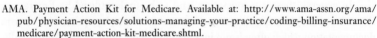

37

CRITICAL CARE BILLING IS NOT LOCATION SPECIFIC

MELISSA W. COSTELLO, MD, FACEP

Case: A 59-year-old female with chronic alcohol abuse presented with a cough and a low-grade fever of 100.5° to the emergency department (ED). The suspicion was that she had pneumonia, but her O_2 saturation was 92% on room air, her blood pressure was 148/92, and her heart rate was 90 with a respiratory rate (RR) of 20. After the x-ray confirmed a right lower lobe pneumonia, she was to be started on a dose of oral antibiotics. An hour after her initial vital signs, she was placed in a standard intermediary care ED room. An hour after that, her BP dropped to 90/60, her heart rate was 110, RR was 28, and fever was 102.4°. She was given a fluid bolus through a recently placed central line, and IV antibiotics were started. Consideration was given for vasopressor support. Arrangements were made for an ICU-level admission. What would be an appropriate level of billing for her care?

E&M Codes 99291 and 99292 are used to bill for critical care services that occur in the outpatient setting or in the adult inpatient setting. These codes (99291 for the first 30 to 74 min and 99292 for each additional 30 min increment) can be billed for the "medical care for a critically ill or critically injured patient."

How is critically ill or injured defined? CPT (Current Procedural Terminology) 2008 defines this as "a critical illness or injury that impairs one or more vital organ systems such that there is a high probability of imminent or life-threatening deterioration in the patient's condition. Critical care involves high complexity decision making to assess, manipulate, and support vital organ system function(s) to treat single or multiple vital organ system failure and/or to prevent further life-threatening deterioration of the patient's condition. Examples of vital organ system failure include, but are not limited to, central nervous system failure, circulatory failure, shock, renal, hepatic, metabolic, and/or respiratory failure."

In general, these are codes that tend to be underutilized by Emergency Physicians (EPs) for several reasons. First and foremost, it requires a bit of extra documentation which often is not included in the documentation. Additionally, a mental shift is required to recognize that the "typical Diabetic Ketoacidosis (DKA)" or the "typical dry septic kid" constitutes critical care in the global world of medicine. EPs tend to discount the complexity and acuity of the care and decision making involved in the care of these types of patients because it is what they do every day. In much the same way a NASCAR driver feels that 80 mi per h is slow, patients who do not necessarily end up in the resuscitation room are not considered for "critical care" by many EPs.

For these reasons, EPs shortchange themselves on the billing. Patients on vasopressors, patients requiring multiple breathing treatments, acute pulmonary edema, ST elevation myocardial infarct (STEMI), acute stroke, trauma activations, unstable overdoses, and sepsis are all examples of patients who should be considered as potential for critical care billing. If the patients meet critical care criteria, the challenge is to provide adequate documentation to support this definition.

Critical care billing is not location specific. It can occur anywhere in the ED, the ICU, the resuscitation room, an urgent care center, the general medicine floor, and even in an ambulance when a physician escorts a transported patient. In hospitals where the EPs respond to cardiac arrests outside the ED, this code can be used when the resuscitation (plus paperwork, etc.) lasts more than 30 min rather than the inpatient consultation codes.

Interestingly, critical care does not have to be continuous and does not have to be all the bedside time. Time can be added up to a total for any calendar day and includes the time for talking with consultants or family, time for reviewing records, labs or imaging studies, and time for doing actual bedside care. It cannot include the time spent doing procedures that are billed separately, and several common critical care procedures are included in the 99291 code.

Included procedures are

- Chest x-rays (71010, 71015, 71020)
- Pulse oximetry (94760, 94761, 94762)
- Blood gases
- Gastric intubation (43752 and 91105)
- Temporary transcutaneous pacing (92953)
- Ventilator management (94656, 94657, 94660, and 94662)
- Vascular access procedures (36000, 36410, 36415, 36540, and 36600)

Common procedures that CAN be billed separately (although cannot be included in the time calculation) include

- Cardiopulmonary resuscitation (CPR) (92950)
- Central venous access (36555 and 36556)
- Arterial line placement (36620)
- Endotracheal intubation (31500)
- Transvenous pacemaker placement (33210)
- Lumbar puncture (62270)
- Ultrasound (Obstetrics (OB), Focused Abdominal Sonography in Trauma (FAST), venous guidance, pneumothorax, and limited cardiac)

Teaching physicians in the academic setting can only charge critical care time for the time actually spent at the bedside or in consultation with a person. The time spent teaching cannot be included, and the teaching physician's note must reflect all of the required elements of time, acuity, and bedside involvement.

When multiple physicians manage the same patient, only one physician can bill 99291 or 99292 for any time segment. It is important to coordinate billing times with consultant physicians to avoid overlaps and overcoding resulting in denial of claims. For example, Dr EP can bill 99291 from 09:00 to 10:00 on a trauma patient and then turn over care to Dr Surgeon who can bill 99291 for his initial care from 10:01 until 11:16 and then 99292 for the 30 min segments that follow.

One of the interesting nuances of E&M coding is the way midnight is handled. At 12:00, a new day begins and critical care time from the day before cannot overlap with the next day. This can be particularly problematic for EPs. For example, if a critically ill patient arrives at 23:40 h and has 40 min of critical care time, 99291 cannot be billed on either side of midnight, given that neither segment lasts for more than 30 min. Although if the care lasted from 23:40 until 00:40, the 99291 can be billed for the postmidnight segment.

In summary, EPs do a lot of critical care and either fail to recognize it as such or fail to document it. A wise billing expert once asked "why would an EP spend an hour saving a life and not spend the extra two minutes documenting to get paid for it?" The important elements essential to billing critical care for the EP are recognition and documentation of severity and time.

SUGGESTED READINGS

Beebe M, Dalton JA, Espronceda M, et al., eds. *CPT 2008, Professional Edition*. Chicago: American Medical Association, 2008;19–21.
McLain T. Tackling four common myths about critical care service codes. *Today's Hospitalist*. 2004;(Aug):4–5.
Vachani A, DeLong P, Manaker S. Documentation and coding of critical care professional services. *Clin Pulmonary Med*. 2003;10(2):85–92.

38

DO NOT RELY ON YOUR STUDENT'S DOCUMENTATION

JULIANNA JUNG, MD, FACEP

Medical students: you teach them, you nurture them, you patiently and lovingly supervise them in all their clinical duties, you guide them in their procedures, and you critique their presentations. You are so proud when you find that their notes are detailed, concise, clear, and accurate. They are even legible! So you cosign with a flourish and move on to the next patient. After all that tender loving care (TLC), who would deny you the right to bill for it? You will get paid, right?

Absolutely not. The Centers for Medicaid and Medicare Services (CMS) have very clear guidelines regarding medical student documentation, and they are very restrictive. These guidelines stem from reform legislation designed to decrease Medicare fraud by ensuring that teaching physicians are personally involved in the care provided by trainees under their direction. The guidelines state

...the documentation of a service by a student that may be referred to by the teaching physician is limited to documentation related to the review of systems and/or past family/social history. The teaching physician may not refer to a student's documentation of physical exam findings or medical decision making in his or her personal note. If the medical student documents services, the teaching physician must verify and redocument the history of present illness as well as perform and redocument the physical exam and medical decision making activities of the service.

That is right: other than review of systems (ROS) and past family/social history, medical student documentation cannot be used for billing. All components of the chart that support billing have to be separately and independently documented by the supervising physician—in this case, the billing physician. The billing physician has to personally repeat and rewrite the History of Present Illness (HPI), exam, and medical decision making, or they will not get paid for the visit. It should be noted that all students are considered equal by the law: from the greenest first year to the most seasoned subintern, if they have not graduated, they are still students according to CMS.

But wait! These guidelines are from CMS and only pertain to Medicare and Medicaid patients, right? Wrong. Private insurance companies have an obvious financial interest in limiting their responsibility for paying claims, and denying payment based on lack of documentation is an easy and foolproof way of doing just that. Therefore, most private insurers have adopted the CMS guidelines as well, so it is unlikely that you will be paid for an inadequately documented visit, regardless of the patient's insurance coverage.

Can you pass on the responsibility to your residents? Yes and no. The resident can independently repeat and rewrite the student's note (so the billing doctor does not have to), but one must ensure that the documentation appropriately references the resident's note. Resident documentation can be used to support billing, provided that the billing physician documents personal involvement with the patient's care and at least briefly notes any key clarifications or changes to the resident's assessment. "Seen and agree" notes are a thing of the past, but it is not necessary to rewrite resident charts the way you must for students.

The bottom line: The billing physician has to independently repeat and rewrite history, physical exam, and medical decision making for all patients evaluated by medical students.

SUGGESTED READING

Medicare Department of Health & Human Services (DHHS). Carriers Manual Centers for Medicare & Medicaid Services (CMS). Part 3—Claims Process, Transmittal 1780: November 22, 2002. Available at: http://www.cms.hhs.gov/Transmittals/Downloads/R1780B3.pdf. Accessed January 9, 2009.

39

KNOW WHAT TO DOCUMENT IN THE REVIEW OF SYSTEMS

STEPHEN G. HOLTZCLAW, MD, FACEP

Just as in other professions, it is not only what you do that is important, but it is also what you document. Documentation in medicine remains of central importance, not only to communicate to other providers but also to provide a basis for reimbursement. Given the importance of documentation, it is surprising that a number of practitioners do not understand how an E&M chart is coded, billed, and ultimately paid.

In 1995 and 1997, the Health Care Financing Administration (HCFA), now the Center for Medicare/Medicaid Services (CMS as of 2003), adopted a system of assessing the clinical content of physicians' charts in relation to each patient interaction. This system is known as the evaluation and management (E&M) of physician services. For emergency medicine, five levels of service were assigned based upon key components of the patient encounter. These key components can be divided into three sections. The first is the subjective data, that is, the data of what patients or their surrogate can tell you about their problem. The second is the objective data, that is, the information you can get from the patient by the physical examination of the patient. The third is the analysis process and the resulting decisions made for the clinical management of the patient. In terms of the HCFA language, these key components are listed in *Table 39.1*.

All of the three components must meet or exceed the stated requirements for a particular level of E&M service. The five levels of service and their appropriate past designations are listed in *Table 39.2*.

For each level of service (E&M) code, HCFS/CMS has determined certain details that must be included in the documentation of each patient encounter

TABLE 39.1	KEY COMPONENTS OF THE HCFA LANGUAGE
History	History of present illness, review of systems, and past/family/social history
Examination	Physical exam appropriate for presenting problem
Medical decision making	Number of management options, complexity of data, and risk of complications

TABLE 39.2	THE FIVE LEVELS OF SERVICE AND THEIR APPROPRIATE PAST DESIGNATION OF E&M OF PHYSICIAN SERVICES	
ASSESSMENT	**LEVEL OF SERVICE**	**E&M CODE**
Brief	1	99281
Limited	2	99282
Intermediate	3	99283
Extended	4	99284
Comprehensive	5	99285

to fulfill the key component requirement. These documentation requirements must be met, and even if the services were delivered, if it was not appropriately documented, the correct E&M code might not be applicable. If the correct elements of the components are not included in the documentation or are limited in their scope, appropriate billing for the actual complexity of the visit will not take place. As a result, a lower level of service will have to be selected. Put another way, each area is coded separately and the chart is coded to the lowest level of the three areas.

There are some helpful hints that should remembered when documenting the level of care in a patient in the emergency department. In particular, with regard to the history, there are three elements that should be addressed: History of Present Illness (HPI), review of systems (ROS), and past, family, social history (PFSH).

- The ROS and PFSH can be recorded by ancillary staff as long as you sign off on the history as agreeing or add your own changes.
- If you cannot obtain a history from the patient, record that you cannot get the history and specify the reason (e.g., coma, unstable, dementia, and respiratory distress). This will cover all elements of the history.
- For the ROS, after you have documented the positives and the pertinent negatives, you may make the statement "all other systems reviewed and negative" if you have indeed assessed these other systems. (Do not use statements such as "not pertinent," "not addressed," and "no other complaints.")

Also keep in mind that if you are writing a note by hand, your note must be legible.

In conclusion, emergency physicians provide a range of services. In order to bill for these services, it is important to understand the documentation requirements for each level of service. In particular, the ROS is one area that must have the appropriate documentation.

SUGGESTED READINGS

AMA. *Payment Action Kit for Medicare*. Available at: http://www.ama-assn.org/ama/pub/
    physician-resources/solutions-managing-your-practice/coding-billing-insurance/medi-
    care/payment-action-kit-medicare.shtml.
AMA. *CPT 2009 Professional Edition*. Chicago: American Medical Association; 2008.
CRS Report for Congress. *Medicare: Payments to Physicians*. Updated January 17, 2008. Avail-
    able at: http://aging.senate.gov/crs/medicare15.pdf.

40

STOP RESISTING CHANGE ... ELECTRONIC HEALTH RECORDS ARE HERE TO STAY!

EDWARD S. BESSMAN, MD, MBA

As determined by The American College of Emergency Physicians, the emergency department (ED) chart or record serves a variety of functions:

1) Medical management
2) Quality improvement
3) Risk management
4) Reimbursement
5) Utilization review
6) Regulatory
7) Research

Accordingly, the ideal ED chart must therefore contain a large number of specific components in order to meet these needs. The "Data Elements for Emergency Department Systems" (DEEDS) specification was developed by the Centers for Disease Control and Prevention in 1997 to serve as a universal foundation for ED charts. DEEDS enumerate several hundred individual data elements that collectively represent a comprehensive ED chart. Although the DEEDS initiative contained representatives from over a dozen different government agencies and medical specialty societies, the specification never caught on. Thus, there exist a wide variety of styles and formats for ED charts with no generally accepted standard. The stakes could not be higher, which calls out for a robust solution. Given the dynamic text and data capabilities of computers, it would seem natural that an electronic medical record (EMR) would be widely adopted.

An EMR (also known as an electronic health record, or EHR) offers a large number of potential benefits. Storage of electronic records requires far less space than paper records. Likewise, an EMR can be retrieved much more quickly than paper and at any location where it is needed. A paper record can comprise a variety of materials from different sources: provider documentation, laboratory results, radiographs, and so forth. All of these can be consolidated in a single EMR. Also, unlike paper records, EMRs can be updated easily and without waste. The value of a templated chart has long been recognized as a way to prompt medical personnel to chart various important elements of the patient's encounter. EMRs are able to embrace and extend this paradigm by giving prompts and cues as the chart is being completed, based on the information that has already been entered. An EMR eliminates the issue of poor legibility and likewise helps to mitigate problems related to nonstandard abbreviations or terminology. This combination of a more complete and legible chart improves reimbursement and patient safety and reduces the risk of professional liability. Furthermore, every step in a patient's care can be logged and tracked in an EMR, greatly facilitating throughput analysis. Additionally, creating customized, legible, and comprehensive discharge instructions is a task made easy by an EMR. Finally, data abstraction for the purposes of public health reporting, care management, quality improvement, research, etc. is greatly facilitated by the use of an EMR.

With all of the stated benefits of using an EMR, the fact that there has not been universal adoption suggests that there is a downside, and indeed there are several potential negatives:

1) Privacy issues are a major concern. While commercially available EMRs take steps to make certain of data security, issues often arise from integrating the system into existing hospital information networks.

2) Lack of standardization is an important issue. There are a plethora of available EMRs as well as hospital information systems. Although there are some dominant companies, there are, as yet, no truly "off the shelf" or "plug and play" solutions. This guarantees implementation problems.

3) Cost is a big barrier to adoption of an EMR. Although it is generally agreed upon that the overall financial impact of an EMR is positive, there are large up-front costs. These include the cost of the software and hardware for the EMR itself; expenses related to infrastructure, which may be substantial in environments with very little preexisting information technology (IT); training IT staff (and often hiring additional staff); developing and implementing interfaces with other electronic systems; customizing the EMR; and training the end users. These start-up costs can easily run upward from several million dollars. Ongoing costs are also not insubstantial.

4) Changeover to an EMR presents the problem of what to do with the preexisting paper records. An ideal solution is to scan the old records and store the digitized images in a database that is linked to the EMR, but this is costly.

5) Staff resistance is a major issue. There is a substantial learning curve even for computer-savvy individuals. Dedicated training is a must. This proves to

be especially problematic in teaching environments where large numbers of individuals rotate through the ED.

6) Adoption of an EMR generally results in decreased productivity and throughput. Although the documentation produced is superior to a paper chart, an EMR is slower. This is particularly so during the start-up phase and is especially troubling to ED staff. After a variable time period, often in the range of several months, productivity will improve but nonetheless there may be a permanent decrement.

In spite of these negatives, the widespread implementation of EMRs is gaining ground. The Office of the National Coordinator for Health Information Technology has encouraged universal implementation by 2014 as a key component of health care quality improvement and patient safety. Furthermore, the Center for Medicare and Medicaid Services plans to tie reimbursement to the use of an EMR, which likely will speed up adoption. A careful consideration of the benefits and obstacles will promote a smoother transition to an EMR in the ED. It seems inevitable that EMR will eventually become the standard documentation method in the future.

SUGGESTED READINGS

National Center for Injury Prevention and Control. *Data Elements for Emergency Department Systems*. Available at: http://www.cdc.gov/ncipc/pub-res/deedspage.htm. Accessed February 28, 2009.

Pollock DA, Adams DL, Bernardo LM, et al. Data elements for emergency department systems, release 1.0 (DEEDS): a summer report. DEEDS Writing Committee. *Ann Emerg Med*. 1998;31:264–273.

Yamamoto LG, Khan A. Challenges of electronic medical record implementation in the emergency department. *Pediatr Emerg Care*. 2006;22(3):184–191.

41

UNDERSTAND THE PURPOSES OF THE EMERGENCY DEPARTMENT CHART AND WHERE TO FOCUS YOUR ATTENTION

EDWARD S. BESSMAN, MD, MBA

The emergency department (ED) chart serves a variety of purposes, besides the obvious one of documenting clinical care. To the practicing emergency physician, the most important uses of the ED chart are for clinical documentation, for generating a bill, and for protecting against a claim of professional negligence.

Although there is no officially prescribed format for an acceptable chart, in fact most charts comprise the same basic elements. This is due to the reimbursement rules put in place by the Center for Medicare and Medicaid Services (CMS) in 1997, which promulgated a formula for determining the proper "evaluation and management (E&M)" billing code. This E&M code is dependent upon a very specific set of elements. Any deviation from the CMS specification results in a lower reimbursement, known as "downcoding."

The descriptors specified by CMS comprise seven major groups:

1) History
2) Physical examination
3) Medical decision making
4) Counseling
5) Coordination of care
6) Nature of presenting problem
7) Time

The first three are the "key components" that determine the E&M code for the ED, and they are further elaborated into six elements:

1) Chief complaint
2) History of present illness
3) Review of systems
4) Past, family, and/or social history
5) General multisystem versus single organ physical examination
6) Complexity of medical decision making

These six elements are further expanded into a varying number of items, the sum of which is used to generate the appropriate E&M code according to a matrix specified by CMS. The prescriptive nature of this specification, coupled as it is to physician reimbursement, has resulted in a de facto format for ED charts. Indeed, one of the major marketing points claimed by virtually every commercially available charting system is how well it maximizes physician reimbursement while simultaneously simplifying the process of meeting the CMS standard.

So from a billing perspective, most ED charts are more than adequate. The question remains as to how well they serve the other two needs. From the standpoint of clinical care, the two most important parts of the chart are the history of present illness and the medical decision making. These two components of the chart are heavily weighted by the CMS reimbursement specification, and thus they are generally well documented by ED providers. However, the emphasis on specific elements of documentation can result in an improved quantity of charting, without a commensurate increase in quality. Thus, although there might be substantial detail, the overall narrative may suffer. Nonetheless, most ED charts that are substantially complete from a CMS billing perspective will be adequate records of the clinical care that was provided.

One of the most important roles of the ED chart is to serve as a record of the thoughts and actions of the ED physician such that it can be used as a defense against a claim of professional negligence or malpractice. For this purpose, the most important components of the chart relate to medical decision making and the formulation of a disposition and, if the patient is discharged, the instructions that were given to the patient or other responsible party at the time of discharge. The key elements of medical decision making consist of the differential diagnosis and the reasoning behind why certain diagnoses were included or excluded. Templated charts and electronic medical records are designed to assist with this process, but the reality is that most records fail to include enough detail to unequivocally substantiate the physician's thought process. Nevertheless, the structure of a generic ED chart will include some aspect of medical decision making because it is a key component of the chart as specified by CMS. Thus, most charts will have adequate, if not optimal, documentation of the medical decision making of the ED physician.

What is striking is that CMS makes essentially no requirement regarding discharge instructions. Consequently, the section devoted to discharge instructions tends to be the least robust part of any ED chart. From a malpractice perspective, however, the instructions given to the patient at discharge represent the most important part of the ED record. The law recognizes that there exist a nearly infinite variety of patient presentations and that an ED physician cannot be held responsible for diagnosing all manner of subtle or rare conditions. Nor should the ED be used for the treatment of long-term conditions. Nonetheless, the standard of care requires that a plan for follow-up and subsequent care be clearly specified to the patient in a language that is appropriate to the patient's ability to understand. This is particularly important in situations where no firm diagnosis could be reached in the ED. Unfortunately, discharge instructions are often peremptory or are a standardized boilerplate that is too generic to be pertinent to the individual patient.

The prudent ED physician will take the time to ensure that patients receive appropriate discharge instructions that adequately indicate what was done, the suspected condition being treated, continuing treatments (if any), recommended follow-up, and reasons for return to the ED. Preprinted or computer-generated instructions are fine as long as they are tailored to the individual patient.

SUGGESTED READINGS

Deutsch LM. Medical Records for Attorneys. American Law Institute-American Bar Association Committee on Continuing Professional Education 2001, 33–35.

1997 Documentation Guidelines for Evaluation and Management Services. Center for Medicare and Medicaid Services. Available at: http://www.cms.hhs.gov/MLNProducts/downloads/MASTER1.PDF. Accessed February 28, 2009.

Wears RL. The chart is dead—long live the chart. *Ann Emerg Med*. 2008;52:390–391.

42

ALWAYS CONSIDER AORTIC DISSECTION IN PATIENTS PRESENTING WITH CHEST PAIN AND ISCHEMIC CHANGES ON ELECTROCARDIOGRAM

TARLAN HEDAYATI, MD AND
STUART P. SWADRON, MD, FRCPC

The complaint of chest pain prompts the emergency physician (EP) to consider a several life-threatening diagnoses. These are usually methodically addressed, one by one, eventually arriving at the final, correct diagnosis. Sometimes, unfortunately, the very tests that the EP depends upon to arrive at the correct diagnosis can erroneously point down a very different path, with catastrophic consequences.

The initial electrocardiogram (ECG) is used to quickly identify any disease processes that require immediate intervention, such an unstable dysrhythmia or evidence or myocardial infarction (MI). The diagnosis of an ST elevation MI (STEMI) by ECG subsequently leads to either activation of the cardiac catheterization laboratory for percutaneous intervention or fibrinolysis, depending on the individual institution. In a significant number of cases, however, patients presenting to the ED with acute aortic dissection (AD) can develop ECG changes consistent with ischemia or infarction, including ST elevation mimicking STEMI.

Thoracic ADs are classified as either Stanford type A (comprising 62% of patients) and the Stanford type B. Stanford type A dissections involve the ascending aorta and are more often managed surgically while type Bs involve the descending aorta. In a Japanese study looking at ECG changes in 89 patients with acute AD, a staggering 55% of type A dissections demonstrated ECG changes, including ST segment depression in 22%, T wave changes in 8%, and ST segment elevation in 8%. The location of the ST elevation was inferior leads (II, III, and aVF) in 75% and high lateral leads (I and aVL) in 25%. Of the type B dissections, 22% had acute ECG changes, but none with ST segment elevation.

The International Registry of Acute Aortic Dissections has been collecting data regarding patients with AD since 1996 and has accumulated data on

464 patients in its first 2 years. Sixty-nine percent of AD patients in this registry demonstrated some ECG abnormality. The most common ECG abnormalities were nonspecific ST/T wave changes (41%), left ventricular hypertrophy (26%), ischemic patterns (15%), and infarction patterns (11%). The ECG changes associated with acute AD are thought to be due to (1) retrograde extension of the dissection causing proximal occlusion of a coronary artery (typically the right) by an intimal flap or compressive hematoma; (2) a shock state, particularly cardiac tamponade; or (3) preexisting coronary artery disease.

If a patient with AD is misdiagnosed as having myocardial ischemia or MI and goes on to receive anticoagulation and/or fibrinolysis, the results can be fatal. In the aforementioned Japanese study, one patient with ST segment depression on ECG received fibrinolysis and died due to cardiac tamponade. According to a study by the European Myocardial Infarction Project, the incidence of acute AD mistakenly treated with fibrinolysis was 0.33%. While this may be considered a relatively rare occurrence, the outcome is almost universally catastrophic for the patients involved.

So, what is the bottom line? Do not ignore the patient's presentation when the ECG shows ischemic changes, even if it appears to be a STEMI. If the pain is ripping or tearing toward the back, one of the upper extremities has lost a pulse, or the mediastinum is very suggestive of AD—it is best to hold fibrinolytics until a more definitive image can be obtained. Many options exist, including computed tomography, transesophageal echocardiography, or even angiography in the catheterization suite. On the other hand, AD is exceedingly unlikely to present with the appearance of an anterior STEMI with reciprocal changes on ECG. In this scenario, delaying reperfusion for STEMI therapy is generally unwarranted unless signs of dissection are obvious.

SUGGESTED READINGS

Hagan PG, Nienaber CA, Isselbacher EM, et al. The International Registry of Acute Aortic Dissection (IRAD): New insights into an old disease. *JAMA*. 2000;283(7):897–903.

Hirata K, Kyushima M, Asato H. Electrocardiographic abnormalities in patients with acute aortic dissection. *Am J Cardiol*. 1995;76:1207–1212.

The European Myocardial Infarction Project Group. Prehospital thrombolytic therapy in patients with suspected acute myocardial infarction. *N Engl J Med*. 1993;329:383–389.

43

REMEMBER TO AGGRESSIVELY MANAGE BLOOD PRESSURES IN PATIENTS WITH ACUTE THORACIC AORTIC DISSECTION

TARLAN HEDAYATI, MD AND
STUART P. SWADRON, MD, FRCPC

Thoracic aortic dissections (ADs) are classified into Stanford types A and B. Stanford type A dissections, which involve the ascending aorta, account for approximately 60% of the total and are surgically managed. Type B ADs involve the descending aorta and are typically medically managed. ADs are considered "acute" if they are of <2 weeks duration.

Hypertension is the most common risk factor associated with AD and is a typical finding in patients diagnosed with AD in the emergency department. It is critically important to measure blood pressure in both arms. If there is a discrepancy, the higher of the two should be used to guide treatment, as it represents the true systemic pressure. Patients with normal or low blood pressures should be assumed to be in shock states secondary to hemorrhage and/or cardiac tamponade until proven otherwise.

Stresses on the aortic wall that lead to dissection are related to both blood pressure and the steepness of the aortic pulse wave. This is known as dP/dt and refers to the speed at which the maximal systolic pressure reaches the aortic root. Factors that increase dP/dt include systolic blood pressure, heart rate, and myocardial contractility. Regardless of the Stanford classification, the immediate therapy for both types of AD is thus aggressive reduction of all three parameters in an effort to prevent progression of the dissection, aortic rupture, and death. The lowest tolerated blood pressure and heart rate that allow for continued cerebral and coronary perfusion is the goal of therapy.

Selection of the antihypertensive agents in AD should be limited to intravenous formulations that allow for rapid, titratable blood pressure and heart rate management.

Nitroprusside is probably the most studied titratable antihypertensive available. It is dosed at 0.25 to 10 μg/kg/min. It is an arterial and venous dilator that reduces both preload and afterload very effectively. Nitroprusside does have its drawbacks though. It can promote baroreceptor activation, causing unwanted tachycardia. For this reason, it should be used in conjunction with a β-blocker to blunt this response. It is photosensitive, requiring the intravenous solution bag and tubing to be wrapped prior to and during administration. Its other drawbacks, nitroprusside resistance (from its activation of the renin-angiotensin-aldosterone system) and cyanide (CN) toxicity, are less relevant in the first few hours and should not prevent its use in the ED setting.

Although emergency personnel are more familiar and comfortable with nitroglycerin through its use in myocardial ischemia, infarction, and heart failure, nitroglycerin is less effective at vasodilation than nitroprusside and, therefore, is a less attractive option in the setting of acute thoracic AD. Like nitroprusside, it should be used with a β-blocking agent to prevent reflex tachycardia. Its dose range starts at 5-10 μg/min as an infusion and titration can occur by increments of 5-20 μg/min every 3-5 minutes.

Fenoldopam is a dopamine-1 agonist that is a selective arteriolar/renal dilator. It is given in a dosage of 0.1 to 0.3 μg/kg/min. It also produces a reflex tachycardia that must be tempered with a β-blocking agent. It can also produce ECG changes including nonspecific T wave changes and ventricular extrasystoles. Like nitroprusside, mild tolerance with prolonged use has been observed.

Nicardipine is a dihydropyridine calcium channel blocker. It is dosed at 5 to 15 mg per h but has a longer half-life of 1 to 4 h relative to other intravenous antihypertensives. It should also be used in conjunction with a β-blocker to prevent tachycardia.

With respect to the β-blockers used in conjunction with the agents listed above, the ability to turn off all antihypertensive agents in an instant may be critical. Esmolol is a very short-acting intravenous β-blocker that most closely fits this description. It is given as an initial bolus of 500 μg/kg followed by an infusion at 50 to 200 μg/kg/min. Labetelol is an effective, combined α- and β-blocking agent that can be administered as a monotherapy in the treatment of AD. It is administered as intravenous boluses of 20 mg every 5 to 10 min, doubling the dose as necessary, and titrated to the desired heart rate and blood pressure (to a maximum dose of 300 mg). However, labetolol "sticks around" for a lot longer than esmolol and is less titratable. In the patient with unstable vital signs, it may be unwise to give agents that cannot be rapidly "dialed down" in the event of severe hypotension with ongoing hemorrhage or cardiac tamponade.

SUGGESTED READINGS

Blumenfeld JD, Laragh JH. Management of hypertensive crises: The scientific basis for treatment decisions. *Am J Hypertens*. 2001;14:1154–1167.

Hagan PG, Neinaber CA, Isselbacher EM, et al. The International Registry of Acute Aortic Dissection (IRAD): New insights into an old disease. *JAMA*. 2000;283(7):897–903.

Shayne PH, Pitts SR. Severely increased blood pressure in the emergency department. *Ann Emerg Med*. 2003;41:513–529.

44

Do not confuse atrial fibrillation with multifocal atrial tachycardia

ERIC J. HEMMINGER, MD

Atrial fibrillation (AF) and multifocal atrial tachycardia (MFAT) are commonly encountered dysrhythmias in the emergency department (ED). Both are characteristically irregular supraventricular rhythms and both may present with common symptoms such as palpitations and syncope. In susceptible patients with underlying heart disease, either rhythm may provoke angina or heart failure, often secondary to a rapid, uncontrolled ventricular response rate that deprives the ventricles sufficient filling time in a shortened diastole. These two entities differ markedly in their etiology, response to antidysrhythmic drugs and cardioversion, and need for long-term anticoagulation. A summary of these differences is provided in *Table 44.1*.

AF is the most common dysrhythmia encountered in clinical practice, and its incidence is increasing as the population ages. The chaotic fibrillatory activity of the atria and subsequent loss of "atrial kick," is often initiated at ectopic foci which originate from the pulmonary veins. Atrial enlargement as

TABLE 44.1	AF VERSUS MFAT—A SUMMARY OF KEY FEATURES	
	AF	**MFAT**
Diagnosis—key features	Irregular atrial fibrillatory waves usually occurring at a rate of ≥375 BPM	Three or more different P-wave morphologies at different rates in one lead
Initial rate-control choice	β-Blocker or calcium channel blocker	Calcium channel blocker
Response to antidysrhythmics	Generally good	Poor
Response to synchronized cardioversion	Good	Poor
Associated pathology	Structural heart disease Thyroid disease	Pulmonary disease
Thromboembolism risk	Well-established risk	Minimal
Amenable to catheter ablation	Yes	No

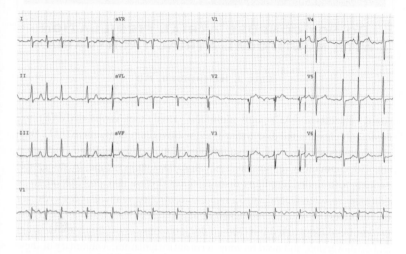

FIGURE 44.1. Atrial fibrillation.

well as underlying disease states such as hyperthyroidism contribute to the dysrhythmogenicity of the atria. Moreover, the presence of AF has an independent association with mortality and heart failure, as well as a well-known risk for thromboembolic events due to stasis of blood flow in the left atrial appendage in particular.

AF can be recognized as the classic "irregularly irregular rhythm," with associated atrial fibrillatory waves. The fibrillatory waves may be course, fine, or barely visible and are often best magnified in lead V1 because of its proximity to the atria. The characteristic feature of fibrillatory waves which differentiate them from more organized atrial events is their *rate*. Electrocardiographic (ECG) atrial events occurring irregularly at a rate of >375 beats per min (which translates to one deflection every 160 ms or four small ECG boxes) are characteristic of AF (*Fig. 44.1*).

MFAT, like AF, is always irregular but less prone to rapid ventricular response. When the ventricular response rate is slower, it is more correctly termed multifocal atrial rhythm. MFAT responds poorly to antidysrhythmic agents and electrical therapy. It is most commonly seen in patients with underlying pulmonary disease, and treatment generally involves therapy for the underlying condition.

MFAT is often mistaken for AF in the ED because both are irregularly irregular supraventricular tachycardias, and AF is overwhelmingly more common. MFAT is characterized by multiple automatic atrial foci which compete with or completely suppress the sinus node as a pacemaker site. By definition, these multifocal atrial foci lead to three or more different P-wave morphologies

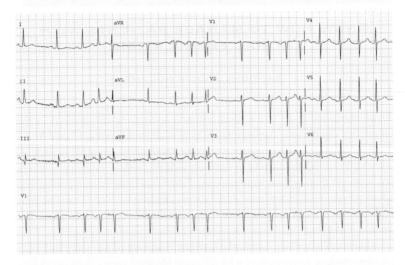

FIGURE 44.2. Multifocal atrial tachycardia.

at different rates in a single ECG lead. As a consequence of the multiform atrial activity, PP, PR, and RR intervals are variable (*Fig. 44.2*). The ventricular rate in MFAT is generally between 100 and 150 beats per min.

SUGGESTED READINGS

Blomström-Lundqvist C, Scheinman MM, Aliot EM, et al. ACC/AHA/ESC guidelines for the management of patients with supraventricular arrhythmias—executive summary. *J Am Coll Card*. 2003;42:1493–1531.

Haissaguerre M, Jais P, Shah DC, et al. Spontaneous initiation of atrial fibrillation by ectopic beats originating in the pulmonary veins. *N Engl J Med*. 1998;339:659–666.

Lloyd-Jones DM, Wang TJ, Leip EP, et al. Lifetime risk for development of atrial fibrillation: The Framingham Heart Study. *Circulation*. 2004;110:1042–1046.

Stewart S, Hart CL, Hole DJ, et al. A population-based study of the long-term risks associated with atrial fibrillation: 20-year follow-up of the Renfrew/Paisley study. *Am J Med*. 2002;113:359–364.

Yurchak PM, Kastor JA, Shine KI. Multifocal atrial tachycardia: Clinical and electrocardiographic features in 32 patients. *N Engl J Med*. 1968;279:344–349.

45

KNOW HOW TO MANAGE PATIENTS WITH ATRIAL FIBRILLATION

SAI-HUNG JOSHUA HUI, MD

Atrial fibrillation (AF) is the most common arrhythmia encountered in the emergency department. Approximately 15% of all strokes in the United States are due to AF. The risk of stroke is increased twofold to sevenfold in patients with AF. Prior ischemic stroke or transient ischemic attack, moderate to severe left ventricle dysfunction, hypertension, diabetes mellitus, female gender, and advanced age are all independent risk factors. The treatment of AF may be generalized into three broad categories: rate control, anticoagulation, and cardioversion. Emergency physicians should be intimately familiar with each.

In clinically stable patients, the first-line treatment of AF with rapid ventricular response is rate control with AV-nodal blocking agents, such as calcium channel blockers, β-blockers, or digoxin. One should always ponder whether tachycardia is due to the underlying AF or due to a secondary cause. The choice of agent depends on physician preference and patient considerations such as underlying comorbidities, contraindications, and potential drug interactions. AV-nodal blockade may cause multiple complications in patients with AF. β-Blockers should be avoided in patients with severe reactive lung disease, as respiratory decompensation can occur. Acute digoxin administration may cause digoxin toxicity in patients with underlying renal insufficiency, hypokalemia, or hypomagnesemia. Digoxin should always be used with caution in patients with chronic renal failure, alcoholism, or on chronic digoxin therapy. Combining agents from different drug classes increases the risk of symptomatic heart block; different classes should only be combined once maximum dosing of one agent fails to achieve successful rate control. Excessive dosing of any of these agents, however, may cause clinical deterioration, particularly in elderly patients or in those with compensatory tachycardia caused by dehydration, blood loss, or sepsis. Finally, AV-nodal blocking agents are contraindicated in the setting of patients with known or suspected Wolf-Parkinson-White syndrome, because of the risk of ventricular fibrillation caused by unimpeded impulse transmission through the accessory pathway.

Cardioversion should only be performed emergently in clinically unstable patients with AF, when the underlying dysrhythmia is considered to be the cause of instability. In this situation, electrical cardioversion is preferred over pharmacologic agents, due to the immediate effect and high success rate. Cardioversion carries a small (1% to 7%) but significant risk of sudden thromboembolism; this risk is highest when the onset of AF is >48 h in duration. According to current guidelines from American College of Cardiology, American Heart Association, and the American College of Chest Physicians, an intravenous heparin bolus should be given immediately prior to or concurrently with cardioversion in noncoagulopathic patients with onset of AF >48 h. In the subset of patients with a clear onset of AF <48 h, cardioversion carries a 0.8% to 0.9% risk of acute stroke; the guidelines are not in agreement regarding anticoagulation in these situations. Unfortunately, studies have consistently shown that these guidelines are not adhered to in the emergency department. It should be noted that even if an echocardiogram demonstrates no evidence of intracardiac thrombus, there is a risk of subsequent thrombus formation after cardioversion. The reason is that the left atrial appendage will undergo a period of stunning with depressed ejection velocity immediately after cardioversion. Therefore, anticoagulation should never be delayed in order to obtain an echocardiogram.

Anticoagulation is indicated in most patients. Unfortunately, heparin is a leading cause of iatrogenic morbidity and mortality. Vigilance is required to avoid potentially devastating bleeding complications. Treatment with low molecular weight heparin is associated with simplified dosing and fewer adverse reactions. In stable patients, the choice of anticoagulation modality should be discussed with either the patient's primary or admitting physician.

SUGGESTED READINGS

Gentile F, Elhendy A, Khandheria BK, et al. Safety of electrical cardioversion in patients with atrial fibrillation. *Mayo Clin Proc*. 2002;77:897–904.

Laguna P, Martín A, del Arco C, et al. Risk factors for stroke and thromboprophylaxis in atrial fibrillation: What happens in daily clinical practice? The GEFAUR-1 study. *Ann Emerg Med*. 2004;44(1):3–11.

Michael JA, Stiell IG, Agarwal S, et al. Cardioversion of paroxysmal atrial fibrillation in the emergency department. *Ann Emerg Med*. 1999;33(4):379–387.

Omran H, Jung W, Rabahieh R, et al. Left atrial chamber and appendage function after internal atrial defibrillation: A prospective and serial transesophageal echocardiographic study. *J Am Coll Cardiol*. 1997;29:131–138.

The Stroke Prevention in Atrial Fibrillation Investigators. Predictors of thromboembolism in atrial fibrillation: II. Echocardiographic features of patients at risk. *Ann Intern Med*. 1992;116:6–12.

Weigner MJ, Caulfield TA, Danias PG. Risk for clinical thromboembolism associated with conversion to sinus rhythm in patients with atrial fibrillation lasting less than 48 hours. *Ann Intern Med*. 1997;126:615–620.

46

Do not confuse Mobitz Type I and Type II Atrioventricular block

Eric J. Hemminger, MD

Atrioventricular block (AVB) has been historically classified as first, second, and third degree in nature. This nomenclature does nothing to highlight the marked differences in etiology, clinical significance, and response to therapy present in this graded description. While first-degree AVB represents delayed conduction through the AV node (not a true block), acquired third-degree AVB represents complete electrical disconnection of the ventricles from the influence of atrial pacemaker activity. The latter should be well recognized by emergency department (ED) physicians as a cardiac emergency requiring stabilization and treatment.

Second-degree AVB by comparison may be physiologically protective and asymptomatic or alternatively highly symptomatic and life-threatening. This seeming dichotomy requires the accurate differentiation of Mobitz I versus Mobitz II type behavior to determine clinical significance. Unfortunately, many physicians fail to discriminate between these two dysrhythmias, perhaps because it is not emphasized in the current American Heart Association protocols.

Mobitz type I AVB, or Wenckebach phenomenon, is the result of decremental conduction at the level of the AV node (*Fig. 46.1*). While this behavior is

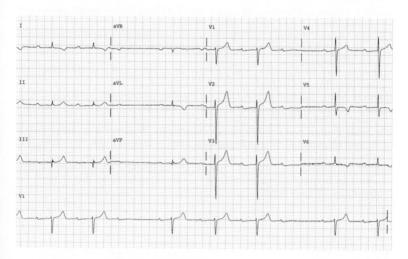

FIGURE 46.1. Mobitz type I AVB.

fairly common, it is rarely symptomatic, or of clinical significance. Wenckebach behavior is generally only pathologic when it occurs at slow atrial rates. In this case, the bradycardia itself may be symptomatic. Mobitz type I AVB is often seen in the setting of an inferior wall myocardial infarction (MI). Treatment with atropine is generally effective, but in an otherwise hemodynamically stable patient, treatment with atropine may worsen ischemia.

Mobitz type I AVB is characterized by a repeating "Wenckebach period," where conduction through the AV node gradually decreases until AV block occurs and the process repeats (*Fig. 46.1*). All of the characteristic ECG features result from this fundamental physiology. It can often be recognized from afar due to the presence of "group beating," that is, a repeat pattern of QRS complexes across the rhythm strip. The following are typical findings in Mobitz type I AVB:

1) Only one beat is dropped in a sequence. Mobitz type I AVB will only rarely result in consecutive dropped beats at very high atrial rates (such as in atrial flutter).
2) The PR interval gradually lengthens with each consecutive beat until a beat is dropped.
3) The RR interval gradually decreases across the Wenckebach cycle, and
4) The RR interval encompassing the dropped beat is less than any two consecutive RR intervals.

Mobitz type II AVB, unlike Wenckebach conduction, results from intermittent conduction failure in the infranodal conduction system (*Fig. 46.2*).

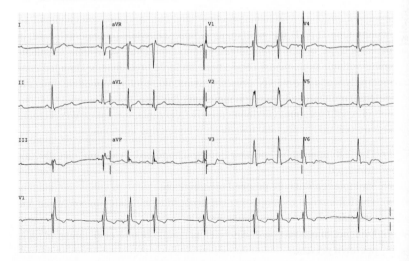

FIGURE 46.2. Mobitz type II AVB. The underlying conduction system disease is evident in the form of a right bundle-branch block.

TABLE 46.1	SUMMARY OF THE KEY FEATURES OF MOBITZ TYPE I AND TYPE II AVB	
	MOBITZ TYPE I	**MOBITZ TYPE II**
Clinical significance	Usually physiologic Usually asymptomatic	Always pathologic Usually symptomatic
Site of AV block	AV node	Infranodal conduction system
Mechanism	Increased vagal tone	Conduction system disease
Pattern	"Group beating"	"Dropped beats"
Dropped beats	Usually single	Multiple consecutive dropped beats possible
PR interval	Prolonged increases with each beat in cycle	Usually normal, constant
RR interval	Shortens with each beat in cycle[a]	Constant[a]
Pause Interval	Always less than the two RR intervals preceding the pause[a]	Compensatory (Pause interval = 2 native RR intervals.)[a]
Response to atropine	Yes	Usually ineffective
Association with other conduction abnormalities	Coincidental	Common
Need for pacemaker	Rarely	Always

[a]May not hold true in the setting of underlying sinus arrhythmia. Not applicable to 2:1 block.

Mobitz type II AVB represents true conduction system disease. It is always pathologic and usually symptomatic. Conduction is an "all or none" phenomenon, without decremental conduction; multiple beats may be dropped consecutively, leading to marked pauses. Pharmacologic interventions are generally ineffective and artificial pacing is indicated (*Table 46.1*).

The ECG features of Mobitz type II AVB contrast those of Wenckebach, and are similarly predictable based on the underlying mechanism:

1) The PR interval is constant in the conducted beats and usually not prolonged.
2) Multiple beats may be dropped consecutively.
3) The RR interval encompassing the dropped beat equals two conducted RR intervals.
4) Evidence of conduction disease such as bundle-branch or fascicular block is not often present.

SUGGESTED READINGS

EEC Committee, et al. American Heart Association guidelines for cardiopulmonary resuscitation and emergency cardiovascular care. *Circulation.* 2005;112(24 Suppl): IV1–203 [Epub 2005 November 28].

Epstein AE, DiMarco JP, Ellenbogen KA, et al. ACC/AHA/HRS 2008 guidelines for device-based therapy of cardiac rhythm abnormalities. *J Am Coll Cardiol.* 2008;51(21):e1–e62.

47

DO NOT CONFUSE ELECTROCARDIOGRAPHIC ARTIFACT FOR DYSRHYTHMIAS

ERIC J. HEMMINGER, MD

The electrocardiogram (ECG) and continuous telemetry monitoring are ubiquitous tools in the emergency department (ED). The ECG often precedes the physical exam when employed as part of a triage protocol to quickly identify life threatening dysrhythmias and ischemia.

Because the ECG is a sensitive instrument that amplifies electrical signals on the order of 1 to 10 mV, it can record electrical artifacts in addition to cardiac electrical activity. The most common artifact recorded on ECG is myoclonic

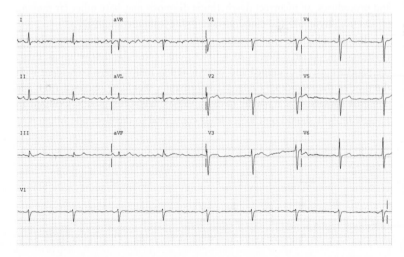

FIGURE 47.1. Tremor artifact mimicking atrial fibrillation. However, P waves are visible and the rhythm is regular.

activity. Parkinson disease, for instance, is particularly prone to cause ECG artifacts as it affects the limbs (the attachment points of the bipolar limb electrodes), causing a resting tremor. The typical parkinsonian tremor of 4 to 6 Hz falls in the very "tachycardic" range of 250 to 300 beats per min. Other common causes of artifact on ECG are interference from other electronic systems or appliances (i.e., intravenous fluid pumps, lithotripsy, etc.) or loose electrodes.

Artifact may render the ECG uninterpretable, leading to a delay in diagnosis and patient care. Secondly, it may lead to the mistaken diagnosis of dysrhthymia. This can be very dangerous. Artifact may be mistaken for both ventricular and atrial dysrhythmias (*Fig 47.1*). It should be difficult to confuse ventricular fibrillation (VF) because VF is a nonperfusing rhythm which leads to pulselessness. Difficulty arises, however, in the case of telemetry monitoring where the "event" may be recorded from afar but not witnessed at the patient's bedside, and the patient is being monitored because he or she has symptoms such as chest pain, syncope, or palpitations.

When artifact is misdiagnosed as a ventricular arrhythmia, it is most often mistaken for ventricular tachycardia (VT). There have been numerous cases where patients have received inappropriate, invasive, and potentially dangerous therapies (including antidysrhythmic drugs, cardiac catheterization, and implantation of internal cardioverter-defibrillators) for ECG artifacts misinterpreted as VT. The majority of these cases involved unwitnessed events on telemetry monitoring. In this scenario, usually only one or two lead tracings are available, which further limits the data available for the physician to make the correct diagnosis. Unsynchronized defibrillation in a patient with a perfusing rhythm may actually induce VF due to an "R-on-T" phenomenon. In addition to unintended therapy and procedures, an incorrect dysrhythmia diagnosis may have other far ranging effects from psychological consequences to life insurance availability.

Besides a high level of scrutiny, there are a few features that may help the emergency physician differentiate artifact from ventricular dysrhythmias. First, the patient must be examined and interviewed as to symptoms coincident with the time of the recording. Collateral information should be obtained from any potential witnesses, if available. Because muscle tremor is usually localized to a single limb, it should only affect leads connected to the electrode which is at

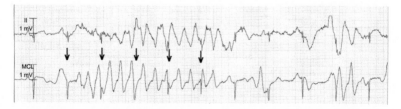

FIGURE 47.2. Two-lead telemetry recording of artifact misdiagnosed as VT. QRS complexes (*arrows*) can be seen "marching through" the artifact.

the site of tremor. A ventricular arrhythmia, in comparison, should generally be visible in all leads. The most important assessment in a case of suspected artifact is the effect on the underlying rhythm. Great scrutiny should be exercised in an attempt to identify potentially obscured QRS complexes which "march through" the background of artifact (*Fig 47.2*). In this exercise, all leads (two leads at a minimum) available to the physician must be examined. The source of artifact should be removed (if possible) and the artifactual recording labeled as such.

SUGGESTED READINGS

Blakeman B, Belusko R, Shah K, et al. Electrocardiographic artifact caused by extracorporeal roller pump. *J Clin Monit*. 1990;6(3):258–259.
Knight BP, Pelosi F, Michaud GF, et al. Clinical consequences of electrocardiographic artifact mimicking ventricular tachycardia. *N Engl J Med*. 1999;341:1270–1274.
Roberts J, Heerdt P, Schiller EC. Life-threatening ECG artifact during extracorporeal shock wave lithotripsy. *Anesthesiology*. 1988;68:477–478.

48

BEWARE OF WOLFF-PARKINSON-WHITE SYNDROME

SAI-HUNG JOSHUA HUI, MD AND
JORGE A. FERNANDEZ, MD, FAAEM, FACEP

Wolf-Parkinson-White (WPW) syndrome is a common cause of ventricular preexcitation and is considered a risk factor for sudden death. Morbidity or mortality may result both directly from underlying dysrhythmias and indirectly from inappropriate treatment. In patients with the WPW syndrome, anomalous embryologic development causes the formation of an accessory atrioventricular (AV) conduction pathway. This accessory pathway does not delay AV conduction like the AV node, so ventricular preexcitation may occur, with the attendant risk of tachydysrhythmia.

The ECG appearance of WPW syndrome is that of a shortened PR interval (<0.12 s) together with a widened QRS complex (>0.10 s) with slurred upstroke. These findings reflect the faster transmission of atrial impulses along the accessory pathway and the slower ventricular depolarization that occurs outside of the His Bundle. However, the ECG may vary from this appearance depending on the distance of the accessory pathway from the AV node. In some cases, WPW may be very difficult to detect based on the surface ECG.

The two most common types of tachydysrhythmia that occur in patients with WPW syndrome are circus movement tachycardia (CMT) and atrial fibrillation (AF). In CMT, there is organized atrial pacemaker activity and regular

QRS complexes. Furthermore, the conduction through the AV node is in the opposite direction of the accessory pathway. In orthodromic CMT, which is the more common subtype, anterograde conduction occurs through the AV node and retrograde conduction occurs through the accessory pathway. Because organized atrial impulses are transmitted through His bundle, a regular, narrow QRS complex is seen. Practically, orthodromic CMT is virtually indistinguishable from paroxysmal supraventricular tachycardia (PSVT) and they can be treated in the same way, with nodal blockade. In antidromic CMT, organized atrial impulses are transmitted anterograde through the accessory pathway and retrograde through the AV node. Ventricular myocytes are depolarized through direct cellular contact rather than through His bundle, so a regular, wide complex QRS is seen. Practically, antidromic CMT is virtually indistinguishable from ventricular tachycardia (VT) and should be treated in the same way, usually with electrical cardioversion. AF is the most dangerous rhythm in patients with WPW syndrome because conduction may bypass the AV node entirely, particularly if AV nodal blocking medications are given. In these cases, extremely rapid atrial rates may be conducted without a refractory period through the accessory pathway, resulting in ventricular fibrillation (VF). Because ventricular depolarization bypasses His bundle, the QRS complex is wide and irregularly irregular in these patients with AF and WPW syndrome.

In general, the safest treatment of wide-complex tachydysrhythmias (antidromic CMT or AF) in patients with WPW syndrome is electrical cardioversion. The American Heart Association also recommends procainamide or amiodarone in these situations; however, there is a paucity of well-controlled studies demonstrating their safety. In fact, there have been numerous case reports documenting poor outcomes when amiodarone has been used to treat AF in patients with WPW syndrome. Because antidromic CMT presents with a wide-complex, regular tachycardia, VT should generally be assumed to be the underlying tachydysrhythmia. Regardless of the underlying cause of wide, regular tachydysrhythmia, synchronized electrical cardioversion is generally safe and effective. When treating orthodromic CMT, which closely resembles PSVT, adenosine is generally accepted as a safe first-line treatment. Longer acting AV-nodal blocking agents should be used with caution: the AV node may be suppressed, favoring transmission through the accessory pathway. Emergency physicians should always carefully analyze a continuous ECG during treatment with adenosine, looking for classic signs of WPW syndrome. If several trials of adenosine fail to convert orthodromic CMT to sinus rhythm, preparations should be made for synchronized electrical cardioversion rather than medical treatment with long acting AV-nodal blocking agents.

From a practical standpoint, emergency physicians should think of WPW syndrome whenever their patients present complaining of palpitations or syncope. Because WPW syndrome is a risk factor for sudden death and for severe iatrogenic complications, it is important to recognize, safely treat, and refer cases to an electrophysiologist for definitive (ablation) therapy. Furthermore, emergency physicians should not hesitate to perform electrical cardioversion in all suspected cases in the setting of a tachydysrhythmia.

SUGGESTED READINGS

AHA. Management of symptomatic bradycardia and tachycardia. *Circulation.* 2005;112:67–77.

Tijunelis MA, Herbert ME. Myth: Intravenous amiodarone is safe in patients with atrial fibrillation and Wolff-Parkinson-White syndrome in the emergency department. *CJEM.* 2005;7(4):262–265.

Yealy D, Delbridge T. Dysrhythmias. In: *Rosen's Emergency Medicine Concepts and Clinical Practice.* 6th ed. Philadelphia, PA: Mosby Elsevier; 2006.

49

NEVER RELY ON THE ELECTROCARDIOGRAM OR CLINICAL INFORMATION TO DISTINGUISH BETWEEN VENTRICULAR TACHYCARDIA AND SUPRAVENTRICULAR TACHYCARDIA WITH ABERRANT CONDUCTION

KIMBALL POON, MD AND AMAL MATTU, MD

The ECG diagnosis of regular, wide-complex tachycardias (RWCT) can be challenging for even the most experienced emergency physicians and cardiologists. The differential diagnosis of the RWCT includes ventricular tachycardia (VT), sinus tachycardia with aberrant conduction (AC), atrial flutter with AC, and supraventricular tachycardia with AC (SVT-AC). Sinus tachycardias with AC and atrial flutter with AC are usually easy to distinguish because of the presence of distinct atrial activity in relation to the QRS complexes on the ECG. However, the distinction between VT and SVT-AC can be very difficult.

If the treating physician is considering the use of AV nodal blocking agents, especially calcium channel blockers, this distinction is critical; these agents, while very effective for SVT-AC, can cause significant hemodynamic compromise and adverse outcomes if administered to patients with VT. On the other hand, the administration of drugs usually used for treatment of VT (e.g., lidocaine, procainamide, amiodarone) to the patient with SVT-AC is considered safe and, in the case of procainamide and amiodarone, often effective. As a result, medical students and resident physicians are classically taught that they should always assume that a RWCT is VT and to treat the rhythm as VT, *not* as SVT-AC. Advance Cardiac Life Support (ACLS) 2000, however, recommends that when physicians are confronted with a RWCT of unknown type, they should "attempt to establish a specific diagnosis" through the use of a 12-lead ECG (p. I-159) and treat accordingly. If the physician concludes that the RWCT is an SVT-AC, traditional medications for SVT may be used. If the physician is incorrect in this determination and the RWCT is actually VT, the results of this treatment can be catastrophic. Given the ACLS recommendation to establish an ECG diagnosis, it is worth evaluating the evidence regarding whether such a determination can be reliably made at all.

Over the past several decades, many electrocardiographers have tried to identify reliable ECG distinctions between VT and SVT-AC. The most famous criteria are from Brugada et al., who in 1991 published a four-step algorithm. The "Brugada" criteria could reportedly distinguish VT from SVT-AC with great accuracy. The algorithm required physicians to evaluate the ECG for (i) absence of an RS complex in all precordial leads, (ii) an RS interval >100 ms in any one precordial lead, (iii) AV dissociation, and (iv) various QRS morphologies in leads V1–2 and V6. The presence of any one of the four criteria was considered diagnostic of VT, whereas the absence of all four criteria ruled out VT in more than 98% of cases—not perfect, but not too bad. Attempts at validating these criteria, however, have been disappointing. Studies by Herbert et al. and Isenhour et al. demonstrated significant problems with interobserver reliability and test accuracy.

In addition to its questionable diagnostic accuracy, the Brugada criteria suffer from being cumbersome; the extensive morphology criteria (step 4) limit convenient application. The Vereckei criteria (2007) are newer, reported to be more accurate, and are the first to incorporate the index of slow conduction. The rationale for this index is that an SVT-AC should still lead to rapid initial activation. In contrast, VT utilizes myocyte to myocyte conduction, hence a slower initial activation. When applied to 450 consecutive cases of RWCT, the Vereckei criteria had significantly better test accuracy than the Brugada criteria; however, these criteria can at times still miss VT. Furthermore, the criteria are cumbersome and have yet to be validated in an ED setting.

So, what is the bottom line for using the ECG to distinguish between VT and SVT-AC? Although the Brugada and Vereckei criteria are useful diagnostic tools, no criteria are foolproof. Failure to diagnose VT can be deadly. If the treating physician incorrectly diagnoses and treats the patient for SVT-AC based on the ECG, there can be disastrous consequences. ACLS 2000's suggestion that the 12-lead ECG and clinical information should be used to "establish a specific diagnosis" is dangerous. Stick with what you learned in medical school and residency: all RWCTs (minus the obvious cases of sinus tachycardia or atrial flutter with AC) should be treated as VT!

SUGGESTED READINGS

American Heart Association. Guidelines for cardiopulmonary resuscitation emergency cardiovascular care. *Circulation*. 2000;102(Suppl I):I–1–I–384.

Brugada P, Brugada J, Mont L, et al. A new approach to the differential diagnosis of a regular tachycardia with a wide QRS complex. *Circulation*. 1991;83(5):1649–1659.

Herbert ME, Votey SR, Morgan MT, et al. Failure to agree on the electrocardiographic diagnosis of ventricular tachycardia. *Ann Emerg Med*. 1996;27(1):35–38.

Isenhour JL, Craig S, Gibbs M, et al. Wide-complex tachycardia: Continued evaluation of diagnostic criteria. *Acad Emerg Med*. 2000;7(7):769–773.

Mattu A. Myths and pitfalls in advanced cardiac life support. www.eMedHome.com, CME article, October 22, 2001. Available at: http://www.emedhome.com/features_archive-detail. cfm?FID = 67.

Vereckei A, Duray G, Szénási G, et al. Application of a new algorithm in the differential diagnosis of wide QRS complex tachycardia. *Eur Heart J*. 2007;28(5):589–600.

50

KNOW THE MIMICS OF VENTRICULAR TACHYCARDIA AND TREAT ACCORDINGLY

CHRISTOPHER MAJOR, MD, FAAEM

In the United States alone, sudden cardiac death occurs approximately 400 thousand times annually. Monomorphic ventricular tachycardia (VT) is thought to precede most events, but up to 20% of patients have alternative etiologies. These include Torsade de Pointes (TDP), hyperkalemia, bypass tracts, toxins, and bundle-branch block.

TDP's incidence and mortality are likely underreported and are unknown. Also known as polymorphic VT, it can be recognized by its ECG presentation of an intermittent bizarre polymorphic appearance. TDP is classically the result of variable repolarization of the myocardium and is typically self-limited; however, it can also deteriorate into ventricular fibrillation. Its causes include the many causes of prolonged QT as well as some non-QT prolonging etiologies. The treatment consists of magnesium to correct the repolarization abnormality and overdrive pacing to nullify it. TDP generally recurs when treated solely with defibrillation. Emergency physicians should suspect medications, low Ca, low Mg, and low K as the cause of most cases of TDP; however, non-QT prolonging causes include ischemia, reperfusion, organic disease, excess catecholamines, and Brugada syndrome.

Another potentially deadly cause of widened QRS is hyperkalemia. In addition to widening of the QRS, hyperkalemia also causes AV nodal blockage, peaked T waves, and P-wave depression and can look very similar to a wide monomorphic VT; in severe cases, it resembles a sine wave. In hyperkalemia, the rate is typically slow and bradycardia might be the most prominent ECG feature. Treatment modalities for hyperkalemia include IV calcium, sodium bicarbonate, insulin and diuretics, nebulized β-agonists, oral sodium polysterene, and hemodialysis.

Bypass tracts, such as Wolff-Parkinson-White (WPW) syndrome, have an incidence up to 3% in the general population and an incidence of sudden death up to 0.6%. Atrial fibrillation in WPW is a very dangerous rhythm. It results in a chaotic irregular, wide complex rhythm. In this setting, synchronized electrical cardioversion is the treatment of choice. Procainamide can also be used in stable patients to decrease impulse transmission along the bypass tract. In the setting of regular, wide complex tachycardia and suspected WPW syndrome, AV nodal blockers can be given safely; however, the administering of these agents in cases of atrial fibrillation with WPW syndrome could be fatal. In sinus rhythm, WPW syndrome may be recognized by a shortened PR interval and δ waves. Because WPW syndrome and other types of bypass tracts are associated with a risk of sudden cardiac death, all cases should be discussed with a cardiologist prior to discharge.

A variety of drugs may widen the QRS. Tricyclic antidepressants widen the QRS and PR intervals. Other sodium channel blockers that may resemble, or cause, monomorphic VT in cases of overdose include cocaine, propranolol, antihistamines, propoxyphene, phenothiazines, chloroquine, quinine, quinindine, procainamide, and disopyramide. Sodium channel blockers generally respond to the high sodium concentration in intravenous sodium bicarbonate. Digoxin may also cause VT, AV block, premature ventricular complexes (PVC's), and other arrhythmias in cases of overdose. Its antidote, digoxin immune Fab (digibind), is generally safe and effective. If the history suggests a toxic cause of widened QRS, bicarbonate or digibind therapy should be strongly considered.

Finally, hemodynamically stable bundle-branch blocks can cause widened QRS intervals. These conduction delays may be a sign of acute pathology, particularly in the setting of other cardiac symptoms. The primary consideration in a new left bundle branch block (LBBB) is myocardial infarction (MI). Cases of MI with acute LBBB fair worse than classic transmural infarctions, and emergent fibrinolysis or percutaneous intervention is indicated in the acute setting. Other causes of LBBB include a pacemaker, cardiomyopathy, structural heart disease, and myocarditis. Right bundle branch block (RBBB) can be caused by pulmonary embolism, right-sided MI, Brugada syndrome, hypertrophic cardiomyopathy and other types of structural heart disease, hypothermia, and certain valvular diseases. Any patient with widened QRS who presents with cardiac symptoms such as syncope, chest pain, or heart failure should be assumed to have underlying cardiac disease.

SUGGESTED READINGS

Darpö B. Spectrum of drugs prolonging QT interval and the incidence of torsades de pointes. *Eur Heart J.* 2001;3(Suppl):K70–K80.

Gupta A, Lawrence AT, Krishnan K, et al. Current concepts in the mechanisms and management of drug-induced QT prolongation and torsade de pointes. *Am Heart J.* 2007;153(6):891–899.

Roden DM. Mechanisms and management of proarrhythmia. *Am J Cardiol.* 1998;82(4A):49I–57I.

51

DO NOT ASSUME ALL PATIENTS WITH ACUTE CORONARY SYNDROMES HAVE CHEST PAIN

SHOMA DESAI, MD

Despite widespread awareness of atypical presentations of myocardial infarction (MI), between 2% and 3% of patients with MI and a similar percentage with non-MI acute coronary syndromes (ACS) are still mistakenly discharged from the emergency department (ED)!

Classically, MI induces retrosternal chest pain, radiating to the neck, shoulder, arms, jaw, and/or epigastrium. The pain is pressure like, burning, squeezing, or heavy and is often associated with shortness of breath, diaphoresis, or nausea.

The American College of Cardiology and the American Heart Association classify high likelihood presentations of ACS to include patients with chest or left arm pain/discomfort reproducing documented angina and a known history of coronary artery disease. Intermediate likelihood presentations include chest or left arm pain/discomfort, age >70 years, male sex, a history of diabetes mellitus, and/or extracardiac vascular disease.

Approximately one quarter to one third of patients with MI have either "silent" or atypical symptoms. Although myocardial ischemia may present asymptomatically or with vague sensations such as weakness or malaise, more common atypical symptoms include dyspnea, presyncope/syncope, diaphoresis, and nausea/vomiting. Brieger et al., using the Global Registry of Acute Coronary Events (GRACE), reported that of 20,881 patients admitted to the hospital with ACS, 8.4% presented without chest pain. The dominant symptom among these patients was dyspnea, which accounted for nearly half. The number of patients presenting with diaphoresis, nausea/vomiting, and presyncope/syncope was 26.2%, 24.3%, and 19.1%, respectively.

One key to accurate diagnosis of patients with atypical presentations of ACS is the identification of particular populations at risk for them. These are well documented in the literature and include women, the elderly (age >70), diabetics, and patients with congestive heart failure.

Delayed diagnosis of ACS in patients without chest pain is correlated with suboptimal medical management. Though these patients are often discovered to have ACS at some point during their hospital stay, they are less likely to receive antiplatelet agents, β-blockers, fibrinolytics, anticoagulants, cardiac catheterization, and statins within 24 h of presentation, as well as throughout their hospital stay. In addition, these patients are less commonly managed in a cardiac care unit or even to receive follow-up with a cardiologist after they are discharged home.

Not surprisingly, missed or delayed diagnosis of ACS is correlated with increased patient morbidity and mortality. Brieger et al. reported a statistically significant increase in the number of complications among atypical patients, including heart failure, dysrhythmias, renal failure, and cardiogenic shock. In fact, mortality rates were 13% in the atypical group as compared with 4.3% in the typical group. Moreover, patients with atypical symptoms tend to be older and have left ventricular failure, potentiating the morbidity associated with ACS.

It is often very difficult to diagnose ACS in patients without chest pain or pressure, and it is simply not possible to achieve a zero percent "miss rate" when it comes to such a common entity. Nonetheless, an awareness of the risk factors and most likely features of these atypical presentations should help reduce the number of patients that are mistakenly sent home from the ED.

SUGGESTED READINGS

Braunwald E, Antman EM, Beasley JW, et al. ACC/AHA guideline update for the management of patients with unstable angina and non–ST-segment elevation myocardial infarction: 2002 summary article. *Circulation.* 2002;106(14):1893–1900.

Brieger D, Eagle KA, Goodman SG, et al. Acute coronary syndromes without chest pain, an underdiagnosed and undertreated high-risk group: Insights from the Global Registry of Acute Coronary Events. *Chest.* 2004;126(2):461–469.

Dorsch MF, Lawrance RA, Sapsford RJ, et al. Poor prognosis of patients presenting with symptomatic myocardial infarction but without chest pain. *Heart.* 2001;86(5):494–498.

52

DO NOT EXCLUDE CARDIAC CAUSES OF CHEST PAIN JUST BECAUSE A PATIENT IS YOUNG

ELISSA SCHECHTER-PERKINS, MD, MPH

During a busy shift, it is easy to underestimate the significance of chest pain (CP) in a young, healthy adult. Dangerous cardiac etiologies of CP in patients under 35 years old include structural heart disease, infection, and atherosclerotic and nonatherosclerotic coronary artery disease (CAD).

Gross structural abnormalities constitute the largest reported etiology of sudden cardiac death (SCD) in young people. Most common is hypertrophic cardiomyopathy (HCM), with a prevalence of 1 in 500 in the general population. Although a subset of patients are symptom free until their death, many people suffering from HCM present with symptoms suggestive of heart failure, including exertional dyspnea and CP. A family history of SCD supports the diagnosis, and auscultation of a murmur in this setting warrants further workup, including an echocardiogram. Other cardiomyopathies, such as dysrhythmogenic right ventricular cardiomyopathy and dilated cardiomyopathy, may also present with CP.

Myocarditis is a potentially lethal cause of CP, involving inflammation of the cardiac tissue. It may be difficult to diagnose because its clinical presentation may be that of a nonspecific viral illness, and CP is not always present. However, when CP is coupled with fever, tachycardia, and respiratory distress, myocarditis should be considered. Chest x-ray (CXR) may show evidence of cardiomegaly or failure, and electrocardiogram (ECG) may reveal ST, T-wave abnormalities, or axis deviation. Though neither CXR nor ECG is particularly sensitive on its own, the use of both together has been found to be sensitive for the detection of myocarditis. Diagnosis is ultimately confirmed by cardiac biopsy.

Nonatherosclerotic etiologies of cardiac ischemia are many in young patients. Cocaine abuse is a widely recognized risk factor for vasospasm and ischemia. There are reports of ischemia resulting from ecstasy (MDMA), methamphetamine, ephedrine and clenbuterol.

Patients with a history of Kawasaki disease (KD) are at increased risk for ACS. Often the history of KD is elusive, either because it was misdiagnosed as a child or long since forgotten. The coronary aneurysms that result from untreated KD lead to calcification and stenosis. In one review, the mean age at presentation of cardiac sequelae was 24.7 years, and symptoms, predominantly CP, occurred during vigorous exercise in 82%.

Another nonatherosclerotic cause of coronary ischemia among young adults is due to congenital coronary artery anomalies. Several anomalies, particularly of the coronary sinus, lead to intermittent obstruction and account for approximately 4% of myocardial infarctions (MIs) in young patients. Although it is unreasonable to expect the EP to make this diagnosis, exertional CP has been noted to precede SCD in these patients and may be sufficient to prompt the EP to pursue further workup and cardiology referral.

Atherosclerotic CAD is a rare but recognized entity in young patients. In the United States, between 4% and 10% of MIs reported occur in patients under the age of 45 years. One prospective study found a 4.7% risk of ACS among patients under age 40 presenting to the ED with CP. Unlike the elderly, young patients with ACS tend to present with classical, rather than atypical symptoms. The task of the EP is to heed those typical symptoms and not dismiss ACS as a possible etiology solely because of the patient's age. Remember that features of patients' acute presentation, not necessarily their age or long-term cardiac risk factors (such as hypertension and cholesterol), determine the likelihood of ACS.

So, what do you need to remember? Be mindful that there are serious cardiac causes of CP in young people. In addition to a careful description of the pain and related symptoms, noting the presence of exertional symptoms, a family history of SCD, a careful exam for a murmur, and a 12-lead ECG and CXR may all assist the EP in picking up one of these important cases.

SUGGESTED READINGS

Burns JC, Shike H, Gordon JB, et al. Sequelae of Kawasaki disease in adolescents and young adults. *J Am Coll Cardiol*. 1996;28(1):253–257.

Choudhury L, Marsh JD. Myocardial infarction in young patients. *Am J Med*. 1999;107(3): 254–261.

Freedman SB, Haladyn JK, Floh A, et al. Pediatric myocarditis: Emergency department clinical findings and diagnostic evaluation. *Pediatrics*. 2007;120(6):1278–1285.

Maron BJ. Hypertrophic cardiomyopathy: A systematic review. *JAMA*. 2002;287(10): 1308–1320.

Schechter E, Hoffman RS, Stajic M, et al. Pulmonary edema and respiratory failure associated with clenbuterol exposure. *Am J Emerg Med*. 2007;25(6):735. e1–3.

Walker NJ, Sites FD, Shofer FS, et al. Characteristics and outcomes of young adults who present to the emergency department with chest pain. *Acad Emerg Med*. 2001;8(7): 703–708.

53

DO NOT FORGET TO CONSIDER "NONTRADITIONAL" RISK FACTORS FOR CORONARY ARTERY DISEASE IN PATIENTS WITH CHEST PAIN

TARLAN HEDAYATI, MD AND JASON GAJARSA, MD

Emergency physicians (EPs) are well versed in "traditional" risk factors for coronary artery disease (CAD) outlined in the Framingham Heart Study, such as hypertension, diabetes, older age, hyperlipidemia, and family history. However, EPs may fail to recognize other "nontraditional" disease processes that are risk factors for coronary ischemia. When a patient presents with symptoms that may represent cardiac ischemia, the presence of these nontraditional risk factors may "tip the balance" and prompt further workup to rule out acute coronary syndromes (ACSs).

HIV AND AIDS

The risk of myocardial infarction (MI) is increased in patients with human immunodeficiency virus (HIV) infection, especially if they are receiving highly active antiretroviral therapy (HAART). Patients with HIV are at higher risk for developing hypertension and dyslipidemia at a young age than the general population, due to effects of the viral infection itself. Additionally, HIV protease inhibitors (PI), the main components of antiviral therapy, cause hyperlipidemia, hyperglycemia, and/or central obesity in up to 60% of patients, thereby increasing cardiovascular risk. In a large study comprised of 26,468 HIV-infected patients, 27% of PI patients developed hyperlipidemia, 27% showed low HDL levels, and 126 patients developed an MI. The incidence of MI increases with longer duration of HAART. While the incidence of MI is relatively low among HIV patients, it is still of clinical significance given the young age of these patients.

KIDNEY DISEASE

Individuals with chronic kidney disease (CKD) are more likely to die of cardiovascular disease (CVD) than to develop renal failure (RF). Patients with CKD have a higher prevalence of arteriosclerosis, left ventricular hypertrophy (LVH), ischemic heart disease, cardiomyopathy, and heart failure as compared to the general population. Additionally, most of the "traditional" risk factors for heart disease, such as diabetes, hyperlipidemia, and LVH are highly prevalent among CKD patients. Furthermore, it appears that as kidney function deteriorates, the risk of CVD and resultant mortality increases. In fact, dialysis patients have a 10 to 30 times higher mortality from CVD when compared to the general population. Therefore, CKD and RF should be considered risk factors for CAD in patients presenting to the ED.

SYSTEMIC LUPUS ERYTHEMATOSUS

Systemic lupus erythematous (SLE) tends to affect premenopausal, young women who are considered a "low-risk" group for CAD. However, the incidence of MI in women aged 35 to 44 years with SLE is 50 times greater than women in age-matched control groups. The mean age of first MI among patients with SLE is 20 years younger than the general population. Significant atherosclerosis and CAD are prevalent among patients with SLE. This premature atherosclerosis may be due to chronic glucocorticoid use, chronic inflammation from SLE, hyperlipidemia (often secondary to glucocorticoid use), coexistent antiphospholipid antibodies, and CKD that results from SLE. To complicate matters, pericarditis, pleuritis, and pulmonary embolism, all of which are relatively common among patients with SLE, can produce symptoms similar to ischemic pain. Therefore, the EP must be cognizant of SLE as an independent risk factor for CAD and evaluate these patients with chest pain in the ED appropriately.

LONG-TERM CORTICOSTEROID USE

Corticosteroids are used successfully in a variety of clinical conditions on a long-term basis, including connective tissue disorders, such as SLE and rheumatoid arthritis, asthma, chronic obstructive pulmonary disease, and transplant recipients. While many of the catastrophic sequelae of these diseases have been curbed by the chronic use of steroids, a relatively large number of these patients go on to suffer cardiovascular events at a higher rate than the general population. Long-term corticosteroid use has been linked to development of hypertension, insulin resistance, hyperlipidemia, obesity, and hypercoagulability, all of which are traditional risk factors for the development of CAD.

SUGGESTED READINGS

Barbaro G, Fisher SD, Giancaspro G, et al. HIV-associated cardiovascular compromise: A new challenge emergency physicians. *Am J Emerg Med*. 2001;19:566–574.

Karrar A, Sequeira W, Block JA. Coronary artery disease in systemic lupus erythematosus: A review of the literature. *Semin Arthritis Rheum*. 2001;30(6):436–443.

Maxwell SR, Moots RJ, Kendall MJ. Corticosteroids: Do they damage the cardiovascular system? *Postgrad Med J*. 1994;70(830):863–870.

Sarnak MJ, Levey AS, Schoolwerth AC, et al. Kidney disease as a risk factor for development of cardiovascular disease: A statement from the American Heart Association councils on kidney in cardiovascular disease, high blood pressure research, clinical cardiology, and epidemiology and prevention. *Hypertension*. 2003;42(5):1050–1065.

Spicker LE, Karadag B, Binggeli C, et al. Rapid progression of atherosclerotic coronary artery disease in patients with human immunodeficiency virus infection. *Heart Vessels*. 2005;20:171–174.

54

DO NOT FORGET ABOUT THE NONCORONARY CAUSES OF ACUTE CHEST PAIN

TARLAN HEDAYATI, MD AND
STUART P. SWADRON, MD, FRCPC

Most emergency physicians (EPs) are extremely vigilant in working up patients with acute chest pain for acute coronary syndromes (ACSs). However, our concern for ACS often leads to "tunnel vision" and a failure to consider other life-threatening causes. Each requires additional imaging studies to confirm, and, because the treatment for each entity is distinct and emergent, each should be considered, if only briefly, in the evaluation and documentation of each case.

AORTIC DISSECTION

Almost all patients with dissection (96%) present with pain. The pain is abrupt in onset in 85% of patients, described as severe/worst ever in 91%, located anteriorly in the chest in 61%, and sharp more often than tearing or ripping. Back pain is reported in about half of all patients. Risk factors for acute aortic dissection (AD) include hypertension, smoking, collagen vascular disease, pregnancy, and inflammatory disorders of the aorta. With retrograde propagation to the coronary vessels, patients may have the electrocardiographic (ECG) findings of an inferior ST elevation myocardial infarction (STEMI). Otherwise, ECG findings in acute AD are nonspecific ST- and T-wave changes.

PULMONARY EMBOLISM

Pulmonary embolism (PE) is the third leading cause of cardiovascular death in North America and is an elusive ED diagnosis. Symptoms include chest pain that may or may not be pleuritic and/or have an abrupt onset, dyspnea, hemoptysis, and syncope. Signs of PE are also nonspecific and include tachypnea, tachycardia, fever, hypoxia, and neck vein distension. Unilateral limb swelling suggests deep vein thrombosis. ECG findings in submassive PE include normal sinus rhythm, sinus tachycardia, and atrial fibrillation or flutter. The classic McGinn–White "S1Q3T3" ECG finding is variably present in 10% to 60% of patients. Other ECG findings such as bundle-branch blocks, p-pulmonale, precordial T-wave inversions, and ST depressions are typically seen with larger PEs but are nonspecific. The only risk factors consistently found in patients with confirmed PE are immobilization, recent surgery, malignancy, and previous thromboembolic disease. Other known risk factors include pregnancy, hormone therapy, and connective tissue disorders.

PNEUMOTHORAX

Pneumothorax is the presence of air in the pleural cavity. Symptoms of pneumothorax include pleuritic chest pain, which is often initially lateral and maximal at onset, and dyspnea. Physical exam findings include tachycardia, tachypnea, hypoxia, decreased breath sounds, and subcutaneous emphysema. Risk factors for developing pneumothorax include chest trauma, previous pneumothorax, Valsalva maneuver, chronic lung disease, acupuncture, and smoking. Although diagnosis of a tension pneumothorax should be clinical, radiographic findings of pneumothorax include a sharp lung edge running parallel to the chest wall, deep lateral costophrenic angle (deep sulcus sign), abdominal quadrant hyperlucency, and/or mediastinal shift. ED ultrasonography is being utilized more frequently in diagnosis with a high sensitivity and specificity.

CARDIAC TAMPONADE

Symptoms of cardiac tamponade are related to the rate at which fluid accumulates in the pericardial sac and the volume of this fluid. Most patients complain of vague chest pain or tightness, dyspnea, or dizziness. Beck's classic triad of chest pain, distended neck veins, and muffled heart tones may not be present if tamponade occurs suddenly and the patient is in a shock state. Pulsus paradoxus, a >10-mm Hg decline in systolic pressure with inspiration, is neither sensitive nor specific for tamponade. ECG findings include decreased voltage or, more rarely, electrical alternans. Tamponade should be suspected in shock patients with recent chest trauma, recent history of percutaneous coronary intervention (PCI), recent cardiac surgery, recent MI resulting in cardiac rupture, or known history of AD. Additionally, a number of disorders can lead to accumulation of pericardial fluid and tamponade including infectious pericarditis, connective tissue disorders, malignancy, and uremia. Cardiac tamponade is readily diagnosed on ED bedside ultrasound.

ESOPHAGEAL RUPTURE

Esophageal rupture typically occurs longitudinally at the left posterolateral aspect of the distal esophagus. Risk factors for esophageal rupture include recent endoscopy, prolonged emesis or retching, increased abdominal pressure due to childbirth, or a history of a caustic burn due to acid or alkali ingestion. Symptoms include pleuritic chest pain worsened with swallowing or neck flexion and dyspnea. Signs include fever, tachycardia, tachypnea, crepitus, and Hamman's crunch. Chest radiographic findings include presence of mediastinal air, subcutaneous air, left pleural effusion, and widened mediastinum. The "V sign of Naclerio," a characteristic x-ray finding, reflects the presence of air along the left border of the aorta and the left diaphragm, forming a "V."

SUGGESTED READINGS

Hagan PG, Nienaber CA, Isselbacher EM, et al. The International Registry of Acute Aortic Dissection (IRAD): New insights into an old disease. *JAMA*. 2000;283(7):897–903.

Hedayati T, Swadron S. The electrocardiogram in selected non-cardiac conditions. In: Mattu A, Barish RA, Tabas JA, eds. *Electrocardiography in Emergency Medicine*. Dallas, TX: American College of Emergency Physicians; 2007:203–221.

Hirata K, Kyushima M, Asato H. Electrocardiographic abnormalities in patients with acute aortic dissection. *Am J of Cardiol*. 1995;76:1207–1212.

Holt BD. Pericardial disease and pericardial tamponade. *Crit Care Med*. 2007;35:S355–S364.

Konstantinides S. Clinical practice: Acute pulmonary embolism. *N Engl J Med*. 2008; 359(26):2804–2813.

Leigh-Smith S, Harris T. Tension pneumothorax-time for a rethink? *Emerg Med J*. 2005; 1:8–16.

Wu JT, Mattox KL, Wall MJ Jr. Esophageal perforation: New perspectives and treatment paradigms. *J Trauma*. 2007;63(5):1173–1184.

55

Beware attributing chest pain to "anxiety" in all patients with recent emotional events

Atman P. Shah, MD, FACC, FSCAI and Jason Gajarsa, MD

Women having a myocardial infarction (MI) tend to present with atypical symptoms (such as nausea, dizziness, and anxiety) more often than men. Moreover, a woman who presents with both anxiety and chest pain is often treated less aggressively than a man with the same risk factors. Furthermore, data show that women under the age of 65 years have a higher mortality after their MI than men of the same age. Chest pain triggered by anxiety or stress should not be immediately treated with antianxiolytics alone; rather, the patient should be thoroughly evaluated for more life-threatening causes of chest pain.

Stressful or exciting circumstances have been shown to trigger MIs. Any severe emotional event ranging from grief at a funeral to anger in traffic can be responsible. A recent study revealed that German males watching the German football team play during the 2006 World Cup doubled their risk of having an acute coronary syndrome (ACS). Additionally, war and earthquakes can trigger emotional responses leading to increased incidence of MIs. Acute emotional duress leads to elevated catecholamine levels which in turn can increase platelet aggregation and cause an unstable intracoronary plaque to rupture.

One well-described syndrome linking emotional events to ACS is the Takotsubo syndrome. Patients with Takotsubo syndrome present with chest pain in the setting of a recent emotional event and have an electrocardiogram (ECG) that is diagnostic for an acute anterior MI (*Fig. 55.1*). Two-dimensional echocardiography will reveal anterior wall hypokinesis, and serum cardiac biomarkers are elevated. However, unlike patients with typical ST segment elevation myocardial infarction (STEMI), patients with Takotsubo syndrome will have coronary angiograms without a culprit lesion. The *sine qua non* of the syndrome is the appearance of the left ventricle "ballooning" seen during the left ventriculogram. This "ballooning" feature of the left ventricle is said to be similar to the type of pots that Japanese fisherman use to catch octopi; thus, the name *takotsubo* (*tako* = octopus and *tsubo* = pot).

Fortunately, the vast majority of patients with the Takotsubo syndrome will normalize their ECG and their left ventricular function within 3 months. The patient should be aggressively managed at the time of his or her clinical presentation according to Advanced Cardiac Life Support (ACLS) guidelines, with aspirin, a β-blocker, an ace inhibitor, clopidogrel, and a statin, as indicated.

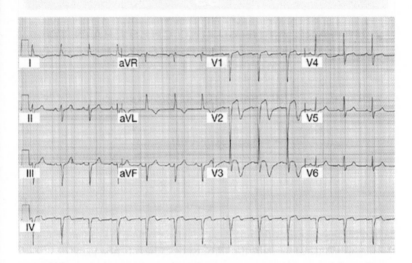

FIGURE 55.1. Twelve-lead ECG of a 56-year-old female presenting with chest pain after attending the funeral of her husband.

If such a patient presents to a hospital without a cardiac catheterization laboratory, the emergency physician will likely have to administer fibrinolytic therapy because the syndrome is indistinguishable from an acute anterior MI on the ECG.

In conclusion, patients presenting with complaints of chest pain in the setting of recent emotional stress should be evaluated within the context of all of their clinical features and risk factors. Physicians should not let their guard down for detecting ACS, even in the face of a clearly stressful emotional event.

SUGGESTED READINGS

Meisel SR, Dayan KI, Pauzner H, et al. Effect of Iraqi Missile War on the incidence of sudden cardiac death in civilians. *Lancet.* 2003;3338:660–661.

Metzl MD, Altman EJ, Spevack DM, et al. A case of Takotsubo cardiomyopathy mimicking an acute coronary syndrome. *Nat Clin Pract Cardiovasc Med.* 2006;3(1):53–56.

Ogawa K, Tsuji I, Shiono K, et al. Increased acute myocardial infarction mortality following the 1995 Great Hanshin-Awaji earthquake in Japan. *Int J Epid.* 2000;29(3):449–455.

Tsuchihashi K, Ueshima K, Uchida T, et al. Transient left ventricular apical ballooning without coronary artery stenosis: A novel heart syndrome mimicking acute myocardial infarction. *J Am Coll Cardiol.* 2001;38(1):11–18.

Vaccarino V, Parsons L, Every N, et al. Sex-based differences in early mortality after myocardial infarction. National Registry of Myocardial Infarction 2 Participants. *NEJM.* 1999;341:217–225.

Wilbert-Lampen U, Leistner D, Greven S, et al. Cardiovascular events during World Cup Soccer. *N Engl J Med.* 2008;358(5):475–483.

Wittstein IS, Thiemann DR, Lima JA, et al. Neurohumoral features of myocardial stunning due to emotional stress. *N Engl J Med.* 2005;352(6):539–548.

56

NEVER RELY ON A SINGLE NEGATIVE OR INDETERMINATE TROPONIN TO RULE OUT ACUTE CORONARY SYNDROMES

JAMES DE LA TORRE, MD, MMM AND
STUART P. SWADRON, MD, FRCPC

Chest pain (CP) accounts for 6 million emergency department (ED) visits annually in the United States. Although missed diagnosis of acute myocardial infarction (AMI) has become less common, it remains an expensive source of malpractice suits filed against emergency physicians (EPs). Missed cases of unstable angina (UA), which may lead to MI and death, remain frustratingly common.

It has become commonplace to order an electrocardiogram (ECG), chest radiograph, and a serum troponin level on every patient presenting to the ED with CP. In fact, this is done in some cases by triage protocol before a physician even sees the patient. However, this reflexive ordering is not without risk.

Cardiac troponin T and I are released into circulation upon ischemic insult to myocardium. During AMI, troponin begins to rise within approximately 6 h and elevated levels are detectable for up to 2 weeks. Troponins are an important tool in evaluating and stratifying patients (both with and without CP) and have important implications with respect to mortality. Although assays differ, troponins have a well-defined range of sensitivity and specificity. *Table 56.1* summarized from Balk et al.'s recent review summarizes the test characteristics of troponin T and I on initial presentation of CP and with serial measurements. Many studies have demonstrated the prognostic utility of detectable troponin levels upon presentation. One *NEJM* study demonstrated that 30-day mortality was significantly higher in patients presenting with AMI and a detectable troponin level. However, an undetectable troponin level does not rule out AMI. Troponin levels may take as many as 6 to 9 h to become detectable and sensitivity does

TABLE 56.1	TEST CHARACTERISTICS OF TROPONIN T AND I ON INITIAL PRESENTATION OF CP AND WITH SERIAL MEASUREMENTS			
	AT PRESENTATION		**SERIAL**	
TEST	**SENSITIVITY**	**SPECIFICITY**	**SENSITIVITY**	**SPECIFICITY**
Troponin I	39 (10–78)	93 (88–97)	90–100	83–96
Troponin T	44 (32–56)	92 (88–95)	93 (85–97)	85 (76–91)

not approach 100% until 12 h post cardiac event. Therefore, an early negative troponin (e.g., <6 h after symptom onset) necessitates a repeat troponin. The precise timing of the second troponin is currently the subject of much debate, and this may depend, in part, on the sensitivity of the specific assay used. Although some authors have suggested that two negative troponins separated by 2 h may be sufficient to rule out MI, others believe that longer intervals are necessary.

Many clinicians use the duration of CP to justify a single troponin "rule out." For example, one might conclude that a single troponin rules out MI in patients in whom CP is >9 or more hours duration. However, it is also important to consider the nature of the symptoms. Ischemic CP may represent a number of different entities, ranging from stable angina to AMI. It may be difficult to distinguish at what point in time UA has become an AMI. For example, 12 h of CP may actually represent 11 h of UA and an MI that began in the past hour. Therefore, in most cases of CP, one troponin leads to another. A large study conducted in 12 American and Canadian EDs demonstrated that using CP duration alone as a criterion for obtaining a single cardiac marker will, in fact, result in missed AMIs.

UA is usually defined as new-onset angina, an increase in the frequency and/or duration of angina, or angina at rest. UA throws a bit of a wrinkle into algorithms for ruling out an ischemic source of CP because it only sometimes results in an elevation of cardiac biomarkers. Even with serial troponins, the sensitivity for UA is only 36%. This may be because ischemia that is sufficient to cause CP or discomfort may not be sufficient to compromise membrane integrity and result in troponin leak. Thus, even with serial negative troponins, there is truly no substitute for obtaining and documenting as accurate a history as possible. UA can be every bit as life threatening as AMI, and current AHA/ACC guidelines for the management of UA share many similarities with those for non-ST elevation MI.

With regard to indeterminate range troponins, it is common for the EP to be told by an internist, "a troponin in the indeterminate range is negative for ACS." However, this statement can be misleading and may result in poor outcomes for patients. The troponin is a single data point. One cannot predict in what direction the troponin will trend. Several studies have shown that patients presenting with indeterminate range troponins have a higher likelihood for adverse events, including AMI and need for invasive cardiac procedures.

So, what is the bottom line? A single troponin does not rule out acute coronary syndrome (ACS). If the decision to use biomarkers to evaluate a patient for MI is made, then at least two troponins spaced in time should be done. Secondly, UA may or may not be accompanied by a detectable troponin leak—go with the total clinical picture. Finally, indeterminate range troponins are misleading and a repeat troponin should be performed to ensure that the level is not rising.

SUGGESTED READINGS

Balk EM, Ioannidis JP, Salem D, et al. Accuracy of biomarkers to diagnose acute cardiac ischemia in the emergency department: A meta-analysis. *Ann Emerg Med.* 2001;37(5):478–494.

Innes G, Christenson J, Weaver WD, et al. Diagnostic parameters of CK-MB and myoglobin related to chest pain duration. *CJEM*. 2002;4(5):322–330.

Kane D, Karras D. Serum markers in the emergency department diagnosis of acute myocardial infarction. *Emerg Med Clin North Am*. 2001;19(2):321–337.

57

DO NOT IGNORE POSITIVE TROPONINS IN A RENAL FAILURE PATIENT

KHAWAR M. GUL, MD

Cardiac troponins (cTn) are well established as specific biomarkers for myocyte injury in the setting of acute coronary syndromes (ACS). In the absence of a major, clinically evident cardiac injury, troponins (cTns) are also found to be elevated in several clinical conditions including renal failure (RF). The 2000 consensus document, updated in 2007 by the American College of Cardiology, American Heart Association, and the European Society of Cardiology, re-defined myocardial infarction (MI). Based on this definition, the measurement of cTn became the new reference standard for diagnosing myocardial injury, replacing creatine kinase-MB (CK-MB).

Research has now demonstrated elevations of cTn in many patients with a large number of acute and chronic conditions or diseases, including pulmonary embolism, perimyocarditis, heart failure, septic shock, chronic obstructive pulmonary disease (COPD), postelectrical cardioversion, and, most notably, chronic RF. Consequently, the interpretation of an elevated cTn level may be challenging.

On one hand, the levels of cardiac biomarkers, including CK, its MB fraction (CK-MB), myoglobin, and cTn are commonly found to be elevated in patients with RF, even in the absence of clinically suspected myocardial ischemia. On the other hand, cardiovascular disease is the most common cause of death in these patients. This clinical quandary should be addressed in a stepwise manner.

The first step is to determine which biomarker is elevated. Elevation of cTn T (cTnT) is seen more frequently than cTn I (cTnI). Both cardiac cTnT and cTnI are specific to heart muscle. However, the first generation of assays used to detect cTnT, cross-reacted with skeletal muscle cTnT. Studies done in patients with RF using the first-generation cTnT assays showed elevations of cTnT in over 70% of patients as compared to only 7% of patients with cTnI elevations. The newer generation assays of cTnT are more cardiac muscle specific but still show elevations in over 50% of patients with no clinical evidence of acute ischemia. This has prompted some to believe that cTnI may be a better cardiac biomarker to assess myocardial necrosis in patients with RF.

The next step is to determine whether the elevation is actually due to myocardial necrosis, and this is not easy. Although various clinical trials have shown the importance of cTn in diagnosis, risk stratification, and treatment of ischemia, most of these trials have excluded patients with renal insufficiency. Additionally, patients with RF presenting with ACS may have atypical presentations. To make matters even more difficult for the clinician, electrocardiogram (ECGs) in patients with RF may be difficult to interpret because of electrolyte disturbances, conduction abnormalities, or left ventricular hypertrophy (LVH).

In patients with suspected ACS, elevation of cTn is associated with adverse outcomes regardless of the degree of renal insufficiency. A recent analysis of 7,033 patients from the GUSTO-IV ACS trial found that the prognostic value of cardiac cTnT was not diminished in patients presenting with renal insufficiency and suspected ACS. These patients should be risk stratified per ACS protocols and should be given β-blockers, antiplatelet therapy, nitroglycerine, and oxygen. Use of antithrombins and glycoprotein IIb/IIIa inhibitors is unclear. Early coronary angiography should be individualized.

Multiple studies have shown the prognostic power of cTn in the setting of renal insufficiency in general. Significant differences in the overall one-year survival was noted for patients with end-stage renal disease (ESRD) and serum cTnT >0.1 ng/mL. Westphal et al. showed that cTnT >0.1 ng/mL was strongly associated with all-cause mortality and cTnT >0.05 ng/mL was associated with fatal cardiovascular disease events. This association was independent of baseline presence of heart disease. All patients with nondetectable cTnT were alive at follow-up. Results from these large trials have shown that cTnT may prove to be a marker of subclinical myocyte damage in patients with RF, either from clinically silent myocardial necrosis or from, perhaps, unrecognized heart failure.

Although the etiology of elevated cTn in RF patients with relatively low suspicion of myocardial ischemia is unclear, it is a reliable biomarker to predict both short- and long-term outcomes, and hence, therapy and disposition decisions in the emergency department. This elevation may reflect subclinical myocardial injury or microinfarcts even in the absence of symptoms. Hence, the ED physician should not dismiss elevated cTn in a RF patient.

SUGGESTED READINGS

Aviles RJ, Askari AT, Lindahl B, et al. Troponin T levels in patients with acute coronary syndromes, with or without renal dysfunction. *N Engl J Med.* 2002;346(26):2047–2052.

Dierkes J, Domröse U, Westphal S, et al. Cardiac troponin T predicts mortality in patients with end-stage renal disease. *Circulation.* 2000;102(16):1964–1969.

Freda BJ, Tang WH, Van Lente F, et al. Cardiac troponins in renal insufficiency: Review and clinical implications. *J Am Coll Cardiol.* 2002;40(12):2065–2071.

Thygesen K, Alpert JS, White HD, et al. Universal definition of myocardial infarction. *J Am Coll Cardiol.* 2007;50(22):2173–2195.

58

DO NOT ASSUME THAT A "NEGATIVE" RECENT ANGIOGRAM DEFINITIVELY RULES OUT ACUTE CORONARY SYNDROME

Atman P. Shah, MD, FACC, FSCAI

Coronary arteriography remains the gold standard for the diagnosis of coronary artery disease. This procedure, performed over one million times each year in the United States, involves the injection of contrast material into the coronary arteries. Using fluoroscopy, stenoses in the coronary arteries are observed. Stenoses >70% of the luminal diameter of the artery usually result in a referral for percutaneous coronary intervention.

In the normal, nonatherosclerotic heart, flow to the myocardium is predominantly regulated by the coronary arterioles, which dilate and constrict as needed. However, as stenoses advance in the epicardial coronary arteries, the arterioles remain constantly dilated to provide flow to the myocardium. In general, once there is a >70% stenosis in an epicardial vessel, arteriolar dilation is no longer able to accommodate for the decrease in flow, and the patient will begin to experience ischemic chest pain with activity. Once the lesion approaches 90% in severity, the patient will begin to suffer ischemic chest pain at rest. The physiologic significance of the 70% lesion was established by Klocke and continues to be the benchmark at which angioplasty is performed.

However, lesions in the epicardial coronary artery may also vary in severity. Lesion severity is calculated by one of two methods. The first, and most commonly used, relies on the cardiologist's estimation of the lesion severity. He or she will visually compare the diameter of the vessel at the location of the tightest stenosis with the diameter of the vessel that is thought to be angiographically normal. The second method to estimate lesion severity is the more objective quantitative coronary angiography (QCA). QCA relies on a computer to analyze and compare the diseased segment to a reference segment to assess the lesion severity. Several studies note that cardiologists routinely overestimate lesion severity compared to QCA.

All appreciable lesions are routinely described in the details of the cardiac catheterization report. However, if there are no epicardial lesions greater than 70%, the procedure may be described "nonobstructive," or even "normal." This can be quite problematic when, for example, a 56-year-old hypertensive male presents to an emergency department with complaints of chest pain and a "negative" recent angiogram. With the history of a recent "negative" angiogram, the emergency physician may dismiss coronary artery disease as a possible etiology of chest pain. This can prove problematic for the following reasons.

First, it is critical to know the time that has elapsed between patient presentation and the angiogram. An angiogram that was negative a few years ago may not be negative now. Studies have shown that lesions can progress in severity by 10% to 20% a year and even faster in diabetics. Also, a patient who presents with chest pain in the 2 weeks following an angiogram must be assessed for a procedural complication such as catheter-induced dissection, which may mimic or precipitate an acute coronary syndrome.

Secondly, the coronary angiogram focuses primarily on stenoses of the large epicardial coronary vessels. Small branches of the epicardial vessels, particularly those < 1.5 mm in diameter, may not be routinely described in reports, as management of lesions in these vessels is purely medical. The microvasculature, principally affected in patients with diabetes, is not visualized at all.

Thirdly, a negative coronary angiogram does not rule out coronary vasospasm as the etiology of the chest pain.

Finally, and most importantly, most ST segment elevation myocardial infarctions result from the rupture of a plaque that occludes far less than a 70% stenosis, typically a 50% lesion, which may have been described as non–flow limiting at the time of the coronary angiogram. It is the nature of the individual plaque, and not the degree of stenosis that results, that determines its likelihood of precipitating an acute coronary syndrome.

In conclusion, the patient who presents with chest pain and a recent "negative" angiogram deserves a more careful look. The patient should be evaluated in the context of the specific details of his or her coronary angiogram and in some cases may need urgent or emergent intervention.

SUGGESTED READINGS

Ambrose JA, Tannenbaum MA, Alexopoulos D, et al. Angiographic progression of coronary artery disease and the development of myocardial infarction. *JACC.* 1988;12:56–62.

Fischer JJ, Samady H, McPherson J, et al. Comparison between visual assessment and quantitative angiography versus fractional flow reserve for native coronary narrowings of moderate severity. *Am J Cardiol.* 2002;90:210–215.

Glaser R, Selzer F, Faxon DP, et al. Clinical progression of incidental, asymptomatic lesions discovered during culprit vessel coronary intervention. *Circulation.* 2005;111(2):143–149.

Klocke FJ. Measurements of coronary blood flow and degree of stenosis: Current clinical implications and continuing uncertainties. *JACC.* 1983;1:31–41.

Sun H, Mori M, Shimokawa H, et al. Coronary microvascular spasm causes myocardial ischemia in patients with vasospastic angina. *JACC.* 2002;39(5):847–851.

59

NEVER ASSUME THAT A RECENT NEGATIVE STRESS TEST DEFINITIVELY RULES OUT ACUTE CORONARY SYNDROME

JAMES DE LA TORRE, MD, MMM
AND STUART P. SWADRON, MD, FRCPC

Many patients who present to the emergency department (ED) have already seen a physician for their chest pain (CP). Many have also had some form of provocative cardiovascular testing, an exercise electrocardiography stress test (EST), nuclear imaging, stress echocardiography, or even cardiac catheterization. There are pitfalls in relying too heavily on previous stress testing, and it is very important to know the limitations of this information.

Exercise electrocardiographic stress testing is common in the evaluation of low-risk patients presenting with CP and as an initial noninvasive strategy for evaluating CP after an appropriate evaluation to rule out acute myocardial infarction (AMI). ESTs use various protocols but share in common a methodology: an attempt to induce and measure cardiac ischemia. Sensitivity and specificity for ESTs are in the range of 68% and 77%, respectively, for single-vessel CAD. These numbers vary in each study, largely due to differences in the patient population being studied. Sensitivity and specificity also increase in the presence of multivessel disease. The prognosis for patients with a "negative EST" is reported to be good with 4-year survival rates as high as 98% to 99%.

A logical extension of the EST is exercise or pharmacological stress nuclear imaging. There are now a variety of different protocols to image the heart using different radiotracers, both at rest and during exercise, in an attempt to unmask ischemia. Resting and exercise images are then compared to define nonperfusing areas of myocardium, reversible perfusion defects, and normal perfusion. *Table 59.1* summarizes the sensitivities and specificities of the most common methods of nuclear cardiac imaging.

A highly positive nuclear study (one demonstrating large reversible perfusion defects) has been shown to predict a high annual event rate (death or MI) of 6% or greater. Patients with known CAD, diabetes mellitus, or a mildly abnormal nuclear study have event rate of 1% to 2% per year. However, a negative or normal cardiac nuclear imaging has a good prognosis with a <1% event rates per year.

Echocardiography can be used to detect wall motion abnormalities, which have been shown to correlate to areas of CAD. In isolation, echocardiography has an unacceptable high false-negative rate for ACS. Stress echocardiography,

TABLE 59.1	SENSITIVITIES AND SPECIFICITIES OF THE MOST COMMON METHODS OF NUCLEAR CARDIAC IMAGING		
		SENSITIVITY (%)	SPECIFICITY (%)
Exercise (treadmill)	Thallium	60–82	65–82
	Tc-99 Sestamibi	82–97	36–90
Adenosine or dipyridamole	Thallium	77–92	75–100
	Tc-99 Sestamibi	81–90	67–72
Dobutamine	Thallium	86–100	36–100
	Tc-99 Sestamibi	80–95	72–80

however, has demonstrated similar test characteristics to nuclear stress testing. The choice of one modality over another is usually a matter of what is available to the ordering clinician.

All forms of cardiac stress testing are designed to detect fixed coronary stenoses, not necessarily in patients at risk for ACS. Unfortunately, ACS frequently arises from unstable lesions that develop in plaques that cause a stenosis of 50% or less of the coronary lumen (so-called nonobstructive lesions). Although a negative stress test does statistically decrease the likelihood that a given patient will have an adverse event in the future, it does not directly assess for or predict the precursor to MI, which is an unstable intracoronary plaque.

Cardiac catheterization is ultimately the gold standard for the diagnosis of flow-limiting cardiovascular disease. So what if a patient with CP, who recently just had a cardiac catheterization, presents to the ED with CP—what risk stratification and prognostic information can the ED physician garner from a negative study or a minimally abnormal one? Recent studies from Italy and the United States have shown a completely normal coronary angiogram to portend an excellent prognosis with a negligible mortality at 10 years. However, other studies have found that a completely normal angiogram only had an event-free rate of 75% and a survival rate of 95% at 3 years. Patients who were at higher risk of events (defined as death, stroke, or reinfarction) were also more likely to be older, have diabetes or depressed ejection fractions. Other studies have suggested coagulopathies, cocaine abuse, and collagen vascular disease were present in MI with normal coronaries. These studies demonstrate that even with a completely normal coronary angiogram, there is still risk for MI.

So, what is the bottom line? When evaluating patients for ACS or AMI, do not rely too heavily on previous negative stress tests. Even a normal cardiac catheterization has its limitations.

SUGGESTED READINGS

Galzio PG, Orzan F, Ferrero PG, et al. Myocardial infarction with normal coronary arteries: Ten-year follow-up. *Ital Heart J.* 2004;5(10):732–738.

Ioannidis JP, Salem D, Chew PW, et al. Accuracy of imaging technologies in the diagnosis of acute cardiac ischemia in the emergency department: A meta-analysis. *Ann Emerg Med.* 2001;37(5):471–477.

Selker HP, Zalenski RJ, Antman EM, et al. ECG exercise stress test. *Ann Emerg Med.* 1997;29(1):33–38.

Terefe YG, Niraj A, Pradhan J, et al. Myocardial infarction with angiographically normal coronary arteries in the contemporary era. *Coron Artery Dis.* 2007;18(8):621–626.

60

REMEMBER TO OBTAIN A RIGHT-SIDED ELECTROCARDIOGRAM IN A PATIENT WITH AN INFERIOR MYOCARDIAL INFARCTION

EMILY A. CARPENTER ROSE, MD

The therapeutic challenge of right ventricular infarction (RVI) associated with inferior myocardial infarction (MI) was first described by Cohn and colleagues in 1974. Until that time, little attention had been given to the role of the right ventricle (RV) in the treatment of MI. Since that first description, much discussion has occurred regarding the importance of early recognition of RVI, as it is associated with increased morbidity and mortality, and often requires unique management.

RVI occurs in up to 50% of inferior MIs, but only about 10% of RVIs are of hemodynamic significance and so often go unrecognized. The vast majority of RVIs are due to right coronary artery (RCA) occlusion, but some emanate the left anterior descending (LAD) artery. Multiple studies have underscored the importance of diagnosing a right-sided infarction as it is a risk factor in itself for increased morbidity and mortality of inferior MIs. More specifically, RVI is associated with an increased incidence of cardiogenic shock, ventricular tachycardia, AV nodal blockade, and death.

In 2004, the American College of Cardiology/American Heart Association (ACC/AHA) task force guidelines recommended obtaining a right-sided ECG in any patient with evidence of inferior wall infarct or ischemia. ST segment elevation (STE) in lead III > II in inferior MIs is suggestive of RV involvement. The right-sided leads to examine include V3R, V4R, V5R, and V6R. The presence of STE of 1 mm or more in any one or combination of these leads in patients with a clinical picture of acute MI is highly sensitive and specific for the diagnosis of RVI, with lead V4R being the most sensitive. Furthermore, attention to the T wave can also help distinguish if the RCA occlusion is a proximal lesion. Patients with proximal occlusion of the RCA have STE of ≥1 mm and a positive T wave in lead V4R. Proximal RCA lesions are important to recognize because these patients are at increased risk for atrioventricular blocks.

At times, STE in leads V1 to V4 caused by RV infarction can be confused with an anteroseptal infarction. The medial RV free wall occupies an anterior location, and thus RVI may also produce anterior lead STE. Typically, this occurs in lead V1 but may occur across the anterior precordial leads resulting in "pseudoanteroseptal" MI. In a patient with STE in leads II, III, and aVF (inferior) and V1 to V5 (anterior), the differential includes either a large LAD lesion or a proximal RCA lesion with concomitant inferior and RV infarcts. Both are of concern, but their initial management and likely complications differ.

The importance of obtaining a right-sided ECG in the emergency department is underscored by the fact that the STE that occurs in lead V4R is often transient. Braat and colleagues found that precordial STE disappeared within 10 h after the onset of chest pain in half of patients with right ventricular involvement.

SUGGESTED READINGS

Braat SH, Brugada P, de Zwaan C, et al. Value of electrocardiogram in diagnosing right ventricular involvement in patients with an acute inferior wall myocardial infarction. *Heart.* 1983;49:368–372.

Greyson CR. Pathophysiology of right ventricular failure. *Crit Care Med* 2008;36:S57–S65.

Levin T. Right ventricular myocardial infarction. UpToDate.com 2008.

Libby P, Bonow RO, Zipes DP, et al., eds. *Braunwald's Heart Disease: A Textbook of Cardiovascular Medicine.* 8th ed. Philadelphia: Saunders; 2008.

Saw J, Davies C, Fung A, et al. Value of ST elevation in lead III greater than lead II in inferior wall acute myocardial infarction for predicting in-hospital mortality and diagnosing right ventricular infarction. *Am J Cardiol.* 2001;87(4):448–450, A6.

Smith SW, Heegaard W, Bachour FA, et al. Acute myocardial infarction with left bundle-branch block: Disproportional anterior ST elevation due to right ventricular myocardial infarction in the presence of left bundle-branch block. *Am J Em Med.* 2008;26:342–347.

Wellens HJJ. The value of the right precordial leads of the electrocardiogram. *N Eng J Med.* 1999;340:381–383.

61

DO NOT FORGET TO APPROPRIATELY MANAGE RIGHT VENTRICULAR ISCHEMIA IN INFERIOR MYOCARDIAL INFARCTION

EMILY A. CARPENTER ROSE, MD

Right ventricular (RV) ischemia in the setting of inferior myocardial infarction (MI) is an independent predictor of mortality. More importantly, RV ischemia and infarction require special management.

The RV is a thin-walled volume pump that directs blood into the lower resistance pulmonary circulation. When ischemic, the RV becomes stiff, dilated, and volume dependent, resulting in reduced filling and diminished right-sided stroke volume. These changes are ultimately transmitted to the left side, with decreased left ventricular (LV) filling and a fall in cardiac output.

RV infarction (RVI) can present similarly to cardiac tamponade or massive pulmonary embolism, with hypotension, jugular venous distension, and clear lung fields. However, hemodynamic compromise develops in only half of all RVIs. Proximal lesions result in larger infarcts and often affect the atrial function, with depressed right atrial contractility, impaired RV filling and performance, and resultant severe hemodynamic compromise. RVIs are associated with an increased risk of atrioventricular (AV) nodal ischemia and blockade, but bradycardia and hypotension are common even with intact AV node function.

Other associated complications of RVI include tachydysrhythmias and ventricular septal rupture. Also, severe right heart dilation and diastolic pressure elevation may stretch a patent foramen ovale, precipitating acute right-to-left shunting. This may manifest as systemic hypoxemia or paradoxic emboli. Severe tricuspid regurgitation may occur secondary to papillary muscle dysfunction or rupture, exaggerating right heart volume overload and low-cardiac output.

Management goals in RVI include improving cardiac filling and stroke volume, maintaining AV synchrony, and cardiac reperfusion. Fluid resuscitation is first-line treatment in patients who do not have evidence of pulmonary edema. Increased vascular volume directly raises the central filling pressure which helps maximize forward flow from the RV. Typically, 1 to 2 L of saline is infused rapidly until the capillary wedge pressure is approximately 15 mm Hg. If central venous monitoring is not available, fluids may be infused with frequent reevaluation of the patient for pulmonary congestion and volume overload.

As cardiac output is dependent on preload, medications that decrease preload should be avoided in RVI. Nitroglycerin, diuretics, and vagal maneuvers can decrease preload and may induce cardiogenic shock. Virtually, all antiischemic agents exert hemodynamic effects. β-Blockers and calcium channel blockers reduce heart rate and depress conduction, thereby increasing the risk of bradyarrhythmias and heart block in chronotropically dependent patients.

Sudden hypotension or bradyarrhythmias can occur even in patients who initially appear well perfused. Conditions that increase RV afterload, such as hypoxia and mechanical ventilation with positive end-expiratory pressure (PEEP), also compromise cardiac output.

Inotropic drugs may be necessary to augment cardiac output when fluid resuscitation is insufficient. Dobutamine is the agent of choice because it may also reduce pulmonary vascular resistance. However, dobutamine also decreases peripheral vascular resistance, and higher doses may induce paradoxical hypotension. For this reason, it may be safest to start with a dopamine infusion in conjunction with dobutamine. Mechanical assist devices such as an intra-aortic balloon pump may be beneficial in patients with refractory hypotension.

Pacing plays an important role in RV dysfunction. Bradyarrhythmias can be hemodynamically devastating as the ischemic RV has a relatively fixed stroke volume and is dependent upon heart rate. AV sequential pacing may be necessary because atrial function also plays a significant role in right heart volume. The ACC/AHA guidelines recommend that AV synchrony should be achieved and bradycardia should be corrected in all patients with a RVI.

Early coronary reperfusion is critical and has been shown to reduce morbidity and mortality. Primary percutaneous intervention has proven to be more successful than fibrinolytics.

RVIs commonly occur in association with inferior infarcts. Emergency physicians should look for RVI by obtaining a right-sided EKG in patients with inferior MIs and be aware of the delicate hemodynamics of RV ischemia.

SUGGESTED READINGS

Goldstein JA. Pathophysiology and management of right heart failure. *J Am Coll Cardiol.* 2002;40:841–853.

Greyson CR. Pathophysiology of right ventricular failure. *Crit Care Med.* 2008;36(1): S57–S65.

Kinn JW, Ajluni SC, Samyn JG, et al. Rapid hemodynamic improvement after reperfusion in right ventricular infarction. *J Am Coll Cardiol.* 1995;26:1230–1234.

Pike R. Right ventricular myocardial infarction. *Can J Cardiovasc Nurs.* 2005;19(3):6–8.

Zehender M, Kasper W, Kauder E, et al. Right ventricular infarction as an independent predictor of prognosis after acute inferior myocardial infarction. *N Engl J Med.* 1993;328(14): 981–988.

62

Do not rely on "reciprocal" changes on the electrocardiogram to diagnose acute ST segment elevation myocardial infarction

Atman P. Shah, MD, FACC, FSCAI and Stuart P. Swadron, MD, FRCPC

At the time of abrupt coronary plaque rupture, if there is complete thrombotic occlusion of the vessel, the patient typically suffers an ST segment elevation myocardial infarction (STEMI). Coronary blood flow to a segment of the myocardium is stopped. The ST elevations (STE) manifest on the surface electrocardiogram (ECG) because the involved area of the myocardium is depolarized incompletely and remains electrically more positive than the uninjured area at the end of depolarization. If revascularization is not achieved in time and the myocardium undergoes necrosis, the balance of the vectorial forces tend to point away from the area, and a wave of negativity, the Q wave, is observed.

An electrode over a part of the myocardium that is infarcting shows STE, whereas an electrode located over uninjured myocardium opposite the infarcted area will reveal ST segment depressions. This is the notion of "reciprocal changes" (i.e., STE in some leads are associated with ST segment changes in other leads).

The presence of reciprocal changes in STEMI can be used to distinguish STEMI from other causes of STE such as benign early repolarization or pericarditis. The classical teaching is that a true STEMI will result in reciprocal changes, while the other conditions will not.

But this is only partly true. The 12-lead ECG is comprised of six limb leads and six precordial leads. Leads I and aVL represent vectors through the lateral wall, while leads II, III, and aVF represent inferior vectors. Einthoven's model shows that a positive force in lead I and aVL will correspond to a negative vector in leads II, III, and aVF. Therefore, STE in lead I and aVL may correspond to ST segment depressions in leads II, III, and aVF and vice versa. However, the precordial leads, V1, V2, V3, V4, V5, and V6, represent vectors on a frontal plane and have no opposite leads in which to exhibit "reciprocal changes." Only if a posterior 18-lead ECG is performed with leads V7, V8, and V9 will anterior STE be matched with ST depressions in the posterior leads. In other words, an anterior STEMI should not be expected to produce "reciprocal changes" in the inferior leads.

Then, why do we see inferior ST segment depressions commonly with an anterior STEMI? These ST depressions in the inferior leads may be a result of the opposite vector causing STE in the lateral leads (e.g., in anterolateral MI).

Alternatively, ST depressions in the inferior leads in the setting of an anterior STEMI can represent ischemia in another segment of the myocardium. This is thus "ischemia at a distance." In either case, ST depressions in the context of a STEMI confer a poor prognosis.

So, the presence of reciprocal changes is not necessary to make the diagnosis of STEMI. But neither is the presence of both ST depressions and STE on the same ECG sufficient. A common pitfall is the misinterpretation of LVH with strain as STEMI during acute presentations for chest pain. In LVH with strain, ST segment elevations are typically seen in leads V1 and V2, whereas ST segment depression is usually seen (in association with asymmetrically inverted T waves) in leads V5 to V6. These specific changes are not the typical reciprocal changes seen in STEMI but rather represent abnormal conduction secondary to subendocardial ischemia.

To make the diagnosis of STEMI, one needs only to observe >1-mm ST segment elevation in two contiguous leads in the setting of symptoms consistent with cardiac ischemia. Whereas reciprocal ST segment changes may heighten suspicion for MI, they are not necessary to make the diagnosis of STEMI.

SUGGESTED READINGS

Chou TC. *Electrocardiography in Clinical Practice*. 4th ed. Philadelphia: W.B. Saunders Company; 1996:121.
Libby P, Bonow RO, Mann DL, et al. *Braunwald's Heart Disease*. 8th ed. Philadelphia: Saunders Elsevier; 2008:1228.
Thygesen K, Alpert JS, White HD. On behalf of the Joint ESC/ACCF/AHA/WHF Task Force for the Redefinition of Myocardial Infarction. Universal Definition of Myocardial Infarction. *Circulation*. 2007;166:2634–2653.

63

DO NOT RELY ON A SINGLE ELECTROCARDIOGRAM TO EVALUATE CHEST PAIN IN THE EMERGENCY DEPARTMENT

JAMES DE LA TORRE, MD, MMM

Since Einthoven invented the first version of the electrocardiogram (ECG) in the early 1900s, its use has become routine in the evaluation of a patient with chest pain (CP). Its utility and prognostic value is rivaled only by a good history and physical exam. However, the ECG has its own set of limitations one needs to be familiar with as an emergency physician.

The ECG is only a snapshot in time of the heart's electrical activity. ECGs may evolve over minutes, and changes can be intermittent and subtle. The sensitivity of the initial ECG for acute myocardial infarction (AMI) in patients presenting with CP is anywhere between 43% and 65%. This sensitivity increases to approximately 83% with serial ECGs. However, up to 1% to 6% of patients ultimately diagnosed with AMI have a normal ECG. A significant percentage, as many as 40% to 50%, may have only nonspecific changes. The bottom line is that if one is suspicious enough about acute coronary syndrome (ACS) to order the ECG, it might not be a bad idea to order a second one. Moreover, an initial normal ECG should not deter an appropriate diagnostic evaluation if there is a clinical suspicion of AMI or an ACS.

Most clinical guidelines mandate that the time to initial ECG in a patient with CP or angina-like symptoms should not exceed 10 min. The most important decision based upon the presenting ECG is the decision to initiate reperfusion therapy with fibrinolytics or percutaneous intervention. But what if the criteria for reperfusion are not present on the initial ECG, only to appear on a repeat ECG? Current guidelines on the timing of repeat ECGs are unclear and ambiguous. The initial presentation of an acute ST segment elevation MI (STEMI) may not be ST elevation but may, in fact, be ST depressions or hyperacute T waves. Q waves in the initial ECG may also pose a diagnostic dilemma for the emergency physician. Again, it is important to stress the dynamic nature of an ECG. Q waves do not necessarily indicate an old infarction and may be present early in the evolving AMI. If one postpones a repeat ECG, valuable time may be wasted, and definitive treatment delayed.

The exact number of ECGs to order is also unclear, but studies have shown that a significant number of patients with initially nondiagnostic ECGs later develop changes consistent with AMI, requiring intervention. Other studies have demonstrated that a significant percentage of patients with missed MI actually had ECGs that were misread. Repeat ECGs may reveal more clearly diagnostic changes that were initially very subtle.

Comparison to old ECGs may also be helpful. Lee et al. showed that using a previously obtained ECG for the evaluation of a patient with CP could avoid unnecessary admissions without sacrificing specificity for AMI. Perhaps the most striking example of a change in management that hinges on the availability of previous ECGs is that which occurs when a patient with left bundle branch block (LBBB) presents with acute CP. If a previous ECG documents the preexistence of LBBB, the patient no longer meets guidelines for reperfusion therapy. To proceed with either fibrinolytics or cardiac catheterization now puts the patient at risk for all of the complications of reperfusion without potential benefit.

So, what is the bottom line? ECG evidence of cardiac ischemia can evolve over time. Relying on one "normal" ECG may lead to a missed diagnosis of AMI and can result in delayed treatment and poor patient outcomes. When evaluating an ECG with nondiagnostic changes, it is important to compare it to previous ECGs, if available. Finally, in the case of a nondiagnostic ECG, if the clinical story is strong enough to indicate one ECG, it should be followed by another.

SUGGESTED READINGS

Lau J, Ioannidis JP, Balk EM, et al. Diagnosing acute cardiac ischemia in the emergency department: A systematic review of the accuracy and clinical effect of current technologies. *Ann Emerg Med.* 2001;37(5):453–460.

Lee TH, Cook EF, Weisberg M, et al. Acute chest pain in the emergency room: Identification and examination of low-risk patients. *Arch Intern Med.* 1985;145(1):65–69.

MacMath T, Fesmire F. The ECG in acute myocardial infarction. *J Emerg Med.* 1988;6: 405–410.

Whitwam W, Smith S. Acute coronary syndromes. *Emerg Med Clin N Am.* 2006;24:53–89.

64

BE WARY OF ELECTROCARDIOGRAM LEAD MISPLACEMENT

ERIC J. HEMMINGER, MD

The assessment and treatment decisions that flow from the electrocardiogram (ECG) are dependent not only on the physician's accurate interpretation but also on the readability and reproducibility of the tracing. The production of an ECG is subject to human error that can affect quality or lead to false diagnoses. Misplacement of ECG leads can occur via two basic mechanisms: (1) incorrect placement of the electrode patches and (2) connection of the ECG cables to the wrong electrode patches.

Proper ECG electrode position is based on specific anatomic landmarks. In some patients, these landmarks, such as the intercostal spaces, may be difficult to identify. In particular, obese patients, females, and patients with thoracic trauma may present a challenge. One common error is to position leads V1 and V2 on the chest higher than the fourth intercostal space. This displacement is commonly seen in women and may lead to the creation of a pseudoinfarction pattern. In a series of patients with no evidence of myocardial infarction at autopsy, premortem ECG demonstrated pathological Q waves (>30 ms duration) in 11%. The majority of these Q waves appeared in the septal leads.

Misplacement of the inferior leads may also lead to the appearance of a pseudoinfarction pattern. In this case, however, it is usually not the electrode position but the position of the heart in the chest that is the source. Because lead III is near the isoelectric axis of the heart, small changes in position can cause marked changes in QRS morphology. Q waves may be seen particularly in patients with a high diaphragm position, and an inferior "infarct" may disappear with changes in respiration. For this reason, an isolated Q wave in lead III is not considered clinically significant.

Another artifact affecting the inferior leads results from placing the leg electrodes on the abdomen. Placement of the leg leads on the hips or lower abdomen amplifies the voltage in the inferior leads, creating ST segment or T wave changes which are "dynamic" if compared with a properly obtained ECG.

ECG abnormalities which result from misconnection of the ECG cables may also be misinterpreted. A common human error is the reversal of left-right orientation. Reversal of the arm lead cables (*Fig. 64.1*) is the most common transposition error. This will result in the following changes to the ECG: (1) lead I is inverted, (2) leads II and III are reversed, and (3) leads aVL and aVR are reversed. These changes in the frontal plane are also seen in dextrocardia, which can be differentiated from arm lead reversal by the loss of normal QRS transition across the precordium. Reversal of the leg leads does not change the ECG appreciably because the electrode positions are close together.

In everyday practice, the most common consequence of lead misplacement is that changes in serial ECGs are misinterpreted as "dynamic changes" and attributed erroneously to ischemia.

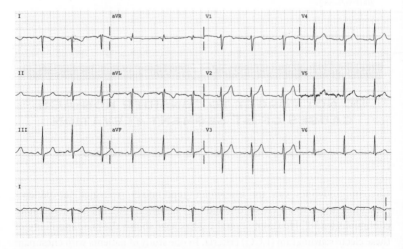

FIGURE 64.1. An ECG demonstrating reversal of the arm lead cables.

TABLE 64.1	**MOST COMMON ECG LEAD PLACEMENT ERRORS**
ECG FINDING	**POSSIBLE LEAD PLACEMENT CAUSE**
Dynamic ST depression or T-wave abnormalities associated with significant QRS voltage changes in the same leads	Suspect change in limb lead proximity to heart
Loss of precordial QRS voltage compared with recent ECG	Suspect unlabeled right-sided ECG
Inverted P wave in lead I	Suspect reversal of the arm lead cables
Lead I, II, or III is nearly isoelectric (flat line)	The right leg cable has been switched with one of the arm cables
Septal Q waves appear in a female patient	Consider misplacement of V1 and V2 electrodes higher than normal
Unusual precordial R-wave transition	Consider misplacement of the precordial electrodes or reversal of two cables

In addition to the examples above, innumerable other alterations in the ECG may occur with lead placement errors. *Table 64.1* summarizes the most common ECG lead placement errors.

SUGGESTED READINGS

Horan LG, Flowers NC, Johnson JC. Significance of the diagnostic Q wave of myocardial infarction. *Circulation*. 1971;43:428–436.
Surawicz B, Knilians TK, eds. Misplacement of leads and electrocardiographic artifacts. *Chou's Electrocardiography in Clinical Practice*. 5th ed. Philadelphia: W.B. Saunders Company; 2001:569–582.

65

DO NOT FORGET TO CONSIDER NON-ACS CAUSES OF ST SEGMENT ELEVATION

KIMBALL POON, MD AND AMAL MATTU, MD

Current guidelines call for immediate reperfusion strategies for patients presenting with typical chest pain and "ST elevation >0.1 mV in two or more contiguous leads." However, several studies have shown the poor specificity of these electrocardiogram (ECG) criteria. In one study of patients with chest pain and ST elevations (STEs), acute myocardial infarction (AMI) was the diagnosis in only 50% to 85% of cases. As a result, the American College of Emergency Physicians qualifies their recommendation to apply to STEs "that are not characteristic of early repolarization or pericarditis, nor of a repolarization abnormality from left ventricular hypertrophy (LVH) or bundle branch block (BBB)." Therefore, it is critical to recognize and systematically exclude other diagnoses prior to making the diagnosis of ST segment elevation myocardial infarction (STEMI).

STE is not a rare finding. In a study of 6,000 healthy, male U.S. Air Force personnel, 90% of patients had > 1 mm STE in a precordial lead, with V2 being the most common. This benign early repolarization (BER) is characterized by an ST segment that is concave upward with occasional notching of the J point. The ST segments of BER are most prominent in leads V2 to V5 and are often accompanied with large T waves.

LVH often leads to deep S waves in V1 to V3. The concomitant repolarization of LVH often leads to an elevation of the J point. Look for evidence of left ventricular strain (ST depression) in inferior and lateral leads to support this diagnosis.

Pericarditis involves the inflammation of the entire epicardium; therefore, the hallmark findings are diffuse STEs that do not follow any coronary distribution. PR depression is found in 50% of cases. The STE is typically concave upward and rarely exceeds 5 mm.

Flutter waves can mimic the appearance of STE (*Fig. 65.1*). Intravenous AV nodal slowing agents can alter the relationship between the QRS complex and the flutter waves, unmasking the true ST segment. If necessary, cardioversion can restore sinus rhythm and permit visualization of an unperturbed ST segment.

Left BBB (LBBB) and right ventricular (RV) pacing lead to a severely distorted pattern of LV repolarization. The ST segments move discordantly, or opposite, to the predominant QRS vector. Therefore, in leads V1 to V3, the deep S wave will be followed by STE. A preexisting LBBB can mask the STE created by AMI. The Sgarbossa criteria have been developed to make the diagnosis of AMI in the presence of LBBB; however, these are far less sensitive than they are specific, and this should not be used to rule out AMI in a patient with LBBB or RV pacing, particularly with suggestive symptoms. In fact, current AHA guidelines continue to recommend immediate reperfusion in patients with symptoms suggestive of AMI and a new or presumed new LBBB on ECG.

Although STE secondary to AMI is a time critical diagnosis, it must be remembered that a number of processes, both pathologic and benign, can lead to STE on ECG. None of the descriptions above are absolute, and in some cases, it simply may be too difficult to distinguish STEMI from more benign causes of STE without serial ECGs or more advanced testing.

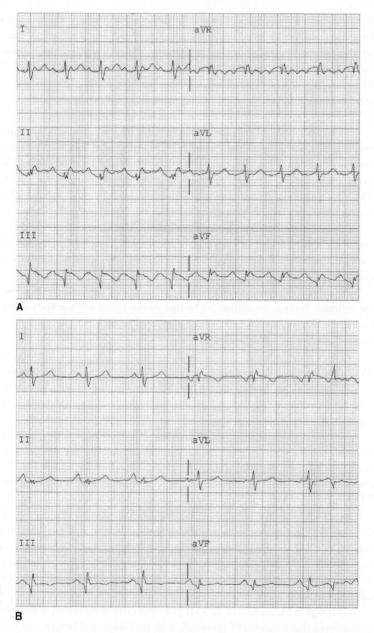

FIGURE 65.1. A: Atrial flutter mimicking an inferior STEMI. B: After cardioversion, the apparent STEMI has resolved. (Courtesy of Kenneth A. Narahara, MD.)

SUGGESTED READINGS

American College of Emergency Physicians. Clinical policy: Critical issues in the evaluation and management of adult patients presenting with suspected acute myocardial infarction or unstable angina. *Ann Emerg Med.* 2000;35:521–525.

Antman EM, Anbe DT, Armstrong PW, et al. ACC/AHA guidelines for the management of patients with ST-elevation myocardial infarction—executive summary. A report of the American College of Cardiology/American Heart Association Task Force on Practice Guidelines (Writing Committee to revise the 1999 guidelines for the management of patients with acute myocardial infarction). *J Am Coll Cardiol.* 2004;44:671–719.

Hiss RG, Lamb LE, Allen MF. Electrocardiographic findings in 67,375 asymptomatic subjects. X. Normal values. *Am J Cardiol.* 1960;6:200–231.

Shlipak MG, Lyons WL, Go AS, et al. Should the electrocardiogram be used to guide therapy for patients with left bundle-branch block and suspected myocardial infarction? *JAMA.* 1999;281:714–719.

Wang K, Asinger RW, Marriott HJ. ST-segment elevation in conditions other than acute myocardial infarction. *N Engl J Med.* 2003;349:2128–2135.

66

KNOW THE ELECTROCARDIOGRAM FINDINGS OF ACUTE MYOCARDIAL INFARCTION IN PATIENTS WITH PACEMAKERS

MATTHEW P. OSTROM, MD

In the United States, nearly 1 million patients suffer from acute myocardial infarction (AMI) annually, a condition which is associated with high morbidity and mortality. Current protocols emphasizing rapid diagnosis and shorter reperfusion times have improved patient outcomes. The prompt recognition of an ST elevation myocardial infarction (STEMI) on a 12-lead electrocardiogram (ECG) is critical as it remains at the center of all reperfusion algorithms.

In 1989, approximately 1 million patients had permanent pacemakers in the United States. More recent estimates suggest that 112,000 pacemakers are implanted annually, and this figure seems only likely to increase. The presence of a right ventricular pacing lead results in a distortion of the normal physiologic depolarization and repolarization due to asynchronous spread of electrical excitation. The resultant ECG manifests a left bundle branch block (LBBB) appearance with discordant ST segments and T waves. The interpretation of ST segments and the diagnosis of STEMI in the setting of a ventricular paced rhythm (VPR) are thus very difficult.

Based on a review of patients with LBBB in the GUSTO trial, Sgarbossa et al. proposed three criteria for the diagnosis of STEMI in patients with

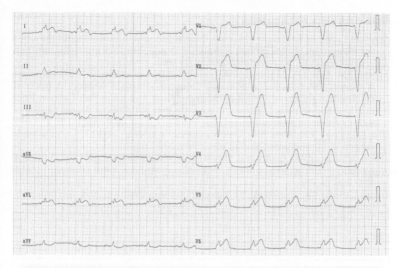

FIGURE 66.1. Acute myocardial infarction in a patient with a pacemaker. Discordant ST-segment elevation of >5 mm can be seen in leads V2 to V3. Concordant ST segment elevation is seen in leads I, avL and V5 to V6.

LBBB: (1) concordant ST-segment elevation (in the same direction as the QRS complex) ≥1 mm, (2) concordant ST-segment depression ≥1 mm in leads V1 to V3, and (3) discordant ST elevation (in the opposite direction of the QRS complex) ≥5 mm. Of the three ECG criteria, discordant ST elevation ≥5 mm was the only one with both relatively high sensitivity (53%) and specificity (88%) for the diagnosis of AMI in the setting of VPR. The other two criteria had acceptable specificity (94% and 82%, respectively) for the diagnosis of AMI but did not meet statistical significance (*Fig. 66.1*).

The low sensitivity of the above criteria has profound implications for patients presenting with AMI who have no "entrance criteria" (ST elevation) into a STEMI pathway and are thus unable to receive the benefit of reperfusion therapy. Similarly, the marginal specificity of the criteria may lead to false assumptions of AMI and unnecessary procedural and bleeding risk. In these cases, a previous ECG with a similar appearance may be especially helpful and prevent the clinician from "pulling the trigger" on reperfusion. Another suggested method of evaluation for STEMI in patients with VPR is the temporary suspension of pacing output using a magnet and an assessment of the native rhythm and ST segments. This method should be used with caution, as the native rhythm may prove to be life threatening (hence the need for the pacemaker!). The use of a positive chronotropic agent such as atropine has also been suggested as a way to increase the native rate above the paced level in an attempt to suppress pacing and assess native ST segments. It seems rather imprudent to employ this final strategy in a patient suspected of having an AMI given the untoward effects of tachycardia in acute ischemia.

The diagnosis of STEMI in a patient with VPR is difficult for even the most astute physicians. There is no single criterion or test that can reliably rule in or rule out an AMI, short of a coronary angiogram. When AMI is strongly suspected based on the clinical presentation and ECG findings, an invasive approach is thus preferable, because it has both diagnostic and therapeutic value.

SUGGESTED READINGS

Bernstein AD, Parsonnet V. Survey of cardiac pacing and defibrillation in the United States in 1993. *Am J Cardiol*. 1996;78:187–196.

Caldera AE, Bryce M, Kolter M, et al. Angiographic signifigance of a discordant ST-segment elevation of ≥ millimeters in patients with ventricular-paced rhythm and acute myocardial infarction. *Am J Cardiol*. 2002;90:1240–1243.

Knott J. Diagnosis of acute myocardial infarct with ventricular paced rhythm. *Emerg Med (Fremantle)*. 2003;15(1):100–103.

Madias JE. The nonspecificity of ST-segment elevation ≥5.0 mm in V1-V3 in the diagnosis of acute myocardial infarction in the presence of ventricular paced rhythm. *J Electrophysiol*. 2004;37:135–139.

Sgarbossa EB, Pinski SL, Barbagelata A, et al. Electrocardiographic diagnosis of evolving acute myocardial infarction in the presence of left bundle branch block. GUSTO-I (Global Utilization of Streptokinase and Tissue Plasminogen Activator for Occluded Coronary Arteries) Investigators. *N Engl J Med*. 1996;334(8):481–487.

Sgarbossa EB, Pinski SL, Gates KB, et al. Early electrocardiographic diagnosis of acute myocardial infarction in the presence of ventricular paced rhythm. GUSTO-I investigators. *Am J Cardiol*. 1996;77(5):423–424.

67

BE AGGRESSIVE WITH INTRAVENOUS NITROGLYCERIN DOSING IN ACUTE CONGESTIVE HEART FAILURE

NICOLAS P. FORGET, MD, DTMH

Acutely decompensated heart failure (ADHF) often requires ICU admission. This need may be decreased with timely intervention and the appropriate use of vasodilators, diuretics, ACE inhibitors, inotropes, and noninvasive ventilatory support. A large consortium of academic leaders in the field, The Heart Failure Society of America, recommends the use of loop diuretics as first-line therapy of ADHF with the addition of nitroglycerin (NTG) as needed. However, in the emergency department setting, NTG has many advantages over furosemide as a first-line agent.

NTG can be administered by multiple routes, including sublingual, oral, transdermal, and intravenous. It takes effect almost immediately, whereas furosemide's diuretic effects begin only after 1 to 2 h. Further, NTG has a very short half-life and can be stopped almost immediately when used intravenously or transdermally. NTG decreases both right and left ventricular filling pressures, systemic and pulmonary vascular resistance, and systemic blood pressure, all while increasing cardiac output. In its early phases of action, within an hour of administration, furosemide actually increases the intravascular volume, and consequently preload and afterload. Although the heart rate generally increases with NTG, this is not usually marked in most patients.

In one recent review, researchers found that NTG is underutilized as a treatment modality for ADHF. Possible barriers to its widespread use may include confusion about its multiplicity of formats and doses, the titration requirements of the intravenous preparation, and very legitimate concerns about hypotension, especially in association with erectile dysfunction drugs such as sildenafil, and right ventricular myocardial infarction. Although not as serious, the high frequency of headache with NTG may prevent some patients and physicians from wanting to use it. NTG-induced headaches usually respond well to common analgesics.

NTG may begin with sublingual spray or tablets, while preparations are being made for initiation of an NTG infusion. However, three sprays of SL NTG over 15 min are mathematically equivalent to an 80 μg per min infusion. Thus, following this up with an NTG infusion that starts at 10 μg per min, as is commonly done and commonly written as a starting dose in nursing manuals, represents, in actuality, a tremendous dose reduction. Furthermore, most protocols call for the infusion to be increased by 10 μg per min every few minutes. At this rate, a dose of 80 μg per min would not be reached for 15 to 20 min. Thus, this standard NTG infusion protocol exposes patients to a period of relative therapeutic nonintervention as the NTG infusion is titrated up. To be conservative, and taking into account the incomplete bioavailability of sublingual NTG, it is reasonable to start an NTG infusion at 40 μg per min and titrate it up by 10 to 20 μg per min every 3 to 5 min, as blood pressure allows.

A number of papers have been published demonstrating the efficacy of high-dose nitrates in the setting of heart failure and pulmonary edema. Emergency physicians should continue to make NTG their first choice in the treatment of ADHF. Initiation of therapy at higher doses, and with more rapid titration than is traditional, is indicated.

SUGGESTED READINGS

Allen LA, O'Connor CM. Management of acute decompensated heart failure. *CMAJ*. 2007;176:797–805.

Cotter G, Metzkor E, Kaluski E, et al. Randomised trial of high-dose isosorbide dinitrate plus low-dose furosemide versus high-dose furosemide plus low-dose isosorbide dinitrate in severe pulmonary oedema. *Lancet*. 1998;351(9100):389–393.

Elkayam U, Roth A, Jumar A, et al. Hemodynamic and volumetric effects of venodilation with nitroglycerin in chronic mitral regurgitation. *Am J Cardiol*. 1987;60(13):1106–1111.

Fromm RE, Varon J, Gibbs LR. Congestive heart failure and pulmonary edema for the emergency physician. *J Emerg Med*. 1995;13:71–87.

Heart Failure Society of America. *Comprehensive Heart Failure Practice Guideline*. Available at: www.heartfailureguideline.org. Accessed June 1, 2008.

Levy P, Compton S, Welch R, et al. Treatment of severe decompensated heart failure with high-dose intravenous nitroglycerin: A feasibility and outcome analysis. *Ann Emerg Med*. 2007;50(2):144–152.

Nashed AH, Allegra, JR, Eskin B, et al. Prospective trial of the treatment of acute cardiogenic pulmonary edema with IV nitroglycerin boluses. *Ann Emerg Med*. 1997;30:382.

Noonan PK, Benet LZ. Incomplete and delayed bioavailability of sublingual nitroglycerin. *Am J Cardiol*. 1985;55:1184–1187.

Sacchetti A, Ramoska E, Moakes ME, et al. Effect of ED management on ICU use in acute pulmonary edema. *Am J Emerg Med*. 1999;17(6):571–574.

Sharon A, Shpirer I, Kaluski E, et al. High-dose intravenous isosorbide-dinitrate is safer and better than Bi-PAP ventilation combined with conventional treatment for severe pulmonary edema. *J Am Coll Cardiol*. 2000;36(3):832–837.

68

AVOID β-BLOCKERS IN COCAINE-ASSOCIATED MYOCARDIAL INFARCTIONS

EMILY A. CARPENTER ROSE, MD

Cocaine is the illicit drug attributed to the most emergency department (ED) visits. Chest pain accounts for 40% of those visits. The occurrence of myocardial infarction (MI) after cocaine use is unrelated to the amount ingested, the route of administration, or the frequency of use.

β-Adrenergic blocker agents (BBs) in MI have been designated as a quality measure in U.S. hospitals because of evidence that they decrease mortality, recurrent ischemic events, reinfarction, ventricular fibrillation, sudden cardiac death, and cardiac rupture. In the setting of cocaine-associated MI, however, their benefit is likely outweighed by their risks.

The mechanism of action of cocaine is complex, and the clinical effects of its metabolites are not entirely known. Cocaine metabolites have varying half-lives and differing cardiovascular effects. Several metabolites are known vasoconstrictors, while others such as ecgonine methylester (EME) may induce cerebral vasodilation.

There are several well-documented mechanisms of cocaine-related chest pain. Cocaine is a sympathomimetic agent that causes an accumulation of catecholamines at the postsynaptic receptor by blocking norepinephrine and dopamine reuptake at the presynaptic adrenergic terminals. This catecholamine surge increases the heart rate, blood pressure, and contractility, which increases myocardial oxygen demand. Second, β-adrenergic stimulation induces coronary artery vasoconstriction and spasm. Coronary artery thrombosis occurs via cocaine-induced platelet stimulation from increased platelet activation and aggregation. This platelet stimulation is the reason why thrombus formation can occur in patients without underlying coronary artery disease. In addition, coronary artery aneurysms are associated with cocaine use, and premature coronary atherosclerosis has been demonstrated in cocaine users.

The mediation of vasoconstriction by β-adrenergic stimulation limits the use of BBs in acute cocaine-associated MIs. According to classic teaching, ischemia can be exacerbated by BBs via the induction of unopposed alpha-adrenergic stimulation, triggering systemic and coronary vasoconstriction which results in worsened ischemia, elevation in blood pressure, and increased myocardial oxygen demand. Even mixed α- and β-adrenergic blockers such as labetalol may carry similar risks because their β-blockade action is stronger than their α-blocking function.

Though decades of research demonstrating the negative effect of β-blockers with acute cocaine intoxication exists, there are still unknowns. No randomized, placebo-controlled trials in cocaine-associated MI have been reported. Instead, therapeutic recommendations are based on animal studies, cardiac catheterizations, observational studies, case series, and case reports.

A recent retrospective study called into question the routine omission of BBs in cocaine-associated chest pain. However, the study by Dattilo et al. considered patients who had a positive urinary toxicology screen for cocaine who were administered BBs during their hospital course. The authors did not control for the duration since last cocaine use. Because cocaine-associated MI typically occurs usually within 3 h of use, and urine drug screens remain positive for 48 h or more after cocaine ingestion, the authors' conclusions must be interpreted cautiously.

Only a small percentage (6% to 14%) of patients with cocaine-related chest pain actually have evidence of MI. Moreover, the mortality of cocaine-associated MI approaches zero. Even if BBs were ultimately proven to be safe in the setting of acute cocaine intoxication, this reduced risk of cocaine-related MI drastically skews the risk-benefit profile of BBs away from their routine use.

In the acute treatment of cocaine-associated MI, the American College of Cardiology/American Heart Association ST elevation MI guidelines are clear. They state "Beta-blockers should not be administered to patients with STEMI precipitated by cocaine use because of the risk of exacerbating coronary spasm."

SUGGESTED READINGS

Dattilo PB, Hailpern SM, Fearon K, et al. Beta-blockers are associated with reduced risk of myocardial infarction after cocaine use. *Ann Emerg Med*. 2008;51:117–125.

Hahn IH, Hoffman RS. Cocaine use and acute myocardial infarction. *Emerg Med Clin N Am*. 2001;19(2):493–510.

Hollander JE. Cocaine intoxication and hypertension. *Ann Emerg Med*. 2008;51:S18–S20.

Hollander JE, Henry TD. Evaluation and management of the patient who has cocaine-associated chest pain. *Cardiol Clin*. 2006;24:103–114.

Lange RA, Hillis LD. Cardiovascular complications of cocaine use. *N Engl J Med*. 2001;345:351–358.

McCord J, Jneid H, Hollander JE, et al. Management of cocaine-associated chest pain and myocardial infarction: A scientific statement from the American Heart Association Acute Cardiac Care Committee of the Council on Clinical Cardiology. *Circulation*. 2008;117:1897–1907.

Morgan JP. Cardiovascular complications of cocaine abuse. UpToDate.com 2008.

Tuncel M, Wang Z, Arbique D, et al. Mechanism of the blood pressure—raising effect of cocaine in humans. *Circulation*. 2002;105:1054–1059.

69

ALWAYS CLARIFY YOUR PATIENTS' UNDERSTANDING OF THEIR OWN CARE

SHARON BORD, MD

Patients often arrive at the emergency department (ED) scared, in pain, and anxious. They hope to leave feeling better with an improved understanding of their illness, be it chronic or acute in nature. Yet, many physicians and scholars wonder how often patients leave the ED frustrated, feeling more confused, and with more questions than when they first arrived.

Studies have shown that patients who understand their diagnosis and the functions of their medications have better perceptions of the quality of communication and are thus more compliant. Patients at a California hospital who were treated and released were questioned on their understanding of their diagnosis, prescribed medications, additional instructions, and plan for follow-up care. Overall, patients correctly identified 59% of their instructions. Of the patients in this study, 63.8% identified the physician as the source for most of the information, and notably this subset had the greatest understanding of their discharge instructions. Engel et al. examined patients' understanding of their ED care in four domains: diagnosis and cause, ED care, post-ED care, and return instructions. Their findings were consistent with prior studies, with 78% of patients being deficient in one domain and 51% being deficient in two or more domains. It is of particular interest that greater than a third of these deficiencies identified (34%) involved post-ED care.

There are certain practice environments and situations where it is especially important to clarify patients' understanding of their care in the ED. Specifically, parents who accompany a sick child to the ED should receive appropriate teaching and instruction. Korsch et al. examined communication in the pediatric ED over 30 years ago, finding that parents were often dissatisfied with the care because they did not have opportunity to express themselves, they noted lack of concern or sympathy from providers, and providers directed most of their talk to the parents rather than to the child. A more recent study that specifically addressed children visiting the ED for asthma corroborated these findings years ago. Parents continue to want more involvement in treatment decisions and more attention paid to their concerns.

Working in an ED, one must care for all individuals who seek care regardless of their race, ethnicity, or language that they speak. Discussing the topic of communication in the ED would not be complete without addressing the issue of language barriers. Non–English speaking patients who were questioned on their care in the ED reported significantly more problems with communication and overall problems with their care and testing. Additionally, only 52% of non–English speaking patients questioned were satisfied with their care, compared with 71% of English speakers. These results stress the importance of diligent communication and review of understanding when discussing medical issues with non–English speakers.

The ED environment oftentimes is not conducive to lengthy discussions with patients explaining what happened during their visit and necessary follow-up. In addition, it is has been shown that patients often leave confused and dissatisfied. "What many patients resent today is their inability to communicate with physicians in a meaningful manner…to have a practical effect on the patient the clinician must have the facility to communicate with him(her)." These words were said at an opening lecture for 3rd year medical students over 30 years ago, but still ring true today. Take the time to ensure effective communication in all four domains: diagnosis and cause, ED care, post-ED care, and return instructions. In particular, when your patients have a good understanding of instructions, both you and your patient can breathe a sigh of relief.

SUGGESTED READINGS

Carrasquillo O, Orav J, Brennan T, et al. Impact of language barriers on patient satisfaction in an emergency department. *J Gen Intern Med*. 1999;14:82–87.

Crane J. Patient comprehension of doctor-patient communication on discharge from the emergency department. *J Emerg Med*. 1997;15:1–7.

Engel KG, Heisler M, Smith DM, et al. Patient comprehension of emergency department care and instructions: Are patients aware of when they do not understand? *Ann Emerg Med*. 2009;53(4):454–461.

Weiss K, Mitchell H, Mohr B. Patient-provider communication during the emergency department care of children with asthma. *Med Care*. 1998;36:1439–1450.

70

BE AN EFFECTIVE TEAMPLAYER: A NURSING PERSPECTIVE

PAULA M. NEIRA, RN, JD, CEN

Emergency medicine and emergency nursing are separate, interdependent professions that must work closely together in order to ensure that each patient receives the highest quality health care in an often stressed, overcrowded, and hectic environment. Enhanced teamwork and choreography between physicians and nurses is vital to avoiding errors and mitigating the consequences of errors that do occur. To that end, there are several areas, from an ED nurse's point of view, on which physicians can focus and evaluate their performance as a team player.

The first area is the very nature of the relationship between the physician and the nursing staff. Gone are the days of the "captain of the ship" approach, whereby the physician bore sole responsibility, and had sole authority, for any care-related decision. This hierarchical approach with nursing being subordinate no longer pertains because of the increased scope and responsibility of nursing practice. Thus, a new way of thinking needs to apply. A more accurate analogy is to liken doctors and nurses to members of a football team—where the doctor is the quarterback. Like a quarterback, the doctor calls the plays, is usually paid better, and has more public accolades but owes his or her success to the players around him or her who must execute the plays, that is, the nurses and ancillary staff. Just as a good blocking tackle is a quarterback's best friend, so too is the nurse the doctor's best friend.

Flowing from this new paradigm is a mutual loyalty. Fostering a sense of loyalty means that nurses will feel empowered to participate as collegial members of the team—sharing their knowledge and perceptions, knowing that their input is valued by the physician. This reduces errors because individuals feel able to point out impending mistakes or question a course of action. A simple act that a physician can do to enhance building loyalty is to demonstrate a willingness to pitch in when something needs to be done for the patient. Just as a quarterback sometimes must throw a block, when all the other players are engaged otherwise, so too must a physician sometimes get a glass of water or take a temperature without asking the nurse to do it. This goes a long way toward creating a team, one that looks out for each other to avoid errors.

The second area where a physician can enhance effective teamwork is to improve his or her time management skills and respect the time constraints which nursing encounters in executing orders. The physician should be efficient in conducting his or her exam and developing the emergency department plan of care. From this, orders should be written in a timely manner and grouped logically. This means not ordering lab work, for example, in a "drip-drip-drip" manner. Nurses plan their interactions to group patient care activities to maximize their efficiency. It is both inefficient and frustrating to have to repeatedly obtain lab work from a patient, not to mention how irritating it is to the patient to be stuck multiple times. Of course, additional testing or treatments are sometimes necessary because of changes in patient condition or the need to perform additional diagnostics.

Other time-related issues are to understand the time it takes to perform an ordered task and to plan for the time it takes to execute an order. It takes but a second to order an IV access to be placed; it may take 30 min to actually do it on a patient with poor vasculature. Further, executing multiple orders on multiple patients takes time. It is counterproductive to ask a nurse "why wasn't this done yet" when the nurse is clearly busy juggling multiple tasks. Also this increases distractions and raises the potential to confuse orders on different patients, leading to medication errors and incorrect treatments being rendered. As an effective team player, if a physician desires a task to be completed sooner, do it yourself or discuss the prioritization with the nurse.

A third, and most important, area where physicians can avoid errors by enhancing teamwork is to improve their team communications. While inter personal communications are discussed elsewhere, communications between team members are vital to effective coordination and patient safety. First and foremost, a physician must hear nurses when they are relaying information about the patient. Take the time to read the nursing notes and nursing assessment. It is the nurse who spends much more time interacting with patients and family members at the bedside. The nurse's observations and assessments can be very valuable in formulating the care plan. Additionally, this demonstrates respect for the nurse's experience and promotes a multidisciplinary approach to patient care.

Open lines of communication between the nurse and the physician are key to avoiding all sorts of errors. Discuss the proposed plan of care and work out a game plan that everyone understands. As the patient progresses through his or her emergency interaction, the physician should keep the nurse informed of test results and the medical decision making thought process. Involving nurses in the decision making utilizes their knowledge and provides for an independent perspective.

Teamwork and clear communication are never more vital than *in extremis* situations. Use closed-loop communications whenever giving verbal orders and in emergent situations. This style of communications, used in aviation and at sea, ensures that both the person giving the orders and the person executing them have a common understanding of the task. This eliminates avoidable errors by highlighting any confusion.

This is but a brief commentary on enhancing physician-nurse team effectiveness and thus lessening the risk of errors. However, physicians can make an immediate impact on improving patient care in whatever setting they practice by embracing their role as quarterback and appreciating their teammates, by being organized and situationally aware about the execution of their orders, and by being effective team communicators.

SUGGESTED READINGS

Arford PH. Nurse-physician communication: An organizational accountability. *Nurs Econ.* 2005;23:72–77.
Beyea S. Improving verbal communication in clinical care. *AORN J.* 2004;79:1053–1054, 1057.

71

BE COGNIZANT OF BIAS

ARJUN S. CHANMUGAM, MD, MBA

There are few activities in this world that have the density of decision making commonly found in the practice of emergency medicine. To compound the issue, the time limitations associated with emergency care are real, ever present, and are about as serious as you can get. Although most emergency physicians are good clinical decision makers in practice, they may be less familiar with the theories underlying the science of decision making. Many of these theories are just beginning to be well articulated in the literature. One area that has received a fair amount of review has to do with bias, more specifically in medicine, diagnostic error.

Everyone makes cognitive errors, some more than others. Is it possible not to be biased in the practice of medicine? Limited studies exist on this topic, but it certainly has been a topic in the mainstream media. In February 2007, Time Magazine had an article entitled "Are Doctors Just Playing Hunches" in which they discussed physician bias in management decisions. It is not just the public that is concerned with biases in medicine, but even the Association of American Medical Colleges has gotten into the act. In Spring 2008, the AAMC put out a report that recommended limiting drug and device makers from offering free material (food, drink, and paraphernalia) to physicians at medical colleges because it might lead to biases among doctors. The basic argument for the pharmaceutical company restriction is based on an information bias. When physicians learn about a medication, they are likely to have greater familiarity with it, and thus feel more comfortable with prescribing it over other drugs, including ones that may be more suitable. As a result, the drug has a greater chance to be recommended to patients by the doctor. This is perhaps one of the more obvious biases, but this informational bias is not the only one that should be considered in our practice. Other cognitive and diagnostic errors abound.

Pat Croskerry, MD, PhD has written extensively about this subject for nearly 20 years. He describes three groups of errors of diagnosis. The first group of errors he considers as no-fault errors—these are errors that are inherently not the fault of the physician but are more associated with imperfect information from the patient. In most cases, the no-fault error is the result of either misleading information or absent information from the patients or their surrogate. Cases involving malingering or refusal of care are examples of the first type of error. The second group of errors has to do with systemic errors. These errors have more to do with conditions of the workplace and include such conditions as overcrowding and delays in laboratory results or radiology results. Finally, the third group of errors is due to "defaults in the physician's thinking. Cognitive errors may range from basic knowledge deficiencies to cognitive dispositions to respond to patients in predictive ways. Cognitive errors may also result from idiosyncratic decision styles…" These cognitive dispositions to respond (CDR) can be considered biases and may be best illustrated by reviewing the following case.

> A 53-year-old male presents with an altered mental status to the ED via public ambulance. It is his third presentation in a week and the second time in 24 h. The paramedics reported that they found him sleeping on a bench, smelling of alcohol—again. He is triaged as "alcohol intoxication" and sent to a stretcher in the hallway. Two 8-h shifts later, it is noticed that he is not responding well to verbal commands. Finally, a head CT scan is ordered which reveals a subdural hematoma.

The physician staff evaluating this patient faced some limitations. The patient was unable to provide any details, and he presented in a similar condition in the past. Nevertheless, there are several CDR that are worth reviewing. The first is one that is called triage cueing, whereby the triage team entered a diagnosis rather than the presenting compliant (alcohol intoxication vs. altered mental status) and the label unduly influenced the physician team. This was followed by a CDR called diagnostic momentum which occurs when a label attached to a patient tends to remain through the course of evaluation. In this case, the patient was labeled as an alcohol intoxicated individual, which may have impeded any other diagnostic considerations. Not pursuing other etiologies can be considered another CDR premature diagnostic closure. Furthermore, there may have been search satisfaction, a likely cause was found to explain his condition so other causes were not entertained, and the physician is satisfied with the current diagnostic impression. There may have been a posterior probability error. This type of error occurs when the past presentations unduly influence the current evaluation; in this case the cause or source of his altered mental status was influenced by his previous ED admission diagnoses, which lead to the physician anchoring to a diagnostic entity. The physician may have suffered from a fundamental attribution error; this cognitive disposition to respond describes a tendency to judge or blame a patient for his or her illness rather than comprehensively evaluate the situation. Finally, there may have been Sutton slip CDR. Willie Sutton was a bank robber who was rumored to have answered a question of why he robbed banks with the quip, "that is where the money is." In the Sutton slip CDR, other nonobvious considerations are ignored, such as that occurred in the above case.

In summary, there are many CDRs; nearly 30 are well described in the literature. Biases, CDR, etc. are part of life of a physician. The problem is not so much associated with the presence of a bias or CDR, it is the failure to recognize them in our decision making process.

SUGGESTED READINGS

Croskerry P. When diagnoses fail. *Can J CME*, November 2003. Available at: http://www.stacommunications.com/journals/pdfs/cme/cmenov2003/diagnoseserrors.pdf

Croskerry P. Diagnostic failure: A cognitive and affective approach. In: *Advances in Patient Safety: From Research to Implementation.* Vol. 1–4, AHRQ Publication Nos. 050021 (1–4). February 2005. Rockville, MD: Agency for Healthcare Research and Quality. Available at: http://www.ahrq.gov/qual/advances/

Wazana A. Physicians and the pharmaceutical industry: Is a gift ever just a gift? *JAMA.* 2000;283:373–380.

72

BEWARE "THE CURBSIDE CONSULT"

ARJUN S. CHANMUGAM, MD, MBA

CASE

A 68-year-old female presents to the emergency department (ED) with a right-sided facial weakness and a history of transient numbness in her left hand. She has no other complaints, but she does have a history of hypertension and diabetes, both of which have been in moderate control over the last few days. Her glucose is 129 and blood pressure is 165/90. The rest of her labs and vital signs are normal. Her head CT scan is negative, but you remain concerned. The neurologist on call has just finished writing a note on one of your colleague's patients. With impeccable timing, you find that perfect moment to broach the subject of your patient. The two of you spend a few minutes casually catching up and eventually, you do discuss your patient. You answer her question about forehead sparring and you both agree that this presentation may be consistent with a Bell palsy (7th nerve/facial nerve peripheral palsy.) She gives you the goodbye smile as she makes her way to the ED exit. You feel comfortable that you got a chance to discuss your patient with her, but as she disappears down the hallway, you think about how you are going to document your curbside consult. Suddenly, you no longer feel as comfortable as you did a minute ago.

A curbside consult can be a meaningful way to get generic information about a disease process. It is an often used mechanism to exchange ideas or discuss a vexing clinical conundrum. However, when managing a specific patient, its utility becomes suspect, its value questionable, and its impact on the patient potentially dangerous. An emergency consultation should involve a written assessment followed by same-visit recommendations or interventions by the consultant who has a specific level of expertise.

In the case discussed above, the diagnostic considerations must include stroke or transient ischemic attack. Did the consultant effectively rule out the stroke considerations, or did she merely state that facial nerve palsy was a possibility? Did she realize that your pleasantly informal conversation was not about a random symptom complex but involved a real live patient that you were seeing in the ED right now? It will never be clear, because in retrospect both you and the consultant will be depending on memory to recall events. When the consultants' recommendations are written contemporaneously, there is little room for ambiguity or miscommunication. In the example above, the consultant did not see or examine the patient. She did not have an opportunity to review the data on the patient. Any decision she rendered would have been based on insufficient information and could lead to a decision that may not be in the patient's interest.

Consults are a necessary part of the practice of emergency medicine. "It is the process by which emergency physicians (EPs) request other specialists (consultants) to participate in the care of the ED patient. By the end of this process, the consultant should provide one of the following recommendations: admit, discharge with or without consultant follow-up, or consult another specialty." Some may be reluctant to get a consult, but one study at a large Army hospital showed that the consult rate for some EPs is nearly 40%.

The bottom line is that consults and referrals are an important part of careful emergency medicine practice. Consults should be well documented and should hopefully aid in the decision process. A curbside consult can leave you empty handed with nothing to support your decision. If you are going to get a consult, get one to protect you, the patient, and the consultant. Leave the curbside consult on the curbside.

SUGGESTED READINGS

Cortazzo JM, Guertler AT, Rice MM. Consultation and referral patterns from a teaching hospital emergency department. *Am J Emerg Med*. 1993;11:456–459.

Lee RS, Woods R, Bullard M, et al. Consultations in the emergency department: A systematic review of the literature. *Emerg Med J*. 2008;25(1):4–9.

Lee RS, Woods R, Bullard M, et al. Consultations in the emergency department: A systematic review of the literature. *Emerg Med J*. 2008;25(1):4–9 [Review].

Woods RA, Lee R, Ospina MB, et al. Consultation outcomes in the emergency department: Exploring rates and complexity. *CJEM*. 2008;10(1):25–31.

73

GIVING BAD NEWS, IT IS BETTER TO BE DIRECT

SHARON BORD, MD

Working in the emergency department can be an unpredictable job. One thing that remains constant is that the role of delivering bad news to patients and their families will fall on the emergency medicine physician. The optimal way to discuss these topics is yet to be determined. Although there are many variations and options for the ideal communication style, a central question remains: is it better to deliver the news in a direct and succinct fashion or is a long drawn-out explanation preferred?

Before this topic can be explored further, it is imperative that we define what is meant by the term "bad news." Ptacek and Eberhardt define bad news as information that "…results in a cognitive, behavioral, or emotional deficit in the person receiving the bad news that persists for some time after the news is received." Another definition states bad news pertains to "a situation where there is either a feeling of no hope, a threat to a person's mental or physical well being, a risk of upsetting an established lifestyle, or where a message is given which conveys to an individual fewer choices in his or her life." Both of these definitions highlight the fact that there are traditional forms of bad news such as telling a family member of a trauma patient that he or she has passed away or is critically injured and less traditional concepts: telling a taxi cab driver who had a seizure that he is now unable to drive.

Discussing these difficult topics can be challenging for providers. The emergency department provides a unique environment, as there is little time to establish rapport with the patients and their family. How the patient and family perceive the discussion of bad news is often hard to judge. Jurkovich et al. set out to explore what family members most value after having been told that their significant other passed away in the emergency department or intensive care unit following trauma. A retrospective survey was administered to 54 family members of 48 patients who had died. The most important features of delivering bad news were judged to be the attitude of the news giver (ranked most important by 72%), clarity of the message, privacy, and knowledge or ability to answer questions. The attire of the news giver, a controversial topic in the emergency department, was ranked as least important being valued by only 3%.

Oftentimes, one is first presented with the task of delivering bad news shortly after he or she begins his or her postgraduate medical training. Residents and physicians have been found in multiple studies to experience discomfort with the psychosocial issues that surround the delivery of unpleasant information. When asked open-ended questions about this topic, residents agreed that using unclear language resulted in confusion and misunderstanding for the patient and their families. One resident said "I never say passed away because I had an episode where someone did not understand what I was saying." Additionally, when physicians watched videotaped consultations of more than 3,000 patients, they felt as if their performance was worse when discussing palliation than when discussing potentially curative treatment.

Research has demonstrated that if bad news is poorly communicated it can cause confusion, long-lasting distress, and resentment, and, if done well, it can assist in understanding, acceptance, and adjustment. Certainty exists that health care workers need additional training to aid in their knowledge and ability to deliver bad, sad, or difficulty news in medicine. Further research is needed to help determine how to best teach someone to be an effective deliverer of bad news and what patients and their family members value most in these challenging situations. It appears that this much is known, that a caring attitude and a succinct and clear message are valuable when delivering bad news.

SUGGESTED READINGS

Dosanjh S, Barnes J, Bhandari M. Barriers to breaking bad news among medical and surgical residents. *Med Educ*. 2001;35(3):197–205.

Fallowfield L, Jenkins V. Communicating sad, bad and difficult news in medicine. *Lancet*. 2004;363:312–319.

Jurkovich G, Pierce B, Pananen L, et al. Giving bad news: The family perspective. *J Trauma*. 2000;48:865–873.

74

KNOW HOW TO PREPARE YOUR EMERGENCY DEPARTMENT FOR PANDEMIC INFLUENZA

MELINDA J. MORTON, MD AND THOMAS D. KIRSCH, MD, MPH

An outbreak of pandemic influenza is the one of the most likely—and most overwhelming—disaster scenarios U.S. emergency departments (EDs) will face in the next decade. Such an event would lead to an estimated 1.9 million American deaths and 10 to 30 million hospitalizations, according to Department of Health and Human Services (HHS) estimates (assuming the strains of influenza were similar in virulence to those seen in the 1918 to 1919 outbreak). These estimates are particularly troubling given the recent report from the Institute of Medicine indicating that hospitals and EDs across the country are already operating at or near peak capacity. The 2003 Severe Acute Respiratory Syndrome (SARS) outbreak in Toronto, which infected 375 people and killed 44, revealed major shortcomings in measures to protect local health care workers, which has been attributed to increasing the death toll.

Several recent survey studies found that in the event of a major disease outbreak, as many as 50% of health care providers may not report to work, largely due to concerns about disease exposure and the need to care for family members during such an outbreak. In order to provide health care in times of heightened need, it will be necessary for hospitals, and EDs in particular, to develop reliable plans and effectively communicate those plans to the staff.

HHS published its Pandemic Influenza Preparedness Plan in November of 2005; more recently, HHS published specific guidelines for influenza planning for general medical clinics and emergency medical transporters. Notably, no official guidelines for EDs and emergency medical providers currently exist, and systematic quantification of ED and emergency provider preparedness for a pandemic influenza or a similar major infectious disease outbreak has not been performed to date.

Because of this deficit in pandemic planning, a novel 15-item pandemic preparedness score for EDs was devised by Morton and Kirsch. This score enables quantification of the preparedness of individual EDs in the United States for an outbreak of pandemic influenza, in relation to published general medical clinic guidelines from the Department of HHS, and other best-practice recommendations in the academic literature. Although not necessarily a comprehensive tool, this score provides quantification of the presence of the major components of pandemic influenza preparedness. The elements of the score are outlined in greater detail in *Table 74.1*, as well as the HHS guidelines for primary care clinics upon which segments of the survey are based.

TABLE 74.1	ELEMENTS OF THE PANDEMIC INFLUENZA/ DISEASE OUTBREAK PREPAREDNESS SCORE

1. Presence of a hospital plan

2. Presence of an ED plan

3. Staffing augmentation plan

4. Surveillance plan

5. Patient triage plan

6. Existence of adequate supplies of personal protective equipment

7. Dissemination of plan to staff

8. Occupational health plan

9. Volunteer management plan

10. Conducting a drill to test the plan

11. Vaccine and antiviral medication triage plan

12. Ventilator triage plan

13. Additional ED space plan

14. Plan to quarantine patients

15. Estimated resource needs for an outbreak

Basic elements of influenza outbreak planning, according to this modified HHS model, include the following major components: (1) Command and control, to include membership on local influenza task forces and presence of communications systems with public health authorities; (2) development and dissemination of a written plan; and (3) components of the written plan. The third component was further divided into the following categories: (a) surveillance and detection, (b) triage and patient flow, (c) personnel (health care providers and staff), (d) supplies and infrastructure, and (e) communications. The personnel category was further divided into the subcomponents of (i) occupational health, (ii) staffing shortages, (iii) credentialing of volunteer providers, and (iv) education and training of health care workers.

Many EDs do not have a written plan, and fewer still have disseminated this plan to their staff. This lack of preparedness could potentially lead to preventable deaths in the event of even a small disease outbreak—as witnessed by the 2003 SARS outbreak in Toronto.

The paucity of care providers during a potential outbreak raises further concerns when many EDs plan to use volunteers or hire temporary staff during a pandemic. It is questionable that these categories of providers will even be available. Not only have prior studies shown that many health care workers will not work during a pandemic, but the widespread nature of the epidemic will mean that all facilities will be attempting to supplement their staff from the same small population of people. It is also unclear that volunteer health workers will respond and place themselves at danger, or have the skills necessary to provide emergency care. In order to combat the projected staffing shortages, it is recommended that EDs maintain large lists of trained professionals and hold quarterly or biannual drills to keep their volunteer providers engaged in community efforts.

CONCLUSIONS

Current data suggest an alarming deficit in preparedness for pandemic influenza and other disease outbreaks in U.S. EDs, according to published guidelines from HHS and other best practice guidelines in the academic literature. These deficits in preparedness appear to be related in part to ED size. ED directors and administrators may benefit from the structured approach to pandemic influenza and other disease outbreak planning.

SUGGESTED READINGS

American College of Emergency Physicians. Nation's Emergency Physicians Present 10-point Plan for Avoiding Mass Casualties from Pandemic Flu Outbreak or Other Disaster. From Testimony of Dr. David Seaburg's testimony before subcommittees of House Committee on Homeland Security, February 8, 2006. Available at: http://www.acep.org/webportal/Newsroom/NR/general/2006/020806.htm

Assessment of States' Operating Plans to Combat Pandemic Influenza. Available at: http://pandemicflu.gov/plan/states/state_assessment.html. Accessed February 11, 2009.

Christian MD, Hawryluck L, Wax RS, et al. Development of a triage protocol for critical care during an influenza pandemic. *CMAJ*. 2006;175(11):1377–1381.

Ehrenstein BP, Hanses F, Salzberger B. Influenza pandemic and professional duty: Family or patients first? A survey of hospital employees. *BMC Public Health*. 2006;6:311.

Emergency Medical Service and Non-Emergent (Medical) Transport Organizations Pandemic Influenza Planning Checklist, U.S. Department of Health and Human Services' Pandemic Flu website. Available at: http://www.pandemicflu.gov/plan/pdf/ems.pdf. Accessed January 22, 2007.

Greenberg MI, Hendrickson RG, CIMERC, et al. Report of the CIMERC/Drexel University emergency department terrorism preparedness consensus panel. *Acad Emerg Med*. 2003;10(7):783–788.

HHS Pandemic Influenza Plan, U.S. Department of Health and Human Services, November 2005. Available at: http://www.hhs.gov/pandemicflu/plan/pdf/HHSPandemicInfluenza Plan.pdf. Accessed January 22, 2007.

Higgins W, Wainright C, Lu N, Carrico R. Assessing hospital preparedness using an instrument based on the Mass Casualty Disaster Plan Checklist: Results of a statewide survey. *Am J Infect Control*. 2004;32(6):327–332.

Institute of Medicine Report, Hospital-Based Emergency Care: At the Breaking Point, June 2006; 14. National Academy of Medicine. Available at: http://books.nap.edu/openbook.php?record_id=11621&page=14. Accessed January 24, 2007.

Irvin C, Cindrich L, Patterson W, et al. Hospital personnel response during a hypothetical influenza pandemic: Will they come to work? *Acad Emerg Med*. 2007;14(Suppl 1):13.

Kick JL, O'Laughlin DT. Concept of operations for triage of mechanical ventialation in an epidemic. *Acad Emerg Med*. 2006;13(2):223–229.

Kwan J. SARS report says Ontario failed health care workers. Reuters News Service, January 9, 2007. Available at: http://today.reuters.com/news/ArticleNews.aspx?type=healthNews&

story ID=2007–01–09T233717Z_01_N09170488_RTRUKOC_0_US-SARS.xml&pageN umber=0&imageid=&cap=&sz=13&WTModLoc=NewsArt-C1-ArticlePage2. Accessed January 22, 2007.

Medical Offices and Clinics Pandemic Influenza Planning Checklist, U.S. Department of Health and Human Services' Pandemic Flu website. Available at: http://www.pandemic-flu.gov/plan/pdf/medofficesclinics.pdf. Accessed January 22, 2007.

Morton MJ, McManus JG, Kelen GD, et al. Emergency department preparedness for pandemic influenza in the US: A survey of medical directors and department chairs. *Ann Emerg Med.* 2008;52(4):S150.

75

LEARN HOW TO INTERACT WITH CONSULTANTS APPROPRIATELY

ARJUN S. CHANMUGAM, MD, MBA

CASE

It is 6:39 PM on a Friday evening. Public ambulance has dropped off a 23-year-old patient who has been struck by a baseball in the right eye. After a thorough and complete evaluation, you determine that the patient has a right orbital blowout fracture without any apparent vision loss or cranial nerve involvement. The patient and his family are requesting a specialist consultation. Because you think it is warranted, you contact the plastic surgeon on call. The ensuing conversation with the surgeon ends prematurely because the surgeon refuses to come in and is upset that he was called. You have negotiated an appointment for the patient the next day at 11:30 AM. Although you feel some relief that you have an appointment for your patient, you have the lingering sentiment that maybe it is true consultants are just mean people…

Consultants are an important part of emergency medicine practice. The proportion of physician consultations in the Emergency Department (ED) ranges from 20% to 60%. As D. Hexter reported in ACEP's risk management publication, "Unfortunately, all emergency physicians, at some time in their practices, probably have experienced an unsatisfactory interaction with a consultant. The causes of these unsatisfactory interactions are many, including everything from personality differences to someone 'just having a bad day' to true disagreements about the appropriateness of care. More worrisome causes include incompetent or impaired consultants. One major source of unhappiness among consultants is the increasing burden of the uninsured and underinsured among emergency department patients." Some say that there is a greater concentration of incivility from consultants in academic centers, because community consultants better appreciate the need for referrals. Regardless of geographic location and type of practice, it seems inevitable that emergency physicians will have at least one less than pleasant experience with a consultant.

Although the literature is sparse on the subject, it appears that most interactions that occur with consultants are handled in a collegial manner. Despite being uncommon, an unpleasant interaction can trigger strong sentiments and force contemplation. Consideration of the quiescent angry gene that becomes unmasked during an ED consult suddenly makes a little more sense. Perhaps there is a secret code that is passed down through generations of consultants to make sure that every tenth consult is unpleasant, making sure that the emergency physicians are happy with the other nine. Fantastic as these theories may seem, most of us who have practiced long enough have witnessed bizarre enough interactions that sometimes we question if maybe these and other such strange theories contain any truth.

Should we have sympathy for the overworked consultant who seems overly perturbed? Is it reasonable to ask for restraint to excuse consultant bad behavior? The merits of such sentiments are debatable and highly dependent on your own battle scars and level of interpersonal generosity. Nevertheless, as sure as you can be that the last IV site that will infiltrate on your hypovolemic patient, you can be sure that you will meet a consultant who is not playing nice in the sandbox. That much is an eventuality; how you negotiate a successful outcome is more variable and more important.

We as emergency physicians are held to a higher standard. We do not have the luxury to return rudeness for rudeness, whether they may be nurses, patients, colleagues, administrators, or other support staff. We have a job to do and frankly, we are too busy to harbor biases that may impair our productivity. Instead, individuals should be treated as honorably as possible, as we advance the agenda that is critical to our professional well-being—the safety of our patients. The issue is not about an individual's character, but rather the focus should be a negotiated outcome for your patient's best interest.

It is always helpful to remember the grade school maxim—pretend you are in the other person's shoes before making judgments. But really, forget judging and simply learn how to negotiate well with others who are reluctant to do anything more for you or your patient. Negotiation is a real skill that must be practiced, honed, and perfected at every opportunity.

There will be times when you meet with what appears to be the "mean" consultant. Resist the urge to judge whether this is true; it is not something that we have luxury to reflect on, especially during a shift. The key is to understand their plight enough to leverage an optimal treatment plan for your patient. If the consultant shows a pattern of inconsideration, unsettled conflicts with consultants should be resolved in accordance with hospital policy. Documentation of unacceptable behaviors with a written review, including a neutral but influential third party, at some later time may be an acceptable course to help minimize their maladaptive behaviors. In the heat of the shift, the paramount consideration is your patients' safety; for that, an objective, neutral and dispassionate assessment of the patient's needs in the context of available resources is key to implementing the optimal treatment plan. Whether there is a dormant angry gene that has suddenly been unmasked makes for interesting discussion, but negotiating an acceptable agreement should be the prime focus.

SUGGESTED READINGS

Hexter DA. *Working With Consultants*. ACEP: Foresight; 2002:53.
Lee RS, Woods R, Bullard M, et al. Consultations in the emergency department: A systematic review of the literature. *Emerg Med J*. 2008;25(1):4–9.
Woods RA, Lee R, Ospina MB, et al. Consultation outcomes in the emergency department: Exploring rates and complexity. *CJEM*. 2008;10(1):25–31.

76

MAKE "CUSTOMER SERVICE" A PRIORITY WHEN WORKING IN THE EMERGENCY DEPARTMENT ... OR YOU'll BE LOOKING FOR A NEW JOB SOON!

EDWARD S. BESSMAN, MD, MBA

Patient satisfaction has been a concern of hospital management for decades, primarily in the context of the "hotel service" aspects of hospital inpatient activities. On the basis of patient satisfaction, as measured in surveys, hospitals could differentiate themselves from their competition and gain market share. With time the process has become more sophisticated and pervasive, but until relatively recently emergency departments received little scrutiny. Likewise, much of the focus in the past has been on hospital personnel, but this too has evolved to include physicians and other providers. An important change has been the widespread public availability of survey results. What used to be a tool for hospital management to fine-tune its service lines is now a report card that individuals can use to select their health care providers and settings. However, the biggest impact will likely be from the coupling of reimbursement to satisfaction scores, a trend that has taken on increased significance with the entrance of the Center for Medicare and Medicaid Services (CMS) onto the scene.

Emergency departments (EDs) and emergency physicians (EPs) have been slow to embrace patient satisfaction for a variety of reasons. A common objection is that the methodology of the survey exaggerates small differences. Most commonly, raw scores for a given institution, representing aggregate patient responses on a five-point scale, are then converted to a percentile ranking of all participating hospitals. Small differences in the raw scores, on the order of a few percent, can lead to enormous differences in the percentile rank. Examining actual patient responses reveals that top performing hospitals receive more 5s (very good) than 4s (good), whereas for lower performers this is reversed. The typical ED objection is that there is nothing wrong with "good." This obscures the fact that most patients, even when not particularly pleased with their experience, are reluctant to give lower scores. Other objections include EDs are crowded with inpatient boarders, the patient population is difficult, the facility is too old or too small, a poor payer mix, and so forth. Often at the root of these comments is the unspoken belief that the mission of an ED is to save lives, not to make patients happy. This belies the fact that many EDs are top performers, in spite of having cramped or old facilities; difficult geographic locations; challenging patient populations; and unfavorable reimbursement environments.

The first step toward improving patient satisfaction is to broaden the focus, as embodied in the concept of "service excellence." At its most basic, emergency medicine is a service industry. Moreover, besides the patients, the emergency physician has many other customers, including families, consultants, and staff (both internal and external to the ED). The idea behind "service" is not that EPs are "servants" or "waiters," but that the patient's perception of the care given is just as important as the quality of the care (if not more so). Patients cannot easily tell whether a given EP practiced quality medicine, but they can easily determine if that person cared. That is where "excellence" comes into play: delivering quality medical care in a way that emphasizes the importance of caring and with the goal of finding and doing those things that elevate everyone's performance. Rather than being a separate program service excellence must be woven into the very fabric of the ED.

The benefits of improved service excellence are manifold. Obviously, patients will be happier. Less obviously, but no less important, staff will be happier; it is a positive feedback loop. EDs with higher patient satisfaction scores are simply more enjoyable places to work. Staff who are happy in their work and feel appreciated by management and by each other are better able to deal with the inevitable problem with patients, without letting it diminish their professionalism. Furthermore, patients who feel that their providers were caring and concerned are much less likely to initiate a malpractice action, independent of the quality of the medical care. For many patients, a good doctor with a bad bedside manner will not get the benefit of the doubt. Finally, as noted above, CMS has initiated a reimbursement plan that takes into account patient satisfaction scores. The program is called the Hospital Consumer Assessment of Healthcare Providers and Systems (HCAHPS). According to this plan, a portion of a hospital's inpatient reimbursement from CMS will be tied to its patient satisfaction scores. Since a majority of inpatient admissions begin in the ED, service excellence in the ED will become important to the hospital's bottom line. Eventually, CMS will tie a portion of ED professional fee reimbursement to patient satisfaction. Those EDs that have not developed robust service excellence programs will see their reimbursements decline. Emergency physicians who do not know and practice the language of service excellence will be at a competitive disadvantage.

SUGGESTED READINGS

CAHPS Hospital Survey. *Centers for Medicare & Medicaid Services*. Baltimore, MD. Available at: http://www.hcahpsonline.org. Accessed February 28, 2009.

O'Cathain A, Coleman P, Nicholl J. Characteristics of the emergency and urgent care system important to patients: A qualitative study. *J Health Serv Res Policy*. 2008;13 (Suppl 2):19–25.

Pines JM, Iyer S, Disbot M, et al. The effect of emergency department crowding on patient satisfaction for admitted patients. *Acad Emerg Med*. 2008;15(9):825–831.

Stelfox HT, Gandhi TK, Orav EJ, et al. The relation of patient satisfaction with complaints against physicians and malpractice lawsuits. *Am J Med*. 2005;18(10):1126–1133.

77

UNDERSTAND DECISION-MAKING FATIGUE AND HOW IT INFLUENCES YOUR OF CLINICAL JUDGEMENT

ARJUN S. CHANMUGAM, MD, MBA

Emergency medicine is unique for many reasons. One of the most singular aspects of this specialty is the density of decision making that must take place during a shift. There are few other situations where a person has to make as many decisions of a significant magnitude as he or she does in an emergency department (ED).

Decision making in the ED is an ongoing process. In many cases, the way emergency physicians make decisions early in a shift is somewhat different than those made at the end of a shift.

Indeed the concept of the shift has at its core the understanding that decision making needs to be transferred to someone else at a given time. The ability of one individual to succeed in high-density decision making is finite. At some point, care of patients must be transferred to someone else with fresh decision-making capability.

Clearly, there are multiple reasons to have shifts in emergency medicine. Well-being issues, intellectual fatigue, and physical demands are all reasons to limit an emergency physician's clinical time and conform to shift work mentality. Shift work in medicine has its origins in emergency medicine. At one point, many other specialists considered the word "shift" a four-letter word. Now, as is so often the case, the paradigm created by emergency medicine is being emulated in other specialties. More and more specialties are adopting mechanisms to ensure that decision makers have a finite time to provide clinical direction before they transfer care to someone else. The recognition that decision making is intellectually and sometimes physically and spiritually taxing is becoming more universal. Intellectual endurance in this model becomes a critical issue, as are strategies to improve and/or sustain that endurance.

With that in mind, it is well worthwhile to consider a shift in three phases—the beginning of a shift, the middle, and the end. Each phase has its own attributes. It may be useful to consider specific strategies for each phase.

At the beginning of the shift, the astute clinical decision maker, the physician, should be well prepared to tackle clinical problems. Two basic recommendations include preparation activities the shift actually begins with. The first strategy would be to prepare oneself mentally prior to starting the shift. Preparation would include mental focusing such that competing non–emergency medicine issues are appropriately compartmentalized to avoid intellectual interference or distraction. The second strategy would be to ensure that proper rest, nutrition, and hydration are obtained before the start of the shift.

In most cases, decision making at the beginning of the shift is usually not overly challenging as compared to the other two phases. This changes by the middle of the shift. The first phase events can influence the second phase depending on how the practitioner views the events. In most cases, by the middle of the shift, fatigue, hunger, and bodily needs should be consciously addressed. Most emergency physicians who work in a busy shift will have to spend a fair amount of time walking and talking, going from place to place verbally communicating with patients, families, nurses, and colleagues. Insensible losses may be accentuated during a shift, and rehydration is the key. According to some reports, the average American is chronically dehydrated, and emergency providers are no exception. Rehydration should be a priority. Light fare foods that can be consumed easily should also be considered. Heavy meals should be avoided as they may cause a postprandial drowsiness.

At the end of shift, clinical decision-making fatigue is likely to be a factor. These are the times that many physicians rely on their training to help sort through decisions, as more intellectual shortcuts are likely to be taken. A conscious effort should be directed toward thoroughness—in both data acquisition and data analysis. A self-reminder to listen carefully to patients and support staff may be helpful. Attention to potential biases should also be considered, as fatigue could make one more subconsciously vulnerable to biases.

Although the above-described strategies are potentially useful for any emergency provider, each individual should know his or her own strengths and weaknesses. Armed with that knowledge, each individual should develop his or her own game plan that addresses his or her unique situation in order to continually improve his or her decision-making endurance.

Emergency medicine is a demanding specialty. The density of decision making is extremely high. With proper attention and phase specific strategies, it may be possible to lessen the effects of decision-making fatigue.

SUGGESTED READINGS

Harrison Y, Horne JA. The impact of sleep deprivation on decision making: A review. *Psychol Appl*. 2000;6(3):236–49.

Kassam KS, Koslov K, Mendes WB. Decisions under distress: Stress profiles influence anchoring and adjustment. *Psychol Sci*. 2009 [Epub ahead of print].

LeBlanc VR. The effects of acute stress on performance: Implications for health professions education. *Acad Med*. 2009;84(10 Suppl):S25–33.

Samkoff JS, Jacques CH. A review of studies concerning effects of sleep deprivation and fatigue on residents' performance. *Acad Med*. 1991;66(11):687–93.

78

UNDERSTAND THE COST OF EMERGENCY DEPARTMENT GRIDLOCK

EDWARD S. BESSMAN, MD, MBA

From a system's perspective, each bed or treatment space in the ED is similar to an assembly line. The difference is that rather than the product (i.e., the patient) moving along a path, in the ED, resources flow around the patient. Both processes, however, are exactly similar in one important respect: if the finished product cannot be "off-loaded" at the end of the line, then the line grinds to a halt. In the case of the ED, if the patient cannot be dispositioned (discharged or admitted) then that bed is out of service for new patients. The resulting gridlock means that incremental patients cannot be accommodated in that treatment space, and the ED becomes overcrowded. Besides the obvious detrimental impact on throughput and patient care, this also results in losing the opportunity to deliver incremental billable services. However, unless this lost opportunity is explicitly accounted for, it remains invisible and the pressure to alleviate gridlock is, from a financial perspective, less compelling.

What is the opportunity cost of ED gridlock? That is, what revenue is foregone by not being able to turn over beds and accommodate incremental patients? A simple way to estimate this would be total revenues divided by total hours, but this is static and insensitive to seasonality and to performance improvements. There are more complex ways reported in the literature (such as estimates of revenue lost by walkouts and ambulance diversion divided by estimates of hours of gridlock) but these are labor intensive and likewise static and insensitive to change. The spreadsheet found in the third reference makes it easy to get a rough idea of the opportunity cost of an hour of gridlock. The inputs are data that are generally available from hospital and professional practice databases: ED census, admission/discharge percentages, and throughput data and charges. The logic behind the formula is based on this: each incremental patient represents a fraction of a discharge and a fraction of an admission. Additionally, each patient likewise represents an incremental charge. Furthermore, the throughput times for admitted and discharged patients are known. Thus, each hour that passes should result in an average charge related to incremental admissions and an average charge for incremental discharges. The sum of those values represents the charges missed when a bed does not turn over. The calculation can be updated as often as desired.

However, regardless of the method used, the cost is substantial, in the range of $300 to $800 per h. Note that it does not matter if the bed is blocked by an inpatient boarder, a consultant delay, or an overlong ED workup: the cost is real and is quantifiable. Furthermore, the costs are additive in that the total cost of gridlock is the sum for each bed that is tied up and out of production. Since most EDs routinely have multiple beds blocked simultaneously, the lost revenue potential is considerable. Conversely, this is the revenue that would become available as a result of efforts made to reduce ED gridlock. From a financial perspective the decision to add incremental resources becomes a straightforward comparison of the cost of the additional resources compared to the revenue captured by the reduction in ED gridlock. Some interventions such as building and staffing inpatient capacity would be quite costly. Others, such as process redesign, require much more modest expenditures. Having a working estimate of the potential revenue that can be recovered is an important foundation for framing the discussion, and this method for calculating the opportunity cost is readily accessible to any ED manager.

Certainly, a complete economic accounting of the costs of ED gridlock and of its potential solutions is quite a bit more involved than this simplified treatment, but the central issue remains: there is a compelling financial argument to be made for solving the problem of blocked ED beds. This is completely in concert with similar arguments made from the perspectives of clinical care and safety. The viability of emergency medicine as a specialty and of EDs as the nation's health care safety net requires that emergency physicians marshal every argument available in order to secure the resources needed for timely and efficient patient care. Neglecting to account for the opportunity cost of ED gridlock lessens the financial pressure to search for a solution.

SUGGESTED READINGS

Bessman E. *ED Gridlock Cost Calculator*. Available at: http://sites.google.com/site/edgridlockcostcalculator/

Falvo T, Grove L, Stachura R, et al. The opportunity loss of boarding admitted patients in the emergency department. *Acad Emerg Med*. 2007;14(4):332–337.

Howell E, Bessman E, Kravet S, et al. Active bed management by hospitalists and emergency department throughput. *Ann Intern Med*. 2008;149:804–810.

79

UNDERSTAND THE DOCUMENTATION REQUIREMENTS OF MIDLEVEL PRACTITIONERS

EDWARD S. BESSMAN, MD, MBA

Increasingly, emergency physicians will find themselves working alongside a physician assistant (PA) or nurse practitioner (NP). Collectively, PAs and NPs are referred to by several different names, including midlevel provider or midlevel practitioner (MLP), physician extender (PE), or nonphysician provider/practitioner (NPP). The Center for Medicare and Medicaid Services (CMS) uses the term NPP.

NPPs are advanced practice clinicians who are authorized to practice medicine under the supervision of a licensed physician. Like physicians, NPPs are granted a license to practice by the individual states. Therefore, the scope of practice, degree of supervision, documentation requirements etc. can vary from state to state. Furthermore, in hospital-based settings such as the Emergency Department (ED), NPPs are generally members of the medical staff and as such are granted privileges by the hospital, which also define their scope of practice. Thus, in any given ED, the degree of autonomy for NPPs in the practice can range from very much to very little. Likewise the skill set can vary considerably; in some EDs NPPs actively manage high acuity patients and do many procedures, whereas in other EDs NPPs primarily see less urgent patients in a "fast track" setting. Consequently, it is important for an emergency physician joining a practice, or an emergency medicine resident on a new rotation, to become familiar with the roles and activities of his or her NPP colleagues.

What are the documentation requirements for NPPs in the ED? There are at least three perspectives that are useful in formulating an answer: statutory, risk management, and reimbursement. Generally, the statutory requirements are clear-cut and are spelled out by the state licensing board and hospital bylaws. In particular, the issue is concurrent oversight and cosignature by the supervising physician versus delayed or even no cosignature. In some states, NPPs may be able to see and treat ED patients independently, doing all of their own charting and without the need for a physician cosignature. Other jurisdictions may require a face-to-face encounter between the emergency physician and the patient with concurrent documentation in the medical record. It is absolutely vital to follow the letter of the law in this regard. Failure to provide concurrent oversight and/or cosignature where such is required, puts the medical licensure of both the NPP and the emergency physician in jeopardy, and is a flagrant malpractice risk.

From a risk management perspective, documentation requirements are much less cut and dry. Certainly, as noted above, any statutory regulations must be followed, but in jurisdictions where there is substantial latitude the question arises of how much concurrent oversight and documentation is reasonable. Risk managers will always say "more is better" when it comes to documentation. The reality is that, in general, NPPs do a better job of documenting clinical care than most physicians. What, then, is gained by additional documentation by the supervising physician? For patients with presentations of low complexity and low risk, probably very little is gained. With more complicated situations and presentations involving greater risk, it makes sense for the NPP to discuss the case with the supervising physician who should then document his or her involvement. Depending on the medical issue at hand, the supervising physician would likely need to see and examine the patient, and of course, write a note. Most ED practices that employ NPPs have evolved guidelines, either formal or informal, that indicate which patients need the concurrent involvement of the supervising physician.

The documentation issue is much more straightforward when it comes to reimbursement. Most third-party payers follow the rules set by CMS: When a patient is seen by an NPP without the direct involvement of the supervising physician, then the charge should be billed under the NPP's name and it will be reimbursed at 85% of the physician fee. If, however, there is "face-to-face" involvement of the supervising physician with the patient and the physician leaves a note, then the bill goes out under the physician's name at 100%. CMS specifies neither what "face-to-face" means nor what constitutes adequate documentation, but it is generally agreed that the supervising physician needs only to speak personally with the patient and write a single line to that effect: "I have seen the patient and agree with the findings" etc. If the supervising physician elicits additional history or examines the patient and documents those findings, then not only can the billing be at 100% but the extra information also can be used to increase the evaluation and management code if appropriate.

It is important not to confuse the supervising physician documentation requirements for NPPs and resident physicians. If there is no attending physician involvement or documentation with a patient seen by an NPP then, as noted above, the charge is submitted at 85%. For a patient seen by a resident physician, if there is no documentation of supervising physician involvement then no bill can be submitted under CMS rules. Another potential source of confusion is that while a resident physician may supervise an NPP from a medical perspective, in general the statutory requirements would not be met; the physician supervisor of the NPP must be an employee of the practice.

SUGGESTED READINGS

Direct Billing and Payment for Non-Physician Practitioner (NPP) Services Furnished to Hospital Inpatients and Outpatients. Center for Medicare and Medicaid Services. Available at: http://www.cms.hhs.gov/Transmittals/downloads/R1168CP.pdf. Accessed February 28, 2009.

Ellis GL, Brandt TE. Use of physician extenders and fast tracks in United States emergency departments. *Am J Emerg Med*. 1997;16:229–232.

Guidelines for Teaching Physicians, Interns, and Residents. Center for Medicare and Medicaid Services. Available at: www.cms.hhs.gov/MLNProducts/downloads/gdelinesteachgresfctsht.pdf. Accessed on February 28, 2009.

80

"Scoop and run" versus "stay and play": Which method is optimal for trauma patients?

Sharon Bord, MD

After an individual has sustained a trauma, time is of the essence. Especially in the case of penetrating trauma or severe hemorrhage, definitive therapy is often needed in the emergency department or operating room. Therefore, it is important to discuss the optimal involvement of field responders in prehospital care; for example, should they "scoop and run" to the hospital or "stay and play" in the field?

Trauma patients have been noted to sustain death in a predictable pattern with 50% occurring at the scene, 30% within a few hours, and the remaining 20% within days or weeks related to sepsis or multiorgan failure. Patients who can be affected by increasing time at the incident or accident scene are the middle 30% who have been noted to decline clinically within the first few hours. This illustrates the concept of the "golden hour" in trauma situations.

Within the United States, it has become standard for trauma patients to be transported by ambulances staffed with individuals trained in advanced life support (ALS) which extends their ability to perform procedures, including intravenous (IV) placement, endotracheal intubation, and cervical spine immobilization, which can become quite time-consuming. The concept of prehospital ALS care was born in 1967, and although it has been shown to be beneficial in patients experiencing cardiac arrest, there has been insufficient data to determine the benefit to the trauma patient. IV access is one such procedure that has been found to significantly prolong scene time, with an effort to obtain access taking anywhere from 2 to 13 additional minutes. It is important to additionally note that following IV access, the amount of fluid that is given en route is oftentimes insignificant. Interestingly, of the crystalloid that is given, only one third will remain in the vasculature.

In Canada, emergency medical services (EMSs) are performed by three contrasting systems: in Montreal, physicians provide ALS care; in Toronto, paramedics provide ALS care; and in Quebec City, emergency medical technicians provide basic life support (BLS) care only. When these three systems were compared, it was found that the overall mortality for trauma patients transported by BLS only was 18% compared to 29% for the ALS group. The study concluded that in urban areas with level 1 trauma centers, there is no benefit to on-site ALS. Another study by Seamon et al. examined patients transported to a level 1 trauma center in Philadelphia who underwent emergency department thoracotomy. Patients who had been transported to the hospital via police or private vehicle had a survival rate to discharge of 17.2% compared with 8.0% for those who were transported by EMS. Patients within the EMS-transported group underwent more prehospital procedures and hence longer transport time to hospital.

However, some ALS skills may be of some benefit to particular subpopulations. Patients who sustained trauma in the rural setting who were transported via ALS, compared with BLS, had a significantly lower death rate. In other reports, endotracheal intubation in the prehospital setting was shown in one study to improve the survival rate from 64% to 74% in patients with blunt injury and a Glasgow Coma Score of 8 or less. Intubation can also improve oxygenation, improve ventilation, and prevent aspiration. There exists concern regarding the complications of field intubation. Stewart et al. showed that paramedic intubation was successful in 90% of patients with cardiac arrest but only 79% of trauma patients. Prehospital intubation has been shown to be most beneficial in head trauma patients, but more research needs to be completed regarding the benefit in other trauma patients.

There are certain groups of patients who deserve special consideration when discussing prehospital interventions. Bickell et al. prospectively studied patients older than 16 years of age who had suffered from penetrating torso trauma with a blood pressure of 90 or less. Within this study, the subset of patients who had received preoperative IV therapy had a trend toward more intraoperative blood loss, an increased length of hospital stay, and decreased survival and discharge rates. Therefore, it was concluded that, contrary to popular belief, IV therapy be withheld in this subset of patients until definitive operative repair.

The concept of the "golden hour" in trauma patients would likely indicate that prehospital "scoop and run" would be most beneficial for trauma patients. However, trauma occurs in many different environments and situations, and the "stay and play" philosophy may be superior at times. Regardless of resuscitation time in the field, when a critically ill trauma patient arrives in the emergency department, remember that time is of the essence and that definitive treatment should be obtained as quickly as possible.

SUGGESTED READINGS

Bickell WH, Wall MJ, Pepe PE, et al. Immediate versus delayed fluid resuscitation for hypotensive patients with penetrating torso injuries. *N Engl J Med.* 1994;331:1105–1109.

Liberman M, Mulder D, Lavoie A, et al. Multicenter Canadian study of prehospital trauma care. *Ann Surg.* 2003;237:153–160.

Liberman M, Mulder D, Sampalis J. Advance or basic life support for trauma: Meta-analysis and critical review of the literature. *J Trauma.* 2000;49:584–589.

Seamon M, Fisher C, Gaugham J, et al. Prehospital procedures before emergency department thoracotomy: "Scoop and run" saves lives. *J Trauma.* 2007;63:113–120.

81

TRANSPORTATION TO THE CLOSEST FACILITY IS NOT ALWAYS BEST FOR THE PATIENT

JULIANNA JUNG, MD, FACEP

"When a patient is seriously ill or injured, time is of the essence—the shorter the transport time, the better." This is a common belief among emergency physician and Emergency medical system (EMS) providers alike, but is it true? A growing body of literature suggests that it is not.

Complex patients requiring specialized care often have better outcomes when they are managed in a facility that has the personnel, equipment, and expertise required to meet their unique needs. Transport of these patients to hospitals lacking adequate resources can result in suboptimal or delayed care, leading to poor outcomes. For example, the National Study on the Costs and Outcomes of Trauma found that severely injured trauma victims are 25% less likely to die if they receive care in a level I trauma center compared to a nontrauma center. Another study found that traumatic brain injury patients transported directly to a trauma center had 50% lower short-term mortality compared to those taken to local hospitals and subsequently transferred.

The benefits of direct transport to specialty centers are not only observed in trauma victims. One study reported lower in-hospital mortality for patients with ST-elevation myocardial infarction (STEMI) who are transported directly to hospitals capable of providing percutaneous coronary intervention (PCI): 2% for those taken to PCI centers compared to 9% for those taken to non-PCI hospitals. A later study demonstrated significantly lower door-to-balloon times among STEMI patients transported directly to a PCI center from the field: 69 min for those taken directly to PCI centers compared to 123 min for those taken to non–PCI centers and subsequently transferred. Eighty percent of those transported directly to PCI centers met the national goal door-to-balloon time of 90 min, compared to only 12% of those transported to the closest facility.

It is a commonly held belief that shorter prehospital transport times lead to better outcomes. However, the mortality benefits described above for trauma and STEMI patients were observed despite longer transport times required for patients taken directly to specialty centers from the field. Even in cardiac arrest, transport time has not been proven to affect mortality. A large multicenter trial recently demonstrated that there is no relationship between longer transport intervals and decreased likelihood of survival. Predictors of survival included witnessed cardiac arrest, bystander CPR, short EMS response time, initial rhythm of ventricular fibrillation, and ventricular tachycardia, but *not* short transport time. Given the growing body of evidence that specialized postresuscitation care may improve outcomes in cardiac arrest, it is possible that arrest victims may benefit from direct transport to a specialty care center, bypassing closer facilities on the way.

In short, the closest facility is not always the best. Specialty care has been shown to positively impact mortality and other key outcomes for severely ill and injured patients, and direct transport to such facilities by EMS can reduce delays and guarantee appropriate care for these patients. The longer transport times that would be required for EMS to take patients to specialty centers do not appear to adversely affect outcomes, even in cardiac arrest.

SUGGESTED READINGS

Hartl R, Gerber LM, Iacono L, et al. Direct transport within an organized state trauma system reduces mortality in patients with severe traumatic brain injury. *J Trauma.* 2006;60(6):1250–1256.

LeMay MR, Davies RF, Dionne R, et al. Comparison of early mortality of paramedic-diagnosed ST-elevation myocardial infarction with immediate transport to a designated primary percutaneous coronary intervention center to that of similar patients transported to the nearest hospital. *Am J Cardiol.* 2006;98(10):1329–1333 [Epub 2006 Sep 28].

LeMay MR, So DY, Dionne R, et al. A citywide protocol for primary PCI in ST-segment elevation myocardial infarction. *N Engl J Med.* 2008;358(3):231–240.

MacKenzie EJ, Rivara FP, Jurkovich GJ, et al. A national evaluation of the effect of trauma center care on mortality. *N Engl J Med.* 2006;354:366–378.

Sasser SM, Hunt RC, Sullivent EE, et al. Guidelines for field triage of injured patients: Recommendations of the National Expert Panel on Field Triage. *MMWR Recomm Rep.* 2009;58(RR-1):1–35.

Spaite DW, Stiell IG, Bobrow BJ, et al. Effect of transport interval on out-of-hospital cardiac arrest survival in the OPALS study: Implications for triaging patients to specialized cardiac arrest centers. *Ann Emerg Med.* 2009;54(2):256–257.

82

RESPECT THE MOUTH, PART I: BEWARE THE PITFALLS IN MANAGING BONY ORAL TRAUMA

GERARD DEMERS, DO, DHSC, MPH

Oral trauma is a common primary or secondary presenting complaint to the ED. Leading injuries resulting in oral trauma include motor vehicle accidents, sports injuries, assaults, physical abuse, or falls. (Think contact with head/face = potential oral trauma.) Oral traumas are often overlooked due to life-threatening injuries to the chest, head, and neck. However, loss of airway and possible aspiration of avulsed teeth are also immediate concerns of oral trauma and need to be addressed accordingly. Later complications of overlooked injuries may result in infection, nonunion of a missed fracture, loss of sensation, malnutrition, and weight loss. These can then lead to cosmetic, functional, and psychological impairment when such injuries are overlooked.

Due to the highly vascular nature of the oral soft tissue, bleeding can significantly obscure the view of the oropharynx. A thorough inspection of soft and bony structures should be completed after stabilization of the patient and after achieving hemostasis. After ABCs, assess the patient for signs of avulsed dentition, lacerations, ecchymosis, and obvious fractures, all of which will require further treatment. Avulsed dentition requires a chest radiograph for possible aspiration if missing teeth cannot be located. A change in facial contour or ecchymosis in the floor of the mouth is a diagnostic sign of a mandibular body or symphysis fracture. Abnormal sensation of the lower lip may be present with a displaced mandibular fracture compressing the inferior alveolar nerve; however, a coherent patient is usually required to get this information. Palpate and range the temporal mandibular joint (TMJ) and mandible (malocclusion is highly suggestive of associated fracture and subluxation). A new TMJ click or pop may be heard with dislocations or bony crepitus/step offs with fractures. (It may also be common in patients with a history of bruxism—you can stop grinding your teeth now...) Get the study before attempting to reduce the dislocation! Film evaluation includes either a panorex (during dentist working hours) or a facial computed tomography (CT). Plain x-rays will miss mandibular fractures. A plain mandibular series including oblique views is not as sensitive but will have to suffice if other modalities are not available. If you identify one fracture, look for more: multiple fractures will be present in over a third of mandibular injuries.

Traumatic dislocations are not subtle and patients present with asymmetric facies, difficulty enunciating and fully closing their mouths. This injury occurs when an open mandible is forced inferiorly, generally resulting in an anterior dislocation. This may occur either unilaterally or bilaterally. The dislocations are not usually associated with significant pain unless fractures are present. Unilateral dislocations involve a tilted mandible and bilateral ones have a bulldog underbite (prognathia). Both versions involve muscle spasm and mechanical obstruction by the articular eminence preventing spontaneous reduction. Conscious sedation, muscle relaxants, or analgesics are usually required for the reduction. There are a variety of reduction techniques available, but the key is to not get stuck with your digits clamped in an oral mousetrap. Please use a bite block before attempting the reduction and get the postreduction films. IF you cannot get the reduction, the patient is likely headed to the operating room.

An important point to remember is do NOT close facial lacerations before treating underlying fractures. Lacerations of gingival mucosa are often associated with occult fractures. The commonly used La Fort classifications of facial fractures are associated with frontal or mandible fractures. Several fracture patterns are not included in this classification system involving the palate, medial maxillary arch, dentoalveolar, and anterior maxillary fractures. The action of facial muscles and the angle of fractures determine whether they will pull together or apart. Indications for surgical correction of mandibular fractures include displacement with unfavorable angle, multiple facial fractures, or bilateral displaced condylar fractures. A single dose of prophylactic antibiotics should be given for fractures, which will decrease the postinjury infection complication rate.

While awaiting definitive management from subspecialists, you must temporarily provide pain relief and begin initial treatment while more definitive intervention is planned. Your responsibilities are to exclude life threats, prevent complications, provide patient comfort, and ensure appropriate and timely follow-up care. Most oral traumas can be discharged to home with outpatient specialty follow-up. Patients with dislocations are instructed to abstain from any wide-open mouth activity. A soft collar may be given to support the reduced TMJ as a comfort measure. Diet is confined to soft bland diet or liquids until their appointment. They should be advised to return to the ER if any signs of expanding hematoma, dysphagia, or airway compromise are seen.

SUGGESTED READINGS

Andreasen J, Jensen S, Schwartz O, et al. A systematic review of prophylactic antibiotics in the surgical treatment of maxillofacial fractures. *J Oral Maxillofac Surg.* 2006;64(11): 1664–1668.

Begum P, Jones S. Towards evidence based emergency medicine: Best BETs from the Manchester Royal Infirmary. Radiological diagnosis of mandibular fracture. *J Accid Emerg Med.* 2000;17(1):46–47.

Bringhurst C, Herr R, Aldous J. Oral trauma in the emergency department. *Am J Emerg Med.* 1993;11(5):486–490.

Buitrago-Tellez C, Schilli W, Bohnert M. A comprehensive classification of craniofacial fractures: Postmortem and clinical studies with two- and three-dimensional computed tomography. *Injury.* 2002;33(8):651–668.

Chan T, Harrigan R, Ufberg J, et al. Mandibular reduction. *J Emerg Med.* 2008;34(4): 435–440.

Gassner R, Tuli T, Häch O, et al. Cranio-maxillofacial trauma: A 10 year review of 9543 cases with 21 067 injuries. *J Cranio-Maxillofacial Surg.* 2003;31(1):51–61.

Howes D, Dowling P. Triage and initial evaluation of the oral facial emergency. *Emerg Med Clin North Am.* 2000;18(3):371–378.

Lee K. Epidemiology of mandibular fractures in a tertiary trauma centre. *J Emerg Med.* 2008;25(9):565–568.

Powers M, Wuereshy F. Diagnosis and management of dentoalveolar injuries. In: Fonseca R, Walker R, Betts N, Barber H, eds. *Oral and Maxillofacial Trauma*, Vol 1. Philadelphia, PA: WB Saunders Co; 1997:419–472.

Tuli T, Haechl O, Berger N, et al. Risk assessment for bone fractures in the cranio-maxillo-facial traumatology in the course of our lifetime. *Int J Oral Maxillofac Surg.* 2007;36(11): 1082–1083.

83

RESPECT THE MOUTH, PART II: BEWARE THE PITFALLS IN MANAGING SOFT TISSUE ORAL TRAUMA

EMILY B. J. OSBORN, MD

Intraoral soft tissue injuries are categorized by location: oropharyngeal, soft palate, lips, tongue, and cheek. Soft tissue injuries are often missed (*you didn't look!*) and, at times, improperly treated. Particularly in the case of trauma, a good oral exam must be done with a bright light inspecting the entire area. Complete a thorough neurovascular exam prior to repairing any lesion. This highly vascularized region bleeds profusely but heals quickly.

When inspecting most intraoral lacerations or avulsions, remember the simple things. Anesthetize the area utilizing nerve blocks, with regional blocks preferred. Tetracaine, adrenaline, and cocaine are safe for minor intraoral lesions. Irrigate to avoid infection, and check for foreign bodies. Anticipate more time for repairs, as suturing in the mouth confines your hand movements. Bite blocks help keep the mouth open during inspection and repairs and keep your fingers from becoming cheese sticks for hungry patients.

Lateral oropharyngeal and soft palate injuries are at risk for neurovascular damage and can be life threatening. Neither the mechanism nor the degree of injury predicts the potential for problems (the dreaded but extremely rare carotid thrombosis). In fact, neurovascular complications may not blossom for days after the inciting injury! Soft palate injuries require treatment in three cases: retained foreign body, through-and-through laceration, and large hanging flaps. Posterior pharyngeal wall injuries are uncommon and difficult to evaluate. Posterior pharyngeal wall injuries with neurologic findings, possible vascular injury, or hemodynamically unstable patients require a CT scan. Major bleeds mandate intubation and surgical consultation. Posterior pharyngeal lacerations rarely lead to retropharyngeal abscess or significant pneumomediastinum. Oropharyngeal and soft palate injuries can usually be treated conservatively and discharged to reliable homes with instructions on infection and airway compromise.

Lip injuries are classified into lacerations and avulsions. Lip lacerations require precise repair. Slight misalignment of even 1 mm will result in a noticeable and deforming scar. You do not want your patients to remember you this way. When the muscle (orbicularis oris) has been interrupted, precise repair is necessary to maintain facial expression and proper speech. For through-and-through lip laceration, closure should be done in a multilayer fashion. The first suture should be at the vermilion-cutaneous border, the most important suture cosmetically. This one determines if your patient curses your name when she applies lipstick. Use magnification during repair for best results. Next, the wet-to-dry mucosal border should be repaired, and lastly, the dry lip and skin. Lower-lip lacerations are best repaired with a mental nerve block and upper-lip repairs with an infraorbital block. Nerve or regional blocks are preferred over direct local anesthesia as they avoid tissue distortion. Lip avulsions are best managed with conservative care and healing by secondary intent.

Most intraoral mucosal lacerations will heal without any treatment at all. Even parotid duct lacerations will heal with salivation stimulation treatment (lemons!) and the patient can be followed up as an outpatient. Repair is necessary when (i) the mucosal laceration is >2 cm, (ii) the laceration is shaped in a way that food particles will become entrapped, or (iii) the laceration causes a flap of mucosal tissue to fall in between the upper and the lower teeth (causing repetitive damage). Small puncture lacerations (<2 cm) heal well without sutures; small through-and-through punctures need sutures only in the facial epidermis. This highly vascularized tissue heals fast! Only absorbable sutures should be used intraorally. Signs or a history of intraoral burns should be referred for immediate care to a burn surgery specialist once the patient is stable.

Management of tongue lacerations has been a topic of controversy until recently. Lamell et al.'s study on tongue laceration management in children found that most tongue lacerations heal well with no repair and without antibiotic treatment. In fact, there is no improvement of outcome when comparing patients with or without repair. Lamell's study included lacerations of all sizes (average 13 mm) in the middle of the tongue that do not gape open at rest. Repair *is* required when (i) bleeding is uncontrolled (after direct pressure, lidocaine with epinephrine, and ice have failed), (ii) large-flap lacerations are observed, or (iii) bisecting or other through-and-through lacerations are observed. These injuries should be repaired using lingual nerve block and 4.0 absorbable sutures and should be discharged with mouthwash and soft diet. In cases of extreme hemorrhage, definitive airway management becomes the priority and should be established immediately (nasotracheal intubation is preferred allowing better access for later oral lesion repair). Complete or partial amputation demands surgical consultation. Frenum lacerations have been regarded as pathognomonic for abuse in children; however, there have been a few documented cases of injury from intubation.

The bottom line is that most intraoral lesions can be treated in the emergency department and heal best with conservative management. For severe injuries, consult your surgical specialist. When repairing intraoral lesions, do not distort your laceration with local anesthesia. Use sutures, not glue. Give tetanus toxoid when appropriate. All patients discharged home should be given instructions on intraoral wound care using saltwater, peroxide, or chlorhexidine gluconate rinses. Lacerations associated with underlying facial fractures or grossly contaminated lacerations should be treated with empiric antibiotics.

SUGGESTED READINGS

Armstrong DB. Lacerations of the mouth. *Emerg Med Clin North Am.* 2000;18(3):471–480.

Banks K, Merlino PG. Minor oral injuries in children. *Mt Sinai J Med.* 1998;65(5–6): 333–334.

Bonadio WA. Safe and effective method for application of tetracaine, adrenaline and cocaine to oral lacerations. *Ann Emerg Med.* 1996;27:396–398.

Brown DJ, Jaffe JE, Henson JK. Advanced laceration management. *Emerg Med Clin N Am.* 2007;25(1):83–99.

Comer RW, Fitchie JG, Caughman WF, et al. Oral trauma: Emergency care of lacerations, fractures and burns. *Postgrad Med.* 1980;85(2):34–37, 41.

Kay SJ, Thomas DW, Shepherd JP. The management of soft tissue facial sounds. *Br J Oral Maxillofac Surg.* 1995;33(2):76–85.

Lamell CW, Fraone G, Casamassimo PS, et al. Presenting characteristics and treatment outcomes for tongue lacerations in children. *Pediatric Dent.* 1999;21(1):34–38.

Lammers R. Principles of wound management. In: Roberts, J, Hedges J, et al., eds. *Clinical Procedures in Emergency Medicine.* 4th ed. Philadelphia, PA: Saunders; 2004.

Marom T, Russo E, Ben-Yehuda Y, et al. Oropharyngeal injuries in children. *Pediatr Emerg Care.* 2007;23(12):914–918.

McHugh TP. Pneumomediastinium following penetrating oral trauma. *Pediatr Emerg Care*. 1997;13(3):211–213.

Randall DA, King DR. Current management of penetrating injuries of the soft palate. *Otolaryngol Head Neck Surg*. 2006;135:356–360.

Rhee ST, Colville C, Buchman SR. Conservative management of large avulsions of the lip and local landmarks. *Pediatr Emerg Care*. 2004;20(1):40–42.

Warabi R, Tanno K, Hirayama S, et al. Occult lacerations to the epiglottis and pharynx by glass fragments. *Am J Emerg Med*. 2008;26(4):518, e1–e3.

Zonfrillo M, Roy AD, Walsh SA. Management of pediatric penetrating oropharyngeal trauma. *Pediatr Emerg Care*. 2008;24(3):172–175.

84

NONTRAUMATIC DENTAL PAIN IS COMMON ... KNOW HOW TO TREAT IT PROPERLY

MICHAEL L. EPTER, DO, FAAEM

A common presenting complaint to emergency departments and urgent care centers is nontraumatic dental pain. An accurate diagnosis of the pathology which causes nontraumatic dental pain is essential since treatment modalities of similar presenting conditions (e.g., tooth eruption, periodontal disease) do not involve universal administration of antibiotics.

Dental pain can occur at the supragingival level (toward the crown) or within the gingival surface. An unclassified cause of dental pain is postextraction pain. This is divided into periostitis and alveolar osteitis. Simply asking the patient, "When was the extraction performed?" will make the diagnosis. The pain associated with periostitis occurs within 24 h of extraction and responds to analgesia. Antibiotics are *not* indicated. By contrast, pain associated with alveolar osteitis (dry socket) occurs 48 to 96 h after extraction and is associated with halitosis and a localized osteomyelitis. Alveolar osteitis treatment includes saline irrigation of the socket and packing with iodoform gauze saturated with a dental paste. A pitfall in the management of alveolar osteitis is failure to obtain an x-ray to identify the persistence of a retained tip of the tooth or foreign body. Since packing changes must occur, dental follow-up is necessary. Antibiotics are *only* indicated in severe conditions with associated systemic signs.

The most common cause of pain at the supragingival level is dental caries. Traditionally, the identification of dental caries is not a diagnostic challenge with careful history taking and physical exam. Patients complain of mild to moderate pain, with hot or cold sensitivity. An examination reveals a pit or fissure on the tooth surface detected with a dental probe. Referral to a dentist, meticulous oral hygiene (chlorhexidine), and analgesia are the only necessary treatments.

A complication of dental caries is the extension of inflammation to the pulp (pulpitis). Similar to dental caries, there is a painful response to thermal stimulus lasting seconds (reversible pulpitis) versus minutes to hours (irreversible pulpitis). Even in the case of irreversible pulpitis, there is no conclusive evidence to suggest the use of an antibiotic.

Gingival causes of pain include tooth eruption, pericoronitis, gingivitis, and periodontitis. In children presenting with dental pain, misdiagnosis of irritation and inflammation associated with tooth eruption versus pericoronitis is a potential diagnostic error which may result in improper management. Pericoronitis is an inflammation of the operculum (gingival tissue associated with the crown of the erupting tooth). The classic association is with the third molar (wisdom tooth). Similar to tooth eruption, erythema and swelling may be present. If no other signs of severe localized (pus able to be expressed from the pericoronal tissue) or systemic symptoms are present, therapy consists of saline irrigation of the pericoronal space. Associated trismus would suggest spread of the infection to the deep parapharyngeal spaces and warrants antibiotics and follow-up within 24 h.

Gingivitis involves erythema, swelling, and inflammation of the gingival tissue with an accumulation of supragingival plaque, which easily bleeds with simple tooth brushing and flossing. Antibiotics are *not* indicated for gingivitis. By contrast, periodontitis also involves gingival inflammation *with* connective tissue loss. This can be identified by the presence of deep gingival pockets and gum recession. Patients may present with a periodontal abscess which requires incision and drainage (I&D) and broad-spectrum antibiotics. In periodontal infections requiring antibiotics, metronidazole is superior or comparable to penicillin in their management. Similarly, metronidazole is the treatment of choice for acute necrotizing ulcerative gingivitis which is characterized by spirochete or anaerobic invasion of nonnecrotic gingival tissue, which has a predilection for the interdental papillae and causes constitutional symptoms along with pain, metallic taste, and halitosis. Penicillin and tetracycline are effective in the management of periodontal disease, but given the increasing recovery of β lactamase–producing bacteria and tetracycline-resistant aerobic and anaerobic strains, their usefulness is limited.

The 2008 consensus recommendations for the placement of patients with a dental complaint on antibiotics for the prophylaxis of infective endocarditis are *ONLY* indicated if there is a manipulation of the gingival or periapical region of the teeth or perforation of the oral mucosa *AND* the patient has a (i) prosthetic heart valve, (ii) previous infective endocarditis, (iii) congenital heart disease, and/or (iv) cardiac transplant with valve regurgitation due to a structurally abnormal valve.

- Antibiotic usage in the management of dental pain is indicated in select patients only and is not a universal treatment.
- Antibiotic choice is important since dental infections are polymicrobial. Traditional teaching has shown penicillin to be the drug of choice. In more fulminant infections, this has been replaced by metronidazole.
- Only a small subgroup of patients requires antibiotic prophylaxis against infective endocarditis. This is a significant change from previous recommendations.

Suggested Readings

Beaudreau RW. Oral and dental emergencies. In: Tintinalli JE, ed. *Emergency Medicine: A Comprehensive Study Guide*. 6th ed. New York: McGraw-Hill; 2004:337–343.

Brook I. Microbiology and principles of antimicrobial therapy for head and neck infections. *Infect Dis Clin N Am*. 2007;21:355–391.

Indresano AT, Haug RH, Hoffman MJ. The third molar as a cause of deep space infections. *J Oral Maxillofac Surg*. 1992;50(1):33–35; discussion 35–36.

Keenan JV, Farman AG, Fedorowicz Z, et al. Antibiotic use for irreversible pulpitis. *Cochrane Database Syst Rev*. 2005;(2):CD004969 [Review].

Loesche WJ. Dental caries and periodontitis: Contrasting two infections that have medical implications. *Infect Dis Clin N Am*. 2007;21:471–502.

Loesche WJ, Giordano JR. Treatment paradigms in periodontal disease. *Compend Contin Educ Dent*. 1997;18:221–232.

Nguyen DH, Martin JT. Common dental infections in the primary care setting. *Am Fam Physician*. 2008;77(6):797–802.

Nishimura RA, Carabello BA, Faxon DP, et al. ACC/AHA 2008 guideline update on valvular heart disease: Focused update on infective endocarditis. A Report of the American College of Cardiology/Amerian Heart Association Task Force on Practice Guidelines. *J Am Coll Cardiol*. 2008;52(23):e1–121.

85

Know how to diagnose and treat the various types of dental trauma

Michael L. Epter, DO, FAAEM

In the management of injuries to the face, the most common injuries to occur (and often the most overlooked/mistreated) are dental injuries. The avoidance of common pitfalls in the management of dental injuries begins with (a) proper classification of the injury sustained to the tooth (e.g., involvement of enamel, dentin, and/or pulp), (b) recognition of the age-defined limits of primary teeth and development of the permanent teeth (since treatment of these injuries varies with age), (c) proper treatment/stabilization of the injury, and (d) pertinent instructions to the patient.

CLASSIFY THE INJURY—LUXATION? FRACTURE? AVULSION?

Luxations are divided into concussions, subluxations, or extrusive, lateral, and intrusive luxations.

Fractures of the teeth are divided into crown fracture (uncomplicated vs. complicated), crown-root fracture, root fracture, and alveolar bone fracture. Along with luxations, crown fractures are the most common type of dental injury. When evaluating the injury, determine if there is pulp exposure. Both types of crown fracture involve the enamel (Ellis I) and dentin (Ellis II) with complicated fractures involving the pulp as well (Ellis III). Pulp exposure is suggested by a pink blush or drop of blood after wiping the tooth.

Crown-root fractures involve the enamel, dentin, and root structure (±) pulp exposure.

Root fractures involve the root of the tooth in a horizontal or diagonal plane with potential mobility and displacement of the coronal segment of the tooth.

Alveolar bone fractures, which are found in association with lateral and intrusive luxations, typically present with mobile segments and associated dislocation.

Avulsions are clinically obvious to the examiner but are the most serious of all dental injuries.

DOES THE INJURY INVOLVE THE PRIMARY TEETH OR PERMANENT TEETH?

There are 20 primary teeth in contrast to the 32 permanent teeth. Primary teeth are smaller, have bulbous crowns, and are often whiter with flat edges than their adult counterparts, which tend to be larger, be cream in color, and have jagged edges on newly erupted teeth. As a general rule, primary teeth begin to shed at 6 years of age with the central incisor/first molar and end at 12 years of age with the canine/second molar.

TREAT/STABILIZE THE INJURY

Uncomplicated Crown Fracture. Primary/Permanent—Place. calcium hydroxide paste over the exposed dentin and cover with enamel-bonded plastic. Alternatives include metal band or foil. Children should be seen by an appropriate specialist as soon as possible secondary to possible pulp contamination.

Complicated C rown Fracture. Primary/Permanent—Minimize contamination and preserve pulp vitality by applying a root canal sealant (e.g., pulpdent, cavet). Do not remove the pulp. Alternatives include application of moist cotton over the exposed pulp and coverage with foil. Complicated crown fractures are a true dental emergency and require immediate attention.

Crown-Root Fracture
Primary/Permanent—Splint.

Root Fracture
Primary—Splint.
Permanent—Reposition the coronal segment of the tooth (if displaced) and splint.

Alveolar Fracture
Primary/Permanent—Reposition (if displaced) and splint.

Concussion
Primary/Permanent—No treatment.

Subluxation
Primary—No treatment.
Permanent—Splint.

Extrusive Luxation
Primary—If <3 mm, reposition or leave the tooth for spontaneous alignment.
Permanent—Reposition the tooth by reinsertion into the tooth socket and splint.

Lateral Luxation
Primary—If there is interference with occlusion, reposition; otherwise, no treatment.
Permanent—Reposition into its original location and splint.

Intrusive Luxation
Primary/Permanent—Treatment is determined by a specialist.

Avulsion
Primary—Do not replace avulsed primary teeth.
Permanent—Do not manipulate the tooth by any other means but the crown. Do not let the tooth dry out. Clean the root surface and remove coagulum from the socket with saline, reimplant immediately, splint, and administer tetanus and antibiotics. Doxycycline is the drug of choice with penicillin in children as an alternative. If treatment is delayed, place the tooth in Hank solution. Similar to STEMI, "time is tooth" and the faster the tooth is replaced, the better the prognosis.

Teeth should be stabilized after an injury with the exception of intrusive luxation. Traditional methods of splinting involve the application of Coe-Pak

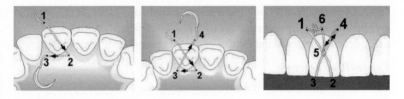

FIGURE 85.1. Stabilizing the teeth.

(periodontal pack). Suturing can also be performed with 2/0 silk in a crisscross pattern (from the palatal soft tissue to the vestibular soft tissue) with a locking horizontal mattress to maintain the position (*Fig. 85.1*).

PERTINENT INSTRUCTIONS

Proper instructions to the patient/family are critical to ensuring the most favorable outcome for dental injuries. Good healing is intimately tied into good hygiene. Utilizing a soft brush with chlorhexidine is recommended. Avoid hot liquids and maintain a soft diet. Patients must have timely follow-up regardless of the injury sustained.

As with all patients who sustain trauma, a stepwise approach is essential to missing potential injuries. Dental injuries represent a unique challenge to the emergency physician. These injuries can cause airway compromise either directly or indirectly (broken tooth fragments in the airway), and errors in their management can lead to long-term endodontic and cosmetic complications.

SUGGESTED READINGS

Amsterdam JT. Oral medicine. In: Marx JA, et al. eds. *Rosen's Emergency Medicine Concepts and Clinical Practice.* 6th ed. 2006;1026–1042.

Flores MT, Andersson L, Andreasen JO, et al. Guidelines for the management of traumatic dental injuries. I. Fractures and luxations of permanent teeth. *Dental Traumatol.* 2007;23:66–71.

Flores MT, Andersson L, Andreasen JO, et al. Guidelines for the management of traumatic dental injuries. II. Avulsion of permanent teeth. *Dental Traumatol.* 2007;23:130–136.

Flores MT, Andersson L, Andreasen JO, et al. Guidelines for the management of traumatic dental injuries. III. Primary teeth. *Dental Traumatol.* 2007;23:196–202.

Lin S, Emodi O, Abu El-Naaj, I. Splinting of an injured tooth as part of emergency treatment. *Dental Traumatol.* 2008;24:370–372.

The Royal Children's Hospital Melbourne: Clinical Practice Guidelines. Available at: http://www.rch.org.au/clinicalguide/. Accessed August 2008.

86

UNDERSTAND THE LIMITATIONS OF COMMON DIAGNOSTIC STUDIES IN PATIENTS WITH NEW-ONSET HEADACHES

ADAM G. FIELD, MD

The major pitfalls in the interpretation of diagnostic studies for potentially life-threatening headaches include the following: failure to appropriately order a CT scan and understand its limitations; failure to perform lumbar punctures (LPs) and correctly interpret the cerebrospinal fluid (CSF) findings; and focus on abnormal studies that may only be indirectly associated with the primary life threat.

The first diagnostic study in evaluating the first or worst headache is typically a noncontrast CT. Several factors affect the sensitivity of the test. If the CT scan is not done with thin cuts (3 mm), a small collection of blood may be missed. Blood and adjacent bone may also be difficult to distinguish. If the patient is anemic with hemoglobin <10 g/dL, the bleed may appear isodense. The sensitivity of a third-generation CT scan for detecting subarachnoid hemorrhage (SAH) is 90% to 98% within the first 24 h of symptoms and decreases to 86% after 1 day, 76% at 2 days, and 58% after 5 days. One recent study demonstrates almost 100% sensitivity with a fifth-generation CT scanner, but most of the recent literature still does not recommend relying solely on a CT to rule out subarachnoid hemorrhage. The sensitivity of CT scan is also reduced in awake and alert patients presumably with smaller bleeds. In one study, minor SAH was not diagnosed by CT scan in 55% of patients and LP was positive in all of them.

LP should be performed in any patient with a negative or inadequate CT whose clinical symptoms suggest SAH. This recommendation is still often not followed in clinical practice. Although LP is an excellent adjunct to the CT scan, especially for diagnosing SAH, it does have some limitations. The classic findings on CSF evaluation with SAH are a red blood cell count that does not diminish from tube 1 to tube 4, elevated opening pressure, and xanthochromia. It is often assumed that a decrease in sequential red blood cell counts suggests a traumatic tap, but this is not necessarily true unless the count decreases to zero. In one study, some patients with SAH demonstrated a 25% decrease in RBC count on sequential counts. If the diagnosis is uncertain, clear CSF from a second puncture one interspace higher than the initial tap would suggest that the initial tap was traumatic. Elevated opening pressure may help to differentiate traumatic tap from SAH and can also be seen with cerebral venous thrombosis, intracranial hypertension, and pseudo tumor cerebri.

The absence or presence of xanthochromia (pink or yellow tint) in the CSF does not absolutely rule in or rule out the possibility of SAH. Xanthochromia represents hemoglobin degradation and is present anywhere from 6 to 12 h after the onset of SAH. The absence of xanthochromia does not rule out the possibility of SAH if the patient presents <12 h or >2 weeks after the onset of headache. Xanthochromia is measured by visual inspection or by spectrophotometry.

Most hospitals measure by visual inspection, which is obviously a much less sensitive test. Xanthochromia from traumatic tap, hyperbilirubinemia, or encephalitis can lead to further unnecessary diagnostic studies.

Additional CSF studies should be considered depending on the clinical scenario, especially if the patient has been in an endemic area or is immuno-compromised. The diagnosis of herpes encephalitis is often delayed even in the presence of new headache, neuropsychiatric symptoms, seizure, appropriate rash, and a lymphocytic pleocytosis. Maintain a low threshold for performing an LP. Less than half of the patients (44%) in one study of patients with bacterial meningitis had the classic symptoms of neck stiffness, fever, and headache.

The evidence suggests that most patients with a normal CT and CSF do not require further studies. This may not be the case in patients with a clinical scenario suggesting carotid or vertebral dissection, cerebral venous sinus thrombosis (CVST), pituitary apoplexy, spontaneous intracranial hypotension, and hypertensive encephalopathy. A negative CT and LP should be followed up by an MRI/MRA, CTA, or cerebral angiogram when clinically indicated. MRA or CTA of the head and neck should be included when there is a suspicion for carotid or vertebral dissection. Magnetic resonance venography (MRV) should be included with the MRI if there is a high clinical suspicion for CVST. CT may be normal in up to 30% of patients with CVST. LP may also demonstrate a lymphocytic pleocytosis and lead the clinician to make a diagnosis of viral meningitis with CVST. Even CT angiography (CTA) or MRI/MRA may miss a symptomatic unruptured aneurysm, cavernous malformation in the cervical spine, or nonaneurysmal bleed. Maintain a high suspicion for unruptured aneurysm, especially with gradual-onset headaches associated with transient ischemic attack (TIA), seizure, or third nerve palsy.

Patients with life-threatening causes of headache may present with multiple other symptoms requiring additional diagnostic testing. Clinicians often develop an anchoring bias to the first positive diagnostic findings which may distract them from the primary life threat. Patients with SAH may present with syncope, triggering an initial cardiac workup. Focusing on findings associated with SAH, such as elevated cardiac enzymes and brain natriuretic peptide (BNP), dysrhythmias, ischemic ECG changes, hyponatremia, and cerebral infarction secondary to vasospasm, may divert the attention from the true life threat. The first diagnosis is not always the correct diagnosis. Be complete in your diagnostic evaluation, but understand the limitations and potential pitfalls of these tests.

SUGGESTED READINGS

Benson P, Swadron S. Empiric acyclovir is infrequently initiated in the emergency department to patients ultimately diagnosed with encephalitis. *Ann Emerg Med.* 2006;47(1):100–105.

Boesiger BM, Shiber JR. Subarachnoid hemorrhage diagnosis by computed tomography and lumbar puncture: Are fifth generation CT scanners better at identifying subarachnoid hemorrhage? *J Emerg Med.* 2005;29(1):23–27.

Davenport R, Sudden headache in the emergency department. *Prac Neurol.* 2005;5:132–143.

Edlow JA, Caplan LR. Avoiding pitfalls in the diagnosis of subarachnoid hemorrhage. *N Engl J Med.* 2000;342:29–36.

Edlow JA, Malek AM, Ogilvy CS. Aneursymal subarachnoid hemorrhage: Update for emergency physicians. *J Emerg Med.* 2008;34(3):237–251.

Heasley DC, Mohamed MA, Yousem DM. Clearing of red blood cells in lumbar puncture does not rule out ruptured aneurysm in patients with suspected subarachnoid hemorrhage but negative head CT findings. *Am J Neuroradiol.* 2005;26:829–824.

Kassell NF, Torner JC, Haley EC Jr, et al. The International Cooperative Study on the timing of aneurysm surgery. 1. Overall management results. *J Neurosurg.* 1990;73:18–36.

Latchaw RE, Silva P, Falcone SF. The role of CT following aneurysmal rupture. *Neuroimaging Clin N Am.* 1997;7:693–708.

Leblanc R. The minor leak preceding subarachnoid hemorrhage. *J Neurosurg.* 1987;66(1): 35–39.

Mace SE. Acute bacterial meningitis. *Emerg Med Clin N Am.* 2008;26(2):281–317.

Morgenstern LB, Luna-Gonzales H, Huber JC Jr, et al. Worst headache and subarachnoid hemorrhage: prospective, modern, computed tomography and spinal fluid analysis. *Ann Emerg Med.* 1998;32:297–304.

Schwedt TJ, Matharu MS, Dodick DW. Thunderclap headache. *Lancet Neurol.* 2006;5: 21–31.

Singer RJ, Ogilvy CS, Rordorf G. Etiology, clinical manifestations, and diagnosis of aneurysmal subarachnoid hemorrhage. *UpToDate.* May 2008. Available at: http://www.uptodate.com.

87

RECOGNIZE THE DANGER SIGNS OF LIFE-THREATENING HEADACHES

ADAM G. FIELD, MD

Approximately 2% of patients presenting to the emergency department with a chief complaint of headache are related to a serious life-, limb-, brain-, or vision-threatening condition. The major pitfalls in the evaluation of a new headache involve missing the danger signs in the history and physical examination, not considering the less common disease processes, and failing to recognize the wide spectrum of disease presentations.

The classic symptom of acute onset of the worst headache of life should trigger the appropriate evaluation for a subarachnoid hemorrhage. Twenty to fifty percent of patients with documented subarachnoid hemorrhage reported a distinct, severe headache days to weeks prior to the index episode of bleeding. Many of these "warning headaches" or sentinel leaks may be associated with other atypical symptoms. They are often misdiagnosed as the flu, viral syndrome, gastroenteritis, and muscle strain. All new abrupt-onset or "thunderclap" headaches, even those of short duration with other atypical features, should be evaluated for subarachnoid hemorrhage (SAH).

The "first time" headache, or a new pattern to an existing chronic headache, requires urgent evaluation. Although focal neurologic deficits may occur with complex migraines, it should not be assumed that these deficits are related to the migraine unless the patient had similar presentations in the past. Maintain a low threshold for diagnostic testing in patients presenting with a change in their chronic headache pattern, especially if they have a history of HIV, immunosuppression, or an underlying malignancy.

A severe headache associated with exertion (cough, valsalva, intercourse, or exercise) should raise concern for carotid dissection, intracranial hemorrhage, or cerebral venous sinus thrombosis (CVST).

Carotid dissection may have additional features of anterior neck pain with anterior circulation neurologic deficits (i.e., Horner syndrome or amaurosis fugax), whereas vertebral dissection may present with posterior circulation deficits (vertebral basilar symptoms) and posterior neck pain. A history of recent neck trauma or manipulation should also be suggestive of this diagnosis. A good headache history should always document the presence of acute or remote trauma. Neurologic deficits may lag hours to days behind the acute onset of pain and lead to a delay in diagnosis.

CVST should be considered with a new headache (either acute or subacute) in the setting of a hypercoaguable condition and a precipitant. These include head trauma, jugular venous catheterization, recent lumbar puncture (LP), pregnancy, surgery, and the use of birth control pills. CVST is sometimes associated with altered mental status, seizures, and focal neurologic symptoms but may present with a "thunderclap" headache and no other symptoms.

New-onset headache in a patient over 50 years of age is a red flag. Older patients have increased incidence of stroke, transient ischemic attack (TIA), acute or chronic subdural hematoma, acute narrow angle glaucoma, and other systemic processes. Inability to ambulate, change in patients' ability to do their activities of daily living, and unstable vital signs are important diagnostic clues to underlying serious pathology. Do not forget the erythrocyte sedimentation rate (ESR), looking for temporal arteritis in patients over the age of 50. Not everyone with temporal arteritis presents with classic unilateral temporal tenderness, jaw claudication, and unilateral blurry vision. Other atypical features may include bilateral blurry vision, occipital tenderness, cough, vague constitutional symptoms, transient ischemic attacks, and vertigo.

Even the most minor visual complaint of "my vision is a little fuzzy" or "I am dizzy doctor" warrants a complete ocular exam including fundoscopy. Papilledema suggests elevated intracranial pressure from a mass lesion, hydrocephalus, or pseudotumor cerebri. Visual acuity should always be documented. Visual field deficits can be associated with pituitary apoplexy, mass lesion, stroke, carotid dissection, or cerebral venous thrombosis. Primary vision problems such as optic neuritis, iritis, and acute narrow angle glaucoma may also present with a chief complaint of headache.

Perform medication reconciliation, especially in the elderly. The use of anticoagulants is associated with more severe intracranial hemorrhage and increases the risk of acute and chronic subdural hematoma. The use of immunosuppressive agents or steroids may trigger a lower threshold to search for CNS and non-CNS infectious etiologies. Relief of headaches with medications or migraine "cocktails" should not be used as a diagnostic tool to rule out more serious intracranial pathology.

Make sure that you take a complete social history. Heavy alcohol use, cigarette smoking, hypertension, cocaine, phenylpropanolamine, and possibly oral contraception may increase the risk of SAH. New headaches in substance abusers may also be related to severe withdrawal symptoms.

Key features of the family history may increase the pretest probability of a serious life-threatening disease. Ask specifically about any history of brain aneurysms. First-degree relatives of patients with SAH have a three to five times increased risk compared to the general population. Multiple family members presenting to the ER within days to hours with similar headaches that resolve rapidly in the ER without intervention may suggest carbon monoxide poisoning.

A complete past medical history is another key component. There is an increased incidence of SAH in patients with polycystic kidney disease, Ehlers-Danlos syndrome, neurofibromatosis, and other collagen vascular disease. Brain abscess should be considered in patients who are immunocompromised or have a history of right to left shunt from cyanotic heart disease or pulmonary arteriovenous malformation (AVM). Preeclampsia may present with headache in the third trimester pregnancy and up to 4 to 6 weeks postpartum.

A complete review of systems is often overlooked in the headache history. Syncope or near syncope, associated with a headache, is particularly concerning for SAH. A new headache associated with confusion, seizures, or new neurological complaints warrants further evaluation. Headaches may also be a symptom of a non-CNS process. Consider infectious etiologies such as pyelonephritis or pharyngitis before subjecting a patient to an unnecessary LP. Profound anemia, hypoxia, or occult malignancy may present with a new-onset headache. A history of paroxysms of hypertension, hyperadrenergic symptoms, and new headaches may suggest pheochromocytoma, hyperthyroidism, or illicit sympathomimetic drug use.

These danger signs are in no way comprehensive, but encourage the clinician to think twice before firing off a quick CT scan in place of a complete history and physical examination.

SUGGESTED READINGS

Cutrer F. Evaluation of headache in the emergency department, *UpToDate*. 2008. Available at: http://www.uptodate.com. Accessed May 31, 2008.

Davenport R. Sudden headache in the emergency department. *Pract Neurol*. 2005;5:132–143.

Edlow JA, Caplan LR. Avoiding pitfalls in the diagnosis of subarachnoid hemorrhage. *N Engl J Med*. 2000;342:29–36.

Edlow JA, Malek AM, Ogilvy CS. Aneurysmal subarachnoid hemorrhage: Update for emergency physicians. *J Emerg Med*. 2008;34(3):237–251.

Locker TE, Thompson C, Rylance J, et al. The utility of clinical features in patients presenting with nontraumatic headache: An investigation of adult patients attending an emergency department. *Headache*. 2006;46(6):954–961.

Rothman RE, Keyl PM, McArthur JC, et al. A decision guideline for emergency department utilization of noncontrast head computed tomography in HIV infected patients. *Acad Emerg Med*. 1999;6(10):1010–1019.

Schwedt TJ, Matharu MS, Dodick DW. Thunderclap headache. *Lancet Neurol*. 2006;5: 621–631.

Seymour JJ, Moscati RM, Jehle DV. Response of headaches to nonnarcotic analgesics resulting in missed intracranial hemorrhage. *Am J Emerg Med*. 1995;13:43–45.

Singer RJ, Ogilvy CS, Rordorf G. Etiology, clinical manifestations, and diagnosis of aneurysmal subarachnoid hemorrhage. *UpToDate*. May 2008. Available at: http://www.uptodate.com.

Stella CL, Jodicke CD, How HY, et al. Postpartum headache: Is your work-up complete? *Am J Obstet Gynecol*. 2007;196(4):318.

Stone JH, Calabrese LH, Hoffman GS, et al. Vasculitis: A collection of pearls and myths. *Rheum Dis Clin North Am*. 2001;27(4):677–728.

88

REMEMBER THESE SIMPLE PEARLS TO HELP IN TREATING CHILDREN WITH NASAL FOREIGN BODIES

ADAM D. FRIEDLANDER, MD

A tracker board with "bead in nose" in room 4 next to "stab wound" in room 5 is the reality of emergency medicine. It just so happens that this juxtaposition of diverse complaints is also what drew most of us to emergency medicine. The art of our craft is to be able to handle both presentations appropriately and efficiently.

Nasal foreign body should be suspected in any child with nasal pain, odor, or discharge, especially when it is unilateral and accompanied by the chief complaint of "She stuck something in her nose." Many methods exist for removing foreign bodies, including the use of forceps, Foley catheters, and suction; however, all of these methods require patient cooperation, or, more realistically, restraint with or without sedation. Additionally, any instrumentation brings with it a risk of pushing the foreign body into the airway, injuring surrounding tissues, and making attempts by a consultant more difficult should you be unsuccessful. Instrumentation does have its place, but if there is an easier, safer, faster way, why not use it?

Several studies have examined such a method, which is less invasive and less painful, improves patient satisfaction, and, above all, works. This method involves the use of positive pressure to expel the foreign body. In one retrospective study of 64 nasal foreign body cases, positive pressure was used in eight cases. In this study, the parent would deliver a rapid puff of air through the child's mouth, while occluding the unaffected nare (an Ambu bag may be used as well). In some cases, several puffs of air were required, but all eight attempts were successful. Another study employed a method which involved the insertion of a tubing connector, one large enough to get a good seal in the unaffected nare, with 15 L of flow. In this study, the positive pressure method was successful in all nine cases in which it was used. Of note, follow-up parental surveys indicated that 100% of parents considered the trauma of the procedure to be less than that of vaccine administration and 80% considered the procedure to be equivalent to a routine oropharyngeal examination. Neither sedation nor restraints were used in any of the cases, and the average time from triage to discharge was 34 min. Even more important is that there were no complications associated with these techniques in either study.

There are, however, certain circumstances in which another "trick of the trade" proves useful. The presence of magnets in the nose, specifically when attracted on opposite sides of the nasal septum, carries a significant risk of necrosis and perforation if not treated quickly, and such necrosis has been documented within hours of such magnets becoming stuck. This usually occurs in the setting of bilateral magnetic (nonpiercing) nose rings. A novel approach to dealing with nasal magnets is discussed in one case report in which a father, who after seeing both an EM physician and two ENT specialists fail at removing magnets from his 13-year-old son's nose, removed the magnets himself with a household pocket magnet while the boy's OR suite was being reserved. This simple and effective method has been further described and merely requires access to a similar magnet, available for $10 or less at many retail stores. The magnet is placed within 1.5 cm of the first magnet in the nare to break the bond between the two offenders across the septum. When the first magnet is attracted to the pocket magnet, the second magnet usually falls out on its own. If it does not, it is removed even more easily than the first, by placing the pocket magnet into the second nare. When passing the magnet into the nare, be sure to apply pressure laterally off of the painful septum to remove the first magnet. Though this method is generally nontraumatic, you should pretreat the nares with 4%

lidocaine and 1:1,000 epinephrine spray to minimize potential bleeding, especially if there is already significant bleeding around the magnet.

While beads and magnets offer unique challenges, button batteries that become lodged in a nostril should raise your blood pressure even more. Up to two thirds of children who insert button batteries into their noses experience septal perforation due to both the leakage of alkaline contents, as well as local currents causing thermal burns, and the production of more alkaline materials via electrolysis. Damage may occur in as little as 3 h, and in one study of 147 nasal foreign bodies, all 14 complications identified were due to button batteries. One child who had been exposed for 24 h had very significant necrosis of her inferior meatus, inferior turbinate, and alar cartilage. The greatest challenge in treating children with button battery foreign bodies can be identifying the button battery. Parents often know that a child has placed something into his or her nose but may not know what the object was. If the foreign body is unknown, it must be addressed as if it is a button battery until proven otherwise. If you are even considering an impacted button battery, you are obligated to remove the object for confirmation (if it is visualized intact with minimal surrounding injury), consult ENT if there is any evidence of leakage of battery contents or evidence of necrosis, or obtain plain radiography emergently if you cannot visualize what may be a button battery. Of course, a plain radiograph cannot definitively show if a foreign body is a battery, but the question here is this: radiolucent or radiopaque? If you are assuming that a foreign body is something benign, and a radiograph shows a round and radiopaque object, you have got some more work to do. If nothing is seen, you are in luck—button batteries are not radiolucent.

Nasal foreign bodies are the perennial subject of humorous jabs at the amusing chief complaints handled by emergency physicians who treat children, but when confronted with this chief complaint, the treatment is not always simple. You will make your life much easier if you remember these three things: try noninvasive removal techniques first, a household magnet can save a nose from necrosis, and while the patient with the stab wound is critical, never ignore the kid with a button battery in his or her nose.

SUGGESTED READINGS

Backlin SA. Positive pressure technique for nasal foreign body removal in children. *Ann Emerg Med*. 1995;25:554–555.

Dane S, Smally AJ, Peredy TR. A truly emergent problem: Button battery in the nose. *Acad Emerg Med*. 2000;7:204–206.

Glynn F, Amin M, Kinsella J. Nasal foreign bodies in children: Should they have a plain radiograph in the accident and emergency? *Ped Emerg Care*. 2004;24:217–218.

Kadish HA, Corneli HM. Removal of nasal foreign bodies in the pediatric population. *Am J Emerg Med*. 1997;15:54–56.

Loh WS, Leong J, Tan HK. Hazardous foreign bodies: Complications and management of button batteries in nose. *Ann Otol Rhinol Laryngol*. 2003;112:379–383.

McCormick SR, Brennan PO, Yassa JG. Magnets and children: An attractive combination? *BMJ* 2000;321(7259):514.

Navitsky RC, Beamsley A, McLaughlin S. Nasal positive-pressure technique for nasal foreign body removal in children. *Am J Emerg Med*. 2002;20:103–104.

Starke L. Easy removal of nasal magnets. *Ped Emerg Care*. 2005;21:598–599.

Tong MC, Van Hasselt CA, Woo JKS. The hazards of button batteries in the nose. *J Otolaryngol*. 1992;21:458–460.

89

KNOW THE PHYSICAL EXAM FINDINGS OF ORBITAL FRACTURES AND KNOW WHEN TO ORDER THE COMPUTED TOMOGRAPHY

CHARLIE GALANIS, MD AND CHRISTOPHER M. SCIORTINO, MD, PhD

In patients presenting with blunt trauma to the midface, do not rely solely on your physical exam to exclude an orbital fracture. Judicious use of radiographic facial imaging and knowing your orbit anatomy will significantly aid in your diagnosis and treatment plan for your patient with facial injuries.

Understanding the anatomy of the bony orbit is the first step in understanding the presentation and management in patients with orbital fractures. Looking way back to anatomy classes, remember the orbit is a complex bony structure composed of seven bones arranged in a conical or pyramidal shape. The orbit is widest anteriorly and narrows dramatically posteriorly with an average depth of 45 to 55 mm. Its contents include the globe, the extraocular muscles, and nerves supplying motor and sensory functions. The optic foramen, located slightly medial at the posterior portion of the orbit, is the hole through which the optic nerve and artery enter the orbit.

Orbital fractures are a prominent fixture in the emergency room for a very simple reason: the thin wall of the orbit makes the structure highly susceptible to fracture. For this reason, all patients with blunt trauma to the face should be viewed as high-risk patients for having suffered an orbital fracture. These fractures most commonly involve the orbital floor and may occur in association with other injuries or as an isolated injury. The most common orbital rim fracture is a zygomaticoorbital fracture classically associated with the lateral orbital wall and infraorbital rim and orbital floor. The most common site of an isolated intraorbital fracture involves the orbital floor medially. The often-described "blowout" fracture occurs when a sudden increase in orbital pressure from trauma leads to fracture displacement of the thin orbital floor and medial orbital wall.

Since orbital fractures are commonly the result of significant force, associated injuries must be suspected. Specifically, intracranial injury, associated facial fractures, and intraocular injury must be investigated.

In general, on examination, most orbital fractures are associated with traumatic ecchymosis, hemorrhage of the subconjunctiva, and periorbital edema. However, as we commented earlier, key physical findings associated with specific orbital fractures can be explained by knowing the orbit's anatomy. Fractures of the anterior orbit are associated with sensory nerve deficits as well as bony step-offs. Fractures of the middle orbit are associated with globe displacement, diplopia, and oculomotor dysfunction. Fractures of the posterior orbit are associated with visual and oculomotor dysfunctions. Keep in mind that these fractures can present in a wide variety of ways or can be completely clinically silent. Orbital fractures' varied presentations decrease the physical exam reliability in a patient with blunt trauma to the face. You risk falsely excluding patients with orbital fractures if your decision is solely on the exam. Instead, base your decision to obtain a thin-cut (3-mm interval) coronal computed tomography (CT) scan of the face on the physical exam findings *or* if you have a high clinical suspicion for fractures based on the mechanism of facial injury, even in the absence of obvious signs or symptoms. In addition to making the diagnosis, an appropriate CT scan allows the surgeon to determine the need for operative intervention as well as plan the surgical approach. Finally, a CT scan also has the advantage of simultaneously evaluating the patient for associated injuries.

All orbital fractures warrant both a surgical and an ophthalmologic evaluation. Visual acuity, pupil reactivity, presence of diplopia, mobility, visual fields, intraocular pressure, and fundoscopic examination are all essential to the proper ocular exam, particularly in cases of suspected associated globe injury. The two major surgical indications for an orbital fracture repair include muscle entrapment and an increased orbital volume. Both of these indications can be confirmed by a CT scan, which again further highlights the importance of this diagnostic modality. In the case of entrapment, the CT illustrates soft tissue incarceration. Entrapment can be additionally corroborated by a positive forced duction examination and the presence of double vision with an abnormal oculomotor exam. In the case of an increased orbital volume >3 mL, a CT scan illustrates the displacement of the globe medially, posteriorly, and inferiorly. Finally, patients with significant orbital hematoma seen on CT may require emergent lateral canthotomy to relieve intraorbital pressure.

In patients presenting with blunt trauma to the midface, do not rely solely on physical exam to exclude an orbital fracture. Orbital fractures may be present in the **absence** of visual field, acuity, or oculomotor deficits. Knowing this, the history and mechanism of the facial injury will be needed to guide your diagnostic evaluation of orbital fractures. Obtaining a thin-cut coronal CT scan of the face will confirm or exclude an orbital fracture, determine the need for urgent intervention, and simultaneously evaluate for associated injuries.

SUGGESTED READINGS

Bord SP, Linden J. Trauma to the globe and orbit. *Emerg Med Clin North Am.* 2008;26(1): 97–123, vi–vii.

Brown DL, Borschel GH. *Michigan Manual of Plastic surgery*, 1st ed. Philadelphia, PA: Lippincott Williams & Wilkins; 2004.

Kaufman Y, Stal D, Cole P, et al. Orbitozygomatic fracture management. *Plast Reconstr Surg.* 2008;121(4):1370–1374.

McCarthy JG, Galiano R, Boutros A. *Current Therapy in Plastic Surgery*. Philadelphia, PA: Saunders Elsevier; 2006.

Thorne CH, Beasley RW, Aston SJ, et al. *Grabb and Smith's Plastic Surgery*. 6th ed. Philadelphia, PA: Lippincott Williams & Wilkins; 2007.

90

NEVER ASSUME THAT A FACIAL FRACTURE IS JUST A "SIMPLE" FACIAL FRACTURE

ALISA GIBSON, MD, DMD

Facial trauma is frequently encountered by the emergency physician. Many of these patients may have relatively benign injuries, often amenable to management as an outpatient. Some fractures of the midface may fall into this group. However, it is important to remember that highly morbid conditions may accompany these fractures, including spinal injury, life-threatening blood loss, vision-ending ocular injuries, and cerebrospinal fistula formation, which could result in meningitis.

In general, trauma above the clavicle should raise suspicion for cervical injury, and midface injuries are no exception. The incidence of concomitant cervical spine injury ranges from 0.3% to 19.3% in the literature. Such injuries are commonly reported as being most frequent in the area of C5 to C7, although damage to any level of the cervical spine can occur. Spinal injury is more common when the cause of maxillofacial trauma is a motor vehicle accident (as opposed to a fall or assault). Such generalizations, however, while noteworthy from a statistical standpoint, mean little when managing an individual patient in the emergency department. The bottom line is that patients with facial fractures need to be in a cervical collar and should be assumed to have a cervical spine injury until proven otherwise.

The significant blood supply to the midface can result in life-threatening hemorrhage, with a reported incidence of 1.4% to 11%. Such severe bleeding is usually attributable to the maxillary artery (which passes within the LeFort fracture borders). It is difficult, if not impossible, to locate the precise origin of the bleeding since it frequently involves both the hard and soft tissues of the midface. As well, since the fractures tend to track in a posterior direction, the damaged vessel may lay within an area too deep to be accessible to the emergency physician. For example, the pterygomaxillary fossa, involved in LeFort fractures, contains the third segment of the internal maxillary artery—a common culprit in severe bleeding. Nasal packing is the treatment of choice and can be lifesaving. While anterior packing is typically sufficient for epistaxis, *posterior* packing is generally required in severe bleeding related to midface fractures. It is important to involve your facial surgeons early, because if the maxilla is mobile, packing may cause further displacement and worsen the bleeding. In these cases, urgent reduction and intermaxillary fixation are required.

Ocular injury is commonly seen with midface fractures (remember, the maxilla, zygoma, ethmoid, and sphenoid bones all form part of the orbit). The incidence of blindness associated with these fractures ranges from 3% to 22%. Most cases are due to globe rupture, but they can also be associated with LeFort II and III complex fractures leading to direct optic nerve injury. Indirect injury (i.e., traumatic optic neuropathy) is more frequently seen and can cause temporary or permanent visual loss. A complete eye exam is mandatory, and maintain a low threshold for early ophthalmology consultation.

Midface fractures may extend into the anterior cranial base. This reminds us of the reason we have all been warned to avoid nasotracheal intubation or nasogastric tubes in their presence. These fractures can put patients at risk for a cerebrospinal fluid (CSF) leak. The leak most commonly occurs at the cribriform plate of the ethmoid bone, associated with naso-orbitoethmoid fractures, or as part of LeFort fractures. Detection of CSF rhinorrhea is not always simple, particularly in cases of trauma when the presence of blood obscures other fluids. First and foremost, you have to *look* for it. A simple bedside test is the "halo" test. CSF separates from blood when it is placed on filter paper, resulting in a central area of blood with an outer ring or halo. This sign does not clinch the diagnosis, as water, saline, and rhinorrhea will also produce a halo when mixed with blood. Analysis for glucose content in the fluid (using glucose oxidase paper) is another common test but is extremely unreliable as nasal secretions have reducing substances which will produce a false-positive result. The current gold standard is the β_2 transferrin assay. If CSF rhinorrhea is confirmed (or highly suspected), a neurosurgical consultation is warranted. Once the diagnosis is made, the biggest management issue facing the EM physician is the use of prophylactic antibiotics. The incidence of meningitis varies wildly in literature, from 4% to 50%. However, there appears to be little support for the use of prophylaxis, with some studies actually showing *higher* rates of meningitis in the groups which received antibiotics. In most cases, the decision will be made by the neurosurgeon.

The next time you see a patient with a midface fracture in the emergency department, keep the following pearls in mind:

Evaluation of the cervical spine for fractures is mandatory
For severe bleeding, pack both the anterior *and* the posterior nasopharynx
Assess and document a complete ophthalmologic exam
Look for a CSF leak (remember the β_2 transferrin test), and tell a neurosurgeon when you find one

SUGGESTED READINGS

Ardekian L, Rosen D, Klein Y, et al. Life-threatening complications and irreversible damage following maxillofacial trauma. *Injury*. 1998;29(4):253–256.

Ashar A, Kovacs A, Khan S, et al. Blindness associated with midfacial fractures. *J Oral Maxillofac Surg*. 1998;56(10):1146–1150; discussion 1151.

Choi D, Spann R. Traumatic cerebrospinal fluid leakage: Risk factors and the use of prophylactic antibiotics. *Br J Neurosurg*. 1996;10(6):571–575.

Clemenza JW, Kaltman SI, Diamond DL. Craniofacial trauma and cerebrospinal fluid leakage: A retrospective clinical study. *J Oral Maxillofac Surg*. 1995;53(9):1004–1007.

Dula DJ, Fales W. The 'ring sign': Is it a reliable indicator for cerebral spinal fluid? *Ann Emerg Med*. 1993;22(4):718–720.

Ellis E III, Scott K. Assessment of patients with facial fractures. *Emerg Med Clin North Am*. 2000;18(3):411–448, vi.

Lalani Z, Bonanthaya KM. Cervical spine injury in maxillofacial trauma. *Br J Oral Maxillofac Surg*. 1997;35(4):243–245.

Lynham AJ, Hirst JP, Cosson JA, et al. Emergency department management of maxillofacial trauma. *Emerg Med Australas*. 2004;16(1):7–12.

Merritt RM, Williams MF. Cervical spine injury complicating facial trauma: Incidence and management. *Am J Otolaryngol*. 1997;18(4):235–238.

Welch KC, Stankiewicz J. *CSF Rhinorrhea*. eMedicine, October 15, 2008. Available at: http://emedicine.medscape.com/article/861126-overview.

91

OPTIMAL MANAGEMENT OF MANDIBLE FRACTURES REQUIRES KNOWLEDGE OF ANATOMY, EPIDEMIOLOGY OF FRACTURE PATTERNS, AND SOUND ASSESSMENT OF ASSOCIATED INJURIES

GERHARD S. MUNDINGER, MD

Do not miss mandible fractures. It pays to know basic mandible anatomy and the epidemiology of mandible fracture locations and patterns (*Figs. 91.1–91.3*). If a mandible fracture is identified, be sure not to miss associated craniofacial injuries.

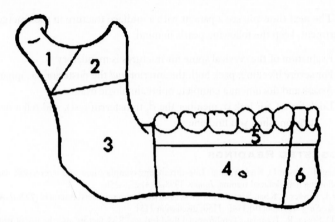

FIGURE 91.1. Mandible anatomy based on common fracture sites. 1. Condylar head and neck; 2. coronoid process; 3. ramus and angle; 4. body; 5. alveolar segment; 6. symphysis. (Adapted from Luyk NH, Ferguson JW. The diagnosis and initial management of the fractured mandible. *Am J Emerg Med*. 1991;9(4):352–359.)

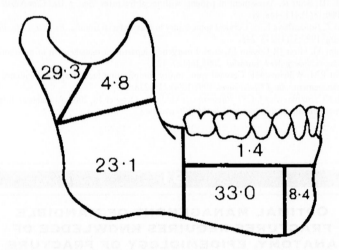

FIGURE 91.2. Distribution of mandibular fractures by percent. (Adapted from Luyk NH, Ferguson JW. The diagnosis and initial management of the fractured mandible. *Am J Emerg Med*. 1991;9[4]:352–359.)

The greatest error to avoid while assessing mandible fractures is violating the ATLS algorithm by focusing on the signs and symptoms of a mandible fracture at the expense of the primary survey.

As always, the advanced trauma life support (ATLS) algorithm applies to trauma patients, and mandible fractures should not be addressed until

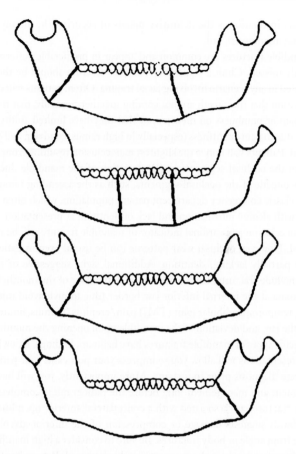

FIGURE 91.3. Common bilateral mandibular fracture patterns. (Adapted from Luyk NH, Ferguson JW. The diagnosis and initial management of the fractured mandible. *Am J Emerg Med.* 1991;9[4]:352–359.)

the primary survey is complete. Generally, mandible injuries (and injuries to the face overall) are not life threatening. The two rare, main exceptions are the occurrence of exsanguination due to facial vessel laceration and airway compromise from facial trauma. These two scenarios should always be considered when assessing any mandible fracture. Bilateral mandible fractures can lead to airway compromise due to prolapse of the central segment. Airway compromise can be temporized in this scenario by bridle wiring around two teeth on either side of the fracture segment or, in the case of a prolapsed medial segment due to bilateral parasymphyseal fractures, with anterior traction on the tongue using a towel clamp or suture. This pulls the prolapsed medial segment anteriorly as an airway-preserving measure.

Of course, intubation is the definitive means of securing the airway if these emergency maneuvers fail.

Mandible fractures are common and appear in predictable patterns yet are commonly missed. Clinical signs of a mandible fracture should be thoroughly investigated in any scenario involving facial trauma. Often, patients will complain of a sensation that their teeth are not coming together normally, that there is an area of pain or numbness on their jaw, or that they have limited ability to open their jaw due to pain or stiffness (especially in high ramus, condylar, and coronoid fractures). Patients will notice the slightest malocclusion resulting from (A) local trauma to the occlusal segments or (B) deviation of the mandible due to fracture sites outside of the occlusal segments, such as the ascending ramus. If you have the classic emergency department patient population, which often includes patients with alcohol intoxication and lack of dentition at presentation, the utility of malocclusion as a cardinal indicator of mandible fracture will be markedly decreased. However, occlusal wear patterns can be useful even in patients with poor (or partially lacking) dentition. Additional signs suggestive of mandible fracture include fractured teeth, ecchymosis in the floor of the mouth, bleeding or hematoma at the internal inferior jaw border (due to mylohyoid injury), jaw swelling, temporomandibular joint (TMJ) pain/crepitus/trismus, limited ability to open the jaw, and deviation of the mandible upon opening the mouth.

Specific types of mandible fractures have hallmark findings. Knowing these classic presentations will allow you to impress your peers and your patient with an accurate diagnosis prior to imaging. More importantly, you will have a plan for treatment and management long before the radiograph is completed. Subcondylar fractures are associated with a contralateral anterior open bite. Lower lip numbness suggests damage or compression of the inferior alveolar nerve resulting from angle or body fractures. Be sure to consider a high mandible fracture in any instance where the inner ear canal is lacerated. Remember that fracture lines are occasionally palpable, leading to an easy diagnosis. Assessment of these signs by visual inspection and bimanual palpation of all areas of the mandible, including the TMJ, is crucial. Mandible fractures can also lead to a painful locked TMJ, which results from subluxation of the condylar head anterior to the glenoid fossa. This dislocation can be corrected with downward pressure on the posterior teeth of the affected side after anesthetizing the lower jaw.

If you suspect or have diagnosed a mandible fracture, be highly suspicious of other craniofacial injuries. Fifty percent of mandible fractures are bilateral and occur in common patterns (*Fig. 91.2*). Forty-three percent are found in occurrence with other craniofacial fractures. Angle fractures are associated with parasymphyseal fractures on the opposite side. Body and angle fractures are usually unilateral. Fractures of the zygomatic arch can impinge medially on the coronoid, clinically mimicking a high mandible fracture. Additionally, there is a strong association between unilateral mandible fractures and high cervical spine injury. A thin-cut (<3 mm/slice) head and face CT with coronal and saggital reconstructions should be ordered on every patient suspected of having a mandible fracture. Do not forget that ramus fractures are commonly missed on CT imaging. If there is tooth involvement in any identified fracture, a panorex image should be obtained to assess tooth and tooth root injury. This is the only situation in craniofacial trauma where thin-cut, multiplanar CT imaging is not the gold standard for bony injury. Beware that panorex imaging alone will result in missed symphyseal/parasymphyseal fractures.

Now that you have reviewed your mandible anatomy, evaluated predictable patterns and findings associated with mandibular fractures, secured the patients airway, evaluated the c-spine and the rest of the face for other injuries, and made the astute diagnosis of an acute mandibular fracture, it is time to call the consultant. A consult to the facial trauma service is always warranted with any mandible fracture. Understanding favorable versus unfavorable fractures will enable you to more effectively communicate the urgency of the consult and anticipate the course of management (*Figs. 91.4* and *91.5*).

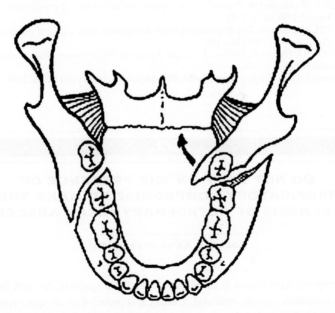

FIGURE 91.4. Favorable (**left**) versus unfavorable (**right**) fractures in the horizontal plane. The *arrow* indicates the vector of destabilizing muscle pull. (Adapted from Luyk NH, Ferguson JW. The diagnosis and initial management of the fractured mandible. *Am J Emerg Med.* 1991;9[4]:352–359.)

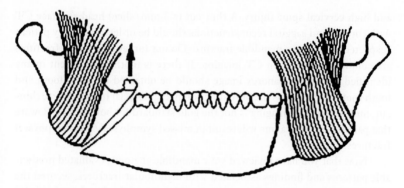

FIGURE 91.5. Favorable (**left**) versus unfavorable fractures in the vertical plane. (Adapted from Luyk NH, Ferguson JW. The diagnosis and initial management of the fractured mandible. *Am J Emerg Med.* 1991;9[4]:352–359.)

SUGGESTED READINGS

Brown DL, Borschel GH. *Michigan Manual of Plastic Surgery.* 1st ed. Philadelphia, PA: Lippincott Williams & Wilkins; 2004.

Hussain K, Wijetunge DB, Grubnic S, et al. A comprehensive analysis of craniofacial trauma. *J Trauma.* 1994;36(1):34–47.

Luyk NH, Ferguson JW. The diagnosis and initial management of the fractured mandible. *Am J Emerg Med.* 1991;9(4):352–359.

McCarthy JG, Galiano R, Boutros A. *Current Therapy in Plastic Surgery.* Philadelphia, PA: Saunders Elsevier; 2006.

Weinzweig J. *Plastic Surgery Secrets.* 1st ed. Philadelphia, PA: Hanley and Belfus; 1998.

92

DO NOT RELY ON THE PRESENCE OF RESPIRATORY COMPROMISE TO MAKE THE DIAGNOSIS OF RETROPHARYNGEAL ABSCESS

COLLEEN ANNA GIBSON, MD

A retropharyngeal abscess is an infection of the deep spaces of the neck that is most commonly seen in childhood. Usually, it is preceded by an upper respiratory tract infection that then tracts posteriorly through the lymphatic system of the nasopharynx into the lymph nodes in the potential space located between the posterior pharyngeal wall and the prevertebral fascia. The majority of these infections are seen in children under age 5. Theoretically, this is because the lymph nodes in the retropharyngeal space atrophy after this age, making infection there much less likely. In adults, retropharyngeal abscess is rare and almost always the result of trauma to the posterior pharynx causing a direct inoculation of infectious material.

Classic teaching is that patients with retropharyngeal abscesses present with signs of respiratory distress and airway obstruction such as stridor, wheezing, tachypnea, and drooling. More current studies, however, demonstrate that these symptoms often do not exist when patients initially present. In fact, signs of airway obstruction are only found in the late stages of disease—long after you should have made the diagnosis. The primary error in the management of retropharyngeal abscesses is not thinking of it until it is too late. Relying on respiratory symptoms or distress to trigger your consideration of this entity will put your patient at considerable risk.

In order for a retropharyngeal abscess to cause respiratory symptoms, the fluctuant mass must occupy enough space to exert a mass effect on the pharynx and trachea. Most patients will have other symptoms long before this occurs. In a recent retrospective review of 64 cases of retropharyngeal abscess, only one patient had stridor and two had wheezing. So if signs of airway compromise are not going to give you the diagnosis until it is progressed to a severe degree, what should you look for? Neck stiffness, limitation of neck movement, fever, sore throat, and a fluctuant neck mass are more sensitive signs of retropharyngeal abscess. A fluctuant mass is very specific for retropharyngeal abscess but will only be visible in about half of cases. Limitation of neck mobility is a historic feature and physical finding that should be actively investigated to help you zero in on the diagnosis. It can present dramatically with torticollis or more subtly, as when a child refuses to move his or her neck in a particular direction during your exam. It is critical that you consider retropharyngeal abscess in any patient with even subtle signs of limitation of neck movement or neck stiffness; otherwise, you may miss this potentially life-threatening illness.

Once the diagnosis is suspected, you must obtain imaging of the neck. Traditionally, the lateral neck radiograph was the most utilized diagnostic imaging modality. Prevertebral space measurements of >7 mm at the level of the second cervical vertebra or >14 mm at the level of the sixth cervical vertebra are consistent with retropharyngeal swelling. Today, the plain neck films are often used as a screening test in patients in whom the diagnosis is not certain. A more definitive study is CT scan because it can localize and quantify the abscess. CT also is helpful in differentiating retropharyngeal cellulitis from abscess. There is also some discussion on using ultrasound of the neck. The advantage of ultrasound is avoidance of radiation and potential ability to do it at a patient's bedside; however, more research is needed in this area before it will replace CT scan as the preferred method of imaging. For now, your best bet is to get the CT scan as soon as possible.

Once you have confirmed that you are dealing with a retropharyngeal abscess, intravenous antibiotics must be initiated. The choice of antibiotics, naturally, is based on the suspected microbes, which vary between different studies, but are a mixture of anaerobic and aerobic bacteria. The ones that are commonly isolated include *Staphylococcus aureus* and *S. epidermidis*, *Streptococcus viridans* and *S. pyogenes*, *Bacteroides*, *Peptostreptococcus*, *Fusobacterium*, *Haemophilus*, and *Klebsiella*. With these microbes in mind, clindamycin should be your first-line antibiotic with cefazolin as an alternative.

Another potential pitfall in evaluation and management of patients with retropharyngeal abscesses is the assumption that all of these patients need surgical drainage. Many studies have demonstrated that patients without signs of airway compromise can be treated with intravenous antibiotics alone. Perhaps we should stop making fun of the ENT doctors who do not want to do surgery; apparently, the literature is on their side for once. That being known, it is still imperative that all of these patients get admitted for IV antibiotics and close observation with ENT determining whether the clinical course warrants surgery. Since this condition, in its early form, can be managed successfully without surgery, it is even more vital for you to recognize a retropharyngeal abscess before airway obstruction and signs of respiratory distress set in. Not only can your vigilance save your patients from emergent airway management, but you can also prevent them from requiring cold steel; two things that the patient and their families will greatly appreciate.

SUGGESTED READINGS

Craig FW, Schunk JE. Retropharyngeal abscess in children: Clinical presentation, utility of imaging, and current management. *Pediatrics*. 2003;111;1394–1398.
Rafei K, Lichenstein R. Airway infectious disease emergencies. *Pediatr Clin N Am*. 2006;53(2): 215–242.
Shah S, Shareif G. Pediatric respiratory infections. *Em Med Clin N Am*. 2007;25(4):961–979, vi.

93

BEWARE EPIGLOTTITIS ... IT IS NOT YET AN EXTINCT DISEASE!

BENJAMIN J. LAWNER, DO, EMT-P

Epiglottitis is an acute inflammation of supraglottic structures. More appropriately termed, "supraglottitis," this acute process can involve the aryepiglottic folds and cause cellulitis of adjacent airway structures. Though there are some conflicting epidemiologic data, epiglottitis seems to preferentially affect men near the fifth decade of life. Prior to the *Haemophilus influenza* vaccine, this disease was most prevalent in younger children. Children may still contract epiglottitis secondary to vaccine failure or noncompliance; however, *H. influenza* is no longer the predominant causative organism. Current pathogens implicated in epiglottitis include *Streptococcus pneumoniae, Staphylococcus aureus*, and β-hemolytic streptococci. Viruses and fungi are rarely implicated in epiglottitis, and cultures from infected tissue should always be obtained.

PRESENTATION

In contrast to the pediatric population, adults usually exhibit a milder form of the disease. An upper respiratory prodrome may herald epiglottitis, and viral syndrome complaints are common. Most adults will complain of a sore throat, odynophagia, and a muffled voice. Hoarseness is uncommon. Occasionally, patients may experience severe pain upon palpation of laryngeal structures. The danger with epiglottitis lies in its potential for rapid progression to airway compromise and subsequent respiratory failure. A cautious, vigilant approach is warranted to guard against decompensation. Indeed, cases of suspected epiglottitis should be admitted to an intensive care setting for observation and intravenous antibiotics.

DIAGNOSIS

The diagnostic gold standard for epiglottitis is laryngoscopy. Aside from visually confirming the presence of an infected epiglottis, this permits the laryngoscopist to obtain cultures that may guide the selection of appropriate antibiotics. For stable patients, indirect laryngoscopy may be attempted. Airway manipulation has the potential to cause respiratory failure via laryngospasm and edema, so providers must remain committed and capable of securing an often difficult airway. Since the risks of laryngoscopy in stable patients may outweigh the potential benefits, it is advisable to start with plain films. Soft tissue films of the neck are approximately 90% sensitive for epiglottitis, but normal films do not exclude disease. Abnormal findings on plain radiography include obliteration of the prevallecular space, epiglottic width >8 mm, aryepiglottic fold <7 mm, and adjacent soft tissue swelling. Epiglottitis is diagnosed clinically when patients are in extremis; do not wait for plain films or fiberoptic laryngoscopy to confirm the diagnosis. Patients with stridor, drooling, and obvious respiratory distress should be prepared for emergent intubation and/or cricothyrotomy. ENT surgeons and anesthesiologists may be of invaluable assistance for critically ill patients (*Fig. 93.1*).

MANAGEMENT

Do not discharge cases of suspected epiglottitis home with short interval follow-up and antibiotics! If the diagnosis of epiglottitis is entertained, the patient should be admitted to an intensive care setting. Antibiotics such as ceftriaxone, cefotaxime, and ampicillin/sulbactam, which are active against

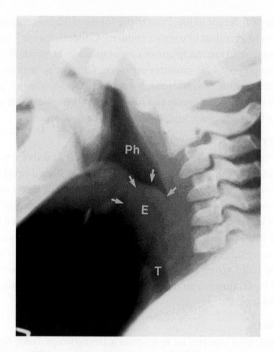

FIGURE 93.1. The "thumb sign"; *arrows* highlight an edematous epiglottis. (Courtesy of Ferri's 2009 Clinical Advisor. St. Louis: Mosby Elsevier; 2009.)

causative bacterial agents, should be promptly initiated. For stable patients, laryngoscopy may be deferred. Ideally, visualization and culture of the epiglottis are attempted in the operating room. For sick and rapidly deteriorating patients, indirect laryngoscopy with fiberoptic devices is contraindicated. Up to 21% of patients with this disease may require emergent and invasive airway intervention. Therefore, intubation should be attempted with a double setup. This particular arrangement brings equipment for both direct laryngoscopy and cricothyroidotomy to the patient's bedside. Laryngoscopy is frequently successful, but the emergency physician needs to prepare for the possibility of securing a surgical airway via cricothyroidotomy. The role of steroids and racemic epinephrine for epiglottis remains unclear. Allow patients to remain in a position of comfort until the swelling and concurrent infection resolve.

COMPLICATIONS AND PITFALLS

Patients with epiglottitis require critical care monitoring. A telemetry floor is an inappropriate disposition since these patients may experience a rapid deterioration in stability. Proximity to advanced airway intervention is crucial. Adult epiglottitis may spread to adjacent structures, and Ludwig angina, abscess, sepsis, and pneumothorax have all been reported. The presence of these conditions does not, therefore, exclude epiglottitis; however, extra-epiglottic manifestations are more likely to occur in the pediatric population. Though blood cultures are of often low yield, close contacts of patients with *H. influenza*–positive diseases should receive prophylaxis with rifampin at 20 mg/kg for 4 days. Since epiglottis may mimic an acute pharyngitis, be sure to discharge patients with instructions that specifically mention the possibility of more severe disease. Patients need to return to the emergency department if they experience worsening odynophagia, drooling, high fever, or increasing respiratory distress.

SUGGESTED READINGS

Alcaide ML. Pharyngitis and epiglottitis. *Infect Dis Clin North Am*. 2007;21(2):449–469.
Bowman KG. *Epiglottitis*. eMedicine.com, December 2006. Available at: www.emedicine.com.
Ferri FF. Epiglottitis. In: *Ferri's 2009 Clinical Advisor*. St. Louis: Mosby Elsevier; 2009.
Marx J. Epiglottitis. In: *Rosen's Emergency Medicine: Concepts and Clinical Practice*. 6th ed. St. Louis: Mosby; 2006.
Tan CK. Adult epiglottitis. *CMAJ*. 2007;176(5):620.

94

RECOGNIZE THE PRESENTATION OF FOREIGN BODY ASPIRATION AND ORDER THE CORRECT DIAGNOSTIC TEST

KIMBERLY A. B. LEESON, MD AND BEN A. LEESON, MD, FACEP

Foreign body aspiration occurs more frequently in small children for several reasons. They lack molars, which prevent them from adequately chewing their food, and have narrower airways. In addition, they talk, laugh, and run about while eating, making accidental aspiration more likely. They also explore the world with their mouths, and may place small objects in their mouths out of shear curiosity. Other times, they are victims of older children or siblings who innocently or maliciously feed inappropriate substances to the baby.

Commonly aspirated items include hot dogs, coins, hard candy, grapes, raisins, balloons, beads, and nuts. For this reason, small foods should be reserved for children of at least 5 years of age and anticipatory guidance is vital to the prevention of this potentially dangerous accident. More than half of aspirations are found in the right main bronchus, since in children it is larger and more linearly aligned with the trachea, making it a direct shot.

Most aspirations occur in children <1 year of age; however, the astute clinician will consider the diagnosis in almost all children who present with respiratory complaints. Medical history is the single most predictive factor in clinical suspicion of foreign body aspiration. Yet frequently, the child cannot or does not provide the key history to assist the emergency physician in getting to the bottom of the problem. Many times the actual ingestion is not witnessed or even noticed, so adult corroboration may be lacking. History is key, but you may not get this important piece of information. Play it safe and consider aspiration in most kids who present with respiratory symptoms.

Foreign body aspiration may present as recurrent cough, wheezing, persistent or recurrent pneumonia, lung abscess, focal bronchiectasis, or hemoptysis. Fever may be present. If the aspiration results in a higher obstruction, stridor, recurrent or persistent croup, and voice changes can occur. The condition can mimic asthma and bronchitis, and even viral syndrome. Up to one third of patients are asymptomatic. Not surprisingly, the clinician can easily overlook the true etiology of symptoms in these patients and fail to order the appropriate workup or consultation that will be curative.

Do not forget your ABC's. Children who can speak or cry and present with coughing, tachypnea, or other mild symptoms may be observed while diagnostic testing takes place. In cases where a child cannot speak or cry, a complete airway obstruction is assumed. Here, the Heimlich maneuver or back blows and chest thrusts in children <1 year of age should be administered without delay.

If the vigilant, meticulous clinician maintains a high degree of suspicion for aspiration, she may consider supportive testing. A cooperative child should undergo an anterior-posterior (AP) expiratory film, which may demonstrate air trapping in the affected lung. Children too young or immature to cooperate can undergo lateral decubitus chest radiography, or an AP film with compression of the abdomen to illicit similar diagnostic evidence. Fluoroscopy and CT scan are additional imaging modalities that may occasionally be helpful.

Consider bronchoscopy early in the workup. Radiographic imaging for this condition has significant limitations. Most aspirated objects are radiolucent, and typical radiographic findings may be subtle to nonexistent. Up to one third of plain radiographs are completely normal, despite the presence of an aspirated foreign body. Midulla found a diagnostic sensitivity of 80% and a specificity of 33% for the presence of a single positive radiographic finding. When present, nonspecific signs of overinflation, atelectasis, and/or opacification of portions of the distal lung that can be seen radiographically can lead the emergency physician (EP) to incorrectly attribute the patient's symptoms to an infectious or reactive airways cause. This diagnostic mistake will undoubtedly result in continued symptomatology and a delay to definitive treatment. If a high probability of foreign body aspiration persists, proceed immediately to bronchoscopy instead of wasting time with radiographic testing.

Medical treatment is largely unnecessary for aspiration. Neither broncho-dilators and corticosteroids nor chest physical therapy and postural drainage should be used to dislodge a foreign body. This may cause the foreign body to move to a more dangerous location and result in a larger airway obstruction. Antibiotics are not indicated in most cases. Rarely, they may be administered after bronchoscopy with corticosteroids, when airway edema and inflammation have been identified.

Foreign body aspiration is a serious condition that can be challenging to identify. Consider the diagnosis of foreign body aspiration in all children with unexplained pulmonary symptoms, including persistent lung infection and new-onset asthma and bronchiectasis. Diagnostic studies have limited utility, and patient symptoms can be vague or nonspecific. Lea found foreign bodies in 45.2% of children with a positive history but with normal physical examination and radiologic studies. Maintain vigilance for this condition in your clinical practice and do not hesitate to consult a pediatric pulmonologist, surgeon, or otolaryngologist for bronchoscopy. Missing an aspirated foreign body delays removal and increases chances of complications such as atelectasis, bronchiectasis, lung abscess, and persistent symptoms.

SUGGESTED READINGS

Bye MR. Airway foreign body. eMedicine.com, last updated: September 13, 2007. Available at: www.emedicine.com/PED/topic286.htm

CDC. Nonfatal choking-related episodes among children-United States, 2001. *MMWR Morb Mortal Wkly Rep.* 2002;51(42):945–948.

Even L, Heno N, Talmon Y, et al. Diagnostic evaluation of foreign body aspiration in children: A prospective study. *J Pediatr Surg.* 2005;40(7):1122–1127.

Midulla F, Guidi R, Barbato A, et al. Foreign body aspiration in children. *Pediatr Int.* 2005;47(6):663–668.

Rovin JD, Rodgers BM. Pediatric foreign body aspiration. *Pediatr Rev.* 2000;21(3):86–90.

Swanson KL. Airway foreign bodies: What's new? *Semin Respir Crit Care Med.* 2004;25(4): 405–411.

Tintinalli JE, Ruiz E, Krome RL, et al., eds. *Tintinalli's Emergency Medicine: A Comprehensive Study Guide.* 6th ed. New York, NY: McGraw-Hill; 2004.

95

USE AN ORGANIZED APPROACH TO MANAGING EPISTAXIS TO MAKE YOUR JOB EASIER

ANDRE' J. MOULEDOUX, JR, MD

Epistaxis is one of the most common ENT emergencies, ranging from self-limited to life-threatening. It is usually classified into anterior and posterior bleeding, with anterior bleeds accounting for 90% to 95% of cases (a significant majority arising from Kiesselbach plexus).

Nose picking ("epistaxis digitorum"), rhinitis, facial trauma, foreign bodies, and intranasal steroids are common causes of anterior bleeds. Patients on warfarin (Coumadin) are at high risk for epistaxis, and massive epistaxis can be the presenting symptom of hereditary hemorrhagic telangiectasia (Osler-Weber-Rendu disease). Alcohol is also a risk factor, while hypertension and aspirin have unclear roles.

ABCs must be a priority in any patient presenting with epistaxis, particularly in trauma patients. Though rare, airway intervention and fluid resuscitation can be necessary. When taking the history, patients can assist by holding pressure over the alae. An emesis basin should be provided, and an anxiolytic can be considered. Some key components of the history include recurrence, known tumors, history of easy bleeding or bruising, and concurrent medical problems (e.g., coronary artery disease (CAD)) that can be exacerbated by blood loss.

The physician must have proper equipment for a thorough evaluation. This equipment includes a head lamp, nasal speculum, and suction (with a Frazier suction tip). Universal precautions (with eye protection) should be utilized as well. Many otolaryngologists suggest two puffs of oxymetazoline to assist with hemostasis. However, lidocaine with epinephrine or 4% cocaine (applied with cotton swabs into the nasopharynx) can be even more effective, as the analgesia they provide can facilitate a detailed patient exam. The patient should be seated in the sniffing position for optimal view. Clots should be removed via suction or by having the patient gently blow his or her nose.

Routine lab studies are usually not indicated. Patients with severe or prolonged bleeding should have a complete blood count (CBC) (to check the hematocrit and the platelet count) and type and screen. Only patients on Coumadin need a prothrombin time (PT) with international normalized ratio (INR) level.

If hemostasis cannot be achieved with compression and an anterior source of bleeding is identified, chemical or electrical cautery is first-line management. Firm pressure with a silver nitrate stick should be applied for 5 to 10 s on a relatively blood-free (as much as possible) surface. However, overzealous cautery should be avoided, and cautery should never be applied to both sides of the nasal septum.

Nasal packing is the next step in management if cautery fails. Nasal tampons or commercial nasal balloon catheters are both effective in achieving tamponade. Gauze packing is also an option, though this method requires more technical expertise and is usually more uncomfortable for the patient. Opioids may be necessary for patient comfort during packing. After placement of a pack, each nare should be checked along with the posterior oropharynx for continued bleeding. If there is persistent bleeding, a contralateral nasal pack should be inserted to provide opposing pressure to the septum. If bleeding continues, then the bleeding is likely from a posterior source.

Balloon catheters are available specifically for posterior bleeds, and Foley catheters have also been used when specific posterior catheters are not available. The anterior nares should be packed as well (in suspected posterior bleeds), as bleeding can be from both anterior and posterior sources, especially in hereditary hemorrhagic telangiectasia. Patients with posterior packs should be admitted for definitive care by an ENT specialist, and patients with anterior packs and multiple comorbidities may require admission as well. Some potential complications from posterior packing include airway compromise from posterior displacement of packing, balloon deflation, and balloon rupture (risk for aspiration if water is in the balloon). On the other hand, the hypothetical "nasopulmonary reflex" is not a risk of posterior packing (i.e., there is no change in pulmonary or cardiac function with posterior packs). Antibiotics should be given for both anterior and posterior packs, though there is a dearth of evidence on antibiotic prevention of toxic shock syndrome or sinusitis.

Thrombogenic foams and gels are new modalities which preliminarily show equivalent efficacy to cautery and packing, and they have decreased patient discomfort; but they have greatly increased the cost. These can be especially useful in patients with hereditary hemorrhagic telangiectasia. Endoscopic arterial ligation and angiographic embolization are alternatives in refractory cases, but these decisions require consultation with an ENT specialist.

Patients on Coumadin with epistaxis should not receive reversal agents unless other modalities fail to stop the bleeding. ENT specialists recommend the lowering of high blood pressures, though there have been no prospective studies demonstrating the efficacy of this practice.

Patients with recurrent bleeds will ultimately need follow-up from an appropriate specialist; for recurrent epistaxis can be a symptom of nasal neoplasm, aneurysm of the head and neck (particularly in patients with previous head or neck surgery), or an undiagnosed bleeding diathesis. Patients with packing (if not admitted) need follow-up with an ENT specialist in 24 to 48 h.

SUGGESTED READINGS

Alter H. Approach to the adult with epistaxis. *UpToDate*, 2008. Available at: www.uptodate. com

Douglas R, Wormald PJ. Update on epistaxis. *Curr Opin Otolaryngol Head Neck Surg.* 2007;15(3):180–183.

Kucik CJ, Clenney T. Management of epistaxis. *Am Fam Physician.* 2005;71(2):312.

Pope LE, Hobbs CG. Epistaxis: An update on current management. *Postgrad Med J.* 2005;81(955):309–314.

96

DO NOT RELY ON A HEAD COMPUTED TOMOGRAPHY TO EXCLUDE SERIOUS CAUSES OF VERTIGO

JAMES A. NELSON, MD, FACEP

Many clinicians are uncomfortable evaluating the vertiginous patient. Although 97% of emergency department patients with vertigo have relatively benign conditions, 3% suffer from a cerebellar stroke. There can be substantial overlap of symptoms between these two, peripheral vertigo and cerebellar infarction.

Many clinicians use head computed tomography (CT) as a means of "ruling out" central causes of vertigo. Do not commit this error! The head CT is only 26% sensitive for acute cerebral infarction and may be even worse or small strokes affecting the posterior circulation.

Separating the serious causes of vertigo from the nonserious causes can be done, but it requires clinical skill. One must know how the common vertigo syndromes present, and one must recognize some red flags that suggest cerebellar infarction.

The most common vertigo syndromes in the emergency department are benign paroxysmal positional vertigo (BPPV), migrainous vertigo, and vestibular neuritis/labyrinthitis. BPPV presents with distinct episodes of vertigo typically lasting less than a minute, provoked by vertical rotation of the head. It is confirmed by characteristic torsional nystagmus on Dix-Hallpike testing. Migrainous vertigo presents in a variable fashion, but the patient should have had similar vertigo episodes in the past, a formal diagnosis of migraine, and a migraine-specific symptom. Headache is present in only 50% of cases.

Vestibular neuritis and labyrinthitis, caused by viral inflammation, are characterized by acute hypofunction of one vestibular labyrinth. The patient feels as if he or she is continually turning his or her head away from the affected side. It is called labyrinthitis when hearing is affected, and vestibular neuritis when it is not.

Cerebellar infarction can present very similarly to vestibular neuritis. A comprehensive neurologic examination including cerebellar examination will identify localizing deficits in 90% of cases of cerebellar infarction. Unfortunately, 10% will present seemingly identical to vestibular neuritis. Three items on physical diagnosis will identify most of these patients.

First, direction-changing nystagmus (also called gaze-evoked nystagmus or multidirectional nystagmus), is a sign of cerebellar infarction. Peripheral nystagmus does not change direction. If the patient's nystagmus changes direction with gaze, a central cause is assumed. The only caveat is that the eyes should not be strained too far laterally, as this causes extraocular muscle fatigue, and the "give way" can be mistaken for nystagmus. Keeping lateral gaze within 30 to 45 degrees is preferred. Among the 10% of patients with cerebellar infarction and no localizing findings, 56% have direction-changing nystagmus.

Second, the inability to walk without support is a sign of cerebellar infarction. Although any patient with vertigo will have a clumsy gait simply from the vestibular symptoms, the patient with vestibular neuritis has an intact central nervous system that integrates information from the proprioceptive and visual systems, enabling ambulation to take place. In contrast, among the 10% of patients with cerebellar infarction and no localizing findings, 71% are unable to walk without support.

Finally, skew deviation is a sign of posterior circulation pathology. If the patient describes a vertical disruption of the visual field, skew deviation is assumed. For example, if the patient looks at a clock, the numbers on one side might be higher than on the other. It reflects a disturbance of some of the vestibuloocular reflexes in the brainstem and cerebellum that allow the visual horizon to be maintained despite head tilting. One study of patients with acute vertigo of unclear cause found that skew deviation had 100% sensitivity for central pathology (most patients had cerebellar infarction or multiple sclerosis).

In summary, when diagnosing the emergency department patient with vertigo, a thorough physical examination is more helpful than a CT scan. This includes examination of gait, assessment of ocular findings, and recognition of skew deviation as a central sign. When the clinician practices these principles, he or she will be able to recognize cerebellar infarction with greater accuracy. When in doubt, consultation with neurology is appropriate, and MRI can be considered either at once or within 24 to 48 h.

SUGGESTED READINGS

Chalela JA, Kidwell CS, Nentwich LM, et al. Magnetic resonance imaging and computed tomography in emergency assessment of patients with suspected acute stroke: A prospective comparison. *Lancet.* 2007;369:293–298.

Lee H, Sohn SI, Cho YW, et al. Cerebellar infarction presenting isolated vertigo: Frequency and vascular topographical patterns. *Neurology*. 2006;67:1178–1183.

Neuhauser H, Lempert T. Vertigo and dizziness related to migraine: A diagnostic challenge. *Cephalalgia*. 2004;24:83–91.

97

DO NOT FORGET ABOUT THE POTENTIALLY SERIOUS COMPLICATIONS OF OTITIS MEDIA

EMILY B. J. OSBORN, MD

In the preantibiotic era, otitis media (OM) and its intracranial complications (meningitis, brain abscess, lateral sinus thrombosis, etc.) caused significant morbidity and even mortality. Now, with antibiotic therapy, these life-threatening illnesses are rare. However, OM can still lead to fatal complications. In most of these cases, this could have been prevented by a careful history and physical examination. *Don't forget to look in the ears*! When a patient presents with meningeal signs or altered mental status, simply examining the ears can narrow the differential dramatically. If you miss a critical finding and the diagnosis is delayed, the patient's attorney will not delay his or her call to you.

OM occurs when fluid accumulates in the middle ear when mucosal inflammation impairs drainage. Infection occurs by eustachian tube reflux. The highest incidence of OM is in children 6 to 12 months old, and their history includes vague symptoms of fever and pain. The best way to diagnose OM is by decreased tympanic membrane mobility. *Learn to use an insufflator*—correct diagnosis is essential to minimize complications!

The treatment of OM remains controversial worldwide. Many countries do not treat OM, approximately half of these infections are viral, and most bacterial infections resolve with the body's own defenses. Others argue treatment of bacterial OM may mask early signs of complications. The most common USA management remains antibiotics and analgesics. Antihistamines and over the counter (OTC) decongestants have no benefit; at most, these will cause drowsiness and dad will get more sleep. Since the era of antibiotics, the morbidity and mortality associated with OM have declined. Amoxicillin remains first-line therapy, but in higher doses, for resistant or recurrent OM, use amoxicillin/clavulanate, cefuroxime, or a macrolide.

When the diagnosis of OM is missed and these patients go untreated, they are at risk for the following complications: OM with tympanic membrane perforation (TMP), chronic suppurative OM, mastoiditis, labyrinthitis, petrositis, cholesteatoma, cranial nerve palsies, cranial osteomyelitis, lateral sinus thrombosis, brain abscess, meningitis, hearing loss, and associated educational disadvantages.

Acute mastoiditis is the most common complication of OM not treated with antibiotics. Do not miss this! Look for an asymmetric auricle, tenderness and erythema in the postauricular region. Mastoiditis is diagnosed with CT or x-rays. Treatment is IV antibiotics, hospital admission, and ENT consult. The increase in *S. pneumoniae* resistance correlates with an increasing need for surgical intervention. Patients in whom infections have stopped prior to intracranial spread can expect full recovery. Missed OM with mastoiditis can spread infection intracranially (in and around the dura), into nerves and vessels, into bony stuctures (petrositis!), and Bezold abscess. Look for Gradenigo syndrome—a triad of suppurative OM, abducens nerve palsy, and deep facial pain. Gradenigo syndrome is treated with IV broad-spectrum antibiotics and surgical drainage. Pott puffy tumor is a rare complication.

OM with TMP requires topical antibiotics—ciprofloxacin or chloramphenicol. Do not make the error of using aminoglycosides as they are ototoxic! When TMP complicates OM, use 1.2% of aluminium acetotartrate eardrops. Topical mupirocin ointment can be used against the ever-spreading methicillin resistant staphylococcus aureus (MRSA). Dry traumatic TMP will heal on its own. Wet traumatic TMP requires prophylactic pseudomonas coverage. Chronic or multiple TMP is a risk for hearing loss, cholesteatoma, and recurrent infections. Patients with any TMP injury, regardless of the cause, should be followed up as an outpatient until healing is verified.

Chronic supportive OM is persistent discharge from the ear over 2 weeks with TMP. Treat by keeping the antibiotic directly on the infection at all times—use an ear wick. Quinolones cost more but alternatives are less effective.

Cranial nerve palsies are a rare complication of OM in which the patient presents with acute OM and ipsilateral facial palsy. Inflammation or infection affects the facial nerve bony canal. Treatment is broad-spectrum antibiotics with myringotomy. Cranial nerve palsies associated with OM are two times more likely to be caused by a bacterial infection than a viral infection. If the patient fails to improve, do not delay CT investigation for deeper infection requiring surgical drainage or debridement.

Lateral sinus thrombosis is still seen as a complication of chronic OM and should be considered in really sick-appearing children. Prior to the advent of operative intervention, lateral sinus thrombosis had a death rate of 100%. Treatment for this complication is thrombectomy; anticoagulation remains controversial.

Suppurative labyrinthitis causes hearing loss, vertigo, imbalance, nausea, and vomiting. It can lead to labyrinthitis ossificans. Bacterial labyrinthitis is still a major cause of all acquired hearing loss. These infections enter the labyrinth through separations caused by cholesteatoma which can be either congenital or result from trauma or infection. A white mass behind the tympanic membrane is suspicious—give anti-Pseudomonal prophylaxis and refer for prompt ENT evaluation.

Remember that an ear infection is not always just an ear infection. Life-threatening complications await those who neglect this crucial part of the physical exam. Taking an extra few minutes to look in the ears and thinking of potential complications will pay off big for you and your patient.

SUGGESTED READINGS

Brinks A, Thomas S. The practice guidelines 'Otitis externa' (first revision) from the Dutch College of General Practitioners: A response from the perspective of general practice. *Ned Tijdschr Geneeskd.* 2008;152(21):1199–1200.

Burston BJ, Pretorius PM, Ramsden JD. Gradenigo's syndrome: Successful conservative treatment in adult and pediatric patients. *J Laryngol Otol.* 2005;119(4):325–329.

Chang P, Kim S. Cholesteatoma—diagnosising the unsafe ear. *Aust Fam Physician.* 2008; 37(8):631–638.

Coleman C, Moore M. Decongestants and antihistamines for acute otitis media in children. *Cochrane Database Syst Rev.* 2007; (2): CD001727. DOI: 10.1002/14651858.CD001727. pub4.

Furukawa M, Minekawa A, Haruyama T, et al. Clinical effectiveness of ototopical application of mupirocin Ointment in methacillin-resistant staphylococcus aureus otorrhea. *Otol Neuroltol.* 2008;29(5):676–678.

Gaio E, Marioni G, De Filippis C, et al. Facial nerve paralysis secondary to acute otitis media in infants and children. *J Pediatr Child Health.* 2004;40(8):483–486.

Greenberg MI, Hendrickson RG, Silverberg M, et al. *Greenberg's Text-Atlas of Emergency Medicine.* Philadelphia, PA: Lippincott Williams & Wilkins; 2004:140–146.

Haydén D. Akerind B, Peebo M. Inner ear and facial nerve complications of acute otitis media with focus on bacteriology and virology. *Acta Otolaryngol.* 2006;126(5):460–466.

Hendley JO. Clinical practice: Otitis media. *N Engl J Med.* 2002;347:1169–1174.

Hoberman A, Paradise JL. Acute otitis media: Diagnosis and management in the year 2000. *Pediatr Ann.* 2000;29:609–620.

Khan A. Potts puffy tumor: A rare complication of mastoiditis. *Pediatr Neursurg.* 2006;42; 125–128.

Leach AJ, Mordris PS, Mathews JD, et al. Compared to placebo, long-term antibiotics resolves otitis media with effusion (OME) and prevent acute otitis media with perforation (AOM-wiP) in a high risk population: A randomized controlled trial. *BMC Pediatr.* 2008;8:23.

Leskinen K, Jero J. Complications of acute otitis media in children in southern Finland. *Int J Pediatr Otorhinolaryngol.* 2004;68(3):317–324.

Unsal EE, Ensari S, Koc C. A rare and serious complication of chronic otitis media: Lateral sinus thrombosis. *Auris Nasus Larynx.* 2003;30(3):279–282.

Woodfield G, Dugdale A. Evidence behind the WHO Guidelines: Hospital care for children: What is the most effective antibiotic regime for chronic suppurative otitis media in children? *J Trop Pediatr.* 2008;54(3):151–156.

Zapalac J, Billings KR, Schwade ND, et al. Suppurative complications of acute otitis media in the era of antibiotic resistance. *Arch Otolaryngol Head Neck Surg.* 2002;128(6):660–663.

98

MANAGE TRAUMATIC EAR INJURIES CAREFULLY TO AVOID COSMETIC AND FUNCTIONAL IMPAIRMENTS

RIZWAN N. TOKHI, MD

AURICULAR HEMATOMAS

Auricular hematomas are the most common complication of blunt ear trauma. They require serious attention as they can result in necrosis of the perichondrium, leading to the cosmetic deformity known as the "cauliflower ear."

They present as dark, nontender, fluctuant collections of blood in the auricle—often as a result of blunt trauma, classically associated with wrestling and boxing injuries.

The hematoma can be aspirated with an 18-guage needle or incised and drained, followed by compressive dressing for 1 week (*Fig. 98.1*), to allow cartilage to readhere to the perichondrium. Ciprofloxacin is recommended for its excellent cartilage penetration. Reexamine patients in 24 to 48 h to prevent recurrence of hematoma.

FOREIGN BODIES

Foreign body impaction is the most common cause of ear trauma in children. Patients may present with pain, bleeding, hearing loss, and in cases of delayed presentation, foul-smelling discharge.

Irrigation is the simplest method of removal—as long as the tympanic membrane is not perforated. Soft or round foreign bodies may be removed by inserting ear curette and rolling outward. Sharp or irregular foreign bodies should be removed with fine alligator forceps. For organic foreign bodies that can expand like beans or nuts, avoid irrigation with water. Removal after dehydration with alcohol is helpful. *Avoid interventions that push the object in further*. Use of procedural sedation may be necessary with some children.

LACERATIONS AND REPAIR

Local anesthesia and use of regional blocks are the primary methods of anesthesia for repair. Use 1% to 2% lidocaine with 1:100,000 epinephrine circumferentially around the auricle in the subcutaneous plane for complete regional anesthesia. The great auricular nerve innervates the medial auricle, lobule, helix, and antihelix. The auriculotemporal nerve innervates the tragus, helical crus, and superior-lateral auricle. To address the conchal bowl, infiltrate widely

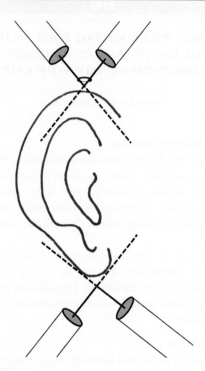

FIGURE 98.1. Auricular hematomas.

around the posterior external auditory meatus to anesthetize sensory branches of CN VII and X (*Fig. 98.2*).

Cleanse the ear thoroughly—chlorhexidine has been found to cause ototoxicity in animal models, so use iodine. The avascular auricular cartilage receives its nourishment from the overlying skin. Minimize debridement to ensure that the repair covers all exposed cartilage. Irrigate copiously with sterile saline. Use 5–0 or 6–0 absorbable sutures for perichondrium and nonabsorbable 5–0 or 6–0 nylon suture for skin. Vertical mattress sutures should be used on helical rim to prevent notching. Instruct patient to cleanse daily with hydrogen peroxide and dress wound with TELFA dressing and antibiotic ointment before discharge. Mastoid and bolster dressings should be used as needed to prevent hematoma/seroma formation. Discharge with ciprofloxacin for 1 week with follow-up suture removal in 5 to 7 days.

TYMPANIC MEMBRANE PERFORATION

Foreign bodies, self-inflicted Q-tip injuries, and barotraumas caused by flight, diving, and explosion can result in hemotympanum and/or tympanic membrane rupture. Avoid eardrops containing gentamicin, neomycin sulfate, or

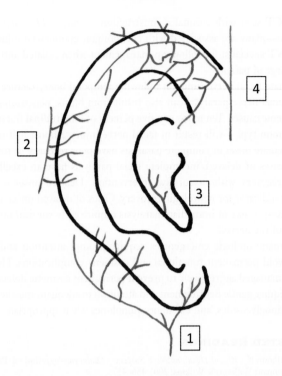

FIGURE 98.2. Nerve locations—*1*, great auricular nerve; *2*, lower occipital nerve; *3*, auricular branch of vagus nerve; *4*, auriculotemporal nerve.

tobramycin—these are ototoxic drugs. Do not irrigate the ear; this can force debris into the middle ear. Postpone swimming until completely healed or up to 6 months. Systemic antibiotic should be used for purulent discharge and diving injuries even in the absence of signs of infection. Use otic suspension for otitis media in the setting of tympanic membrane rupture.

TEMPORAL BONE FRACTURE AND FACIAL NERVE INJURIES

Patients who suffer from craniofacial trauma can sustain temporal bone fractures. The temporal bone houses many vital structures, including the cochlear and vestibular end organs, the facial nerve, the carotid artery, and the jugular vein. Presenting signs of injury include Battle sign, raccoon eyes, nystagmus, hemotympanum, otorrhea, CSF rhinorrhea, ear canal laceration, and facial weakness on affected side. *Do not miss this diagnosis*—studies have shown between 35% and 85% of these patients will suffer hearing loss. Other associated complications include facial nerve paralysis, CSF fistula, and meningitis.

Use CT scan with coronal reconstruction to image. *These injuries rarely occur alone*—many are associated with concomitant craniofacial injuries. Consult an ENT specialist for follow-up management when isolated and considering discharge of patient.

Evaluate facial nerve function following temporal bone fracture. Trauma-induced facial nerve paralysis can also result from burns, penetrating injuries, and iatrogenic causes. Ten to twenty-five percent of longitudinal fractures—the most common type—will result in facial nerve injury. Almost half of patients with immediate onset of complete paralysis have poor recovery of function. In contrast, cases of delayed/incomplete facial paralysis have an excellent prognosis for recovery without surgical intervention. Delayed onset is the most important indicator for neurologic recovery. Cases of delayed onset are treated conservatively. Cases of immediate paralysis require early surgical intervention for repair of the nerve.

Traumatic otologic emergencies require prompt attention and management to avoid permanent functional and cosmetic complications. Hematomas should be managed aggressively to prevent permanent cosmetic defect, and lacerations require gentle debridement and attention to adequate anesthesia. Avoid topical aminoglycosides, and use fluoroquinolones when appropriate.

SUGGESTED READINGS

Bailey B, Calhoun K. *Atlas of Head and Neck Surgery—Otolaryngology*. 2nd ed. Philadelphia, PA: Lippincott Williams & Wilkins; 2001:456–457.

Davidson TM. Ambulatory healthcare pathways for ear nose, and throat disorders. UCSD Otolaryngology—Head & Neck Surgery. Available at: http://drdavidson.ucsd.edu/Portals/0/Ambuindex.htm. Accessed July 28, 2006.

Gmyrek R. *Local Anesthesia and Regional Nerve Block Anesthesia*. eMedicine.com, 2004. Available at: www.emedicine.com/derm/topic824.htm

Lalwani A. Diseases of external ear. In: *Current Diagnosis & Treatment in Otolaryngology-Head & Neck Surgery*. Philadelphia, PA: McGraw-Hill; 2004.

Roberts JR, Hedges J, eds. *Clinical Procedures in Emergency Medicine*. 4th ed. Philadelphia, PA: WB Saunders; 2003:1299–1300.

Tintinalli JE, Kelen GD, Stapczynski JS, eds. *Emergency Medicine: A Comprehensive Study Guide*. 6th ed. New York, NY: McGraw-Hill; 2004:1470.

Kislevsky VE, Prepageran N, Michael Hawke, et al. Ear trauma: Investigating the common concerns. *Can J Diagn*. 2003;52:111. Available at: http://www.stacommunications.com/journals/diagnosis/archive2003.html

99

Pediatric sinusitis: It is not necessary to give antibiotics to every kid with a runny nose

Jacob Poulsen, MD

It seems like every kid between the ages of 3 months and 10 years has a runny nose. You do not want to be known as "that doc" who hands out antibiotics to kids, like candy on Halloween, every time a child sneezes or tugs at his or her ears. Unfortunately, it can be difficult to distinguish between a viral rhinosinusitis, allergy, and acute bacterial sinusitis. Indeed, allergy or cold often precede the development of acute bacterial sinusitis, as the swelling of the nasal tissues obstructs the osteomeatal complex and allows stasis within the sinus cavity. The pathophysiology is similar to that of acute otitis media, with *Streptococcus pneumonia*, *Haemophilus influenza*, and *Moraxella catarrhalis* being the most common cause of infection. *Staphylococcus aureas*, *Pseudomonas aeruginosa*, and fungal infections may be seen in the immunocompromised. The ethmoid and maxillary sinuses develop shortly after birth, whereas the sphenoid sinus develops at 3 to 5 years and the frontal sinus around 8 years of age, so do not expect to see a frontal sinusitis in a 3 year old.

The most common symptoms of sinusitis include cough, nasal drainage, and fever. The common signs are purulent nasal drainage, facial tenderness, and swelling. Suspect nasal foreign body if the purulent nasal drainage is limited to one nostril. Sinus transillumination is not reliable in children under 10 years of age and should not be relied upon to make the diagnosis of sinusitis. The American Academy of Pediatrics (AAP) defines acute bacterial sinusitis as severe or persistent infection of the paranasal sinuses <30 days of duration (persistent is characterized in most studies as >10 days, and many clinicians follow "the 10-day rule"). The ED evaluation should also focus on the potential complications of sinusitis including epidural or orbital abscesses, periorbital cellulitis, meningitis, and cavernous sinus thrombosis. These complications are rare; however, one must take caution when the patient in question is immunocompromised. Radiologic studies including CT and plain films (including Water view to evaluate the maxillary sinus) should be reserved for those cases in which a complication is suspected, as the diagnosis of acute bacterial sinusitis is primarily clinical.

Currently, the AAP consensus guidelines recommend antibiotics as the primary treatment of bacterial sinusitis. Amoxicillin at 45 mg/kg bid is an acceptable start in a patient population with a low prevalence of resistant *S. Pneumo*. If resistance is high, or the patient fails to improve after 3 days of therapy, then amoxicillin/clavulanate or a second-generation cephalosporin can be used. Ceftriaxone IV or IM can be given to the child with uncontrolled vomiting. Macrolides are the next line of treatment for those with penicillin allergy; however, with increasing resistance of *S. Pneumo* to macrolides, clindamycin may be a reasonable alternative. Antibiotics should be used for 10 to 21 days or 7 days after symptoms have resolved. Decongestants are not recommended for the treatment of acute sinusitis in children.

In summary, suspect acute bacterial sinusitis in a child with symptoms of cough, fever, and nasal drainage for at least 10 days. Use CT if you suspect that the child may have an extension of infection to other structures. Antibiotics may shorten the duration of the illness and prevent complications, but most children will eventually recover on their own, so it is okay to be a little stingy. Admit patients who are immunocompromised or who have developed a serious complication; otherwise, a 3-day follow-up is a reasonable time frame. Refer the patient to an ENT specialist if the patient has had multiple treatment failures or in the case of a serious infection in an immunocompromised patient.

SUGGESTED READINGS

American Academy of Pediatrics. Subcommittee on Management of Sinusitis and Committee on Quality Improvement. Clinical practice guideline: Management of sinusitis. *Pediatrics.* 2001;108(3):798–808.

Holt KR, Cuenca MM, Cuenca PJ, et al. Acute pediatric sinusitis and "the 10-day rule." Pediatric Emergency Medicine Practice. February 2006. Available at: http://www.ebmedicine.net/Pediatric-Emergency-Medicine-Practice-articles.html

Otten FW, Grote JJ. The diagnostic value of transillumination for maxillary sinusitis in children. *Int J Pediatr Otorhinolaryng.* 1989;18(1):9–11.

Wald ER. Microbiology of acute and chronic sinusitis in children. *J Allergy Clin Immunol.* 1992;90(3 Pt 2):452–456.

100

THE NONTRAUMATIC RED EYE: IT IS NOT ALWAYS CONJUNCTIVITIS

DAVID FARMAN, MD

The red eye is a common complaint but is one that leads to significant anxiety among physicians faced with treating it. Barriers to successful diagnosis include lack of familiarity with the tools of diagnosis (namely, the slit lamp and tonometers) as well as a tendency to prematurely close the diagnosis on benign or self-limited diseases.

Before anchoring on the diagnosis of conjunctivitis, there are three questions the physician must answer.

1) Is the eye painful? By definition, conjunctivitis is not painful.
2) Is the vision normal? Conjunctivitis does not cause a change in visual acuity. *Every* ocular complaint should have a visual acuity recorded in the chart. If the patient's vision is not at baseline, it must be explained.
3) Is the cornea normal? Defects in the cornea can cause a red eye that looks like conjunctivitis, but the treatment and follow-up required can be vastly different.

In answering these questions, the physician must have a plan of attack. For the nontraumatic red eye, these maxims should be followed: (1) If it is red, *stain it*; (2) If it hurts, *get pressures*.

As in most medical complaints, the history provides much useful information. Does everyone at work have the same painful eye problem? (Think epidemic keratoconjunctivitis [EK].) Does the patient have the history of an autoimmune disorder? (Think iritis or scleritis.) Has the patient had a history of eye trauma in the past or severe farsightedness? (Think angle-closure glaucoma.) Does the patient have a history of oral ulcers? (Think herpes.)

STAIN IT

If the patient complains of a red eye, the physician must inspect the cornea. This is done by applying a local anesthetic (1% tetracaine) to the eye, followed by the application of fluorescein. In the absence of a slit lamp, a Wood lamp may be used to inspect the eye's surface. Of the causes of the nontraumatic red eye with corneal irregularities, there are only four major culprits: EK, UV keratitis, herpes, and zoster.

Both epidemic and UV keratitis have similar appearances: multiple punctate lesions on the cornea. The patient's history will often be indicative: large groups of close contacts with the same symptoms in EK and welding/snow blindness in the latter. Pain control for these entities with PO narcotics or topical NSAIDS is paramount. The addition of topical antibiotics has not proven to be beneficial but has become the standard of care. Patients with both these complaints should recover spontaneously with minimal complications.

On the other hand, herpes keratitis can be ocularly devastating, and the physician must always be suspicious. Historic teaching describes dendrites visible on the cornea, but in the early stages, the lesions may only be punctate. The cornerstone of treatment is topical antiviral drops with or without the addition of an oral agent, in conjunction with ophthalmological consultation. The treatment of shingles is the opposite: oral therapy to treat the shingles, with or without topical therapy, in conjunction with Ophthalmology. Medical management and close follow-up are the standard of care. Consult an antimicrobial guide for dosing.

All lesions to the cornea, nontraumatic or otherwise, should be given ophthalmology follow-up within 24 h.

GET PRESSURES

If the patient is complaining of pain, as he or she would in the above cases, eye pressures should be obtained since ocular pain can also be indicative of elevated intraocular pressure (IOP >20 mm Hg). Commercially available tonometry pens or applanation devices can aid the physician in obtaining this information in seconds. However, keep in mind that the tonometry pens tend to *under*estimate higher pressures.

If the pressures are very high (50 to 70), one must be concerned for angle-closure glaucoma. The patient will often report a sudden onset of symptoms, including severe pain, headache, and nausea. The eyeball will be firm to the touch and often demonstrate a fixed/dilated pupil. In conjunction with an ophthalmologist, topical β-blockers, topical steroids, and IV acetazolamide should be given to lower the IOP. One hour later, pilocarpine should be given. The patient will likely need admission to the hospital for surgical correction, as blindness may result.

Higher pressures may also be seen in iritis and scleritis (iritis' cousin). Both are often autoimmune in nature and have more of a gradual onset. The buzzwords "perilimbic hyperemia," "consensual photophobia," and "cells and flare" are often used in describing iritis. However, "cells and flare" may be more accurately described as "bits of sparkle" in a "smoky" background when one looks behind the cornea into the anterior chamber. Both iritis and scleritis are quite painful. The redness in the eye of a patient with iritis is greatest around the corneal edges (perilimbic hyperemia), whereas a patient with scleritis will have perilimbic sparing. Both diseases are treated the same and require topical steroid drops, with the addition of a cycloplegic for pain control in iritis. Both require urgent ophthalmology follow-up within 24 h. Do not forget to look for a hypopyon in the anterior chamber of patients with iritis, your consultants will be impressed.

CONCLUSION

If a patient presents with a nontraumatic red eye, the physician must be prepared to use the available tools to make the proper diagnosis. If it is red, stain the cornea to insure that it is not something sight threatening, like herpes. If it hurts, get pressures to guarantee that the patient is not suffering from iritis or acute glaucoma. Always explain an abnormal visual acuity.

And after all this, if you still think it is conjunctivitis, prescribe them the *cheapest* topical antibiotic that they are not allergic to, send them out the door, and tell them to come back or see an eye specialist if it is not getting better in 48 h.

SUGGESTED READINGS

Alteveer JG, McCans KM. The red eye, the swollen eye and acute Vision loss: Handling non-traumatic eye disorders in the ED. *Emergency Medicine Practice*. 2002:4(6).

Birinyi F, Mauger T. Opthalmologic conditions. In: Knoop KJ, Stack LA, Storrow AM, eds. *Atlas of Emergency Medicine*, 2nd ed. New York, NY: McGraw-Hill. 2002.

Calder LA, Falasubramanian S, Fergusson D. Topical nonsteroidal anti-inflammatory drugs for corneal abrasions: Meta-analysis of randomized trials. *Acad Emerg Med*. 2005:12(5): 467–473.

Flynn CA, D'Amico F, Smith G. Should we patch corneal abrasions? A meta-analysis. *J Fam Pract*. 1998;47(4):264–270.

Gaynor BD, Margolis TP, Cunningham ET Jr. Advances in diagnosis and treatment of herpetic uveitis. *Int Opthalmol Clin*. 2000 Spring;40(2):85–109.

Leibowitz HM. The red eye. *N Engl Med*. 2000;343(5):345–351.

Michael JG, Hug D, Dowd MD. Management of corneal abrasion in children: A randomized clinical trial. *Ann Emerg Med*. 2002;40(1):67–72.

Peak D, Chisholm C, Knoop K. Opthalmologic trauma. In: Knoop KJ, Stack LA, Storrow AM, eds. *Atlas of Emergency Medicine*, 2nd ed. New York, NY: McGraw-Hill. 2002.

Sheikh A, Hurwitz B. Antibiotics versus placebo for acute bacterial conjunctivitis. *Cochrane Database Syst Rev*. 2007;(4):CD001211. DOI: 10.1002/14651858.CD001211.pub2.

Shovlin JP. Orbital infections and inflammations. *Curr Opin Opthalmol*. 1998;9(5):41–48.

101

MANAGE EYELID LACERATIONS WITH EXTREME CAUTION

AMY MAY ZHENG, MD, MPHIL

We have all heard the phrase "put that stick down or you'll poke your eye out," but sadly, most patients do not heed the warning and frequently present to the emergency department with eyelid lacerations. In one study, ocular or orbital injuries were found in 16% of patients with major trauma. Inappropriately managed lacerations of the eyelid can cause chronic complications, including excessive tearing, scarring, corneal ulceration, improper lid function, and blindness.

Even though eyelid injuries can be some of the most nausea-inducing injuries, a diligent emergency physician must remember to start with taking a good history and perform a detailed ophthalmologic examination. This exam can be the most difficult part of the patient evaluation since most emergency physicians skipped their rotation in ophthalmology. Attention can be directed toward repairing eyelid lacerations only after serious injuries such as globe rupture, traumatic glaucoma, hypema, and orbital wall fracture with entrapment are ruled out.

Many simple eyelid lacerations can be repaired primarily by emergency physicians using good wound care techniques. This can be done with copious irrigation, debridement of devitalized tissue, and closure of the laceration using 6–0 nonabsorbable suture. Be careful not to strangulate the wound in your excitement as you are not sewing in a chest tube but rather performing a precision repair. Excessive tension can cause eyelid retraction. Take extra care on the placement of the sutures and suture ends. They can cause irritation and abrasion on the delicate eye structure if not properly performed. Due to the excellent vascularity of the eye area, delay in the closure of eyelid wounds up to 36 h can still result in good cosmetic outcome.

Do not attempt to suture wounds involving the upper or lower lid margins. These should be referred to a specialist for repair within 24 h. Further more, damage to the tarsal plates frequently accompany deep eyelid injuries which require a layered closure by an opthalmologist. Complications of improper repair can lead to corneal scarring and vision loss. If these problems occur, it is better they happen under a consultant's license than yours!

Injury medial to the puncta should raise concern for canalicular injury. If the diagnosis is in doubt, instill some fluorescein dye. If the lacrimal system is disrupted, the dye will fail to disappear. Once this injury is discovered, the ophthalmologist will need to place a stent in the cannaliculus to maintain patency while the wound is healing. While waiting for the arrival of the consultant, you can place iced saline gauze over the medial canthus to decrease edema. A canalicular injury should be repaired within 24 to 48 h after injury because it will be harder to identify the lacerated ends once granulation has started.

Emergency physicians must also accurately diagnose eye lids injuries involving the orbital septum. Any upper eyelid wound, where periorbital fat is visible, requires exploration by an ophthalmologist. Remember, this is not an abdominal stab wound that gets explored, so do not stick a Q-tip inside the wound and poke at the globe. Trauma to the orbital septum puts the patient at risk for injury to the levator palpebrae muscle. Even in the absence of any visible fat, horizontal lacerations on the upper lid accompanied by ptosis are assumed to be levator palpebrae muscle damage until proven otherwise. Your local ophthalmologist needs to achieve hemostasis before closure of the septum, in order to reduce the risk of retrobulbar hematoma.

Be afraid, be very afraid if the eyelid wound appears to be small. Ask the patient about penetrating trauma. The innocent appearance of narrow eyelid wounds may cause the emergency physician to overlook the possibility of globe trauma. If, after instillation of fluroscein, there is a waterfall effect (Seidel sign), then an ophthalmologist needs to be consulted for globe rupture. Do not attempt to use the Tono-Pen on a ruptured globe or vitreous humor will squirt out—this is fine for a horror movie, but a truly poor form in patient care. If there is any concern for retained foreign body in the eye, a CT scan of the orbits should be ordered.

Although Fido may be "man's best friend," he is not beyond taking a good bite out of your eyelid. Animal bites are a common cause of eyelid injury, often involving the lacrimal structures. As with all wounds, patients should be assessed for their tetanus status and given rabies prophylaxis when appropriate. High pressure irrigation is imperative to decrease the bacterial load and please, anesthetize your patients BEFORE you irrigate their wound. Patients with high risk lacerations should be given antibiotic prophylaxis. These include cuts >8 h old, deep punctures (especially if it is from a cat bite), need for surgical repair, and patients with underlying medical problems which may compromise wound healing. Amoxicillin-Clavulanate (Augmentin) is a good choice for both cat and dog bites. For patients with penicillin allergies, clindamycin plus ciprofloxacin or trimethoprim-sulfamethoxazole is a good alternative drug for dog bites, whereas doxycycline is the preferred alternative for cat bites.

When a patient arrives in the emergency department with an eyelid injury, obtain an accurate history, perform a good ophthalmologic exam, conduct a thorough wound exploration, and have a low tolerance for seeking specialist help. Attention to detail and an understanding of what injuries require ophthalmologic consult will prevent permanent disfigurement and visual impairment for your patients.

SUGGESTED READINGS

Brown DJ, Jaffe JE, Henson JK. Advanced laceration management. *Emerg Med Clin North Am.* 2007;25:83–99.

Chang EL, Rubin PA. Management of complex eyelid lacerations. *Int Ophthalmol Clin.* 2002;42(3):187–201.

Della Rocca DA, Ahmad SM, Della Rocca RC. Direct repair of canalicular lacerations. *Facial Plast Surg.* 2007;23:149–155.

Gilbert DN, Moellering RC Jr, Eliopoulos GM, et al. *The Sanford Guide to Antimicrobial Therapy.* 37th ed. Sperryville, VA: Antimicrobial Therapy; 2007.

Hogg, NJ, Horswell BB. Soft tissue pediatric facial trauma: A review. *J Can Dent Assoc.* 2006;72(6):549–552.

Poon, A. McClusky PJ, Hill DA. Eye injuries in patients with major trauma. *J Trauma.* 1999;46(3):494–499.

Reifler D. Management of canalicular laceration. *Surv Ophthalmol.* 1991;36:113–132.

Rhatigan M, Taylor RH. A potentially life-threatening upper eyelid laceration. *Injury.* 1996;27(3):229–230.

Slonim CB. Dog bite-induced canalicular injury: A review of 17 cases. *Ophthal Plast Reconstr Surg.* 1996;12(3):218–222.

Stefanopoulos PK, Tarantzopoulou AD. Facial bite wounds: Management update. *Int J Oral Maxillofac Surg.* 2005;34:464–472.

102

Do not discharge headache without thinking Temporal Arteritis

Jonathan Larson, MD

History

The first known case of temporal arteritis (TA) was in 1890. A patient was referred for "red streaks on his head" that were painful and prevented him from wearing his hat. The red streaks proved to be swollen temporal arteries, which over time became firm and pulseless. Today, the prevalence of TA is <1%. Needless to say, prevalence increases with age and TA is rare below the age of 50. Patients 50 years and older with a headache (HA) should be considered to have TA until proven otherwise by history and physical exam. TA left undiagnosed or unconsidered may lead to blindness and other complications.

Signs and Symptoms

The physical exam in a patient with TA is frequently unremarkable. Ultimately, you must integrate multiple clinical factors in order to optimize diagnostic and therapeutic strategies for patients with suspected TA. Despite the variability in presenting symptoms, three physical exam findings increase the lik elihood of TA:

1) Jaw claudication—quadruples the likelihood of TA. Jaw claudication refers to pain in the proximal jaw near the temporomandibular joint that develops after a brief period of chewing, especially food requiring vigorous mastication. In one study, jaw claudication was one of two historical features with likelihood ratios (LRs) of sufficient power to be useful to clinicians. Jaw claudication had the highest positive LR of 4.2. While somewhat insensitive (34%), it is a relatively specific feature for TA.

2) Diplopia—doubles the likelihood of TA. In one study of 170 patients with TA, 85 (50%) had ocular symptoms to include visual loss (97.7%), amaurosis fugax (30.6%), diplopia (5.9%), and eye pain (8.2%). The diplopia was often transient, variable, and sometimes not associated with motility examination abnormalities. The diagnosis of TA should be considered in all patients older than 50 years with unexplained or transient diplopia.

3) Temporary artery abnormality—doubles the likelihood of TA. Abnormalities of the temporal arteries include tenderness, reduced or absent pulsation, erythema, nodularity, or swelling detected by light palpation just anterior and slightly superior to the tragus of the ear. Following the temporal artery

pulse anteriorly along the temples and comparing it with the contralateral side help detect findings that may be remarkably focal. Among physical examination findings, beaded, prominent, or enlarged arteries confer the highest positive LRs of any clinical or laboratory feature and substantially increase the probability that a patient with suspected TA will have positive biopsy results.

The American College of Rheumatology developed a standard for clinicians when considering the diagnosis of TA (TA when three of five criteria are met):

- Age of onset ≥50 years old.
- New onset of localized HA.
- TA tenderness or decreased pulsation.
- Erythrocyte sedimentation rate (ESR) >50 mm per h.
- Abnormal artery biopsy.

Unfortunately, virtually all individual physical exam features demonstrate poor sensitivity, and the lack of any feature on history or physical examination does not effectively rule out TA in patients older than 50 years. Age is an important factor in determining the likelihood of TA. Clinical criteria most strongly suggestive of TA include jaw claudication, C-reactive protein (CRP) above 2.45 mg/dL, and an ESR of 47 mm per h or more, in that order.

MANAGEMENT

The most useful laboratory finding is a normal ESR, which makes TA unlikely. A low or normal level is more likely to rule out disease than a high value is likely to rule in disease. The mean value for patients with disease was 88 mm per h. Some literature found CRP >2.45 mg/dL to be more sensitive (100%) than ESR (92%) for detection of TA. ESR combined with CRP gave the best specificity (97%). Despite this, it should be emphasized that the diagnosis of TA is a clinical diagnosis and that laboratory results alone should not be relied on for diagnosis. Bilateral temporal artery biopsy is the GOLD STANDARD for diagnosis of TA; unilateral biopsy has a sensitivity of 86% (negative biopsy does not always exclude the diagnosis).

TREATMENT

The most feared complication of TA is vision loss, unilateral and ultimately bilateral. The emphasis must be on early diagnosis and treatment of these patients at risk for catastrophic visual outcomes. Many clinicians choose to treat patients they have referred for biopsy with corticosteroids pending biopsy results. Oral corticosteroids remain the mainstay of treatment of TA. Most studies recommend an initial dose of oral prednisone of 1.0 to 1.5 mg/kg/day (60 to 100 mg per day). However, many clinicians recommend IV therapy (250 mg methylprednisolone, four times daily for 3 to 5 days) in patients with visual loss resulting from TA. Regardless of the ESR, patients with high clinical suspicion for TA should be treated with steroids.

SUMMARY

Catch TA early, you may save your patient's sight. You will miss TA if you fail to consider the diagnosis in your patients over 50 years with HAs, vision changes, or temporal artery abnormalities. If your patient has symptoms suspicious for TA, order an ESR and CRP. If after history and physical exam TA still sits atop your differential diagnosis, then refer your patient for emergent temporal artery biopsy. As you fill out the emergent referral, pull out your prescription pad to write a prescription for steroids to cover your patient in the interim. Failure to do so could mean the difference between night and day for the remainder of your patient's life.

SUGGESTED READINGS

Gabriel SE, O'Fallon WM, Achkar AA, et al. The use of clinical characteristics to predict the results of temporal artery biopsy among patients with suspected giant cell arteritis. *J Rheumatol*. 1995;22:93–96.

Gur H, Rapman E, Ehrenfeld M, et al. Clinical manifestations of temporal arteritis: A report from Israel. *J Rheumatol*. 1996;23:1927–1931.

Hayreh SS, Podhajsky PA, Raman R, et al. Giant cell arteritis: Validity and reliability of various diagnostic criteria. *Am J Ophthalmol*. 1997;123:285–296.

Lee AG. Temporal arteritis: A clinical approach. *J Am Geriatr Soc*. 1999;47(11):1364–1370.

Nusser JA. Which clinical features and lab findings increase the likelihood of temporal arteritis. *J Fam Pract*. 2008;57(2):119–120.

Smetana G, Shmerling R. The rational clinical examination: Does this patient have temporal arteritis? *JAMA*. 2002;287:92–101.

Widico CR, Newman DH. Does this patient have temporal arteritis? *Ann Emerg Med*. 2005;45(1):85–87.

103

UNDERSTAND THE DIFFERENCES IN RESUSCITATION OF THE SEVERELY HYPOTHERMIC PATIENT

SONIA Y. JOHNSON, MD

Accidental hypothermia can happen year-round and in any climate. Patients who present to the emergency department (ED) with severe hypothermia (temperature <30°C) require important modifications to their management, particularly if they develop cardiac arrest. Therapeutic modalities used in normothermic patients can be detrimental to a severely hypothermic patient with globally depressed organ function.

Aggressive rewarming strategies should be initiated emergently. When verifying the patient's temperature, be aware that erroneous temperature readings may result from axillary measurements, esophageal probe readings with heated inhalation, and rectal probes inserted into cold feces. Severely hypothermic individuals will need active rewarming. Caution is advised to avoid the *afterdrop* phenomenon, which occurs if the periphery is warmed before thermostabilization, causing colder blood from the extremities to return to the core and drop the body's temperature further.

The myocardium becomes particularly irritable with severe hypothermia. Excessive movement of the patient or direct cardiac manipulation by procedures, that is, internal jugular and subclavian line placement, CVP catheter placement, or intracardiac transvenous pacing, should all be avoided as they may precipitate malignant dysrhythmias. Although there has been concern about endotracheal (ET) intubation also precipitating arrhythmias, multiple studies have shown it to be safe. Thus, the threshold for intubating these patients should be the same as in other patients, based on their mental and respiratory status.

With severe hypothermia, serum electrolytes should be evaluated frequently. If the patient is found to be hyperkalemic, it is particularly important to note that hypothermia will enhance cardiac toxicity and alter the ECG changes that we normally associate with hyperkalemia. Patients with potassium of 10 mEq/L or above have an ominous prognosis. Coagulopathies are also expected with hypothermia, as the activated clotting factors are functionally depressed by the cold. There is no need to transfuse clotting factors; rewarming is sufficient. It is also important to seek and treat intoxication and underlying disease, as these are the leading causes of urban accidental hypothermia.

The Osborn (J) wave seen on the ECG is potentially diagnostic of hypothermia and typically appears at temperatures below 32°C. J wave abnormalities become more pronounced with a decline in core temperature and can appear to simulate myocardial injury, which has led to the erroneous use of fibrinolytics.

As cold exposure induces diuresis, hypothermic patients will be dehydrated. Cold water immersion and alcohol intoxication will further enhance this *cold diuresis*. Warmed intravenous crystalloid is indicated; however, as the cardiac function is depressed, one should be sure to look for early signs of heart failure to avoid precipitating cardiogenic pulmonary edema.

Although basic life support (BLS) management remains the same, advanced cardiac life support (ACLS) management of hypothermic patients who develop cardiac arrest differs considerably from management of normothermic arrest. Hypothermic patients in cardiac arrest have been known to tolerate hours of cardiopulmonary resuscitation (CPR) with complete recovery. Since the hypothermic heart is poorly responsive to cardioactive drugs, pacers, and defibrillation, rapid active rewarming is paramount. A trial of defibrillation is only recommended for ventricular fibrillation (VF) and pulseless ventricular tachycardia (VT) for a maximum of three shocks. Once the body temperature reaches 30°C, defibrillation can be attempted again. As bradycardia may be physiologic, pacing is generally unnecessary unless it persists after rewarming.

Pharmacologic manipulation of blood pressure and pulse should be avoided for a number of reasons. Since most drugs' efficacy is temperature dependent, overmedication may be needed to achieve therapeutic response. Drug clearance will also be poor as renal and liver functions are depressed. Ultimately, when the patient is rewarmed, these drugs can potentially reach toxic levels. There have been a number of animal studies and case reports suggesting that pharmacologic therapies may have a role for some patients with hypothermia and ventricular fibrillation, but the evidence remains unclear. Therefore, intravenous drugs are not recommended at temperatures <30°C and should be given at increased intervals and in smaller doses when the core temperature is >30°C.

If the patient arrests, continue CPR and attempt a trial of defibrillation if VF or pulseless VT is present. Avoid drug therapies until core temperature reaches >30°C. Although mortality is high for patients with severe hypothermia, those who survive may have full neurological recovery, so emergent, aggressive treatment is essential.

SUGGESTED READINGS

American Heart Association. Emergency Cardiac Care Guidelines. Part 8: Advanced challenges in resuscitation. Section 3: Special challenges in emergency cardiac care. *Circulation* 2000;102:I-229–I-232.

Kempainen RR, Brunette DD. The evaluation and management of accidental hypothermia. *Respir Care* 2004;49:192–205.

Silfvast T, Pettila V. Outcome from severe accidental hypothermia in southern Finland—A 10 year review. *Resuscitation* 2003;59:285–290.

Wira CR, Becker JU, Martin G, et al. Anti-arrhythmic and vasopressor medications for the treatment of ventricular fibrillation in severe hypothermia: A systematic review of the literature. *Resuscitation.* 2008;78(1):21–29 [Epub 2008 Apr 10]. Doi:10.1016/j.resuscitation.2008.01.025.

104

KNOW THE BASICS OF REWARMING AND RESUSCITATION OF HYPOTHERMIC PATIENTS

BJORN C. WESTGARD, MD, MA

The management of hypothermic patients can be extremely challenging particularly of those who are unstable and severely hypothermic. Rewarming and basic resuscitation are the primary goals of therapy, but additional awareness of common and potentially self-correcting physiologic abnormalities will help avoid inappropriate interventions in caring for the hypothermic patient.

Hypothermia is defined as a core temperature <35°C. Moderate and severe hypothermia are <32°C and <28°C, respectively. Extremely low measurements and peripheral vasoconstriction render oral and axillary temperatures inaccurate in hypothermic patients; therefore, the use of a low-reading rectal thermometer is required. Moderate and severe hypothermia require further continuous invasive monitoring. Though a variety of probes have been used, bladder monitoring is the easiest and most reasonable estimate of core temperature.

Resuscitation should involve rewarming, volume replacement, cardiovascular support, and continuous monitoring. Hypothermia severely decreases metabolism, with corresponding depression of CNS, cardiac, respiratory, renal, and other functions. This leads to lethargy, hypotension, bradycardia, hypoventilation, and cold diuresis resulting in a shocklike state. Yet, a hypothermic patient's vital signs, clinical appearance, and biochemical markers may not be true indicators of survivability. Vital signs should be carefully assessed, and any suggestion of life should prompt rewarming and resuscitation. Even asystole should prompt attempts to revive and rewarm, remembering that a patient is not dead until he or she is warm and dead. Only after a patient's core temperature has been rewarmed to 32°C for at least 30 min can death be declared.

Rewarming methods may be passive or active, external, or internal. Mild hypothermia requires passive rewarming, making sure that a patient is warm, dry, covered, and allowed to shiver. Moderate hypothermia requires active external rewarming, using heating blankets, forced air, radiant heat, or warm immersion. Simple internal rewarming with heated fluids through peripheral lines may also be useful. In severe hypothermia, active internal rewarming should be instituted early along with other methods. Available internal techniques include warm fluid lavage of the chest via chest tubes or thoracotomy, peritoneal lavage, continuous arteriovenous rewarming, and cardiopulmonary bypass. Care should be taken to avoid aggravating the irritable myocardium during invasive procedures such as central line or chest tube placement for internal methods, as this may result in a terminal dysrhythmia.

While rewarming is begun, assessment and resuscitation should be started. Intubation should be carried out if necessary and ACLS protocols initiated, with the expectation that cardiopulmonary arrest may be refractory until a patient has been rewarmed. Due to vasoconstriction, decreased metabolism, and thus unreliable absorption, medications administered peripherally may cause delayed effects or toxicity. As a result, it is important to understand that prolonged paralysis may occur with the use of neuromuscular blockers. ACLS medications are also less effective at temperatures <30°C. Defibrillation, transcutaneous pacing, and antiarrhythmics such as bretylium, amiodarone, and lidocaine may be used, but have shown mixed results in studies. Many dysrhythmias are refractory but spontaneously convert with rewarming. Hemodynamic instability should also be managed by volume resuscitation with normal saline. Blood products may be considered for blood loss or significant anemia. Vasopressors such as epinephrine, norepinephrine, and dopamine may be considered, though they have also shown variable effectiveness in hypothermic patients, occasionally even precipitating paradoxical hypotension and dysrhythmias.

It is important to recognize that other abnormalities are common but may not require aggressive management. Acidosis, coagulopathy, and abnormal glucose and potassium levels are all common findings in hypothermia. Acidosis should generally be corrected to a pH of 7.4, though excessive correction may worsen the condition. Coagulopathy is common and will usually improve with rewarming. However, signs of trauma or ongoing hemorrhage should prompt aggressive correction with blood products. Hypoglycemia should obviously be addressed, but correction of hyperglycemia may require high doses of insulin and predispose a patient to severe hypoglycemia upon rewarming. Hypokalemia or hyperkalemia can be present; attempts to remedy small variations may lead to large changes on rewarming, the signs of which may be masked by hypothermia. All of these abnormalities warrant frequent monitoring during resuscitation and rewarming, with an understanding that overcorrection is possible.

There are many difficulties in caring for hypothermic patients, but timely institution of rewarming and resuscitation are paramount. Consideration of the following points should mitigate against complications in the care of these patients:

- Interventions aimed at rewarming and resuscitation should be instituted with an understanding of their risks
- Cardiovascular instability and laboratory abnormalities may be resistant to conventional therapy until the patient is rewarmed.
- Acid-base, electrolyte, and hematologic abnormalities should be anticipated and managed in severe cases

SUGGESTED READINGS

Brunette DD, McVaney K. Hypothermic cardiac arrest: An 11 year review of ED management and outcome. *Am J Emerg Med.* 2000;18:418–422.

Corneli H. Hot topics in cold medicine: Controversies in accidental hypothermia. *Clin Pediatr Emerg Med.* 2001;2:179–191.

Hanania NA, Zimmerman JL. Accidental hypothermia. *Crit Care Clin.* 1999;15:235–249.

Petrone P, Kuncir EJ, Asensio JA. Surgical management and strategies in the treatment of hypothermia and cold injury. *Emerg Med Clin North Am.* 2003;21:1165–1178.

105

DO NOT CAUSE FURTHER TISSUE INJURY DURING THE MANAGEMENT OF FROSTBITE

BENJAMIN S. OROZCO, MD

Frostbite is a cold-induced injury that results in direct tissue damage. Errors in management can directly contribute to tissue damage. Alternatively, proper management may reduce tissue damage and possibly result in better outcomes such as reduced amputation rates. The most commonly affected body parts are the fingers, toes, ears, nose, and cheeks, but any surface or an entire extremity can be subject to frostbite. Frostbite is the direct result of tissue damage initiated by ice crystals in intracellular and extracellular spaces and the resulting inflammation, microvascular occlusion, cellular necrosis, and even gangrene of affected tissues. Similar to thermal burns, frostbite may manifest in varying degrees. First-degree frostbite is superficial epidermal freezing, resulting in anesthesia of affected skin with surrounding edema. Second-degree frostbite extends deeper into the dermis, resulting in blister formation within 24 h with clear or opaque nonhemorrhagic fluid. Third-degree frostbite leads to hemorrhagic blistering within 24 h and progresses to eschar over the ensuing weeks. Fourth-degree frostbite includes deep tissue and/or bone involvement and results in tissue necrosis and possibly gangrene. Such severe frostbite may not blister as tissues may not be reperfused. Remediation of this injury pattern involves rapid rewarming and restoration of blood flow to the affected area. However, this approach may precipitate core temperature afterdrop. Thus, any patient with an acute cold injury should first be evaluated and have treatment initiated for hypothermia! Unlike hypothermia, frostbite is generally a cause of morbidity rather than mortality. Patients with previous cold injury, Raynaud's, tobacco use, peripheral vascular disease, extremes of age, intoxication, altered mental status, mental illness, or any other condition that compromises behavioral adaptation, circulation, or thermoregulation have higher risk of frostbite and complications thereof.

Rewarming can be complicated by thermal burns if done improperly or carelessly. Fires, heaters, and other unregulated mechanisms of rewarming should be avoided. The method of choice is submersion in 40°C to 42°C water until completely thawed. During rewarming, reperfusion injury inevitably results, but it can be mitigated minimally with ibuprofen orally and aloe vera (a topical thromboxane inhibitor). Some also advocate pentoxifylline (Trental), which increases red blood cell deformity, and prophylactic penicillin. Reperfusion injury is exacerbated by repeated freeze and thaw, so thaw should not be attempted until the patient is no longer at risk of reexposure. The frostbitten tissues are easily subject to mechanical trauma, and care should be taken to avoid any unneeded motion or movement of affected tissue. Do not allow patients to vigorously rub or massage frostbitten tissues. Pain with rewarming is inevitable and opioid analgesia is generally indicated.

There are no clear guidelines on management of the extensive bullae that may result from second- or third-degree frostbite. A conservative approach includes debriding nonhemorrhagic bullae that impede motion and only aspirating large hemorrhagic bullae. However, some advocate debridement of all bullae. As in thermal burns, there is risk of secondary infection so all dressings should be managed in sterile fashion. Tetanus has been reported in victims of frostbite so tetanus prophylaxis guidelines should be followed. Care should be taken to use nonadherent dressings that are interposed between digits to prevent tissue maceration.

In cases where significant amputation is likely, intra-arterial thrombolytics may be of benefit if given within the first 24 h. In one retrospective study, they were able to completely avoid proximal amputation and reduce the digital amputation rate from 41% to 10%. As with most tPA indications time to initiation of treatment is important; therefore, early consultation with a burn surgeon is warranted.

Delayed amputation, often >1 month post injury, has been the standard of care as overly aggressive amputation may prematurely remove viable tissues. Technetium (Tc)-99 scintigraphy can be a useful measure of the extent of tissue injury and response to therapy. It is not clear if it can be used to indicate early amputation. The role of hyperbaric oxygen has not yet been clearly determined.

In summary, the emergency physician must play an active role in mitigating the tissue damage in frostbite without contributing to it further.

KEY POINTS

Do

- Thaw the affected tissues promptly with warm water.
- Administer ibuprofen orally and use aloe vera topically.
- Follow tetanus prophylaxis guidelines.
- Dress frostbitten tissues with nonadherent dressing to prevent maceration.
- Consider penicillin and pentoxifylline for severe frostbite.
- Consult a burn surgeon early, particularly with cases of severe frostbite that might benefit from tPA.

Do not

- Overlook hypothermia; be mindful of core afterdrop.
- Rewarm carelessly and cause thermal burns.
- Thaw until the risk of refreeze is eliminated.
- Rub, massage, or unnecessarily move frostbitten tissues.
- Debride unnecessarily.
- Amputate as viability is not easily assessed early on.

Suggested Readings

Bhatnagar A, Sarker BB, Sawroop K, et al. Diagnosis, characterisation and evaluation of treatment response of frostbite using pertechnetate scintigraphy: A prospective study. *Eur J Nucl Med Mol Imaging*. 2002;29(2):170–175.

Bruen KJ, Ballard JR, Morris SE, et al. Reduction of the incidence of amputation in frostbite injury with thrombolytic therapy. *Arch Surg*. 2007;142(6):546–551; discussion 551–543.

Murphy JV, Banwell PE, Roberts AH, et al. Frostbite: Pathogenesis and treatment. *J Trauma*. 2000;48(1):171–178.

Petrone P, Kuncir EJ, Asensio JA. Surgical management and strategies in the treatment of hypothermia and cold injury. *Emerg Med Clin North Am*. 2003;21(4):1165–1178.

106

BEWARE SNAKEBITE INJURIES INCLUDING THE ONES THAT INITIALLY HAVE BENIGN PRESENTATIONS

JEFFERSON G. WILLIAMS, MD, MPH

A patient presenting with a bite from a venomous snake may be a rare occurrence in many U.S. emergency departments. The number of true incidence of venomous snake bites is probably several thousand, and those bites cause approximately 5 to 10 deaths per year. Many snake bites or presumed bites are "occult injuries," that is, no snake actually seen, or the species is not identified as venomous or nonvenomous. Also, up to 25% of bites from venomous snakes are "dry bites" (i.e., no venom injected). Any snake bite victim, or the patient in whom a venomous snake bite is on the differential diagnosis, must undergo admission or extended observation in the emergency department (8 to 12 h) in order to determine the correct and safe disposition.

Indigenous venomous snakes in the United States are essentially limited to the crotalid family (copperheads and rattlesnakes). Venom from crotalids causes local necrosis, coagulopathy, and occasional hypotension. Rarely, a patient in the United States will present with a coral snake bite. Coral snakes belong to the Elapid family and have neurotoxic venom that may cause delayed-onset symptoms. Victims may initially present with minimal local symptoms. Over a period of several hours, systemic symptoms such as tremor, general weakness, nausea and vomiting, and progressive lethargy may develop.

The definitive treatment of true venomous snakebites (specifically crotalids) is CroFab. CroFab, or FabAV, is the newer of two available antivenoms that facilitates an antigen-antibody reaction to inactivate the venom. Antivenom can be expensive and can have serious side effects including anaphylaxis. However, research suggests that anaphylaxis is less of a risk than previously thought when using the newer FabAV antivenom. In true venomous bites, antivenom may need to be given in large volumes due to a large venom burden or recurrent or delayed-onset systemic effects of the bite. The initial dose of FabAV is usually 4 to 6 vials to establish initial control of the envenomation. However, anywhere from the initial dose to 30 or 40 vials may be necessary for adequate treatment. In addition, crotalid antivenom should always be given in an ICU setting with monitoring and medication to treat an acute hypersensitivity reaction at the bedside. Furthermore, in rare patients, digit or extremity amputation or fasciotomy may still be indicated for bites refractory to antivenom.

On the other hand, bites from nonvenomous snakes, "dry bites," and occult injuries with puncture wounds that are likely not snake bites may be discharged to home. These patients should receive local wound care, and a tetanus booster if indicated. It is also appropriate to check baseline laboratory studies in these patients, including complete blood count with platelets, coagulation profile, and electrolytes with renal profile. These results will be important for comparison at the end of an observation period or obviously necessary to trend in the event of an envenomation.

However, after extended observation to ensure that signs and symptoms of envenomation do not occur, snake bite victims or patients with occult puncture wounds may be sent home. All patients in whom a crotalid bite is suspected should be observed for at least 8 h due to the possibility of delayed manifestations of envenomation. All patients in whom a coral snake bite is a possibility should be observed for at least 12 h, as these patients can develop delayed toxicity which can be rapidly fatal.

Snake bite treatment occupies the entire range of emergency department disposition plans, from discharging to home after a dry bite to admitting to the ICU for continued crotalid antivenom or in the case of compartment syndrome to the operating room for fasciotomy. In addition, appropriate snake bite treatment may evolve over an extended period of several hours. For example, the risk- and cost-benefit ratios of antivenom may preclude its initial use depending on the clinical circumstances, that is, minimal-local or no-systemic effects of known envenomation, or a bite from a low-risk species. On the other hand, antivenom administration may need to be repeated at large volume doses if the clinical situation worsens.

Always observe patients complaining of "snake bite" for several hours, do not forget to draw basic labs to help determine disposition, and be sure to frequently reassess these patients while they are in your emergency department!

SUGGESTED READINGS

Corneille MG, Larson S, Stewart RM, et al. A large single-center experience with treatment of patients with crotalid envenomations: Outcomes with and evolution of antivenin therapy. *Am J Surg*. 2006;192(6):848–852.

Gold BS, Dart RC, Barish RA. Bites of venomous snakes. *N Engl J Med*. 2002;347(5): 347–356.

Hall EL. Role of surgical intervention in the management of crotaline snake envenomation. *Ann Emerg Med*. 2001;37:175–180.

Lavonas EJ, Gerardo CJ, O'Malley G, et al. Initial experience with crotalidae polyvalent immune Fab (ovine) antivenom in the treatment of copperhead snakebite. *Ann Em Med*. 2004;43(2):200–206.

107

KNOW THE SYMPTOMS OF ACUTE MOUNTAIN SICKNESS AND REMEMBER THAT DESCENT IS THE ONLY DEFINITIVE TREATMENT

COLLEEN BIRMINGHAM, MD

Many in today's society enjoy a multitude of outdoor activities such as hiking, skiing, and rock climbing which expose them to high altitude settings and their associated risks. The most benign of these risks is an illness known as acute mountain sickness (AMS) that presents with largely nonspecific symptoms at altitudes which are relatively commonplace to the modern traveler. AMS has been defined as the presence of headache in an unacclimatized person who has recently arrived to an altitude of 2,500 m or more plus the presence of one or more of the following symptoms: anorexia, nausea, vomiting, insomnia, dizziness, or fatigue. In reality, these diagnostic criteria are very easily met given that the peak summits of many U.S. ski resorts are at 2,000 to 3,500 m.

The signs and symptoms of AMS usually develop within 8 to 24 h of arriving at altitude. The associated headache tends to be throbbing, bilateral, frontal, and worse with exercise. While the exact pathogenesis of this headache is not known, hypoxia is thought to be a major contributing factor. At an altitude of merely 3,000 m, the barometric pressure and inspired PO_2 are only 70% of the sea level value, sometimes causing relative hypoxia in otherwise well people. Additionally, the periodic breathing that occurs in most people while sleeping at altitudes above 4,000 m may exacerbate symptoms due to even lower levels of oxygen in the blood after apneic episodes.

The definitive management of AMS involves descent to a lower altitude with a descent of only 500 to 1,000 m, usually leading to resolution of symptoms. If descent is not possible, a portable hyperbaric chamber or low flow oxygen (1 to 2 L per min) generally alleviates symptoms. Finally, pharmacologic interventions should be considered in moderate AMS and include acetazolamide, dexamethasone, or both drugs until symptoms resolve. Importantly, patients should not ascend to a higher altitude until symptoms have completely resolved. While AMS may present as seemingly innocuous headache and fatigue, continued ascent can lead to the deadly high altitude cerebral edema (HACE). At altitudes over 5,000 m, ascents of as little as 200 m have precipitated HACE in those suffering from moderate AMS.

HACE is clinically defined as the onset of ataxia, altered consciousness, or both in someone suffering from AMS or high altitude pulmonary edema (HAPE).

Though the incidence of HACE is hard to quantify, it may be as high as 1% to 2% in people ascending above 4,500 m. Early neurological manifestations may include mood changes or hallucinations and can progress to drowsiness, lethargy, stupor, coma, and death due to brain herniation if the patient is not treated. While the overall presentation in HACE tends to be one of a global encephalopathy, focal findings such as cranial nerve palsies also occasionally manifest due to elevated intracranial pressure. As such, the pathophysiology is thought to be a severe manifestation on the spectrum of that proposed for AMS; cerebral vasodilatation, limited cerebral autoregulation, and elevated pressures in the microcirculation contribute to the formation of cerebral edema. Additionally, some suggest that hypoxia-induced changes in the blood-brain barrier contribute to failed autoregulation and thereby accelerate the development of HACE.

Just as it is critical to halt further ascent in the setting of AMS, immediate descent or evacuation is imperative in the setting of HACE. The abovementioned dexamethasone and oxygen are routinely administered when possible but these are not definitive treatments. A portable hyperbaric chamber may also be used as a temporizing measure until transport is arranged. Following descent, care is largely supportive and patients may continue to manifest some symptoms of HACE, commonly ataxia, for days to weeks before they enjoy a full recovery. Occasionally, patients do suffer persistent neurological damage after prolonged or severe cases of HACE.

The other potential harbinger of HACE, HAPE, also deserves a few words given its own potential morbidity and mortality. This disease is a form of noncardiogenic pulmonary edema which generally affects young, healthy persons often at or above a particular threshold altitude. Clinically, it presents as insidious cough, dyspnea which does not respond to rest and seems out of proportion to exertion, cyanosis, and possibly even hemoptysis. It is thought to be due to exaggerated hypoxic vasoconstriction and associated pulmonary artery hypertension in the setting of decreased nitric oxide production which leads to leakage from capillary beds. A severe disease in its own right, HAPE has an overall mortality rate of 11%. Similar to AMS and HACE, the initial treatment of HAPE includes supplemental oxygen and prompt descent. Sublingual or oral nifedipine may also be given as an adjunctive treatment in severe cases and CPAP/BiPAP should be considered prior to endotracheal intubation in the setting of impending respiratory failure. Importantly diuretics and vasodilators should be avoided in HAPE, as these interventions are not helpful and may cause worse outcomes in patients with underlying dehydration.

SUGGESTED READINGS

Hackett PH, Roach RC. High altitude illness. *N Engl J Med.* 2001;345(2):107–114.

Hackett PH, Yarnell PR, Hill R, et al. High-altitude cerebral edema evaluated with magnetic resonance imaging: Clinical correlation and pathophysiology. *JAMA.* 1998;280(22): 1920–1925.

Harris S. Altitude illness-cerebral syndromes. eMedicine.com; April 16, 2008. Available at: http://www.emedicine.com/EMERG/topic22.htm. Accessed July 30, 2008.

Richardson D., ed. High altitude illness. In: *Harwood Nuss' Clinical Practice of Emergency Medicine*. 4th ed. Lippincott Williams & Willines; 2005:1760.

Roach RC, Bartsch P, Oelz O, et al. Lake Louise AMS Scoring Consensus Committee: The Lake Louise acute mountain sickness scoring system. In: Sutton JR, Houston CS, Coates G., eds. *Hypoxia and Molecular Medicine*. Burlington VT: Queen City Press; 1993:272.

West JB, American College of Physicians, American Physiological Society. The physiologic basis of high-altitude diseases. *Ann Intern Med*. 2004;141(10):789–800.

108

DO NOT OVERRESUSCITATE THE PATIENT WITH HEATSTROKE

MORGAN SKURKY-THOMAS, MD

Severe heat injury can result in devastating multisystem failure and cardiovascular collapse in both elderly and young. While much of the care for these patients is intuitive and straightforward (aggressive cooling and supportive care), fluid resuscitation of the heatstroke patient is an area in which mistakes can easily be made.

Heatstroke represents the most severe end of a spectrum of heat injury. Milder heat injury (heat cramps and heat exhaustion) are primarily due to depletion of salts and water and respond well to passive cooling and oral or IV hydration.

In heatstroke, the same underlying issues exist, but the body's regulatory mechanisms have failed. The clinical picture of heatstroke is similar to heat exhaustion but with more marked hyperthermia (usually >40.5°C) and marked CNS dysfunction, which is the hallmark of heatstroke.

It seems intuitive that if gentle fluid resuscitation is the cornerstone of treating mild heat illness (heat cramps and heat exhaustion), then aggressive fluid resuscitation should be the key to treatment of heatstroke. However, there is ample data that overaggressive fluid resuscitation of the heatstroke patient has the potential to cause significant harm.

First of all, the heatstroke patient is usually nearly euvolemic. While these patients will often be hypotensive and appear markedly hypovolemic, in fact they have simply shunted their blood flow to the skin in an attempt to dissipate heat. Marked peripheral dilatation leads to a relative hypovolemia, but this is a distributive issue, rather than true volume depletion. As the patient is actively cooled, peripheral vasoconstriction rapidly shunts this volume back to the central circulation. While sweating and insensible losses will have led to some volume loss, in multiple series of carefully monitored heatstroke patients, the average volume requirement in the first 4 h of treatment is between 1,000 and 1,200 mL and very rarely exceeds 2,000 mL. Barring other coexisting processes, almost no heatstroke patient will be depleted more than 2 L.

In addition to being already euvolemic, the heatstroke patient may have cardiac pump dysfunction that makes them unable to deal with any fluid overload. There is evidence from pathologic, echocardiographic, radionucleotide, and physiologic studies that suggest that there is at least temporary myocardial suppression or dysfunction in heatstroke patients. Even in young, healthy patients, cardiac output, especially right-sided cardiac output, can be significantly impaired.

Thus, rather than being markedly dehydrated as one might expect, we can see that the heatstroke patient is actually in danger of fluid overload. If the patient is given 3, 4, or 5 L of fluid in the first hours of resuscitation and then cooled, forcing more volume to rapidly return to the central circulation, this volume overload in combination with myocardial pump dysfunction can lead to heart failure, pulmonary edema, and further decompensation.

How, then, should resuscitation of the heatstroke patient be approached? First, the central component must be rapid cooling. The best combination of practicality and rapid cooling is probably offered by water mist and fans for evaporative cooling. Core temperature should be continuously monitored and the patient cooled rapidly to 39°C, at which point active cooling should be stopped to avoid overshooting. As this cooling occurs, the hemodynamic derangements of heatstroke should resolve. Moderate fluid resuscitation should be given simultaneously, averaging 1 to 2 L total in the average patient. It has been suggested that this fluid resuscitation can best be guided by monitoring central venous pressure (CVP), and discontinued once CVP has become normal or elevated.

If hemodynamics do not respond to this regimen, pressor or inotrope therapy should be initiated instead of giving further fluid resuscitation. It has been proposed that dopamine or dobutamine may represent the best pressor therapy for the critical heatstroke patient, as the inotropic effects may overcome some of the myocardial suppression seen in this disease.

Of course, there will be exceptions, and there will be patients with multiple concurrent processes (e.g., the septic patient from a very hot apartment) who will require much more aggressive fluid resuscitation. Treatment should be tailored to the individual patient, and fluids should not be withheld in patients who are facing imminent cardiovascular collapse.

Remember to be judicious with your fluid resuscitation of the patient with heat illness.

SUGGESTED READINGS

Seraj MA, Channa AB, al Harthi SS, et al. Are heat stroke patients fluid depleted? Importance of monitoring central venous pressure as a simple guideline for fluid therapy. *Resuscitation.* 1991;21(1):33–39.

Tek D, Olshaker JS. Heat illness. *Emerg Med Clin North Am.* 1992;10:299–310.

Vicario S. Heat illness. In: Marx JA, Hockberger RS, Walls RM, et al., eds. *Rosen's Emergency Medicine, Concepts and Clinical Practice.* 6th ed. Philadelphia, PA: Mosby Elsevier; 2006.

109

SMOKE INHALATION: THERE IS MORE TO TREATMENT THAN JUST SECURING THE AIRWAY

KRISTIN COCHRAN, MD

In the victim of smoke inhalation, considering the need for intubation is always first. However, despite having a patent/protected airway and regular, clear respirations without the appearance of cyanosis, the victim of smoke inhalation may not be adequately transporting and utilizing oxygen in his or her tissues due to concomitant carbon monoxide (CO) and/or cyanide poisoning.

CO impairs the ability of hemoglobin not only to bind oxygen but also to off-load oxygen to tissues and inhibits utilization of oxygen in tissues by inhibiting oxidative phosphorylation. In the victim of smoke inhalation who is also suffering from cyanide poisoning, this problem is compounded by the fact that cyanide further inhibits oxidative phosphorylation such that even the oxygen that is received by the tissues cannot be utilized. The end result of these processes is anaerobic metabolism producing lactic acid and metabolic acidosis.

Cyanide poisoning and CO poisoning are often difficult to detect on initial exam, because as previously stated, patients will often not appear cyanotic. This is both because hemoglobin will take on a red hue whether bound to oxygen or CO, and due to the decreased utilization of oxygen at the tissues, both oxy-hemoglobin and carboxyhemoglobin will build up and provide a red to pink tone in perfused tissues. The classic "cherry red" appearance often associated with both poisonings, however, is only present in a minority of cases. Additionally, standard pulse oximeters will not differentiate oxyhemoglobin from carboxyhemoglobin and will read a high saturation although oxyhemoglobin content in the blood may actually be low. The physician must maintain a high suspicion for CO and cyanide poisoning in all suspected victims of smoke inhalation despite normal pulse oximetry and the absence of cyanosis on exam.

Although cyanide levels are not attainable acutely, carboxyhemoglobin levels can be measured from arterial or venous blood. An anion gap acidosis may also be recognized on a basic chemistry panel. If possible, a central venous PO_2 measurement allows the physician to calculate a venous-arterial PO_2 gradient, which in the case of smoke inhalation complicated by CO and cyanide may be narrowed due to decreased utilization of oxygen in peripheral tissues.

CO, aside from its effects on oxygen delivery, can also directly damage myocardium, and acute myocardial injury has been found in over one third of all cases of moderate to severe CO poisoning. Therefore, the physician should not forget to obtain an ECG and cardiac enzymes in the victim of smoke inhalation.

Because of the pathophysiology discussed above, the victim of smoke inhalation, if not requiring intubation, should be placed on 100% oxygen by non-rebreather mask. This allows oxygen to compete with CO for hemoglobin binding. For certain victims of carbon monoxide poisoning, namely those with CO level >25 (or 20 if pregnant), pregnancy with fetal distress, loss of consciousness, pH of <7.1, or evidence of end organ ischemia, hyperbaric oxygen therapy is indicated; however, these criteria are still controversial. In victims of fires and smoke inhalation, however, recognize that there may be a multitude of factors contributing to the patient's loss of consciousness, fetal distress, acidosis, or organ ischemia such as trauma or perfusion. Regardless, it is important to keep these indications in mind.

Antidotal treatment of isolated cyanide poisoning classically involves binding cyanide to produce a more readily excreted molecule by administering 50 mg/kg of hydroxocobalamin or by providing sulfur donors to the enzyme that transforms cyanide to its excreted form by administering 1.65 mL/kg of IV sodium thiosulfate, and inducing methemoglobinemia to competitively bind cyanide and reduce its binding to cytochrome complexes in the oxidative phosphorylation chain. However, in victims of smoke inhalation who are likely also suffering from CO poisoning, inducing methemoglobinemia by giving amyl nitrite or sodium nitrite is contraindicated because it further impairs oxygen delivery to tissues.

In summary, always think about CO and cyanide poisoning in association with smoke inhalation. Detect lactic acidosis, myocardial injury, administer high flow 100% oxygen, and remember special considerations for treating concomitant CO and cyanide in the case of smoke inhalation.

SUGGESTED READINGS

Bozeman WP, Myers RA, Barish RA. Confirmation of the pulse oximetry gap in carbon monoxide poisoning. *Ann Emerg Med.* 1997;30(5):608–611.

Hampson NB, Dunford RG, Kramer CC, et al. Selection criteria utilized for hyperbaric oxygen treatment of carbon monoxide poisoning. *J Emerg Med.* 1995;13(2):227–231.

Kao LW, Nanagas KA. Carbon monoxide poisoning. *Emerg Med Clin North Am.* 2004;22(4):985–1018.

Shusterman D, Alexeeff G, Hargis C, et al. Predictors of carbon monoxide and hydrogen cyanide exposure in smoke inhalation patients. *J Toxicol Clin Toxicol.* 1996;34(1):61–71.

110

REMEMBER THAT "ATYPICAL" PRESENTATIONS OF ACUTE CORONARY SYNDROME ARE TYPICAL IN ELDERLY PATIENTS

JAN M. SHOENBERGER, MD, FAAEM, FACEP

Although patients 65 years of age and older represent approximately 13% of the population of the United States, they account for half of all hospital admissions and 80% of deaths for acute coronary syndrome (ACS). As every emergency physician knows, emergency department (ED) diagnosis of ACS in this group of patients can be challenging. There are many potential pitfalls, but three of the most common are in history gathering, interpretation of symptoms, and electrocardiogram (ECG) analysis.

Elderly patients who are ultimately diagnosed with ACS are more likely to present with something other than chest pain as their chief complaint on presentation to the ED. They may complain of fatigue or shortness of breath without chest pain. This may have to do with a higher rate of long-standing diabetes in this age group or it may be more related to the presence of other comorbidities. Some elderly patients may have baseline dementia or other cognitive disorders that make it more difficult for them to express symptoms. A study published in *JAMA* in 2000 showed that patients who were ultimately diagnosed with acute myocardial infarction (AMI) and who presented without chest pain, were more likely to be older, have diabetes, be female, be of a nonwhite racial/ethnic group, and have a prior history of congestive heart failure and stroke. Moreover, those patients who do not have chest pain as a presenting symptom are at increased risk for delays in seeking medical attention, less aggressive treatments and in-hospital mortality.

Even when an elderly patient presents with chest pain, diagnosis can be a challenge. A large study published in 1989 reviewed over 7,000 patients who presented to the ED with chest pain. The goal of the study was to examine differences in presentation between older and younger patients. Elderly patients ultimately diagnosed with AMI were significantly less likely to have features considered typical for AMI than younger patients. They were less likely to be male and less likely to have radiation of pain to the jaw, neck, left arm, or left shoulder. In some ways, however, the older patients were more likely to have more "typical" presentations. They were more likely to have preexisting coronary artery disease and to describe their pain on presentation as "worse than prior angina or similar to a prior AMI."

Older patients are more likely to have preexisting ECG abnormalities such as left bundle-branch block or paced rhythms. This clearly makes their ECGs more difficult to interpret for acute events. They also present more frequently without ST segment elevation.

The elderly patient with AMI or an ACS is at higher risk for poor outcome. This may be due to both delay in diagnosis with a resultant decrease in aggressive therapies and the fact that older age is associated with structural and physiologic changes that predispose patients to adverse outcomes. These include preexisting abnormalities of left ventricular function, a decrease in systemic vascular compliance, an increase in left ventricular mass index, and altered neurohormonal and autonomic responses.

The combination of atypical symptoms, delayed presentation, and nondiagnostic ECGs can make the diagnosis of ACS in the elderly patient difficult. Although there is no magic solution to make these diagnoses easy, an awareness of how the elderly differ in their presentations can help the clinician avoid some of the more common pitfalls.

SUGGESTED READINGS

Canto JG, Shlipak MG, Rogers WJ, et al. Prevalence, clinical characteristics and mortality among patients with myocardial infarction presenting without chest pain. *JAMA.* 2000;283(24):3223–3229.

Gillum BS, Graves EJ, Wood E. National hospital discharge survey. *Vital Health Stat 13.* 1998;(133):i–v, 1–51.

Mehta RH, Rathore SS, Radford MJ, et al. Acute myocardial infarction in the elderly: Differences by age. *J Am Coll Cardiol.* 2001;38(3):736–741.

Solomon CG, Lee TH, Cook EF, et al. Comparison of clinical presentation of acute myocardial infarction in patients older than 65 years of age to younger patients: The multicenter chest pain study experience. *Am J Cardiol.* 1989;63(12):772–776.

111

ABDOMINAL PAIN IN THE ELDERLY PATIENT ... BE AFRAID ... BE VERY AFRAID!

WILLIAM K. MALLON, MD, FAAEM, FACEP

Abdominal pain is a common emergency department (ED) problem for elderly patients, accounting for approximately 5% of all ED visits in patients over 65 years old. About half of these patients are admitted to the hospital and as many as one third will require a surgical intervention during their hospital stay. Another sobering statistic: the mortality for geriatric abdominal pain is approximately 10%, which is similar to that of ST-elevation myocardial infarction.

The ED evaluation of the elderly patient with abdominal pain is complex, imaging-intense, and time-consuming. In the young, patients with undifferentiated abdominal pain are often discharged without a specific final diagnosis (nonspecific abdominal pain) after a limited evaluation with close follow-up. This approach in elderly patients is problematic and the emergency physician (EP) should consider a more complete evaluation for most elderly patients with abdominal pain.

Diagnostic difficulties abound with the elderly abdominal pain patient. The history of present illness may be limited in the patient with a previous stroke, Alzheimer's dementia, Parkinson's disease, or age-related dementia. The past medical history may be expansive and difficult to review. Medication lists are longer for these patients and drug-pathology interactions can confuse clinicians. Steroids, nonsteroidal anti-inflammatory drugs (NSAIDs), and acetaminophen can mitigate the febrile response more easily in elderly patients, and nonverbal manifestations of pain may be easily overlooked. β-Blockers can blunt tachycardia and a normal blood pressure could be "relative hypotension" for many elderly patients. These diagnostic challenges predictably result in delays in both diagnosis and surgical intervention. Nonetheless, the incidence of surgical disease is very high. Even appendicitis can be a challenging diagnosis; the perforation rate in the elderly is much higher compared with younger adults.

Imaging studies are almost always needed in the evaluation of abdominal pain in the elderly and computed tomography (CT) is the modality of choice. New scanners can do angiographic studies, are highly sensitive for any perforated viscus, and allow for increased diagnostic certainty (from 36% to 77%). Nonetheless, among the important life-threatening diagnoses that must be considered are mesenteric ischemia, acalculous cholecystitis, sepsis, and omental infarct, all of which can be "CT-negative" and therefore represent major pitfalls for the clinician who relies only on CT to rule out serious pathology. Bedside ultrasound by the EP to evaluate the aorta, kidney, and gallbladder can also be useful, and formal ultrasound studies can provide greater detail for a wide array of diagnoses.

The most common specific diagnoses made are biliary tract disease (12%) and small bowel obstruction (12%). Constipation and irritable bowel syndrome are overdiagnosed and overtreated in the elderly and should be considered only after a thorough evaluation has not revealed other pathologies.

Variables associated with adverse outcomes in the elderly include hypotension, abnormal plain films, leukocytosis, and abnormal bowel sounds, but most physical examination findings are not helpful in identifying patients with adverse outcomes.

In summary, it is a mistake to dismiss abdominal pain in the elderly patient as due to a functional or benign condition without a more complete evaluation. The EP must be vigilant for vascular emergencies, perforated viscus, malignancies, and biliary disease (including acalculous cholecystitis), which are all more common and more dangerous in the elderly.

SUGGESTED READINGS

Bugliosi TF, Meloy TD, Vukov LF. Acute abdominal pain in the elderly. *Ann Emerg Med.* 1990;19(12):1383–1386.

Laurell H, Hansson LE, Gunnarsson U. Acute abdominal pain among elderly patients. *Gerontology.* 2006;52(6):339–344.

Marco CA, Schoenfeld CN, Keyl PM, et al. Abdominal pain in geriatric emergency patients: Variables associated with adverse outcomes. *Acad Emerg Med.* 1998;5(12):1163–1168.

Martinez J, Mattu A. Abdominal pain in the elderly. *Emerg Med Clin North Am.* 2006;24(2): 371–388.

Morley JE. Constipation and irritable bowel syndrome in the elderly. *Clin Geriatr Med.* 2007;23(4):823–832.

Yeh EL, McNamara RM. Abdominal pain. *Clin Geriatr Med.* 2007;3(2):255–270.

112

CONSIDER THYROID DISORDERS IN THE ELDERLY

WILLIAM K. MALLON, MD, FAAEM, FACEP

Thyroid disorders are common in the elderly both as a cause of emergency department (ED) presentation and as an important comorbidity impacting ED management. Hypothyroidism affects 5% to 20% of women and 3% to 8% of men and is more common in Caucasian populations with high iodine intake. In geriatric populations, these percentages can *double*. Increasingly, medications are implicated in hypothyroidism, with lithium, amiodarone, sedative-hypnotics, and cytokines frequently identified as contributing or causal factors. Autoimmune thyroid gland destruction, radioiodine therapy (with inadequate replacement), and thyroid surgery are also causes of hypothyroidism.

Hyperthyroidism is a more difficult diagnosis in the elderly because atypical and "apathetic" presentations without overt clinical signs of thyrotoxicosis are more common. A goiter may not be present either. This is in contrast to younger patients, where thyrotoxicosis and storm are more clinically apparent. Laboratory testing is frequently required to facilitate diagnosis in the elderly and a delay in diagnosis is common. Finally, euthyroid sick syndrome (ESS) with an increased reverse T3 has been associated with decreased survival in the elderly. The importance of ESS for ED care is currently not known.

Emergency physicians (EPs) must decide when to commence a thyroid evaluation in the ED. While most investigators recommend against routine screening for thyroid disease in the elderly, because inpatient mortality has been associated with thyroid disease in geriatric patients and atypical presentations are common, liberal testing is recommended by some. A rapid, third-generation ultrasensitive thyroid stimulating hormone (TSH) test is now available with a rapid turnaround time in many EDs. A TSH is the most useful test and will usually allow diagnosis of both hypothyroidism and hyperthyroidism.

Liberal testing for thyroid disorders is indicated in patients taking amiodarone because the incidence of thyroid disorders associated with this drug is high. Although amiodarone can precipitate thyrotoxicosis, particularly in iodine-deficient areas, it is more likely to cause hypothyroidism in iodine-sufficient areas.

Thyrotoxic periodic paralysis with associated hypokalemia is an emergent complication of hyperthyroidism that can be seen in the elderly. The elderly patient who presents to the ED with acute weakness should have a serum potassium level checked and if low, a TSH should be considered to diagnose this disorder.

Treating hypothyroidism or myxedema coma with intravenous (IV) thyroxine is critical to patient survival but must be combined with ventilation, warming, fluids, and corticosteroids. The combination of IV thyroxine with vasopressors is potentially dangerous and dysrhythmias can result. Administration of IV thyroxine should thus be undertaken slowly (300 to 500 μg over 20 to 30 min) and vasopressors should be discontinued as soon as possible.

In the treatment of thyrotoxicosis, β-blockade, the mainstay of therapy, can be dangerous as well. Cardiac arrest and cardiovascular collapse have been tied to β-blocker therapy and have led to recommendations that short-acting, titratable β-blockers, such as esmolol, be employed.

Table 112.1 illustrates the broad landscape of conditions associated with thyroid disorders. These conditions may lead to the diagnosis of an endocrinopathy or may precipitate acute decompensation of an endocrinopathy.

TABLE 112.1	DISORDERS ASSOCIATED WITH THYROID DISORDERS
HYPOTHYROIDISM	**HYPERTHYROIDISM**
Amiodarone therapy	Amiodarone therapy
Lithium	Acute abdomen
Sedative-hypnotics	Cholestatic jaundice
Depression	Atrial fibrillation
Hypothermia	Apathetic thyrotoxicosis
Congestive heart failure	Stimulant drugs
Vitamin B_{12} deficiency	Blunt neck trauma
Viral infection	Viral infection
Radioablation (I-131)	Neck surgery

Bidirectional thinking from an associated illness back to the underlying thyroid disorder is an important aspect of assessing the elderly. Moreover, awareness of just how common thyroid problems are in geriatric populations can help the EP avoid missing their diagnosis and treatment.

SUGGESTED READINGS

Brunette D, Rothong C. Emergency department management of thyrotoxic crisis with esmolol. *Am J Emerg Med*. 1991;9(3):232–234.

Campbell AJ. Thyroid disorders in the elderly: Difficulties in diagnosis and treatment. *Drugs*. 1986;31(5):455–461.

Duggal J, Singh S, Kuchinic P, et al. Utility of esmolol in thyroid crisis. *Can J Clin Pharmacol*. 2006;13(3):e292–e295.

Forestier E, Vinzio S, Sapin R, et al. Increased reverse T3 is associated with shorter survival in independently-living elderly. *Eur J Endocrinol*. 2009;160(2):207–214 [Epub 2008 Nov 10].

Hofmann A, Nawara C, Ofluoglu S. Incidence and predictability of amiodarone-induced thyrotoxicosis and hypothyroidism. *Wien Klin Wochenschr*. 2008;120(15–16):493–498.

Laurberg P, Andersen S, Bulow Pedersen I, et al. Hypothyroidism in the elderly: Pathophysiology, diagnosis and treatment. *Drugs Aging*. 2005;22(1):23–38.

Pimentel L, Hansen KN. Thyroid disease in the ED: A clinical and laboratory review. *J Emerg Med*. 2005;28(2):201–209.

Ursella S, Testa A, Mazzone M, et al. Amiodarone-induced thyroid dysfunction in clinical practice. *Eur Rev Med Pharmacol Sci*. 2006;10(5):269–278.

Wartofsky L. Myxedema coma. *Endocrinol Metab Clin North Am*. 2006;35(4):687–698.

113

DO NOT MISS THE OCCULT HIP FRACTURE IN ELDERLY PATIENTS

ALEXANDER A. KLEINMANN, MD AND
RALPH J. RIVIELLO, MD, MS, FACEP

Hip fractures are a commonly encountered diagnosis in the emergency department (ED). Risk factors for hip fracture include white race, female gender, and advanced age. Mortality is high—up to 36% at 1 year. In addition, there is an association between delay to definitive treatment (operative reduction) and higher mortality. The significant incidence of *occult* hip fractures—fractures which are missed by plain x-rays—is thus of critical importance to the emergency physician. Fractures that are undisplaced and thus more likely to be invisible on plain films will become displaced after such a patient is inadvertently discharged, dramatically increasing the risk of avascular necrosis of the femoral head and other complications of hip fracture, most notably death.

Pitfalls that may foil a correct diagnosis of hip fracture include failure to ask about the mechanism of injury or to recognize subtle signs of trauma to the hip or knee. Importantly, negative examination findings regarding tenderness to palpation, FABER (flexion, abduction, external rotation) range of motion testing, pain with axial loading, limb shortening, straight leg raise test, and neurological deficit are notorious for misleading the clinician. Patients with nondisplaced fractures may not exhibit any of these findings. In patients with risk factors for hip fracture and even seemingly trivial trauma, the inability to ambulate or an antalgic gait with pain referable to the hip is a sufficient reason to pursue the workup beyond negative plain films.

One of the first review articles on the subject published in 1992 included an algorithm for detecting occult hip fractures. They suggested that patients with suspected hip fractures and negative radiographs be instructed to rest and not bear weight on the affected hip for 1 week. They further recommended that patients return for repeat plain films in 1 week. If repeat plain films were positive or the patient continued to be symptomatic after 1 week, further imaging with CT, MRI, or bone scan was suggested.

In the past decade, there has been a paradigm shift aimed at identifying occult hip fractures earlier. CT, MRI, and bone scans are all diagnostic options for further study of the patient with clinical suspicion for fracture and negative plain films. Bone scans have been reported to have a sensitivity of 93% and specificity of 95% within 3 days of injury. However, a bone scan provides only a qualitative result; it may show increased uptake in a metabolically active area that was already suspicious for fracture. Furthermore, it does not delineate the anatomy well enough to guide surgical management and it is not readily available in the ED setting.

CT and MRI are both more promising, but MRI clearly appears to be the superior of the two. In a small prospective study comparing CT and MRI in patients with negative plain x-rays, CT missed an occult fracture in four of six cases detected by MRI. Although CT is more readily available than MRI and can be considered as an alternative, the clinician must recognize that negative CT imaging cannot exclude hip fracture. MRI is considered a gold standard for the identification of occult hip fractures.

The bottom line is that if you suspect that a patient has a hip fracture despite negative plain films, you should try to obtain an MRI to confirm the diagnosis. If not available immediately, admit the patient and keep them non–weight bearing until you can obtain an MRI. If a CT is performed and is negative, then MRI should be subsequently obtained to exclude the diagnosis.

SUGGESTED READINGS

Alba E, Youngberg R. Occult fractures of the femoral neck. *Am J Emerg Med.* 1992;10(1):64–68.

Hossain M, Barwick C, Sinha AK, et al. Is magnetic resonance imaging (MRI) necessary to exclude occult hip fracture? *Injury.* 2007;38(10):1204–1208.

Lubovsky O, Liebergall M, Mattan Y, et al. Early diagnosis of occult hip fractures MRI versus CT scan. *Injury.* 2005;36(6):788–792.

Perron AD, Miller MD, Brady WJ. Orthopedic pitfalls in the ED: Radiographically occult hip fracture. *Am J Emerg Med.* 2002;20(3):234–237.

114

RECOGNIZE THAT ELDERLY PATIENTS ARE AT HIGH RISK FOR FALLS

JAN M. SHOENBERGER, MD, FAAEM, FACEP

Between 1993 and 2003, emergency department (ED) visits in the United States for patients aged 65 to 74 years increased by 34%. If this trend continues, ED visits for the 65- to 74-year-old group could nearly double from 6.4 million visits to 11.7 million visits by 2013. In this population, falls are a serious health concern. Although most falls do not result in serious injury, they have a major effect on quality of life due to restriction of activities for fear of falling. One in five falls requires medical attention and 1% to 2% result in hip fracture. Unintentional injuries are the fifth most common cause of death in the elderly population. Because ED practitioners are seeing more and more elderly patients, recognition of those at high risk for falls at home in order to aid in prevention of falls and modification of risk for falls should be part of the ED care of these patients.

In a recent evidence-based review by Carpenter, seven risk factors for fall were identified. These risk factors include medications (specifically, benzodiazepines, phenothiazines, and antidepressants), dementia, residual stroke sequelae, Parkinson's disease, difficulty rising from a chair, previous falls, and fear of falling. Recognizing that patients with dementia, gait instability, stroke-related neurologic deficits, and previous falls are at extremely high risk for future falls at home may help ED practitioners assist in injury prevention.

ED-initiated fall screening has been recommended, although at this point in time, there has not been any evidence of a successful ED-based intervention to prevent falls in the United States. In Europe, however, fall-related mortality has decreased 4.3% during the last decade, presumably because of proactive fall-prevention programs. A British trial examined a multidisciplinary secondary fall-prevention strategy for patients found to be at risk in the ED. In the study, patients over age 65 who had experienced a fall were randomized to an intervention group or usual care. The intervention group underwent a detailed medical and occupational therapy assessment with referral to relevant services if indicated. The authors demonstrated a 20% absolute risk reduction for falls in the intervention group in the year following the ED visit. Whether this type of program is feasible in U.S. EDs remains to be determined.

In 1997, Baraff et al. published an ED practice guideline for the management of falls in elderly patients. This guideline contains several common sense recommendations that ED-based health care providers can make to their patients to aid in fall prevention. These include

- **Exercise** (simple stretching, strengthening, and balance training)
- **Calcium and vitamin D** (preventing osteoporosis)
- **Medications** (avoiding sleep aids and benzodiazepines, and consulting with primary physician to determine whether medications can be reduced)
- **Footwear** (shoes with low heels and large contact with the ground such as smooth-soled sneakers are best)
- **Home hazard review** (night lights, handrails/safety strips in bath, and securing loose rugs and removing objects that are difficult to see)
- **Vision screening**
- **Avoidance of alcohol** (no more than one or two drinks a day if any)

It may not be reasonable to expect the ED personnel to review all of these points verbally with all elderly patients at risk. However, having a handout in the ED available that contains these recommendations, along with a listing of community resources (such as places with exercise programs for the elderly, low cost optometry, etc.), is a good way to help educate patients about fall prevention and to document these efforts. Speaking with family members about concerns regarding future fall risk and the things they can do to help may also be of benefit.

SUGGESTED READINGS

American Geriatrics Society, et al. Guideline for the prevention of falls in older persons. *J Am Geriatr Soc*. 2001;49(5):664–672.

Baraff LJ, Della Penna R, Williams N, et al. Practice guideline for the ED management of falls in community-dwelling elderly persons. *Ann Emerg Med*. 1999;30(4):480–492.

Carpenter CR. Evidenced-based emergency medicine/rational clinical examination abstract. Will my patient fall? *Ann Emerg Med*. 2009;53(3):398–400 [Epub 2008 May 23].

Close J, Ellis M, Hooper R, et al. Prevention of falls in the elderly trial (PROFET): A randomized, controlled trial. *Lancet*. 1999;353(9147):93–97.

Petridou ET, Dikalioti SK, Dessypris N, et al. The evolution of unintentional injury mortality among elderly in Europe. *J Aging Health*. 2008;20(2):159–182.

Roberts DC, McKay MP, Shaffer A. Increasing rates of Emergency Department visits for elderly patients in the United States, 1993 to 2003. *Ann Emerg Med*. 2008;51(6):769–774.

115

DO NOT MISTAKE DELIRIUM FOR DEMENTIA IN THE ELDERLY

DOHWA KIM, MD

Delirium is a common problem in geriatric patients and remains underrecognized in various clinical settings. Additionally, the pathophysiology of delirium remains poorly understood. Approximately one third of patients 70 years or older admitted to a medical service suffer from delirium. One half of these are delirious on admission to the hospital. There is clear evidence that delirium is strongly associated with poor outcomes, including an increased risk of nosocomial infection, prolonged hospitalization, greater need for post-acute nursing home placement, and death.

According to the Diagnostic and Statistical Manual-IV of the American Psychiatric Association (DSM-IV), delirium is defined as a change in cognition with a disturbance in attention that develops over a short period of time and is usually caused by general medical conditions (*Table 115.1*).

Delirium remains a clinical diagnosis, based on observations and information from collateral sources. The DSM-IV criteria may be difficult to apply in acute clinical settings such as the emergency department (ED). The Confusion Assessment Method (CAM) may be more clinically useful in the ED setting. With appropriate understanding and training, this method of

Table 115.1	**DSM-IV Diagnostic Criteria for Delirium Due to a General Medical Condition**

- Disturbance of consciousness (i.e., reduced clarity of awareness of the environment) with reduced ability to focus, sustain, or shift attention

- A change in cognition (such as memory deficit, disorientation, language disturbance) or the development of a perceptual disturbance that is not better accounted for by a preexisting, established, or evolving dementia

- The disturbance develops over a short period of time (usually hours to days) and tends to fluctuate during the course of the day

- There is evidence from the history, physical examination, or laboratory findings that the disturbance is caused by the direct physiological consequences of a general medical condition

Table 115.2	**The Confusion Assessment Method**

The diagnosis of delirium requires the presence of features 1 and 2 and either 3 or 4

1. Acute change in mental status and fluctuating course

2. Inattention

3. Disorganized thinking

4. Altered level of consciousness

assessment can achieve more than 95% sensitivity and specificity in diagnosing delirium (*Table 115.2*).

The differential diagnosis of delirium includes dementia, depression, and acute psychiatric syndromes. However, these syndromes can coexist and dementia is one of the strongest and most consistent risk factors for delirium. Twenty-five to fifty percent of delirious patients have been found to have dementia, and the presence of dementia increases the risk of delirium by a factor of two to three. Thus, a common diagnostic issue in the ED setting is whether a newly presenting confused elderly patient has dementia, delirium, or both. To make this determination, the physician must know the patient's baseline mental status. This will be most likely obtained from family members, caregivers, or others who know the patient. In addition, the time course of the development of mental status change is essential to make the diagnosis of delirium.

All patients with diagnosed delirium require a careful history including the time course of the changes in mental status and their association with other symptoms, physical examination, and focused laboratory testing. There are multiple etiologies (*Table 115.3*) of delirium in the elderly. Because medications are the most common and treatable cause of delirium, a careful medication history including prescription, over-the-counter and herbal medication,

---

TABLE 115.3   **COMMON ETIOLOGIES OF DELIRIUM**

- Acute cardiac events (e.g., myocardial infarction, congestive heart failure, and arrhythmia)

- Acute pulmonary events (e.g., asthma, chronic obstructive pulmonary disease, pulmonary embolism, hypoxemia, and hypercarbia)

- Bed rest

- Drug withdrawal (e.g., sedatives and alcohol)

- Fluid or electrolyte disturbances including dehydration, hyponatremia, and hypernatremia

- Infections

- Intracranial events (e.g., stroke, bleeding, and infection)

- Medications

- Severe anemia (hematocrit < 30%)

- Uncontrolled pain

- Urinary retention and fecal impaction

- Use of indwelling devices

- Use of restraints

---

and nutritional supplements is imperative. Nearly every class of medications has the potential to cause delirium in the elderly, but medications commonly causing delirium include narcotics, sedative-hypnotics, and drugs with anticholinergic action such as tricyclic antidepressants, antihistamines, antipsychotics, anticonvulsants, and antiparkinsonian agents. Alcohol and other drugs of abuse should also be sought.

Prompt treatment of the underlying etiology remains the cornerstone of management. Multiple contributing factors are often present, so the workup should not be terminated because a single "cause" is identified. The management of delirium requires an interdisciplinary team approach by physicians, nurses, family members, and other health care professionals who are involved in the care of the patient. The delirious patient may need to be admitted to a monitored setting, depending on the level of agitation and possible underlying causes.

SUGGESTED READINGS

American Psychiatric Association. *The Diagnostic and Statistical Manual of Mental Disorder.* 4th ed., Text revision. Washington, DC: American Psychiatric Association; 2000:143.

Cox DR, Oakes D. *Analysis of Survival Data.* New York, NY: Chapman and Hall; 1984.

Inouye SK, van Dyck CH, Alessi CA, et al. Clarifying confusion: The confusion assessment method. *Ann Intern Med.* 1990;113(12):941–948.

Rakel RE, Bope ET. *Conn's Current Therapy, 2001: Latest Approved Methods of Treatment for the Practicing Physician.* Philadelphia, PA: W.B. Saunders Company; 2001:1145.

116

DO NOT FORGET THAT NEGLECT IS A TYPE OF ELDER ABUSE

DIANA C. SCHNEIDER, MD AND WESLEY S. WOO, MD

Emergency departments (ED) are often the first point of contact within the medical system for elder maltreatment (EM) victims. Types of EM frequently cited include physical abuse, neglect, self-neglect, financial abuse, and psychological abuse. Although physical abuse is the most apparent form of EM, neglect is the most prevalent form. Elder neglect accounts for over 60% of all EM reports made to Adult Protective Services annually and likely accounts for the majority of EM cases that are not reported.

Neglect is defined as the failure of a caregiver to provide basic care, typically assistance with the activities of daily living. In contrast to self-neglect, this definition necessarily involves a person with whom the victim has an established relationship. Elder neglect has been associated with certain victim characteristics, including dementia, depression, and other mental illnesses. Interestingly, abuser risk factors may be better predictors of EM than victim attributes. These risk factors include alcoholism, legal difficulties, psychiatric disease, and deviant behaviors. The presentation of neglect is often subtle, and even the most common chief complaints of elderly patients in the ED (i.e., falls, dehydration, and failure of self-care) can be signs or symptoms of neglect. In elderly patients with severe cognitive and/or communication impairment, neglect may present with nonspecific behavioral changes or physical exam findings (*Table 116.1*). Signs that should arouse suspicion of possible neglect include a delay in seeking care for an injury, failure to seek medical care, poor hygiene, pressure sores, dehydration, and malnutrition. Given the absence of specific forensic markers for neglect, the American Medical Association recommends that physicians routinely screen elderly patients for EM.

Once neglect is suspected, the emergency physician's goal is not to determine whether neglect was intentional or unintentional. The focus should be on the identification, documentation and treatment of injuries, as well as the disposition of the patient to a safe environment.

TABLE 116.1	SIGNS OF NEGLECT IN THE ELDERLY
BEHAVIORAL CHANGES	**PHYSICAL SIGNS**
Faking seizures	Decubitus ulcers
Elective mutism	Poor hygiene
Refusing to eat	Poor nutrition
Aggressive behavior	Weight loss
Withdrawal	Unkempt toenails
Lack of compliance with medical regimen	Filthy living conditions
	Unclean clothing or bedding
	Lack of hearing aids, dentures, and eyeglasses
	Overexposure to the elements

The identification of neglect involves several key steps. The interview of the patient and caregiver should be conducted separately in a nonjudgmental manner. Documentation must be done carefully using specific dates and the victim's own words as much as possible. Sketches of any lesions on physical exam (a body map) are helpful. Medical photography is often even better evidence, as long as the chain of custody is maintained (i.e., place photographs immediately into the medical record when possible). A head-to-toe physical examination with emphasis on the head and neck, skin, feet, and neurological and musculo-skeletal systems should be performed. A complete blood count, basic chemistry panel, urine analysis, and a chest x-ray can be used to screen for evidence of malnutrition, dehydration, and rib fractures.

The disposition of the neglect victim often depends on the patient's decisional capacity. If a patient has the capacity, he or she cannot be forced into another social situation against his or her will. If the neglect victim demonstrates signs of reduced capacity, the emergency physician must ensure that the patient is removed from the neglectful living situation (e.g., hospital admission or placement) until they can receive a complete assessment.

Reporting of abusers is not dependent upon a victim's disposition, and once neglect is suspected, the patient's case should be reported to Adult Protective Services and/or other appropriate authorities. Oftentimes, the neglect victim may not want the case reported due to reasons such as embarrassment, fear of retaliation, and fear of being uprooted from his or her home. Nonetheless, reporting of suspected elder abuse and neglect is mandatory in most states. For the victim who will not accept assistance, the health care team can still aid in the development of a safety plan or additional resources within the home.

SUGGESTED READINGS

Fulmer T, Paveza G, Vandeweerd C, et al. Neglect assessment in urban emergency departments and confirmation by an expert clinical team. *J Gerontol*. 2005;8:1002–1006.

Geroff A, Olshaker JS. Elder abuse. *Emerg Med Clin North Am*. 2006;24:491–505.

Kleinschmidt KC. Elder abuse: A review. *Ann Emerg Med*. 1997;30:463–472.

Strasser S, Fulmer T. The clinical presentation of elder neglect: What we know and what we can do. *J Am Psychiatr Nurses Assoc*. 2007;12(6):340–349.

Tatara T. *Suggested State Guidelines for Gathering and Reporting Domestic Elder Abuse Statistics for Compiling National Data*. Washington DC: National Aging Resource Center On Elder Abuse (NARCEA); 1990.

117

DO NOT BE AFRAID TO TREAT PAIN IN ELDERLY PATIENTS AGGRESSIVELY

JAN M. SHOENBERGER, MD, FAAEM, FACEP

Pain is one of the most frequent reasons patients present to an emergency department (ED) for care. Many studies have demonstrated that care providers in the ED often provide inadequate analgesia. This has been shown to be particularly true in elderly patients.

In 1996, Jones et al. published one of the first studies looking at age as a risk factor for inadequate analgesia in the ED. Patients who had sustained isolated long-bone fractures and were either older than 70 years of age or aged 20 to 50 years were studied. The study found that nonelderly patients were more likely than elderly patients to receive ED pain medication (80% vs. 66%) and received it in a shorter period of time (mean, 52 vs. 74 min). The younger patients were more likely to receive narcotics and they received a higher equivalent dose than the elderly patients. This pattern of oligoanalgesia in elderly patients with acute (and chronic) pain has been demonstrated in other studies as well.

There are several possible explanations for why elderly patients who suffer from painful conditions might be undertreated. One reason is that elderly patients often refuse pain medication when offered. They may not want to have their judgment clouded. They may sense an imminent loss of independence upon learning that they have fractured a hip, for example. In these situations where elderly patients are attempting to be stoic and continue to refuse pain medication, ED care providers may consider offering alternative pain control such as a femoral nerve block.

Physicians may also be concerned about the potential for drug-drug interactions in elderly patients with multiple comorbidities. ED care providers are often faced with a patient with a bag full of medications or a patient who cannot

TABLE 117.1	GUIDELINES FOR ACUTE PAIN MANAGEMENT IN THE ELDERLY

1. Elderly patients should be asked regularly about pain. Whenever possible, the intensity of pain should be assessed quantitatively (e.g., numerical rating scale) to avoid misunderstanding.

2. In patients with fractures, target analgesia to times of likely patient movement, such as before radiographs or admission to the hospital.

3. Use opiates with a short half-life (e.g., morphine, hydromorphone, and fentanyl)

4. Use adjunctive medications (e.g., acetaminophen and antiemetics) to improve pain control; may allow a lower opiate dose or counteract side effects.

5. Patients with moderately severe to severe pain should have their opioid analgesics given intravenously. The patients can be given small serial doses of IV opioids to safely and effectively relieve pain.

6. Use analgesic drugs correctly. "Start low and go slow" remains the best rule. Achieve adequate doses and anticipate side effects (e.g., anticholinergic symptoms, respiratory depression, and nausea).

7. Non-steroidal anti-inflammatory drugs (NSAIDS) should be prescribed cautiously in patients with preexisting renal disease, heart failure, hypertension, peptic ulcers, or bleeding disorder.

Source: Adapted from Jones JS, Johnson K, McNinch M. Age as a risk factor for inadequate emergency department analgesia. *Am J Emerg Med*. 1996;14(2):157–160.

remember all of the names of his or her long list of medications. Adverse drug events in this age group are common and often result in hospitalization. The fear of hypotension, cardiac depression, and side effects may cause ED caregivers to think twice (and then forget) about giving parenteral narcotic analgesia, even when indicated.

Another barrier to adequate pain control may be the ability to assess pain in the elderly patient with underlying dementia or cognitive disorders. Questions about the level of pain or pain score may go unanswered by patients with aphasia or dementia. This hindrance to communication may lead to underestimation of pain. In patients with these conditions, pain is best assessed by nonverbal methods such as those used with pediatric patients. The Faces Pain Scale or other such tool might be more appropriate than numeric scores.

The *Table 117.1* summarizes guidelines for acute pain management in the elderly.

SUGGESTED READINGS

Fletcher AK, Rigby AS, Heyes FL. Three-in-one femoral nerve block as analgesia for fractured neck of femur in the emergency department: A randomized, controlled trial. *Ann Emerg Med*. 2003;41(2):227–233.

Fosnocht DE, Swanson ER, Barton ED. Changing attitudes about pain and pain control in emergency medicine. *Emerg Med Clin North Am*. 2005;23(2):297–306.

Jones JS, Johnson K, McNinch M. Age as a risk factor for inadequate emergency department analgesia. *Am J Emerg Med*. 1996;14(2):157–160.

Neighbor ML, Honner S, Kohn MA. Factors affecting emergency department opioid administration to severely injured patients. *Acad Emerg Med*. 2004;11(12):1290–1296.

Pautex S, Michon A, Guedira M, et al. Pain in severe dementia: Self-assessment or observational scales? *J Am Geriatr Soc*. 2006;54(7):1040–1045.

Rupp T, Delaney KA. Inadequate analgesia in emergency medicine. *Ann Emerg Med*. 2004;43(4):494–503.

Won AB, Lapane KL, Vallow S, et al. Persistent nonmalignant pain and analgesic prescribing patterns in elderly nursing home residents. *J Am Geriatr Soc*. 2004;52(6):867–874.

118

BE VERY CAREFUL WITH MEDICATION DOSING IN THE ELDERLY PATIENT

JAN M. SHOENBERGER, MD, FAAEM, FACEP

Pharmacokinetics and pharmacodynamics change with age. As patients grow older, they have decreased lean body mass, decreased total body water, and an increased proportion of body fat. These changes in body composition lead to a decreased volume of distribution and an increase in plasma concentration of drugs. Clinicians must appreciate these differences in age-related drug metabolism and prescribe accordingly.

Clearance by all renal routes (glomerular filtration and tubular reabsorption and secretion) decreases with age and is lower in women than in men. It is important to note that significantly decreased creatinine clearance can be present in elderly patients even when they have a normal serum creatinine measurement. This is illustrated by review of the Cockroft-Gault formula for calculation of creatinine clearance (CrCl):

$$CrCl\,(mL/min)\ =\ \frac{(140 - age\,[years] \times weight\,[kg])}{creatinine\,(mg/dL) \times 72}$$

(The result should be multiplied by 0.85 for women to account for lower skeletal muscle mass.)

The plasma concentration of a drug is inversely related to its volume of distribution. The volume of distribution is in turn dependent on the water (extracellular) space and fat stores of the body. The volume of hydrophilic drugs therefore decreases, and equal doses as would be given in a younger patient will result in higher plasma concentrations in the older patient. This is the case with drugs such as aspirin, famotidine, lithium, warfarin, digoxin, propranolol, and ethanol. Use of diuretics may reduce the extracellular (or water) space further, leading to exacerbation of the problem.

Hepatic metabolism in the elderly may also be affected. This depends on lifestyle, genotype, hepatic blood flow, hepatic disease, hepatic size, and interactions with other medications. It may be reduced up to 30% to 50% in elderly patients. Drug metabolism in the liver occurs in two phases. Phase I reactions occur through the cytochrome P450 system which either clears drugs or allows oxidation and drug activation. This occurs more slowly with age and leads to changes in the serum concentration and activity levels of certain drugs. Inhibitors of the P450 system will cause an increase in the serum concentration by impairing clearance. Medications that induce the P450 system will lead to decreased levels of medications that are metabolized by this system. Phase II reactions include metabolism by acetylation, sulfonation, conjugation, and glucoronidation and these are typically minimally affected in the elderly patient.

Serum protein concentration also decreases with age. This is especially true with respect to the albumin levels in frail or malnourished patients. Lower albumin levels mean less binding sites for protein bound medications, resulting in higher serum concentrations. If normal excretion and clearance are occurring, more rapid clearance of the drug may occur. Increased levels could occur if excretion or clearance is altered. Competitive inhibition for protein binding sites by drugs can lead to displacement of one drug by another. An important example of this phenomenon occurs with the coadministration of aspirin and warfarin, where aspirin increases the unbound fraction of warfarin.

In emergency settings, pharmacist or geriatrician input is not usually available and exact weight measurements and serum creatinine levels are not known prior to initiating some medications. For the most part, loading doses of parenteral medications do not need to be adjusted. It is the subsequent doses that need to be more carefully considered to prevent unintentional overdosing.

When dealing with a titratable drug in an elderly patient who may be at risk for decreased drug clearance, start with a smaller initial dose than would be given to a younger adult (e.g., 50%). The dose should then be titrated to a defined therapeutic response.

One helpful mnemonic that may help emergency providers remember the specific patient groups where drug dosing needs to be carefully reviewed is "CLOCK." This stands for

C, CNS disease
L, Liver disease
O, Old age
C, Children
K, Kidney disease

Patients in these high-risk groups often require lower doses of drug (particularly sedative/hypnotics or narcotics). In the case of older patients, some authors have suggested that "geriatric dose" packaging, similar to pediatric dose packaging, might help decrease unintentional overdosing in emergency settings.

SUGGESTED READINGS

Blanda M. Pharmacologic issues in geriatric emergency medicine. *Emerg Clin N Am.* 2006;24:449–465.

McLean AJ, Le Couteur DG. Aging biology and geriatric clinical pharmacology. *Pharmacol Rev.* 2004;56(2):163–184.

Schwartz JB, The current state of knowledge on age, sex and their interactions on clinical pharmacology. *Clin Pharmacol Ther.* 2007;82(1):87–96.

Turnheim K. When drug therapy gets old: Pharmacokinetics and pharmacodynamics in the elderly. *Exp Gerontol.* 2003;38(8):843–853.

119

BE AWARE OF THE DANGERS OF POLYPHARMACY IN THE ELDERLY

EDUARDO BORQUEZ, MD

Elderly patients represent a special and vulnerable population in the emergency department (ED). As the elderly population increases, so too will the frequency and complexity of their presentations to the ED. Currently, elders represent 15% to 19% of ED visits and that figure is projected to increase. Persons aged over 65 years use one third of all prescription medications, and over 40% use five or more different medications per week. Twelve percent use over 10 medications per week. The causes of this trend seem fairly obvious. Combination therapies for many common diseases such as hypertension, diabetes, and hyperlipidemia have been promoted. With the development of a few common diseases over the years, the medication list lengthens. With each additional medication, the initial low risk of a drug reaction increases. To compound this further, there is the temptation to treat a side effect (such as dyspepsia) with the addition of yet another medication. Lastly, elderly patients have an increased incidence of cognitive deficits and decreased social support that may lead to medication errors. Recognizing the potential for polypharmacy and adverse drug events (ADEs) is thus becoming increasingly important.

This combination of factors has predictable consequences. ADEs have been shown to occur in about one third of the elderly population per year, with 10% of those ADEs requiring an ED visit. However, many ADEs have been shown to be both predictable and preventable. Once the potential pitfalls of polypharmacy have been identified, solutions begin to emerge.

First, clinicians should have in their mind a short list of high-risk medications that are red-flagged when elicited on history and before prescribing. The high-risk drugs have been found to be independent risk factors for ADEs include opiates, antipsychotics, antibiotics, antiepileptics, and antidepressants.

Second, the sheer number of medications any given patient is taking has not surprisingly been found to be associated with ADEs. The risk and benefit to starting multidrug combination therapy for a given disease should be weighed carefully. If multidrug therapy for a single problem is found to be necessary, then combination or extended release formulations should be considered. In the ED environment, the same principles are operant; if a single medication will suffice, this should be tried before a combination, especially for drugs commonly associated with ADEs.

Third, each new prescription should take into account the entire medication list for possible interactions and to formulate the most simple overall administration schedule possible. No prescription should be added in isolation. In the ED, it is wise to document that the patient's current medications were reviewed as part of the medical decision making involved with the case.

Fourth, communicating with the patient regarding treatment goals may allow for further simplification of regimens. That is to say, as life expectancy decreases, the goals of a medication regimen may shift to treating symptoms, not disease prevention. Many of these issues will be at the forefront of the primary physician's (or geriatrician's) mind. Therefore, if any changes to the regimen are contemplated in the ED, communication with the primary team is crucial. Occasionally, additional resources, such as the involvement of a social worker or case worker, may be required to ensure that a *necessarily* complex medication regimen is adhered to.

Lastly, remember to keep polypharmacy issues, new medications, and side effects in the differential diagnosis when an elderly patient presents with any complaint. Even when it is important to address other critical diagnoses first, the role of medications should be considered.

SUGGESTED READINGS

Birnbaumer D. The elder patient. In: Marx JA, Hockberger RS, Walls RM, eds. *Rosen's Emergency Medicine: Concepts and Clinical Practice*. 6th ed. St. Louis, MO: Mosby; 2006.

Field TS, Gurwitz JH, Avorn J, et al. Risk factors for adverse drug events among nursing home residents. *Arch Int Med*. 2001;161(13):1629–1634.

Gurwitz JH. Polypharmacy: A new paradigm for quality drug therapy in the elderly? *Arch Intern Med*. 2004;164(18):1957–1959.

Hanlon JT, Schmader KE, Koronkowski MJ, et al. Adverse drug events in high risk older outpatients. *J Am Geriatr Soc*. 1997;45(8):945–948.

Kaufman DW, Kelly JP, Rosenberg L, et al. Recent patterns of medication use in the ambulatory adult population of the United States: The Slone survey. *JAMA*. 2002;287(3):337–344.

Kroenke K. Polypharmacy: Causes, consequences, and cure. *Am J Med*. 1985;79(2):149–152.

120

TREAT ACTIVELY BLEEDING ITP PATIENTS WITH PLATELETS, IVIG AND STEROIDS

ANGELA P. CORNELIUS, MD AND KIMBERLY A. B. LEESON, MD

Idiopathic thrombocytopenia purpura (ITP) is an uncommon disorder that can contribute to significant bleeding problems in the emergency department (ED). ITP is an autoimmune disorder caused by antiplatelet antibodies. These antibody-coated platelets are destroyed, leading to platelet counts below 150,000. ITP has both acute and chronic forms, and the precise underlying mechanism is unknown.

The chronic form predominates in adults and the incidence is 58 to 66 cases per million. This disease typically strikes women of childbearing age. The symptoms range from mild bruising to acute severe hemorrhage. In adults, the onset is insidious and the diagnosis often made incidentally.

Acute-onset ITP occurs mainly in children, following an immunization or viral syndrome. The incidence is 4 to 5.3 per 100,000. In 80% to 85% of children, this condition resolves without treatment within 6 months. Acute ITP is often heralded by the appearance of purpura and bruising over 24 to 48 h. Fifteen to twenty percent of symptomatic children will develop chronic ITP.

ITP is a diagnosis of exclusion made by looking at the history, physical exam, complete blood count (CBC), and peripheral blood smear. The differential diagnosis includes pseudothrombocytopenia, leukemias, inherited thrombocytopenias, myelodysplasia, liver disorders, trauma, and alcoholism. Additional testing should be undertaken to rule out other causes. Thrombocytopenia should be confirmed by a citrate test to rule out pseudothrombocytopenia from ethylenediaminetetraacetic acid (EDTA) medium. The blood smear should be examined for signs of other causes of thrombocytopenia. If the above tests do not show atypical features or are not suggestive of an alternative diagnosis then no further testing is needed. If the peripheral smear shows atypical features then bone marrow exam is often warranted.

While the exact mechanism underlying ITP may be unclear, the emergency management of ITP is not. The emergency physician must act to stop or limit active bleeding from the GI or GU tract into the CNS or onto the bed of any patient with ITP. Always send a type and screen on these patients immediately. Administer high-dose platelet transfusions coupled with high-dose steroids and intravenous immunoglobulin (IVIG) in critically ill patients, but steer clear of platelet administration in the absence of active hemorrhage. Steroids and IVIG have been shown to help decrease the platelet destruction seen in this disorder. When treating a patient with known ITP in the ED, always inquire about their personal treatment regimen and contact their hematologist early in the evaluation process. If he or she is on steroids or has had a splenectomy, thoroughly explore for sources of opportunistic infection. Chemotherapy is also commonly used for those resistant to standard treatment, so do not neglect the effects, both therapeutic and deleterious, of these powerful medications.

Long-term treatment has been addressed by many organizations, including the American Society of Hematology (ASH) and the British Journal of Haematology (BJH). Much of the literature from both groups is based on anecdotal evidence and not clinical trials. These two guidelines differ greatly in their treatment recommendations. The ASH position bases treatment primarily on platelet levels with symptoms representing a secondary determinant. *Table 120.1* summarizes these ASH guidelines.

The BJH outlines a treatment regimen dictated by clinical situation and recommends treatment only when absolutely necessary. The BJH cites a 2001 review that showed that many treated patients died of infection than bleeding. The recommended "safe" levels of platelets are shown in *Table 120.2*. The BJH suggests a watch and wait policy for children with acute ITP. They cite

TABLE 120.1	AMERICAN SOCIETY OF HEMATOLOGY GUIDELINES		
	PLATELET LEVELS	**SYMPTOMS**	**TREATMENT**
Children	>30,000	Asymptomatic or minor purpura	None
	<20,000	Significant mucous membrane bleeding	IVIG or steroids
	<10,000	Minor purpura	IVIG or steroids
Adults	>50,000	Asymptomatic or mild purpura	None
	<50,000	Significant mucous membrane bleeding or bleeding risk factors	IVIG or steroids
	<20,000–30,000	Asymptomatic	IVIG or steroids

TABLE 120.2	SAFE PLATELET GUIDELINES FROM THE BRITISH SOCIETY OF HAEMATOLOGY	
PROCEDURE	RECOMMENDED SAFE PLATELET LEVELS
Dentistry	$>10 \times 109/L$
Extractions	$>30 \times 109/L$
Regional dental block	$>30 \times 109/L$
Minor surgery	$>50 \times 109/L$
Major surgery	$>80 \times 109/L$

numerous studies that show that >80% of children have no significant bleeding and will recover within 6 to 8 weeks without treatment. This source cautions the clinician about treating children solely based on their platelet level or cutaneous manifestations, as they frequently have no or mild symptoms, even with very low platelet counts. Reserve treatment for children with significant bleeding. Many children in the United States, when treated, are treated preferentially with IVIG rather than steroids due a better side-effect profile.

As an emergency physician, you should be prepared to treat any significant bleeding episode promptly with platelets, steroids, and IVIG but should be willing to withhold treatment if there are only mild cutaneous symptoms. Also be very aware of the opportunistic infections that can occur due to the immunosuppression caused by the treatments for this entity. Caution parents and children to avoid activities associated with a high risk of trauma. Return precautions for physician reevaluation after any trauma should be strongly recommended. Consider involving a hematologist early in the patient's ED course.

SUGGESTED READINGS

George JN, Woolf SH, Raskob GE, et al. Idiopathic thrombocytopenic purpura: A practice guideline developed by explicit methods for the American Society of Hematology. *Blood*. 1996;88:3–40.

Li X, Hou M. Management of adult idiopathic thrombocytopenic purpura. *Clin Adv Hematol Oncol*. 2008;13:237–254.

Provan D, Newlanda, Norfolk D, et al. Guidelines for the investigation and management of idiopathic thrombocytopenic purpura in adults, children and in pregnancy. *Br J Haematol*. 2003;120:574–596.

Shad, AT, Gonzalez CE, Sandler SG. Treatment of immune thrombocytopenic purpura in children: Current concepts. *Paediatr Drugs*. 2005;7:325–336.

121

RECOGNIZE THROMBOTIC THROMBOCYTOPENIC PURPURA AND DO NOT GIVE THE "KNEE-JERK" PLATELET TRANSFUSION

CRAIG A. MANGUM, MD AND DAVID STORY, MD

Thrombotic thrombocytopenic purpura (TTP) is a disease with devastating outcomes if not properly recognized and treated. The emergency physician must recognize this entity and avoid some potentially dangerous errors in its management. TTP consists of a pentad of symptoms which include (1) fever, (2) altered mental status or neurologic disturbances, (3) renal abnormalities, (4) thrombocytopenia, and (5) microangiopathic hemolytic anemia. Memorize those five criteria for your boards but do not forget, like all "classic" diagnostic criteria in medicine, all five of the classic symptoms will not be uniformly present upon presentation. Do not be fooled by this. In fact, in the clinical setting it may be more prudent to look for the triad of thrombocytopenia, schistocytosis, and an elevated lactate dehydrogenase (LDH) level. The symptoms and signs of end organ damage (renal and neurologic disturbances) are often late manifestations of the disease, so do not hold your breath.

Recent studies show that the pathophysiology centers on a deficiency of ADAMTS-13, a von Willebrand factor–cleaving protease, which allows for platelet aggregation and microvascular thrombosis. These thrombotic events are systemic and trigger the clinical symptoms seen, including platelet depletion, hemolytic anemia (via shearing factors on the erythrocytes), and tissue infarction. Both familial and acquired forms of this disease exist, although in the emergency department setting, the diagnostic dilemma will revolve around the acquired form, as patients with the familial form have carried the diagnosis since childhood.

This disease is prevalent during pregnancy, specifically around the peripartum period. A common error of emergency medicine (EM) physicians is to mistake this disease entity for preeclampsia (HELLP) syndrome. Do not fall into this trap as the treatments are vastly different. With TTP platelet counts are lower, around the 20,000/mm³ range. With preeclampsia and hemolysis, elevated liver enzymes, low platelets (HELLP), platelets are typically below 100,000/mm³. If the degree of liver dysfunction is substantial, the coagulation profile (prothrombin time (PT), partial thromboplastin (PTT), international normalized ratio (INR)) may be affected in HELLP syndrome, but remains unaffected in TTP.

Avoid the error of responding to the thrombocytopenia of TTP with a knee-jerk platelet transfusion. Platelet transfusion has been shown to exacerbate the disease process by fanning the flame of platelet coagulation, resulting in aggravated end organ damage and a poorer patient outcome. Empiric platelet transfusion will undoubtedly please our lawyer friends, and might just allow the patient to live in your house, with your dog. However, only in the setting of life-threatening bleeding should platelets be transfused.

The current preferred treatment for TTP consists of plasma exchange. Survival rates reach 80% to 90% with plasma exchange. Given that plasma exchange is not available to most emergency departments; plasma infusion is a good alternative for you to remember. Cappo et al. showed that high-dose (25 to 30 mL/kg) plasma infusion is a useful alternative first-line therapy until plasma exchange can be arranged. High-dose glucocorticoid treatment may be beneficial in the chronic treatment of TTP by diminishing the production of antibodies against the metalloprotease, but there is no benefit in the acute setting.

In summary, TTP is a disorder characterized by systemic microvascular thrombosis that causes platelet depletion, hemolytic anemia, and end organ dysfunction. Platelet counts are severely affected, usually below $20,000/mm^3$. The disease process classically consists of fever, altered mental status, renal dysfunction, thrombocytopenia, and hemolytic anemia; however, for diagnostic purposes, the triad of low platelet count, schistocytes on peripheral blood smear, and an elevated LDH should raise the clinician's suspicion for TTP, and treatment should be instituted immediately. It may seem "intuitively obvious" to treat the thrombocytopenia with platelet transfusion, but it must be remembered that this could exacerbate the thrombosis in the vascular system and is only appropriate in the setting of life-threatening bleeding. The accepted treatment for TTP in the acute setting involves infusion of fresh frozen plasma, or better yet, emergent plasma exchange if available.

SUGGESTED READINGS

Bonnar J, Dunlop W. *Recent Advances in Obstetrics and Gynaecology*. London, UK: RSM Press; 2003.

Cappo P, Bussel A, Charrier S, et al. High-dose plasma infusion versus plasma exchange as early treatment of thrombotic thrombocytopenic purpura/hemolytic-uremic syndrome. *Medicine (Baltimore)*. 2003;82(1):27–38.

Furlan M, Robles R, Galbusera M, et al. von Willebrand factor-cleaving protease in thrombotic thrombocytopenic purpura and the hemolytic-uremic syndrome. *N Engl J Med*. 1998;339(22):1578–1584.

Harkness DR, Byrnes JJ, Lian EC, et al. Hazard of platelet transfusion in thrombotic thrombocytopenic purpura. *JAMA*. 1981;246(17):1931–1933.

Moake JL. Thrombotic microangiopathies. *N Engl J Med*. 2002;347:589–600.

Sadler JE. Von Willebrand factor, ADAMTS13, and thrombotic thrombocytopenic purpura. *Blood*. 2008;112(1):11–18.

Sadler JE, Moake JL, Miyata T, et al. Recent advances in thrombotic thrombocytopenic purpura. *Hematol Am Soc Hematol Educ Prog*. 2004:407–423.

Sibai BM. Imitators of severe preeclampsia. *Obstet Gynecol*. 2007;109(4):956–966.

122

BEWARE ACUTE CHEST SYNDROME IN THE PEDIATRIC PATIENT

ADAM D. FRIEDLANDER, MD

One of the scariest presentations in any emergency department is that of a pediatric patient with respiratory failure secondary to acute chest syndrome (ACS). Though the treatment of this critically ill patient is somewhat algorithmic at the outset, preventing progression to this stage is not always as clear, especially for those unfamiliar with the management and complications of sickle cell disease (SCD). Fortunately, the advent of modern therapies has lead to more patients surviving to adulthood. In fact, 50% survive beyond the fifth decade of life, and it is adult patients who are at a higher risk of death from ACS.

ACS is defined as a new infiltrate on chest x-ray accompanied by at least one of the following: chest pain, cough, abnormal lung sounds, tachypnea, or fever. ACS is the most common cause of hospitalization and death in patients with SCD. As in any vasoocclusive crisis of SCD, hydration and pain control are important, but there are other necessary adjuvant therapies, including incentive spirometry, antibiotics, bronchodilators, supplemental oxygen, and occasionally, blood transfusion, that will improve your ACS patient's morbidity and mortality.

Multiple studies support the importance of aggressive therapy in ACS, which often includes anticipating the development of ACS in any patient admitted for an SCD-related diagnosis. In one study of ACS patients, nearly half were admitted for diagnoses other than ACS, and 72% were admitted for vasoocclusive crises. Most importantly, of those not admitted with ACS, radiographic and clinical findings of ACS appeared a mean of 2.5 days after admission. It is because of this that all patients with SCD-related diagnoses at presentation must be treated as though they are in the prodrome stage of ACS. In patients who either present with or eventually develop ACS, those younger than 10 years most commonly present with chief complaints of wheezing, cough, and fever, while older patients most commonly present with pain in the arms and legs and dyspnea. If these patients hit your department, aggressive therapy to prevent progression to ACS is as important as the subcutaneous heparin and proton pump inhibitors (PPIs) that you are prescribing to your ever increasing population of patients "boarding" in the emergency department.

Any patient with an SCD-related diagnosis in your emergency department requires incentive spirometry and frequent monitoring for pulmonary disease. If the diagnosis of ACS is confirmed, then incentive spirometry must be continued, supplemental oxygen added as needed, and bronchodilators and antibiotics initiated. First-line antibiotics should be broad spectrum, including a third-generation cephalosporin to cover *Streptococcus pneumoniae, Haemophilus influenzae*, and *Klebsiella pneumoniae* and a macrolide to cover *Mycoplasma pneumoniae* and *Chlamydia pneumoniae*. The most common pathogens isolated in ACS are *C. pneumoniae, M. pneumoniae*, and respiratory syncytial virus (RSV). In addition, bronchodilator therapy should be added even in patients without evidence or history of pulmonary pathology aside from ACS. ACS alone should make you assume that airway hyperreactivity is present. Roughly, one in five of these patients will have an improvement in their respiratory status with bronchodilators.

The next key to ACS treatment is transfusion, which improves oxygenation in patients with ACS. Both simple and exchange transfusion achieved similar results with regard to oxygenation, but knowing how and when to transfuse is just as important as knowing that it is the key to treating ACS. How, then, do you make your decision? In certain cases of very mild disease and in the absence of hypoxia and respiratory symptoms, transfusion may be deferred. However, routine, early transfusion is crucial for all ACS patients at high risk for the development of severe complications, especially adults with cardiac disease and severe limb pain at presentation. Also, patients with severe anemia, thrombocytopenia, and/or multilobar infiltrates should receive simple transfusion before respiratory distress inevitably develops.

To answer the question of when to use simple versus exchange transfusion, simple transfusion is appropriate in patients with relatively mild episodes of ACS in the setting of a relatively severe anemia. Exchange transfusion is best reserved for patients whose condition is rapidly worsening or who have only a mild anemia compared to their baseline. The rationale is that simple transfusion in SCD patients in the setting of mild anemia will increase their risk of stroke and worsened vasoocclusive disease as raising the hematocrit raises blood viscosity. This is another reason that in certain settings of mild disease, mild anemia, and no respiratory symptoms or hypoxia, transfusion should be deferred, not only because it may not be necessary, but because the risks of transfusion, particularly simple transfusion in the setting of mild anemia, outweigh the benefits.

A final pearl, which is often not mentioned in a discussion of SCD and ACS, is that there is increased risk for ACS in patients with asthma and that "early and effective" asthma therapy reduces morbidity and mortality from pulmonary complications of SCD in these patients. In other words, despite your best efforts at not becoming a primary care physician, you must discuss optimal asthma management with your SCD patients. If you are debating initiating or changing asthma therapy in one of your patients because of repeated exacerbations on his or her current regimen (or lack thereof), the decision should be a no-brainer if the patient has SCD.

SUGGESTED READINGS

Bernard AW, Yasin Z, Venkat A. Acute chest syndrome of sickle cell disease. *Hosp Physician.* 2007;44:15–23.

Knight-Madden JM, Forrester TS, Lewis NA, et al. Asthma in children with sickle cell disease and its association with acute chest syndrome. *Thorax.* 2005;60(3):206–210.

Platt OS. The acute chest syndrome of sickle cell disease. *N Engl J Med.* 2000;342: 1904–1907.

Platt OS, Brambilla DJ, Rosse WF, et al. Mortality in sickle cell disease—life expectancy and risk factors for early death. *N Engl J Med.* 1994;330:1639–1644.

Vichinsky EP, Neumayr LD, Earles AN, et al. The national acute chest syndrome study group. Causes and outcomes of the acute chest syndrome in sickle cell disease. *N Engl J Med.* 2000;342:1855–1865.

Wayne AS, Kevy SV, Nathan DG. Transfusion management of sickle cell disease. *Blood.* 1993;81:1109–1123.

123

TREAT TUMOR LYSIS SYNDROME AGGRESSIVELY

POOJA KHANDELWAL, MD

Tumor lysis syndrome (TLS) is defined as a spectrum of metabolic derangements seen after rapid lysis of tumor cells and release of cellular products into the bloodstream. The abnormalities seen are

1) Hyperuricemia
2) Hyperkalemia
3) Hyperphosphatemia
4) Hypocalcemia
5) Uremia
6) Acute renal failure and death

Most common errors in management of TLS are

1) Failure to recognize risk
2) Failure to hydrate adequately
3) Failure to distinguish between preventative and definitive treatment

TLS can occur spontaneously in certain tumor types with high cellular turnover rates but usually occurs 12 to 72 h after the initiation of cytoreductive therapy. It is therefore important to order screening labs which include serum potassium, phosphorus, calcium, uric acid, and lactate dehydrogenase (LDH)

TABLE 123.1	RISK FACTORS FOR DEVELOPING TLS
Type of Malignancy	Burkitt Lymphoma Lymphoblastic lymphoma Diffuse large cell lymphoma Acute lymphoblastic leukemia Solid tumors with high proliferative rates and rapid response to therapy
Tumor burden/extent of disease	Bulky disease (>10 cm) LDH >(2× Upper limit of normal) WBC (>25,000/μL)
Renal function	Preexisting renal failure Oliguria
Baseline uric acid	Serum/plasma uric acid >450 μmol/L (7.5 mg/dL)
Effective and rapid cytoreductive therapy	Disease specific, varies according to tumor type

in all patients with predisposing malignancies to rule out existing spontaneous TLS. In instances where initial labs are normal, the criteria mentioned in *Tables 123.1 to 123.3* should guide the physician in anticipating the likelihood of developing TLS.

Best management of TLS is prevention. Aggressive hydration is the mainstay of adequate prevention; however, a common error is the addition of potassium in the fluids. This can be potentially fatal and should be avoided under all circumstances. For pediatric patients, 200 mL/kg/d, if <10 kg, or 2 to 3 L/m²/d of intravenous quarter normal saline or 5% dextrose is the fluid of choice. For adults, the IV rate should be at twice the maintenance rate. Urine output should be maintained within a range of 4 to 6 mL/kg/h if <10 kg or 80 to 100 mL/m²/h. The specific gravity of urine should be <1.010. Typically, due to potential exacerbation of electrolyte abnormalities, the use of diuretics should be avoided. Recognition of causes of preexisting renal failure, which include tumor related urinary tract obstruction, hypercalcemia, and renal vasoconstriction associated with adenosine release from neoplastic cells, is important since these will need to be corrected prior to the initiation of chemotherapy.

A common practice in management of TLS is administration of sodium bicarbonate to alkalinize the urine, which helps in the excretion of uric acid. Alkalinization of urine is now not recommended for the management of TLS especially with concomitant use of allopurinol, as it can cause precipitation of the xanthine metabolites in the renal tubules, due to altered solubility, leading to obstructive uropathies.

TABLE 123.2	CAIRO-BISHOP CLASSIFICATION OF LABORATORY TLS

Uric acid >476 μmol/L or 8 mg/dL or 25% increase from baseline values

Potassium >6.0 mmol/L or 6 mg/L or 25% increase from baseline values

Phosphorus >2.1 mmol/L for children or >1.45 mmol/L for adults or 25% increase from baseline values

Calcium <1.75 mmol/L or 25% decrease from baseline values

Two or more changes within 3 days before or 7 days after cytotoxic therapy define TLS. Clinical TLS is defined as laboratory TLS + one or more of the following: increased serum creatinine (1.5 times >upper limit of normal), cardiac arrhythmias/sudden death, and seizures.

TABLE 123.3	EVALUATION OF PATIENT RISK FACTORS
Low risk	Clinical judgment and monitoring
Medium risk	Hydration plus initial management with allopurinol. If hyperuricemia develops, start rasburicase
High risk	Hydration plus initial management with rasburicase

Allopurinol is not recommended for the treatment of TLS in situations of elevated uric acid levels or established TLS. Allopurinol serves to prevent formation of uric acid and does not help in the clearance of the existing high uric acid levels. In such instances, Rasburicase is the drug of choice and is dosed at 0.1 to 0.2 mg/kg in 50 mL of normal saline IV over 30 min for 1 to 7 days. It is also the drug of choice in high-risk pediatric patients, as a part of prevention.

Always rule out glucose-6-phosphate deficiency prior to starting rasburicase, as it is a contraindication to starting the drug. In acute situations, involvement of a nephrologist to start dialysis should not be delayed. The decision to continue or hold chemotherapy while the patient has ongoing TLS needs to be determined by the oncologist and is a case-by-case decision.

SUGGESTED READINGS

Coiffier B, Altman A, Pui CH, et al. Guidelines for management of pediatric and adult tumor lysis syndrome: An evidence based review. *J Clin Oncol.* 2008;26(16):2767–2768.

Ho VQ, Wetzstein GA, Patterson SG, et al. Abbreviated rasburicase dosing for the prevention and treatment of hyperuricemia in adults at risk for tumor lysis syndrome. *Support Cancer Ther.* 2006;3(3):178–182.

124

SEARCH DILIGENTLY FOR THE SOURCE OF FEVER IN PATIENTS WITH NEUTROPENIA

JANSEN M. TIONGSON, MD

When evaluating and treating a patient with neutropenic fever (NF), investigate all possible sources of infection and analyze the current absolute neutrophil count. You do not have to admit every single patient with NF. You can save the patient and hospital time and money.

NF with an overall 15% to 30% mortality rate is defined by the 2002 Infectious Disease Society of America (IDSA) guidelines as a single oral temperature >38.3°C or a febrile state >38°C over at least 1 h and absolute neutrophilic count <500 or <1,000 with a predicted nadir of <500 in the ensuing 24 to 48 h. Although other causes such as drug-induced neutropenia can cause NF, nearly two thirds can be attributed to an infectious process, most notable are bacterial infections which constitute 85% to 90% of the infectious etiology.

When evaluating the patient with possible NF, a complete history and physical exam are warranted. You must ask the patient when the last chemotherapy treatment took place, what type of chemotherapeutic drug was used, and, if known, what the intensity of the regimen was. These associated treatments can potentially lead to NF even without a source of infection. Also, do not ignore that viral infections, blood transfusion products, and even the malignancy itself could be the source of fever. When performing the physical exam, it is important not to dismiss doing a perirectal exam as a history of hemorrhoids places the neutropenic patient, especially those with leukemia, at high risk. Be cautious, however, when performing a digital rectal exam as it could potentially make them bacteremic. Moreover, cancer patients may not show the classic signs of inflammation (erythema, pain, and swelling) as those with neutropenia often have impaired inflammatory responses. Cultures must be obtained from each port, lumen, peripheral vein line, and orifice of the patient. Despite obtaining pancultures, no microorganisms could be isolated in 49% of children and 38% of adults with NF. After obtaining the complete blood count (CBC) (with a differential), appropriate calculation of the absolute neutrophil count (ANC) should be undertaken and should be compared with previous counts, if available, to determine not only the chronicity of the neutropenia but also the severity of neutropenia which influences the final disposition. The longer duration of the neutropenia puts the patient at greater risk with nearly 100% of patients developing an infection within 7 days of ANC <500. The American Society of Clinical Oncology has stratified patients into risk groups based on calculated

ANC. An ANC of 1,000 to 1,500 puts the patient at slight risk, while 500 to 1,000 at moderate risk and <500 at severe risk. This stratification can ultimately affect whether a patient is discharged or admitted.

It is clinically accepted that patients with NF are treated empirically with broad-spectrum antibiotics, whether utilizing an aminoglycoside + antipseudomonal β-lactam ± vancomycin or monotherapy with ceftazidime or cefepime. Broad-spectrum coverage should be implemented in the patient with neutropenia if there is a single oral elevated temperature >38.5°C or 3 elevations >38 during a 24-h period. Remember that even if the patient has no fever upon presentation, the circadian variability of thermal regulation can alter the patient's actual temperature. Empirical fungal therapy should also be considered if a neutropenic patient remains febrile after 1 week of antibiotics or has recurrent fever.

Until recently, standard policy for all NF patients has warranted hospitalization for treatment with a mean duration of hospital stay of 6 to 7 days. However, recent publications are challenging the status quo. In a Cochrane database analysis in 2004, there was no statistical difference in the mortality rate between IV and oral antibiotics with an RR of 0.83. Treatment failure is also similar at RR of 0.94. As such, oral antibiotics may potentially be offered to a patient who is at low risk for mortality. Nijhuis et al. (2002) showed that 78% of fevers in inpatients and 77% in outpatients resolved without modification of the initial regimen, with a mortality rate of 2% and 4%, respectively. Appropriate risk stratification, using a current ANC, can help determine proper disposition. Moreover, the American Society of Clinical Oncology deems the following as high risks for NF, thus warranting admission: (a) inpatients with fever while developing neutropenia, (b) outpatients requiring acute hospital care for problems beyond neutropenia and fever, and (c) stable outpatients with uncontrolled cancer. Low-risk febrile NF patients can potentially receive oral fluoroquinolones after receiving one dose of IV monotherapy and discharged to home with appropriate follow-up.

Not every NF patient needs inpatient admission. Escalante et al. (2004) studied two outpatient antibiotic pathways utilizing oral ampicillin/clavulanate (500 mg) and ciprofloxacin (500 mg) or IV ceftazidime (2 g) and clindamycin (600 mg) every 8 h in order to estimate successful response to outpatient treatment in low-risk NF patients. After studying 257 febrile episodes in 191 patients, they report that 205 (80%) of febrile episodes successfully responded to outpatient treatment and only 52 (20%) needed hospitalization. Outpatient treatment in low-risk patients can be utilized as this study highlights the minimal associated morbidity and mortality. Treating them as outpatients not only saves a bed in already overcrowded inpatient hospitals but also saves patients' money that would be used for hospitalization and treatment as well as allows them to be in the comfort of their own homes for improvement.

As ED physicians, we have fear of sending these patients home, but do not be afraid. If you obtain all the proper information and evaluate them accordingly, you will know what to do. However, if you are considering outpatient treatment, consultation with the patient's oncologist and assurance of very close follow-up are critical.

Ultimately, take the fever in a cancer patient very seriously. Use the skills you learned in medical school and perform a thorough physical examination. Order as many tests and cultures as you need to find the source so you or their oncologist can adjust their treatments accordingly. Do not forget to calculate the ANC. After all, they do not call it neutropenic for nothing. Remember that not every cancer patient needs to be admitted. A lot of them will appreciate you taking the time and effort to see if they are eligible to be treated as outpatients.

SUGGESTED READINGS

American Society of Clinical Oncology. Update of recommendations for the use of hematopoietic colony-stimulating factors: Evidence-based clinical practice guidelines. *J Clin Oncol*. 1996;14(6):1957–1960.

Escalante CP, Weiser MA, Manzullo E, et al. Outcomes of treatment pathways in outpatient treatment of low risk febrile neutropenic cancer patients. *Support Care Cancer*. 2004;12(9):657–662.

Oude Nijhuis CS, Daenen SM, Vellenga E, et al. Fever and neutropenia in cancer patients: The diagnostic role of cytokines in risk assessment strategies. *Crit Rev Oncol Hematol*. 2002;44(2):163–174.

Perrone J, Hollander JE, Datner EM. Emergency department evaluation of patient with fever and chemotherapy-induced neutropenia. *J Emerg Med*. 2004;27(2):115–119.

Pizzo PA. Management of fever in patients with cancer and treatment-induced neutropenia. *N Engl J Med*. 1993;328(18):1323–1332.

Pizzo PA, Robichaud KJ, Wesley R, et al. Fever in the pediatric and young adult patient with cancer: A prospective study of 1001 episodes. *Medicine*. 1982;61(3):153–165.

Tamura K. Clinical guidelines for the management of neutropenic patients with unexplained fever in Japan: Validation by the Japan Febrile Neutropenia Study Group. *Int J Antimicrob Agents*. 2005;26(Suppl 2):S123–S127.

Vidal L, Paul M, Ben dor I, et al. Oral versus intravenous antibiotic treatment for febrile neutropenia in cancer patients: A systematic review and meta-analysis of randomized trials. *J Antimicrob Chemother*. 2004;54(1):29–37.

125

ADMINISTER ANTIBIOTICS EARLY TO NEUTROPENIC PATIENTS WITH A FEVER

STEPHEN YUAN-TUNG LIANG, MD

Neutropenia remains a common complication of chemotherapy, radiation, and primary hematologic malignancy. With increasing duration and severity of neutropenia comes a greater risk of serious infection and bacteremia. Considered an oncologic emergency, neutropenic fever is defined as an absolute neutrophil count of <500 or <1,000 cells/mm³ with an anticipated decline below 500 cells/mm³ over the next 48 h in the presence of a single temperature of ≥38.3°C (101°F) or a persistent temperature of ≥38.0°C (100.4°F) for more than 1 h. Almost half of all patients presenting to the emergency department with neutropenic fever have an infection, established or occult. Therefore, we must assume that every patient with neutropenic fever has an acute and potentially life-threatening infection until proven otherwise.

Empiric antibiotic therapy in neutropenic fever (*Table 125.1*) has dramatically reduced the mortality of this disease over the past half century. Prompt

TABLE 125.1	EMPIRIC ANTIBIOTIC THERAPY FOR FEBRILE NEUTROPENIA

Monotherapy:

- Cefepime
- Ceftazidime
- Imipenem
- Meropenem
- Piperacillin-tazobactam

Two-drug therapy: Monotherapy agent + aminoglycoside

- Gentamicin
- Tobramycin
- Amikacin

Adjunct therapy:

- Vancomycin

broad-spectrum intravenous antibiotic therapy takes precedence over any further diagnostic evaluation of the patient with documented neutropenic fever once blood culture specimens have been obtained. While no specific time frame exists in the literature for antibiotic administration, I recommend treating neutropenic fever as early as possible, with some institutions striving for a door-to-antibiotic time of 30 min or less. All patients presenting to the emergency department with neutropenic fever should be admitted for intravenous antibiotics and further observation. Given the high risk of occult infection with neutropenia, the same treatment philosophy should apply even to afebrile patients, especially those presenting with respiratory complaints, abdominal pain, mental status change, or other signs or symptoms of infection.

In the last 20 years, the spectrum of infectious organisms in neutropenic fever has shifted from Gram-negative bacilli (*Pseudomonas aeruginosa*, *Escherichia coli*, and *Klebsiella* species) toward Gram-positive organisms (*Staphylococcus aureus*, *S. epidermis*, and *Streptococcus* species). Whenever possible, antibiotic therapy should be based upon local and institutional microbial epidemiology and patterns of drug resistance. Guidelines established by the Infectious Diseases Society of America in 2002 currently recommend either empiric monotherapy with a broad-spectrum intravenous antipseudomonal cephalosporin (cefepime or ceftazidime) or carbapenem (imipenem or meropenem). The antipseudomonal β-lactam, piperacillin-tazobactam, has also become a widely accepted monotherapy for neutropenic fever since the publication of these guidelines. Addition of an aminoglycoside (gentamicin, tobramycin, or amikacin) should be considered in the critically ill and septic patient where *P. aeruginosa* or resistant Gram-negative bacteria are suspected. Vancomycin, a glycopeptide antibiotic, should be added in clinically apparent catheter-related infection, skin and soft tissue infection, severe mucositis, documented Gram-positive bacteremia, known colonization with methicillin-resistant *S. aureus*, or hemodynamic instability. In order to prevent further antibiotic resistance, the empiric use of vancomycin is otherwise not recommended. When a vancomycin-resistant Gram-positive infection is feared, the use of linezolid, daptomycin, and quinupristin-dalfopristin should be considered in consultation with an infectious disease specialist, as guidelines for the use of these agents in neutropenic fever do not yet exist.

Empiric therapy with antiviral drugs (acyclovir, valacyclovir, or famciclovir) is indicated in febrile neutropenic patients with cutaneous or mucous membrane lesions consistent with herpes simplex or varicella-zoster virus infection, as these lesions frequently serve as portals for bacterial and fungal infection. Likewise, antifungal therapy (fluconazole) is warranted in cases of oral and esophageal candidiasis. Fungal sinusitis concerning for mucormycosis should prompt immediate treatment with intravenous amphotericin B. In the absence of obvious signs of viral or fungal disease, the emergency physician should not worry about empiric coverage of these opportunistic infections in the emergency department.

As care of the cancer patient shifts increasingly toward the ambulatory setting, emergency physicians will play a vital role in the management of neutropenic fever. Early recognition, appropriate microbiological evaluation including prompt blood culture sampling, and timely empiric antibiotic therapy are crucial to taming a disease with a historically high rate of morbidity and mortality.

SUGGESTED READINGS

Bodey GP, Buckley M, Sathe YS, et al. Quantitative relationships between circulating leukocytes and infection in patients with acute leukemia. *Ann Intern Med*. 1966;64:328–340.

Hughes WT, Armstrong D, Bodey GP, et al. 2002 Guidelines for the use of antimicrobial agents in neutropenic patients with cancer. *Clin Infect Dis*. 2002;34:730–751.

Perrone J, Hollander JE, Datner EM. Emergency department evaluation of patients with fever and chemotherapy-induced neutropenia. *J Emer Med*. 2004;27:115–119.

Viscoli C, Varnier O, Machetti M. Infections in patients with febrile neutropenia: Epidemiology, microbiology, and risk stratification. *Clin Infect Dis*. 2005;40:S240–S245.

126

DO NOT UNDERDOSE FACTOR REPLACEMENT IN PATIENTS WITH HEMOPHILIA EMERGENCIES

CRAIG A. MANGUM, MD

Hemophilia is a coagulation disorder that is relatively rare. However, it is common enough that you, as an emergency physician, need to know what to do when it walks through your doors on a busy night. Errors made by emergency physicians in managing this disease are potentially devastating and can be easily avoided by remembering a few things.

Classic hemophilia, or hemophilia A, is a deficiency of factor VIII, whereas hemophilia B is a lack of factor IX. These patients will present to the emergency department with a wide array of complications. Hemophilia can be broken down into mild, moderate, and severe forms of the disease depending on the amount of factor present in the patient's plasma. The patient or patient's family may have this information. Factor levels <1% are considered severe hemophilia, whereas those with mild disease have 5% to 25% plasma factor levels. However, in the absence of this information, you must assume the worst; treat your patient aggressively, as if he has severe hemophilia.

Just like the disease itself, the types of bleeds experienced by hemophiliacs can be broken down into mild, moderate, and severe. Early hematomas, light mucosal bleeding, and early hemarthrosis are considered *mild*. Expanding hematomas, persistent hemarthrosis, and epistaxis can be categorized as *moderate* bleeds. Intra-abdominal, intracranial, oropharyngeal/airway, and other life-threatening bleeding are considered *severe*, as you might imagine. Do not make the mistake, however, of underestimating the mechanism of injury. Most injuries, especially any head trauma however seemingly trivial, should be considered to have the potential to result in a severe bleed and be treated as such.

Spontaneous bleeding has been reported in all forms of hemophilia but is obviously more common in those with the severe form. Trauma is of particular concern in this patient population as it usually heralds a bleed. Pay close attention to the hemophiliac presenting after even a seemingly minor trauma, as well as his twin who just arrived after a major motor vehicle crash, as both types of mechanisms have been shown to cause clinically significant hemorrhage.

Not always are the bleeds immediately evident and can be delayed. In fact, traumatic intra-abdominal bleeding has been reported 4 weeks after initial injury. Do not make the error of "brushing off" the injury that occurred a week or two ago.

Recombinant factor is the mainstay of therapy. The dosing for recombinant factor can seem tricky but is actually quite easy to remember. Whether administering human or recombinant factor, the dose doubles with increasing severity of the bleed. The dose should match the severity of the bleed. While administering too much factor for minor injuries is simply a waste of money and product, the opposite mistake is potentially lethal. The guidelines for factor replacement are summarized in *Table 126.1*.

If the appropriate factor preparation is not available, DDAVP or desmopressin can be given. Desmopressin is convenient in that it can be administered with good efficacy by way of IV, subcutaneously, or via intranasal spray. Activated factor VII has also shown some promise in treating acute bleeds in the hemophiliac patient.

TABLE 126.1	**GUIDELINES FOR FACTOR REPLACEMENT**	
TYPE OF HEMORRHAGE	**RECOMBINANT FACTOR VIII DOSE (U/KG)**	**RECOMBINANT FACTOR IX DOSE (U/KG)**
Minor	10–20 (12.5)	20–30 (25)
Moderate	15–30 (25)	25–50 (50)
Severe	30–50 (50)	50–100 (100)

In summary, remember that the hemophiliac patient deserves your undivided attention, no matter how minor the trauma or pain at first glance may appear. Forgetting that distant trauma may be the reason for the patient's complaint is a potentially serious mistake. Attempt to categorize the type of bleed and dose the factor accordingly, but when in doubt, assume the worst and replace to 100% clotting activity (50 U/kg of factor VIII or 100 U/kg of factor IX). Inadequate dosing of factor just costs money and doesn't get the job done! DDAVP and factor VII are also of benefit when needed.

SUGGESTED READINGS

Mannucci PM, Ruggeri ZM, Pareti FI, et al. 1-Deamino-8-d-arginine vasopressin: A new pharmacological approach to the management of haemophilia and von Willebrands' diseases. *Lancet*. 1977;1(8017):869–872.

Revel-Vilk S, Blanchette VS, Sparling C, et al. DDAVP challenge tests in boys with mild/moderate haemophilia A. *Br J Haematol*. 2002;117(4):947–951.

Roberts HR, Monroe DM, White GC. The use of recombinant factor VIIa in the treatment of bleeding disorders. *Blood*. 2004;104(13):3858–3964.

Samaiya A, Gupta S, Chumber S, et al. Blunt abdominal trauma with delayed rupture of splenic hematoma in a hemophiliac patient. *Hemophilia*. 2001;7(3):331–334.

127

DO NOT OVERTEST OR UNDERTREAT PATIENTS WITH VASOOCCLUSIVE PAIN CRISES SECONDARY TO SICKLE CELL ANEMIA

ROBERT J. SOBEHART, MD

The diagnosis of sickle cell vasoocclusive pain crises is rarely a dilemma; however, treating these events can present a significant challenge to the emergency physician. Sickle cell patients are an immunocompromised, chronically ill group who suffer from acute painful crises and struggle with chronic pain issues. Despite their susceptibility to infections and other severe disease, pain crises account for about 90% of hospital admissions. Physicians employ myriad diagnostic and treatment modalities to manage these vasoocclusive episodes with varying degrees of success. Rapid and adequate pain control in the emergency department (ED) is the goal of both the patient and physician, so let us take a look at the evidence regarding the proper diagnostic workup and expert treatment of vasoocclusive pain episodes.

The most commonly performed tests on patients with sickle cell pain crises include a complete blood count (CBC), reticulocyte count, and a search for occult infection. Chest and abdominal painful crises are excluded from this discussion because they provide a significantly greater diagnostic dilemma than simple extremity pain crises. Pollack et al. (1991) studied the use of screening chest x-ray and urinalysis in sickle cell pain crises without fever. Occult infection was found in 10% of patients using this strategy. In 2006, Bernard et al. (2006) reviewed the utility of routine CBC and reticulocyte counts in a meta-analysis of small studies. They found no evidence to support their routine use. Screening chest x-ray and urinalysis should be performed in all patients with simple vasoocclusive pain crises to detect occult infection, while other tests should be reserved for the more complicated presentations of sickle cell disease.

Oxygen and intravenous (IV) fluids are also classically thought of as important interventions in vasoocclusive sickle cell pain crises. This strategy is not validated in the literature. There are no studies that specifically compare providing supplemental oxygen versus placebo. Hydration is used similarly but has not been studied. Steinberg presented guidelines for management of acute pain crises in 1999 but did not mention oxygen in the algorithm and suggested fluid replacement by either oral or IV is adequate. In the absence of compelling evidence, it seems unnecessary to hydrate the well hydrated or oxygenate the already well oxygenated. You should focus on early, ample, and appropriate analgesia first and reserve oxygen and hydration for the hypoxic and volume-depleted patient!

Sickle cell patients have chronic pain with superimposed acute vasoocclusive pain crises. They are usually instructed on the outpatient treatment of their pain crises and only come to the ED after failure of outpatient management. They are often thought of as "drug seekers" due to narcotic tolerance. Only a minority of sickle cell patients fit this description, and while it adds to the complexity of their care, it should not deter us from treating their pain with narcotics early and often!

No single study has comprehensively evaluated pain management strategies for vasoocclusive pain crises. In a 2008 Cochrane review, Dunlap and Bennett (2006) tried to compile the limited available data. Opioid analgesics are safe and effective if used in the correct dosing—beginning at 0.1 mg/kg of morphine or morphine equivalent and titrating to effect. One small study found ketorolac to be equivalent to meperidine, but it was found to be synergistic in other studies. Prednisone has even been studied with some benefit, but limited data exist on its long-term side effects and efficacy. There are benefits to patient-controlled analgesia (PCA) pumps beginning early in the ED, which include decreased total amount of opioid, decreased perceived pain by patients, and trends toward decreased length of stay. The combination of nonsteroidal anti-inflammatories and narcotics treat vasoocclusive pain very well, so use them early and often!

So, what is the bottom line for treating sickle cell vasoocclusive pain episodes? Screen for infection with a urinalysis and chest x-ray, and reserve other testing for the more complicated crises. The vast majority of these patients are not "drug seekers" and have a legitimate reason for pain.

Fluids and oxygen may make YOU feel good, but they do not make the patient feel good, so treat the pain up front with a combination of opioid analgesics and nonsteroidal anti-inflammatory medications! Use the correct dosing of opioids (at least 0.1 mg/kg of morphine or its equivalent—even in kids!). Evaluate their pain within 20 min of the first dose and have rescue analgesia ready if necessary. If they only respond minimally to two or three doses of adequate analgesia, they will need to be admitted. Do not be afraid to initiate PCA in the ED.

SUGGESTED READINGS

Bernard AW, Venkat A, Lyons MS. Best evidence topic report: Full blood count and reticulo-cyte count in painful sickle cell crisis. *Emerg Med J.* 2006;23(4):302–303.

Dunlap RJ, Bennett KC. Pain management for sickle cell disease. *Cochrane Database Syst Rev.* 2006;19(2):CD003350.

Melzer-Lange MD, Walsh-Kelly CM, Lea G, et al. Patient-controlled analgesia for sickle cell pain crisis in a pediatric emergency department. *Pediatr Emerg Care.* 2004;20(1):2–4.

Okomo U, Meremikwu MM. Fluid replacement therapy for acute episodes of pain in people with sickle cell disease. *Cochrane Database Syst Rev.* 2007;18(2):CD005406.

Pollack CV. Emergencies in sickle cell disease. *Emerg Med Clin North Am.* 1993;11(2):365–378.

Pollack CV Jr, Jorden RC, Kolb JC. Usefulness of empiric chest radiography and uri-nalysis testing in adults with acute sickle cell pain crisis. *Ann Emerg Med.* 1991;20(11):1210–1214.

Stienberg MH. Management of sickle cell disease. *N Engl J Med.* 1999;340(13):1021–1030.

van Beers EJ, van Tuijn CF, Nieuwkerk PT, et al. Patient-controlled analgesia versus continu-ous infusion of morphine during vaso-occlusive crises in sickle cell disease, a randomized controlled trial. *Am J Hematol.* 2007;82(11):955–960.

128

RULE OUT MALIGNANT SPINAL CORD COMPRESSION IN ALL CANCER PATIENTS PRESENTING WITH BACK PAIN

MICHAEL MCLAUGHLIN, MD

Malignant spinal cord compression (MSCC) from spinal epidural metasta-ses (SEM) is a devastating complication of cancer. It can lead to significant impairment of neurologic function, and thus, can severely degrade quality of life. Despite advanced imaging techniques and treatment options, studies indicate that more than half of patients are not diagnosed until unable to walk independently. By recognizing at-risk patients, imaging appropriately, initiating early treatment, and involving the appropriate consultants, you can minimize neurologic deterioration in patients with this disease.

Approximately 5% of patients who die from cancer experience MSCC. Any malignancy can cause MSCC, but the majority of cases are from breast, prostate, and lung cancers, each of which accounts for 15% to 20% of cases. Other common culprits are non-Hodgkin lymphoma, multiple myeloma, and kidney cancer. MSCC occurs in children as well with nearly the same frequency as adults although, the cancers responsible differ between the two age groups. The majority of cases of MSCC occur in patients with known malignancy. However, 20% of cases present as the initial manifestation of malignancy, making the diagnosis more challenging. For the emergency physician, any patient with cancer presenting with back pain must be assumed to have SEM until proven otherwise.

Ninety percent of patients with MSCC complain of back pain. Approximately 60% of SEM are found in the thoracic spine, 30% in the lumbosacral spine, and 10% in the cervical spine. Unfortunately, back pain alone cannot differentiate between patients with MSCC and without MSCC. One study did identify several independent risk factors for MSCC: inability to walk, increased deep tendon reflexes, compression fractures on spine radiographs, bone metastases present, bone metastases diagnosed more than 1 year before, and age <60. Patients with none of these risk factors had a 4% risk of MSCC compared to 87% for those patients with five risk factors.

A thorough neurologic exam must be performed and documented. The degree of neurologic impairment before treatment is by far the best predictor of posttreatment function. Weakness is present in 60% to 85% of patients. Sensory deficits may be present; however, sensory levels do not accurately predict the level of spinal cord involvement. Bowel and bladder disturbances (typically overflow urinary incontinence) are present in about half of patients at the time of diagnosis but are unlikely to occur without weakness in MSCC. A postvoid residual urine volume >100 mL is diagnostic of urinary retention.

If MSCC is a concern, MRI must be performed emergently. MRI is the test of choice. CT myelography is done in patients with contraindications to MRI. Studies have shown that plain radiographs and clinical examination alone are not adequate in identifying SEM in patients with malignancy. MRI altered treatment decisions in 53% of patients compared to plain radiographs and examination alone. Back pain alone should prompt MRI investigation in these patients with known cancer. Even without symptoms of radiculopathy or myelopathy, the risk of SEM in cancer patients with back pain is 30%. Multiple SEM are identified in 25% to 39% of patients with MSCC when the entire spine is imaged. Therefore, the MRI should be performed on the entire spine, not just the symptomatic area.

Corticosteroids have been shown to improve ambulation outcomes in patients with MSCC compared to placebo. The role of corticosteroids in patients without neurologic deficits is less clear. Dexamethasone has been studied most extensively in MSCC. The exact dosing remains a controversy. Higher doses are associated with more side effects and no definite improvement in functional outcomes. Exact dosing would have to be confirmed amongst the treatment team, but a proposed regimen is 10 mg (by any route) as a bolus followed by 4 mg four times daily.

Definitive treatment of MSCC involves either radiation therapy or surgery, or perhaps both. The exact indication for each is beyond the scope of the emergency physician. It is recommended that all patients with MSCC have consultations with a spine surgeon, radiation oncologist, and medical oncologist. All will require admission. If these specialties are unavailable, the patient will require emergent transfer to a facility with these capabilities.

In summary, MSCC is a devastating complication of malignancy. Delays in diagnosis are common. It involves the thoracic spine roughly 60% of the time. Prostate, breast, and lung cancers are most frequently associated. Any cancer patient presenting with back pain or neurologic deficit requires emergent evaluation with MRI or CT myelography if MRI is contraindicated. This should be done immediately in the ED, not after admission to the hospital or as an outpatient. The entire spine should be imaged. If MSCC is confirmed, begin dexamethasone and arrange admission and consultation with spine surgery, radiation oncology, and medical oncology.

SUGGESTED READINGS

Cook AM, Lau TN, Tomlinson MJ, et al. Magnetic resonance imaging of the whole spine in suspected malignant spinal cord compression: Impact on management. *Clin Oncol (R Coll Radiol)*. 1998;10(1):39–43.

Husband DJ, Grant KA, Romaniuk CS. MRI in the diagnosis and treatment of suspected malignant spinal cord compression. *Br J Radiol*. 2001;74(877):15–23.

Kienstra GE, Terwee CB, Dekker FW, et al. Prediction of spinal epidural metastases. *Arch Neurol*. 2000;57(5):690–695.

Levack P, Graham J, Collie D, et al. Don't wait for a sensory level–listen to the symptoms: A prospective audit of the delays in diagnosis of malignant cord compression. *Clin Oncol (R Coll Radiol)*. 2002;14(6):472–480.

Loblaw DA, Perry J, Chambers A, et al. Systematic review of the diagnosis and management of malignant extradural spinal cord compression: The Cancer Care Ontario Practice Guidelines Initiative's Neuro-Oncology Disease Site Group. *J Clin Oncol*. 2005;23(9):2028–2037.

Maranzano E, Latini P, Beneventi S, et al. Radiotherapy without steroids in selected metastatic spinal cord compression patients: A phase II trial. *Am J Clin Oncol*. 1996;19:179–183.

Prasad D, Schiff D. Malignant spinal-cord compression. *Lancet Oncol*. 2005;6(1):15–24.

Schiff D. Spinal cord compression. *Neurol Clin*. 2003;21(1):67–86, viii [Review].

Schiff D, O'Neill BP, Suman VJ. Spinal epidural metastasis as the initial manifestation of malignancy: Clinical features and diagnostic approach. *Neurology*. 1997;49(2):452–456.

Talcott JA, Stomper PC, Drislane FW, et al. Assessing suspected spinal cord compression: A multidisciplinary outcomes analysis of 342 episodes. *Support Care Cancer*. 1999;7(1): 31–38.

129

CONSIDER COMMUNITY-ACQUIRED METHICILLIN-RESISTANT *STAPHYLOCOCCUS AUREUS* WHEN TREATING SKIN AND SOFT TISSUE INFECTIONS

MICHAEL P. MALLIN, MD

The rise of community-acquired methicillin-resistant *Staphylococcus aureus* (CA-MRSA) has drastically changed the treatment of patients with acute skin and soft tissue infections (SSTIs) presenting to the emergency department. CA-MRSA has risen as a cause of SSTI from 29% in 2001 to 64% in 2004. A single strain of MRSA called USA 300 is responsible for up to 97% of these SSTIs. USA 300 harbors a virulence not seen in hospital-acquired MRSA. Luckily, however, USA 300 and other strains of CA-MRSA, although virulent, are still fairly susceptible to common, cheap antibiotics. The emerging resistance to these antibiotics, however, is complicated and actively changing.

The treatment of choice for CA-MRSA abscesses is blatantly clear. Incision and drainage (I&D) is the primary intervention for all abscesses regardless of the bug suspected. Unfortunately, the common medical belief that I&D is a definitive treatment for SSTI was rooted in a time before CA-MRSA. Currently, there exists no conclusive research that CA-MRSA abscesses can be managed with I&D treatment alone. CA-MRSA is a more virulent bacterium than Staph and Strep and thus prior research regarding I&D treatment alone may not be applicable to this new bug. Nevertheless, several recent articles have suggested that I&D treatment alone applies to CA-MRSA also. For example, to make his argument for I&D alone, Greg Moran references, in his landmark CA-MRSA paper, an article by Fridkin in 2005. This paper indeed found no significant change in treatment outcomes for addition of antibiotic coverage to I&D therapy. However, the same paper found that I&D was not a significant predictor of treatment failure in the same population. Other research indicates that patients with suspected MRSA abscesses should also be started on antibiotics with CA-MRSA coverage. Ruhe et al. (2007) recently demonstrated antibiotic coverage to be the only independent predictor for determining treatment failure in a 492-subject study comparing different treatments for SSTI. In their group treated with I&D alone, they noted a 13% treatment failure. For this reason, suspected CA-MRSA abscesses should receive empiric antibiotic coverage, especially if the patient is immunocompromised, diabetic, has systemic symptoms, or has surrounding cellulitis.

While it is clear that CA-MRSA has taken over as the predominate bacteria causing abscesses, data are less clear regarding the organism involved in basic cellulitis. Strep has traditionally been indicated as the predominate strain; however, recent data suggest that CA-MRSA may be the culprit in up to 50% of basic cellulitis infections. For this reason and due to the high virulence of USA 300, basic cellulitis presenting to the emergency department should receive treatment for typical Gram-positives and CA-MRSA. The days of Ancef and probenecid are effectively over.

Outpatient antibiotic regimens for covering CA-MRSA cellulitis and cutaneous abscesses are complicated and changing readily (*Fig. 129.1*). The most commonly prescribed antibiotics for oral CA-MRSA coverage include TMP-SMX, clindamycin, tetracyclines, and linezolid. Of these oral antibiotics, TMP-SMX is the most attractive due to its near 100% susceptibility rate. It is important to note, however, that treatment for CA-MRSA is dose specific and should be treated with TMP-SMX DS 2 tabs twice per day. Clindamycin was a good choice early in the emergence of CA-MRSA. However, inducible resistance has continued to emerge and currently 49% to 76% of CA-MRSA strains carry the ability to methylate the binding site for clindamycin, known as

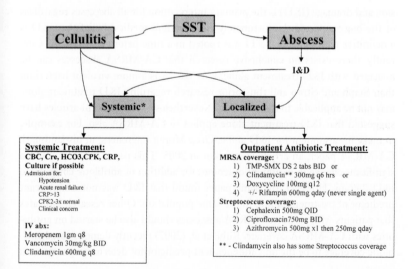

FIGURE 129.1. Soft tissue treatment regime.

"induced resistance." This resistance will not be found by typical susceptibilities received with bacteria cultures. Instead, a *D* test must be specifically ordered and performed by the laboratory. Despite this high rate of inducible resistance, clindamycin remains an attractive alternative due to its *Streptococcus* coverage for use in cellulitis and its ability to halt protein synthesis, giving it a theoretical advantage in the treatment of systemic CA-MRSA infections. The resistance patterns to clindamycin are geographical at this time, thus the practitioner should know his or her local resistance patterns before prescribing it.

Tetracyclines such as doxycycline or minocycline are another family of CA-MRSA antibiotics with diminished susceptibility in the past several years. A recent study in Boston describes a new strain of CA-MRSA, USA 300–0247. This new strain carries a 74% resistance to tetracyclines such as doxycycline. Typical resistance patterns seem to be on the range of 10% to 15% resistance countrywide. Again, just as with clindamycin, local resistance patterns should be established prior to prescribing tetracyclines.

Patients with evidence of sepsis should be admitted. Do not overlook systemic symptoms such as hypotension, fever, hypothermia, or tachycardia. For instance, when admission is equivocal or the patient has any systemic symptoms, basic blood work may be obtained to help determine the need for admission. The Infectious Disease Society of America (IDSA) *Practice Guidelines for the Diagnosis and Management of Skin and Soft-Tissue Infections* recommends admission if a patient is found to be hypotensive, have an elevated creatinine, low serum bicarbonate, creatine phosphokinase (CPK) of 2 to 3 times normal, or a c-reactive protein (CRP) of >13. For these patients, it is of utmost importance to obtain a culture and begin broad-spectrum antibiotics.

SUGGESTED READINGS

Fridkin SK, Hageman JC, Morrison M, et al. Methicillin-resistant *Staphylococcus aureus* disease in three communities. *N Engl J Med*. 2005;352:1436–1444.

Han LL, McDougal LK, Gorwitz RJ, et al. High frequencies of clindamycin and tetracycline resistance in methicillin-resistant *Staphylococcus aureus* pulsed-field type USA300 isolates collected at a Boston ambulatory health center. *J Clin Microbiol*. 2007;45(4):1350–1352.

Moellering RC. Current treatment options for community-acquired methicillin-resistant Staphylococcus aureus infection. *Clin Infect Dis*. 2008;45:1032–1037.

Moran GJ, Amii RN, Abrahamian FM, et al. Methicillin-resistant Staphylococcus aureus in community-acquired skin infections. *Emerg Infect Dis*. 2005;11(6):928–930.

Phillips S, MacDougall C, Holdford DA. Analysis of empiric antimicrobial strategies for cellulitis in the era of methicillin-resistant *Staphylococcus aureus*. *Ann Pharmacother*. 2007;41(1):13–20.

Ruhe JJ, Smith N, Bradsher RW, et al. Community-onset methicillin-resistant *Staphylococcus aureus* skin and soft-tissue infections: Impact of antimicrobial therapy on outcome. *Clin Infect Dis*. 2007;44:777–784.

Stevens DL, Bisno AL, Chambers HF, et al. Practice guidelines for the diagnosis and management of skin and soft-tissue infections. *Clin Infect Dis*. 2005;41(10):1373–1406.

130

DIAGNOSE AND TREAT NECROTIZING SOFT TISSUE INFECTIONS QUICKLY

JOSEPH J. DUBOSE, MD, FACS

Necrotizing soft tissue infections are characterized by fulminant destruction of the tissue. Patients may present with systemic signs of toxicity, a sequela associated with a high mortality rate. While there are many types of infectious processes, depending upon the clinical features, most have similar pathologies. Regardless of the location and clinical presentation, all cases of necrotizing soft tissue infections require early diagnosis and appropriate treatment. Aggressive interventions, including early surgical therapy, are paramount to the successful treatment of this entity.

True risk factors have not been identified for necrotizing soft tissue infection, although conditions including drug use, diabetes mellitus, obesity, and immunosuppression are commonly associated. Key clinical features, however, should raise suspicion. These include the presence of systemic findings (fever, tachycardia, and hypotension) and signs and symptoms such as tense edema outside the involved skin, disproportionate pain, blisters/bullae, crepitus, and subcutaneous gas. Even with these fairly specific findings, the sensitivity for detecting necrotizing infections is only 10% to 40%. Given the case that the fatality rate for necrotizing fasciitis is approximately 25%, clinical suspicion must remain high, and aggressive efforts must be made to rule out the diagnosis.

Necrotizing fasciitis, one of the most commonly encountered forms of necrotizing soft tissue infection, exists in two clinical subtypes. Type I is a mixed infection caused by aerobic and anaerobic bacteria. It most commonly occurs after surgical procedures and in patients who are immunocompromised due to diabetes, peripheral vascular disease, or other chronic diseases. The Type II variant refers to a monomicrobial infection caused most commonly by group A streptococcus and frequently occurs in patients without chronic medical diseases. Type II infections due to other organisms such as *Clostridium* have also been described. Community-acquired methicillin-resistant *Staphylococcus aureus* (CA-MRSA), in particular, represents an emerging concern for these types of infections.

Regardless of the suspected type or clinical presentation, the diagnosis of necrotizing fasciitis must always be suspected in suspicious soft tissue infections. Although risk stratification with laboratory parameters has been proposed, this practice may prove time intensive and result in a dangerous delay in diagnosis. Imaging modalities such as soft tissue x-rays, computed tomography, and MRI may prove useful if there is gas in the tissues but more often will show only nondescript soft tissue swelling. Direct surgical exploration remains the only reliable modality to rapidly and effectively determine the presence of soft tissue infection. For this reason, immediate surgical consultation should be sought in all cases in which necrotizing infections are suspected.

Prompt surgical exploration facilitates early diagnosis as well as therapeutic debridement and the biopsy of material for appropriate cultures. In conjunction with aggressive surgical debridement, early empiric antibiotic therapy should be initiated promptly. Given the range of causative organisms, broad-spectrum coverage with clindamycin and high-dose penicillin was once considered the mainstay of initial coverage. The potential involvement of clindamycin-resistant methicillin-resistant *S aureus* (CR-MRSA) and other resistant organisms, however, is an emerging concern for these types of infections. If CA-MRSA is suspected, the regimen should include vancomycin or other agents with specific activity against this organism. It is advisable that prompt infectious disease consultation be sought, particularly for serious infections. The Infectious Disease Society of America guidelines, most recently revised in November 2005, serve as an excellent resource in guiding initial empiric therapy based on the type and severity of infection. In all cases, local sensitivity testing and culture results should be utilized to appropriately guide continued therapy.

In patients presenting with rapidly progressive cases, shock is a common presenting symptom. Appropriate hemodynamic support should be aggressive in these settings, with the judicious use of fluids, transfusion, and pressors as required for resuscitation. The guidelines developed by the Surviving Sepsis campaign serve as an excellent, evidence-based tool to guide the resuscitation of these septic patients. The use of high-dose immunoglobulins should also be considered, as the mortality associated with intractable hypotension and necrotizing infection is very high; and it has been demonstrated that the use of intravenous immunoglobulin (IVIG) may improve survival in for severe infections.

In summary, the most rapid and effective diagnosis of necrotizing soft tissue infections is by surgical exploration. Immediate surgical consultation should be sought in all patients for whom this diagnosis is expected. Early empiric antibiotic therapy should also be initiated as soon as possible, in conjunction with prompt infectious disease consultation for severe cases. Patients presenting in shock should be treated with adequate resuscitation, as outlined by the guidelines of the Surviving Sepsis campaign. The use of IVIG should also be considered for severe infections, as early data suggest that this therapy may improve survival in this setting. The use of other treatment modalities, including hyperbaric oxygen therapy, may also have utility in select cases, although the employment of this latter modality may not be clinically feasible in an unstable, severely ill patient.

SUGGESTED READINGS

Anaya DA, Dellinger EP. Necrotizing soft-tissue infection: Diagnosis and management. *Clin Infect Dis*. 2007;44:705–710.

Darenberg J, Ihendyane N, Sjolin J, et al. Intravenous immunoglobulin G therapy in streptococcal toxic shock syndrome: A european randomized, double-blind, placebo-controlled trial. *Clin Infect Dis*. 2003;37:333–340.

Miller LG, Perdreau-Remington F, Rieg G, et al. Necrotizing fasciitis caused by community-associated methicillin-resistant staphylococcus aureus in Los Angeles. *N Engl J Med*. 2005;352:1445–1453.

Norrby-Teglund A, Muller MP, Mcgeer A, et al. Successful management of severe group A streptococcal soft tissue infections using an aggressive medical regimen including intravenous polyspecific immunoglobulin together with a conservative surgical approach. *Scand J Infect Dis*. 2005;37:166–172.

Wong CH, Wang YS. The diagnosis of necrotizing fasciitis. *Curr Opin Infect Dis*. 2005;18: 101–106.

131

UNDERSTAND POSTEXPOSURE PROPHYLAXIS FOR HIV IN THE EMERGENCY DEPARTMENT

HANS BRADSHAW, MD

To avoid confusion over how to care for patients potentially exposed to human immunodeficiency virus (HIV), it helps to categorize exposures as either occupational or nonoccupational events. From here, guidelines exist for either scenario to direct you further. The Centers for Disease Control and Prevention (CDC) and the American College of Emergency Physicians have treatment recommendations for occupational postexposure prophylaxis (PEP). Similarly, the U.S. Department of Health and Human Services and the American Academy

TABLE 131.1	EXPOSURE TYPE RISK LEVEL	
RISK LEVEL	**EXPOSURE TYPE**	**DESCRIPTION**
Low	Needlestick or mucous membrane/nonintact skin contact	Solid needles, superficial injuries, or few drops of body fluid
High	Needlestick or mucous membrane/nonintact skin contact	Deep punctures, used large-bore hollow needles, visible blood on the device, or major body fluid splash

of Pediatrics have treatment recommendations for nonoccupational PEP. This discussion is specific to occupational exposures and summarizes how to avoid errors in patient therapy based on reviews of these guidelines.

Potential Errors: Understand what constitutes an exposure, initial treatments, transmission risks, and HIV testing considerations.

Occupational exposures of health care providers (HCP) to infectious material such as blood, tissue, or body fluids (not including feces, nasal secretions, saliva, sweat, tears, urine, and vomit) through percutaneous injury, mucous membrane contact, or nonintact skin contact are concerning for possible HIV transmission especially if it involves you. Immediately wash percutaneous and nonintact skin injuries with soap, alcohol, or water and irrigate mucous membranes with water or saline. The risk of HCP contracting HIV from an HIV-infected patient is low. Prospective studies show an HIV transmission risk with no PEP of 0.3% for percutaneous exposures, 0.09% for mucous membrane exposure, and 0.1% for nonintact skin. PEP reduces these risks by 80% if started within 24 to 36 h. Rapid testing should be performed if the HIV status of the source is unknown. HCP need to be tested too, which can be quite traumatizing from personal experience.

Potential Errors: Categorize exposure and source risk levels.

The CDC therapy guidelines hinge on determining the risk levels of exposure type and source HIV status (*Tables 131.1* and *131.2*).

Potential Errors: Determine if HIV PEP is necessary, pregnancy considerations, and when to start treatment and for how long.

Armed with risk level information, you can now direct specific therapy (*Fig. 131.1*). The inside information is that a negative source HIV status (confirmed within 2 h with a rapid test) regardless of exposure risk and unknown source with low-risk exposures require no antiretroviral therapy. However, any positive source HIV status requires PEP regardless of risk-exposure level. Patients exposed to the HIV positive source get a three-drug therapy regimen unless the positive source HIV status is class 1 and there was low risk exposure, then patients get a two-drug regimen. Do not forget to obtain pregnancy tests on women before starting PEP due to possible fetus toxicity, and if pregnant, consider consultation with an HIV guru and high-risk obstetrician. PEP is started ideally within 2 h and definitely within 36 h after the event. The duration of treatment is 4 weeks.

TABLE 131.2	SOURCE HIV POSITIVE RISK LEVEL
RISK LEVEL	**CRITERIA**
Class 1	Asymptomatic, low viral load <1,500 RNA copies/mL
Class 2	Symptomatic, AIDS, acute seroconversion, or high viral load

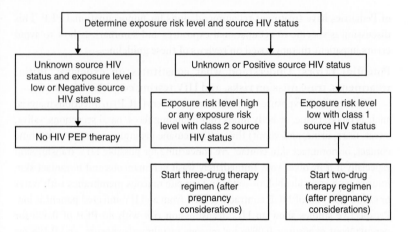

FIGURE 131.1. Therapy recommendations for potential occupational HIV exposure.

Potential Errors: Determine which drugs to use for HIV PEP.

There are three classes of drugs that independently interrupt the normal HIV life cycle: the nucleoside and nucleotide reverse transcriptase inhibitors (NRTIs), the nonnucleoside reverse transcriptase inhibitors (NNRTI), and the protease inhibitors (PIs). NRTIs interfere with the action of reverse transcriptase. NNRTIs bind to reverse transcriptase and block RNA- and DNA-dependent DNA polymerase activity. PIs block HIV protease, an enzyme that establishes HIV infectivity. Initial preferred treatment regimens include 2 NRTIs + 1 PI, 2 NRTIs + 2 PIs, or 2 NRTIs and 1 NNRTI. For low-risk exposures, use a combination NRTI drug tenofovir/emtricitabine (TDF 300 mg/FTC 200 mg) one tablet daily. For high-risk exposures, use Tenofovir/Emtricitabine (TDF 300 mg/FTC 200 mg) one tablet daily plus a combination PI drug lopinavir/ritonavir (LPV/r) two tablets twice daily. For high-risk exposures in patients who want a once-daily dosing regimen, use Tenofovir/Emtricitabine (TDF 300 mg/FTC 200 mg) plus NNRTI atazanavir (ATV 300 mg) plus NNRTI ritonavir (RTV 100 mg). Drugs to avoid for PEP are NRTI Abacavir (ABC) and NRTI Nevirapine (NVP) because of life-threatening side effects during the first few weeks of treatment.

Potential Errors: Arrange follow-up once treatment has begun.

Once the dust has settled, issues arise with therapy monitoring and compliance. The party line to exposed patients needs to include HIV screening performed at baseline, 6 and 12 weeks, and at 6 months after exposure to track possible seroconversion typically occurring within 3 months. Patients on PEP need complete blood count with differential, hepatic function, and renal function tests at baseline and 2 and 4 weeks to monitor for drug toxicity after starting PEP. Patients treated with a PI need to be monitored for hyperglycemia. Ensure that the follow-up you arrange for the patient will provide them with these critical resources.

SUGGESTED READINGS

American College of Emergency Physicians Board of Directors-ACEP Policy Statement, Bloodborne Infections in Emergency Medicine, revised and approved April 2004. Available at: www.acep.org/practres.aspx?id=29130. Accessed October 15, 2008.

Ehrenkranz PD, Ahn CJ, Metlay JP, et al. Availability of rapid human immunodeficiency virus testing in academic emergency departments. *Acad Emer Med*. 2008;15:144–150.

Hammer SM, Eron JJ Jr, Reiss P, et al. Antiretroviral treatment of adult HIV infection: Recommendations of the International AIDS Society-USA panel. *JAMA*. 2008;300(5): 555–570.

Havens PL. Postexposure prophylaxis in children and adolescents for nonoccupational exposure to human immunodeficiency virus. *Pediatrics*. 2003;111:1475.

Panlilio AL, Cardo DM, Grohskopf LA, et al. Updated U.S. Public Health Service guidelines for the management of occupational exposures to HIV and recommendations for postexposure prophylaxis. *MMWR Recomm Rep*. 2005;54:1–17.

Smith DK, Grohskopf LA, Black RJ, et al. Antiretroviral postexposure prophylaxis after sexual, injection-drug use, or other nonoccupational exposure to HIV in the United States: Recommendations from the U.S. Department of Health and Human Services. *MMWR Recomm Rep*. 2005;54:1–20.

132

ALWAYS PRESCRIBE A MULTI-DRUG REGIMEN FOR HIV POSTEXPOSURE PROPHYLAXIS

LORI ANN STOLZ, MD

Emergency physicians are at the frontlines of treating health care workers, survivors of sexual assault, and others who have had a potential exposure to bloodborne pathogens. Though the rates of transmission are low (0.3% for needlestick exposures, 0.1% for vaginal intercourse, and 0.5% for anal intercourse), when the source is known to be HIV positive, use of HIV postexposure prophylaxis (PEP) has been shown to decrease transmission by 81%. The decision to initiate prophylaxis for an HIV exposure can be daunting and includes assessing the risk of the exposure type (needlestick, blood splash on mucosa, and sexual contact), the time since exposure (<72 h or not), and the HIV status of the source (most often unknown). Then, you must decide which drugs to start as prophylaxis, the choices commonly being foreign and with potentially serious toxicity. Luckily, the CDC has published guidelines that do just that.

These guidelines have changed over time, however, and although originally zidovudine monotherapy was sufficient, this is no longer the case. One important pitfall to avoid is prescribing monotherapy. The evidence substantiating multidrug regimens is based on the successful decrease of viral load in HIV-infected individuals, the theoretical benefit of using drugs that work at different stages in the viral replication cycle, and the growing resistance to antiretrovirals among the HIV-positive population. Unfortunately, no clinical trials exist or will likely be done on this subject for several reasons. First, seroconversion is so infrequent that enormous trials would be necessary for statistical reasons, and second, the ethicality of conducting such a study is questionable. Despite the current recommendations against monotherapy, one retrospective study found that zidovudine monotherapy continued to be frequently prescribed even after the 1998 CDC guidelines recommending against monotherapy were published. Seven percent of emergency practitioners surveyed in 2001 stated that they were still prescribing zidovudine monotherapy. In no instance, by any current standards, is monotherapy acceptable.

Now that it is established that a multidrug regimen must be used, there is the question of a three-drug versus a two-drug regimen. CDC guidelines recommend a three-drug regimen in all cases of sexual, injection drug use, and other nonoccupational exposures. For occupational exposures, cases are subdivided into those where the HIV status of the source is either known to be positive or is unknown. For patients whose exposure source is known to be HIV positive, use triple therapy. For patients whose exposure source has an unknown HIV status, use two-drug regimen.

There is evidence that a three-drug regimen is being overprescribed for occupational exposures. A survey of ED practitioners by Merchant and Keshavarz (2003) found that respondents would prescribe a three-drug regimen 55% of the time in an occupational exposure to an unknown HIV status source. The CDC reports that between 1994 and 2008, 45.8% of unknown HIV status occupational exposures were given triple therapy. The concern in these situations is unnecessarily increasing the risk of toxicity. Up to 75% of PEP users experience toxicity and/or side effects, which are known to be more severe in those on triple therapy. The CDC's registry of 448 health care workers, who received PEP early in its use, shows that 53% who were prescribed PEP stopped taking it midcourse. Half of these discontinuations were related to side effects. Even though we know that a three-drug regimen is more toxic than a two-drug choice and that toxicity leads to discontinuation of the regimen, there is no study showing greater discontinuations among those who receive a three-drug versus two-drug regimen. There is also no evidence that fewer drugs lead to increased treatment adherence. Bassett et al. (2004) attempted to circumvent the issue of recruiting large numbers of study participants and created a decision model. Using current knowledge of transmission rates from known exposure sources, resistance rates, drug toxicity, and discontinuation, they evaluated 100,000 cases. In this model, when the source was known to be HIV positive, two-drug therapy resulted in fewer transmissions than three-drug therapy. One can only assume that this would be equally true in a situation where the source had unknown HIV status.

For occupational exposures, save three-drug regimens for cases when the source is known to be HIV positive. Exposures from unknown sources should receive a two-drug regimen. There are some challenging situations when choosing the proper drug regimen is beyond the knowledge base of an emergency physician. For these, get a consultant. Options include consultation with infectious disease specialists and calling the health department or the National Clinicians' PEPline. This is a free, 24 h service for clinicians uncertain about whether to prescribe and how to prescribe PEP. They can be reached at 1-888-448-4911.

SUGGESTED READINGS

Bassett IV, Freedburg KA, Walensky RP. Two drugs or three? Balancing efficacy, toxicity, and resistance in postexposure prophylaxis for occupational exposure to HIV. *Clin Infect Dis.* 2004;39:395–401.

Calfee DP. Prevention and management of occupational exposures to human immunodeficiency Virus (HIV). *Mt Sinai J Med.* 2006;73(6):852–856.

Cardo D, Culver D, Cielsielski C, et al. A case-control study of HIV seroconversion in health care workers after percutaneous exposure. *N Engl J Med.* 1997;337(21):1485–1490.

Centers for Disease Control and Prevention. The HIV postexposure prophylaxis registry, 1999. Available at: http://www.cdc.gov/ncidod/hip/blood/PEPRegistry.pdf. Accessed August 18, 2008.

Merchant RC, Becker BM, Mayer KH, et al. Emergency department blood or body fluid exposure evaluations and HIV postexposure prophylaxis usage. *Acad Emerg Med.* 2003;10(12):1345–1353.

Merchant RC, Keshavarz R. HIV postexposure prophylaxis practices by US ED practitioners. *Am J Emerg Med.* 2003;21(4):309–312.

Panlilio AL, Cardo DM, Grohskopf LA, et al. Updated U.S. Public Health Service guidelines for the management of occupational exposures to HIV and recommendations for postexposure prophylaxis. *MMWR.* 2005;54(RR09):1–17.

Smith DK, Grohskopf LA, Black RJ, et al. Antiretroviral postexposure prophylaxis after sexual, injection-drug use or other nonoccupational exposure to HIV in the United States. *MMWR.* 2005;54(RR02):1–28.

Young TN, Arens FJ, Kennedy GE, et al. Anitretroviral post-exposure prophylaxis (PEP) for occupational HIV exposure. *Cochrane Database Syst Rev.* 2007;1. DOI: 10.1002/14651858.CD002835.pub3.

133

EARLY RECOGNITION AND INTERVENTION FOR SYSTEMIC INFLAMMATORY RESPONSE SYNDROME AND SEPSIS ARE VITAL

BRYAN BUCHANAN, MD AND BEN A. LEESON, MD, FACEP

Sepsis is within a spectrum of syndromes describing the body's response to overwhelming infection via the release of inflammatory mediators. Sepsis is the number one cause of death in noncardiac ICUs, with 750K cases yearly and a mortality rate of up to 60%. The most common sources of infections leading to sepsis are pneumonia, urinary tract infection (UTI), abscess, cellulitis, and ear/throat infections. Systemic inflammatory response syndrome (*SIRS*; introduced in 1992) involves at least two of the following: elevation or depression in body temperature, tachypnea with elevated $PaCO_2$, tachycardia, and an acutely elevated or depressed white count with bandemia. The precision of these parameters is not as important as early recognition that this process is occurring and the rapid assessment of the severity; sepsis requires acute intervention and can be rapidly fatal. A patient with SIRS and a confirmed microbiological cause is *septic* and can deteriorate to *severe sepsis*. Severe sepsis involves failure of one or more organs, hypotension, acidosis, and acute respiratory distress syndrome. The end stage of this process is *septic shock* whose cardinal sign is a blood pressure not responsive to fluid boluses. Granted, septic shock is easier to diagnose than SIRS but is much, much harder to treat.

SIRS is a term that encompasses the first stages of the body's systemic inflammatory response. It is a direct result of cascades of cytokines and chemical mediators, the purpose of which is to prepare the body to face an impending catastrophic insult from any condition that can degrade to shock such as hypovolemia, infection, ischemia, or anaphylaxis. These defenses are intended to preserve organ perfusion, mobilize defenses against infection and physical injury, and accelerate the body's metabolism for quick action. The rapid recognition of this response profoundly affects patient survival. Rangel-Fausto et al. found that there is a stepwise, progressive decline in survival through the spectrum of sepsis, and for each further step toward shock, the patient risks a poorer outcome. The difference in mortality made by recognizing and treating SIRS versus treating at the point of shock is as high as 62%!

Early recognition of SIRS relies on the clinician's awareness of the criteria leading to its diagnosis and a high index of suspicion. Be aware that some of the cardinal symptoms of SIRS can be masked by the medications that patients take: β-blockers can cause spuriously low heart rate, and the influences of immunosuppressive agents and drug-drug interactions must be taken into account. Patients at the extremes of age may not exhibit typical diagnostic criteria for SIRS. The most sensitive sign across age groups, though not the most specific, may be an elevated respiratory rate.

Early goal-directed therapy is a checklist shown to decrease in-hospital mortality by an incredible 16% in SIRS/sepsis patients. Begin fluid resuscitation with crystalloid or colloid equivalent immediately for all hypotensive patients, "fill the tank." If the tank is full, but the pressure is not responding, then the patient is in shock and it is time for pressors. A urinary catheter is placed so that a goal urine output of >0.5 mL/kg can be reliably measured. Also, sending labs early on to elucidate the cause of the SIRS is crucial. Basic labs; cardiac enzymes; a baseline lactate, thorough cultures of blood, urine, and wounds; and a procalcitonin level to help elucidate an infectious cause can all be helpful. However, some patients need empiric antibiotics automatically: neutropenic patients, asplenic patients, and of course, those who are rapidly progressing toward frank sepsis. Imipenem, meropenem, or a fluoroquinolone, plus vancomycin if methicin resistant Staphylococcus aureus (MRSA) is suspected, are good choices. Linezolid is as effective as it is expensive, so save your administration some chest pain by starting with vancomycin. Especially, virulent organisms like *Pseudomonas aeruginosa* are usually double covered, as are infections in immunocompromised patients. Patients need deep vein thrombosis (DVT) prophylaxis according to your institution's preference and stress ulcer prophylaxis with famotidine 20 mg IV each night. All protocol-driven interventions need to be monitored, and any change in the patient's condition requires one to start from the beginning and assess problem areas. Lastly, although activated protein C and steroids have been shown to help patients in severe sepsis, they have little to no role in the management of SIRS.

Pitfalls in the management of sepsis can be divided into those which occur within in the first 6 h and those that occur after 6 h. Within the first 6 h of recognition, the patient ought to be aggressively hydrated with crystalloid unless coexistent lung injury exists. Often, patients do not receive the full amount of fluids that they require within this time frame, or patients become fluid overloaded due to unrecognized comorbid acute lung injury (ALI) or adult respiratory distress syndrome (ARDS). "Source control" in the context of infectious emergencies has become a hot topic as of late. Source control refers to the process of discovering and initiating focused treatment on the nidus of the patient's infection early on in treatment. Culture thoroughly including urine and lines; two blood cultures are needed at least one of which is percutaneous. Rapid initiation of broad-spectrum antibiotics within 1 h of presentation is considered the standard of care. In one recent study, 46% of providers neglected to order lactate levels. Lactate is a helpful guide for immediate initiation of resuscitation (>4 mg/dL) and can predict mortality. So, do not forget to send a lactate!

TABLE 133.1	EARLY GOAL-DIRECTED THERAPY
SEPSIS RESUSCITATION BUNDLE (<6 H)	**SEPSIS MANAGEMENT BUNDLE (<24 H)**
1. Serum lactate	1. Low-dose steroids for septic shock
2. Blood cultures	2. Activated protein C
3. Broad-spectrum antibiotics (1 h)	3. Tight glucose control <150 mg/dL
4. Volume resuscitation w/wo pressors	4. Inspiratory plateau maintained <30 cm H_2O
a) Minimum of 20 mL/kg crystalloid bolus	
b) Apply pressors if pressure refractory hypotension to maintain a MAP > 65	
5. In septic shock: CVP > 8 mm Hg and SvcO₂ > 65%	

CVP, central venous pressure; MAP, mean arterial pressure; SvcO₂, central venous oxygen saturation.

After 6 h, the main pitfalls involve lack of planning for the patient's ICU stay: steroids for the patient at risk for adrenal insufficiency, activated protein C, serial serum lactate levels, planning for tight glycemic control, and maintenance of low volume ventilation with adequate positive end expiratory pressure (PEEP) are all important interventions that may go unnoticed. With bed shortages occurring all too frequently, patients will likely spend more time in the ED. Therefore, it becomes vital that we recognize the need for and take responsibility for these later interventions. The idea of "sepsis bundles" has gained popularity, to prevent oversights (*Table 133.1*). Lastly, consider the diagnosis of sepsis in all infected patients who warrant admission, and never forget, "if you didn't document it, you didn't do it!"

In summary, sepsis is a spectrum of syndromes that describe the body's response to overwhelming infection. Quick recognition of SIRS, initiation of ample fluid resuscitation, judicious use of pressors, source control, and planning for the patient's ICU stay and road to recovery are crucial to the skillful management of these patients. Good luck!

SUGGESTED READINGS

Burdette SD. Systemic inflammatory response syndrome. eMedicine, 16 August, 2007. Available at: http://www.emedicine.com/med/topic2227.htm. Accessed October 2, 2008.

Dellinger RP, Levy MM, Carlet JM, et al. Surviving sepsis campaign: International guidelines for management of severe sepsis and septic shock. *Crit Care Med.* 2008;36(1):296–327.

Marshall JC, Maier RV, Jimenez M, et al. Source control in the management of severe sepsis and septic shock: An evidence-based review. *Crit Care Med.* 2004;32(11 Suppl):S513–S526.

Marx JA, Hockberger RS, Walls RM, eds. *Rosen's Emergency Medicine: Concepts and Clinical Practice.* 6th ed. Philadelphia, PA: Mosby; 2006.

Raghavan M, Marik PE. Management of sepsis during the early "golden hours." *J Emerg Med.* 2006;31(2):185–199.

Rangel-Frausto Ms, Pittet D, Costigan M, et al. The natural history the systemic inflammatory response syndrome. *JAMA*. 1995;273(2):117–123.

Rivers E, Nguyn B, Havstad S, et al. Early goal-directed therapy in the treatment of severe sepsis and septic shock. *N Eng J Med*. 2001;345(19):1368–1377.

Shapiro NI, Howell MD, Talmor D. Serum lactate as a predictor of mortality in emergency department patients with infection. *Ann Emerg Med*. 2005;45(5):524–528.

Schlichting D, McCollam JS. Recognizing and managing severe sepsis: A common and deadly threat. *South Med J*. 2007;100(6):594–600.

Surviving Sepsis Campaign, Institute for Healthcare Improvement. Severe sepsis bundles. Institute for Healthcare Improvement, 2005. Available at: http://www.ihi.org/ihi. Accessed September 1, 2008.

Talan DA, Moran GJ, Abrahamian FM. Severe sepsis and septic shock in the emergency department. *Infect Dis Clin North Am*. 2008;22(1):1–31.

Tintinalli JE, Kelen GD, Stapczynski JS, et al. eds. *Emergency Medicine: A Comprehensive Study Guide*. 65th ed. New York, NY: McGraw-Hill; 2003.

134

ADMINISTER FLUIDS AGGRESSIVELY IN PATIENTS WITH SEPTIC SHOCK

J. MICHAEL WILSON, MD, MPH

Severe sepsis affects an estimated 750,000 people in the United States annually. Thanks to the Surviving Sepsis Campaign and early goal-directed therapy (EGDT), mortality has dropped from 50% to 30% over recent years. However, mistakes still occur and must be corrected. Making a few critical changes to your practice will decrease morbidity and save the life of your septic patient.

First, identify the septic patient early. Second, draw a baseline lactate level prior to giving fluids and then follow it through the resuscitation. Third, once the severely septic patient is identified, place a central line for central venous pressure (CVP) monitoring and an arterial line. Finally, aggressively resuscitate the patient with IV fluids. Of all these, failure to give adequate IV fluids, thus moving to the use of pressors too early, is the most common and most deadly mistake in sepsis management.

The first goal of EGDT is to "fill the tank" and restore preload to the heart. If the patient's systolic blood pressure (SBP) is below 90 after a fluid challenge of 2 L OR the initial lactate is ≥4 and there are 2 or more systemic inflammatory response syndrome (SIRS) criteria present, then the patient is septic and aggressive fluid resuscitation must be continued. To monitor your progress, a central venous (CV) catheter must be placed in the superior vena cava targeting a CVP of 8 to 12 mm Hg (12 to 15 mm Hg if the patient is intubated). This step is often neglected for a myriad of reasons. The central line must be placed. Lack of a CVP measurement can lead to underresuscitation with IV fluids and premature initiation of pressors. The femoral vein approach is not appropriate for measuring an accurate CVP so a superior approach either through the subclavian or through the internal jugular vein should be secured. Currently, there is no clear data that support the specific use of a pulmonary artery (PA) catheter over a properly placed central line, so any available line is acceptable.

Be prepared to use large amounts of fluids to resuscitate the truly septic patient. Again, the most common mistake is the use of vasopressor and ionotropic agents without adequate intravascular volume. It is not uncommon to use 6 to 10 L of crystalloid during the initial resuscitation phase. In the original EGDT study by Rivers et al., the EGDT group received an average of 5 L of crystalloid in the first 6 h, with an additional average of 8.6 L per patient from hours 6 to 72. The type of fluid used, be it crystalloid or colloid, can be left to the discretion of the clinician. There is no firm data that show one to be more effective than the other. The SAFE (Saline versus Albumin Fluid Evaluation) study showed albumin to be as safe and equally effective as crystalloid. Note that 1 L of normal saline (NS) will add about 275 mL to the plasma volume, where the same amount of 5% albumin will add 500 mL to the plasma volume. In patients who present septic with low CVPs as well as pulmonary edema, albumin could help reach the target CVP with less volume.

There are multiple variables that should be continually monitored during the initial resuscitation phase that will help gauge the progress and effectiveness of the treatment. The current Surviving Sepsis Campaign 2008 guidelines recommend fluid administration via a fluid challenge technique of 1,000 mL of crystalloid or 300 to 500 mL of colloid over 30 min with repeated evaluation of overall hemodynamic status after each challenge. If hemodynamic improvement falls off with continued increase in CVP, the amount of fluid administration should be decreased. Additionally, persistently elevated or rising lactate levels are an indication of ongoing tissue hypoperfusion and ischemia. Other parameters that are monitored include pH, base deficit, and urine output. Over time, pH should continue to rise toward normal, the base deficit should trend down, and urine output should improve. If substantial improvement in these variables is not appreciated in the first hours of presentation, the patient is likely still hypovolemic and in need of additional fluids.

Mortality from sepsis remains high, even when treated early and aggressively. Therefore, early identification of the septic patient, following serial lactate levels, placement of a CV catheter, and liberal use of IV fluids to restore CVP are paramount concepts but are often overlooked in the care of the septic patient (*Fig. 134.1*). The most common cardinal sin of sepsis management is the restriction of IV fluids and premature initiation of ionotropic/vasopressor agents. Changing this practice alone will make a significant difference in the mortality of your patients.

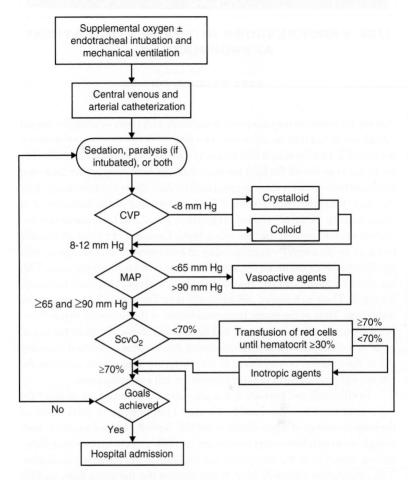

FIGURE 134.1. Care of the septic patient.

SUGGESTED READINGS

Dellinger RP, Levy MM, Carlet JM, et al. Surviving sepsis campaign: International guidelines for management of severe sepsis and septic shock: 2008 [published correction appears in *Crit Care Med*. 2008;36:1394–1396]. *Crit Care Med*. 2008;36:296–327.

Otero RM, Nguyen HB, Huang DT, et al. Early goal–directed therapy in severe sepsis and septic shock revisited: Concepts, controversies, and contemporary findings. *Chest*. 2006;130(5):1579–1595.

Nguyen BH, Rivers EP, Abrahamian FM, et al. Severe sepsis and septic shock: Review of the literature and emergency department management guidelines. *Ann of Emer Med*. 2006;48(1):28–54.

Rivers E, Nguyen B, Havstad S, et al. Early goal–directed therapy in the treatment of severe sepsis and septic shock. *N Engl J Med*. 2001;345:1368–1377.

135

USE VASOPRESSORS IN THE SEPTIC PATIENT APPROPRIATELY

GREG GARDNER, MD

Patients presenting to the emergency department with systemic infection present a challenge in that they are often at death's door or in various stages of meandering toward it. Determining which patient you are dealing with and how badly they are trying to go toward the light can be a challenge. Some may appear somewhat stable and then suddenly crash in a mad dash for the unknown, others slowly circle the drain. Recently, much guesswork has been taken out of the management of septic patients, with goal-oriented resuscitation guidelines. Goal-oriented resuscitation was the spawn of the "Surviving Sepsis Campaign" in which all available literature on the subject was reviewed by an international panel of experts, with specific recommendations on therapy and treatment end points being made. This has created a "goal-oriented" algorithmic, aka "cookbook," approach to managing sepsis. There is, however, still ambiguity regarding some of the resuscitative techniques. Most of the recent recommendations of the Surviving Sepsis Campaign are a mix of expert opinion and limited data, especially when the use of pressors is concerned. To date, no convincing data have been produced regarding any of the common pressors used in the emergency department, and thus the efficacy and possible harm of these pressors are still a guessing game.

To effectively use pressors in a septic patient, one must keep in mind the objective of this intervention and how it plays a role in sepsis. A quick review of the pathophysiology of sepsis should be helpful. Basically, sepsis is a state of shock brought on by an inflammatory process and is usually a mix of hypovolemia (dehydration, especially in the very young and the elderly) and systemic vasodilation. This combination ultimately leads to hypotension (for the sepsis folks, an SBP <90 mm Hg, MAP <65 mm Hg, is considered hypotensive), tissue hypoperfusion, and an imbalance of oxygen supply and demand which leads to more inflammation, additional hypotension, and a vicious downward spiral ensues. The goal of resuscitation is to restore oxygen supply to meet the demand. This is accomplished first by airway management (if no oxygen gets in, none can be delivered), then volume resuscitation using both colloid and crystalloid solutions (to restore volume and oxygen carrying capacity), and lastly, restoration of perfusion pressure and cardiac output by the use of pressors to maintain perfusion to vital organs.

Goal-oriented resuscitation removes much of the guesswork regarding what intervention to do and when to employ it. A "cookbook" approach allows one to employ effective interventions, in proper order, to achieve an end point.

The use of pressors is the last step in the goal-oriented management of sepsis. Using them before other interventions are completed will render them ineffective. The main function of pressors is vasoconstriction to decrease vascular space and increase perfusion pressure. This works synergistically with fluid resuscitation. If the patient's tank is not full and his or her pump is not primed, you will be flogging a dried out, wilted horse. Therefore, it is very important that the patient has, or is receiving, adequate crystalloids and/or colloids prior to starting norepinepherine or dopamine. Normal saline or lactated Ringer's should be used to increase central venous pressure to a target of 6 to 13 mm Hg. Blood transfusions are used as necessary for a target hemoglobin of 7 to 9 g/dL.

After the tank is full, the question becomes which pressor to use and how much to give. To date, no specific pressor has been named as THE pressor of choice in sepsis; however, dopamine and norepinephrine have been named as the pressors to reach for in the management of sepsis. Previously, norepinephrine has been frowned upon as being inferior, often cited as causing extensive end-organ damage secondary to hypoperfusion from overconstriction; however, no hard evidence has been produced to substantiate this claim. In fact, many authors acknowledge a glaring lack of quality evidence regarding the efficacy of specific pressors in general. One small cohort study looked specifically at norepinephrine, in association with other factors, and found an association with the use of norepinephrine and favorable patient outcomes. Acknowledging the limitations of the study design, it appeared that norepinepherine had a positive effect on patient outcome. Given these findings "levophed and leave 'em dead" may not be true. Similarly, dopamine was once theorized to have a renal protective effect at low doses; however, no quality evidence supporting this has ever been produced, and some data refute this notion. If the patient has a SBP >90 and still has signs of hypoperfusion (decreased cap refill, narrowing pulse pressure), dobutamine can be added to the regimen for inotropic support to increase cardiac output and systemic oxygen delivery. Other pressors such as epinephrine, phenylephrine, and vasopressin are not recommended.

Start low and go slow when using pressors. Both dopamine and norepinephrine are known to have complications such as acute renal failure and extremity gangrene when given in high doses. In very critical patients, large doses of pressors may be necessary to maintain vital organ perfusion; however, this may be associated with significant comorbidities as mentioned previously. If the patient survives, it is best to use just enough to get the job done. The "goal" as stated in the Surviving Sepsis Campaign is a MAP >65 mm Hg as measured by direct arterial monitoring. Arterial lines should be used to monitor SBP instead of peripheral monitoring. Peripheral measurements of pressure may give an inaccurate representation of actual systemic perfusion pressures, and the use of an arterial line to titrate pressor dosage is a much closer and more accurate way of monitoring patient response to therapy.

Lastly, care should be taken with patients who present with comorbities, specifically cardiac comorbidities such as coronary artery disease (CAD). Norepinephrine is a predominately α agonist which means its actions will be mostly isolated to the peripheral vasculature, which translates to moderated cardiac stimulation and myocardial oxygen consumption. Dopamine has both α and β_1 effects. Theoretically, low-dose dopamine (2.5 to 5 μg/kg/min) has a vasodilatory effect on renal, splanchnic, and coronary vasculatures. At increasing doses, however, β agonist activity predominates and results in increased cardiac stimulation, which may be good in some patients but may cause problems in patients with underlying CAD. Increasing cardiac activity will increase oxygen demand and may result in demand outstripping supply, adding an MI onto the patient's list of problems. Again, a "start low and go slow" approach may avoid this. Careful consideration to the physiology and needs of the patient must be considered. For example, a patient with atrial fibrillation and rapid ventricular response (RVR), that is, hypotensive as a result of systemic inflammatory response and an unstable heart rate, may benefit from the use of phenylepherine until the tachycardia can be resolved. The pure α agonist activity of phenylephrine may raise blood pressure while avoiding exacerbation of the RVR from the β effects of dopamine and norepinephrine. No protocol or cookbook can handle every situation; risk versus benefit analysis and clinical judgment are key.

In summary, pressors are used in septic patients after the tank is full and oxygen carrying capacity is restored. Norepinephrine and dopamine are the pressors of choice with dobutamine used for increased inotropic support if necessary. Any patient started on pressors needs to be monitored by direct arterial catheterization. Start low and go slow with the pressor dosage, titrating to a target MAP of 65 mm Hg. Comorbidities such as CAD should be taken into account, and the risk benefit of pressor therapy should be weighed before treatment is initiated.

SUGGESTED READINGS

Beale RJ, Hollenberg SM, Vincent JL, et al. Vasopressor and inotropic support in septic shock: An evidence-based review. *Crit Care Med.* 2004;32(11 Suppl):S455–S465.

Dellinger RP, Levy MM, Carlet JM, et al. Surviving Sepsis Campaign: International guidelines for management of severe sepsis and septic shock: 2008. *Crit Care Med.* 2008;36(1): 296–327.

Katz DV, Troster EJ, Vaz FA. Dopamine and kidney in sepsis: A systematic review. *Rev Assoc Med Bras.* 2003;49(3):317–325 [Epub 2003, November 5].

Martin C, Viviand X, Leone M, et al. Effect of norepinephrine on the outcome of septic shock. *Crit Care Med.* 2000;28(8):2758–2765.

Müllner M, Urbanek B, Havel C, et al. Vasopressors for shock. *Cochrane Database Syst Rev.* 2004;(3):CD003709.

Myburgh JA. Catecholamines for shock: The quest for high-quality evidence. *Crit Care Resusc.* 2007;9(4):352–356.

Sevransky JE, Nour S, Susla GM, et al. Hemodynamic goals in randomized clinical trials in patients with sepsis: A systematic review of the literature. *Crit Care.* 2007;11(3):R67.

136

TREAT INFLUENZA WITH THE PROPER ANTIVIRALS

KATHERINE M. HILLER, MD, FACEP

Influenza is an important disease in the fall and winter months. Every year, on average, 5% to 20% of the population is infected. In nonpandemic years, in the United States alone, influenza results in at least 36,000 deaths and 200,000 hospitalizations. Complications from influenza infection include pneumonia, sinusitis, otitis media, and coinfection with other bacterial pathogens. Time lost from work and hospitalization add to the burden of disease. Epidemics occur yearly, and pandemics occur approximately every 10 to 20 years, during which the morbidity and mortality can triple.

While vaccination greatly reduces infection, rates of vaccination have historically been low. Once infection occurs, there are two types of antiviral treatments for influenza, the adamantanes (amantadine and rimantadine), which work against influenza A only, and the neuraminidase inhibitors (oseltamivir and zanamivir), which are effective against both influenza A and influenza B. These agents reduce the duration of symptoms but are largely limited by how quickly they are given. Though there are little data on antiviral treatment and complications related to influenza, some studies suggest that antiviral medications decrease pneumonia and hospital admissions by 50% in patients with influenza.

Effectivity of antiviral agents depends greatly on the timing of treatment. The sooner you give them, the better the reduction in symptom duration. If started >48 h after the onset of symptoms, antivirals do not decrease the duration or severity of symptoms. Therefore, do not give antivirals to patients who present 48 h after symptom onset.

During the 2005–2006 influenza epidemic, there was a 92% resistance of influenza A (H_3N_2) to the adamantanes. In practice, resistance is lower, it is seen in about one third of patients who are treated with amantadine or rimantadine, but it develops rapidly—within the first 2 to 3 days of treatment. Do not use amantadine or rimantadine for the routine treatment of influenza at all. While resistance to zanamivir and oseltamivir has also been demonstrated in vitro; in practice, resistance to these agents seems less of a problem. For these reasons, it is okay to use the neuraminidase inhibitors for treatment and prophylaxis of influenza instead.

Zanamivir is an inhaled drug for patients 5 years and older. Oseltamivir is an oral drug for patients 1 year and older. Both are given twice daily for

5 days. For patients with renal insufficiency, oseltamivir is given only once daily. Pediatric dosing for oseltamivir is weight based. There are no data regarding the safety or efficacy of the neuraminidase inhibitors in pregnancy (i.e., they are class C agents); therefore, they should be used only when the potential benefit to the mother and fetus outweighs the risk.

Prophylactic treatment of immunosuppressed patients or household contacts of patients with influenza with a neuraminidase inhibitor prevents influenza in some cases, until these patients can be vaccinated. Treat these patients with a neuraminidase inhibitor after exposure until 2 weeks after vaccination.

In summary, do not treat influenza with antivirals after the first 48 h of illness because it does not improve either the duration or the extent of illness. Even when started within 48 h, antivirals only reduce the duration of symptoms by 1 day. Do not use amantadine or rimantadine because resistance to these agents is extremely high. Zanamivir is approved for patients over age 5, and oseltamivir is approved for patients over age 1. Both agents are class C in pregnancy.

SUGGESTED READINGS

Centers for Disease Control and Prevention (CDC). High levels of adamantane resistance among influenza A (H3N2) viruses and interim guidelines for use of antiviral agents—United States, 2005–06 influenza season. *MMWR Morb Mortal Wkly Rep.* 2006;55(2):44–46.

Cooper NJ, Sutton AJ, Abrams KR, et al. Effectiveness of neuraminidase inhibitors in treatment and prevention of influenza A and B: Systematic review and meta-analyses of randomised controlled trials. *Br Med J.* 2003;326(7401):1235.

Fiore AE, Shay DK, Broder K, et al. Prevention and control of influenza: Recommendations of the Advisory Committee on Immunization Practices (ACIP), 2008. *MMWR Recomm Rep.* 2008;57(RR-7):1–60.

Jefferson T, Demicheli V, Rivetti D, et al. Antivirals for influenza in healthy adults: Systematic review. *Lancet.* 2006;367(9507):303–313.

Kaiser L, Wat C, Mills T, et al. Impact of oseltamivir treatment on influenza-related lower respiratory tract complications and hospitalizations. *Arch Intern Med.* 2003;163(14): 1667–1672.

137

DO NOT WAIT FOR A PETECHIAL RASH OR SIGNS OF MENINGITIS TO CONSIDER INVASIVE MENINGOCOCCAL DISEASE

CLAYTON P. JOSEPHY, MD

Among infectious emergencies, invasive meningococcal disease (IMD) is possibly the scariest. *Neisseria meningitidis* (MC), the bacterial pathogen responsible for IMD, is the leading cause of bacterial meningitis in children and young adults in the United States and is the second most common community-acquired adult bacterial meningitis. Mortality in IMD remains very high in spite of appropriate therapy, ranging from as high as 20% in all-comers to 50% in those with meningococcemia and disseminated disease.

MC is an aerobic Gram-negative encapsulated bacteria transmitted by respiratory secretions. It presents most commonly as meningitis, but the diagnosis is elusive. Early symptoms often mimic those of benign viral syndromes, including fever (94%), nausea and vomiting (76%), drowsiness (81%), headache (40%), pharyngitis (23%), and myalgias (84%). Unlike viral syndromes, these patients will progress to a degree of illness severity far beyond that typically seen with more benign diagnoses. Unfortunately, relying on the classic presentation of hemorrhagic rash (50%), photophobia and meningismus (27% to 35%), and altered mental status (10%) will identify only those in the late stages of the disease.

This disease kills healthy young people and moves fast, so keep it in mind. You should have a low threshold for panculturing (CSF) and initiating antibiotics therapy in anyone suspicious. A large sample showed that severe infection, including profound bacteremia, sepsis, altered mental status, and seizures, can present in <24 h from onset of malaise.

Do not forget about coagulation catastrophes in these patients. IMD is known for its propensity to induce profound disseminated intravascular coagulation and purpura fulminans, which result from an acquired protein C deficiency. These manifestations of IMD carry a mortality rate as high as 50% to 80% in some series and can occur in as many as 15% to 20% of cases. Therapy includes aggressive replacement of coagulation factors, platelets, and whole blood as guided by coagulation studies. Interestingly, literature guiding the decision of when and how to replace blood products in disseminated intravascular coagulation (DIC) is exceedingly scarce. There is literature that suggests that protein C concentrate and antithrombin III replacement may provide mortality benefit for DIC associated with IMD; however, compelling randomized controlled trials have yet to support this as standard of care. Be afraid, draw coagulation studies, and have blood products on call.

Therapy of IMD begins with the basics. Airway management and hemodynamic support are the mainstay, complemented by prompt administration of broad-spectrum antibiotics, early goal-directed therapy for sepsis, and careful attention to markers of end organ perfusion. Most known isolate of MC are susceptible to penicillin, and in patients with positive MC blood cultures or CSF analysis, penicillin (PCN) at 250,000 IU is given every 6 h. This does not apply to the ED. These results will not be rapidly available. In all suspected cases of IMD, empiric antibiotic therapy should include ceftriaxone at 2 g IV (covering *S. pneumoniae* and *H. influenzae*) and vancomycin 1 g IV (covering resistant *Streptococcus* species). And do not let the inpatient folks talk you into holding off on antibiotics until cultures are available.

A critical action in the management of IMD is the identification of exposures and chemoprophylaxis for those at risk. Preventing an epidemic is perhaps one of the most important parts of our job. Those at risk include household contacts, persons in day care exposed to an index case, direct exposure to index case (kissing, sharing utensils, etc.), and health care professionals who are near the airway (i.e., intubation). Prophylaxis is accomplished with a single dose of ciprofloxacin 500 mg PO, except in children and pregnant women, in whom ceftriaxone 125 mg IM (<12 years old) or 250 mg IM (>12 years old) is the best choice (16), unless, of course, you are unlucky enough to live and work in certain counties in North Dakota, where ciprofloxacin has been ineffective.

In summary, IMD continues to be a devastating disease and carries an extremely high mortality and morbidity. Identifying IMD in those with nonspecific "viral" symptoms can be a diagnostic challenge. Know who is at risk, and be wary of rapidly progressive and severe symptoms. Do not wait for petechiae and sudden inflammatory response syndrome (SIRS); obtain CSF and blood cultures in suspicious cases who are hemodynamically stable, and use antibiotics judiciously. Identify sepsis and treat it aggressively with crystalloid, vasopressors, and blood products in the case of coagulation catastrophes. While protein C and antithrombin III are not ready for prime time, keep your eyes out for emerging literature. Administer empiric vancomycin and ceftriaxone quickly. Treat the exposed, including yourself and your resuscitation team members who may have had contact with oral secretions, with single-dose ciprofloxacin or IM ceftriaxone and, as always, pay meticulous attention to universal precautions.

SUGGESTED READINGS

Alberio L, Lammle B, Esmon CT. Protein C replacement in severe meningococcemia: Rationale and clinical experience. *Clin Infect Dis.* 2001;32(9):1338–1346.

American Academy of Pediatrics. Meningococcal disease prevention and control strategies for practice based physicians. *Pediatrics.* 1996;97(3):404–412.

Apicella MA. Neisseria meningitidis. In: Mandell GL, Douglas RG, Benner JE, et al., eds. *Principles and Practice of Infectious Disease*. 5th ed. Philidelphia, PA: Churchil-Livingstone; 2000:2228–2241.

Centers for Disease Control and Prevention. Meningococcal disease. In: Atkinson W, Wolfe S, Hamborsky J, et al., eds. *Epidemiology and Prevention of Vaccine-Preventable Diseases*. 11th ed. Washington, DC: Public Health Foundation; 2009.

Durand ML, Calderwood SB, Weber DJ, et al. Acute bacterial meningitis in adults. *N Engl J Med*. 1993;328(1):21–28.

Edwards MS, Baker CJ. Meningococcal infections. In: Mcmillen JA, DeAngelis CD, Feigin RD, et al., eds. *Oski's Pediatrics: Principles and Practice*. 3rd ed. Philadelphia, PA: Lippincott Williams & Wilkins; 1999:980–984.

Ferguson, LE, Hormann MD, Parks DK, et al. Neisseria meningitidis: Presentation, treatment and prevention. *J Pediatr Health Care*. 2002;16(3):119–124.

Fijnvandraat K, Peters M, Derkx B, et al. Endotoxin induced coagulation activation and Protein C reduction in meningococcal septic shock. *Prog lin Biol Res*. 1994;388:247–254.

Fourrier F, Chopin C, Huart JJ, et al. Double-blind, placebo controlled trial of antithrombin III concentrates in septic shock with disseminated intravascular coagulation. *Chest*. 1993; 104:882–888.

Fraser A, Gafter-Gvili A, Paul M, et al. Antibiotics for preventing meningococcal infections. *Cochrane Database Syst Rev*. 2006;(4):CD004785 [Review].

Giraud T, Dhainaut JF, Schremmer B, et al. Adult overwhelming meningococcal purpura: A study of 35 cases, 1977–1989. *Arch Intern Med*. 1991;151:310–316.

Havens PL, Garland JS, Brook MM, et al. Trendsin mortality in children hospitalized with meningococcal infections, 1957–1987. *Ped Infect Disease J*. 1989;8:8–11.

Kienast J, Juers M, Wiedermann CJ, et al. Treatment effects of high dose antithrombin without concomitant heparin in patients with severe sepsis with or without disseminated intravascular coagulation. *J Thromb Hemost*. 2006;4(1):90–97.

Thompson MJ, Ninis N, Perera R, et al. Clinical recognition of meningococcal disease in children and adolescents. *Lancet*. 2006;367(9508):397–403.

White B, Livingstone W, Murphy C, et al. An open-label study of the role of adjuvant hemostatic support with protein C replacement therapy in purpura fulminans associated meningococcemia. *Blood*. 2000;96:3719–3724.

138

MANAGE MENINGITIS QUICKLY AND AGGRESSIVELY: PART I

DIANA A. HANS, DO AND ERIC D. KATZ, MD, FAAEM, FACEP

Meningitis is an inflammation of the membranes that surround the central nervous system. The dura, arachnoid, and pia mater are affected. It is absolutely essential to realize that meningitis is a clinical diagnosis, and antibiotic treatment must be initiated before any workup is completed. During a patient's emergency department course, there are numerous points where an EM physician can get into trouble. First, however, a short review of the common organisms that can cause meningitis is provided.

The use of the *Haemophilus influenzae* type b conjugate vaccine has shifted the frequency of various bacteria that are responsible for community-acquired bacterial meningitis. Today, the leading cause of bacterial meningitis after the neonate stage is *Streptococcus pneumoniae*, followed by *Neisseria meningitides* and *Listeria monocytogenes*. Also, nosocomial meningitis is today a contributor among adult cases. In general, bacterial meningitis can occur at any age in otherwise healthy individuals.

The clinician must have a thorough understanding of the presenting signs and symptoms. If a high index of suspicion exists, the patient must be treated empirically. Signs and symptoms include fever, nuchal rigidity, altered mental status, lethargy, and headache. Studies consistently report that the vast majority will have at least one of the above mentioned findings. Other findings include Brudzinski and Kernig signs. Patients can also present with photophobia, sore throat, and a rash. A classic petechial rash is most commonly seen with *N. meningitides* but can also occur with *S. pneumoniae* and other bacteria. In general, adverse outcome and increased mortality have been observed in people over age 60 and in patients who initially presented with seizure activity or severely altered mental status.

A common mistake is to delay treatment until blood work, cerebrospinal fluid analysis, or computed tomography (CT) results are available. It is true that the definitive diagnosis is often not revealed until a lumbar puncture is performed. However, initial treatment is the same regardless of the ultimate diagnosis. The reason we want to identify the specific organism is to modify our empirical antibiotic regimen. It also serves to keep statistics current and to better allow the Center for Disease Control (CDC) to analyze trends.

There is an ongoing debate over whether a CT scan should be performed prior to lumbar puncture. In general, this should be done if the patient has focal neurological signs, papilledema, or is in a state of coma. On the other hand, the yield of CT scan is very low in the absence of such findings. Again, antibiotics should be given first, even if the clinician decides to obtain a head CT prior to lumbar puncture.

Even though we have a much better understanding of the disease today, and newer antibiotics have been introduced, it is interesting to note that during the past 35 years, overall case fatality rates have remained high at 20% to 25%. Bacterial meningitis is a rapidly fatal infection, and empirical intravenous antibiotic treatment is appropriate and necessary. Currently, using corticosteroids as an adjunct treatment is hotly debated. Early reports stated that steroids did not affect overall mortality. It was soon recognized, however, that they decrease complications associated with bacterial meningitis, especially hearing loss. Other sequelae include brain damage, learning disabilities, and mental retardation. In 2007, the *Cochrane Database of Systematic Reviews* stated that the use of corticosteroids in community-acquired bacterial meningitis reduces mortality, hearing loss, and other neurological complications in both children and adults. As a result, dexamethasone is the drug of choice to be given prior to, or with the first antibiotic dose.

Prophylaxis for close contacts of patients with meningococcal meningitis is currently recommended. Close contacts include members of the same household or day care and those with direct contact with oral secretions (may include EMS or ED personnel). Current regimens for prophylaxis include single-dose ciprofloxacin or rifampin 600 mg PO q12h for 4 doses. Respiratory isolation is recommended for all suspected meningitis patients. Antibiotic errors in the management of bacterial meningitis are reviewed in a separate chapter and will therefore not be covered here.

SUGGESTED READINGS

Cabral D, Flodmark O, Farrell K, et al. Prospective study of computed tomography in acute bacterial meningitis. *J Pediatrics*. 1987;111:201–205.

Center for Disease Control and Prevention. Division of Bacterial and Mycotic Diseases. Available at: http://www.cdc.gov/ncidod/dbmd/diseaseinfo/meningococcal-g.html. Accessed October 15, 2007.

Drumheller B, D'Amore J, Nelson M. A simple clinical decision rule to predict bacterial meningitis in patients presenting to the emergency department. *Ann Emerg Med*. 2007;50(3):S10.

Durand M, Calderwood S, Weber D, et al. Acute bacterial meningitis in adults: A review of 493 episodes. *N Engl J Med*. 1993;328:21–28.

Menaker J, Martin IB, Hirshon JM. Marked elevation of CSF white blood cell count: An unusual case of Streptococcus pneumoniae meningitis, differential diagnosis, and a brief review of current epidemiology and treatment recommendations. *J Emerg Med*. 2005;29(1):37–41.

Pizon A, Bonner M, Wang H, et al. Ten years of clinical experience with adult meningitis at an urban academic medical center. *J Emerg Med*. 2006;31(4):367–370.

Quagliarello V, Scheld W. Treatment of bacterial meningitis. *N Engl J Med*. 1997;336: 708–716.

Rosenstein N, Perkins B, Stephens D. Meningococcal disease. *N Engl J Med*. 2001;344: 1378–1388.

Schuchat A, Robinson K, Wenger J, et al. Bacterial meningitis in the United States in 1995. *N Engl J Med*. 1997;337:970–976.

Swartz M. Bacterial meningitis: A view of the past 90 years. *N Engl J Med*. 2004;351: 1826–1828.

van de Beek D, de Gans J, McIntyre P, et al. Corticosteroids for acute bacterial meningitis. *Cochrane Database of Sys Rev*. 2007;(1):CD004405.

139

MANAGE MENINGITIS QUICKLY
AND AGGRESSIVELY: PART II

NATHANIEL ARNONE, MD

To avoid making errors in the management of acute meningitis which could result in potentially devastating sequelae, we must make a rapid clinical diagnosis of acute meningitis, obtain studies capable of identifying the pathogenic organism, and choose and rapidly administer appropriate empiric antibiotic therapy. We should be aware that antibiotic administration before lumbar puncture may prevent ultimate identification of the pathogenic organism. One study has shown sterilization of CSF culture only 2 h after antibiotics in meningococcal meningitis and 4 h after antibiotics in pneumoccocal meningitis. Despite the potential for interfering with the ultimate CSF culture results, the administration of appropriate empiric antibiotics should be done *emergently*. Neither the American College of Emergency Physicians nor the Infectious Disease Society of America has published a clinical policy guideline advocating a specific door to antibiotic time. For obvious reasons, there will never be a controlled, prospective, randomized clinical trial to quantify the amount of delay in antibiotics that causes a worsened clinical outcome. Suffice to say, your patient with acute meningitis should receive antibiotics as soon as possible.

Appropriate antibiotic therapy is initially based on the predominate pathogens in the patient's demographic group, as well as local antibiotic resistance patterns. Know your hospital's antibiogram and the antibiotic resistance patterns in your community. When it comes to empiric therapy for acute meningitis, embrace your inpatient colleagues' stereotype of emergency physicians: Go big. Go broad-spectrum. Let the admitting physician narrow the spectrum and tailor the antibiotics in an intellectual manner when it is safe (and easier) to do so—after the cultures and sensitivities are finalized.

For neonates <1 month of age, the predominant organisms responsible for acute bacterial meningitis are *Streptococcus agalactiae, Escherichia coli, Listeria monocytogenes*, and *Klebsiella* species. Note that ceftriaxone is not used in this age group, because it can displace bilirubin bound to albumin leading to unsafe levels of serum bilirubin in neonates. Additionally, a warning was added by the FDA in 2007 because of deaths in neonates who received ceftriaxone in conjunction with calcium-containing products. Therefore, you should cover this group empirically with ampicillin plus cefotaxime or ampicillin plus an aminoglycoside. Herpes simplex virus (HSV) is another important and potentially devastating pathogen in this age group that should not be forgotten. If there is a maternal history of HSV, any suspicious skin lesions, or the lumbar puncture is suggestive of HSV meningitis, acyclovir should be added.

For children 1 to 23 months old, the usual bacterial suspects are *Streptococcus pneumoniae, Neisseria meningitidis, Haemophilus influenzae, S. agalactiae*, and *E. coli*. You should cover this group empirically with vancomycin plus ceftriaxone or cefotaxime.

For patients 2 to 50 years of age, the common bacteria are *S. pneumoniae* and *N. meningitidis*. Empiric treatment for this group is with vancomycin plus ceftriaxone or cefotaxime.

For adults over 50 years of age, the common bacteria are *S. pneumoniae, N. meningitidis, L. monocytogenes*, and aerobic Gram-negative bacilli. Empirically, treat this patient group with vancomycin plus ceftriaxone or cefotaxime. If there is a recent history of aerobic Gram-negative bacilli infection (such as *Pseudomonas aeruginosa*), cefepime should be used instead of the third-generation cephalosporin.

For patients with intracranial instrumentation (ventriculoperitoneal shunt, penetrating head trauma, recent neurosurgery), the common bacteria are *Staphylococcus aureus*, coagulase-negative staphylococci, and aerobic Gram-negative bacilli. Empiric treatment is with vancomycin plus cefepime, vancomycin plus meropenem, or vancomycin plus ceftazidime.

As a result of the success of the HiB vaccine, *S. pneumoniae* has become the most common organism in acute meningitis in the United States, and there is an increasing prevalence of penicillin-resistant and cephalosporin-resistant strains. Accordingly, vancomycin has been recommended as a first-line addition to empiric therapy for all children older than 1 month by the American Association of Pediatrics and for adults by the Infectious Diseases Society of America. Because of concern that adjunct therapy with dexamethasone may decrease the amount of vancomycin that crosses the blood-brain barrier, some experts also recommend adding rifampin for penicillin-/cephalosporin-resistant *S. pneumoniae*; however, there are no clinical trials which demonstrate a clear benefit, and it is *not* recommended as a first-line empiric therapy.

Appropriate treatment of acute meningitis by the emergency physician requires more than writing an order for a shot of ceftriaxone and a phone call to the admitting service. Know the appropriate empiric antibiotics for each age group and initiate them early. Do not wait for lab or radiology results to begin treatment. Be aware of the increasing prevalence of resistant strains of *S. pneumoniae* as well as local patterns of resistance of other organisms in your community. Avoiding these potential errors is crucial in the expert management of this uncommon but potentially devastating disease.

SUGGESTED READINGS

American Academy of Pediatrics. Pneumococcal infections. In: Pickering LK, Baker CJ, Long SS, et al. eds. *Red Book: 2006 Report of the Committee on Infectious Diseases*. 27th ed. Elk Grove Village, IL: American Academy of Pediatrics; 2006.

FDA Alert 9/07. Information for healthcare professionals: Ceftriaxone. Available at: http://www.fda.gov/CDER/DRUG/InfoSheets/HCP/ceftriaxone.htm. Accessed August 15, 2008.

Kanegaye JT, Soliemanzadeh P, Bradley JS. Lumbar puncture in pediatric bacterial meningitis: Defining the time interval for recovery of cerebrospinal fluid pathogens after parenteral antibiotic pretreatment. *Pediatrics*. 2001;108(5):1169–1174.

Tunkel AR, Hartman BJ, Kaplan SL, et al. Practice guidelines for the management of bacterial meningitis. *Clin Infect Dis*. 2004;39:1267–1284.

140

DO NOT BE MISLED BY THE TRADITIONAL MYTHS OF DIARRHEA

DILLON ROACH, MD

Feces, poop, kaka, turd, dung, crap, and any other four letter words you can think of to identify bowel movements are not the topic of choice for most people to start a conversation. However, for all of us who live in the emergency department pits, this topic is something that we encounter daily as an introduction conversation with a new patient. In fact, there are an estimated 211 to 375 million cases of diarrhea in the United States each year (1.4 per person per year). It is the second most common reason to miss work and causes about 900,000 hospitalizations and 6,000 deaths in the United States each year and over 24 million deaths worldwide. Let us take a closer look at the "not-so-funny-if-you-have-it" topic of diarrhea, review current treatment recommendations, and dispel several of the myths regarding treatment of acute infectious diarrhea in adults.

DIARRHEA: THE STRAIGHT POOP

Some authors state that diarrhea is defined as having more than three stools exceeding 200 g in total weight. In reality, since none of us weigh our stool, it is simply defined as more frequent stools with lesser consistency. Typically, the majority of diarrhea cases are viral or self-limited, occur during the winter months, last <24 h, and require no treatment other than supportive care with oral rehydration. Medical intervention can become necessary if diarrhea is more severe, lasts longer than one day, and is with patients who have fevers with blood and/or pus in the stools.

CAUSES OF DIARRHEA

Beyond acute infectious diarrhea, there are several other causes of diarrhea and specific patient populations to consider. Hiking or camping can expose individuals to parasites. Do not forget to review the patients history of recent antibiotic use or hospitalization which increases the risk of infection with *Clostridium difficile*. Some other causes of diarrhea to consider include organo-phosphate poisoning, laxative overuse, chemotherapy, pancreatic insufficiency, irritable bowel syndrome (IBS), and inflammatory bowel disease (IBD). Additionally, patients who are immunocompromised are more susceptible to other causes of diarrhea than a healthy patient and often require a more extensive evaluation.

PHYSICAL EXAM

When evaluating a patient with diarrhea, hydration status and the abdominal examination are the most valuable portions to include as you complete your assessment. What is the severity of the patient's dehydration and will he or she need IV rehydration or simple oral rehydration therapy (ORT)? On the abdominal exam, try to determine if there are other causes for the patient's abdominal pain and diarrhea and always consider diagnosis such as appendicitis, IBD, or diverticulitis. Lastly, everyone's favorite portion of the physical exam, the rectal exam, aka "welcome to the ER," is unfortunately necessary to determine if the patient is hemoccult positive or to evaluate if he or she has a fecal impaction.

Beyond the basics, it is important to be informed about two main myths surrounding diarrhea treatment, so you do not fall victim to these pit falls.

Myth 1. *Antimotility agents should not be used because it slows down the body's defense mechanism and makes humans more susceptible to enteric infection.* This myth was started after a 1963 study on guinea pigs that were infected with *Shigella* toxin; half of the group was given opium to slow intestinal motility. The researchers found that an increased percentage of the guinea pigs given opium died. Another study done on humans approximately 10 years later perpetuated this myth. This study, containing only 25 patients with four treatment arms, concluded that patients who were infected with Shigellosis and given Lomotil (diphenoxylate and atropine) might have had increased risk of invasive infection.

Myth 2. *Antibiotics should be avoided in the treatment of infectious diarrhea because it can prolong the shedding of Salmonella.* This fear arose from a 1969 study that found *Salmonella* excretion was prolonged by 1 to 2 days if the patient was given antibiotics. The study resulted in physicians not treating people who could be infected with *Salmonella*, eventually leading to not treating anyone with diarrhea. There has also been some concern about treatment of children with *E. coli*

O157 and increasing the rate of Hemolytic Uremic Syndrome, which has lead to physicians not wanting to treat adults with antibiotics as well.

CUTTING THROUGH THE CRAP

In the last 20 years, there have been multiple studies that have shown it is safe to use both antibiotics and antimotility agents for the treatment of acute infectious diarrhea in immunocompetent adult patients. Cumulatively, these studies outline that you can decrease the frequency of stools and shorten the duration by as much as 1 to 3 days depending on the infection. Most of these studies were done using ciprofloxacin or trimethoprim/sulfamethoxazole and loperamide. There have been several studies that show that ciprofloxacin is superior to and has less resistance than trimethoprim/sulfamethoxazole and is therefore considered a first-line therapy. In more severe cases or in patients refractory to loperamide, the combination of diphenoxylate and atropine may be helpful. "Even though most infectious diarrheas are self-limited, because of the inconvenience and occasionally life-threatening nature of the disease, we recommend ciprofloxacin treatment for all patients believed to have infectious diarrhea who do not have a contraindication to antimicrobial treatment." We also recommend the use of loperamide, because along with antibiotic treatment, it has clearly been shown to shorten the duration of illness (*Table 140.1*).

Remember the bottom line, do not fall into the trap of the myths regarding nontreatment of diarrhea. Ciprofloxacin and loperamide are good. And lastly, I will leave you with one more bit of advice: while conducting your exam, wear a glove.

TABLE 140.1	DIARRHEA TREATMENTS	
GENERIC NAME	**TRADE NAME**	**DOSAGE**
Ciprofloxacin	Cipro	500 mg PO single dose or 500 mg PO BID for 3 d
Trimethoprim/ sulfamethoxazole	Bactrim, Septra	160/800 mg (DS dose) PO for single dose or DS dose PO BID for 3 d
Loperamide	Imodium	4 mg initially, then 2 mg after each unformed stool to a maximum of 16 mg/d
Diphenoxylate and atropine	Lomotil	Two tablets or 10 mL PO QID
Bismuth subsalicylate	Pepto Bismol	30 mL or two tablets q30 min for 8 doses × 2 d Prophylaxis: two tablets with each meal and qhs

SUGGESTED READINGS

Cullen N. Constipation. In: Marx JA, Hockberger RS, Walls RM, et al., eds. *Rosen's Emergency Medicine: Concepts and Clinical Practice.* 6th ed. Philadelphia, PA: Mosby; 2006:237–242.

Ericsson CD, DuPont HL, Mathewson JJ, et al. Treatment of traveler's diarrhea with sulfamethoxazole and trimethoprim and loperamide. *JAMA.* 1990;262(2):257–261.

Sadosty AT, Hess JJ. Vomiting, diarrhea, and constipation. In: Tintinalli JE, Kelen GD, Stapczynski JS, et al., eds. *Emergency Medicine: A Comprehensive Study Guide.* 6th ed. New York, NY: McGraw-Hill;2003:551–559.

Thielman NM, Guerrant MD. Acute infectious diarrhea. *N Engl J Med.* 2004;350(1):38–47.

141

TOXIC SHOCK SYNDROME: DO NOT HESITATE—RESUSCITATE

CHRISTOPHER M. SCIORTINO, MD, PhD AND CHARLIE GALANIS, MD

Toxic shock syndrome (TSS) is classically thought of to be the result of superabsorbent tampons. Although up to half of *Staphyloccus*-related cases are associated with menstruation, lack of such history does not exclude the diagnosis. Infectious sources range vastly and include nasal/pharyngeal and surgical wounds, osteomyelitis, mastitis, burns, postpartum vaginitis, undrained abscesses, and diabetic ulcers. Further, an infectious source may not be apparent. Suspect the diagnosis in any patient who presents with a high fever, hypotension, signs of multiple organ dysfunction, and a potential unidentified infectious source.

TSS refers to hypotension and multiple organ dysfunction attributed to an infection with an exotoxin producing strain of *Staphylococcus aureus*. This results in the release of superantigens such as IL-1 and tumor necrosis factor. Infections with an exotoxin-producing strain of group A *Streptococcus* (GAS) can result in a similar clinical sequela, and it is termed steptococcal toxic shock syndrome (STSS). Although TSS and STSS have separate infectious agents and clinical outcomes, the initial diagnostic and treatment strategies are similar. The incidence of TSS in the United States is estimated to be 1 to 2 cases/100,000 and is higher in women. The mortality rate is reported to be between 3% and 5%. The true incidence of STSS is not known but is estimated between 10 and 20 cases/100,000. The mortality rate is reported to be 30% to 75%. Both forms of TSS have a recurrence rate approaching 40%.

Tables 141.1 and *141.2* outline the clinical criteria for the diagnosis of TSS and STSS, respectively. Fever and hypotension are typical for both TSS and STSS. The majority of patients with TSS will have a diffuse

TABLE 141.1	STAPHYLOCOCCAL TSS	
Fever	≥38.9°C	
Hypotension	*Adults*: Systolic blood pressure ≤90 mm Hg or orthostatic hypotension	
	Children <16 y: Systolic blood pressure less than the 5th percentile for age	
Rash	Macular erythroderma	
Desquamation	1–2 weeks after onset of symptoms (palms and soles)	
Microbiology	Negative cultures; no elevation in antibody titers to Rocky Mountain spotted fever, leptospirosis, or rubeola	
Multiple organ impairment (2 or more of the following)	Renal	Creatinine and/or BUN twice the upper limit of normal for age or greater than twofold elevation over baseline level Sterile pyuria
	Coagulopathy	Platelets ≤100,000/mm³ DIC: ↑ clotting times, ↓ fibrinogen, ↑ fibrin degradation products
	Hepatic	AST, ALT, or total bilirubin levels > twice the upper limit of normal for age *Preexisting hepatic disease*: Greater than twofold increase over baseline
	Musculoskeletal	Myalgia or CPK levels ≥ twice the upper limit of normal
	GI	Emesis or diarrhea
	Mucous membrane inflammation	Oropharynx, cunjunctiva, vagina
	CNS	Disorientation, delirium (not present without hypotension and/or fever)

ALT, alanine transaminase; AST, aspartate transaminase; DIC, disseminated intravascular coagulopathy.

macular erythematous "sunburn" rash. Rash is less typical in STSS. The rash desquamates after 10 to 14 days, especially on the palms and soles. Up to half of patients with TSS may have a strawberry tongue. STSS will most often present with pain overlying the site of infection. Laboratory studies may demonstrate a leukocytosis with bandemia as well as results typical of underlying organ dysfunction. Imaging studies may reveal a site of undrained abscess but oftentimes will be negative.

TABLE 141.2	**STREPTOCOCCAL TSS**	
Hypotension	*Adults*: Systolic blood pressure ≤90 mm Hg or orthostatic hypotension	
	Children <16 y: Systolic blood pressure less than the 5th percentile for age	
Multiple organ impairment (2 or more of the following)	Renal	*Adults*: Creatinine ≥2 mg/dL
		Children: Creatinine ≥ twice the upper limit of normal for age
		Preexisting renal disease: Greater than twofold elevation over baseline creatinine level
	Coagulopathy	Platelets ≤100,000/mm³
		DIC: ↑ clotting times, ↓ fibrinogen, ↑ fibrin degradation products
	Hepatic	AST, ALT, or total bilirubin levels > twice the upper normal limit for age
		Preexisting hepatic disease: Greater than twofold increase over baseline
	ARDS	Diffuse pulmonary infiltrates Hypoxemia in the absence of cardiac failure
	Cutaneous	Generalized erythematous macular rash that may desquamate
	Soft tissue	Necrotizing fasciitis, myositis, or gangrene
Microbiology	Isolation of GAS	*Probable*: Clinical criteria AND isolation of GAS from a nonsterile site
		Confirmed: Clinical criteria AND isolation of GAS from a normally sterile site

ARDS, acute respiratory distress syndrome; DIC, disseminated intravascular coagulopathy; GAS, group A *Streptococcus*.

Treatment of TSS in the ED requires appropriate fluid resuscitation, hemodynamic support, intravenous (IV) antibiotics, source control (if possible), and early medical or surgical consultation. Place patients in critical care bed with continuous telemetry and frequent vital sign acquisition. As with any critically ill patient, securing the airway is of prime importance. Patients can present with acute respiratory distress syndrome or in extremis and require intubation. Utilize supplemental oxygen to maximize end-organ oxygenation. Obtain early and adequate IV access; this may require central venous access. Patients may be fluid seeking and may require both high rate of IVF infusion and multiple fluid boluses to maintain adequate blood pressure. Vasopressors may also be required for hemodynamic support. Foley catheter placement allows for accurate measurement of urine output in the hemodynamically labile patient. Patients who require ongoing resuscitation should also have an arterial line placed for close hemodynamic monitoring and frequent lab draws.

Although patients may present with classic toxic shock due to Staph or Strep, it is important to remember that the etiological agent will not be identified during their stay in the ED. Selection of antibiotics should include coverage for Staph and strep and requires broad-spectrum coverage if the diagnosis is at all in question. Further, consideration of MRSA and resistant strains of GAS must be included in the antibiotic selection. An initial broad-spectrum regime could include a β-lactam with lactamase inhibitor such as piperacillin-tazobactam and MRSA coverage such as vancomycin or linezolid. Clindamycin can be used in TSS for treatment and is often added empirically as a toxin inhibition. However, its use as monotherapy is not recommended as strains of clindamycin-resistant MRSA and GAS have been identified.

Clearing the infectious source, if possible, will reduce the toxin burden. Keep in mind the possibility of a retained tampon or contraceptive device. Patients with surgical wounds may have undrained fluid collections or retained pieces of packing material. Diabetic patients may have an ulcer or wound that they are unaware of secondary to neuropathy. The dialysis patient may have an infected AV fistula or central line. It is therefore of great importance to perform a thorough physical examination that includes removal of all wound dressings, exploration of all wounds, and performance of a pelvic examination when appropriate.

The need for early consultation cannot be overstated. Patients may require urgent or emergent surgery for debridement or exploration. Medical patients may require ongoing ICU resuscitation and invasive hemodynamic monitoring. Early consultation also works to minimize the time to transfer and brings the team that will continue to care for the patient on line early. TSS is an infrequent disease but one with potentially high mortality. Recognition of the sequela of TSS is key to the initiation of resuscitation, source control, appropriate antibiotic therapy, and surgical or medical consultation. The ED team takes the lead role in leading the initial care of these patients and can have a positive impact on the clinical outcome.

SUGGESTED READINGS

Hajjeh R, Reingold A, Weil A, et al. Toxic shock syndrome in the United States: Surveillance update, 1979–1996. *Emerg Infect Dis.* 1999;5(6):807–810.

Lamani TL, Darenberg J, Luca-Harari B, et al. Epidemiology of severe Streptococcus pyogenes disease in Europe. *J Clin Microbiol.* 2008;46(7):2359–2367.

McCormick JK, Yarwood JM, Schlievert PM. Toxic shock syndrome and bacterial superantigens: an update. *Ann Rev Microbiol.* 2001;55:77–104.

Parsonnet J, Deresiewicz R. Shaphylococcal infections. In: Fauci AS, Braunwald E, Kasper DL, et al., eds. *Harrison's Principles of Internal Medicine.* New York, NY: McGraw-Hill; 2008.

Wessels M. Streptococcal and enterococcal infections. In: Fauci AS, Braunwald E, Kasper DL, et al., eds. *Harrison's Principles of Internal Medicine.* New York, NY: McGraw-Hill; 2008.

142

DO NOT GIVE PROPHYLACTIC ANTIBIOTICS FOR LOW-RISK PROCEDURES ... THE RISK OF ANAPHYLAXIS MAY BE GREATER THAN THE RISK OF ENDOCARDITIS!

SAJID HUSSAIN SHAH, MD

Practices for prophylaxis of infective endocarditis have been very variable. The treatment rationale has largely been based on retrospective case-control and descriptive studies. It should be noted that no prospective randomized controlled trial has ever been carried out evaluating the efficacy of antibiotic prophylaxis in infective endocarditis. Prophylactic antibiotics for the prevention of infective endocarditis have largely been administered to patients based on traditional teaching and practical dogma. Guidelines by various different authorities in the past have often been confusing, complicated, and ambiguous. Current evidence is beginning to suggest that the risk of infective endocarditis from individual procedures is small when compared to the cumulative bacteremia caused by routine daily activities. For example, activities such as tooth brushing have been estimated to cause bacteremia thousands to millions of times greater than a single tooth extraction. It is estimated that 1 in 46,000 patients is at risk of infective endocarditis from dental procedures without prior antibiotics. This risk decreases to 1 in 150,000 with the use of antibiotics. With such a high number needed to be treated, it has been suggested by some that the use of prophylactic antibiotics, with the small but real risk of anaphylaxis, may be as dangerous as beneficial for patients. Indeed, 15 to 25 people per million suffer a fatal anaphylactic reaction from administration of a single, prophylactic dose of antibiotic!

To clarify and simplify the situation, in 2007, the AHA published consensus guidelines addressing the issue of prophylactic antibiotics in infective endocarditis. These guidelines now recommend antibiotic prophylaxis for only high-risk cardiac patients with (1) prosthetic cardiac valves, (2) previous infective endocarditis, (3) unrepaired congenital heart disease, (4) congenital heart disease repaired with prosthetic material in the last 6 months, (5) repaired congenital heart disease with defects at the repair site, or (6) cardiac transplant patients who develop valvulopathy.

Antibiotic prophylaxis is recommended for dental procedures involving gingival or periapical tooth manipulation or perforation of oral mucosa. Patients with the above cardiac conditions undergoing respiratory tract, infected skin, skin structure, or musculoskeletal tissue procedures should also receive prophylaxis. The current guidelines no longer recommend prophylaxis for patients undergoing gastrointestinal or genitourinary procedures.

Penicillins are the first choice of antibiotics in infective endocarditis prophylaxis. Oral amoxicillin (2 g) should be given 30 to 60 min prior to the procedure. Intramuscular or intravenous ampicillin (2 g), ceftriaxone (1 g), or cefazolin (1 g) may be used if the patient is unable to take medication orally. Give clindamycin (600 mg), clarithromycin (600 mg), azithromycin (500 mg), or cephalexin (2 g) to patients with penicillin allergies. However, extra caution must be taken when administering cephalosporins in patients with a penicillin allergy due to the small but significant risk of cross-reactivity.

So what does today's emergency physician need to take home from all this? Give prophylactic antibiotics only to high-risk cardiac patients with a history of previous infective endocarditis, prosthetic valves, or congenital heart disease. Do not give prophylactic antibiotics for common procedures such as esophagogastroduodenoscopy, cystoscopy, or even Foley catheter insertion. If an antibiotic is indicated, make sure you administer the most appropriate drug, bearing in mind any allergies or other restrictions the patient may have. Remember that even a single dose of an antibiotic can be harmful when given inappropriately or incorrectly.

SUGGESTED READINGS

Ahlstedt S. Penicillin allergy-can the incidence be reduced? *Allergy*. 1984;39:151–164.

Duval X, Alla F, Hoen B, et al. Estimated risk of endocarditis in adults with predisposing cardiac conditions undergoing dental procedures with or without antibiotic prophylaxis. *Clin Infect Dis*. 2006;42(12):e102–e107.

Roberts GJ. Dentists are innocent! "Everyday" bacteremia is the real culprit: A review and assessment of the evidence that dental surgical procedures are a principal cause of bacterial endocarditis in children. *Pediatr Cardiol*. 1999;20(5):317–325.

Wilson W, Taubert KA, Gewitz M, et al. Prevention of infective endocarditis: Guidelines from the American Heart Association: A guideline from the American Heart Association Rheumatic Fever, Endocarditis, and Kawasaki Disease Committee, Council on Cardiovascular Disease in the Young, and the Council on Clinical Cardiology, Council on Cardiovascular Surgery and Anesthesia, and the Quality of Care and Outcomes Research Interdisciplinary Working Group. *Circulation*. 2007;116(15);1736–1754.

143

CONSIDER ENDOCARDITIS EARLY AND TREAT APPROPRIATELY

ZACHARY STURGES, MD

Infective endocarditis (IE) remains an elusive diagnosis for the emergency physician (EP). No definitive guidelines exist for ED risk stratification of patients with fever and suspicion of endocarditis, and many decisions to pursue the diagnosis rest on the history alone. Of the diagnostic criteria available, the Duke criteria are proven to be the most sensitive and should be used in place of older criteria such as the von Reyn. The Duke criteria include (1) positive blood cultures, (2) positive echo findings, and (3) physical exam findings such as fever, embolic phenomena, and end-organ dysfunction. Review the specifics, especially the weird exam findings, and know them when considering the diagnosis. Are you looking at a chest x-ray or a head CT with multiple cavitary lesions? Think IE and work it up as such. Furthermore, IE should be kept in the differential diagnosis of any fever without a source as bacteremia and IE have been shown to comprise a small but significant number of ED patients presenting with fever alone. Patients with prosthetic valves and fever without source deserve admission, antibiotics, and aggressive screening for bacteremia given their high probability of developing endocarditis.

Since the Duke criteria rely heavily on blood culture positivity, do not skimp on these. A single positive blood culture for coagulase-negative Staph ruins everyone's day. A recent retrospective study found that if only two blood cultures are obtained, 10% of bacteremias go undetected. The sensitivity of a single blood culture for bacteremia is 85% to 95%, and this climbs to 95% to 100% for two and, finally, 99% to 100% for three sets. Make it foolproof: always get two cultures immediately (15 to 20 mL of blood from two separate sites) along with your initial blood work and then another two cultures 1 h later. Following this system with every patient negates the confounders of recent antibiotic therapy and skin contaminants while providing plenty of data for the inpatient team.

Once cultures are obtained, immediately begin broad-spectrum antimicrobial therapy. Antibiotic therapy reduces embolic events, and the earlier the initiation, the earlier the benefit is seen. Only if the disease process appears indolent can these be withheld and only in consultation with the admitting service. Appropriate empiric antibiotic coverage includes initially nafcillin (12 g/24 h) or ceftriaxone (2 g/24 h) and gentamicin (3 mg/kg/24 h). If intravenous drug use (IVDU) is present or if the patient is allergic to penicillin, vancomycin (30 mg/kg/24 h) is added. Rifampin is added as a synergistic antibiotic if prosthetic material is involved. Finally, due to the high mortality of fungal endocarditis, IVDU or immunocompromised patients should have amphotericin B (5 mg/kg/d) added. Do not underdose antibiotics, do not use single agents, and do not hesitate to cover zebras—let the infectious disease specialists peel off coverage.

If you as the EP are performing bedside echocardiography to assess for vegetations, be skeptical of your findings. No data exist on the sensitivity of EP-performed transthoracic echocardiogram (TTE), but commonly cited sensitivities for vegetations seen by other practitioner's TTEs vary between 60% and 70%. In light of this poor sensitivity, absence of vegetations on TTE cannot rule out the diagnosis, and the EP should not rely on this test to do so. Admission for transesophageal echocardiogram (TEE) (sensitivity 95 + %) and appropriate antimicrobial therapy are warranted.

Historically, anticoagulation has been theorized as an adjunct in reducing embolic events related to IE. However, multiple recent studies, including the recent executive summary by the American College of Chest Physicians, recommend against this practice as it offers no benefit. There is no role for anticoagulation in the EP's management of IE. Reversal of warfarin anticoagulation is necessary if signs of embolic stroke are present due to the possibility of hemorrhagic transformation.

In summary, the EP must keep endocarditis in the differential for febrile patients and initiate a broad, thoughtful workup before initiation of antimicrobial therapy in these patients. Scour the chart for any mention of prosthetic valves, ask about IVDU, and consider prior seeding of the blood stream during surgical and dental interventions. Then, obtain your cultures and get high-dose antibiotics on board before getting the patient upstairs.

SUGGESTED READINGS

Baddour LM, Wilson WR, Bayer AS, et al. Infective endocarditis: Diagnosis, antimicrobial therapy and management of complications: A statement for healthcare professionals from the committee on rheumatic fever, endocarditis, and Kawasaki disease, council on cardiovascular disease in the young, and the councils on clinical cardiology, stroke and cardiovascular surgery and anesthesia, American Heart Association. *Circulation.* 2005;111(23):e394–e434.

Dickerman SA, Abrutyn E, Barsic B, et al. The relationship between the initiation of antimicrobial therapy and the incidence of stroke in infective endocarditis: An analysis from the ICE Prospective Cohort Study (ICE-PCS). *Am Heart J.* 2007;154(6):1086–1094.

El-Ahdab F, Benjamin DK Jr, Wang A, et al. Risk of endocarditis among patients with prosthetic valves and *Staphylococcus aureus* bacteremia. *Am J Med.* 2005;118(3):225–229.

Evangelista A, Gonzalez-Alujas MT. Echocardiography in infective endocarditis. *Heart.* 2004;90(6):614–617.

Gur H, Aviram R, Or J, et al. Unexplained fever in the ED: Analysis of 139 patients. *Am J Emerg Med.* 2003;21(3):230–235.

Lee A, Mirrett S, Reller LB, et al. Detection of bloodstream infections in adults: How many blood cultures are needed? *J Clin Microbiol.* 2007;42(11):3546–3548.

Rutledge R, Kim BJ, Applebaum RE. Actuarial analysis of the risk of prosthetic valve endocarditis in 1,598 patients with mechanical and bioprosthetic valves. *Arch Surg.* 1985;120(4):469–472.

Salem DN, Stein PD, Al-Ahmad A, et al. Antithrombotic therapy in valvular heart disease—native and prosthetic: The Seventh ACCP Conference on Antithrombotic and Thrombolytic Therapy. *Chest.* 2004;126(3 Suppl):457S–482S.

Sandre RM, Shafran SD. Infective endocarditis: Review of 135 cases over 9 years. *Clin Infect Dis.* 1996;22(2):276–286.

144

DO NOT MISS THE DIAGNOSIS OF CATHETER-RELATED BLOODSTREAM INFECTION

CHRISTINE T. TRANKIEM, MD, FACS AND HOUMAN SAEDI, MD

A catheter-related bloodstream infection (CRBSI) is defined as bacteremia/fungemia in a patient with an indwelling intravascular catheter with at least one positive blood culture obtained from a peripheral vein, clinical manifestations of infection (i.e., fever, chills, and/or hypotension), and no apparent alternative source for the bloodstream infection. Bloodstream infections are considered to be associated with a central line if the line was in use during the 48-h period before the development of the bloodstream infection. If the time interval between the onset of infection and device use is >48 h, there should be compelling evidence that the infection is related to the central line. Having said that, a sick patient presenting to the emergency department with SIRS or sepsis and a central venous catheter in place should be assumed to have a CRBSI until proven otherwise and treated promptly and aggressively as such.

Consideration of CRBSI should be a three-pronged approach: prevention, identification, and treatment.

PREVENTION IS THE BEST CURE

The best strategy regarding CRBSI is to prevent its occurrence. Prevention begins at the time of central line insertion. The current guidelines from the Institute for Healthcare Improvement suggest the use of the central line bundle whose five key components are listed below:

1) Hand hygiene: Yes, the school nurse was right. Washing your hands really does kill germs. Interestingly, many practitioners who place central lines miss performing this most basic and crucial first step.

2) Maximal barrier precautions upon insertion: This includes both you and your patient. For you: hat, eye protection, mask, sterile gown, and sterile

gloves. For your patient: sterile drapes which cover the patient from head to toe. This usually requires opening a large sterile drape in addition to the smaller one included in standard kits.

3) Chlorhexidine skin antisepsis: Chlorhexidine has been proven to be more effective than betadine-type preparations for skin antisepsis.

4) Optimal catheter site selection, with the subclavian vein as the preferred site for nontunneled catheters: The subclavian vein site is associated with fewer CRBSIs than the internal jugular vein and femoral vein positions.

5) Daily review of line necessity with prompt removal of unnecessary lines: If the patient does not require central access, get it out! Place adequate peripheral lines and remove the central line.

LOOK AT THE PATIENT

Identifying a CRBSI is the next step. The catheter skin insertion site should be inspected for signs of infection. (Do you remember from medical school calor, rubor, dolor, and tumor? These were bad back then and are still bad now.) "Every site, every day": Every central line site should be inspected on a daily basis. Even without obvious stigmata at the catheter skin insertion site, the diagnosis of CRBSI must be entertained in any patient with signs and symptoms of sepsis who has a central venous catheter. (Crash course → Sepsis in a nutshell. It's "SIRS with a source": Temperature too high or too low; WBC too high, too low, or bandemia; tachycardia; tachypnea or hypocarbia; known or presumed source of infection.) Additional signs of sepsis from CRBSI include chills, low serum albumin, acute renal failure, and urinary tract infection.

GET THE BLOOD

To confirm the diagnosis of CRBSI, obtain two or more blood cultures. A minimum of one culture from the catheter port and one from a peripheral site (ideally two peripherally) should be collected simultaneously and labeled appropriately, as earlier positivity of blood cultures drawn from catheters versus from peripheral sticks is very predictive of catheter-related sepsis. Specimen collection should be completed prior to implementing any antibiotic therapy, as this order of events maximizes the prospect of a positive culture of the organism causing the sepsis. Administering antibiotics before collecting blood cultures might prevent the ultimate recovery of a causative organism.

GET BUGS AND THEN GIVE DRUGS

As soon as a diagnosis of CRBSI has been made, treatment is the next step. After quickly obtaining blood cultures, treatment with broad-spectrum antibiotics must follow within 2 h of presentation to the emergency room. Initial choices must include broad-spectrum antibiotics and should cover Gram-positive and

Gram-negative organisms. Failure to give a drug that is active against the causative organism has a direct and negative effect on the outcome.

GET IT OUT!

The final and somewhat self-evident step in the initial treatment of CRBSI is that the central venous catheter should be removed if suspected as the source of sepsis. Its tip and the portion of the catheter directly underlying the skin entry site should be sent for culture.

SUGGESTED READINGS

Blot F, Schmidt E, Nitenberg G, et al. Earlier positivity of central venous versus peripheral blood cultures is highly predictive of catheter-related sepsis. *J Clin Microbiol*. 1998;36: 105–109.

Chaiyakunapruk N, Veenstra DL, Lipsky BA, et al. Chlorhexidine compared with povidone-iodine solution for vascular catheter-sire care, a meta-analysis. *Ann Intern Med*. 2002;136(11):792–801.

Dellinger RP, Levy MM, Carlet JM, et al. Surviving Sepsis Campaign: International guidelines for management of severe sepsis and septic shock: 2008. *Crit Care Med*. 2008;36(1): 296–327.

Ibrahim EH, Sherman G, Ward S, et al. The influence of inadequate antimicrobial treatment of bloodstream infections on patient outcomes in the ICU setting. *Chest*. 2000;118:146–155.

Lorente L, Henry c, Martin MM, et al. Central venous catheter-related infection in a prospective and observational study of 2,595 catheters. *Crit Care*. 2005;9(6):R631–R635.

O'Grady NP, Alexander M, Dellinger EP, et al. Guidelines for the prevention of intravascular catheter-related infections. Appendix A, CDC Guideline. *MMWR*. 2002;51(RR10):27–28.

Smith-Elekes S, Weinstein MP. Blood cultures. *Infect Dis Clin North Am*. 1993;7:221–234.

145

DETERMINE DECISION-MAKING CAPACITY BEFORE ALLOWING A PATIENT TO REFUSE CARE

JAN M. SHOENBERGER, MD, FAAEM, FACEP

Patients refuse care relatively frequently in the emergency department (ED). In these cases, the clinician must make a determination of the patient's decision-making capacity. If patients have the capacity to refuse care, they may simply be discharged against medical advice (AMA). If not, they may, in some cases, be treated against their will. Thus, the ability to assess decision-making capacity is a fundamental skill for anyone who evaluates patients in the ED.

Larkin et al. recently published a review on this important topic for emergency physicians. They outline four criteria that must be satisfied in order to establish adequate decision-making capacity. The patient must demonstrate the ability to

1) Receive information
2) Process and understand information
3) Deliberate
4) Make, articulate, and defend choices

Decision-making *capacity* is unlike *competency*. *Competency* is a legal conclusion that is court determined. It represents a more static (even permanent) entity. In contrast, decision-making capacity is something that varies as a function of the host and environmental factors over time. A patient who is determined to be impaired with respect to decision-making capacity may be competent for one decision and not another, depending on the seriousness and implications of the decision in question. If a patient disagrees with the recommendations of his or her physician but is nonetheless determined to have capacity, that decision must be respected.

Clear communication must be ensured when a patient expresses a desire to refuse care that an emergency provider deems necessary. Patients may not understand what is being explained, and the clinician may not understand what the patient is trying to express. The provider has an ethical obligation to take the time to explain the situation fully. If there is any question of a communication barrier, adequate measures, including the use of translators and/or other health care professionals to assist patients to understand the significance of their decision, may be necessary. Even when patients are deemed to lack decision-making capacity and thus not in a position to refuse care, good communication may help the providers create a plan with which patients will cooperate.

In the event that a patient is determined to lack capacity, a surrogate decision maker should be sought out whenever possible. Circumstances may prohibit this depending on the urgency of the situation. If the patient has a written advance directive or health care proxy, these should be followed and any named surrogates should be contacted to aid in resolution of the situation. Family members should also be contacted. If time permits, many hospitals also have ethics committees who may also be of assistance. Only when none of these options exist or circumstances prohibit taking time to explore these options, the treatment should proceed against the patient's wishes.

If there are no resources to aid the clinician in decision making on behalf of the patient, a "best-interest" standard should be used. This means that the clinician should do what a reasonable person would want to be done under the same circumstances. Once a decision is made, the reasons for the decision must be clearly documented in the medical record.

In terms of legal ramifications, one question that emergency care providers should ask themselves when faced with these cases is "if I should end up on the witness stand, can I say that I did what I thought was best for my patient who lacked decision-making capacity?" Conversely, "would I rather say that I did what the law required even though it might cause my patient to have an adverse outcome?" Both questions direct clinicians to act in the patient's best interest at all times.

Although it is an essential skill for everyday emergency medicine practice, the determination of decision-making capacity is complex and involves judgment and experience. One helpful guide to assist the clinician in these cases is the "DECISION" mnemonic:

*D*etermine need to establish decision-making capacity

*E*nsure voluntary ability to communicate

*C*orrect reversible environmental, metabolic, mental, toxicological and physical challenges to decision-making capacity

*I*nvestigate affect and cognition using standardized tests of competency, when appropriate

*S*urvey patient goals, values, and fears

*I*ntegrate information gathered to determine understanding of alternatives and foreseeable consequences

*O*penly communicate your assessment with patients and health care advocates, if present

*N*ote essential elements of decision-making capacity or its impairment in the medical record

SUGGESTED READINGS

Larkin GL, Marco CA, Abbott JT. Emergency determination of decision-making capacity: Balancing autonomy and beneficence in the emergency department. *Acad Emerg Med.* 2001;8(3):282–284.

Palmer RB, Iserson KV. The critical patient who refuses treatment: An ethical dilemma. *J Emerg Med.* 1997;15(5):729–733.

Simon JR. Refusal of care: The physician-patient relationship and decision-making capacity. *Ann Emerg Med.* 2007;50(4):456–461.

146

DO NOT IGNORE THE NURSING NOTES

MICHAEL A. SILVERMAN, MD

Whether it is an attorney pursuing a malpractice case, an expert witness, or a community medical director, one of the first steps to evaluating a bad outcome, or even a complaint, is to review the case and put together a timeline of the patient's care. The medical director does not just review the physician's component of the chart; they will review the entire chart. Contained within the chart will be a triage note and nursing notes, as well as other potential items, such as an EMS run sheet and an order sheet showing the times that orders were entered and completed. The importance of the nursing notes cannot be underestimated, especially when it comes to showing the course of the visit. Ongoing vital signs; communication with the patient, family members, and the physician; as well as the nurse's own assessment are included in the nursing notes. Most often, the nursing notes will show a concordance with the physician evaluation and assessment, lending support for the care that the physician provided. Other times, they can potentially show the physician in a bad light.

Nursing notes are used for many functions. The nurses are the ones who ask many of the Joint Commission–mandated questions, such as inquiries about the threat of physical violence or TB risk. Nursing notes contain vital signs, and most hospitals have the nurses at least initiate a medical reconciliation form. Nurses also perform assessments and interventions that get documented. Finally, nurses document observations. They will also document communication with patients, their visitors, and the physician.

Although, the triage assessment was initially designed to be a very quick process, it can now involve numerous questions and extensive history taking. In many hospitals, the physician can get the majority of the history of present illness and past medical history just from the nursing triage sheet. The physician can then perform his or her own history and confirm what the nurse has documented. Throughout the course of the ED evaluation, the nurse will add to his or her nursing notes, adding comments on patient condition, such as vital signs or peak flows after a nebulizer. In many cases, the nurses notes contain information regarding pain or other symptoms as well as tests and other interventions that the care team may be waiting for before disposition can be made.

In the absence of thorough and complete nursing notes, the hospital and staff are more vulnerable to a lawsuit. The nursing literature has numerous articles that discuss documentation and how it can prevent a lawsuit. It is believed that many times it is a nursing act of omission that contributes to a lawsuit, such as failure to do timely and adequate assessments, to follow-up on tests or treatments, or to notify a physician in a timely fashion about a significant abnormality.

There are also certainly times where the physician disagrees with the nursing assessment or other documented information. First, the doctor should not approach the nurse and ask him or her to change his or her assessment. After all, this was the nurse's assessment at the time. However, doctors can write a note adjacent to the nursing documentation that says that the current history, fact, or assessment is different from their interpretation. Physicians can also write in their own assessment referencing the nursing documentation and then account for the discrepancy.

Many doctors cringe when they hear a nurse say, "just so you know." Physicians are often cautious when they know that the chart will then read "MD aware." However, such documentation is part of a nurses job. It is then physicians' job to decide what to do with that information. It may mean writing an order for pain medicine or documenting the pertinent information on the medical record with a plan to monitor. Nonetheless, it is these types of communication between the nurse and doctor that can make a difference in patient care. If a doctor is initially unapproachable, how likely is it that the nurse will come back to the doctor when a patient is starting to have a bit of respiratory distress? Nurses, after being yelled out previously to let the medicines do their job, may sit back and wait, only to then find the patient in severe respiratory distress a short time later. Had the nurse notified the physician to intervene earlier, perhaps the mild respiratory distress could have been handled before symptoms became worse.

It is potentially an unrealistic expectation that the physician will review the entire nursing note on every patient. However, the physician must be aware of critical events in the patient care environment and should make a habit of reviewing key parts of the nursing note, including ongoing vital sign monitoring, rhythm strips, pain levels, and any new complaints, particularly prior to discharge.

Many people go into emergency medicine because of the team environment. The communication between the physician and the nurse, whether written or verbal, is a critical component of the team functioning at its highest level and will likely help improve patient care and help prevent possible litigation.

SUGGESTED READINGS

Patel PB, Vinson DR. Team assignment system: Expediting emergency department care. *Ann Emerg Med*. 2005;46(6):499–506 [Epub 2005 Sep 1].

Zimmermann PG. Preventing lawsuits by noting and acting on key aspects in a patient's condition. *Orthop Nurs*. 2008;27(1):31–35.

147

INFORMED CONSENT SHOULD BE HONORED IN THE EMERGENCY DEPARTMENT WHENEVER POSSIBLE

ARJUN S. CHANMUGAM, MD, MBA

Over 40 years ago, the concept of informed consent was introduced into the U.S. case law. It has since become the standard principle to guide medical treatment. Its foundation lies in both the law and bioethics. Despite the emphasis informed consent has on a national and societal basis, informed consent to treatment is not an absolute right, as there are exceptions. Notably, in situations where immediate treatment is required to prevent death or serious harm to a patient, care may be provided without first obtaining informed consent. Such an exception provides a very convenient and necessary exclusion which is especially relevant in emergency medicine. However, it should not be used as a license for emergency physicians to suspend one of their primary obligations to patients—that is to inform their patients about their treatment alternatives and to explicitly obtain permission for treatment.

The exception for informed consent has its place for a significant number of emergency department patients; for this population, there is little concern about the lack of informed consent. This applies to any patient in extremis, any patient who requires immediate stabilization, any patient who is too ill to effectively communicate, and any patient who is unable to communicate because of an acute need. For all other patients, the doctrine of informed consent must be applied, because of its legal implications and its moral obligations.

The doctrine of informed consent has well-established legal implications. It serves as a vehicle for establishing duties of disclosure and for financially compensating patients for injuries suffered as a result of failure to disclose information about a treatment. How does this affect the practicing physician? Ignoring informed consent can result in legal action that is based on two different theories of liability—battery and negligence. Battery is the intentional, nonconsensual, and offensive touching of the patient by the physician. The concept of battery has to do with patients' physical integrity against unwanted invasion. Negligence has more to do with the physician's unintentional failure to satisfy a professional standard of care which in the case of informed consent has been to provide significant relevant information about the risks and complications of potential treatment interventions or other interventions. The basic elements that need to be present to prove negligence with regards to informed consent are the following:

1) The physician had a duty to disclose information regarding a treatment or intervention.
2) The physician did not disclose that information (breach of duty).
3) The treatment or intervention resulted in harm to the patient.
4) Harm was the materialization of undisclosed information about that risk.
5) The patient would not have consented to the treatment had the patient been given the necessary information about the risk.

Although there are legal implications of informed consent, the moral obligations are also considerable. Some claim that the ethic of informed consent has its origins in the post–World War II era. After the Nuremberg trials, there were 10 standards that were articulated regarding physicians' responsibility for human subject experimentation. In this setting of heightened human rights, the concept of voluntary informed consent became firmly established. In 1957, the term informed consent found its way from case law into the medical community. It became the basis for medical ethics and fostered further debate about decisional authority. Ultimately, the moral foundation of informed consent rests on two essential values, patient well-being and patient autonomy. Providing patients with the necessary information and options allows patients to decide what is best for them based on their individual values, beliefs, and traditions. This has the dual function of fostering well-being and enhances each patient's sovereign decision-making right.

The essence of informed consent rests on three basic features. The patient must have the mental capacity to understand the options given to him or her and the ability to make an informed reasonable decision based on his or her individual beliefs and values. Second, the patient must be presented the options along with the background information so that the patient has the necessary information to make a reasoned decision. Finally, the patient must feel comfortable such that there is no element of coercion or duress that will impede a freely made decision.

Informed consent is the basis of physician-patient relationship. Although emergency physicians are often expected to intervene as quickly as possible to stabilize some patients without obtaining informed consent, it is not an excuse to suspend the informed consent standard. There is widespread understanding that some emergency patients are not capable of giving informed consent because of their condition. On the other hand, there is also awareness that many emergency department patients are capable of giving informed consent. Furthermore, some authors are quick to point that many emergency department patients do not have a true emergency and thus should benefit from the full informed consent concept. Honoring the principals of informed consent as much as possible in the ED goes a long way in preserving the integrity of the doctor-patient relationship.

SUGGESTED READING

Moskop J. Informed consent in the emergency department. *Emerg Med Clin North Am.* 1999;17(2):327–340.

148

KNOW THE LAWS FOR CONSENT OF MINORS AND ADOLESCENTS IN THE EMERGENCY DEPARTMENT

JAN M. SHOENBERGER, MD, FAAEM, FACEP

Minors frequently present to the emergency department (ED) for care without their parents. A 1991 study in Michigan found that 3% of visits by minors to EDs were unaccompanied, and some sources believe this number to be higher. Unaccompanied minors may be brought to the ED by emergency medical services or by babysitters or other caretakers. They may also present without their parents because they are seeking care for complex psychosocial issues like sexually transmitted infections or pregnancy.

In the case of minors unaccompanied by parents, there are pitfalls related to consent issues. In general, minors require parental consent for medical procedures. There are several exceptions, however. An exception is made in the case of emergencies because a delay in care may jeopardize the minor's health.

The definition of "emergency care" in these situations may include not only life-threatening illnesses but also the treatment of pain and interventions that have the potential to prevent disability. In cases where there is no time for consent, emergency physicians are expected to act in the child's best interest and proceed with treatment that would be deemed reasonable. Consent is also not required for the initial evaluation and stabilization of a minor.

Another exception to required parental consent is for the treatment of certain conditions. Many states allow minors to seek medical care for treatment related to sexually transmitted infections, contraception, pregnancy, mental illness, and drug/alcohol abuse. States differ in the specific ages and conditions for which minors may seek care without parental consent. In cases where state law is not clear, courts have acknowledged the "mature minor" rule. Under this rule, a minor (usually an adolescent) may be deemed by the physician as capable of giving the same degree of consent as an adult and therefore may consent to treatment, provided that the treatment is low risk. The process by which the physician obtains informed consent is the same as would be followed in the case of an adult. The adolescent must demonstrate understanding of the risks and benefits of the various treatment options. The age that is most commonly agreed upon as having capacity to make decisions and consent to treatment is 14 years of age.

Emancipated minors are another category of minors who do not need parental consent. These are adolescents who do not live at home and are self-supported. Pregnant or married minors also are considered to be emancipated, as are those in the military or those who have been declared emancipated by the court. The exact definition of an emancipated minor varies somewhat from state to state.

If an emergency physician cares for an adolescent minor without parental consent, physician-patient communications are confidential. Thus, if the parent of an adolescent were to inquire as to the nature of the visit or wanted any information, the physician would not be able to reveal any information without the consent of the patient. In situations involving drug or alcohol abuse, sexually transmitted infections, pregnancy, or mental illness, adolescents should, however, be encouraged to talk with their parents or guardian so that they have the possibility of obtaining the much needed parental support. The American Medical Association endorses the concept of confidential health care for adolescent patients. They state,

> When in the opinion of the physician, parental involvement would not be beneficial, parental consent or notification should not be a barrier to care....The same confidentiality will be preserved between the adolescent patient and physician as between the parent (or responsible adult) and the physician.

SUGGESTED READINGS

Baren JM. Ethical dilemmas in the care of minors in the emergency department. *Emer Med Clin North Am.* 2006;24(3):619–631.

Gans JE, ed. *Policy Compendium on Confidential Health Services for Adolescents.* Chicago, IL: American Medical Association; 1993.

Holden A. Minors' right to consent to medical care. *JAMA.* 1987;57:1099–1101.

Jacobstein CR, Baren JM. Emergency department treatment of minors. *Emerg Med Clin N Am.* 1999;17(2):341–352.

Keshavarz R. Adolescents, informed consent and confidentiality: A case study. *Mt Sinai J Med.* 2005;72(4):232–235.

Treloar DJ, Peterson E, Randall J, et al. Use of emergency services by unaccompanied minors. *Ann Emerg Med.* 1991;20(3):297–230.

Weddle M, Kokotailo P. Adolescent substance abuse: Confidentiality and consent. *Pediatr Clin North Am.* 2002;49(2):301–315.

149

KNOW WHAT IS IN YOUR CONTRACT

TERRENCE W. BROWN, MD, JD, MS

One of the most eagerly anticipated and anxiety-provoking milestones of the soon-to-be attending physician as well as the seasoned emergency physician is the auspicious signing of the next employment contract. Physicians approach this process with a range of emotions, varying degrees of preparation, and often scant attention to details. Some hire attorneys who handle almost every aspect of the negotiation process and meticulously review and revise each contract draft prior to committing to a signed document. A few may just briefly glance over their contracts once, only to make sure if the name, hours, and compensation seem about right. Most physicians hope that by at least carefully reading each contract provision, with an eye toward a tweak here and there, they will protect their interests as they transition to practice. Whichever approach you choose, there are some key aspects of the contracting process to bear in mind to protect your most important asset—you—as you embark on the next phase of your career.

Contract law is a complex field. The key elements of any employment contract are designed to minimize any confusion regarding the respective duties, rights, and responsibilities of each party to the contract and are particularly important when a dispute arises. Most litigation is not the result of one party's attempt to unscrupulously deprive the other party of his or her rights and equity. Although this does happen, most litigation is the consequence of an agreement that did not clearly reflect both parties' views of their respective obligations and an inadequate attention to the contract details such that each parties' views are memorialized in clear, unambiguous terms prior to signing.

There a few key aspects of physician contracts that deserve special attention, as they are frequent sources of confusion and potential litigation:

1) What is Your Employer's Business Organization Form?

If you have not yet thought strategically about your prospective employer's legal business structure, now is the time to start, as each business entity form implicates differing financial benefits and legal risks for you when you sign on as an employee. You may face vastly different personal and tax liabilities based on whether your employer is a partnership, corporation, limited liability company, or government entity, and these obligations may differ according to what status you have when you first start practicing with them. If you are signing on as a partner with a financial "buy in," be aware you are also buying into the firm's legal and financial obligations, unless you specially ask for an "indemnification" provision that protects you from costs incurred prior to your sign on. As a partner, you will be liable for the acts of the partnership that do not involve medical decision making, including billing fraud, Medicare violations, and state and federal regulatory sanctions. Employees of the above organizations may be entitled to some basic protections under law (albeit in many states only minimal ones) that independent contractors do not have. Be aware that for tax purposes, in particular, the mere recital of your role as "independent contractor" does not necessarily mean the Internal Revenue Service (IRS) will recognize you as such. If your contract is structured in a way more closely resembling the typical employer-employee relationship, you may end up with tax consequences you did not anticipate.

2) How Do You Become a Full Member of Your Employer's Organization?

A frustrating realization that may present after investing some years and sweat equity with your practice group is that the "easy" path promised to full partner or shareholder status is in fact fraught with unanticipated obstacles. Does your contract spell out a specific time limit after which you are entitled to buy in as a member of your group? Does it spell out explicitly the milestones you must reach along the way? Contract provisions that state you are "eligible" to join an organization or that the key players will "consider" your application to join once you hit certain benchmarks are not equivalent to a contractual obligation to extend an offer. If a sure path to partner or shareholder is important to you, make sure that your contract provides explicitly for such a path and that any prerequisite conditions (hours worked, revenue earned, administrative contributions made) are spelled out clearly in your contract.

3) What Kind of Malpractice Protection Does Your Contract Provide?

Most employers offer paid malpractice coverage. Find out which of the two major types of coverage you will have. An "occurrence" policy covers you for claims made against you no matter when the claim is made. A "claims made" policy covers claims made only during a specified term—usually up to when your employment ends; a "tail" policy is used to cover any claims made after you leave. Your employer has no obligation to provide you with tail coverage unless it is expressly provided for in your contract, and your contract might have a clause that requires you to pay for this coverage if you resign or if you breach your contract. Make sure that your contract specifically states the kind of coverage your employer is providing, including what the maximum payout per claim limits are. If you have doubts about your employer's ability to protect you from future liability, ask for a proof of coverage document to review and ask that it be made part of the contract if you find it satisfactory.

4) What If You Want to End Your Employment?

Few physicians think (or want) to plan for ease of exit from their first job (or even subsequent jobs) and are often surprised at the financial and legal implications of even the most amicable of separations. With the oft-quoted reality that almost one half of new attendings will change positions within just 3 years after graduation, it is imperative to consider how that first contract will dictate just how easy (or painful) the first career transition might be. Resignation may set in motion contractual events that are unexpected and disadvantageous to the physician, including loss of past and present bonuses, relinquishment of shares, forfeit of hospital privileges, and in the case of partnerships, payment to the firm for future liabilities.

The contract may regulate the means by which you can terminate your employment and will most certainly provide for the means by which the employer can terminate you. Find out how much notice the employer must give you before ending your employment and what, if any, due process the contract grants you as a means of fixing whatever problems led to this point. Most contracts are "at will," meaning you can be terminated for any reason, without cause. Unless you are working for a government entity, you are not entitled by law to any due process in such cases, and any notice prior to termination is required only to the extent that your contract provides for it. Most terminations that occur "for cause" do not allow for practical notice, such as in the case of commission of fraud, felony, loss of license or credentials, or disability. Terminations "without cause" generally should be bilateral and allow reasonable notice for both parties—notice provisions vary from 30 to 90 days.

5) Should I Ever Sign a Contract With a Restrictive Covenant?

A restrictive covenant, or "noncompete" clause, is a legal protection sought by business organizations seeking to limit the ability of a former employee to compete with the organization after his or her contract ends and the employee takes up practice elsewhere. Courts have been ambivalent about enforcing restrictive covenants, typically finding them enforceable only when they are found to be narrowly tailored to protect the organization's business interests and if they are seen to be reasonable in geographic scope and length of time. A typical non-compete clause might read: "Employee agrees not to take a position within 25 mi of Employer for a period of 3 years after termination." Such a clause effectively locks you out of your current market and, depending on your contract, may do so even if you are terminated involuntarily. Although ubiquitous in physician contracts, restrictive covenants have a limited logic in emergency medicine; patients do not choose emergency departments based on what attending is working.

Typically, such clauses in emergency medicine contracts are drafted by a group practice concerned that its employees may form a separate group and compete directly to "steal" their former practice's hospital contract. Such an eventuality does not require an overly broad restrictive covenant, and if a potential employer insists on one, this should prompt you to investigate what troubles are brewing in your future job market that make such a clause so important. Do not be lulled into the oft-stated myth that "restrictive covenants are rarely enforced." While this may be true in your future geographic market, it does not protect you from the costs of litigation should an employer choose to enforce a contract provision you have already signed. Ultimately, as with any contract provision, the decision to accept such a restriction boils down to what you stand to gain in return and involves the art of negotiation.

6) Am I Ready to Sign?

There are a number of great resources available to you as you begin the contracting process. Most state medical societies offer some degree of free advice about general issues unique to their health care environment. Many law firm web pages publish helpful tips, including case law updates, on physician contract issues. The American Medical Association offers an excellent online publication, "Contracts—What You Need to Know," that provides a comprehensive review of the basic provisions of a good contract, as well as advice to consider during the negotiation process. The Emergency Medicine Residents' Association's "Contract Issues for Emergency Physicians" is a useful primer on both contract negotiation and drafting with an emphasis on issues common to the emergency medicine practitioner. No such resource is a substitute, however, for professional legal counsel. Just as you would not (hopefully) curbside your cardiologist colleague to read a pelvic ultrasound to rule out ectopic, do not rely on the casual advice of your cousin, the criminal defense attorney, in making a contract decision. Health care law issues vary significantly from state to state, and a lawyer with contracts experience in your future home state can identify the unique legal landmines lurking in your contract. Familiarizing yourself ahead of time with the essential elements of the contract negotiation and signing process can help you work with your attorney, as a team, to ensure that your particular interests are protected.

SUGGESTED READINGS

American Medical Association. Contracts: What you need to know. The American Medical Association Young Physicians Section. March, 1997. Available at: http://www.ama-assn.org/

George J. Contract law: It's only as good as the people. *Emerg Med Clin North Am.* 2004;22(1):217–224.

Lowry JW. Covenants not to compete in physician contracts: Recent trends defining reasonableness at common law. *J Leg Med.* 2003;24(2):215–232.

Wood JP, Rapp MT, Shufeldt JJ, eds. *EMRA Contract Issues for Emergency Physicians.* 2nd ed. Irving, TX: Emergency Medicine Residents' Association; 2007.

150

KNOW YOUR RESPONSIBILITY FOR "LEFT WITHOUT BEING SEEN" PATIENTS

MICHAEL A. SILVERMAN, MD

In the United States, there are about 5,000 emergency departments (EDs). In a recent survey study, crowding in the ED was found to be pervasive with multiple factors contributing to this phenomenon. These factors affecting crowding in the ED include patient hospital bed shortages, insufficient availability of ED examination beds, shortages in RN staff, increasing medical acuity, and, of course, increasing patient volume. The full impact of crowding and its implications for health care delivery have yet to be well described. However, there is a growing body of literature to suggest that there may be increased risks of harm to patients resulting from impaired communication and diminished access to care, all leading to possible increases in morbidity and mortality.

One of the consequences of increased crowding is patients leaving the ED without being fully evaluated or at least screened. For whatever reasons, the tolerance of patients to wait for hours has become somewhat limited. Twenty years ago, it would have been unheard of for patients to call 911 when they were already in an ED waiting room. Waits of 12 or more hours in EDs as a result of crowding has caused increased public scrutiny; in the 21st century, ED waiting room patients calling 911 to ask for help has occurred. More importantly, increased reports of patients suffering significant injury secondary to delay of care—or worse dying in the ED waiting room—has raised the awareness of the medical community and the public alike. As the average wait for care in an ED has increased, the possibility that patients' tire of waiting and leave the ED without having an appropriate evaluation also increases. The manner in which

EDs handle wait times and patient's who leave without being seen (LWBS) can impact liability, patient safety, and hospital finances.

The Emergency Medical Treatment and Active Labor Act has had a huge impact on EDs. It was passed in 1986 as part of the Combined Omnibus Budget Reconciliation Act and is often referred to as the COBRA law, or EMTALA. (In 1989, an amendment removed the word "Active" from the official name of the statute.) The statute only applies to "participating hospitals" which are defined as hospitals who accept payment from the Department of Health and Human Services, Center for Medicare and Medicaid Services. This essentially means every hospital in the United States except for maybe the Shriners Hospital and many military hospitals. The key provision associated with this chapter topic is as follows: any patient who comes to an ED requesting examination or treatment for a medical condition must be provided with an appropriate medical screening examination to determine if he or she is suffering from an emergency medical condition. If an emergency medical condition exists, then the patient must be stabilized or transferred to another hospital. In other words, EDs are required to comply with providing a medical screening exam to all who present to the ED. Depending on the state, the institution, and the triage model, this may be done by a physician, midlevel provider, or in some cases, a nurse.

Once the triage has been completed, having a policy and procedure in place that can ensure continued monitoring of patients who are waiting is necessary. While the best case scenario is that the doctor is aware of all of the patients in the waiting room, the reality is that, in most cases, this task falls to the charge nurse. Triage assessments must be reliable so that patients wait no more than what is considered a medically appropriate time. Vital signs should be reevaluated on a regular basis while patients are in the waiting room. (The Joint Commission recommends following your own established protocol, though many hospitals use two hours as a guideline.) Patients with a change in vital signs or a change in symptoms should be reassessed and have their triage level adjusted appropriately.

There is no doubt that in the court of public opinion, the hospital bears some responsibility when someone dies in the waiting room after a prolonged wait. Was the triage assessment appropriate based on the chief complaint and vital signs? Did the wait time exceed the national standards for that triage level? Were reassessments performed on a regular basis? These are questions that need answering when reviewing the individual case.

Due to prolonged waits, a small percentage of patients may leave prior to being seen in the ED and forfeit their right to a medical screening exam. Every physician has probably been aware of patients who left within the first 15 min of a wait, though usually patients will wait several hours before making the decision to leave.

Patients are allowed to leave prior to being fully evaluated. However, the ED has the responsibility to make sure that these patients are cognitively appropriate. In other words, patients who are allowed to leave should have no evidence of intoxication, psychosis, or delirium such as the patient who is postictal after a seizure. Patients must be able to make an informed decision about the risks of leaving prior to their screening exam. Some patients will present back to the triage or charge nurse and will announce that they are leaving. The hospital health care professional, whether it is a nurse or physician, should document the patient's mental status and his or her refusal to wait for a medical screening exam.

Emergency physicians have long been taught that they are responsible for patients who are waiting in the waiting room. To some extent, they may actually be responsible for the patients who choose not to wait as well.

SUGGESTED READINGS

ACEP. After the medical screening exam: Non-emergent care and the ethics of access in the emergency department. *Practice Resources*. Available at: http://www.acep.org/practres. aspx?id = 30112

Moskop JC. Informed consent in the emergency department. *Emerg Med Clin North Am.* 1999;17(2):327–340.

Strickler J. EMTALA: The basics. *JONAS Healthc Law Ethics Regul.* 2006;8(3):77–81; quiz 82–83.

Twanmoh JR, Cunningham GP. When overcrowding paralyzes an emergency department. *Manag Care.* 2006;15(6):54–59.

www.emtala.com. A resource for current information about the Federal Emergency Medical Treatment and Active Labor Act, also known as COBRA or the Patient Anti-Dumping Law.

151

MAINTAIN A PROPER BALANCE BETWEEN PATIENT CARE AND COOPERATION WITH LAW ENFORCEMENT OFFICERS

JAN M. SHOENBERGER, MD, FAAEM, FACEP

Law enforcement officers are frequently present in the emergency department (ED). They may be present at the request of the staff to provide protection from a potentially violent visitor or patient. They also may be escorting a patient to the ED from an accident or crime scene or seeking information about patients who were transported by ambulance. Officers may want to interview patients in the ED or collect evidence. In any of these scenarios, emergency care providers must keep in mind some important pitfalls.

Clinicians must be careful not to violate either the Health Insurance Portability and Accountability Act (HIPAA) or their fundamental duty to protect patient privacy when interacting with officers who are seeking information. Information should not be shared with the police without permission from the patient.

Officers often seek to obtain immediate access to patients in the ED. This may delay or interfere with patient evaluation and treatment or potentially worsen the condition of an unstable patient. This should be unacceptable to any health care provider; the patients' best interest should always be kept in mind.

If the police wish to interview a patient in the ED and if they will not interfere with immediate patient care needs, this should be communicated to the patient. Patients may decide for themselves whether or not they choose to speak with the police and what information is released. If a patient agrees, the physician has the responsibility to monitor the patient and to stop the interview if his or her clinical or mental condition begins to deteriorate. In the case of children or patients with surrogates, the police should not be allowed access until parents or surrogates have been contacted and informed.

Intoxicated patients, those with altered mental status, or those with underlying cognitive limitations deserve special mention. If the physician feels they are not capable of participating or consenting to a police interview, he or she should advise the police that the interview might be compromised. If the officer wishes to proceed and believes that there is valuable information that can be gained, surrogates or physicians may decide to allow the interview to proceed. If the patients' capacity is in question, psychiatric consultation may be advisable.

Physicians may be asked to assist the police either directly (by asking questions) or indirectly (by encouraging patients to cooperate). Police officers and physicians have different roles and obligations to the patient, and this is particularly true if the patient is a suspect in a criminal case. Physicians have a duty to respect patient privacy and play a role that involves assumed trust on the part of the patient. The police do not have such a relationship with the patient/suspect and no such duty to protect confidentiality or privacy.

The American College of Emergency Physicians (ACEP) policy statement regarding law enforcement information gathering in the ED states

> The American College of Emergency Physicians believes that the physician-patient relationship requires that the confidentiality of protected health information be maintained. Emergency physicians should adhere to federal and state laws addressing privacy and confidentiality. Except when legally required, information about a patient should not be released without permission from the patient or surrogate decision maker. When necessary, the presence of law enforcement or security officials without patient consent is appropriate to ensure the safety of patients and staff. Documentation of law enforcement interactions with the patient may include

audio or video recordings. Without all parties' consent, these recordings should not include any physician-patient or staff-patient communication or interaction.

In addition to this policy, individual institutions may have additional applicable policies, and these can be helpful to guide physicians in their interactions with police. Individual states also have laws that apply to specific situations, such as the collection of blood in suspected impaired driving cases. ED staff should not obstruct the police in carrying out their responsibilities under the law.

When the police are present in the ED, they should not visualize or listen to the care of other patients. Although they frequently proceed unaccompanied through an ED, they should ideally be treated like any visitor in the department and their business in the department should be limited to the specific patient they seek to contact.

The relationship between the police and physicians need not be antagonist; but both parties have a job to do that is bound by separate legal and ethical obligations. It is in the best interest of all parties that professional boundaries be respected on both sides.

SUGGESTED READINGS

Jones PM, Appelbaum PS, Siegel DM. Law enforcement interviews of hospital patients. *JAMA.* 2006;295(7):822–825.
Law enforcement information gathering in the emergency department. *American College of Emergency Physicians.* Available at: http://www.acep.org/practres.aspx?id = 29538. Accessed November 23, 2008.
Moskop JC, Marco CA, Larkin GL, et al. From Hippocrates to HIPAA: Privacy and confidentiality in emergency medicine – part II: Challenges in the emergency department. *Ann Emerg Med.* 2005;45(1):60–67.

152

NEVER TALK TO YOUR PATIENT'S LAWYER UNLESS YOUR OWN LAWYER IS PRESENT

STEPHEN G. HOLTZCLAW, MD, FACEP

The emergency department (ED) can be a challenging place for both patients as well as providers. There are multiple factors that make it difficult for the emergency physician to provide care, including but not limited to time constraints, resource limitations, overcrowding issues, lack of longitudinal access of care, and specialist availability. Patients often have unrealistic expectations as to the course of their diagnosis and treatment, and many patients present with high-acuity illness. Additionally, the ED is an operationally complex environment of triage, consultations, admission, and discharge. This perpetual cycle of hand-offs and care transfer amplifies the difficulty in establishing and maintaining a continuous relationship with patients. The net result is that patients may seek legal counsel regarding some element of their care in the ED.

Medical errors in the ED are a fact of life. Given the complexity of the working environment and the very nature of episodic care, the likelihood of an error occurring at some point exists. Not all errors result in poor patient outcome. Nevertheless, this too may serve as impetus for a patient to contact a lawyer.

WHEN YOU DO GET A CALL FROM A PATIENT'S LAWYER, SHOULD YOU TALK TO HIM OR HER?

The short answer is No! You should not talk to him or her. The first step is to stop and evaluate the situation. There are some preliminary considerations that should be addressed. For instance, consider your insurance policy and recognize that insurance carriers need to be involved as early as possible. In many cases, the first step you should take is to contact your insurance carrier and ask for a lawyer to represent you. This can be a critical step, because with some insurance policies, they become void if you do not contact the insurance company within a specified, and often short, period of time! Also, check your employment contract, you may be required to notify other individuals including someone from the ED group, the hospital legal office, or some other office.

If a patient has contacted a lawyer, it is likely that they are considering a suit. If you speak to the lawyer, anything you say can be held against you and possibly admitted into evidence. Some lawyers may call and say they are only gathering facts about the case and you are not the target. *Do not fall for this*! In many cases, they are looking for any admissions or potentially inaccurate statements you may make. You should only speak to the patient's lawyer if your lawyer is sitting next to you or has reviewed your situation and clears you to speak without counsel present. Similarly, if you are asked to give a deposition in a legal case or state board of medicine inquiry where you are not the defendant, be sure to contact your insurance carrier/lawyer first. The goal here is to protect you from being a target down the line. In other words, you do not want to say anything that will turn you into a defendant.

Once you learn of a potential lawsuit, do not discuss the case with anyone but your lawyer. It is tempting to "run the case by" a colleague or codefendant. This is more than a confidentiality issue, because the plaintiff's lawyer will ask you if you have discussed the case with anyone. If so, they will subpoena everyone you spoke to and ask them what you said! Additionally, do not discuss the case with the patient or the patient's family for the same reason.

In summary, emergency medicine is a specialty that has many inherent difficulties. Medical errors can occur. It seems likely that at some point in your career, a patient's lawyer may contact you. If that does happen, do not talk to the lawyer without taking some important first steps: contact your insurance company; make sure that you have notified all the right people and offices as stipulated by your emergency medicine practice policy. The bottom line: make sure you have proper legal counsel before you talk to any plaintiff's attorney.

SUGGESTED READINGS

Dodge AM, Fitzer SF. *When Good Doctors Get Sued: A Guide for Defendant Physicians Involved in Malpractice Lawsuits.* Oregon: BookPartners; 2001.

Fish R, Ehrhardt M, Fish B. *Malpractice: Managing Your Defense.* 2nd ed. Saddlebrook, NJ: Medical Economics Books; 1990.

Kachalia A, Gandhi KT, Puopolo AL, et al. Missed and delayed diagnoses in the emergency department: A study of closed malpractice claims from 4 liability insurers. *Ann Emerg Med.* 2007;49(2):196–205.

153

THOROUGHLY UNDERSTAND THE EMERGENCY MEDICAL TREATMENT AND LABOR ACT

ROBERT R. MARSHALL, JR, MBA

The Emergency Medical Treatment and Labor Act (EMTALA), enacted in 1986, was intended to ensure public access to emergency service, including active labor, regardless of ones ability to pay. Hospitals are obligated to provide a medical screening examination (MSE) to anyone who comes to the emergency department presenting with an emergency medical condition. Stabilizing treatment must be provided prior to discharge, according to the hospital's capability, or transfer to a higher level of care. EMTALA is also referred to as the Emergency Medical Treatment and "Active" Labor Act. Both are correct. The word "Active" was deleted to further clarify a more broad definition of labor.

TRIAGE IS NOT THE MEDICAL SCREENING EXAMINATION

MSE must be done by individuals, usually a physician, determined to be qualified by the hospital's bylaws. Additionally, the MSE is that which is reasonably performed, including ancillary testing to determine if an emergency medical condition exists. MSEs may be performed in the triage area and may be done parallel to the triage process. Medical screening exams can take the place of triage, but stand-alone nurse triage does not satisfy the requirement for a medical screening exam.

Medical Screening Exam Is Not Always Done in the Emergency Department

Medical screening exams can be done in other departments as hospital policy. For example, many hospitals send patients in active labor immediately to labor and delivery. Additionally, patients with minor burns, in some cases, may go directly to the burn unit. In both of these cases, the unit receiving the patient performs the medical screening exam. There must be an agreement that provides clear guidance on who is responsible for the medical screening exam as a matter of policy.

EMTALA Requirements Are not Exclusive to Patients Presenting to the Emergency Department

Emergency services do not need to be provided in the emergency department. Individuals presenting to any location on the hospital property and seeking emergency treatment are entitled to a medical screening exam under EMTALA. The medical screening exam can occur at any location within the hospital, as long as the patient is accompanied by qualified medical personnel; there is a medical reason to move the patient; and all patients with similar medical conditions are treated in the same manner.

EMTALA Requirements Are Not Limited to the Property Inside the Hospital

In fact, hospital property can include an entire medical campus. Generally, hospital property is defined as the physical area immediately adjacent to hospital buildings or the physical area located within 250 yards of main hospital buildings. Patients seeking emergency services are entitled to a medical screening exam. Again, all patients with similar conditions are to be treated in the same manner. Patients are expected to be treated by qualified medical personnel within the hospital and not transferred until after stabilized.

Ravenswood Hospital—This hospital was fined $40,000 when it refused to treat a patient in an alley proximal to the emergency department. The patient, who was suffering from gunshot wounds and left there by friends, was eventually wheeled to the emergency department by police after hospital personnel would not come to his aid. He died of his injuries. The hospital had a policy of not allowing hospital personnel to leave hospital grounds. While this case occurred prior to the 250-yard rule, it emphasizes the meaning of "coming to the emergency department."

EMTALA ALSO APPLIES TO PATIENTS ARRIVING BY GROUND OR AIR TRANSPORT

In a 2008 appeals court decision, it was determined that a patient en route to a hospital by a nonhospital owned ambulance is protected by EMTALA. The United States' first Circuit Court of Appeals sided with the nineth Circuit Court when it determined the patient has "come to the hospital" when the hospital is notified by the ambulance by radio or telephone that the patient is en route. In this case, paramedics were asked for insurance information. When it was not given, the conversation was abruptly terminated. The paramedics determined this as a refusal to accept the patient.

EMTALA DOES EXTEND TO OTHER SPECIALISTS THROUGH ITS ON-CALL PROVISION

In 1998, CMS (HCFA, Health Care Financing Administration renamed Centers for Medicare and Medicaid Services) clarified its intent on on-call physicians. Emergency departments must be proactively aware of which physicians are available to treat and stabilize individuals with emergency medical conditions. Further, hospital policies should specify responsibilities of on-call physicians to respond.

EMTALA MAY APPLY IN FOLLOW-UP CARE SITUATIONS

Generally speaking, once a patient is discharged and stable, EMTALA no longer applies. The operative phase is stable. However, patients must be given a plan for appropriate follow-up care with the discharge instructions. Emergency departments have the responsibility to refer patients to providers that will provide follow-up care. If they believe patients will not get care, there is an obligation to provide a referral to a provider that will provide care.

Conclusion. In summary, EMTALA has several provisions, the central one focusing on the need to provide an MSE. Patients do not have to present to the ED for EMTALA to apply but can be anywhere on the hospital property, indeed even within 250 yards of the medical campus. EMTALA does extend to other specialists. Each ED should have clear policies regarding its on-call specialists.

SUGGESTED READINGS

Centers for Medicare and Medicaid Service (CMS). http://www.cms.hhs.gov/emtala/.

Frew SA. Ambulance eedirect ruling from 1st circuit. Federal Court upholds EMTALA in ambulance radio denial case. MedLaw.com, May 16, 2008. Available at: http://www.med-law.com/healthlaw/EMTALA/courtcases/ambulance-redirect-ruling-from-1st-circuit.shtml.

Moy MM. *The EMTALA Answer Book*. New York: Aspen Publishers; 2005.

[No author noted]. Special note—What is the 250-yard rule and how does it affect these issues? Available at: http://www.emtala.com/250yard.htm.

www.EMTALA.com.

www.MEDLAW.com.

154

UNDERSTAND THE BASICS OF MEDICAL MALPRACTICE IN ORDER TO AVOID IT

PAULA M. NEIRA, RN, JD, CEN

Emergency medicine is one of medicine's most litigated practices. The Department of Health and Human Services estimated that between $60 and $108 billion are added to health care costs each year due to medical liability costs (Lynch, 2008). Every emergency department (ED) provider and nurse, to some degree, practices defensively—whether by ordering an additional test or spending extra time on documentation—in the hopes of staving off what appears to be an inevitable negligence lawsuit. Obviously, the best way to counter the threat of litigation is to avoid negligence in the first place. Doing so includes understanding the applicable legal standards, recognizing high-risk activities and vulnerabilities, and communicating clearly what actions were taken on the patient's behalf.

The ED physician should recognize that medical negligence (malpractice) lawsuits often result from poor outcomes and the human desire to place blame. Some people cannot accept that outcomes are sometimes poor despite every best effort. However, do not think that all lawsuits are frivolous. Real cases of malpractice occur; those cases usually quickly settle before trial. Of the cases that do go to trial, the defendant practitioner prevails the majority of the time (PIAA, 2005).

Malpractice cases sound in tort law, an area of civil liability. The burden of proof lies with the plaintiff, who must prevail by a *preponderance of the evidence*. This means that the plaintiff must tip the scale of justice ever so slightly in his or her favor in order to win at trial. This is a much lower standard of proof than the criminal standard, *beyond a reasonable doubt*. It is the reason that O.J. Simpson was found not guilty of murder but held liable for millions in a wrongful death suit. To prove a medical negligence claim, four elements must be established:

- Duty/standard of care
- Breach
- Causation
- Damages

The standard of care is now generally a national standard that is applicable to all physicians in whatever setting they practice, whether a rural hospital or an urban trauma center. With the advent of modern communication technology, the past regional standards are obsolete. Also note that every time a department establishes a policy or procedure, it establishes a standard of care. Breach means that the standard of care was not met. This is determined based on an objective *reasonable man* standard. In short, this means that one must practice in the same manner as a reasonable and prudent provider with the same training and experience would. It does not mean that one must practice to the highest standard of medicine but rather to a lower, common standard. This breach of the standard of care must then be the cause of the injury claimed, and there must be legally recognizable damages.

With an understanding of the legal standards, the physician should next recognize that there are certain situations and activities where the risks of alleged negligence are heightened. Some of these situations arise from the patient's presenting complaint, be it chest pain, abdominal pain, or an emergent obstetrical complaint. Others arise from the environment in which ED physicians work. Malpractice risks increase later in the day, often when the department is the most chaotic; later in the shift, when physicians may be more fatigued; and as a result of shift work (Kuhn, n.d.). Additionally, during shift changes and whenever care is being handed off, for example admission or transfer, the risk of malpractice increases due to the potential for miscommunication (Kuhn, n.d.). The vast majority of ED-related malpractice claims allege misdiagnoses or a failure to diagnose which arise from allegations of failure to order appropriate diagnostic testing, failure to appreciate test results, failure to perform adequate history and physical exam, and/or failure to obtain an appropriate consultation (Glauser, 2008). Further, there is an additional, increasingly alarming trend to allege negligence because of the delay in making a diagnosis or initiating a treatment. Making a correct diagnosis and ordering the proper intervention may no longer be enough, you now have to do so quickly.

The resulting question becomes, "How do I avoid these pitfalls?" Other than ensuring that you are properly rested and the proper attention to detail is being given to each patient, the most salient item that a physician can address is communication. That includes communicating appropriately with the patient and his or her family, the nurse, and peers. *Document these communications clearly in the medical record.*

Communicating with the patient includes taking a thorough medical history and documenting it. Use direct quotes when possible, particularly if the patient is agitated or starts the interaction with threats of litigation. Patient communication includes addressing delays in care, updating the patient on the status of tests, and thoroughly discussing test results with the patient and the plan of follow-up care. Make the patient a partner in this plan and document his or her concurrence with the plan. In doing this, the physician shows respect for the patient, builds a relationship, however brief, and lets the patient know that the physician is willing to listen to his or her concerns. These strategies can go far to lessen the risks of litigation (Hickson & Jenkins, 2007).

Nurse-physician communication involves including the nurse in your decision-making process. Ask questions, discuss ordered tests, and ask for input. Nurses will often save a doctor from potential malpractice. Also, listen when the nurse provides test results, shares patient observation data, or documents assessments in the chart, which should be read as a routine practice. Nurses are well educated on the importance of documenting communication; notes that say, "Dr. Smith notified of [fill in the blank]" are commonplace.

Because hand offs and consultations are major situations giving rise to claims of negligence, having appropriate communications with other providers is vital. Whether coming on or going off shift, ensure that a proper review of the patient's status is held. A standard form of communications such as SBAR (Situation-Background-Assessment-Recommendation) should be used. SBAR was developed to improve the quality of hand off communications (Institute for Healthcare Improvement, n.d.).

If it is not documented, it is not done. This adage is indoctrinated in all health care practitioners who document in the medical record. Your documentation should be clear and concise. It should include all communications and acknowledgment of test results and consultations. Document the patient's response to ordered interventions. Because negligence allegations often arise from a claim that a physician failed to order a test, study, or consult, document your rationale for not doing something to demonstrate that it was considered and rejected as opposed to being simply omitted or overlooked.

To conclude, here are some final words of guidance should the efforts to avoid litigation fail and a lawsuit is filed.

- However tempting, do not write any addendums in the medical record to further explain your actions—such additions generally do more harm than good to your defense.

- Do not discuss the case with colleagues outside of the peer review process, which often has legal protections against discovery and use at trial. A conversation in the cafeteria is fair game for discovery and you will be asked by the plaintiff's attorney if you discussed the case.

- At deposition, do not get into a struggle of egos with counsel—take it as a given that both of you are highly educated professionals. Do not let the plaintiff's counsel make you lose your composure.

- Wait a bit before answering questions to allow your lawyer time to raise an objection.

- If you are unsure of a question, ask for it to be repeated. If you do not know, do not guess—"I don't recall" is a legitimate response.

- Answer the question you are asked and do not volunteer information—the answer to the question, "Do you recall the weather yesterday?" is "Yes" or "No"; it is not, "It was raining."

- Stay involved as an active member of your defense team. But, remember that the lawyer is the specialist in law; you are the specialist in medicine.
- Keep up your morale because litigation can be a drawn-out process. And remember that it often has nothing to do with you as a doctor or as a person.

SUGGESTED READINGS

Glauser J. The etiology of malpractice [Electronic version]. *Emerg Med News.* 2008;30(7):6–7.

Hickson GB, Jenkins AD. Identifying and addressing communication failure as a means of reducing unnecessary malpractice claims [Electronic version]. *North Carolina Med J.* 2007;68(5):362–364.

Institute for Healthcare Improvement. SBAR technique for communication: A situational briefing model. Available at: http://www.ihi.org/IHI/PatientSafety/SafetyGeneral/Tools/SBARTechniqueforCommunicationASituationalBriefingModel.htm. Accessed February 16, 2009.

Kuhn W. *Malpractice and Emergency Medicine.* University of Georgia School of Medicine. n.d. Available at: http://www.mcg.edu/som/clerkships/EM/PracticeIssues/Malpractice%20and%20Emergency%20Medicine.pdf. Accessed February 15, 2009.

Lynch M. Cost of malpractice insurance forcing doctors to leave high-risk specialties: Lawyers benefit from huge damage awards. *Concord Monitor.* March 13, 2008. Available at: http://www.concordmonitor.com/apps/pbcs.dll/article?AID = /20080313/OPINION/803130304&template = page2. Accessed February 15, 2009.

Physicians Insurers Association of America (PIAA). Data sharing project: outcomes of malpractice cases closed in 2004. 2005. Retrieved from: http://www.piaa.us/pdf_files/2006_AMASmarrSHORT.pdf.

155

UNDERSTAND THE HEALTH INSURANCE PORTABILITY AND ACCOUNTABILITY ACT—THE PRIVACY RULE

ROBERT R. MARSHALL, JR, MBA

The Health Insurance Portability and Accountability Act of 1996 (HIPAA) establishes a privacy rule that sets standards for the "privacy of individually identifiable health information." Health information that is protected is referred to as "protected health information" (PHI), and organizations subject to the privacy rule are referred to as "covered entities." HIPAA is enforced by the Office for Civil Rights, which is within the United States Department of Health and Human Services (HHS). The privacy rule is just one of five rules covered under HIPAA. The intent of the privacy rule is to protect the individual's health information while at the same time allowing the flow of information needed to care for the individual. Striking a balance between the two is easier said than done.

Compliance professionals agree that HIPAA, designed to protect privacy rights of individuals, can be difficult to implement. Creating a culture of privacy—emphasizing infrastructure, avoiding incidental disclosures, and working closely with external organizations—can help mitigate risk. However, there is considerable misunderstanding and lack of agreement or consensus when it comes to specific issues. HHS has offered a summary of the privacy rule on their Web site. Even with guidelines, the obvious becomes seemingly complicated with rules and regulations. For example, after hurricane Katrina, HHS issued a two-page set of privacy guidelines. While well intentioned, it is questionable whether the guidelines helped or hindered the provision of care.

The creation of an environment of care that is effective and ethical and that respects the privacy concerns of patients and families is fundamental to what health care providers do. There is a long-standing obligation among health care professionals to uphold patients' privacy and confidentiality, especially among emergency medicine providers. These obligations and sense of duty are not new and indeed have ancient origins.

WHAT IS A HIPAA VIOLATION?

Information from the privacy rule itself and from the 22-page summary published by HHS can be further summarized into three questions or tests.

1) Is the information considered Individually Identifiable Health Information (IIHI)?

   IIHI may be summarized as individually identified past, present, or future physical or mental health condition or payment for provision of health care including demographics.

   Example: ED status boards and trackers that display ED wait times, ED census, room numbers, color codes, and icons are generally not considered IIHI.

2) Does the information fall under the privacy rule's definition of "PHI"?

   Protected health information is IIHI that is transmitted or maintained in electronic media or in any other form or media. If it is not IIHI, it is not PHI.

3) Has there been "reasonable safeguards" applied to ensure compliance with the "minimum necessary" standard?

   The minimum necessary standard is perhaps the most important and most useful test for the emergency department. The minimum necessary standard states,

   > when using or disclosing protected health information... a covered entity must make reasonable efforts to limit protected health information to the minimum necessary to accomplish the intended purpose of the use, disclosure, or request.

Example: The severity of a patient's condition may be considered PHI. However, reasonable safeguards are in place by including that information as an Emergency Severity Index (ESI), the meaning of which is unknown to the general public. Knowledge of the ESI of patients is considered minimally necessary to manage the care of patients effectively.

CONCLUSION

The HIPAA privacy rule is relatively new and untested, and there remains much confusion regarding what is and what is not an HIPAA violation. Even when applying the tests above, reasonable people will disagree. Better definitions of health information, reasonable safeguards, and minimally necessary will eventually develop. Concerns for the privacy rule should never get in the way of providing ethical and effective care to patients. The Department of HHS' Office of Civil Rights is very clear when they say the privacy rule is "not intended to impede … customary and essential communications and practices and, thus, does not require that all risk of incidental use or disclosure be eliminated to satisfy its standards."

Health care institutions and organizations are free to establish rules, guidelines, policies, and procedures. Some organizations will establish offices that exclusively deal with HIPAA issues to come into compliance with the HIPAA privacy rule. There are many guidelines and summaries available on the Internet, including the HHS' Office for Civil Rights Web site which is dedicated to HIPAA. Since there may be varying opinions on the privacy rule, it is important to understand your department and the institution's policies and procedures regarding privacy and HIPAA.

SUGGESTED READINGS

Avoid a HIPAA emergency in your organization's emergency department. Strategies for Health Care Compliance; June 11, 2006. Available at: http://www.hcpro.com/CCP-57952–237/ Avoid-a-HIPAA-emergency-in-your-organizations-emergency-department.html.

Moskop JC, Marco CA, Larkin GL, et al. From Hippocrates to HIPAA: Privacy and confidentiality in emergency medicine–Part I: Conceptual, moral, and legal foundations. *Ann Emerg Med*. 2005;45(1):53–59.

United States Department of Health and Human Services. Business Associates [45 CFR 164.502(e), 164.504(e), 164.532(d) and (e)]. OCR HIPAA Privacy, December 3, 2002 Revised April 3, 2003. Available at: http://www.hhs.gov/ocr/privacy/hipaa/understanding/coveredentities/businessassociates.pdf.

United States Department of Health and Human Services. HIPAA Privacy Rule and Public Health: guidance from CDC and the U.S. Department of Health and Human Services (The Privacy Rule 45 C.F.R. § 160.103). *MMWR*. April 11, 2003;52:1–12. Available at: http://www.cdc.gov/mmwr/preview/mmwrhtml/m2e411a1.htm.

United States Department of Health and Human Services: Office for Civil Rights. Hurricane Katrina Bulletin: HIPAA Privacy and Disclosures in Emergency Situations, September 2, 2005. Available at: http://privacyruleandresearch.nih.gov/pdf/HurricaneKatrina.pdf.

United States Department of Health and Human Services. Summary of the HIPAA Privacy Rule rev. 05/03. Available at: http://www.hhs.gov/ocr/privacy/hipaa/understanding/summary/index.html.

156

ACID-BASE: A NORMAL ANION GAP DOES NOT EXCLUDE ACIDOSIS

SAMIT DESAI, MD

The evaluation of the anion gap has long held importance as a proxy measure for acidosis. In the emergency department, the calculation ($Na^+ - [\ Cl^- + HCO_3^-\ ]$) is often performed to aid in critical decision making with regards to a patient's acid-base condition. However, a "normal" anion gap may not always effectively rule out acidosis.

In line with the law of electroneutrality, for every cation there must be an anion. Herein lies the value of the anion gap. The anion gap represents the quantity of unmeasured anions. This primarily consists of albumin and phosphate among others.

There are multiple mechanisms and pathways by which acidosis may arise. A common approach to analyzing acidosis involves classification into wide anion gap acidosis and normal anion gap acidosis. In the wide anion gap acidosis state, the buffering provided by serum bicarbonate for the newly created hydrogen ions is counterbalanced by the formation of anions that go unmeasured. This increase in unmeasured anions is responsible for the elevated anion gap. With a normal anion gap acidosis, the decline of bicarbonate due to buffering is balanced by an increase in serum chloride. The anion gap will not widen in these circumstances, and focusing only on the anion gap and not the clinical picture will lead to missed diagnoses. Diarrhea, renal tubular acidosis, and considerable normal saline administration are a few situations that produce a normal anion gap acidosis.

Apart from the normal anion gap acidosis, the anion gap will not always be elevated despite the presence of unmeasured anions. There is often a delay in the development of an elevation in the anion gap by processes that typically induce a wide anion gap acidosis. This delay will often falsely lead to the conclusion that a normal anion gap acidosis exists or that no acidosis exists whatsoever. There exist many studies that suggest that the application of the anion gap to screen for lactic acidosis in particular for emergency department patients has poor sensitivity. Using a normal level of 6 mmol/L, the sensitivity for detection of lactic acidosis improves substantially. The specificity, however, declines significantly. The utility of the anion gap as a sole screening test for acidosis may have limited application for certain types of acidosis.

Finally, the calculation and determination of what constitutes a normal anion gap are often done in error. The normal values of the anion gap range from approximately 8 to 10 mmol/L. However, the normal range may vary according to the patient. It is important, when possible, to ascertain the steady-state anion gap. Theoretically, in states of hypoalbuminemia, the expected normal anion gap should be lower due to the decrease in concentration of the primary constituents of the anion gap, albumin, or phosphate. There are formulas that may help you correct the gap appropriately. However, despite correction, one study suggests that the sensitivity for detecting lactic acidosis remains insufficient.

The anion gap continues to remain a vital and readily accessible element in a physician's assessment of a patient's acid-base status. With knowledge of the underlying physiology and thus its limitations as a screening tool, a physician can accurately make the necessary decisions to help care for patients.

SUGGESTED READINGS

Adams BD, Bonzani TA, Hunter CJ. The anion gap does not accurately screen for lactic acidosis in emergency department patients. *Emerg Med J*. 2006;23:179–182.

Dinh CH, Ng R, Grandinetti A, et al. Correcting the anion gap for hypoalbuminemia does not improve detection of hyperlactatemia. *Emerg Med J*. 2006;23:627–629.

Fauci AS, Braunwald E, Kasper DL, et al., eds. *Harrison's Principles of Internal Medicine*. 17th ed. New York: McGraw Hill; 2008.

Figge J, Jabor A, Kazda A, et al. Anion gap and hypoalbuminemia. *Crit Care Med*. 1998;26: 1807–1810.

Iberti TJ, Leibowitz AB, Papadakos PJ, et al. Low sensitivity of the anion gap as a screen to detect hyperlactatemia in critically ill patients. *Crit Care Med*. 1990;18:275–277.

Levraut J, Bounatirou T, Ichai C, et al. Reliability of anion gap as an indicator of blood lactate in critically ill patients. *Intensive Care Med*. 1997;23:417–422.

Mikulaschek A, Henry SM, Donovan R, et al. Serum lactate is not predicted by anion gap or base excess after trauma resuscitation. *J Trauma*. 1996;40:218–222; discussion 2224.

Nicolaou DD, Kelen GD. Acid-base disorders. In: Tintinalli JE, Kelen GD, Stapczynski JS, et al., eds. *Emergency Medicine: A Comprehensive Study Guide*. New York: McGraw-Hill; 2004:149–159.

157

ADMINISTRATION OF NORMAL SALINE IS THE TREATMENT FOR HYPONATREMIA

EMILIE J. B. CALVELLO, MD, MPH

The discovery of hyponatremia in the clinical setting is frequently met with the administration of normal saline despite the multitude of etiologies that may cause hyponatremia. This common error is based on the misunderstanding that hyponatremia must be due to a decrease of total body sodium. In reality, the body has more complicated adaptive mechanisms, and therefore the practitioner's understanding must be more nuanced for appropriate patient care. In the most basic form, hyponatremia may be due to a sodium issue, a water issue, or a sodium and water issue. Appropriate treatment requires determination of where the abnormality lies.

Hyponatremia is defined as sodium that is <135. Significant aberrations from this norm must be reconfirmed by repeat laboratory analysis. While the clinical manifestations and treatment are outside the scope of this chapter, patients are frequently more symptomatic at values <120 mEq/L with neurologic manifestations likely at sodium concentrations <113 mEq/dL. It should be noted that the symptoms of hyponatremia are related not only to the absolute serum sodium concentration but also to the rate of change of the sodium concentration value.

One of the first steps in the evaluation of hyponatremia should begin with the measurement of the serum osmolality (*Fig. 157.1*). This measured value must then be compared with the calculated value from the following equation:.

$$\text{Serum osmolality} = 2\,Na^+ + glucose/18 + BUN/2.8$$

Hypertonic hyponatremia occurs when there are large amounts of solutes that are confined to the extracellular space. This can occur most commonly with hyperglycemia or administration of exogenous agents such as mannitol or glycerol. Isotonic hyponatremia occurs when there is factitiously low sodium reported secondary to laboratory analysis of a sample with hyperproteinemia (Waldenstrom macroglobulinemia, multiple myeloma) or hyperlipidemia.

The most common clinical encounter is in the patient with hypotonic hyponatremia. Once this state is identified, the next step of diagnosis is reevaluation of the history and physical examination as these will suggest the volume status of the patient. Hypotonic hypovolemic patients may be further differentiated into extra renal and intrinsic renal losses by measurement of the UNa^+. If the UNa^+ is <10 mEq/L, it confirms extrarenal losses that can usually be

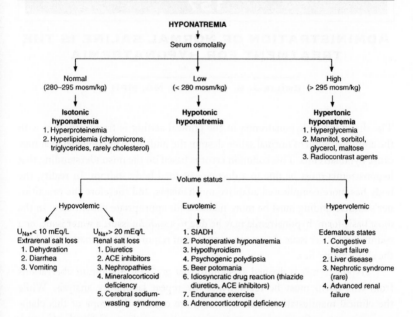

FIGURE 157.1. Algorithm for the evaluation of hyponatremia. (Reprinted with permission from McPhee SJ, Papadakis MA. *Current Medical Diagnosis and Treatment.* 48th ed. New York: McGraw Hill; 2009. Available at: http://www.accessmedicine.com. © The McGraw-Hill Companies, Inc.)

identified by the history. Urine Na >20 mEq/L suggests renal salt loss that can be due to a number of different etiologies (diuretics, intrinsic renal disease, mineralocorticoid deficiency, etc.). Hypotonic euvolemic patients most frequently have syndrome of inappropriate antidiuretic hormone (SIADH); however, this is a diagnosis of exclusion after consideration of thyroid disease, adrenal insufficiency, and psychogenic polydipsia. SIADH itself has multiple etiologies including central nervous system disease, pulmonary disease, neoplasia, and drugs. Finally, hypovolemic hyponatremia includes the edematous states, which include congestive heart failure, liver cirrhosis, and renal failure.

Appropriate treatment is dependent on both the rapidity in the change in serum sodium and the etiology of hyponatremia. For the patient in coma or seizure, it is appropriate to consider administration of 3% (514 mEq/L) saline with a goal of increasing the serum sodium 1 to 2 mEq/L/h. Hypertonic hyponatremia does not require any treatment beyond treatment of the underlying disorder in the case of hyperglycemia. Isotonic hyponatremia also does not require treatment as it is primarily present as facticious hyponatremia secondary to limitations in laboratory analysis. Hypotonic hypovolemic hyponatremia secondary to extrarenal losses is the only state that may be treated with normal saline fluid resuscitation with strict attention to only increasing the rise in Na by 0.5 mEq per h. Hypotonic euvolemic hyponatremia should prompt a search for underlying processes as well as fluid restriction. Hypotonic hypervolemic hyponatremia should be managed by salt and water restriction often coupled with diuretics.

In summary, evaluation of hyponatremia requires the careful consideration of history and physical examination combined with the measurement of serum osmolality. Treatment with normal saline should only be considered for hypotonic hypovolemic hyponatremia.

158

DO NOT FIND OUT THAT YOUR PATIENT IS HYPOGLYCEMIC ON THE COMPUTED TOMOGRAPHY SCANNER

ZHANNA LIVSHITS, MD AND ANDREW STOLBACH, MD

Hypoglycemia is easy to diagnose … if you think of it. The "classic" hypoglycemic patient presents with both autonomic and neuroglycopenic symptoms. Autonomic symptoms, as a result of catecholamine release, include tremor, tachycardia, and diaphoresis. The neuroglycopenic symptoms result from the effects of glucose deprivation in the brain: confusion, seizures, and coma. Unfortunately, many patients do not present in a "classic" fashion. Hypoglycemia should be considered in patients with any neuropsychiatric abnormality, including focal neurologic deficits.

Some patients fail to recognize their own hypoglycemia. Well-controlled diabetics are less likely than others to recognize the onset of hypoglycemia. Patients who are taking β-blockers may not have significant autonomic symptoms, making the diagnosis unclear for the clinician and the patient alike.

In some patient populations, clinicians might fail to consider hypoglycemia. Obtain a blood glucose level on the intoxicated person on the hallway stretcher. Alcoholic patients are especially prone to hypoglycemia, since ethanol inhibits gluconeogenesis and eventually depletes glycogen stores. Because hypoglycemia may cause a focal neurological deficit, check the glucose level before you send your hemiplegic "rule out CVA" to the computed tomography scanner.

Once you have obtained a bedside glucose measurement, be careful when interpreting it. Hypoglycemia is both a clinical and a laboratory diagnosis. In one study, poorly controlled diabetics first developed symptoms at a mean glucose of 78 mg/dL, while nondiabetics became symptomatic at a mean glucose of 53 mg/dL. Your diabetic with a numerically "normal" glucose may well be hypoglycemic.

Many providers undertreat hypoglycemic patients. The treatment for hypoglycemia is intravenous dextrose, followed by a meal. The adult patient should receive 0.5 to 1 g/kg of intravenous 50% concentrated dextrose ($D_{50}W$); children should receive 25% concentrated dextrose solution ($D_{25}W$), and infants 10 % ($D_{10}W$). Because the standard "amp" of D_{50} has 25 g of dextrose, almost all adult patients should get more than one syringe. Each one of those "amps" has merely 100 cal. The initial bolus should be followed by a meal. If the patient can eat, feed him or her. A meal will provide hours of sustained-release calories.

Dextrose infusions may be necessary for patients who cannot eat or who overdose on a longer acting form of insulin. When ordering the infusion, remember that D_5 is not a glucose replacement solution. Each 1 L bag of D_5 contains 50 g of glucose, or 200 cal. Administering this solution at a rate of 100 mL per h would deliver an insignificant 20 cal per h to the patient! A better choice is to prepare a 10% dextrose solution and supplementing with D_{50}. Another option is to administer 20% dextrose, but this should be given through a central venous catheter to avoid venous injury.

Glucagon is often administered intramuscularly to hypoglycemic patients who do not have intravenous access. Glucagon requires adequate glycogen stores to be effective and thus may not be effective in children, the elderly, and in patients with decreased metabolic reserve due to alcoholism or chronic illness. Because glucagon is only a temporizing measure and provides no benefits over dextrose alone, there is no role for glucagon in management of hypoglycemia for patients with intravenous access.

Patients using short-acting insulin may be discharged if they do not require further treatment for hypoglycemia over a 4- to 6-h observation period (*Table 158.1*). Because the kinetics of insulin are not predictable in overdose, patients with intentional overdoses should be admitted. In one case of lente insulin overdose, hypoglycemia did not occur until 18 h after the overdose. Similarly, patients with renal failure, hepatic failure, or unexplained hypoglycemia should be admitted.

What is the take home point? You cannot diagnose hypoglycemia if you do not think of it. Hypoglycemia may manifest with any neuropsychiatric abnormality and may be present even with a "normal" blood glucose. Once you identify hypoglycemia, the proper management is not merely an "amp" of D_{50} and discharge home. Patients should be fed a meal, and select patients should be admitted. If you cannot identify the cause of hypoglycemia, the patient is safer in the hospital.

TABLE 158.1	INSULIN TYPES WITH ONSET AND DURATION OF ACTION INCLUDING PEAK RESPONSE		
INSULIN	ONSET OF ACTION (H)	DURATION OF ACTION (H)	PEAK GLYCEMIC RESPONSE (H)
ULTRASHORT ACTING			
Lispro (Humalog)	0.25–0.5	<5	0.5–2.5
SHORT ACTING			
Regular	0.5–1	5–8	2.5–5
Insulin aspart	0.25	18–24	0.75–1.5
INTERMEDIATE ACTING			
Lente	3–4	18–24	6–14
NPH	2–4	18–24	6–14
LONG ACTING			
Insulin glargine	1.1	24	2–20
Ultralente	6–10	20–36	8–20

SUGGESTED READINGS

Andrade R, Mathew V, Morgenstern MJ, et al. Hypoglycemic hemiplegic syndrome. *Ann Emerg Med*. 1984;13:529–531.

Blohmé G, Lager I, Lönnroth P, Smith U. Hypoglycemic symptoms in insulin-dependent diabetics. A prospective study of the influence of beta-blockade. *Diabetes Metab*. 1981;7(4):235–238.

Bosse GM. Antidiabetics and hypoglycemics. In: *Goldfrank's Toxicologic Emergencies*. 8th ed. New York: McGraw-Hill; 2006:749–763.

Boyle PJ, Scwartz NS, Shah SD, et al. Plasma glucose concentrations at the onset of hypoglycemic symptoms in patients with poorly controlled diabetes and in nondiabetics. *N Engl J Med*. 1988;318:1487–1492.

Malouf R, Brust JC. Hypoglycemia: causes, neurological manifestations, and outcome. *Ann Neurol*. 1985;17:421–430.

McKenney JM, Goodman RP, Wright JT Jr. Use of antihypertensive agents in patients with glucose intolerance. *Clin Pharm*. 1985;4(6):649–656.

Munck O, Quaade F. Suicide attempt with insulin. *Dan Med Bull*. 1963;10:139–141.

Seibert DG. Reversible decerebrate posturing secondary to hypoglycemia. *Am J Med*. 1985;78:1036–1037.

Spiller HA, Schroeder SL, Ching DS. Hemiparesis and altered mental status in a child after glyburide ingestion. *J Emerg Med*. 1998;16:433–435.

Verschoor L, Wolffenbuttel BH, Weber RF. Beta blockade and carbohydrate metabolism: Theoretical aspects and clinical implications. *J Cardiovasc Pharmacol*. 1986;8(Suppl 11): S92–S95.

Wallis WE, Donaldson I, Scott RS, et al. Hypoglycemia masquerading as cerebrovascular disease (hypoglycemic hemiplegia). *Ann Neurol*. 1985;18:510–512.

159

DO NOT FORGET ABOUT OCTREOTIDE FOR SOME PATIENTS WITH HYPOGLYCEMIA

ZHANNA LIVSHITS, MD AND ANDREW STOLBACH, MD

Do not forget that you can use octreotide as an antidote for sulfonylurea induced hypoglycemia. Sulfonylureas potentiate the release of endogenous insulin from the pancreatic β-cells. Sulfonylureas have a long duration of action and, most concerning to the emergency physician, often have delayed onset of action. There are reports of patients taking sulfonylureas and developing hypoglycemia 16 h later! For this reason, patients who develop hypoglycemia while taking a sulfonylurea and any child who may have taken a sulfonylurea need to be observed for at least 24 h (*Table 159.1*).

The initial management of sulfonylurea-associated hypoglycemia is the same as that for any hypoglycemia—administer intravenous dextrose and then feed the patient. Unfortunately, recurrent hypoglycemia is a problem in patients

TABLE 159.1	ORAL HYPOGLYCEMICS	
DRUG GENERIC NAME	**DRUG TRADE NAME**	**DURATION OF ACTION (H)**[a]
SULFONYLUREAS		
First Generation		
Acetohexamide	Dymelor	12–18
Chlorpropamide	Diabenese	24–72
Tolazamide	Tolinase	16–24
Tolbutamide	Orinase	6–12
Second Generation		
Glimepiride	Amaryl	24
Glipizide	Glucotrol	16–24
	Glucotrol XL	
Glyburide	Micronase	18–24
	Glynase	
	DiaBeta	

[a]Duration of action is for therapeutic doses in adults and will be greater following an overdose in children.

with sulfonylurea-induced hypoglycemia because sulfonylureas potentiate endogenous insulin release. So, every time you administer dextrose, the patient's pancreas releases more insulin, resulting in recurrent hypoglycemia. When you respond to the recurrent hypoglycemia by giving more dextrose, the pancreas creates more insulin and—you get the picture.

The resulting cycle may be impossible to break without octreotide. Octreotide is a somatostatin analog that inhibits pancreatic insulin secretion. In other words, octreotide prevents hypoglycemia, even sulfonylurea-associated hypoglycemia. Case reports demonstrate its efficacy in patients with glipizide, glyburide, gliclazide, or tolbutamide overdose. In a controlled trial of patients with sulfonylurea-induced hypoglycemia, the octreotide group had higher mean glucose levels at 4 to 8 h than those who received standard therapy alone. The investigators probably could have eliminated all recurrent hypoglycemia in the octreotide group if they had repeated the octreotide dose at 6 h as is recommended by some textbooks.

The suggested dose of octreotide is 50 μg subcutaneously every 6 h for adults and 4 to 5 μg/kg/d divided in 6 h intervals for children. Side effects, which might include nausea or diarrhea, are almost never observed when octreotide is given in this manner. Because sulfonylureas may have a long duration of action, octreotide should be continued for 24 h.

SUMMARY POINTS

When you see your next hypoglycemic patient, take a careful medication history. If he or she is taking a sulfonylurea medication, admit the patient no matter how good the patient looks after you correct the glucose level, because you cannot reliably tell who will develop another episode of hypoglycemia. For the same reason, admit any child who may have ingested a sulfonylurea. If hypoglycemia recurs after you initially correct the patient's glucose, administer octreotide. This safe medication will save you time and save the patient from yet another episode of hypoglycemia.

SUGGESTED READINGS

Bosse GM. Antidiabetics and hypoglycemics. In: *Goldfrank's Toxicologic Emergencies*. 8th ed. New York: McGraw-Hill; 2006:749–763.

Boyle PJ, Justice K, Krentz AJ, et al. Octreotide reverses hyperinsulinemia and prevents hypoglycemia induced by sulfonylurea overdose. *J Clin Endocrinol Metab*. 1993;76:752–756.

Braatvedt GD. Octreotide for the treatment of sulfonylurea induced hypoglycemia in type 2 diabetes. *N Z Med J*. 1997;110:189–190.

Fasano CJ, O'Malley G, Dominici P, et al. Comparison of octreotide and standard therapy versus standard therapy alone for the treatment of sulfonylurea-induced hypoglycemia. *Ann Emerg Med*. 2008;51:400–406.

Fleseriu M, Skugor M, Chinnappa P, et al. Successful treatment of sulfonylurea-induced prolonged hypoglycemia with use of octreotide. *Endocr Pract*. 2006;12(6):635–640.

Graudins A, Linden C, Ferm R. Diagnosis and treatment of sulfonylurea-induced hyperinsulinemic hypoglycemia. *Am J Emerg Med*. 1997;15:95–96.

Howland MA. Octreotide. In: *Goldfrank's Toxicologic Emergencies*. 8th ed. New York: McGraw-Hill; 2006:770–773.

Hung O, Eng J, Ho J, et al. Octreotide as an antidote for refractory sulfonylurea hypoglycemia. *J Toxicol Clin Toxicol*. 1997;35(5):540.

Krentz AJ, Boyle PJ, Justice KM, et al. Successful treatment of severe refractory sulfonylurea-induced hypoglycemia with octreotide. *Diabetes Care*. 1993;16:184–186, 189–190.

McLaughlin SA, Crandall CS, McKinney PE. Octreotide: An antidote for sulfonylurea induced hypoglycemia. *Ann Emerg Med*. 2000;36:133–138.

Mordel A, Sivilotti MLA, Old AC, et al. Octreotide for pediatric sulfonylurea poisoning. *J Toxicol Clin Toxicol*. 1998;36:437.

Quadrani DA, Spiler HA, Widder P. Five-year retrospective evaluation of sulfonylurea ingestion in children. *J Toxicol Clin Toxicol*. 1996;34:267–270.

160

DO NOT JUST FOCUS ON THE GLUCOSE IN PATIENTS WITH DIABETIC KETOACIDOSIS

SAMIT DESAI, MD

Diabetic ketoacidosis represents one of the more common and potentially dangerous endocrinologic emergencies we face. With the incidence of diabetes rising, we will continue to see its presence more often in our daily practice. With the pathology so well appreciated, it is imperative that a provider has a sound understanding on how best to reverse its course.

Diabetic ketoacidosis represents a disease state characterized by hyperglycemia, dehydration, and ketoacidosis. The underlying defect is an inability of the pancreas to produce sufficient insulin to meet the body's metabolic demands. The result is a cascade of up-regulation of counter-regulatory hormones such as glucagon, catecholamines, and glucocorticoids. This process, if left unchecked, may spiral out of control resulting in significant morbidity and even mortality.

Once diagnosed with diabetic ketoacidosis, the mainstay of treatment revolves around rehydration, insulin administration, electrolyte monitoring and repletion, and treatment of the underlying etiology. To understand the end points of treatment, one must first be aware of the pathophysiology. When noncompliant with insulin therapy or in a stressed state, such as myocardial infarction or infection, the body responds with a counter-regulatory response marked by the release of cortisol, catecholamines, and glucagon. These hormones are catabolic and result in an increased serum glucose concentration to support an increased metabolic demand. In patients with relative or complete insulin deficiency, the metabolic demand cannot be met as glucose is unable to enter cells and serve as a fuel source. Without an appropriate substrate, the body begins the process of lipolysis, ultimately leading to the production of ketones, specifically β-hydroxybutyrate and acetoacetate. These ketones represent unmeasured strong acids that elevate the anion gap inducing a metabolic acidosis. It is this acidosis coupled with increasingly profound dehydration that is responsible for death from diabetic ketoacidosis.

The kidneys begin spilling glucose into the urine due to a phenomenon known as osmotic diuresis. As this process continues and hyperglycemia persists, dehydration worsens. The glomerular filtration rate decreases secondary to the poor perfusion, leading to even higher levels of hyperglycemia. The result is total body volume depletion and, in particular, intracellular dehydration.

The central tenets of diabetic ketoacidosis resuscitation involve appropriate fluid hydration, estimated at 2 L of normal saline over the first 2 h, and the initiation of an insulin drip (0.1 U/kg/h). The patient's volume status must be monitored closely, and further administration of fluid may be dosed accordingly. Inadequate fluid resuscitation and monitoring may lead to a worsening of the acidosis and shock state.

The insulin drip must remain until there is a clearing of the anion gap. It is assumed that once the anion gap has closed there is no longer a production of ketones and ketonemia. The body has now met its metabolic demand after the administration of insulin and the subsequent shift of glucose into cells.

It is important to note that the serum glucose concentration will begin to drop with fluid administration alone. This is due to the improving glomerular filtration rate as well as the increased responsiveness of tissues to insulin now that perfusion has improved. Again, the fundamental problem present with diabetic ketoacidosis is the body's starvation and inability to use glucose as substrate. A declining serum glucose value does not tell a physician whether or not the starvation has resolved, only the resolution of ketone production will. Therefore, the recommendation in the treatment of diabetic ketoacidosis is to counterintuitively add dextrose to fluid when the serum concentration has dipped to 250 to 300 mg/dL. When the anion gap has closed, representing the cessation of ketone production, dextrose administration, as well as insulin drip therapy, may be stopped. It is at this point that the patient can be transitioned to subcutaneous insulin therapy.

Finally, the third essential component of effective management of diabetic ketoacidosis is serum potassium control. The serum potassium level may vary from low to high depending upon the degree of ketoacidosis and hyperglycemia involved. There are two processes that affect the serum potassium. Due to the hyperglycemia-induced osmotic diuresis, the kidneys filter potassium. Over time, the body will have a total body potassium deficit. However, depending on the amount of acidemia, the serum potassium may be paradoxically elevated. With excess hydrogen ion in the serum, the H^+-K^+ pump will shift intracellular potassium to the extracellular compartment. It is impossible to know where the level will be along the continuum. Prior to insulin therapy, a serum potassium level must be checked. An electrocardiogram is important to note any dysrhythmias from an altered potassium level. In a similarly counterintuitive intervention as in the addition of glucose in the face of hyperglycemia, potassium repletion must be considered once the serum level approaches 5.0 to 5.5 mEq/L. This is due to total body potassium depletion and the concurrent hypokalemic effects of continued insulin therapy. The key point is that serial potassium levels should be monitored frequently.

Among the few true endocrine emergencies, diabetic ketoacidosis is a disease state whose process is well-known. With an essential understanding of the underlying pathophysiology, the physician can methodically reverse a process that would otherwise lead to a serious outcome. Mind the gap!

SUGGESTED READINGS

American Diabetes Association. Introduction: Clinical practice recommendations 2002. *Diabetes Care*. 2002;25(S1):S1–S2.

Fauci AS, Braunwald E, Kasper DL, et al., eds. *Harrison's Priciples of Internal Medicine*. 17th ed. New York: McGraw Hill; 2008.

Kitabchi AE, Nyenwe EA. Hyperglycemic crises in diabetes mellitus: Diabetic ketoacidosis and hyperglycemic hyperosmolar state. *Endocrinol Metab Clin N Am*. 2006;35(4):725–751.

Kwon KT, Tsai VW. Metabolic emergencies. *Emerg Med Clin N Am*. 2007;25(4):1041–1060.

Lebovitz HE. Diabetic ketoacidosis. *Lancet*. 1995;345:767.

Tintinalli JE, Kelen GD, Stapczynski JS, et al., eds. *Emergency Medicine: A Comprehensive Study Guide*. 6th ed. New York: McGraw-Hill; 2004.

161

DO NOT RELY ON ORTHOSTATIC VITAL SIGN TESTING FOR DIAGNOSING DEHYDRATION

ARJUN S. CHANMUGAM, MD, MBA

Most of us learned about the value of orthostatic hypotension (OH) in medical school. It is a time-honored measurement that is supposed to yield important information about a patient's ability to manage the change in blood distribution when changing positions. It is important to keep in mind that it is a physical finding and not a diagnosis, although sometimes the lines get blurred between the two. The other confounding effect is that it may be accompanied by symptoms or it could be asymptomatic.

The definition of OH is a fall of systolic blood pressure of at least 20 mm Hg or a fall of diastolic blood pressure of within 3 min of standing. The problem with this definition is that a good percentage of elderly patients (by some estimates, nearly 50%) will meet these criteria.

Some authors have suggested that there are several kinds of OH, an initial OH and a delayed OH. The initial OH occurs before 1 to 3 min of the normal type OH. Delayed OH occurs after 3 to 10 min but can happen later. It is described well in the neurology literature. Both the initial and the delayed OH have important implications but are not generally used in the emergency department (ED). It should be noted that the initial OH is somewhat common in young adults with a reported incidence of 3.6% and could be a common cause of presyncope and syncope. A clear history of immediacy of symptoms within 5 to 10 s after standing and an accompanying 40 mm Hg systolic drop and/or 20 mm Hg diastolic drop are required for consideration of this entity.

There are several predisposing factors for OH. One factor that most emergency physicians are familiar with is dehydration. Also on the list of predisposing factors are deconditioning, nutrition, and aging. Of course, there is another very important predisposing factor and that is medications, especially tricyclic antidepressants, antihypertensives, diuretics and vasodilators.

The important causes of OH include autonomic neuropathy, pure autonomic failure, and Parkinson disease. Multiple system atrophy, some forms of dementia, brainstem lesions, and spinal cord injury are also important causes of OH.

In the ED, as in most places, common things are common. Dehydration is a contributing factor to many patients' health status. According to the Nutrition Information Center in New York, the average American is chronically dehydrated and consumes only 4.6 servings of water per day. The National

Resource Council estimates that the average person needs between 9 and 12 cups of water per day based on a caloric expenditure of 2,200 to 2,900 cal per day. It seems to make sense that a significant percentage of patients who present to the ED will have a component of dehydration. Having a sensitive indicator of dehydration would be a useful diagnostic weapon in the ED.

The measurement of OH gives the emergency physician yet another diagnostic data point. In a specialty that is driven by empiric interventions, one more bit of evidence can only be helpful. OH can be a valuable tool in many cases, but its results have to be interpreted very carefully, because many disease states cause it and multiple factors contribute to it.

In summary, OH is a useful physical finding, especially when associated with symptoms. Contributing factors of OH include dehydration, deconditioning, nutrition, medications, and aging. Causes of OH include autonomic neuropathy and other neurological conditions. It can be a useful tool in the ED, but its interpretation must take into account other factors than just volume depletion.

SUGGESTED READINGS

Robertson D. The pathophysiology and diagnosis of orthostatic hypotension. *Clin Auton Res.* 2008;18(Suppl 1):2–7 [Epub Mar 27, 2008].
Survey of 3003 Americans, Nutrition Information Center, New York Hospital-Cornell Medical Center (April 14, 1998).
Vaddadi G, Lambert E, Corcoran SJ, et al. Postural syncope: Mechanisms and management. *Med J Aust.* 2007;187(5):299–304 [Review].

162

HYPERGLYCEMIC HYPEROSMOLAR NONKETOTIC SYNDROME: BE AFRAID ... BE VERY AFRAID!

SAMIT DESAI, MD

When evaluating a patient in the midst of a hyperglycemic crisis, all too often the major focus rests on whether or not a ketoacidosis exists. This line of thinking may lead to the misdiagnosis and the subsequent mismanagement of an equally worrisome and potentially more dangerous hyperglycemic state, hyperglycemic hyperosmolar nonketotic syndrome (HHNS).

The definition of HHNS by the American Diabetes Association (ADA) is as follows: (1) serum glucose >600 mg/dL, (2) plasma osmolality >315 mOsm/kg,

(3) serum bicarbonate >15, (4) pH >7.3, and (5) negative or mildly positive serum ketonemia. From this definition, it is clear that HHNS does share certain characteristics with diabetic ketoacidosis in its presentation. For one, both syndromes have an elevated serum glucose. The severe intravascular volume depletion present is a direct result of osmotic diuresis, a function of hyperglycemia, and the kidneys' inability to reabsorb filtered glucose. As the diuresis takes hold, renal function declines and hyperglycemia worsens. Volume depletion may manifest in a lactic acidosis as well as severe electrolyte disturbances, particularly involving potassium. Furthermore, many of the same precipitants of diabetic ketoacidosis lead to the development of HHNS. Infection, myocardial infarction, and medical noncompliance all may induce the condition.

HHNS is thought to be similar to diabetic ketoacidosis in its pathophysiology with one major exception. The body does not undergo lipolysis necessary for the formation of ketoacids. A number of hypotheses, from elevated insulin levels inhibiting lipolysis to a lack of a counter-regulatory hormone response, abound. However, the exact mechanism remains unclear. As a result, the wide anion gap acidosis secondary to ketone formation seen with diabetic ketoacidosis does not exist. This represents the fundamental difference between the two syndromes.

One added complication is the elevated plasma osmolality. With HHNS, the serum glucose is often markedly higher than that seen with diabetic ketoacidosis. With glucose as one of the primary determinants of plasma osmolality, many patients with HHNS may exhibit some degree of altered mental status, presumably a result of the elevated plasma osmolality. Of note, serum glucose concentration is one marker the ADA uses to distinguish the two hyperglycemic syndromes.

HHNS tends to develop over a longer period of time as its clinical presentation is insidious. It is often seen in the elderly and those whose access to free water is limited. The inability to replenish ongoing fluid losses leads to worsening of the condition. It is the very patients who are predisposed to HHNS, those with significant comorbidities and poor substrate, who lend to its relatively high mortality. In fact, HHNS has reported mortality rates up to 15%. Compare that with the approximately 4% mortality seen with diabetic ketoacidosis.

The management of HHNS is similar to that of diabetic ketoacidosis, fluid rehydration and insulin administration with close monitoring of electrolytes. Treatment differs in that the end points are rehydration and slow normalization of glucose as opposed to hydration and closure of the anion gap with diabetic ketoacidosis.

HHNS represents a clinically important hyperglycemic crisis. Without knowledge of its pathophysiology and the aggressive intervention that is necessary, there remains potential for serious morbidity and even mortality.

SUGGESTED READINGS

American Diabetes Association. Hyperglycemic crises in patients with diabetes mellitus. *Diabetes Care.* 2002;25(S1):S100.

Centers for Disease Control and Prevention. *National Diabetes Fact Sheet: National Estimates and General Information on Diabetes in the United States.* Atlanta: U.S. Department of Health and Human Services, Centers for Disease Control and Prevention; 1997.

Tintinalli JE, Kelen GD, Stapczynski JS, et al., eds. *Emergency Medicine: A Comprehensive Study Guide.* 6th ed. New York: McGraw-Hill; 2004.

163

KNOW THE 3-PRONGED TREATMENT OF HYPERKALEMIA: STABILIZE, REDISTRIBUTE, AND REDUCE

JOHN W. BURGER, MD

Hyperkalemia is a common electrolyte abnormality encountered in the emergency department. Prompt recognition and appropriate management of hyperkalemia is critically important as elevated potassium levels can disrupt normal cardiac conduction leading to fatal arrhythmias. The risk of developing EKG changes and potential life-threatening arrhythmias is based not just on the absolute plasma concentration but also on the rate of rise of potassium in the extracellular space. In general, serum concentrations of potassium >5.5 mEq/L can be associated with clinical symptoms, though some patients can have dangerously high concentrations of serum potassium with no evidence of classic EKG changes until very late in their course.

Ultimately, the management of hyperkalemia depends on the correction of the patient's underlying disorder. However, several therapeutic modalities can be utilized to treat hyperkalemia in the acute setting. Because these treatments vary in mechanism of action, time of onset, and duration, it is useful to divide them into three categories: those that stabilize the cardiac membrane, those that redistribute total body potassium, and those that reduce total body potassium.

MEMBRANE STABILIZATION

The first step in the management of hyperkalemia, specifically in the setting of EKG changes, is the administration of intravenous calcium. Hyperkalemia increases cardiac excitability by altering the resting membrane potential of the myocyte. As the potassium level rises, T waves become peaked, the QT interval shortens, and the PR interval gets longer. Eventually the QRS complex widens with flattening of the P wave and the EKG takes on a "sine wave" appearance that can degenerate into ventricular fibrillation or asystole. Calcium directly antagonizes the effect of hyperkalemia by altering the myocyte's activation threshold leading to membrane stabilization. Improvements in EKG findings occur 1 to 3 min after administration with effects lasting 30 to 60 min.

Either calcium gluconate or calcium chloride can be used to treat hyperkalemia. Calcium chloride has three times the amount of calcium per 10 mL compared to calcium gluconate but is more caustic to the veins and surrounding tissue in the event of IV infiltration. Calcium gluconate is the preferred choice if the patient only has peripheral IV access, whereas calcium chloride is preferred if the patient has central venous access.

Normally, 10 mL of 10% calcium gluconate can be given over the span of 2 to 3 min. Caution must be used when giving calcium to patients taking digoxin as intravenous calcium can potentiate the myocardial toxicity of digoxin. If membrane stabilization is essential in this subgroup of patients, then the calcium should be added to 100 mL of 5% dextrose solution and given very slowly over 30 min.

REDISTRIBUTION

The next step in management is to drive potassium out of the plasma and into the intracellular space. Insulin and albuterol are able to do this by enhancing the activity of the Na-K ATPase pump responsible for the active transport of potassium. Because the mechanism by which insulin activates this pump differs from the β_2 activation offered by albuterol, it is thought that using these two therapies in conjunction with each other has an additive potassium lowering effect. Since they produce a transient effect, insulin and albuterol may have to be given in multiple doses over time.

Typically, a bolus of 10 U of IV insulin is administered concurrently with 50 mL of 50% dextrose solution to prevent hypoglycemia. The onset of action occurs within 15 to 30 min and lasts 2 to 4 h. This results in a 0.5 to 1 mEq/L drop in plasma potassium concentration. Patients who are already hyperglycemic would not benefit from the coadministration of glucose. In fact, elevated glucose in the setting of diabetic ketoacidosis often leads to extracellular shifting of potassium and elevated serum potassium levels despite normal or depleted total body potassium levels. In this case, correction of the underlying metabolic derangement with insulin and fluids is usually enough to shift potassium back into the cells and correct the hyperkalemia.

Administration of 10 to 20 mg of nebulized albuterol in 4 mL of saline has also been shown to decrease potassium concentrations by 0.5 to 1 mEq/L. The onset of action occurs in <30 min and duration of action lasts about 90 min.

Elevation of serum pH is another potential mechanism to shift potassium intracellularly. Sodium bicarbonate can be used as a treatment option in the setting of a severe acidemia, though its role as a first-line agent in the general treatment of hyperkalemia has come into question.

REDUCTION

A definitive treatment of hyperkalemia is removal of potassium from the body. This can be achieved by decreasing intestinal absorption with cation exchange resins such as Kayexalate, increasing renal excretion with loop diuretics, or directly removing extracellular potassium from the blood by means of hemodialysis.

Cation exchange resins bind potassium in the colon in exchange for sodium and can be dosed every 4 to 6 h. The oral dose is 15 to 30 g mixed with 60 to 120 mL of 20% sorbitol solution and takes about 4 to 6 h to work. Sorbitol is given to decrease the risk of constipation as prolonged transit time can lead to concretion of resin and abdominal perforation. However, some reports indicate that the addition of sorbitol itself can lead to perforation and intestinal necrosis in certain patient populations. In general, it is best to avoid oral administration of cation exchange resins in patients with impaired intestinal mobility if at all possible.

Loop or thiazide diuretics can be used in patients with preserved renal function as a way to lower potassium levels by increasing renal excretion. Like cation exchange resins, it can take hours for any appreciable change in serum potassium to occur. Given that most patients with hyperkalemia will have some form of abnormal renal function, the response to diuretic may be limited. Always remember that in an emergent situation, hemodialysis is the only way to definitely remove potassium from the body.

KEY POINTS

Recognition of true hyperkalemia is essential. When initiating therapy be mindful of the possibility of psueudohyperkalemia as lysis of red cells in the specimen can cause falsely elevated potassium levels. If the patient is stable with no EKG changes, then it is usually worthwhile to recheck the potassium level prior to treatment to avoid iatrogenic hypokalemia. However, do not wait for laboratory data to come back before giving calcium if significant EKG changes are present. Remember that therapies aimed at stabilization of the cardiac membrane have no effect on potassium levels and that redistribution efforts are temporizing measures aimed at causing a transient decrease in potassium levels. The goal is to provide enough time so that other measures aimed at reducing overall potassium levels can take effect. One of the most important interventions in the management of life-threatening hyperkalemia is hemodialysis to remove potassium from the body.

SUGGESTED READINGS

Allon M, Dunlay R, Copkney C. Nebulized albuterol for acute hyperkalemia in patients on hemodialysis. *Ann Intern Med.* 1989;110:426–429.

Allon M, Shaklin N. Effect of bicarbonate administration on plasma potassium in dialysis patients: Interactions with insulin and albuterol. *Am J Kidney Dis.* 1996;28:508–514.

Ho-Jung K, Sang-Woong H. Therapeutic approach to hyperkalemia. *Nephron.* 2002; 92:33–40.

Hollander-Rodriguez J, Calvert J. Hyperkalemia. *Am Fam Physician.* 2006;73:283–289.

Kamel KS, Wei C. Controversial issues in the treatment of hyperkalemia. *Nephr Dial Transplant.* 2003;18:2215–2218.

Parham W, Mehdirad A. Hyperkalemia revisited. *Tex Heart Inst J.* 2006;33:40–47.

Rogers F, Li S. Acute colonic necrosis associated with sodium polystyrene sulfonate (Kayexalate) enemas in a critically ill patient: Case report and review of the literature. *J Trauma.* 2001;51:395–397.

Szwelip HM, Weiss J, Singer I. Profound hyperkalemia without electrocardiographic manifestations. *Am J Kidney Dis.* 1986;7:461–465.

164

KNOW WHICH THYROID FUNCTION TESTS TO ORDER (AND WHAT THEY MEAN!)

EMILIE J. B. CALVELLO, MD, MPH

Hyperthyroidism and hypothyroidism are common illnesses encountered in the emergency department (ED). These disorders can contribute to other disease states, or they can be the primary cause of the patient's ED presentation. Despite the prevalence of thyroid disorders, thyroid function is often a secondary or sometimes even a neglected consideration in the ED patient. In the critically ill patient, the determination of thyroid function can play an important role in determining the correct treatment plan.

Diagnosis of thyroid disease can only be made with a clear understanding of the normal thyroid physiology. Regulation and synthesis of thyroid hormone from the thyroid are mediated by thyroid simulating hormone (TSH). TSH stimulates multiple pathways within the thyroid gland via the TSH receptor ultimately leading to the increased production and release of thyroxine (T_4) and triiodothyronine (T_3). T_4 and T_3 both have direct negative feedback effects on the pituitary release of TSH. Regulation of TSH is also mediated by the hypothalamic thyroid releasing hormone. Once T_4 and T_3 are released into circulation, the majority of the hormones are protein bound via thyroid binding globulin (70%), albumin (15%), and transthyretin (10%). The plasma concentrations of T_4 are approximately 90 times that of T_3, although T_3 is the significantly more active hormone. T_4 serves as a prohormone for T_3 via deiodination in the plasma to produce 80% of the circulating T_3 hormone (*Fig. 164.1*).

Ultimately, thyroid hormone controls a number of metabolic processes leading to the various manifestations of hypo- and hyperthyroid states. In the

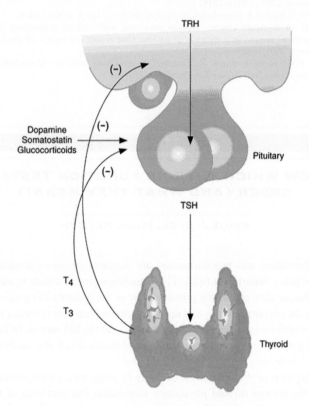

Hypothalamus

TRH

(-)

Dopamine
Somatostatin
Glucocorticoids

(-)

(-)

Pituitary

TSH

T₄

T₃

Thyroid

FIGURE 164.1. Thyroid hormone metabolism. (Reproduced with permission from Molina PE. *Endocrine Physiology.*, 2nd ed. New York: McGraw-Hill, http://www.accessmedicine.com. © The McGraw-Hill Companies, Inc.)

ED, one must have a high clinical suspicion for both hypo- and hyperthyroidism in those patients who present with appropriate symptoms. Measurements which are available for quantification by the lab are TSH, serum T_4/T_3, and free T_4/T_3. Serum T_4 and T_3 measure both bound and unbound moieties which confounds the interpretation of these values as drugs, and illness can alter the concentration of binding proteins. Free T_4 and T_3 more appropriately measure what is physiologically available for cell use. Free T_4 is most frequently what is measured as the free T_3 measurements have not proven to have significant clinical utility. Notably, in the severely critically ill patient, thyroid function tests are uniformly low even when primary thyroid pathology is not present. Surprisingly, thyroid hormone replacement therapy has not been shown to be of benefit in these patients.

TABLE 164.1	THYROID FUNCTION TESTS AND DISEASE STATES	
CLINICAL STATE	TSH	FREE T$_4$
Primary hypothyroidism	↑	↓
Subclinical hypothyroidism	↑	normal
Hyperthyroidism	↓	↑
Subclinical hyperthyroidism	↓	normal
Central hypothyroidism	↓ or normal	↓
TSH-mediated hyperthyroidism	↑ or normal	↑

For all ED patients in whom alterations in the thyroid hormone axis are suspected, both a TSH and a free T$_4$ should be sent. Most ED practitioners are familiar with primary hyper- and hypothyroid states such as Grave disease, toxic multinodular goiter, iodine intake, thyroiditis, autoimmune etiologies, etc. While the majority of thyroid hormone alterations are caused by primary pathology, deviation in the TSH alone cannot be interpreted to suggest etiology. A free T$_4$ must be included to establish the less common diagnoses of secondary hypothyroidism or TSH-mediated hyperthyroidism from primary thyroid pathology. Secondary hypothyroidism refers to a deficit in thyroid hormone secondary to a disorder of the hypothalamic-pituitary portal circulation, hypothalamus, or the pituitary itself. The causes of secondary hypothyroidism stem from pituitary pathology (apoplexy, mass lesion, infarction, etc.) or hypothalamic pathology (mass lesion, infection, infiltrative lesions, trauma, and radiation). TSH-mediated hyperthyroidism manifests with the classic history and physical exam findings of hyperthyroidism but is usually caused by overproduction of TSH from pituitary adenomas. Rarer abnormalities are due to aberrations in the receptors responsible for the negative feedback of T$_3$ to the pituitary also manifesting as hyperthyroid states with elevated TSH. For a summary of expected laboratory measurements for given disease states, see *Table 164.1*.

In summary, while primary thyroid disorders are the most common presentations of thyroid disease states, laboratory evaluation must include both a TSH and a free T$_4$ so as not to miss potentially life-altering diagnoses.

SUGGESTED READINGS

Becker RA, Vaughan GM, Ziegler MG, et al. Hypermetabolic low triiodothyronine syndrome of burn injury. *Crit Care Med*. 1982;10:870–875.

Brent GA, Hershman JM. Thyroxine therapy in patients with severe nonthyroidal illnesses and low serum thyroxine concentration. *J Clin Endocrinol Metab*. 1986;63:1–8.

Molina P, ed. Thyroid gland. In: *Endocrine Physiology*. 2nd ed. New York: McGraw Hill; 2006.

165

UNDERSTAND THE LIMITATIONS OF TESTING FOR URINARY KETONES AND SERUM ACETONE

SUSAN MARIE PETERSON, MD AND ARJUN S. CHANMUGAM, MD, MBA

Urine and serum ketones are commonly used in order to determine the diagnosis of diabetic ketoacidosis (DKA), alcoholic ketoacidosis (AKA), and salicylate ingestion. However, there are important caveats to the use of both urine and serum ketone tests that clinicians must be aware of in order to treat patients appropriately.

β-Hydroxybutyrate and acetoacetate are the two primary ketones produced by the liver in response to low levels of glucose, providing an alternative energy source to the brain and stimulating insulin production. Ketones are normally produced at a ratio of 1:1 (β-hydroxybutyrate:acetoacetate), but in illnesses such as DKA, AKA, and salicylate poisoning, the ratio often increases to over 3:1. Having a quantitative measure of ketone bodies present can be a useful indication of the severity of disease.

Currently, the only means of assessing the presence of ketones in the serum and urine is the nitroprusside test. Its great limitation is that it only indicates whether acetoacetate is present, and hence false negatives are possible, particularly with the urine test which is a simple qualitative test. The serum nitroprusside test is semiquantitative, utilizing dilutions of acetoacetate. A sample is tested for acetoacetate; if it is positive, then the sample is diluted in half or 1:2 and tested again. If the first dilution is positive, then a second dilution is obtained yielding a 1:4 dilution which is tested. Until the sample tests negative for acetoacetate, the sample will continue to be diluted as described. A dilution of 1:16 indicates more severe disease than a dilution of 1:8. The 1:8 sample only had acetoacetate in it after 3 dilutions, whereas the 1:16 sample had acetoacetate in it after 4 dilutions (1, 1:2, 1:4, 1:8, 1:16).

The nitroprusside test is a good initial screen; however, it gives no indication of the presence of β-hydroxybutyrate. The urine test is further limited as it only provides a qualitative measure. In addition, the nitroprusside test may also be associated with false positives in the presence of common drugs such as captopril, bucillamine, N-acetylcysteine, dimercaprol, and other drugs containing free sulfhydryl compounds secondary to the urinary production of compounds such as mesna. Acetone may also be detected using this test, creating false positives for conditions such as isopropyl alcohol ingestion.

Furthermore, in conditions such as DKA, the serum nirtroprusside test may mislead clinicians into thinking that patients are not initially improving. When patients receive insulin, there is an initial decrease in ketone bodies as well as a conversion of β-hydroxybutyrate to acetoacetate. Because of this conversion, the serum nitroprusside test may make it seem as though the acetoacetate level is at a sustained high level when in fact the total number of ketones and the actual β-hydroxybutyrate level may have decreased. As a result, in order to gain a better appreciation of ketone level, clinicians typically resort to tracking a patient's progress using the anion gap. Narrowing of the anion gap is indicative of improvement and can be done quickly and inexpensively and does not have selective ketone problem associated with the nitroprusside assay. It should be noted that a new serum quantitative β-hydroxybutyrate test is now commercially produced but may not be universally available from institution to institution.

In summary, the urine nitroprusside test used to indicate the presence of ketones is a qualitative test for only one of the major ketones, acetoacetate, and as a result may have false negatives. In addition, false positives are possible in the presence of commonly used medications such as captopril. Serum nitroprusside tests are more useful because the semiquantitative nature gives a better indication of severity of disease; however, when determining insulin regimens using the anion gap or a quantitative serum, β-hydroxybutyrate test is a more accurate indicator of a patient's progress.

SUGGESTED READINGS

Csako G, Elin RJ. Unrecognized false-positive ketones from drugs containing free-sulfhydryl groups. *JAMA.* 1993;279(13):1634.

Davidson M. Diabetic detoacidosis and hyperosmolar nonketotic syndrome. In: *Diabetes Mellitus: Diagnosis and Treatment.* 4th ed. Philadelphia: WB Saunders Co; 1998:159–164.

Laffel L. Ketone bodies: A review of physiology, pathophysiology and application of monitoring to diabetes. *Diabetes Metab Res Rev.* 1999;15:412–426.

166

UNDERSTAND THE ROLE OF MAGNESIUM IN THE TREATMENT OF HYPOKALEMIA

JOHN W. BURGER, MD

PRINCIPLES OF POTASSIUM REPLETION

There are two basic mechanisms of hypokalemia: increased excretion of potassium and movement of potassium into the intracellular space. Treatment of hypokalemia ultimately depends on correcting the underlying cause, but this may not be entirely possible in the acute setting. Until the underlying cause is fixed, it is no great surprise that patients who are losing potassium continue to need replacement.

In general, administration of 10 mEq of potassium chloride will correspond to a 0.1 mEq/L increase in serum potassium. The preferred route of replacement in large part depends on the severity of the hypokalemia. Patients who have potassium levels <2.5 mEq/L, who are severely symptomatic, or who have evidence of EKG changes should receive intravenous replacement of potassium. There are patients who present with a low potassium who will have a total body potassium depletion. These patients require significant amounts of potassium, because the cells in the body have given up their intracellular stores to compensate for a low serum potassium. The standard dose in patients with peripheral access is 10 mEq per h. Those receiving more than 20 mEq per h of potassium require central venous access as well as cardiac monitoring since a rapid rise in potassium can lead to arrhythmias. Patients who have potassium levels between 2.5 and 3.5 mEq/L and exhibit little to no symptoms can usually be managed with oral replacement therapy. The recommended dose of oral potassium given at any one time is 40 to 60 mEq. Higher doses are not tolerated well because of the propensity for gastrointestinal (GI) upset and vomiting.

REFRACTORY HYPOKALEMIA

While the principles of potassium repletion in patients who are hypokalemic seem straightforward, simply giving a fixed amount of exogenous potassium may not be enough to correct the presenting deficit. This could be attributed to the fact that the amount of potassium being wasted is greater than the total amount being administered. However, when the potassium level does not rise as expected despite adequate treatment, it may signify the presence of a refractory hypokalemia. The first step in approaching hypokalemia that does not respond to treatment is to check a magnesium level. Magnesium deficiency often accompanies hypokalemia. Until the magnesium level is corrected, the hypokalemia will be very difficult to reverse.

The exact mechanism of how low magnesium levels lead to refractory hypokalemia is unclear. One theory suggests that magnesium deficiency can impair cellular uptake of potassium by affecting the Na-K ATPase pump. Another theory proposes that a lack of magnesium increases potassium excretion by altering specific potassium channels in the kidney. Regardless of the mechanism, magnesium levels should be checked in patients requiring urgent or emergent potassium replacement. While hypomagnesemia can certainly exacerbate hypokalemia, magnesium deficiency by itself is seldom the underlying cause driving the hypokalemia. A low magnesium level can explain why the potassium level is difficult to fix but does not answer why the level was abnormal in the first place.

MAGNESIUM REPLACEMENT

In the acute setting, magnesium replacement is best achieved via intravenous administration of magnesium sulfate. The normal range of serum magnesium is 1.7 to 2.2 mg/dL. For magnesium levels ranging >1.3 mg/dL, 1 to 2 g of magnesium sulfate should be given over 30 to 60 min. For levels <1 mg/dL, 3 to 4 g of magnesium sulfate can be given over a span of 2 h.

Magnesium plays a role in mitigating other electrolyte abnormalities beyond just that of potassium. Magnesium also plays a key role in maintaining calcium balance. Low magnesium level can aggravate hypocalcemia rendering it refractory to replacement efforts. In this case, magnesium deficiency is thought to impair calcium regulation by inhibiting the release of parathyroid hormone.

KEY POINTS

Hypokalemia can be a life-threatening emergency like any other electrolyte abnormality. Be sure to recheck levels after the commencement of exogenous potassium replacement as aggressive treatment puts patients at risk for iatrogenic hyperkalemia. Any patient receiving a rapid infusion or large amount of potassium should be placed on a cardiac monitor due to the possibility of arrhythmias. Magnesium plays an important role in repletion of both potassium and calcium. If hypokalemia or hypocalcemia do not respond to initial treatment, consider the possibility of magnesium deficiency. Remember, hypomagnesemia can make the situation worse but is rarely the causative agent. After correcting the magnesium deficiency, continue to investigate other potential reasons for the electrolyte derangement.

SUGGESTED READINGS

Al-Ghamdi S, Cameron E, Sutton R. Magneium deficiency: Pathophysiologic and clinical overview. *Am J Kidney Dis*. 1994;24:737–752.

Gennari F. Hypokalemia. *N Engl J Med*. 1998;339:451–458.

Huang C, Huo E. Mechanism of hypokalemia in magnesium deficiency. *J Am Soc Nephrol*. 2007;18:2649–2652.

Tintinalli J, Kelen G, Stapczynski J. *Emergency Medicine: A Comprehensive Study Guide*. 6th ed. New York: McGraw-Hill;2003:172–177.

2005 American Heart Association Guidelines for Cardiopulmonary Resuscitation and Emergency Cardiovascular Care. Part 10.1: Life-threatening electrolyte abnormalities. *Circulation*. 2005;112:IV-121–IV-125.

167

USE VENOUS RATHER THAN ARTERIAL BLOOD GAS MEASUREMENTS

SAMIT DESAI, MD

The arterial blood gas is a lab test that is often regarded as fundamental. The question of whether a venous blood gas may be sufficient in lieu of an arterial blood gas has been a source of controversy for years. This discussion will not focus on the clinical need of the blood gas but instead on whether or not a venous blood gas is an acceptable replacement for the time-honored arterial blood gas.

Three questions need answering to help solve this dilemma. First, does evidence suggest that there is a reasonable and reliable degree of accuracy between the two samples with regard specifically to pH and the partial pressure of carbon dioxide (an assumption is made that the partial pressure of oxygen will range wildly depending on the state of oxygen extraction)? Second, does pulse oximetry serve as an adequate surrogate for the arterial blood gas in determining the patient's oxygenation status? And finally, and maybe most importantly, which test better represents the information that is necessary for patient care?

We will, for a moment, assume the widely held belief that the arterial blood gas is held in higher regard than the venous blood gas. Does the pH correlate between the two types of tests? There have been a number of studies that have sought to establish what degree of difference exists between arterial and venous samples. For pH, in particular, a study performed on patients with diabetic ketoacidosis yielded a mean difference of 0.03. Yet another study, this time evaluating patients across a broad-spectrum of illness, resulted in a mean difference of 0.04. One study to refute this reliable difference in pH was among patients in cardiac arrest. It is arguable, however, that the pH of a patient in cardiac arrest carries little significance.

The partial pressure of carbon dioxide in the setting of respiratory distress is yet another reason why a blood gas is often obtained. A number of studies have demonstrated an increase in the venous partial pressure of carbon dioxide to be on average 6 mm Hg. Admittedly, the agreement was not as consistent as that seen with pH, and a screening cutoff of 45 mm Hg was suggested to demonstrate 100% sensitivity in the detection of hypercarbia. As expected, as the venous partial pressure of carbon dioxide rises, the specificity for detecting hypercarbia increases.

What is the need for a partial pressure of oxygen when a reliable pulse oximetry reading gives you more information about the patient's cellular oxygen delivery? Pulse oximetry has near widespread acceptance for its ability to accurately portray arterial hemoglobin saturation with oxygen. One study suggests that a pulse oximeter reading is within 2% to 5% of a recorded arterial blood gas oximetry reading provided that the actual arterial value falls within the range of 70% to 100%. Furthermore, it is thought that the amount of oxygen that a cell receives is a function of cardiac output, level of hemoglobin, and the *oxygen saturation of that hemoglobin*. Therefore, unless there is reason to suggest an inaccurate pulse oximetry reading, an arterial blood gas need not be obtained to solely assess oxygenation status. Examples of cases during which the pulse oximeter may be suspect include extremely poor peripheral perfusion, methemoglobinemia, and carbon monoxide poisoning.

Thus, the argument can be made, with evidence in hand, that the venous blood gas, combined with pulse oximetry, may serve as a substitute for the arterial blood gas. Further, the lynchpin in the argument against the arterial blood gas rests on the rejection of the notion that the arterial blood gas carries greater clinical significance than the venous blood gas. If our focus rests on resuscitation at the cellular level, should we not record values after cellular metabolism is accounted for? In regard to the partial pressure of carbon dioxide, it is the venous value that the lung must dispense of and not the arterial value. This line of thinking would place more value on venous pH and partial pressure of carbon dioxide than arterial values.

The arterial blood gas hurts. There is evidence that the venous blood gas not only provides accurate measurement of clinically relevant values but may also serve as a more significant indicator of a patient's condition.

SUGGESTED READINGS

Brandenburg MA, Dire DJ. Comparison of arterial and venous blood gas values in the initial emergency department evaluation of patients with diabetic ketoacidosis. *Ann Emerg Med.* 1998;31(4):459–465.

Jensen LA, Onyskiw JE, Prasad NG. Meta-analysis of arterial oxygen saturation monitoring by pulse oximetry in adults. *Heart Lung.* 1998;27:387–408.

Kelly AM. Venous pCO(2) and pH can be used to screen for significant hypercarbia in emergency patients with acute respiratory disease. *J Emerg Med.* 2002;22(1):15–19.

Tintinalli JE, Ruiz, Krome RL, et al., eds. *Emergency Medicine: A Comprehensive Study Guide.* 6th ed. New York: McGraw-Hill; 2004.

168

DO NOT DISCOUNT THE COMPLAINTS OF "FREQUENT FLIERS"

EDUARDO BORQUEZ, MD

Frequent users of the emergency department (ED), often pejoratively (and inappropriately) referred to as "frequent fliers," have gained increasing interest in emergency medicine. They are a complex and diverse population. While the definition of what constitutes a frequent user of the ED ranges from as few as three to more than twelve annual visits, some authors have chosen the more vague but generally agreed-upon definition of patients whom the staff know by name. Although they represent less than one in ten patients (8%), they account for over a quarter (28%) of ED visits in some studies.

In the minds of many emergency physicians, this percentage may be perceived as being much higher. As a sometimes very vocal minority, frequent users of the ED are often categorized as intractable and difficult patients. To add fuel to the fire, intense scrutiny on the problem of ED crowding has focused the attention of some administrators on what they perceive as unnecessary visits. Studies in the early 1990s showed that nearly half of patients (43%) visiting EDs had illnesses or injuries that could have been dealt with in a nonemergent setting.

With these facts in mind, many have hypothesized that frequent ED users are responsible for "inappropriate" visits that cause undue strain on the system. However, several facts contradict this commonly held belief. First, several studies have shown that the vast majority of frequent ED users have both insurance (84%) and primary care physicians (81%). Even more surprisingly, it has been found that patients without a usual (non-ED) source of care were *less* likely to be frequent users! Moreover, in contrast to common belief, frequent users tend to be as sick as or sicker than patients who use the ED less frequently. Finally, repeat patients have higher rates of hospital admission, higher mortality and higher rates of mental illness, as well as lower socioeconomic status.

This situation presents a recipe for a myriad of pitfalls when dealing with a patient labeled as a "frequent flier." Familiarity with the ED staff may cause undue reassurance that the current presentation does not represent the actual acute disease. Additionally, an associated mental illness may mask the recognition of true medical disease.

When considering these challenges in caring for frequent ED users, several potential solutions emerge. First, clinicians need to recognize the *increased* likelihood of acute disease and exacerbations of chronic illnesses in repeat patients. The clinician should have a *heightened*, not decreased, concern for underlying medical conditions in repeat patients with psychiatric complaints. Second, when dealing with frequent ED users, the clinician should be aware of the risk factors that may contribute to a potentially difficult patient-physician relationship. These risk factors include mental illness, personality disorder, secondary gain issues, and the suspicion of malingering. The frequent ED user may evoke feelings of "anger, self-doubt, and frustration" on the part of the nursing staff and physician.

Fortunately, there are proven management strategies that have been shown to help in these situations. Some experts recommend strategies such as empathizing with patients and acknowledging the frustration they must feel regarding the chronic nature of their disease. Setting reasonable goals with the patient at the beginning of the ED visit has also been shown to help. Using case management to create a multidisciplinary plan for repeat visitors has been shown to result in both clinical and cost-effectiveness.

If recent trends in emergency medicine continue, frequent users will compose an increasing percentage of the ED patient population. Emergency physicians should become fluent in the challenges that this special population faces.

SUGGESTED READINGS

Emergency Departments. *Unevenly Affected by Growth and Change in Patient Use*. Washington, DC: US General Accounting Office; 1993.

Harrison D. The difficult patient. In: *Rosen's Emergency Medicine: Concepts and Clinical Practice*. 6th ed. St. Louis: Mosby, Inc.; 2006.

Hunt KA, Weber EJ, Showstack JA. Characteristics of frequent users of emergency departments. *Ann Emerg Med*. 2006;48(1):1–8.

Okin RL, Boccellari A, Azocar F, et al. The effects of clinical case management on hospital service use among ED frequent users. *Am J Emerg Med*. 2000;18(5):603–608.

Ruger JP, Richter CJ, Spitznagel EL, et al. Analysis of costs, length of stay, and utilization of emergency department services by frequent users: Implications for health policy. *Acad Emerg Med*. 2004;11(12):1311–1317.

Shumway M, Boccellari A, O'Brien K, et al. Cost-effectiveness of clinical case management for ED frequent users: Results of a randomized trial. *Am J Emerg Med*. 2008;26(2):155–164.

Sun BC, Burstin HR, Brennan TA. Predictors and outcomes of frequent emergency department users. *Acad Emerg Med*. 2003;10(4):320–328.

Williams ER, Shepherd SM. Medical clearance of psychiatric patients. *Emerg Med Clin North Am*. 2000;18(2):185–198.

169

BE VIGILANT FOR PHYSICAL ABUSE AND NEGLECT

MARY SADEGHI, MD AND JORGE A. FERNANDEZ, MD, FAAEM, FACEP

Because emergency physicians are on the front lines of caring for outpatient victims of trauma, it is incumbent on them to make the diagnosis of physical abuse or neglect, whether it be from child maltreatment, elder abuse, or intimate partner violence (IPV). Emergency physicians may be the only health care practitioners involved in their patients' care. On the other hand, it is also important not to misdiagnose abuse in cases of accidental trauma.

Each year in the United States, women experience 4.8 million intimate partner–related physical assaults and rapes. Despite this alarming figure and published guidelines by the American Medical Association recommending that all women routinely be questioned about abuse, many emergency physicians fail to routinely ask their female patients about domestic abuse. There are several historical and physical exam findings that are suggestive of IPV abuse, including, but not limited to, injuries indicating a defensive posture, a central pattern of injury, injuries inconsistent with the patient's explanation, multiple injuries in various stages of healing, and substantial delay between the time of injury and the presentation for treatment. In busy and chaotic emergency departments, physicians may fail to consider IPV in cases that are not clearly obvious. Unfortunately, if emergency physicians rely on diagnosing IPV only when it is obvious, they will miss a substantial number of cases. When diagnosing IPV, the main goal should be to ensure the safety of the victim and her children and to provide the patient with information about her risks and options. Mandatory reporting of cases is controversial, and laws vary in each state.

Abuse and neglect may be one of the least recognized and reported causes of morbidity and mortality in the elderly population. More than 33,000 elderly patients were treated for assault-related injuries in the United States in 2001. However, in a national survey of emergency physicians, only 31% reported having elder abuse protocols and only 50% of suspected elder abuse cases were reported. Some of the barriers to the reporting are unfamiliarity with available resources and mandatory reporting laws, fear of time constraints, and concern for offending the patient.

In contrast to IPV and elder abuse, emergency physicians are generally more diligent when it comes to child maltreatment. Despite significant public health efforts, child maltreatment is still a significant cause of morbidity and mortality; in 2006, more than 1,500 children died from abuse and neglect. It is imperative that emergency physicians obtain a detailed history from caregivers and look for inconsistency between the history and the extent and pattern of injuries. The physical examination should note the child's overall appearance and interaction with the caregiver. Classic physical findings in child abuse are subdural hematomas, skull fractures, retinal hemorrhage, abdominal trauma, bruising on the trunk or genitals, human bites, atypical burns, and certain fractures that rarely occur in accidental trauma.

The misdiagnosis and subsequent reporting of child abuse can be devastating to families. Physicians should remember to consider alternative causes such as atypical fractures from osteogenesis imperfecta, osteopenia, and congenital syphilis. Impetigo, staphylococcal scalded skin syndrome, and atopic dermatitis can commonly be mistaken for burns. Bruises in various stages of healing, or with underlying hematomas, can be the first presentation of hemophilia, idiopathic thrombocytopenic purpura (ITP), leukemia, or vasculitis. Physicians must also be aware of various cultural practices, such as cupping or coining, which can cause bruises or burns.

When in doubt of the diagnosis of abuse, it is best to admit patients for further medical and social services evaluation, as the consequences of missed diagnosis of abuse could be fatal.

SUGGESTED READINGS

Abbot J. Assault-related injury: What do we know, and what should we do about it? *Ann Emerg Med*. 1998;32:363–366.

Flitcraft A, Hadley S. *Diagnostic and Treatment Guidelines on Domestic Violence*. Chicago, IL: American Medical Association; 1992.

Heider TR, Priolo D, Hultman CS, et al. Eczema mimicking child abuse: a case of mistaken identity. *J Burn Care Rehabil*. 2002;23(5):357–359.

Jain AM. Emergency department evaluation of child abuse. *Emerg Med Clin North Am*. 1999;17(3):575–593.

Jones JS, Veenstra TR, Seamon JP, et al. Elder mistreatment: National survey of emergency physicians. *Ann Emerg Med*. 1997;30(4):473–479.

Kleinschmidt KC. Elder abuse: A review. *Ann Emerg Med*. 1997;30(4):463–472.

National Center for Health Statistics. *Center for Disease Control and Prevention*. 2006. Available at: http://www.cdc.gov.

Rodriguez MA. Screening and intervention for intimate partner abuse: Practices and attitudes of primary care physicians. *JAMA*. 1999;282:468–474.

Salber PR. Intimate partner violence and abuse. In: *Emergency Medicine: A Comprehensive Study Guide*. 6th ed. New York: McGraw-Hill Companies Inc.; 2004.

Walter AJ. Misdiagnosis of abuse. *CMAJ*. 2003;169(7):651–652.

Zachary MJ, Mulvihill MN, Burton WB, et al. Domestic abuse in the emergency department: Can a risk profile be defined? *Acad Emerg Med*. 2001;8(8):796–803.

170

BE CERTAIN TO PROTECT PATIENTS OR THIRD PARTIES FROM HARM

MARY LOUISE MARTIN, MD AND
JORGE A. FERNANDEZ, MD, FAAEM, FACEP

There are several situations in emergency medicine that require a notification of public health officials or law enforcement personnel. Emergency physicians must be intimately aware of these laws, which may vary from state to state. Often, the duty to protect patient or family confidentiality may be overridden by the duty to protect citizens or society from harm.

The duty to warn third parties of imminent harm is an infamous example. In 1974, the courts of California ruled that a psychologist was negligent for not notifying Tatiana Tarasoff of the death threat that his patient had made against her. At the time, there was no legal precedent that mandated a health care professional to warn and protect third parties. Unfortunately, despite police notification and a subsequent 2-week incarceration, the patient murdered Ms Tarasoff, and the psychologist was successfully sued by her family. In 1976, the California Supreme Court upheld the original court decision and ruled that health care professionals had a duty to protect third parties from a foreseeable danger of violence from their patients. This ruling has been challenged by many in the health care community as compromising the basic core of the physician-patient relationship. Although two states have ruled against Tarasoff laws, it has been upheld in most circumstances. Furthermore, its scope has often been extended beyond the original intent. Therefore, emergency physicians should know the legal statutes in their respective states.

Suspected child or elder neglect or abuse is another situation where a physician's duty to protect is explicitly mandated by law. In these circumstances, all states are in agreement. The issue of mandatory reporting in cases of intimate partner violence is more controversial. When a violent weapon is used, most states mandate reporting. However, in other settings of intimate partner violence, there is more variation among states. Notably, the American College of Emergency Physicians (ACEP) and the American Medical Association have adopted a policy against mandatory reporting of intimate partner violence due to unclear scientific evidence of patient benefit.

There are numerous diagnoses that require mandatory reporting to appropriate authorities. Any condition that may cause recurrent lapses of consciousness, such as seizure or syncope, is reportable. Furthermore, there are numerous infectious diseases that require mandatory public health reporting. Physicians must become familiar with the diseases that require mandatory reporting to public health officials in their state.

The emergency physician's role in his or her duty to protect third parties can be safely met by adhering to the following guidelines. First, the prompt stabilization of the patient should be the initial priority. The duty to protect includes maintaining the safety of everyone in the emergency department. In the case of violent patients, there is a duty to protect hospital staff by the use of physical and/or chemical restraints. Once everyone in the emergency department has been stabilized and protected, the physician may extend the duty to protect to third parties outside the department. In cases of potential dangerous behaviors, psychiatric consultation should be obtained. If a threat to third parties is explicitly made, law enforcement personnel should be notified in most situations. As with any other high-risk situation, thorough documentation is necessary. A description of the patient's threats and behaviors must be detailed in the medical record. Efforts to involve psychiatry and law enforcement as well as all attempts to notify potential victims should also be documented.

The application of the emergency physician's duty to protect third parties carries many ethical dilemmas, and each case should be evaluated on an individual basis. The use of the best medical practices for the patient should always accompany appropriate actions that address concerns for the well-being of others. The ACEP Code of Ethics states, "Respect patient privacy and disclose confidential information only with consent of the patient or when required by an overriding duty such as the duty to protect others or to obey the law." Remember to always familiarize yourself with the individual state laws that govern your practice.

SUGGESTED READINGS

[No authors listed]. Code of ethics for emergency physicians. *Ann Emerg Med*. 2004;43(5): 686–694.

Knopp RK, Satterlee PA. Confidentiality in the emergency department. *Emerg Med Clin N Am*. 1999;17(2):385–396.

Moskop JC, Marco CA, Larkin GL, et al. From Hippocrates to HIPAA: Privacy and confidentiality. *Ann Emerg Med*. 2005;45(1):53–67.

Pointer JE, Small LB. Emergency physicians' duty to warn and protect. *J Emerg Med*. 1986;4:75–78.

Rosen P, O'Connor M. The practice of medicine vs. the practice of law. *J Emerg Med*. 1986;4:67–68.

171

UNDERSTAND THE DANGERS ASSOCIATED WITH TASER INJURIES

SAI-HUNG JOSHUA HUI, MD AND JORGE A. FERNANDEZ, MD, FAAEM, FACEP

TASER (Thomas A. Swift Electric Rifle, TASER International, Scottsdale, AZ) is the brand name for a line of stun gun devices that incapacitate subjects by inducing transient neuromuscular paralysis through a transmission of 2 to 3 amps and 50,000 V of electricity in 10 μs pulses lasting a total of 5 s. The device has gained immense popularity among law enforcement personnel over the past two decades. According to its manufacturer, approximately 11,000 police departments in the United States and 115,000 private citizens own TASER devices. The devices are considered weapons and are therefore not regulated by the U.S. Food and Drug Administration as medical devices. Numerous deaths and morbidities have been associated with the use of the TASER, in both lay press and peer-reviewed research publications. Nevertheless, there are also numerous studies defending the safety of the devices. Because individuals who are "TASERed" are frequently brought for medical evaluation, emergency physicians should be aware of the potential complications associated with TASER use in order to avoid missing serious associated injuries.

Although patients may not be forthcoming or may be unable to relate an accurate history, it is important to recognize underlying illness, toxicity, and injury. Patients are frequently agitated or combative. Dehydration and mixed drug intoxication with phencyclidine (PCP), cocaine, amphetamines, and alcohol commonly occur in these patients. Not surprisingly, rhabdomyolysis and transient hyperkalemia are frequently observed. Whether patients actually develop rhabdomyolysis as a result of TASER application is controversial, because agitated delirium itself may be responsible in the reported cases.

There are numerous traumatic complications following TASER use. Blunt injury to the head, cervical spine, pelvis, and extremities may result because of postural muscle paralysis. The TASER barbs themselves may cause penetrating injuries. TASER barbs measure <1 cm, are shaped like a small fishhook, and travel at a speed of approximately 170 ft per s. There are case reports of open globe injury or intracranial penetration. They may become lodged in any body part, and physicians should consider deep injury underlying the site of any embedded barb.

There is currently considerable controversy regarding the association of TASERs with ventricular fibrillation and sudden cardiac death. Conflicting results and conclusions have been drawn from hundreds of studies. In most animal and human studies, troponin elevations were not seen in healthy subjects despite multiple TASER shocks. In many reported cases, ventricular arrhythmia and sudden death may have occurred secondary to underlying predisposition toward tachydysrhythmia, which was aggravated by agitation, intoxication, and hyperkalemia. Interestingly, in one patient with an implanted pacemaker, a TASER shock resulted in myocardial capture and stable ventricular tachycardia; however, there was no adverse outcome.

The American College of Emergency Physicians has not published a clinical policy regarding the management of TASER injuries. Although few recommendations can be made based on evidence, the common sequelae outlined above should help the practitioner know what to look for. In general, patients with persistent altered sensorium upon ED arrival should be placed onto a cardiac monitor. Whether to obtain an ECG or serial troponins remains controversial; nevertheless, some emergency practitioners routinely advocate these tests in all patients following TASER shock. The measurement of creatine kinase and urinalysis are helpful to rule out rhabdomyolysis, but again, blanket recommendations for these are difficult to make based on the available evidence. Careful examination of the site of barb implantation should be undertaken in each case.

SUGGESTED READINGS

Amnesty International. United States of America Excessive and Lethal Force? Amnesty International's Concerns About Deaths and Ill-treatment Involving Police Use of Tasers; 2004. Available at: http://www.amnestyusa.org/countries/usa/Taser_report.pdf.

Cao M, Shinbane JS, Gillberg JM, et al. Taser-induced rapid ventricular myocardial capture demonstrated by pacemaker intracardiac electrograms. *J Cardiovasc Electrophysiol.* 2007;18(8):876–879.

Jauchem J, Sherry C, Fines D, et al. Acidosis, lactate, electrolytes, muscle enzymes, and other factors in the blood of Sus scrofa following repeated TASER® exposures. *Forensic Sci Int.* 2006;161(1):20–30.

Ng W, Chehade M. Taser penetrating ocular injury. *Am J Ophthalmol.* 2005;139(4):713–715.

Ordog GJ, Wasserberger J, Schlater T, et al. Electronic gun (Taser) injuries. *Ann Emerg Med.* 1987;16(1):73–78.

Rehman T, Yonas H, Marinaro J. Intracranial penetration of a TASER dart. *Am J Emerg Med.* 2007;25(6):733.e3–e4.

Sanford JM, Jacobs GJ, Roe EJ, et al. Two patients subdued with a taser(R) device: Cases and review of complications. *J Emerg Med.* Apr 23, 2008 [Epub ahead of print.]

TASER International. X26 and M26 products specification. Available at: http://www.taser. com

Walter R, Dennis AJ, Valentino DJ, et al. TASER X26 discharges in swine produce potentially fatal ventricular arrhythmias. *Acad Emerg Med.* 2008;15(1):66–73.

172

MAINTAIN A LOW THRESHOLD TO PERFORM ARTHROCENTESIS IN PATIENTS WITH SWOLLEN JOINTS

JESSICA HERNANDEZ, MD

The patient with a complaint of an acutely swollen joint is a frequent clinical presentation and can pose a diagnostic challenge to the physician. The differential diagnosis is extensive and it can be difficult to distinguish among them without thorough investigation. Such likely entities include, but are not limited to, rheumatoid arthritis, gout, pseudogout, septic arthritis, and synovitis. Of these, it is critical that the physician does not miss a diagnosis of septic arthritis as it is deemed a medical emergency and carries significant morbidity and mortality for the patient. Unfortunately, history, physical exam, and basic laboratory tests are not enough to definitively rule out septic arthritis. It is imperative that clinicians maintain a low threshold for performing arthrocentesis in patients presenting with an acute swollen joint to minimize delay in the diagnosis and treatment of septic arthritis.

Septic arthritis is a rapidly destructive microbial infection of the joint space synovial tissue. Common portals of entry include hematogenous, contiguous (i.e., osteomyelitis, cellulitis), and direct violation of the joint space (i.e., traumatic, iatrogenic). The usual suspects include streptococcus, staphylococcus, and Gram-negative bacteria. The human body's own inflammatory response to the bacteria causes the destruction of cartilage and joint structures. Identified risk factors include a history of rheumatoid disease, diabetes, prosthetic joints, IV drug use, alcoholism, and skin ulcers. Septic arthritis classically presents as an acutely swollen, hot, tender joint accompanied with restriction of movement and fever.

The gold standard for the diagnosis of septic arthritis is arthrocentesis with analysis of joint aspirate (culture, WBC with differential, and Gram stain). Criteria most useful in supporting a diagnosis of septic arthritis in the acute setting include a high WBC joint aspirate, >90% polymorphonuclear cells, and positive Gram stain. Treatment should be initiated as soon as possible to avoid permanent joint destruction and, in some instances, death. In addition to appropriate antibiotic therapy (should be tailored to the specific organism stained or cultured), the patient will likely require arthroscopy or arthrotomy to thoroughly wash out the infected joint. Even in cases where appropriate treatment is promptly initiated, there remains a significant risk of morbidity and mortality to the patient.

Unfortunately, historical facts can falsely reassure the clinician that septic arthritis is unlikely and arthrocentesis is unnecessary. Case in point, a history of rheumatoid arthritis or other systemic joint disease may sway the physician to attribute the diagnosis to an acute flare of the patient's primary disorder. However, a prior inflammatory joint condition places patients at an increased risk for the development of septic arthritis. Another pitfall to avoid is in regard to the widely held misconception that septic arthritis is a monoarticular entity when, contrary to this belief, studies have shown that it can often present as polyarticular. Additionally, the various entities that cause arthropathies manifest similarly, and it is difficult to confidently rule out septic arthritis based on a history and physical exam alone.

It is also important for the physician to recognize that although septic arthritis can present as a systemic inflammatory infection, many patients may not have fever or an elevated peripheral white count. Synthesizing 14 studies involving 6,242 patients, the sensitivity of fever was 57%. The sensitivity of an elevated peripheral WBC was 48% in one study and 75% in another.

Aspiration of purulent fluid and positive cellular analysis are most helpful in distinguishing septic arthritis from similarly presenting entities in the acute setting. A review article by Margaretten et al. (2007) in the *JAMA* clinical exam series concluded that arthrocentesis with analysis of joint WBC and polymorphonuclear cells is a requirement when assessing the probability of septic arthritis before culture results are available.

The risks associated with arthrocentesis are minimal, while the risks associated with a missed diagnosis of septic arthritis can be devastating. Some relative contraindications to arthrocentesis include bacteremia, attempts by physicians not trained in the procedure, overlying cellulitis or severe dermatitis, severe coagulopathy, and an uncooperative patient. The development of iatrogenic septic arthritis is a rare complication, and efforts should be made to avoid entering through the infected soft tissue. However, even in these instances, if the suspicion for septic arthritis is high, joint aspiration is still indicated. Coumadin therapy is not a contraindication to arthrocentesis.

Because septic arthritis is a medical emergency that manifests with nonspecific features, maintain a low threshold for arthrocentesis in patients presenting with swollen joints.

TAKE HOME POINTS

- The clinician must consider and rule out septic arthritis in patients with a nontraumatic acutely swollen joint.
- Septic arthritis will cause rapid joint destruction and, in some instances, death.
- Arthrocentesis with Gram stain and culture is absolutely necessary for the definitive diagnosis of septic arthritis.
- Purulent joint fluid, an elevated joint WBC, and elevated joint polymorphonuclear cells are most helpful for the diagnosis before culture results become available.
- A history of joint disease increases the risk for the development of septic arthritis.
- Fever, elevated peripheral WBC, and elevated ESR are nonspecific findings, and lack of these factors does not rule out septic arthritis.

SUGGESTED READINGS

Coakley G, Mathews C, Field M, et al. BSR & BHPR, BOA, RCGP and BSAC guidelines for the management of the hot swollen joint in adults. *Rheumatology (Oxford).* 2006;45(8):1039–1041.

Levine M, Siegel LB. A swollen joint: Why all the fuss? *Am J Ther.* 2003;10(3):219–224.

Li SF, Cassidy C, Chang C, et al. Diagnostic utility of laboratory tests in septic arthritis. *Emerg Med J.* 2007;24:75–77.

Li SF, Henderson J, Dickman E, et al. Laboratory tests in adults with monoarticular arthritis: Can they rule out a septic joint? *Acad Emerg Med.* 2004;11(3):276–280.

Margaretten ME, Kohlwes J, Moore D, et al. Does this adult patient have septic arthritis? *JAMA.* 2007;297:1478–1488.

Mathews CJ, Coakley G. Septic arthritis: Current diagnostic and therapeutic algorithm. *Curr Opin Rheumatol.* 2008;20(4):457–462.

173

DO NOT ASSUME THAT SYNOVIAL FLUID ANALYSIS IS 100% ACCURATE FOR THE DIAGNOSIS OF SEPTIC ARTHRITIS

JENNIFER BAINE, MD AND LALEH GHARAHBAGHIAN, MD

INTRODUCTION

The differential diagnosis for monoarticular joint pain includes septic arthritis. Delayed diagnosis can lead to permanent joint disability and even mortality. For this reason, a high clinical suspicion must be maintained for patients with atypical presentations or lab findings that are not classically diagnostic.

HISTORY AND PHYSICAL EXAM

The chief complaint is often monoarticular joint pain (usually lower extremity) that is worse with movement and associated with edema and warmth, although polyarticular pain and upper extremity septic arthritis may occur. Children may stop using the affected limb. Underlying joint disease, such as rheumatoid arthritis, gout, or osteoarthritis, are predispositions to developing septic arthritis. Immunocompromised patients, such as those with HIV or those on chemotherapeutic and chronic corticosteroid therapy, may not have significant pain and may also have minimal warmth and edema. Patients with chronic reactive arthritis may have pain in one joint out of proportion to pain in other joints.

Atypical joints must be considered in IV drug users, as these patients can develop septic arthritis in sternoclavicular, sacroiliac, and manubriosternal joints.

Patients with septic arthritis tend to have normal vital signs except for a fever; however, a fever cannot be relied upon for the diagnosis of septic arthritis. These patients hold the joint still in a position of maximum comfort, relaxing the joint capsule and enlarging the joint space. In the hip, flexion, abduction, and external rotation enlarge the joint space, and in the knee, 30 degrees of flexion is the position of maximal comfort. During examination, the joint is extremely painful to palpation and with movement, both active and passive. An effusion should be palpable and the overlying skin may be warm and erythematous. In the deep joints—the hip and shoulder—effusion may not be obvious.

LABORATORY RESULTS

Joint aspiration is warranted with a suspicion of septic arthritis. The synovial fluid is typically sent for Gram stain and culture, crystal analysis, WBC count and differential, and glucose. Ideally, the offending organism is present by Gram stain and then cultures can direct antibiotic therapy. A recent meta-analysis reviewed the components of a typical clinical evaluation to identify best indicators of septic arthritis and found that the most useful rapid tests of joint aspirate are WBC count and percentage of polymorphonuclear (PMN) cells. Synovial fluid with a bacterial infection is typically described as cloudy, low in glucose with WBC count of >50,000 cells/mm, >90% of which as PMN cells.

The greatest pitfall in the evaluation of septic arthritis is the erroneous elimination of the diagnosis with a negative synovial fluid analysis. Even though joint fluid culture is the gold standard diagnostic test, the results of Gram stain and culture are negative in as high as 25% of septic arthritis cases. If suspicion for septic arthritis remains high, the clinician should consider synovial tissue biopsy which may reveal an organism in the setting of a negative fluid culture. Gram stain and cultures may be negative early in the course of the infection, secondary to poor culturing technique or delay in culturing, with fastidious organisms or in the presence of leukocytes which have engulfed the bacteria. Blood and urine cultures should be obtained and potentially repeated with a high clinical suspicion of septic arthritis. Another potential pitfall with synovial fluid interpretation is removal of septic arthritis from the differential diagnosis upon a joint aspirate revealing crystals. Though crystals may increase the relative weight of gout and other diseases on the differential, crystals may also be present in a septic joint and therefore do not rule out the diagnosis of septic arthritis.

So how can the emergency physician avoid missing a septic joint? Given that a miss has the potential to cause permanent disability or even mortality, it is critical to keep septic arthritis on the differential in the setting of negative synovial analysis. Clinical suspicion should guide the emergency physician more than any diagnostic test—all of which have been proven to be fallible. In many settings, pursuing the diagnosis by more advanced studies such as synovial tissue biopsy may not be feasible; yet, one should consider treating empirically and send joint fluid culture for potential antibiotic therapy guidance.

SUGGESTED READINGS

Kocher MS, Zurakowski D, Kasser JR. Differentiating between septic arthritis and transient synovitis of the hip in children: An evidence-based clinical prediction algorithm. *J Bone Joint Surg*. 1999;81:1662–1670.

Margaretten ME, Kohlwes J, Moore D, et al. Does this adult patient have septic arthritis? *JAMA*. 2007;297(13):1478–1488.

Scherping SC, Aaron AD. Orthopedic infections. In: Wiesel SW, Delahay JN, eds. *Essentials of Orthopedic Surgery*. 3rd ed. New York, NY: Springer; 2007.

Shah K, Spear J, Nathanson LA, et al. Does the presence of crystal arthritis rule out septic arthritis? *J Emerg Med*. 2007;32:23–26.

Siva C, Velazquez C, Mody A, et al. Diagnosing acute monoarthritis in adults: A practical approach for the family physician. *Am Fam Physician*. 2003;68(1):83–90.

Zink B. Bone and joint infections. In: Marx JA, Hockberger RS, Walls RM, eds. *Rosen's Emergency Medicine: Concepts and Clinical Practice*. 6th ed. Philadelphia, PA: Mosby-Elsevier; 2006.

174

IF ONLY JOINT DISEASE WAS CRYSTAL CLEAR ... CRYSTAL ARTHROPATHIES DO NOT PRECLUDE A SEPTIC JOINT

AMRITHA RAGHUNATHAN, MD

Joint pain is a common chief complaint and is associated with many disorders. Gout and pseudogout are crystal-induced arthropathies causing atraumatic monoarticular joint pain. However, an acute attack of monoarticular gout or pseudogout can be clinically indistinguishable from septic arthritis. A prior history can increase the likelihood, but it has been shown that long-standing arthropathy increases the probability of developing septic arthritis. Fever, leukocytosis, redness, swelling, and an inability to bear weight or range the joint can also be present in both cases. Infection can cause cartilage and joint destruction if untreated. Therefore, an arthrocentesis and synovial fluid analysis must be considered even in patients with known, previously diagnosed arthritis. The presence of crystals does not exclude a concomitant septic joint. Synovial fluid analysis should include a total leukocyte count and differential, Gram stain and culture, and crystal analysis (*Table 174.1*).

Unfortunately, there have been multiple cases of culture-proven septic arthritis in patients with leukocyte counts <50,000. The higher the leukocyte count, and the greater the proportion of neutrophils, the higher the probability of septic arthritis. Culture results are the gold standard for diagnosis.

BASIC FACTS ON GOUT AND PSEUDOGOUT

Epidemiology. The prevalence of gout is between 2.7 and 8.4 patients per 1,000 individuals. Twenty percent of patients with a family history will develop the disease. The average age of those affected with pseudogout is 72.

TABLE 174.1	SYNOVIAL FLUID ANALYSIS	
DIAGNOSIS	WBC COUNT	PMN (%)
Noninflammatory	<2,000	<50
Inflammation	2,000–50,000	<75
Infectious	>50,000	>75

Pathophysiology. Gout and pseudogout attacks are due to severe joint space inflammation by crystals. Gout is caused by monosodium urate monohydrate crystals and pseudogout by calcium pyrophosphate dihydrate (CPPD) crystals. In gout, hyperuricemia from a high-purine diet, renal disease, medications, or a metabolic disorder and supersaturated serum results in uric acid deposition in the joint. However, hyperuricemia is mostly asymptomatic. Other risk factors include obesity, alc ohol intake, and recent trauma or surgery. The majority of people with CPPD deposition are asymptomatic. Crystal formation may be due to an increase in calcium or pyrophosphate. Hemochromatosis, hypothyroidism, hyperparathyroidism, hypomagnesemia, hypophosphatemia, and joint trauma increase the risk.

Clinical Manifestations. Swelling, redness, and severe pain in the affected joint are most common. The classic joint in gout is the first metatarsophalangeal joint. In pseudogout, it is the knee. Chronic gout or pseudogout often results in tophi formation, crystal deposits in soft tissue and joints, if untreated. A low-grade fever may be present, but high fever, chills, and malaise are not present in gout or pseudogout and are more likely to occur with septic arthritis.

Diagnosis. The cornerstone of diagnosis is arthrocentesis, with fluid analysis under polarizing microscopy. Negatively birefringent crystals (urate crystals) are seen within a neutrophil in patients with an acute gout flare with a sensitivity and specificity of 85% and 100%, respectively. In pseudogout, positively birefringent crystals (CPPD crystals) are seen. CPPD crystals are more difficult to detect as they are smaller and more polymorphic. In order to increase the sensitivity, care must be taken to examine the fluid immediately after arthrocentesis.

While uric acid levels are often ordered, they are not helpful, as hyperuricemia is present in many asymptomatic people, and others can develop acute gout with normal or low serum urate levels.

Imaging is not necessary. Patients may have evidence of a joint effusion, soft tissue swelling, bone erosions, or tophi on plain radiographs. In pseudogout, CPPD crystal deposition appears as radiodensities. This disease also causes degenerative changes, and often subchondral cysts, osteophyte formation, and intra-articular osteochondral bodies are seen.

Treatment. A typical attack resolves within a few weeks even without treatment. However, it is important to avoid the chronic consequences. The first course of action is to address all modifiable risk factors—in the case of gout, obesity, alcohol intake, diuretic use, and diet, and in the case of pseudogout, electrolyte abnormalities. For acute flares, the therapeutic options are nonsteroidal anti-inflammatory drugs (NSAIDs), colchicine, and corticosteroids. Colchicine is for acute treatment and for prophylaxis. It inhibits the inflammatory response to crystals, but not in response to bacterial products. For patients with contraindications or resistant disease, glucocorticoid therapy is a possibility. In terms of long-term prevention, allopurinol, a urate-lowering drug, is used. It is not used for treatment of an acute gout flare.

SUMMARY

Gout and pseudogout are the most common crystal arthropathies causing mono-articular disease. NSAIDs and colchicine are the primary therapeutic agents used for acute flares, and colchicine and allopurinol are used for prophylaxis. However, while the history and physical exam may strongly suggest a crystal arthropathy, septic arthritis can be clinically indistinguishable. Arthrocentesis should be performed on all patients with acute, atraumatic, severe joint pain with fever, redness, or swelling. Following that, the practitioner may exclude septic arthritis and proceed with treatment for crystal arthropathy.

SUGGESTED READINGS

Bleyer AJ, Hart TC. Genetic factors associated with gout and hyperuricemia. *Adv Chronic Kidney Dis.* 2006;13(2):124–130.

Campion EW, Glynn RJ, DeLabry LO. Asymptomatic hyperuricemia: Risks and consequences in the normative aging study. *Am J Med.* 1987;82(3):421–426.

Choi HK, Atkinson K, Karlson EW, et al. Purine-rich foods, dairy and protein intake, and the risk of gout in men. *N Engl J Med.* 2004;350(11):1093–1103.

Craig MH, Poole GV, Hauser CJ. Postsurgical gout. *Am Surg.* 1995;61(1):56–59.

Eggebeen AT. Gout: An update. *Am Fam Physician.* 2007;76(6):801–808.

Gordon C, Swan A, Dieppe P. Detection of crystals in synovial fluids by light microscopy: Sensitivity and reliability. *Ann Rheum Dis.* 1989;48(9):737–742.

Harrington L, Schneider JI. Traumatic joint and limb pain in the elderly. *Emerg Med Clin N Am.* 2006;24(2):389–412.

Jones AC, Chuck AJ, Arie EA, et al. Diseases associated with calcium pyrophosphate deposition disease. *Semin Arthritis Rheum.* 1992;22(3):188–202.

Lawrence RC, Helmick CG, Arnett FC, et al. Estimates of the prevalence of arthritis and selected musculoskeletal disorders in the United States. *Arthritis Rheum.* 1998;41(5):778–799.

Lin KC, Lin HY, Chou P. Community based epidemiological study on hyperuricemia and gout in Kin-Hu, Kinmen. *J Rheumatol.* 2000;27(4):1045–1050.

Martel W, McCarter DK, Solsky MA, et al. Further observations on the arthropathy of calcium pyrophosphate crystal deposition disease. *Radiology.* 1982;141(1):1–15.

Mcgillicuddy DC, Shah KH, Friedberg RP et al. How sensitive is the synovial fluid white blood cell count in diagnosing septic arthritis? *Am J Emerg Med.* 2007;25:749–752.

[No author listed]. Guidelines for the initial evaluation of the adult patient with acute musculoskeletal symptoms. American College of Rheumatology Ad Hoc Committee on Clinical Guidelines. *Arthritis Rheum.* 1996;39(1):1–8.

Park YB, Park YS, Lee SC, et al. Clinical analysis of gouty patients with normouricaemia at diagnosis. *Ann Rheum Dis.* 2003;62(1):90–92.

Schlesinger N, Schumacher R, Catton M, et al. Colchicine for acute gout. *Cochrane Database Syst Rev.* 2006;(4):CD006190.

Shah K, Spear J, Nathanson LA, et al. Does the presence of crystal arthritis rule out septic arthritis? *J Emerg Med.* 2007;32(1):23–26.

Wilkins E., Dieppe P, Maddison P, et al. Osteoarthritis and articular chondrocalcinosis in the elderly. *Ann Rheum Dis.* 1983;42(3):280–284.

175

KNOW THE CAUSES OF BACK PAIN THAT KILL PATIENTS

MISHA KASSEL, MD AND LALEH GHARAHBAGHIAN, MD

Back pain is a common chief complaint in emergency departments, accounting for 1% of emergency department visits. It is an extremely common problem, and 70% to 90% of individuals have debilitating back pain during their lifetime. While the vast majority of these visits are benign in origin, it is critical to identify emergent causes of back pain that, if missed, can quickly lead to severe disability and death. A thorough yet focused history and physical exam can help identify these rare but critical causes of back pain (*Table 175.1*).

AORTIC DISSECTION

Aortic dissection is classically thought of as chest pain that radiates to the back; it can also present as back pain alone and has a mortality rate >90%, if undiagnosed. Important historical findings that suggest dissection include sudden-onset severe pain and associated nausea, vomiting, or anxiety. Physical exam findings that suggest aortic dissection are unstable vital signs, unequal upper extremity blood pressure, new-onset aortic insufficiency murmur, and diaphoresis. Hypertension is common.

TABLE 175.1	PHYSICAL EXAMINATION RED FLAGS
PHYSICAL EXAM FINDINGS	**CONCERN**
Fever, writhing in pain	Infection
Anal sphincter laxity, incontinence or residual postvoidal volume >100 mL, perianal/perineal sensory loss, bilateral neurologic deficit	Epidural compression (classically cauda equine syndrome)
Motor weakness, abnormal reflexes	Epidural compression or herniated disc
Positive straight or cross straight leg test	Herniated disc
Bone tenderness	Infection, fracture
Hypertension, unequal upper extremity blood pressure	Aortic dissection
Pulsatile abdominal mass, decreased lower extremity pulses	AAA

ABDOMINAL AORTIC ANEURYSM

Similar to aortic dissection, it is not classically thought to present with back pain and if missed has a very high mortality. Important historical findings for abdominal aortic aneurysm (AAA) are pain radiating to the back and potentially syncope. Physical exam findings suggestive for AAA are pulsatile abdominal mass, diminished lower extremity pulses, or abdominal bruit. If suspicion is high for AAA and the patient is unstable, it is important to remember that a rapid bedside ultrasound is both sensitive and specific and can quickly screen for AAA.

INFECTIOUS

Both spinal epidural abscesses and vertebral osteomyelitis are rare yet present primarily with back pain. History of a recent infection is common, especially pneumonia or urinary tract. Other historical findings that suggest an infectious source of back pain are past medical history of diabetes, immunocompromised state, chronic renal failure, cancer, recent spinal or genitourinary surgery or trauma, and intravenous drug use. Physical exam findings of fever, bony tenderness, signs of sepsis, night pain, unremitting pain (even when lying flat), and undesired weight loss should all raise suspicion for an infectious source of back pain. Focal neurologic findings are usually late in the clinical course. Due to difficulty in diagnosing these diseases, MRI is the diagnostic test of choice if these red flags are present.

SPINAL CORD COMPRESSION (CAUDA EQUINA SYNDROME AND SPINAL FRACTURE WITH CORD IMPINGEMENT)

Complete spinal cord compression is easy to identify; the challenge for emergency physicians is recognizing partial compression and early signs and symptoms. Epidural compression can occur rarely from herniated discs but also from malignancies, abscesses, hematomas, and fractures. Historical findings include urinary and/or bowel incontinence, bilateral leg pain and weakness, and saddle anesthesia. Physical exam findings include urinary retention with overflow incontinence, perianal/perineal anesthesia, and lower extremity stiffness. Evaluation of rectal tone, lower extremity weakness, and perianal sensation must be performed, and the specific findings depend on the level of cord compression. It is critical to recognize that these signs may be subtle upon the initial presentation.

CANCER

History of previous cancer is an important risk factor as 80% of cancer patients who seek medical care for back pain have spinal metastasis. Other historical findings that suggest cancer are weight loss, night pain, age >50 or <18, and continuous pain not relieved by lying flat or rest. Examination findings consistent with a possibility of a cancerous etiology of back pain are spinal tenderness,

TABLE 175.2	HISTORICAL RED FLAGS
HISTORY	**CONCERN**
Age >50	Tumor, AAA, fracture
Age <18	Congenital anomaly, tumor, discitis
History of cancer	Metastasis
Major trauma, minor trauma (elderly), corticosteroid use	Fracture
Immunocompromised, IV drug use	Infection
Fever, unexplained weight loss, night sweats, pain >6 weeks, unremitting pain	Malignancy, infection
Saddle anesthesia, severe or progressive neurologic deficit, incontinence	Epidural compression
Diaphoresis, nausea	Aortic dissection

lymphadenopathy, and signs of cancer elsewhere (prostate, breast). Delayed presentations may be associated with signs of spinal cord compression.

FRACTURE

Historical risk factors are age >50, history of osteoporosis, trauma (may be minimal in the elderly), corticosteroid use, cancer, and female gender (*Table 175.2*). Spinal tenderness on physical exam is suggestive of a fracture. Be cautious in the multiple-injured trauma patient, as spine fractures can easily be missed in the presence of painful distracting injuries.

CONCLUSION

Back pain is not always benign in origin! The emergency physician must consider the patient's age and medical history and should be wary of a complaint of back pain if any additional signs or symptoms are present that do not correlate with a simple muscular injury. These include hematuria, weakness, paresthesias, urinary retention, urinary and/or bowel incontinence, fever, and history of cancer.

SUGGESTED READINGS

Bentz S, Jones J. Towards evidence-based emergency medicine: Best BETs from the Manchester Royal Infirmary. Accuracy of emergency department ultrasound scanning in detecting abdominal aortic aneurysm. *Emerg Med J.* 2006;23(10):803–804.

Bradley WG Jr. Low back pain. *AJNR Am J Neuroradiol.* 2007;28(5):990–992.

Della-Giustina D, Coppola M. Thoracic and lumbar pain syndromes. In: Tintinalli JE, Kelen GD, Stapczynski JS, et al., eds. *Emergency Medicine: A Comprehensive Study Guide.* 6th ed. New York, NY: McGraw-Hill; 2003.

Henschke N, Maher CG, Refshauge KM. Screening for malignancy in low back pain patients: A systematic review. *Eur Spine J.* 2007;16(10):1673–1679.

Henschke N, Maher CG, Refshauge KM. A systematic review identifies five "red flags" to screen for vertebral fracture in patients with low back pain. *J Clin Epidemiol.* 2008;61(2):110–118.

Herbert M, Lanctot-Herbert M. Low back pain. In: Mahadevan SV, Garmel GM, eds. *An Introduction to Clinical Emergency Medicine.* 1st ed. New York, NY: Cambridge University Press; 2005.

Manning WJ. *Clinical Manifestations and Diagnosis of Aortic Dissection.* UpToDate.com. Available at: http://www.uptodate.com/patients/content/topic.do?topicKey = ~bVyysQkaR.3H.r.

Rodgers KG, Jones JB. Back pain. In: Marx JA, Hockberger RS, Walls RM, eds. *Rosen's Emergency Medicine: Concepts and Clinical Practice.* 6th ed. St. Louis, MU: Mosby; 2006.

Wheeler SG, Wipf JE, Staiger TO, et al. *Approach to the Diagnosis and Evaluation of Low Back Pain in Adults.* UpToDate.com. Available at: http://www.uptodate.com/patients/content/topic.do?topicKey=~NAN/sJQ3H1JYcr&selectedTitle=1~150&source=search_result.

176

ALWAYS CONSIDER CAUDA EQUINA SYNDROME IN PATIENTS WITH LOW BACK PAIN

JONATHAN LARSON, MD

Nearly, all adults experience low back pain at some point in their life. Unfortunately or fortunately, 85% of isolated low back pain is idiopathic. Among patients with low back pain, 4 out of 10,000 will have Cauda equina syndrome (CES). CES should be excluded on every patient with a chief complaint of low back pain by accurate history, physical exam, and/or diagnostic testing.

The cauda equina, or *horses tail*, is the collection of nerve roots caudal to the termination of the spinal cord. CES occurs when these nerve roots are compressed. The most common causes of CES include massive disc herniation, or epidural/spinal processes to include hematoma, abscess, or tumor.

HIGH YIELD HISTORY

1) Is this a systemic disease causing the pain? Does the patient have a history of cancer/malignancy or associated signs such as unexplained/unintended weight loss. In 96% of spinal metastases, back pain is the initial symptom.

2) Is the patient an injection drug user? Placing the patient at a higher risk for spinal infectious processes.

3) Recent trauma? A potential inciting event for disc herniation or spinal fracture.

4) Does the severity of the pain increase with recumbency? A concerning sign of a more insidious cause of low back pain.

5) How long has the patient been experiencing symptoms? Subacute pain raises a red flag as 80% to 90% of patients' symptoms resolve by 4 to 6 weeks if the back pain is due to a benign, self-limiting etiology.

6) Does the pain radiate? Sciatica raises a concern for herniated disc or nerve root inflammation. Most (95%) herniation occurs at the L4-L5 or L5-S1 intervertebral discs, thereby impinging on the L5 or S1 nerve roots, and in close anatomic proximity to the cauda equina.

7) Any urinary or fecal incontinence? This must be considered CES until proven otherwise. A large postvoid residual (>100 mL) in the presence of back pain suggests significant neurologic compromise.

Signs and Symptoms

CES is commonly associated with a triad of signs and symptoms including saddle anesthesia, loss of bowel or bladder function, and lower extremity weakness. The first presenting symptom of CES is usually low back pain. Upward of 70% of patients with CES report a history of chronic back pain. Inquire regarding perceived saddle anesthesia (numbness in the perineum, genitals, buttocks, and posterosuperior thighs), as it holds a sensitivity of approximately 75% for CES. Is there bladder or bowel dysfunction? The most common finding in CES is urinary retention with overflow incontinence with a sensitivity of 90% and a specificity of 95% for CES.

Lower extremity motor and sensory loss is another common finding in the setting of CES. Lower extremity weakness is present in 60% to 85% of patients with CES. The majority of patients are not ambulatory at diagnosis due to weakness or severe pain with ambulation.

Targeted Physical Exam

The straight leg test is essential in assessing for sciatica. Proper execution of the test is integral in concert with an accurate interpretation of exam findings. A positive test reproduces the symptoms of sciatica with pain that radiates below the knee, not merely back or hamstring pain.

Patients and physicians alike would prefer to skip over the digital rectal exam, but you must assess the patient's rectal tone, as anal sphincter tone is decreased in 60% to 80% of cases of CES. While you are down there, assess for perineal sensation.

If warranted by history and physical findings, obtain a postvoid residual. Urine catheterization showing significant volume with little or no urge to void signifies clinically significant urinary retention. The absence of a large postvoid residual essentially excludes CES, with a negative predictive value of 99.99%.

Management

Plain radiography has no role in excluding CES. Emergent MRI of the spine is the gold standard in evaluating for CES. MRI is more sensitive for infection, metastatic cancer, and neural tumors. If your clinical suspicion for neoplasm is high, consider imaging the entire spine as 10% of patients with vertebral metastases have additional silent epidural metastases.

Labs are of limited utility in the acute, clinical workup of CES. Drawing a complete blood count (CBC), sed rate (ESR)/c-reactive protein (CRP), and urine analysis (UA) is reasonable.

Treatment of CES aims to relieve pain and swelling. Recommendations include dexamethasone 10 mg IV or Solumedrol 125 mg IV to minimize progression of vasogenic edema and compression.

If the emergent MRI reveals CES, emergent consultation with the appropriate surgical service is indicated.

Common Pitfalls. If you are in the ER and hear "doc, my tail hurts," do not look for the zebra's tail; look for the horse's tail. Although CES is rare, you must consider it in your differential diagnosis of patients presenting with back pain; failing to do so may lead to dire consequences for you and your patient. Assess and document the patient's rectal tone, saddle sensation, and—if necessary—postvoid residual. If the history and physical exam leave you pondering CES, then order the MRI, as it remains the gold standard for excluding this debilitating source of back pain.

SUGGESTED READINGS

Atlas SJ, Deyon RA, Patrick DL, et al. The Quebec Task Force classification for Spinal Disorders and the severity, treatment, and outcomes of sciatica and lumbar spinal stenosis. *Spine (Phila Pa 1976)*. 1996;21(24):2885–2892.

Della-Giustina D. Emergency department evaluation and treatment of back pain. *Emerg Med Clin North Am*. 1999;17(4):877–893.

Della-Giustina D, Coppola M. Thoracic and lumbar pain syndromes. In: Tintinalli JE, Kelen GD, Stapczynski JS, et al., eds. *Emergency Medicine: A Comprehensive Study Guide*. 6th ed. New York, NY: McGraw-Hill; 2003.

Deyo R, Weinstein J. Primary care: Low back pain. *N Engl J Med*. 2001;344(5):363–370.

Deyo RA, Rainville J, Kent DL. What can the history and physical examination tell us about low back pain? *JAMA*. 1992;268:760–765.

Small SA, Perron AD, Brady WJ. Orthopedic pitfalls: Cauda equina syndrome. *Am J Emerg Med*. 2005;23:159–163.

Winters ME. Management of patients with acute back pain in the ED. In: Mattu A, Goyal D, eds. *Emergency Medicine: Avoiding the Pitfalls & Improving the Outcomes*. Hoboken, NJ: Wiley; 2007:33–38.

177

NEVER MISS COMPARTMENT SYNDROME: PEARLS AND PITFALLS OF EVALUATION

ZULEIKA LADHA, MD

Compartment syndrome develops when there is an increase in pressure within a closed anatomical space, such as with injury to the muscles enclosed within dense fascial sheaths. Injury can result from intrinsic damage to the muscle or from external compressive forces. The unyielding fascial sheaths are unable to expand to accommodate the swelling associated with tissue insult. This compromises perfusion of the contained muscular and nervous tissues and leads to ischemic damage and necrosis. Rhabdomyolysis, renal failure, postischemic contractures, or limb loss may subsequently occur. Compartment syndrome most commonly occurs in the extremities, specifically in the leg and the forearm, but it can be found in any muscle group that is enclosed by fascia, such as the back or the buttock.

Although 75% of compartment syndrome cases result from fracture, it is important to recognize that soft tissue and vascular injuries can lead to this condition as well. In a study of 164 patients in the United Kingdom, 69% involved a fracture (half involving the tibial shaft) but 31% had soft tissue injury without a fracture. Crush injuries, infection, snakebites, arterial injuries, circular constrictive dressings, burns, prolonged immobilization, intravenous infiltration, and exertion are also other important causes of compartment syndrome. Patients with coagulopathies, such as hemophiliacs or those on coumadin, are at increased risk of developing compartment syndrome after even a minor insult such as peripheral venipuncture.

Plain radiographs are essential for the diagnosis of underlying fractures. The degree of damage to bone will also provide a qualitative assessment of the magnitude of the forces that caused the injury. Comminuted, displaced, and open fractures usually require a significant mechanism of injury. It is a mistake to think that an "open" fracture is under less pressure because the compartment is open to the outside. In fact, in one series, compartment syndrome was more common with open than closed fractures.

The diagnosis of compartment syndrome is primarily clinical. It is imperative that the emergency physician recognizes compartment syndrome in its earliest stages so that intervention can occur before the onset of permanent injury. The five "Ps" of pain, parasthesia, pallor, paralysis, and pulselessness have been classically described but are late findings and more consistent with an arterial injury to the extremity. Pain out of proportion to clinical exam has been highlighted as the earliest and most consistent finding. A patient who requires repeated or increasing doses of narcotic pain medication than one would expect for a given injury should be closely evaluated for compartment syndrome. The pain that patients with compartment syndrome often describe is difficult to localize and is dull or aching in quality. It is exacerbated by passive stretching and not relieved by immobilization. The individual compartment may be tense and tender upon palpation. Sensory exam of the nerves that traverse the suspected compartment may reveal a decrease in two–point discrimination.

Comatose or altered patients with extremity trauma should be closely observed for signs of compartment syndrome as they are unable to accurately indicate their pain levels. Have a low threshold to check compartment pressures in these patients. A common misstep is to assume that compartment syndrome can be ruled out by the presence of strong distal pulses. Decreases in distal pulses and capillary refill time are extremely late findings and they are associated with significant necrosis and irreversible injury to the enclosed tissues.

A recent meta-analysis by Ulmer of 104 studies on the diagnosis of compartment syndrome from 1966 to 2001 found that each of the commonly used clinical diagnostic parameters (pain, paralysis, parasthesias, and pain with passive stretch) has a sensitivity between 13% and 19%. Thus, serial examinations in the setting of a high clinical suspicion are necessary to diagnose compartment syndrome, especially in those patients with equivocal findings.

Compartment pressures should be measured in patients with suspected compartment syndrome. It is generally agreed that normal compartment pressures are below 10 mm Hg. Fasciotomy is recommended at tonometer tissue readings above 30 to 40 mm Hg. Pressures in this range have been associated with significant ischemia and irreversible tissue damage.

The definitive treatment for acute compartment syndrome is emergent fasciotomy, yet there are other measures that an emergency physician can take to reduce morbidity. Removal of constrictive dressings alone can reduce compartmental pressures by 25 mm Hg. Intravenous hydration to maintain urine output can prevent the complication of rhabdomyolysis. Placing the effected extremity at the level of the heart is thought to maximize both arterial perfusion and venous return (raising the extremity above the heart "to reduce swelling" may be deleterious). Anticoagulants and steroids have not been proven to be useful and are not recommended.

TAKE HOME POINTS

- Pain out of proportion to expectation and increasing use of analgesia out of proportion to expectation for the injury should immediately raise the suspicion of compartment syndrome.

■ Although compartment syndrome is most commonly associated with extremity fractures, think about this diagnosis in patients with significant soft tissue (e.g., crush injury) and vascular injuries.

■ Measure tissue compartment pressures to diagnose compartment syndrome.

SUGGESTED READING

Konstantakos EK, Dalstrom DJ, Nelles ME, et al. Diagnosis and management of extremity compartment syndrome: An orthopaedic perspective. *Am Surg.* 2007;73(12):1119–1209.

Matsen FA III, Winquist RA, Krugmire RB Jr. Diagnosis and management of compartmental syndromes. *J Bone Joint Surg Am.* 1980;62(2):286–291.

McQueen MM, Gaston P, Court-Brown CM. Acute compartment syndrome: Who is at risk? *J Bone Joint Surg Br.* 2000;82(2):200–203.

Perron AD, Brady WJ, Keats TE. Orthopedic pitfalls in the ED: Acute compartment syndrome. *Am J Emerg Med.* 2001;19(5):413–416.

Ulmer T. The clinical diagnosis of compartment syndrome of the lower leg: Are clinical findings predictive of the disorder? *J Orthop Trauma.* 2002;16(8):572–577.

178

CONSIDER OCCULT HIP FRACTURE IN PATIENTS WITH HIP PAIN AND INABILITY TO WALK EVEN IF PLAIN FILMS ARE NEGATIVE

JAMES M. MATERN, MD, MPH

Hip fracture is one of the most common orthopedic injuries seen by emergency physicians, especially in the elderly. It includes fractures of the femoral head and neck, trochanteric fractures, intertrochanteric fractures, and subtrochanteric fractures. The incidence of hip fractures is about 250,000 to 300,000 cases annually and is expected to rise as the population ages. Hip fracture is two to three times more common in women, and there is a higher prevalence in white populations.

Hip fracture is a diagnosis that carries a high morbidity and mortality, with estimates of 1 year mortality ranging from 15% to 25%. Of those who survive 6 months, only 50% of patients will return to their prefracture level of ability to perform their activities of daily living. Delayed recognition of hip fracture can increase morbidity and mortality. Patients can suffer from unnecessary pain, nonunion of the fracture, and avascular necrosis, leading to a rapid decline in quality of life.

Most hip fracture patients do not present with a diagnostic dilemma. The typical presentation is an elderly person with the inability to walk after a fall. They may have shortening and external rotation of the affected leg and may frequently have a complaint of pain, especially with movement of the affected hip.

Plain radiographs of the affected hip often confirm clinical suspicion and reveals evidence of hip fracture; however, hip fracture can be missed with plain radiographs. The incidence of missed hip fracture on initial plain radiographs is estimated at 2% to 9%. Due to the limitations of plain radiographs, especially in nondisplaced hip fractures, it is important to obtain further imaging of the affected hip if clinical suspicion remains high. One sign that should be used to prompt further imaging is the patient having the inability to walk or walking only with severe difficulty. MRI is the diagnostic study of choice in these patients. If MRI is unavailable, bone scanning may also be used. Bone scanning has significant limitations and drawbacks in that current recommendations support waiting 2 to 3 days before obtaining the study to optimize the chances of detecting a fracture. MRI has been shown in several studies to have up to 100% sensitivity for diagnosing hip fracture; bone scanning has had up to a 98% sensitivity.

In summary, due to the high morbidity and mortality of hip fractures, it is important to recognize the possibility of hip fracture among those patients with negative or inconclusive plain radiographs. Inability to walk in the setting of hip pain should prompt further imaging, especially in elderly patients. Should plain radiographs fail to reveal a diagnosis, MRI is the diagnostic study of choice. Patients with high suspicion of hip fracture should be admitted to the hospital until a definitive diagnostic imaging study can be obtained.

TAKE HOME POINTS

- Plain radiographs will miss 2% to 9% of hip fractures.
- If the patient with hip pain is unable to walk, admit the patient for further imaging.
- The imaging modality of choice for an occult hip fracture is MRI.

SUGGESTED READINGS

Alba E, Youngberg R. Occult fractures of the femoral neck. *Am J Emerg Med*. 1992; 10(1):64–68.

Brunner LC, Eshilian-Oates l, Kuo TY. Hip fractures in adults. *Am Fam Physician*. 2003; 67(3):537–542.

Conway WF, Totty WG, McEnery KW. CT and MRI imaging of the hip. *Radiology*. 1996; 198(2):297–307.

Mlinek EJ, Clark KC, Walker CW. Limited magnetic resonance imaging in the diagnosis of occult hip fractures. *Am J Emerg Med*. 1998;16(4):390–392.

Parker MJ. Missed hip fractures. *Arch Emerg Med*. 1992;9(1):23–27.

Perron AD, Miller MD, Brady WJ. Orthopedic pitfalls in the ED: Radiographically occult hip fracture. *Am J Emerg Med*. 2002;20(3):234–237.

Rogers FB, Shackford SR, Keller MS. Early fixation reduces morbidity and mortality in elderly patients with hip fractures from low impact falls. *J Trauma*. 1995;39(2):261–265.

Zuckerman JD. Hip fracture. *N Engl J Med*. 1996;334:1519–1525.

179

ADMIT ALL HIGH-RISK PATIENTS WITH TRANSIENT ISCHEMIC ATTACK

SAI-HUNG JOSHUA HUI, MD

The incidence of transient ischemic attack (TIA) in the United States is estimated at 240,000 per year. The definition of TIA is currently in flux. Previously, TIA was defined as a thromboembolic event causing focal neurological deficits lasting <24 h. Recently, however, the time frame for TIA has been dramatically reduced to <1 h. If neurological deficits persist longer than 1 h, the patient has frequently suffered a stroke as evidenced by objective findings on advanced neuroimaging modalities, such as magnetic resonance (MR). Moreover, for those patients whose symptoms last more than 1 h or do not rapidly improve within 3 h, only 2% to 15% return to baseline neurologically within 24 h. TIA and stroke should thus be considered as two different points on a continuum of disease.

The word *transient* in TIA is actually misleading: it fails to convey the risk that the TIA patient has of suffering a full-fledged stroke in very near future. A 2000 study by Johnston et al. showed that 10.5% of patients presenting to the emergency department (ED) went on to experience a stroke within 90 days; half of those patients did so within 48 h. Another study estimated the 7-day risk of stroke in patients suffering a first-ever TIA to be 8%.

It can be very tempting to discharge the TIA patient with a very minimal workup, especially in the setting of a completely normal neurological examination. By the time the emergency physician (EP) sees the patient, symptoms have generally resolved.

So which patients presenting to the ED with a TIA need to be admitted? To answer this question, we need to know which patients are at the highest risk of developing a stroke in the near future. In 2005, Rothwell et al. derived and validated the "ABCD" scoring system (*Table 179.1*). Characteristics of TIA that correlated with an increased risk of stroke included unilateral weakness and aphasia. The total score was used to estimate the risk of stroke in 7 days after the onset of TIA. With a score of 6, the 7-day risk of stroke was found to be 31.4%;

TABLE 179.1	ABCD SCORING SYSTEM	
RISK FACTOR	**POINTS**
Age ≥60 y	1
Blood pressure (systolic >140, diastolic >90)	1
CLINICAL FEATURES	
■ Unilateral weakness	2
■ Speech disturbance without weakness	1
■ Other features (e.g., unilateral numbness)	0
DURATION OF SYMPTOMS	
■ ≥60 min	2
■ 10–59 min	1
■ <10 min	0

a score of 5, 12.1%; and a score of 4 or less was 0% to 4%. As of 2008, multiple prospective and retrospective validation studies have confirmed the prognostic value of the ABCD rule.

A study by Johnston et al. in 2007 attempted to estimate the risk of stroke at 2 days. Their scoring system (called "ABCD²") adds diabetes to the previous "ABCD" system, allotting a single additional point for diabetes. Using this modified scoring system, 21%, 45%, and 34% patients were identified as high (score of 6 to 7), medium (score of 4 to 5), and low risk (score of 0 to 3), respectively. High-risk patients had an 8.1% risk of stroke at 2 days, 11.7% at 7 days, and 17.8% at 90 days. The ABCD² study still remains to be validated by additional studies—these are currently underway.

Current thinking on TIA will continue to evolve with advances in neuroimaging and further studies. Although the prediction rules for stroke after TIA are not yet as rigorous as other decision rules in emergency medicine, they can still serve as important tools to help identify patients at particularly high risk, prompting admission and more urgent evaluation for preventable causes of stroke, such as mural emboli and carotid stenosis.

The bottom line: Consider admission in any TIA patient with significant high-risk features for an early stroke.

SUGGESTED READINGS

Albers GW, Caplan LR, Easton JD, et al. Transient ischemic attack–proposal for a new definition. *N Engl J Med*. 2002;347(21):1713–1716.

Johnston SC, Gress DR, Browner WS, et al. Short term prognosis after emergency department diagnosis of TIA. *JAMA*. 2000;284(22):2901–2906.

Johnston SC, Rothwell PM, Nguyen-Huynh MN, et al. Validation and refinement of scores to predict very early stroke risk after transient ischaemic attack. *Lancet.* 2007;369(9558): 283–292.

Lovett JK, Dennis MS, Sandercock PA, et al. The very early risk of stroke after a first transient ischaemic attack. *Stroke.* 2003;34(8):e138–e140 [Epub 2003 July 10].

Rothwell PM, Giles MF, Flossmann E, et al. A simple score (ABCD) to identify individuals at high early risk of stroke after transient ischaemic attack. *Lancet.* 2005;366(9479):29–36.

Sciolla R, Melis F, SINPAC Group. Rapid identification of high-risk transient ischemic attacks: Prospective validation of the ABCD score. *Stroke.* 2008;39(2):297–302.

180

ADMIT PATIENTS WITH ACUTE GUILLAIN-BARRÉ SYNDROME TO MONITORED BEDS

MATTHIEU DE CLERCK, MD

Guillain-Barré syndrome (GBS) is an immune-mediated inflammatory attack on peripheral myelin sheaths or, in some cases, on the peripheral axon itself, often triggered by a recent infection. GBS is characterized by progressive symmetric ascending muscle weakness, paralysis, and hyporeflexia, with or without sensory or autonomic symptoms. The progression of weakness and paralysis can be rapid (hours to days) or prolonged (days to weeks) and usually reaches a plateau by 2 to 4 weeks. While most patients recover completely by 12 months, GBS carries a 5% mortality rate secondary to complications. The most immediately life-threatening complications include respiratory failure, cardiac dysrhythmia, and cardiac failure secondary to autonomic dysfunction. Failure to anticipate these complications may result in mistaken triage of GBS patients to an unmonitored setting.

Presenting symptoms of GBS can be quite variable, including paralysis, subjective weakness, or merely paresthesias. Because of these often subtle findings, the diagnosis of GBS is frequently delayed. A retrospective case series of 20 patients with GBS presenting to the emergency department (ED) by McGillicuddy found a wide variety of chief complaints, weakness being the chief complaint in 14 patients and paresthesia the sole complaint in four patients. Furthermore, of these 20 cases, only five were diagnosed on their initial presentation, while 13 cases had seen anywhere from two to four physicians prior to being correctly diagnosed. The diagnosis of GBS should be entertained in all patients presenting with ascending paralysis, muscle weakness, or disappearance of deep tendon reflexes.

Hypoxia secondary to respiratory muscle weakness is the most common cause for ICU admission in GBS, occurring in approximately 33% of patients. The mean duration of mechanical ventilation after intubation is 18 to 29 days. Ventilation becomes compromised as the progression of weakness decreases inspiratory effort, effective expiratory force, and the ability to protect the airway. Respiratory failure can progress rapidly in GBS and is best addressed at an early stage to avoid emergency intubation or respiratory arrest. Although many patients will not require mechanical ventilation in the ED, admitted GBS patients will need serial monitoring of respiratory function as the course of their disease progresses. Such monitoring can realistically only be provided in an ICU or telemetry setting.

Autonomic dysfunction commonly occurs in GBS as demyelination and axonal damage affect sympathetic and parasympathetic nerves, including the vagus and splanchnic nerves. Approximately 65% of patients with GBS will be affected by some form of dysautonomia, ranging from bladder and bowel dysfunction to cardiac dysrhythmias and labile blood pressure. While urinary and bowel dysfunction alone require specific care, it is the dysrhythmias, bouts of paroxysmal hypertension, and orthostatic hypotension that merit admission to a monitored setting. Sudden swings in blood pressure occur in 5% to 10% of patients, with paroxysmal hypertension and orthostatic hypotension being the most commonly recognized dysautonomia. Hypertensive and hypotensive episodes in GBS patients carry the same risks as in non-GBS patients but with the added challenge of being extremely labile and sensitive to interventions. The incidence of specific cardiac dysrhythmias is not well documented but such events can be disastrous. The full spectrum of bradydysrhythmias and tachydysrhythmias has been described in association with GBS. Patients requiring mechanical ventilation and those with volatile blood pressure and heart rates appear to be at higher risk for developing cardiac dysrhythmias.

In summary, GBS is a peripheral neuropathy that can progress rapidly with life-threatening consequences. Sequelae such as autonomic instability, dysrhythmias, and progressive respiratory failure are common and should be anticipated.

SUGGESTED READINGS

Bradley WG, Dardoff RB, Fenichel GM, et al. *Neurology in Clinical Practice: Principles of Diagnosis and Management.* Philadelphia, PA: Elsevier; 2004.

Chalea JA. Pearls and pitfalls in the intesive care management of Guillain-Barré syndrome. *Seminars Neurol.* 2001;21(4):399–405.

McGillicuddy DC, Walker O, Shapior MI, et al. Guillain-Barré syndrome in the emergency department. *Annal Emerg Med.* 2006;47(4):390–393.

Mehta S. Neuromuscular disease causing acute respiratory failure. *Resp Care.* 2006;51(9): 1016–1021.

Pheiffer G, Schiller B, Krause J, et al. Indicators of dysautonomia in severe Guillain-Barré syndrome. *J Neurol.* 1999;246(11):1015–1022.

Zochodne DW. Autonomic involvement in Guillain- Barré syndrome: A review. *Muscle Nerve.* 1994;17(10):1145–1155.

181

BEWARE OF THE COMORBIDITIES AND COMPLICATIONS OF ACUTE STROKE

THOMAS M. MAILHOT, MD, FAAEM

Stroke is a leading cause of morbidity and mortality in the United States. When patients present to the emergency department (ED) with strokelike symptoms, the emergency physician (EP) is faced with a difficult decision: to give tissue plasminogen activator (tPA) or not to give tPA. This decision is important, but there are other interventions that may be equally important in preventing morbidity and mortality.

Stroke unit care was begun in the 1990s in order to improve outcomes, providing a specialized, multidisciplinary team focusing on acute and rehabilitative care. According to the American Stroke Association, "the magnitude of the benefits of stroke unit care is comparable to that of intravenous tPA." Furthermore, while only a small subset of stroke patients are eligible for fibrinolytics, all stroke patients benefit from the specialized care of a stroke unit.

As patients stay for longer periods of time in the ED awaiting inpatient hospital beds, EPs are being confronted with the need to begin elements of acute stroke care that, in the past, would have been deferred to the inpatient admitting service. Initiating these treatments in the ED can prevent morbidity and mortality, as well as shorten hospital length of stay. Supportive care and treatment of acute complications in the management of stroke include the prevention, recognition, and treatment of hypoxia, myocardial infarction, deep vein thrombosis (DVT), pulmonary embolism, infections such as urinary tract infections and aspiration pneumonia, dehydration, poor nutrition, skin breakdown, and metabolic disorders.

Preventing hypoxia is a cornerstone of neurological resuscitation. Stroke victims often have diminished airway reflexes due to bulbar palsies as well as depressed levels of consciousness. Such patients may require intubation to secure the airway and prevent the devastating complication of aspiration pneumonia. Even without intubation, steps to prevent aspiration pneumonia should be implemented early in the care of the stroke patient: elevate the head of the bed to 30 degrees and keep the patient *nil per os* (npo) until a speech and swallowing evaluation has been completed. Supplemental oxygen may be needed to ensure adequate brain oxygenation, especially in the setting of hypoventilation and atelectasis. Oxygen therapy is not without its own toxicity however, particularly with prolonged oxygen concentrations over 50%, so supplemental oxygen should be titrated to use the minimum amount necessary. Current guidelines suggest a goal oxygen saturation of at least 92% in stroke patients.

Hyperthermia is consistently associated with worsened outcomes in stroke. The presence of fever mandates an aggressive search for a cause, such as pneumonia, urinary tract infection, or endocarditis. Pneumonia (frequently from aspiration) is a leading cause of mortality in stroke patients. Any infection should be promptly treated and fevers should be treated with antipyretics and other cooling measures as necessary.

Stroke victims are at high risk of developing both DVT and decubitus ulcers due to limited mobility. DVT prophylaxis can be accomplished by using sequential compression devices on the legs. Heparin should be avoided in the acute setting due to the risk of hemorrhagic conversion of the stroke. Decubitus ulcers are not often considered by EPs, but these are a growing concern as patients are boarded in the ED for longer periods of time. Most ED gurneys have thin mattresses that are not designed for the prevention of pressure ulcers. Furthermore, although nursing guidelines recommend repositioning patients every 2 h, this is often not feasible in a busy ED. Regardless of these obstacles, any efforts on the part of ED staff to address ulcer prevention may lead to better patient outcomes. Particularly, susceptible areas for skin breakdown in the supine patient include the sacrum and heels.

Glucose control is an important component of stroke care. Hypoglycemia can produce focal neurological signs mimicking a stroke, thus all presumed stroke patients must have their serum glucose measured promptly upon presentation. Hypoglycemia can also directly lead to brain injury, and in stroke patients who are npo, this represents a real threat to recovery. Frequent serum glucose measurements will identify mild hypoglycemia before it becomes a problem. Hyperglycemia is also associated with higher mortality in stroke. Blood sugar levels above 200 mg/dL should be treated with insulin.

Hypertension is a common finding in stroke patients, and controversy exists regarding its treatment in the acute setting. Although stroke victims with severely elevated blood pressure have worse outcomes than normotensive patients, no clinical benefit is seen in patients who receive antihypertensive therapy acutely. Hypotension is also associated with worsened outcomes in stroke and should be avoided. A prudent approach seems to be to reduce outside stimulation, empty the bladder, and treat pain, and severely elevated blood pressure will diminish without dropping dangerously. Precipitous lowering of blood pressure with antihypertensive agents should be avoided.

As patients wait longer and longer to be admitted to ward or critical care beds, the burden of acute stroke care is shifting to the ED. By paying attention to these small but important aspects of care, EPs can reduce the morbidity and mortality of stroke and decrease the length of stay in the hospital.

SUGGESTED READINGS

Adams HP Jr, del Zoppo G, Alberts MJ, et al. Guidelines for the early management of adults with ischemic stroke. *Stroke*. 2007;38(5):1655–1711 [Epub Apr 12, 2007].

Greer DM, Funk SE, Reaven NL, et al. Impact of fever on outcome in patients with stroke and neurologic injury: A comprehensive meta-analysis. *Stroke*. 2008;39(11):3029–3035. Epub Aug 21, 2008.

Roquer J, Rodriquez-Campello A, Gomis M, et al. Acute stroke unit care and early neurological deterioration in ischemic stroke. *J Neurol*. 2008;255(7):1012–1027 [Epub Jun 2, 2008].

Williams LS, Rotich J, Qi R, et al. Effects of admission hyperglycemia on mortality and costs in acute ischemic stroke. *Neurology*. 2002;59(1):67–71.

182

DO NOT MISS A CEREBRAL VENOUS THROMBOSIS

DAVID T. WILLIAMS, MD, FAAEM

Cerebral venous thrombosis (CVT) was first diagnosed at autopsy over 150 years ago and was initially thought to be universally fatal. Angiography revealed a range of disease severity, and heparin anticoagulation was first proposed as treatment in 1941. Today, heparin has become the first-line treatment for CVT even in the setting of hemorrhagic infarction. Mortality is now as low as 10%. As imaging technology advances, CVT as an etiology for headache, seizure, and stroke is being recognized with increasing frequency.

With mild disease severity, the emergency physician (EP) is challenged clinically because headache is frequently the only presenting symptom. The onset of venous outlet obstruction headache has been described as acute, subacute, or chronic; and gradual or thunderclap. It may mimic migraines, be intermittent, bandlike in nature, and localized or general. Some patients have visual complaints, such as pulsations or peripheral visual field loss, and there is a predisposition for thrombophilia or hypercoagulable states. One differentiating sign for the EP is that papilledema occurs in the majority of CVT cases, detectable by fundoscopy. Unlike other forms of venous thromboembolism, the d-dimer laboratory assay has not proven itself useful in ruling out CVT. Although d-dimer is elevated in most cases, a negative test does not rule out the disease, even in low-risk patients.

When it presents only with headache and papilledema, CVT is clinically indistinguishable from idiopathic intracranial hypertension (IIH) (also known as pseudotumor cerebri). Although these diseases appear to be pathophysiologically related, underlying CVT should be considered prior to making the diagnosis of IIH. Patients at particular risk for CVT include those recently started on certain medications (e.g., doxycycline and oral contraceptives), those with chronic or active ear or mastoid infections, those with thrombophilia or hypercoagulable risk factors, and those with intrapartum or puerperal associated symptoms.

Although the diagnosis of CVT can be made with computed tomography (CT) imaging, CT may miss as many as 30% of cases. If CVT is strongly suspected based on the severity of presentation or the appearance of evolving neurological signs, emergent MR, specifically with MRV (magnetic resonance venography) adjuncts, will usually reveal the diagnosis. The American College of Emergency Physicians includes a statement that suspicion of CVT warrants emergent MR/MRV imaging in its most recent clinical policy on the management of acute headache in the emergency department.

In the more severe range of disease, CVT may be considered in a patient with seizures, altered mental status, papilledema, and CVT risk factors. Moreover, the neurologic deficits seen in CVT do not conform to the typical cerebral arterial distribution of arterial stroke. Imaging may suggest the diagnosis of CVT when edema or hemorrhagic infarcts are not in common hypertensive locations but occur bilaterally and at the gray-to-white matter junctions, suggesting venous congestion and back pressure.

So what is the bottom line for not missing CVT? The diagnosis can occur in a range of clinical settings from headache to seizure to stroke. In the mild form of the disease, CVT presents as a venous outlet obstruction headache but may be seen on CT. The diagnosis should be aggressively pursued with emergent MR and MRV adjuncts when CVT risk factors are present. In the more severe forms of the disease, the diagnosis is suggested when intracerebral hemorrhage and clinical symptomatology do not correlate anatomically. In either case, specialty consultation should be sought; in addition to heparin, some cases may require emergent interventional radiologic and neurosurgical interventions.

SUGGESTED READINGS

Agostoni E. Headache in cerebral venous thrombosis. *Neurol Sci.* 2004;25(Suppl 3): S206–S210 [Review].

American College of Emergency Physicians (ACEP). Clinical policy: Critical issues in the evaluation and management of patients presenting to the emergency department with acute headache. *Ann Emerg Med.* 2002;39(1):108–122.

Bousser MG. Cerebral venous thrombosis: Diagnosis and management. *J Neurol.* 2000; 247(4):252–258.

Cumurciuc R, Crassard I, Saroy M, et al. Headache as the only sign of cerebral venous thrombosis: A series of 17 cases. *J Neurol Neurosurg Psychiatry.* 2005;76(8):1084–1087.

Ferro JM, Canhão P, Stam J, et al. Prognosis of cerebral vein and dural sinus thrombosis results from the International Study on Cerebral Vein and Dural Sinus Thrombosis (ISCVT). *Stroke.* 2004;35(3):664–670.

Friedman DI, Jacobson DM. Diagnostic criteria for idiopathic intracranial hypertension. *Neurology.* 2002;59(10):1492–1495.

Lalive PH, de Moerloose P, Lovblad K, et al. Is measurement of D-dimer useful in the diagnosis of cerebral venous thrombosis? *Neurology.* 2003;61(8):1057–1060.

Leker RR, Steiner I. Isolated intracranial hypertension as the only sign of cerebral venous thrombosis. *Neurology.* 2000;54(10):2030.

Stam J. Thrombosis of the cerebral veins and sinuses. *N Engl J Med.* 2005;352(17):1791–1798 [Review].

Stam J, De Bruijn SF, DeVeber G. Anticoagulation for cerebral sinus thrombosis. *Cochrane Database Syst Rev.* 2001;(4):CD002005.

183

DO NOT BE FOOLED BY THE MIMICS OF STROKE

SHOMA DESAI, MD

Stroke is usually easily diagnosed in the emergency department by signs and symptoms of an acute neurological deficit corresponding to a particular vascular distribution. But in the age of fibrinolytic therapy for an early stroke, the recognition of conditions that mimic stroke is crucial. Misadministration of fibrinolytics to patients with a stroke mimic exposes them to unnecessary risks of life-threatening intracerebral hemorrhage.

The term "stroke mimic" refers to any nonvascular cause of neurological symptoms and signs. The differential diagnosis includes seizure (postictal deficits), toxic-metabolic disturbances, tumor, infection, complex migraine, peripheral nerve palsy, trauma, and conversion disorder. Approximately 19% of patients presenting with what appears to be an acute stroke, in fact, have a stroke mimic.

The most common of these is unrecognized seizure. Seizures occur as a result of excessive neuronal stimulation; in some cases, it is a manifestation of a structural or metabolic abnormality. Generalized tonic-clonic seizures and, occasionally, complex partial seizures result in postictal states, traditionally a transient period of confusion, decreased level of consciousness, and/or agitation. The postictal period can be further complicated by the presence of sensory deficits or motor weaknesses (Todd paralysis). This period of altered level of consciousness, aphasia, sensory, and/or motor deficits may be easily confused with stroke. Clues to this diagnosis can be found in the patient's previous medical records or via witnesses to prehospital seizure activity. Although acute stroke occasionally does present with seizures, it is more likely that seizures are secondary to an old stroke in a given patient presenting with both a neurological deficit in a cortical vascular distribution and a seizure.

Metabolic derangements of serum glucose, calcium, and sodium can cause focal neurological deficits. Hypoglycemia (blood glucose <45 mg/dL), in particular, is known for producing dense neurological signs occasionally in the setting of a relatively preserved level of consciousness. Due to the availability of point-of-care glucose testing and rapid reversibility with dextrose infusion, all patients should be assessed and treated for hypoglycemia upon arrival to the emergency department.

Central nervous system (CNS) tumors commonly present with a slow, progressive onset of symptoms. Less frequently, however, these disorders present with an unclear timeline or with acute neurological deficits. Tumors, or their resulting mass and edema effects, are often, but not always, visible on CT. Their presence precludes the use of fibrinolytics.

Infection, both systemic and CNS in origin, can also lead to stroke-like signs and symptoms. Though sepsis from any source can lead to cerebral involvement, Hand et al. (2006) reported a prevalence of pulmonary infections among their septic causes of stroke mimics. Brain abscess should be considered in any immunocompromised patient with acute neurological deficits, especially in the context of fever, leukocytosis, or head or neck infection (e.g., sinusitis). Noncontrast CT may provide evidence of CNS infection with signs of edema, air-fluid levels, intracerebral gas, and bony erosions signifying osteomyelitis. Herpes simplex encephalitis deserves special mention as its predilection for the temporal lobes leads to symptoms of hemiparesis, aphasia, and visual field deficits. MR will frequently give more information; LP should be avoided in the setting of focal deficits until after imaging.

Complex migraine is a stroke mimic that is extremely difficult to diagnose. Though the patient may have motor, sensory, or visual deficits as part of his or her migraine aura, hemiplegic migraines present with motor deficits lasting hours to days, even in the absence of headache in some cases! Clues to this diagnosis include previous episodes and a family history. To further frustrate matters, patients with migraine are at higher risk of stroke.

Peripheral nerve palsies are often mistaken for stroke in the emergent setting. These disorders may be difficult to differentiate from central deficits. The most common peripheral nerve palsy encountered by emergency physicians is Bell's palsy (peripheral cranial nerve VII deficit). Ischemia to the supranuclear pons region may cause nearly identical weakness in the contralateral face but usually can be distinguished by the preservation of upper facial motor strength (due to bilateral central innervation).

Trauma causing intracranial hemorrhage may present with stroke symptoms and signs. In these cases, a good clinical assessment and CT imaging can usually distinguish the two. Multiple sclerosis (MS) is a central demyelinating disease that may also mimic stroke. Classic presentations of MS (e.g., optic neuritis, acute transverse myelitis, internuclear ophthalmoplegia) or a previous diagnosis of MS will help facilitate this diagnosis. Finally, functional stroke, or conversion disorder, should be considered as a diagnosis of exclusion.

Stroke mimics are common, so they should be considered routinely. If they are not, appropriate therapies will be unnecessarily delayed and potentially harmful fibrinolytic therapy will be inappropriately administered.

SUGGESTED READINGS

Hand PJ, Kwan J, Lindley RI, et al. Distinguishing between stroke and mimic at the bedside: The brain attack study. *Stroke*. 2006;37(3):769–775.
Huff J. Stroke mimics and chameleons. *Emerg Med Clin N Am*. 2002;20(3):583–595.
Libman RB, Wirkowski E, Alvir J, et al. Conditions that mimic stroke in the emergency department: Implications for acute stroke trials. *Arch Neuro*. 1995;52(11):1119–1122.

184

DO NOT CONFUSE CENTRAL AND PERIPHERAL SEVENTH CRANIAL NERVE PALSIES

SAI-HUNG JOSHUA HUI, MD

The facial or seventh cranial nerve (CN7) innervates the muscles of facial expression, provides sensation for the anterior two thirds of the tongue, and provides the efferent limb of the corneal reflex. Patients with CN7 palsy present with unilateral facial droop, the vast majority of which are peripheral lesions. When examining such a patient, it is crucial to identify whether the deficit is due to a central or peripheral lesion because this dictates the urgency of the treatment. In CN7 palsy, the lesion is deemed to be anatomically central when the lesion lies above the motor nuclei in the pons. Causes of central CN7 palsy include tumors, multiple sclerosis, and thromboembolic events like stroke and TIA, which may require more emergent evaluation and treatment. In peripheral CN7 palsy, the lesion is anatomically below the nuclei in the pons. There are a myriad of causes, including infection, trauma, and other idiopathic causes. In general, peripheral CN7 palsies do not require emergent treatment. Therefore, when examining any patient with a facial droop, identifying the correct anatomical location of the lesion, or simply deciding whether the lesion is central or peripheral, is extremely important. Mistaking a central cause of CN7 palsy as a more benign peripheral cause is a grave error that may result in poor patient outcomes. Mistaking a peripheral cause of CN7 palsy as a central cause occurs much more frequently and leads to unnecessary testing in the emergency department.

In order to differentiate a central from a peripheral lesion on physical exam, the EP must understand the essential anatomy of CN7. Dedicated nerves from both contralateral and ipsilateral hemispheres innervate the frontalis and orbicularis oculi muscles. By contrast, the lower two thirds of facial muscles are only innervated by the ipsilateral hemisphere. Thus, in the case of a central lesion such as a cortical stroke, the forehead muscles and eye closure movements will be preserved (forehead sparing) as the deficit from one hemisphere is compensated by innervation from the opposite hemisphere. In addition, ischemic causes of facial droop will almost always be associated with other neurological findings such as unilateral hemiparesis of the extremities or other cranial nerve palsies. Large tumors affecting CN7 at the cerebellopontine angle are likely to involve other adjacent cranial nerves originating from the pons, such as the abducens (CN6) and vestibulocochlear (CN8) nerves.

What are the physical examination findings for peripheral CN7 palsies? The forehead muscles will not be spared because the lesion lies below the pons, interrupting the dedicated nerves that contain innervation from both hemispheres. As a result, the entire half of the face will be weakened or paralyzed, *including* the forehead muscles.

In summary, the diagnosis of a peripheral CN7 palsy should be made only after a central lesion is excluded. Detailed neurological examination is required in both cases, paying particular attention to forehead movement. If the forehead muscles are spared, the facial droop has a central cause, and a neurologist should immediately be consulted if a thromboembolic event is suspected. Do not send a patient with facial droop home with prednisone and acyclovir until you have performed a detailed neurological examination! The presence of any additional cranial nerve palsies, hemiparesis, or hemisensory loss requires further investigation.

SUGGESTED READING

Stettler B, Pancioli A. Brain and cranial nerve disorders. In: Marx JA, Hockberger RS, Walls RM, eds. *Rosen's Emergency Medicine: Concepts and Clinical Practice.* 6th ed. Philadelphia, PA: Mosby; 2006.

185

DO NOT CONFUSE ELEVATED BLOOD PRESSURE PLUS HEADACHE FOR TRUE HYPERTENSIVE ENCEPHALOPATHY

THOMAS M. MAILHOT, MD, FAAEM

Poorly controlled hypertension is a common finding in patients presenting to the emergency department (ED), with as many as 30% of ED patients presenting with a blood pressure >140/90. Faced with an excessively elevated blood pressure, many emergency physicians (EPs) feel compelled to give medications in an attempt to acutely lower the pressure to a more "acceptable" number. This compulsion to act is often unnecessary and even dangerous. It is important for the EP to distinguish between poorly controlled hypertension (for which no *emergent* treatment is needed) and hypertensive emergencies, which are true threats to life.

Hypertensive emergencies involve acute end-organ damage. Although most of these emergencies have easily recognizable symptoms (chest pain in myocardial infarction or aortic dissection, shortness of breath in acute pulmonary edema, and headache in subarachnoid hemorrhage), because it is rare and less clearly defined, hypertensive encephalopathy is less familiar to most EPs.

The classic triad of hypertensive encephalopathy consists of hypertension, altered mentation, and papilledema. Hypertension must be severe (mean arterial pressure or MAP > 150 mm Hg), exceeding the ability of the brain to autoregulate cerebral perfusion pressure. This results in cerebral hyperperfusion and edema. Altered mentation may manifest as disorientation or confusion, decreased level of alertness, coma, or seizure activity. Visual symptoms and vomiting may also occur. Symptoms of hypertensive encephalopathy can be quite subtle, making a careful and complete neurological examination of the utmost importance. This should include an assessment of mental status, cranial nerves, strength, sensation, reflexes, gait, and cerebellar testing.

Headache is a common complaint in the setting of elevated blood pressure and may accompany the neurological symptoms and signs of hypertensive encephalopathy. However, isolated headache in the absence of altered mental status is not suggestive of hypertensive encephalopathy.

If hypertensive encephalopathy is suspected, an aggressive attempt to lower the blood pressure acutely should be undertaken. Severely elevated blood pressure should be lowered with intravenous, titratable antihypertensive agents. The most quoted goal is to decrease the MAP by 20% to 25% over about 30 min. If the blood pressure drops too rapidly, the drug can be titrated down or discontinued immediately. Recommended agents include nitroprusside, nicardipine, labetolol, esmolol, and fenoldopam.

On the other hand, if no hypertensive emergency exists (i.e., no end-organ damage is occurring acutely), there is no benefit to emergently lowering the patient's blood pressure. There may, in fact, exist a very real harm in precipitously lowering the blood pressure in these patients who merely have uncontrolled hypertension. Cerebral blood flow is under strict autoregulation, adapting to changes in systemic blood pressure to ensure adequate cerebral perfusion. In patients with chronic hypertension, the autoregulatory system adapts to higher baseline pressures, making the brain less tolerant of drops in blood pressure. In such patients, a rapid reduction in blood pressure can produce cerebral ischemia and infarction.

A common scenario occurs when a patient presents to the ED with a headache and is incidentally discovered to have an elevated blood pressure. If no other symptoms or signs suggest a hypertensive emergency, treatment should be directed toward controlling the patient's headache with analgesics. This treatment alone will often produce a mild reduction in blood pressure and will do so in a much safer way than would an antihypertensive agent.

Elevated blood pressure is a common finding among ED patients, with the majority of such patients requiring no specific treatment in the ED. It is the task of the EP to make sure that no hypertensive emergency is occurring. It is also important to bring elevated blood pressure readings to the attention of the patient and ensure that proper follow-up readings and management occur if hypertension exists. But resist the urge to treat a number alone, especially with aggressive IV agents, because in the absence of a hypertensive emergency, you can do more harm than good.

SUGGESTED READINGS

Gardner CJ, Lee K. Hyperperfusion syndromes: Insight into the pathophysiology and treatment of hypertensive encephalopathy. *CNS Spectr.* 2007;12(1):35–42.

Hoekstra J, Qureshi A. Management of hypertension and hypertensive emergencies in the emergency department: The EMCREG-International Consensus Panel Recommendations. *Ann Emerg Med.* 2008;51(3):S3–S38.

Shayne PH, Pitts SR. Severely increased blood pressure in the emergency department. *Ann Emerg Med.* 2003;41(4):513–529.

186

DO NOT FORGET TO CONSIDER SUBCLINICAL STATUS EPILEPTICUS

MATTHIEU DE CLERCK, MD

Nonconvulsive status epilepticus (NCSE) is defined as a behavioral or cognitive change from baseline for at least 30 min with EEG evidence of seizure. NCSE is not characterized by the typical tonic-clonic movement of convulsive status epilepticus but often has similar brain wave activity and neurologic sequelae. Subtle status epilepticus (SSE) and status epilepticus in the comatose or paralyzed patient are important entities to recognize and terminate.

SSE, also referred to as subclinical status epilepticus, is a form of NCSE that arises from generalized convulsive status epilepticus (GCSE) that has either been undertreated, thus blunting the muscular response to epileptic CNS discharge, or not treated at all, with eventual cessation of motor activity secondary to progressive CNS insult. When the clinical signs that usually prompt physicians to treat seizure (i.e., tonic-clonic movements) are no longer present, the patient's CNS continues to experience the damaging effects of epileptic discharges. The incidence of SSE following treatment of GCSE is significant, estimated at 14% to 25%. The signs of SSE are correctly termed "subtle": a prolonged postictal state (>30 min to 1 h), postictal confusion, agitation or aggression, hallucinations, and lethargy. Motor findings consist of nystagmoid jerks or deviations of the eye and focal twitches of eyelid, face, jaw, or trunk. Autonomic responses caused by a catacholamine surge include hypertension, tachycardia, dysrhythmia, hyperglycemia, and tremulousness. Such findings should be actively sought out by the EP; missing these clinical clues that indicate persistent SE leads to undertreatment of seizure activity and likely increased morbidity and mortality. EEG commonly is the only clear manifestation of underlying CNS discharge in SSE.

A second form of NCSE arises in the comatose or paralyzed patient. Patients may arrive in the emergency department comatose secondary to severe status epilepticus or to another CNS insult. The challenge in diagnosing SE in these patients is that they most often have no overt manifestation of seizure activity. Towne et al. (2000) conclude from a prospective study of 236 comatose patients that 8% of comatose patients without clinical signs of seizure showed EEG seizure activity. The authors argue that NCSE is an underrecognized cause of coma and that EEG should be routine in the evaluation of comatose patients. Others report an even higher incidence of up to 34% of NCSE in ICU patients with coma of unclear etiology. Patients arriving to the ED in SE are often pharmacologically paralyzed and intubated for airway protection. Once sedated and/or paralyzed, overt seizure manifestations will be blunted or completely masked. Again, EEG may be the only manifestation of underlying CNS discharge.

Mortality estimates for NCSE vary widely, ranging from 3% to 60%. This wide range reflects the underlying causes of the seizures and comorbidities of these patients. Morbidity from prolonged CNS discharge in NCSE results from permanent brain damage but, likewise, has been difficult to quantify.

A recent clinical policy on the management of ED seizure patients by the American College of Emergency Physicians recommends emergency EEG in seizure patients with persistent altered consciousness, refractory status epilepticus, pharmacologically managed sedation, NCSE/SSE, and coma. The policy recognizes the use of EEG in the detection of GCSE that may have progressed into SSE. Obtaining an EEG in most EDs, unfortunately, is a formidable challenge: most hospitals will have limited hours in which an EEG can be obtained, let alone interpreted. Simpler bispectral index monitoring systems, which require only a few leads, may prove suitable for use by the ED staff but are not yet in widespread use. In the absence of an EEG to guide sedation and anticonvulsant therapy, paralysis should be avoided whenever possible, so that, at a minimum, physical signs of SSE are not masked.

SUGGESTED READINGS

ACEP Clinical Policies Committee, Clinical Policies Subcommittee on Seizures. Clinical policy: Critical issues in the evaluation and management of adult patients presenting to the emergency department with seizures. *Ann Emerg Med*. 2004;43(5):605–625.

Bradley WG, Dardoff RB, Fenichel GM, et al. *Neurology in Clinical Practice: Principles of Diagnosis and Management*. Philadelphia, PA: Elsevier; 2004.

DeLorenze RJ, Waterhouse EJ, Towne AR, et al. Persistent nonconvulsive status epilepticus after the control of convulsive status epilepticus. *Epilepsia*. 1998;39(8):833–840.

Kaplan P. Assessing the outcomes in patients with nonconvulsive status epilepticus: Nonconvulsive status epilepticus is underdiagnosed, potentially overtreated, and confounded by comorbidity. *J Clin Neurophysiol*. 1999;16(4):341–352.

Meierkord H, Holtkamp M. Non-convulsive status epilepticus in adults: Clinical forms and treatment. *Lancet Neurol*. 2007;6:329–339.

Towne AR, Waterhouse EJ, Boggs JG, et al. Prevalence of nonconvulsive status epilepticus in comatose patients. *Neurology*. 2000;54(2):340–345.

Wasterlain CG, Treiman DM. *Status Epilepticus: Mechanisms and Management*. Cambridge, MA: The Mit Press; 2006.

187

DO NOT MISTAKE SEIZURES FOR SYNCOPE

THOMAS M. MAILHOT, MD, FAAEM

A transient loss of consciousness is a common reason for presentation to the emergency department (ED). Possible causes include both seizure and syncope, and an attempt to differentiate the two is necessary in order to appropriately guide the workup. The evaluation of syncope is geared toward identifying a dangerous (especially cardiac) cause, including myocardial ischemia, dysrhythmia, and valvular or structural cardiac disease. In order to rule out the life-threatening causes of syncope, a significant number of such patients are admitted for inpatient testing. By contrast, seizure patients can more often be discharged home from the ED after a limited workup. Attributing a loss of consciousness to seizure rather than syncope can therefore be dangerous.

Differentiating a seizure from syncope is difficult for many reasons. Oftentimes, there are no witnesses to the event, or if witnesses are present, they may not be available for questioning. Both seizure and syncope result in a loss of consciousness during the event, and patients are often unable to recall what happened immediately preceding the event. Both disorders may be preceded by a sensation of dizziness. Syncope may be accompanied by myoclonic jerks resulting from brain hypoxia, resembling a seizure activity. A seizure may occur without any tonic or clonic movements (atonic seizure). Even more confusing is the fact that seizures may occasionally lead to dysrhythmias that, in turn, may cause syncope. Furthermore, physicians may draw disparate conclusions regarding patient histories and physical examinations. In one study of 118 patients with either syncope or seizure, physicians interpreting identical patient data came to the same conclusion only 31% of the time.

A history is widely held to be the most helpful factor in distinguishing syncope from seizure. Tongue biting is more likely to be present with seizure activity than with syncope. Hoefnagels et al. (1991) found the best discriminatory finding to be postictal confusion, making seizure five times more likely than syncope. Other historical features suggestive of syncope include lightheadedness, sweating, prolonged standing, precipitants such as micturition, pain or exercise, and complaints of chest pain or palpitations. Features that point to a seizure include a sense of déjà vu, aphasia, an aura, or an epigastric "rising" sensation. Urinary incontinence occurs in both conditions and does not add any diagnostic value. The presence of head trauma is similarly unhelpful.

A history should also be obtained from any available witnesses. If necessary, witnesses should be solicited by telephone for their description of the event. If witnesses report pallor and sweating prior to the event (even if myoclonic jerking ensues), syncope is probable. If witnesses report aphasia, head turning, posturing, and postevent delirium, a seizure is likely.

Sheldon et al. (2002) proposed a questionnaire-based scoring system to assist clinicians in predicting a diagnosis of syncope or seizure. In this scoring system, each of several historical factors is assigned a point value: tongue biting (2 points), déjà vu (1), associated emotional stress (1), head turning during the event (1), unresponsiveness/unusual posture/limb movement/amnesia (1), confusion after the event (1), lightheaded spells (−2), sweating before the event (−2), and event associated with prolonged sitting or standing (−2). A total point score of 1 or greater suggests a seizure; if the score is <1, the likelihood is syncope. This scoring system correctly diagnosed 94% of patients and was 94% sensitive and 94% specific in identifying seizures.

On physical examination, bradycardia and hypotension point to syncope as the etiology of the loss of consciousness. Any focal neurological abnormality is more consistent with a seizure than syncope.

Laboratory parameters may suggest an etiology for the loss of consciousness. Lactate levels rise transiently during seizures due to local muscle hypoxia, and measurement of serum lactate shows promise in helping clinicians distinguish syncope from a seizure. One study comparing venous lactate levels in patients with generalized seizure activity and patients with syncope found that a lactate level >2.5 mmol/L was 73% sensitive and 97% specific for generalized seizures. Creatine kinase (CK) may also be a useful test. An elevated CK level measured 3 h after loss of consciousness has a sensitivity of 80% and a specificity of 94% in diagnosing a seizure.

It can be exceedingly difficult to classify a single transient loss of consciousness as either syncope or a seizure. In cases where doubt exists, it may be best not to label the patient as having definitely suffered either syncope or a seizure but to acknowledge that diagnostic uncertainty remains.

SUGGESTED READINGS

Hazouard E, Dequin PF, Lanotte R, et al. Losing consciousness: Role of the venous lactate levels in the diagnosis of convulsive crises. *Presse Med.* 1998;27(13):604–607.

Hoefnagels WA, Padberg GW, Overweg J, et al. Transient loss of consciousness: The value of the history for distinguishing seizure from syncope. *J Neurol.* 1991;238(1):39–43.

Libman MD, Potvin L, Coupal L, et al. Seizure vs. syncope: Measuring serum creatine kinase in the emergency department. *J Gen Intern Med.* 1991;6(5):408–412.

Sheldon R, Rose S, Ritchie D, et al. Historical criteria that distinguish syncope from seizures. *J Am Coll Cardiol.* 2002;40(1):142–148.

188

DO NOT OVERLOOK THE CENTRAL CAUSES OF VERTIGO

YIAN (MICHAEL) CHENG, MD

Vertigo, the sensation of illusory movement, is a common complaint that merits careful scrutiny. It represents a wide range of overlapping symptoms and a differential diagnosis spanning from benign to life-threatening diseases.

Balance is principally managed by the peripheral vestibular system, central vestibular nuclei, cerebellum, and eighth cranial nerve. Central causes of vertigo are much more concerning and include vertebrobasilar insufficiency, acoustic neuromas, multiple sclerosis, infection, and intoxications. Of these, vertebrobasilar insufficiency is the most important for the emergency physician. Posterior circulation stroke syndromes leave permanent debilitating deficits and carry a high mortality rate (7% to 20%), even with aggressive neurosurgical and medical intervention.

Classically, vertigo manifests in two ways. Peripheral causes of vertigo tend to have a sudden onset, are paroxysmal in nature, have associated hearing loss or tinnitus, have nystagmus suppressed with visual fixation, and have unidirectional postural instability with an intact ability to walk. Central causes typically have a gradual onset, are constant in nature, have no associated hearing loss/tinnitus, have nystagmus not suppressed with fixation, and have postural instability with frequent falls while walking.

Unfortunately, none of these findings can be relied upon completely to distinguish peripheral from central causes of vertigo, although an amalgamation of these factors can help direct the diagnosis. In contrast to the classic presentation of central vertigo, posterior circulation vascular ischemia may often be sudden in onset with associated severe vertigo but improve within a week and resolve within several weeks to months. While posterior circulation stroke is often associated with dysarthria, dysphagia, dysmetria, dysdiadochokinesia, and ataxia, as well as descending motor or sensory deficits, patients with inferior cerebellar strokes may present with few symptoms beyond vertigo, nystagmus, and postural instability. Interestingly, nystagmus elicited through oft-cited physical exam tests is unreliable for establishing peripheral vertigo. The Dix-Hallpike test has an estimated sensitivity of 79% and specificity of 75%. Similarly, the side-lying test has a sensitivity of 90% and specificity of 75%.

Given these limitations, how can one most promptly and dependably differentiate peripheral from central causes of vertigo? More importantly, how do we identify posterior circulation ischemia? Place an emphasis on the patient's age and vascular risk factors (diabetes, prior strokes, cardiac disease, and hypertension). Although cerebellar, cranial nerve, motor, or sensory deficits in patients are all red flags that should direct further workup, the absence of these signs cannot definitively exclude a central process, especially in light of stroke risk factors and vertigo that lasts longer than a few minutes. While the time course of central vertigo may mimic the characteristic sudden onset of peripheral vertigo, symptoms that last only seconds are likely peripheral. Recurrent transient symptoms (usually <30 min but more than a few seconds), on the other hand, may suggest ischemic disease. Nystagmus that is vertical or multidirectional, is worsened with fixation, and changes directions with altered direction of gaze should also further increase suspicion for a central cause of vertigo.

There is currently no validated clinical decision rule for imaging patients with suspected central vertigo. Should the patient's history and exam increase your suspicion for a central etiology, a neurological consultation and magnetic resonance (MR) are both indicated, although computed tomography is still a useful first step to rule out hemorrhage and edema associated with large infarcts. If MR for stroke is negative, it may reveal other causes of central vertigo such as a mass lesion or multiple sclerosis.

SUGGESTED READINGS

Halker RB, Barrs DM, Wellik KE, et al. Establishing a diagnosis of benign paroxysmal positional vertigo through the dix-hallpike and side-lying maneuvers: A critically appraised topic. *Neurologist*. 2008;14(3):201–204.

Hornig CR, Rust DS, Busse O, et al. Space-occupying cerebellar infarction. Clinical course and prognosis. *Stroke*. 1994;25(2):372–374.

Hotson J, Baloh R. Acute vestibular syndrome. *N Engl J Med*. 1998;339(10):680–685.

Kase CS, Norrving B, Levine SR, et al. Cerebellar infarction: Clinical and anatomic observations in 66 cases. *Stroke*. 1993;24(1):76–83.

189

DO NOT RELY ON PLAIN X-RAYS OR COMPUTED TOMOGRAPHY TO RULE OUT SPINAL CORD COMPRESSION

EDUARDO BORQUEZ, MD

Nontraumatic spinal cord compression (SCC) is rare, but it is a "do not miss" diagnosis in emergency medicine. Compression may result from a variety of processes, including infectious, neoplastic, skeletal, and hemorrhagic. Examples of SCC include spinal epidural abscess (SEA), disc herniation, spinal epidural hematoma (SEH), and primary or metastatic tumors.

Making a diagnosis of SCC presents several challenges. Firstly, the disease is rare (SEA occurs in 1 in 10,000 hospitalized patients per year, SEH occurs in 1 in 1 million per year). Secondly, the presentation may be insidious. The signs and symptoms are insensitive and often subtle and nonspecific. For instance, in SEA, over 25% of patients will *not* have back pain as a presenting complaint, the majority will *not* be febrile, and over 75% will *not* have tenderness to palpation over the spine. Thirdly, a huge number of patients are considered to have risk factors that place them at risk for the development of compression syndromes. For SEA, risk factors include diabetes, alcoholism, immunocompromised status, and any current infection. For SEH, coagulopathy is an important risk factor. Each of these processes can mimic each other, and one can be a risk factor for another (i.e., disc herniation can predispose one to infection, and tumors can predispose one to bleeding). In neoplastic disease, up to 10% of people with cancer first present with spinal metastasis, and 10% of patients with known cancer will be diagnosed with spinal metastasis in their lives. Lastly, back pain is a common complaint in the ED, and identifying the very few with serious pathology from a huge number of patients presents obvious difficulties.

Given the scope of the problem, the liberal use of imaging may at first seem attractive. Plain films and computed tomography (CT) are the most readily available modalities, and it may therefore be tempting to get these images either as a "first pass" or in lieu of magnetic resonance (MR). CT (and to a lesser degree, plain x-ray) is excellent in showing boney abnormalities. While this may be of some importance in the long term to the patient (for instance, a lytic malignant lesion), these abnormalities seldom need to be identified emergently in the patient without trauma. Plain films and CT are not helpful in excluding cord compression. The sensitivity of CT for SEA is as low as 33%. These modalities may show findings that are *associated with* conditions that cause cord compression, such as disk space narrowing or boney lytic lesions, but their absence does not rule out the coexistence of cord compression. CT *with myelography* is useful in ruling out compression, with sensitivities similar to MR (>90%). However, CT with myelography may require the injection of contrast media into the subarachnoid space proximally via the lateral C1,2 approach or cisternal puncture in addition to the usual L3/L4 approach—not a trivial detail.

One may be left with the impression that almost every patient with back pain needs to be worked up for a compressive lesion. Given the rarity of the disease and the significant resources involved in obtaining an emergent MR, this is not possible. With the sheer number of patients presenting to the ED with back pain this would also bring any department to a grinding halt. Even if one did have unlimited resources, a small randomized trial using rapid MR as the *initial* imaging modality for low back pain has shown it to be cost-*in*effective.

To avoid missing the diagnosis of SCC, it is critical to identify those few patients with *rapidly progressive neurologic deficits* that need emergent MR imaging and immediate neurosurgical consultation. In addition, patients who are at especially high risk, even without neurological findings, such as intravenous drug users, those with a history of malignancy, coagulopathy, and those with night pain or constitutional symptoms, should also be considered for further workup. Unlike the insensitive clinical features described above, erythrocyte sedimentation rate has a sensitivity >90% for SEA and is helpful in ruling out this diagnosis. The most significant errors are failure to include the diagnosis of SCC in the differential diagnosis in the first place, failure to document a complete neurologic examination and why further workup was not undertaken, and false reassurance by normal plain films and/or CT.

SUGGESTED READINGS

Darouiche RO. Spinal epidural abscess. *N Engl J Med*. 2006;355(19):2012–2020.
Jarvik JG, Maravilla KR, Haynor DR, et al. Rapid MR imaging versus plain radiography in patients with low back pain: Initial results of a randomized study. *Radiology*. 1997;204(2):447–454.
Perron AD, Huff JS. In: Marx JA, Hockberger RS, Walls RM, eds. *Rosen's Emergency Medicine: Concepts and Clinical Practice*. 6th ed. St. Louis: CV Mosby;2006;1683–1687.
Reihsaus E, Waldbaur H, Seeling W. Spinal epidural abscess: A meta-analysis of 915 patients. *Neurosurg Rev*. 2000;23(4):175–204.

190

DO NOT RELY SIMPLY ON COMPUTED TOMOGRAPHY TO RULE OUT SUBARACHNOID HEMORRHAGE

STUART P. SWADRON, MD, FRCPC

Subarachnoid hemorrhage (SAH) is one of the "can't miss" diagnoses in emergency medicine. Although there are only approximately 30,000 cases diagnosed each year in the United States, the high mortality and devastating sequelae of SAH make every case important.

Most headaches that present to the emergency department do not require an evaluation for SAH. Headaches that should arouse suspicion are those that are new or different than any previous headaches in their quality and severity and those that are sudden and maximal at onset.

As the technology of neuroimaging improves, there is a temptation among many clinicians to believe that the role for lumbar puncture (LP) and cerebrospinal fluid analysis to rule out SAH has been eliminated. Unfortunately, this is not true, and missing a diagnosis of SAH by relying on a computed tomography (CT) scan is difficult to defend based on the available evidence.

SAH may present with a sentinel or "warning" leak prior to a more devastating bleed that results in severe neurological signs or coma. This is the ideal time to make the diagnosis, as it provides a window of opportunity for the neurosurgeon to find the source of the SAH (usually a saccular cerebral artery aneurysm) and treat it, either surgically or by interventional radiological techniques. Once a more major bleed has occurred, the prognosis is much worse, and it may even be too late for intervention. Sensitivities approaching 100% for CT to detect SAH are often derived (and quoted by some clinicians) by working backward from a group of patients in whom a final diagnosis has already been established, often only after a major bleed. In the group of patients with sentinel leaks, the amount of blood in the CSF might be very small, and the sensitivity of CT in these patients is lower.

Small bleeds may be very subtle indeed and beyond the threshold of detection of CT. In some instances, these may only be detected by a neuroradiologist. Remember that a neuroradiologist, not a general radiologist, was considered the reference standard to rule out intracranial bleeding on CT in the landmark stroke trial that established fibrinolytics as a therapy for ischemic stroke. LP, on the contrary, will pick up even microscopic amounts of bleeding and can effectively rule out even the smallest sentinel leaks.

In addition, even the most modern CT scanner becomes less sensitive for SAH with each passing hour after symptom onset. One week after symptoms begin, the sensitivity for CT is no better than 50%. At one week, an LP, which can detect both red blood cells as well as the xanthochromia caused by their breakdown, is still virtually 100% sensitive.

In every recent series that has looked at the question, all but one have revealed several cases of SAH that were detected only on LP; even with a retrospective reading, the CT was negative for blood. The percentage is not huge (around 2% to 7% of cases), but it is persistent.

Some have suggested that noninvasive angiography, such as CT or MR angiography, be used in the place of LP. While these studies definitely have a role in the evaluation of SAH, they are by no means a panacea to rule out the diagnosis. Aside from their expense (and additional radiation, in the case of CT angiography), these modalities are actually less sensitive than LP for the detection of SAH—they may miss small aneurysms. More importantly, simply because an aneurysm is detected on angiography does not guarantee that it was the cause of the patient's symptoms. Because the prevalence of saccular aneurysms is approximately 2% (and higher in older patients), many aneurysms will be incidental findings. In the worst case, in the absence of a positive LP to confirm acute bleeding, this may lead to unnecessary neurosurgery, as the rate of bleeding of unruptured, asymptomatic aneurysms is very small over a patient's lifetime.

Many emergency physicians document that patients "refuse" an LP when the subject is broached during the workup of SAH. This may be the case, but we should also be clear with our patients that with a suggestive history only a negative LP can reliably rule out this deadly diagnosis.

Suggested Readings

Al-Shahi R. Subarachnoid haemorrhage. *Br Med J.* 2006;333:235–240.
Edlow JA, Caplan LR. Avoiding pitfalls in the diagnosis of subarachnoid hemorrhage. *N Engl J Med.* 2000;342:29–36.

191

GIVE APPROPRIATE ANTIBIOTICS TO PATIENTS WITH MENINGITIS AND MENINGOENCEPHALITIS

MONICA KUMAR, MD

Meningitis, the result of inflammation of the leptomeninges, has an annual incidence of 4 to 6 per 100,000 cases. It can present as an acute, subacute, or chronic disease. Bacterial causes most typically present acutely, within a 24-h period. While viral and fungal presentations are more insidious, they should also be considered. Alteration in consciousness commonly indicates meningoencephalitis, resulting from an inflammatory response, and portends a worse prognosis. Due to the potential for grave outcomes, bacterial meningitis requires emergent treatment by the emergency physician (EP).

Meningitis and meningoencephalitis should be treated with antibiotics as soon as they are suspected. Some EPs mistakenly withhold antibiotics until after the lumbar puncture (LP) is done in the hope of obtaining a more reliable cerebrospinal fluid (CSF) culture. However, acute bacterial meningitis is rapidly progressive, and any delay in treatment may worsen outcomes. Moreover, performance of an LP may be significantly delayed while awaiting results of head computed tomography (CT) or laboratory data (such as a platelet count and coagulation studies) or if the patient needs to be stabilized before undergoing the procedure. Although CSF cultures may become sterile in as little as 1 to 2 h after antibiotics, a diagnosis can frequently be obtained through polymerase chain reaction (PCR) analysis of the CSF, a technique that is viable despite the prior administration of antibiotics. Blood cultures should also be drawn prior to administering antibiotics because 50% to 75% of bacterial meningitis cases will have positive blood cultures, allowing the causative organism to be identified.

Because of the many different etiologies of meningoencephalitis, choosing the appropriate antibiotic coverage for patients often presents a challenge. Typical bacterial causes of meningitis vary predictably according to age (*Table 191.1*), allowing the EP to initiate empiric treatment before confirmatory test results are available. Additional patient factors discernible through history and physical examination may lead to a broadening or change of antibiotics given. Therefore, to determine the most appropriate therapy for meningoencephalitis, the EP must extrapolate an empiric treatment based on the patient's age and known or suspected underlying conditions.

While age is usually known or easily estimated, patients' underlying conditions may not be, particularly if they have altered mental status and are unable to

TABLE 191.1	TYPICAL BACTERIAL CAUSES OF MENINGITIS ACCORDING TO AGE	
AGE RANGE	**CAUSATIVE ORGANISMS**	**RECOMMENDED ANTIBIOTICS**
Neonates (<30 d)	GBS, *Listeria*, GNR, HSV	Cefotaxime + Ampicillin ± Acyclovir
Children (1–23 mo)	*S. pneumo, Neisseria, H. flu, E. coli*	Cefotaxime/Ceftriaxone + Vancomycin
Children (2–18 y)	*S. pneumo, Neisseria*	Cefotaxime/Ceftriaxone + Vancomycin
Adults (18–50 y)	*S. pneumo, Neisseria*	Cefotaxime/Ceftriaxone + Vancomycin
Elderly (>50 y)	*S. pneumo, Neisseria, Listeria*	Cefotaxime/Ceftriaxone + Vancomycin + Ampicillin

GBS, Group B Streptococci; GNR, Gram-negative rods; HSV, Herpes simplex virus; *S. pneumo, Streptococcus pneumoniae; Neisseria, Neisseria meningitidis; H. flu, Haemophilus influenzae.*

provide any history. In the setting of known or suspected immunocompromise (including AIDS, chronic alcoholism, or medical disease), ampicillin should also be added to cover *Listeria*.

In any age range, if there is CSF leak, recent trauma to the central nervous system (CNS), or a history of neurosurgery, some sources suggest replacing ceftriaxone with a fourth-generation cephalosporin such as cefepime. This is to improve coverage for *Staphylococcus aureus* and aerobic Gram-negative bacteria such as *Pseudomonas* and *Propionibacterium acnes*.

In neonates, a maternal history of genital herpes should prompt empiric acyclovir. If there are any focal neurological findings, including alteration of consciousness or seizure, the diagnosis of meningoencephalitis is likely. Although it does not necessarily need to be administered empirically prior to the LP, the combination of a negative Gram stain on the LP and meningoencephalitis should lead to the subsequent initiation of acyclovir in addition to standard antibiotic therapy.

So, what is the bottom line for EPs in the treatment of suspected acute meningitis and meningoencephalitis? Once the disease is suspected, draw a blood culture and administer antibiotics first and then proceed with diagnostics such as head CT and LP. Tailor the antibiotics to the individual patient, taking into account the patient's age and comorbidities. Taking these considerations into account will allow the EP to stay on the right track while the precise etiology of the meningitis is still being determined.

SUGGESTED READINGS

Benson PC, Swadron SP. Empiric acyclovir is infrequently initiated in the emergency department to patients ultimately diagnosed with encephalitis. *Ann Emerg Med.* 2006; 47(1):100–105.

Fitch MT, Abrahamian FM, Moran GJ. Emergency department management of meningitis and encephalitis. *Infect Dis Clin N Am.* 2008;22:33–52.

Kanegaye JT, Soliemanzadeh P, Bradley JS. Lumbar puncture in pediatric bacterial meningitis: Defining the time interval for recovery of cerebrospinal fluid pathogens after parenteral antibiotic pretreatment. *Pediatrics.* 2001;108(5):1169–1174.

Mace S. Acute bacterial meningitis. *Emerg Med Clin N Am.* 2008;38:281–317.

van de Beek D, de Gans J, Tunkel AR, et al. Community acquired bacterial meningitis in adults. *N Engl J Med.* 2006;354(1):44–53.

192

USE FIBRINOLYTICS FOR STROKE WITH CARE

ARTI GEHANI, MD

The decision to administer fibrinolytics in the treatment of acute ischemic stroke can be a very challenging one for the emergency physician (EP). In 1995, the National Institute for Neurological Disorders and Stroke (NINDS) published a sentinel study marking a new era in stroke management. The study concluded that patients with ischemic stroke presenting within 3 h of symptom onset had a 30% chance of recovering most or all of their neurological functions in 3 months if treated with tissue plasminogen activator (tPA). On the other hand, the same study also reported a nearly 10-fold increased risk of life-threatening intracerebral hemorrhage (ICH) with tPA (6.4% vs. 0.6%).

Many EPs are appropriately reluctant to administer fibrinolytics if a clearly defined protocol is not in place and adequate support services (neuroradiology, neurology, and/or neurosurgery) are lacking at their center. Lawsuits have been pursued against EPs for both administering and not administering fibrinolytics under various circumstances.

So, what is the current recommendation regarding fibrinolytics in stroke? In 2000, the American Heart Association (AHA) made fibrinolysis in stroke a Class I ("definitely recommended") therapy for patients who meet *all* inclusion criteria. A patient failing to meet *any* of the inclusion criteria is thus ineligible for fibrinolysis. The AHA guidelines were updated in 2007; however, the recommendation that physicians strictly adhere to the established inclusion criteria has not changed.

The most critical of the AHA guidelines is that fibrinolytics are only indicated for patients presenting within 3 h of symptom onset. Symptom onset is defined as the last time the patient or family member witnessed that individual to be symptom free. If a neurologic deficit is discovered upon awakening, symptom onset is considered as the time that the patient went to sleep. If the patient's symptoms are initially mild but then progress, then symptom onset is nevertheless considered the time that the patient first noticed symptoms. Many clinicians and researchers have attempted to broaden the time frame for fibrinolytic therapy to up to 6 h after symptom onset, often with disastrous results. However, a recent study by Hacke et al. (2008) showed a clinical benefit in stroke patients treated with fibrinolysis for up to 4.5 h from symptom onset. Results of this latest study will likely trigger renewed debate on the appropriate time frame for fibrinolysis, but currently, EPs should adhere to the 3-h window recommended by the AHA.

Another important AHA guideline states that fibrinolytics are contraindicated if neurological symptoms are minor or resolving spontaneously. Resolving symptoms often represent either a transient ischemic attack (TIA) or a nonischemic cause of neurological deficit. The NIH Stroke Scale (NIHSS) is one tool that is used to define a patient's neurologic deficit. In the NINDS trial, patients needed to have a "deficit measurable on the NIHSS" in order to be eligible for fibrinolysis. Patients with NIHSS scores <2 are more likely to completely recover from their deficit without any therapy, and the increased risk of ICH in these patients with the use of tPA greatly outweighs the benefit of improving their minor symptoms. Conversely, patients with NIHSS scores >20 ("moderate to severe" stroke symptoms) are more likely to incur permanent neurological deficits. Despite a concomitant increased risk in ICH in these patients, the benefit of potential neurological recovery may outweigh the risk of ICH from fibrinolysis. Unfortunately, the AHA does not have a defined NIHSS score value below or above which fibrinolytics are contraindicated.

A documented discussion of these risks and benefits with the patient and family members prior to the decision may assist the EP if the decision is later challenged. In one study, nearly 16% of charts for patients who received fibrinolytics did not have documented informed consents from either patients or their family.

The bottom line is that EPs should follow a very strict protocol for inclusion and exclusion of patients for fibrinolytic therapy that includes the availability of appropriate consultation services. Fibrinolytics should not be given outside of the 3-h window or to any patient who has minor or resolving symptoms. Finally, patients receiving fibrinolytics (or their surrogates) should be informed in advance about the potential risks, benefits and alternatives of this therapy. This should be clearly documented in the medical record. EPs should know in advance how and where to transfer patients for higher levels of care if there is an adverse outcome with fibrinolysis.

SUGGESTED READINGS

Adams HP Jr, del Zoppo G, Alberts MJ, et al. Guidelines for the early management of adults with ischemic stroke: A guideline from the American Heart Association/American Stroke Association Stroke Council, Clinical Cardiology Council, Cardiovascular Radiology and Intervention Council, and the Atherosclerotic Peripheral Vascular Disease and Quality of Care Outcomes in Research Interdisciplinary Working Groups: The American Academy of Neurology affirms the value of this guideline as an educational tool for neurologists. *Stroke*. 2007;38(5):1655–1711 [Epub Apr 12, 2007].

Hacke W, Kaste M, Bluhmki E, et al. Thrombolysis with alteplase 3 to 4.5 hours after acute ischemic stroke. *N Engl J Med*. 2008;359(13):1317–1329.

Weintraub MI. Thrombolysis (tissue plasminogen activator) in stroke: A medicolegal quagmire. *Stroke*. 2006;37(7):1917–1922 [Epub May 25, 2006].

[No author listed]. Tissue plasminogen activator for acute ischemic stroke. The National Institute of Neurological Disorders and Stroke rt-PA Stroke Study Group. *N Engl J Med*. 1995;333(24):1581–1587.

193

Do not withhold radiologic imaging in pregnancy when it is necessary for the diagnosis

Maura Kennedy, MD

Pregnant patients and physicians often worry about and avoid exposing a fetus to ionizing radiation from radiologic studies such as computed tomography (CT) and plain radiographs. Much of this anxiety stems from evidence that fetuses exposed *in utero* to radiation from the atomic bombs in Hiroshima and Nagasaki had higher rates of prenatal death, microcephaly, mental retardation, malformation, and increased rates of childhood cancer compared to children who were not exposed to radiation *in utero*.

The effect of ionizing radiation depends on the gestational age at which the fetus is exposed and dose of radiation absorbed by the fetus. The dose of radiation absorbed is measured in rads (or the standard international unit Grey; 1 rad = 0.01 Grey). Information regarding the effects of radiation exposure on developing fetuses has been extrapolated from observation studies of survivors of the atomic bombings and the Chernobyl nuclear power plant accident, from case control and cohort studies of pregnant women exposed to diagnostic or therapeutic radiation, and from animal studies (*Table 193.1*).

Fetal malformation is more likely to occur if the fetus is exposed to radiation during weeks 2 to 8 of pregnancy, when organogenesis occurs. The central nervous system undergoes extensive development and is most sensitive to radiation during weeks 8 to 15 of pregnancy; there is a gradual decrease in sensitivity from week 15 to 25. There is no evidence of mental retardation from radiation exposure before week 8 and after week 25 of pregnancy.

If the fetus is outside the field of view (for instance in an ankle radiograph), the fetus will have very minimal radiation exposure; the exposure may be further limited by using lead shielding. When the fetus is directly in the field of view, the dose absorbed depends on the distance from the source, the thickness through which the radiation passes before reaching the fetus, and the dose of

TABLE 193.1	RELATIONSHIP OF IONIZING RADIATION DOSE AND TIME OF EXPOSURE TO MALFORMATION	
MALFORMATION	GESTATIONAL AGE FOR GREATEST RISK (WEEKS POSTCONCEPTION)	ESTIMATED THRESHOLD DOSE TO CAUSE MALFORMATION
Mental retardation	8–15	0–8 wk post conception: none 8–15 wk post conception: 6–31 rad 16–25 wk post conception: 25–28 rad 25+ wk post conception: >50 rad
Diminished IQ	8–15	10 rad
Microcephaly	8–15	>2,000 rad
Other malformation (skeletal, genital, etc.)	3–11	>20 rad

radiation administered. Radiologists can often modify radiographic techniques to decrease the dose administered.

An exposure to <5 rad of ionizing radiation has not been demonstrated to cause an increase in malformation or fetal loss (*Table 193.1*) regardless of gestational age of the fetus and is routinely used as the limit of recommended ionizing radiation exposure during pregnancy. There are no diagnostic procedures that equal or exceed 5 rad of radiation (*Table 193.2*). While exposure to 1 to 2 rad of ionizing radiation *in utero* may increase background leukemia rates 1.5 to 2.0 times over background incidence, given the low background incidence of leukemia, approximately 2,000 fetuses would need to be exposed to diagnostic radiation to cause one additional case of leukemia.

Neither ultrasound nor magnetic resonance imaging (MRI) exposes the fetus to ionizing radiation. There are no documented adverse effects from pre-natal exposure to either modality. When diagnostically feasible, ultrasound or MRI should be preferentially utilized in diagnostic imaging of pregnant women, instead of a modality that involves exposure to ionizing radiation. For instance, MRI can be utilized to diagnose appendicitis, and ultrasound can be used to evaluate for deep vein thrombosis or genitourinary pathology.

If a diagnostic radiology procedure involving ionizing radiation is medi-cally indicated to appropriately care for the pregnant patient, it should be performed. The likelihood of harm from not performing indicated imaging

TABLE 193.2	APPROXIMATE RADIATION DOSE TO FETUS FROM STANDARD RADIOLOGIC PROCEDURES	
PROCEDURE	**FETAL EXPOSURE (RAD)**	
Chest x-ray (2 view)	<0.001	
Abdominal film (single view)	0.1	
Hip film (single view)	0.2	
Barium enema or small bowel series	2–4	
CT scan of head or chest	<1	
CT scan of abdomen and lumbar spine	3.5	
CT pelvimetry	0.25	

outweighs potential harm to the fetus. Position statements from the numerous organizations including the American College of Obstetricians and Gynecologists and the International Commission on Radiological Protection emphasize that the radiation exposure from a single diagnostic radiology procedure does not result in harmful fetal effects.

In summary, when caring for the pregnant patient, attempts should be made to choose diagnostic imaging modalities that avoid ionizing radiation exposure. If no such alternative exists, and performing a diagnostic study is medically indicated and would alter patient care, it is acceptable to perform diagnostic studies that involve exposure to ionizing radiation. Attempts should be made to minimize the dose absorbed by a fetus. Patients should be reassured that there is no evidence that radiation exposure from a single diagnostic study results in harmful fetal effects.

SUGGESTED READINGS

American College of Obstetricians and Gynecologists. Guidelines for Diagnostic Imaging During Pregnancy, ACOG Committee Opinion No. 299. *Obstet Gynecol*. 2004;104: 647–651.

De Santis M, Di Gianantonio ED, Straface G, et al. Ionizing radiations in pregnancy and teratogenesis: A review of the literature. *Reprod Toxicol*. 2005;20(3):323–329.

International Commission on Radiological Protection. *Pregnancy and Medical Radiation. ICRP Publication 84*. Oxford: Pergamon Press; 2000.

Kennedy A. Assessment of acute abdominal pain in the pregnant patient. *Semin Ultrasound CT MR*. 2000;21(1):64–77.

McCollough CH, Schueler BA, Atwell TD, et al. Radiation exposure and pregnancy: When should we be concerned? *Radiographics*. 2007;27(4):909–918.

194

AVOID PLACING PRESSURE ON THE UTERINE FUNDUS WHEN ATTEMPTING TO REDUCE A SHOULDER DYSTOCIA DURING EMERGENCY DELIVERY

HOLLY SCHRUPP-BERG, MD

An emergency delivery is one of the most anxiety-producing procedures for emergency care providers. While the vast majority of deliveries proceed without difficulty, emergency physicians must be prepared to deal with unexpected complications. One of the most feared is a shoulder dystocia. Defined by the American College of Obstetrics and Gynecology (ACOG) as a delivery that "requires additional obstetric maneuvers following failure of downward traction on the fetal head to effect delivery of the shoulders," a shoulder dystocia puts the infant and mother at risk of significant complications. The most common complications are maternal postpartum hemorrhage and high-degree lacerations. Infants are at risk for fractures, brachial plexus trauma, and hypoxic brain injuries from umbilical cord compression.

A shoulder dystocia represents a size imbalance between the fetal shoulders and the maternal pelvic inlet, typically an impaction of the fetal anterior shoulder against the maternal pubic symphysis. Less commonly, it can occur from wedging of the posterior shoulder against the maternal sacral promontory. The basic risk factors for a shoulder dystocia include abnormal maternal pelvic anatomy, gestational diabetes (resulting in fetal macrosomia), postdates pregnancy, and forceps- or vacuum-assisted vaginal delivery. Overall incidence of a shoulder dystocia increases with birth weight.

A shoulder dystocia is often first recognized when the fetal head delivers then retracts suddenly against the maternal perineum. This phenomenon, known as the "turtle sign," reflects the wedging of the anterior shoulder against the symphysis. It is diagnosed when standard downward pressure fails to deliver the shoulder. When attempting to reduce a shoulder dystocia, it is imperative that you avoid the natural tendency to apply fundal pressure. Direct pressure on the uterine fundus may further worsen the impaction and increases the risk of uterine rupture.

In the event you encounter a dystocia, the first move is to call for help. Have someone alert available obstetrics staff and assign a nurse to assist you with additional maneuvers. The first reduction technique recommended by most experts and ACOG is the McRoberts maneuver. Accomplished by acutely flexing the maternal thighs up against her abdomen, the maneuver effectively increases the diameter of the pelvis, allowing the posterior shoulder to push over the sacrum and rotate the impacted shoulder. With successful application of the maneuver, the shoulders should deliver with normal downward traction. In a retrospective study of 250 shoulder dystocias by Gherman et al., the researchers noted successful reduction with the McRoberts maneuver in 42% of patients. Over half of the dystocias were resolved with a combination of McRoberts maneuver and suprapubic pressure or episiotomy.

Suprapubic pressure is a technique commonly used in conjunction with the McRoberts maneuver. Applied from the side of the mother and directed posterior, the intent is to force the fetal anterior shoulder under the symphysis. Some authors suggest a cyclic pressure, similar to cardiopulmonary resuscitation compressions, to help dislodge the wedged shoulder.

While the McRoberts maneuver and suprapubic pressure frequently relieve a shoulder dystocia, some will necessitate the introduction of internal rotation techniques. Both the Woods corkscrew and Rubin maneuvers attempt to reduce the bisacromial distance by abducting or adducting the shoulders internally. In the Woods corkscrew, the practitioner places pressure on the anterior surface of the posterior shoulder, thus abducting the posterior shoulder. The Rubin maneuver, or reverse Woods, requires posterior pressure on the most accessible part of the fetal shoulder to attempt adduction. It may be helpful to push the fetal presenting part proximally into the pelvis to help facilitate rotation. Of note, while it is generally accepted that a shoulder dystocia is a bony impaction and thus an episiotomy should not be a routine part of therapy, if patients require internal rotation maneuvers, it may be required to allow the practitioners' hands enough room to complete the manipulation.

The Gaskin maneuver, or the "all-fours" technique, is another safe and easy method for the reduction of a shoulder dystocia. Have the patient turn over, positioning herself on her hands and knees, and apply gentle downward traction. Some studies using x-ray pelvimetry report an increase of the pelvic diameter by up to 20 mm. This position is also compatible with the use of the internal rotation measures mentioned previously.

In the case that the above maneuvers are unsuccessful in reducing a dystocia, there are last resort techniques, including intentional clavicle fracture, and the Zavanelli maneuver that are best performed with the assistance of an anesthesiologist and obstetrician.

SUGGESTED READINGS

ACOG Committee on Practice Bulletins-Gynecology, The American College of Obstetricians and Gynecologists. ACOG practice bulletin clinical management guidelines for obstetrician-gynecologists. Number 40, November 2002. *Obstet Gynecol.* 2002; 100(5 Pt 1):1045–1050.

Geary M, McParland P, Johnson H, et al. Shoulder dystocia – is it predictable? *Eur J Obstet Gynecol Reprod Bil.* 1995;62:15–18.

Gherman RB, Chauhan S, Ouzounian JG, et al. Shoulder dystocia: The unpreventable obstetric emergency with empiric management guidelines. *Am J Obstet Gynecol.* 2006;195:657–672.

Gherman RB, Goodwin TM, Souter I, et al. The McRoberts' maneuver for the alleviation of shoulder dystocia: How successful is it? *Am J Obstet Gynecol.* 1997;176:656–661.

Gherman RB, Tramont J, Muffley R, et al. Analysis of McRoberts' maneuver by X-ray analysis. *Obstet Gynecol.* 2000;95:43–47.

Gobbo R, Baxley EG. Shoulder dystocia. In: ALSO: *Advanced Life Support in Obstetrics Provider Course Syllabus.* Leawood, KS: American Academy of Family Physicians; 2000.

Gross TL, Sokol RJ, Williams T, et al. Shoulder dystocia: A fetal-physician risk. *Am J Obstet Gynecol.* 1987;156:1408–1418.

195

REMEMBER TO CONSIDER PERIPARTUM CARDIOMYOPATHY IN PREGNANT PATIENTS WITH SHORTNESS OF BREATH

DARRYL V. CALVO, MD

Shortness of breath is a common complaint often associated with physiologic changes that occur during a normal pregnancy. As the diaphragm is elevated by a gravid uterus, functional residual capacity decreases but tidal volume can increase up to 30% to 40%. This results in a paradoxical lowering of PCO_2 due to increased minute ventilation and a subjective sense of dyspnea. However, in the emergency department, attributing symptoms of shortness of breath or dyspnea to a gravid uterus alone can be a pitfall leading to missed diagnosis of an ominous underlying condition.

Dyspnea associated with pregnancy is usually mild, does not affect normal physical activities, does not occur at rest, and does not significantly worsen with advancing gestational age. When these symptoms are present, more serious causes of dyspnea should be suspected, such as pulmonary embolism, valvular disorders, preeclampsia, and cardiomyopathies including peripartum cardiomyopathy.

Peripartum cardiomyopathy should be suspected in a pregnant patient who presents with shortness of breath. Typical signs and symptoms of heart failure, such as orthopnea, pulmonary edema, and peripheral edema, can result for this type of dilated cardiomyopathy. Peripartum cardiomyopathy specifically is a rare but potentially fatal condition of idiopathic heart failure defined as a left ventricular ejection fraction of <45% and occurs between the last month of pregnancy and up to 5 months postpartum. The mortality rate from this condition ranges from 25% to 50% with death usually occurring from associated arrhythmia, congestive heart failure, or thromboembolic diseases due to a clot formation in these hypodynamic chambers. In the later stages of the disease, this diagnosis is not subtle, but in the early stages, the signs and symptoms of heart failure could be easily masked by signs and symptoms of normal pregnancy. For example, peripheral edema, jugular vein distention, mild tachycardia, shortness of breath, and an S3 heart sound can be normal findings in pregnancy and can mask the suspicion of a cardiac disease.

The evaluation of a pregnant patient with shortness of breath can begin with a simple chest x-ray and an EKG looking for things such as cardiomegaly or arrhythmias. A bedside echocardiogram can also be a useful tool and can easily screen for pericardial effusion or hypodynamic myocardium. B-type natriuretic peptide (BNP) levels are an especially good screening tool for ruling out heart failure in the pregnant patient who presents with shortness of breath. Resnik et al. (2005) found that in normal pregnancies, mean BNP levels remain <20 pg/nL throughout gestation and suggest that levels <20 effectively rule out heart failure as a cause of symptoms. Those patients with elevated BNPs should be evaluated further with echocardiography looking for cardiac chamber dilation, decreased ejection fraction, and thrombus formation in the cardiac chambers. Even in patients in whom pulmonary embolism is diagnosed, a BNP level may be helpful as cardiomyopathy with thrombus formation can lead to thromboembolic phenomena such as pulmonary embolus, stroke, or limb and mesenteric ischemia.

The bottom line is to use caution when quickly attributing shortness of breath in a pregnant patient to the pregnancy. The normal physiology of the pregnant patient can mask a cardiac disease, so have a low threshold to screen these patients for heart failure as cardiomyopathy can be easily missed.

TAKE HOME POINTS

- Mild dyspnea in pregnancy can be normal but can also hide a serious underlying pathology.
- The normal physiologic changes of pregnancy can mimic those of heart failure.
- A BNP level is a simple and effective method to screen for heart failure due to peripartum cardiomyopathy.

SUGGESTED READINGS

Resnik JL, Hong C, Resnik R, et al. Evaluation of B-type natriuretic peptide (BNP) levels in normal and preeclamptic women. *Am J Obstet Gynecol.* 2005;193(2):450–454.
Sliwa K, Fett J, Elkayam U. Peripartum cardiomyopathy. *Lancet.* 2006;368(9536):687–693.

196

KNOW THE INDICATIONS AND CONTRAINDICATIONS FOR METHOTREXATE THERAPY IN ECTOPIC PREGNANCY

ASHLEIGH HEGEDUS, MD

Ectopic pregnancy is not an infrequent emergency department (ED) diagnosis, with reports that it may be present in up to 18% of women with ED chief complaints of first-trimester vaginal bleeding, abdominal pain, or both. Ectopic pregnancy can cause significant morbidity and mortality if not treated appropriately and is still the primary cause of maternal death in the first trimester. Medical management of ectopic pregnancy with methotrexate is increasingly more common in practice and can be safe and highly efficacious in the proper setting. As a result, it may be tempting to treat all ectopic pregnancies with methotrexate instead of calling a late-night gynecologic or surgical consult; however, not all patients are good candidates for methotrexate. Individual patient factors such as hemodynamic stability and patient medical problems must be taken into consideration prior to using methotrexate.

Hemodynamic stability must be the first consideration when deciding appropriate treatment for your ectopic pregnancy patient. A patient who is in shock, has persistent tachycardia or orthostatic hypotension despite resuscitation, or who has a rigid abdomen is concerning for a ruptured ectopic, and immediate surgical consultation is indicated. In patients who are hemodynamically stable, factors leading to failure of methotrexate therapy have been carefully described. The most common dosing of methotrexate for ectopic pregnancy is a single intramuscular dose of 50 mg/m^2 of body surface area, as calculated on the day that the patient receives the dose of methotrexate. One 1999 study evaluated patient clinical factors and the efficacy of this dose of methotrexate in hemodynamically stable patients. Specifically, factors such as serum concentrations of human chorionic gonadotropin (hCG) and progesterone, size and volume of the mass, fetal cardiac activity, and the presence of free fluid were investigated. It was concluded that the most important predictive factor for failure of treatment with methotrexate was a high hCG level. Although no guidelines have been set forth, in this study of 350 ectopic pregnancies, 94% with an initial hCG of <10,000 mIU were successfully treated with methotrexate. The data suggest that hCG level may be used to screen out patients in whom methotrexate may not be successful. Other studies have since shown that low initial levels of progesterone and the absence of cardiac activity may also be factors suggesting potential successful treatment of an ectopic pregnancy with methotrexate.

Methotrexate acts through inhibiting DNA synthesis and repair and cell regulation. It acts systemically at the sites of most rapid division and growth, including trophoblastic cells, bone marrow, buccal and intestinal mucosa, and respiratory mucosa. As a result, methotrexate use can be dangerous in women with known blood dyscrasias such as bone marrow hypoplasia, leukopenia, thrombocytopenia, or gastrointestinal or pulmonary disease. Furthermore, methotrexate is hepatotoxic and renally cleared, and it should not be used in patients with liver or renal disease. Prior to the use of methotrexate, it is recommended that creatinine, liver transaminases, and a complete blood count are used as a screening for these medical problems and that these levels be rechecked approximately 1 week after the treatment to assess for signs of toxicity secondary to methotrexate. Women who are breast-feeding should also not be given methotrexate because it is passed into breastmilk.

Lastly, patients who will undergo medical management of ectopic pregnancy with methotrexate must also be considered to be reliable patients with good follow-up plans. It is imperative to have close follow-up to monitor for signs of hemodynamic instability or for treatment failure. Furthermore, a known complication of methotrexate for tubal pregnancies is abdominal pain, which is thought to be possibly due to the tubal abortion. If a patient's pain does not resolve with over-the-counter analgesics, the patient needs to be reevaluated for potential surgical treatment.

The key to using methotrexate therapy in ectopic pregnancies is remembering that methotrexate is not indicated in all patients. It should not be considered in patients who are hemodynamically unstable, have multiple medical problems or are breast-feeding, or do not have a good follow-up. In patients with high initial hCG levels, it may be considered, but data have indicated that there is a higher failure rate, and it may be prudent to consider consultation for surgical management in this case.

SUGGESTED READINGS

American College of Obstetricians and Gynecologists. ACOG Practice Bulletin No. 94: Medical management of ectopic pregnancy. *Obstet Gynecol.* 2008;111(6):1479–1485.

Lipscomb GH, McCord ML, Stovall TG, et al. Predictors of success of methotrexate treatment in women with tubal ectopic pregnancies. *N Engl J Med.* 1999;341:1974–1978.

Lipscomb GH, Stovall TG, Ling FW. Nonsurgical treatment of ectopic pregnancy. *N Engl J Med.* 2000;343(18):1325–1329.

Mol F, Mol BW, Ankum WM, et al. Current evidence on surgery, systemic methotrexate and expectant management in the treatment of tubal ectopic pregnancy: A systematic review and meta-analysis. *Hum Reprod Update.* 2008;14(4):309–319.

Nama V, Manyonda I. Tubal ectopic pregnancy: Diagnosis and management. *Arch Gynecol Obstet.* 2009;279(4):443–453.

197

KNOW THE COMPLICATIONS OF INFERTILITY TREATMENT

ERINE OI MING FONG, MD

With the increasing prevalence of assisted reproductive therapies (ARTs), it is important to recognize complications that occur more frequently than in naturally conceived pregnancies. Two major complications to be aware of in ART pregnancies include ovarian hyperstimulation and heterotopic pregnancies.

Ovarian hyperstimulation syndrome (OHSS) is a potentially life-threatening complication of ART. OHSS occurs when ovarian stimulation surpasses the goal, resulting in an excessively large number of follicles (generally >20). The use of gonadotropins in ART causes the majority of cases, though it can also occur with the use of clomiphene. The prevalence of clinically significant OHSS is estimated to be 0.5% to 5% of medically stimulated ovarian cycles. Presenting symptoms of OHSS include abdominal pain, distention, malaise, nausea, vomiting, constipation/diarrhea, dark urine, dyspnea, edema, and altered mental status. Symptoms result from hypertrophic ovaries and subsequent overproduction of ovarian hormones and vasoactive substances such as VEGF, cytokines, and angiotensin. Ovaries may enlarge to >12 cm and have a high risk of rupture, hemorrhage, and torsion. Increased vasoactive substances cause increased vascular permeability and may lead to ascites, hydrothorax, and/or edema. This fluid accumulation depletes intravascular volume by third spacing, resulting in multiorgan failure in the most severe cases.

Physical examination of patients with OHSS may reveal increased abdominal girth, abdominal tenderness, and edema. Abdominal/pelvic ultrasound (US) is indicated in women who present to the emergency department (ED) with any of the symptoms above and a history of ART. In patients with OHSS the US will likely show enlarged ovaries measuring 5 to 12 cm, with multiple follicular cysts and ascites. US will also assist in evaluating for hemorrhage and ovarian torsion. If clinical suspicion is high after a nondiagnostic US, a CT may provide additional information; however, the risk of radiation should be considered if fertilization has occurred. A basic metabolic panel should also be obtained to evaluate for hyponatremia and renal impairment caused by the intravascular volume depletion that these patients experience. For patients with dyspnea, pulmonary manifestations of severe OHSS such as pneumonia, pulmonary embolism (PE), hydrothorax, atelectasis, and acute respiratory distress syndrome (ARDS) should be suspected and a chest x-ray should be obtained. ARDS in OHSS is rare but has a high mortality rate if not recognized and managed appropriately. A high index of suspicion should be maintained for PE, because of the hypercoagulable state associated with OHSS. Ten percent of patients with OHSS will have a thrombotic event.

In general, treatment of OHSS is supportive. With mild OHSS, patients have abdominal pain, nausea, and enlarged ovaries. Close follow-up with Ob/Gyn is appropriate for these patients. In moderate OHSS, patients will also have vomiting and/or diarrhea as well as ascites indicated on US. Severe OHSS will additionally show clinical evidence of ascites, hydrothorax, hemoconcentration, coagulopathy, renal dysfunction, hepatic dysfunction, and/or thromboembolism. Hospital admission is necessary for moderate to severe OHSS. Liver function test (LFTs), basic metabolic panel (BMP), complete blood count (CBC), and coagulation should be monitored. Medical therapy is aimed at maintaining effective circulating volume by shifting fluid back into the intravascular space. Due to the risk of acute intra-abdominal hemorrhage, pelvic exam should be avoided in moderate to severe OHSS. Patients diagnosed with OHSS should be managed in consultation with an obstetrician or reproductive medicine specialist.

Another potentially life-threatening complication of ART is ectopic pregnancy and in particular heterotopic pregnancy. A heterotopic pregnancy is one in which gestation occurs at two or more implantation sites with at least one being extrauterine. A heterotopic pregnancy occurs in 1 in 30,000 spontaneous pregnancies, but is increased to 1 in 100 pregnancies conceived by ART. With in vitro fertilization specifically, embryo placement near the tubal ostia, excessive force or volume during embryo transfer, and transfer of multiple embryos may contribute to the increased risk of heterotopic pregnancies. Early diagnosis is imperative but can be challenging. Case series reveal that patients with heterotopic pregnancies often present with hypovolemic shock due to tubal rupture. To avoid missing this life-threatening condition in the ED, extrauterine pregnancies (EUPs) should still be ruled out after recognizing an intrauterine pregnancy. A comprehensive US must be obtained to evaluate for the presence of an EUP or findings such as free fluid, adnexal mass, and pelvic mass which are highly suggestive of an EUP. Obstetrical consultation should be obtained early in the evaluation of any patient suspected of having an EUP and certainly if a heterotopic pregnancy is diagnosed, as the most common method of management is surgical.

With the increasing availability and use of ART, it is important to be familiar with its possible complications. While common complications of pregnancy must still be considered in women using ART who present to the ED, physicians should also maintain a high level of suspicion for OHSS and heterotopic pregnancies.

SUGGESTED READINGS

Braude P, Rowell P. Assisted conception. III–problems with assisted conception. *Br Med J.* 2003; 327(7420):920–923.

Budev MM, Arroliga AC, Falcone T. Ovarian hyperstimulation syndrome. *Crit Care Med.* 2005;33(10 Suppl):S301–S306.

Childs AJ, Royek AB, Leigh TB, et al. Triplet heterotopic pregnancy after gonadotropin stimu-
lation and intrauterine insemination diagnosed at laparoscopy: A case report. *South Med
J.* 2005;98(8):833–835.
Dumesic DA, Damario MA, Session DR. Interstitial heterotopic pregnancy in a woman
conceiving by in vitro fertilization after bilateral salpingectomy. *Mayo Clin Proc.*
2001;76(1):90–92.
Mukhopadhaya N, Arulkumaran S. Reproductive outcomes after in-vitro fertilization. *Curr
Opin Obstet Gynecol.* 2007;19(2):113–119.

198

BEWARE OF POSTPARTUM HEADACHES

CHANDLER H. HILL, MD

Headache is a common complaint in the postpartum period. Up to 39% of postpartum women reported headache symptoms in the month following delivery. In women with known headache disorders, symptoms often improve during pregnancy and worsen after delivery, likely secondary to the effect of estrogen on increasing pain tolerance. The patient with postpartum headache presents a challenge to the emergency physician. While the etiology of head-ache in many of these patients may be benign, there are at least two conditions that are life threatening and difficult to differentiate from less serious ones. In a recent study of 381 patients with postpartum headache, the most com-mon diagnoses were tension (38%), migranous (26%), musculoskeletal (11%), and migraine (9%). However, central venous sinus thrombosis (CVST) and late-onset eclampsia are rare but serious causes of headache in the postpartum women that should be considered by the emergency physician.

CVST is the spontaneous thrombosis and occlusion of cerebral sinuses. Postpartum women are at higher risk for this disease due to hypercoaguability. CVST is a rare disorder, with an incidence of about 0.6 per 100,000 per year or 1 in 3,000 pregnancies. Headache is the usual presenting symptom and can occur acutely in the first hours to days after delivery or up to 6 weeks post-partum. Symptoms that should raise suspicion of venous thrombosis include worsening of pain with sitting up, throbbing pain, nausea and vomiting, leth-argy, and focal neurologic symptoms.

Unfortunately, a computed tomography (CT) is not sufficient to rule out venous sinus thrombosis. While head CT may show abnormalities including intracranial hemorrhage (ICH) or cerebral infarction, in a recent retrospective review 7 of 22 head CTs in patients with this disease were completely normal. The most sensitive diagnostic studies for the postpartum patient who has symptoms consistent with CVST are MRA and MRV. Clearly, not all women who have a headache after pregnancy need this expensive and time-consuming workup. However, if the patient has progressing headaches, a reduced level of consciousness, any focal neuro signs, seizures, papilledema, or concerning findings on head CT (ICH or ischemia), the MRA and MRV should be obtained. The treatment for CVST, while controversial, has traditionally been heparin initially and anticoagulation with coumadin for up to 6 months.

A second dangerous and easy to overlook cause of headache in the postpartum period is late-onset preeclampsia. Preeclampsia is a disease that results in widespread vasospasm leading to the classic findings of hypertension, peripheral edema, and proteinuria. Cerebral vasospasm can present with headache and progress to eclamptic seizures, coma, and death. Eclampsia is responsible for 15% of maternal mortality. Traditionally, eclampsia is seen as a disease of pregnancy and the treatment is delivery of the fetus. However, in a recent review of 89 cases of ecclampsia, over 30% developed in the postpartum period. Even more concerning is that only 5 of these 29 cases had been previously diagnosed during pregnancy with preeclampsia. Most postpartum preeclampsia presents within 48 h of delivery, though it can occur up to 4 weeks later.

Classic symptoms of cerebral vasospasm in preeclampisia are a severe headache with nausea and visual changes. This can progress to altered mental status and ultimately seizure. Classic signs of preeclampsia may be present, including blood pressure over 140/90, proteinuria, and peripheral edema. Unfortunately, some women present with headache and no other signs of preeclampisa. Again, as with sinus venous thrombosis, initial head CT may be normal. MRI may show findings consistent with eclampsia and is the test of choice to rule out the disease when suspicion is high enough. If a patient with postpartum headache has other signs of preeclampsia, if MRI findings are consistent with preeclampsia, or if you are highly suspicious of preeclampsia even without these findings, the patient should be started on magnesium in consultation with an obstetrician.

Headache is a common postpartum complaint. The large majority of patients need no further treatment other than pain control and reassurance. However, remember these points to avoid misdiagnosis of a life-threatening headache.

TAKE HOME POINTS

- Consider preeclampsia/eclampsia or CVST in any postpartum patient with
  - Severe or worsening headaches
  - Visual disturbances
  - Seizures

- Papilledema
- Altered mental status
- Abnormal neurologic exam
- Workup should minimally include a urine analysis (UA) and blood pressure measurement to evaluate for preeclampsia.
- A normal head CT is not sufficient to rule out these serious processes.
- MRI is the study of choice to look for signs of eclampsia and CVST.

SUGGESTED READINGS

Fink JN, Mcauley DL. Cerebral venous sinus thrombosis: A diagnostic challenge. *Intern Med J*. 2001;31:384–390.

Dziewas R, Stogbauer F, Freund M, et al. Late onset postpartum eclampsia: A rare and difficult diagnosis. *J Neurol*. 2002;249:1287–1291.

Chames MC, Livingston JC, Ivester TS, et al. Late postpartum eclampsia: A preventable disease? *Am J Obstet Gynecol*. 2002;186(6):1174–1177.

Goldszmidt E, Kern R, Chaput A, et al. The incidence and etiology of postpartum headaches: A prospective cohort study. *Can J Anesth*. 2005;52(9):971–977.

199

DO NOT FORGET TO CONSIDER NONOBSTETRIC CAUSES OF ABDOMINAL SYMPTOMS IN A PREGNANT PATIENT

COLLEEN C. KNIFFIN, MD

Pregnant women commonly present to the emergency department complaining of abdominal pain, nausea, or vomiting. Although these symptoms are often related to the pregnancy, clinicians must remember to also consider the common nonobstetric causes. Many of these conditions are relatively benign (e.g., round ligament pain, constipation, and gaseous distension). However, several nonobstetric causes of abdominal symptoms may be life threatening to the mother and fetus. Of the estimated 6 million pregnancies in the United States each year, between 0.2% and 1.0% will be complicated by a nonobstetric condition, requiring urgent or even surgical intervention, and most of these present as abdominal pain, nausea, or vomiting. Early suspicion for a nonobstetric etiology, specifically appendicitis, cholecystitis, bowel obstruction, and pancreatitis, can help to avert unnecessary maternal morbidity and fetal loss.

Appendicitis is the most common nonobstetric surgical emergency in pregnant patients. The incidence is the same as in the nonpregnant population, but the rate of perforation is significantly higher (43% vs. 4% to 19% in the nonobstetric population). This increase may reflect delay in diagnosis or hesitancy to operate on a pregnant woman. There are a few points to remember when considering whether a woman with abdominal symptoms may have appendicitis. First, remember that appendicitis occurs with equal frequency in each trimester. Second, the appendix may be progressively displaced both cephalad and laterally as the uterus expands. By 24-week gestation, the appendix is usually just superior to the right iliac crest, and late in the pregnancy, it may be closer to the gallbladder than to McBurney point. Keep in mind, however, that this commonly held belief has been challenged by a recent prospective study that found that the location of the appendix changed in only 23% of pregnant patients. Regardless, the most common and reliable symptom of appendicitis in the pregnant patient remains right lower quadrant pain. Third, it is important to understand that the growing uterus displaces the abdominal wall and peritoneum away from the abdominal viscera. This results in difficulty localizing the pain on exam, a decrease in the somatic sensation of pain, and often results in delayed development of peritoneal signs. On the other hand, separation of the peritoneum from the appendix may, in some cases, facilitate diffuse peritonitis as the omentum is unable to wall off the inflamed appendix before it perforates. Finally, remember that pregnant patients with appendicitis may not develop fever, leukocytosis, or tachycardia. This blunted inflammatory response is thought to be due to elevated maternal levels of pregnancy-related steroids. -

Cholecystitis is the second most common surgical condition in pregnant patients. The clinical presentation of cholecystitis is almost identical in pregnant and nonpregnant women, with the exception of Murphy sign which is less common in pregnant women. Keep in mind that the usual differential diagnosis for right upper quadrant pain should be expanded in the pregnant patient to also include acute fatty liver of pregnancy, HELLP syndrome, preeclampsia, and acute appendicitis. Lab values are less indicative in pregnant women with cholecystitis. Elevated direct bilirubin and transaminase levels may support the diagnosis just as in the nonpregnant patient. However, serum alkaline phosphatase and leukocyte counts are less helpful as they are commonly increased during pregnancy.

Bowel obstruction is the third most common indication for nonobstetric laparotomy during pregnancy. Approximately 60% to 70% of cases are caused by adhesions, but, unlike the general population, 25% are the result of volvulus. Bowel obstruction incidence increases as the pregnancy progresses with most cases occurring in the third trimester. As the uterus, cervix, and adnexa share the same visceral innervation as the lower ileum, sigmoid colon, and rectum, distinguishing between pain of gynecologic origin and that of gastrointestinal origin is quite difficult. However, the typical symptoms of intestinal obstruction are unchanged in the pregnant woman and include crampy abdominal pain, obstipation, and nausea/vomiting. Unfortunately, the mortality rate of intestinal obstruction is much higher during pregnancy than in the general population.

Acute pancreatitis occurs most commonly late in the third trimester or in the early postpartum period and in most cases is caused by cholelithiasis. Management is usually nonoperative and is similar to management of any other patient with pancreatitis. The typical symptoms are as in nonpregnant women and include severe epigastric pain, nausea, vomiting, and occasionally fever. Elevation in serum lipase is a reliable diagnostic test.

In summary, when evaluating a pregnant patient remember that not all abdominal symptoms are obstetric in origin. Do not forget that anatomic and physiologic changes of pregnancy can affect both clinical presentation as well as laboratory test results. If you remember these points and maintain a high index of suspicion for serious nonobstetric causes of abdominal symptoms, you are more likely to make the right diagnosis and offer the best treatment for the mother and the fetus.

SUGGESTED READINGS

Dietrich CS, Hill CC, Hueman M. Surgical diseases presenting in pregnancy. *Surg Clin North Am.* 2008;88(20):7–8.
Hodjati H, Kazerooni T. Location of the appendix in the gravid patient: A re-evaluation of the established concept. *Int J Gynaecol Obstet.* 2003;81(3):245–247.
Kilpatrick CC, Monga M. Approach to the acute abdomen in pregnancy. *Obstet Gynecol Clin North Am.* 2007;33:389–402.
Parangi S, Levine D, Henry A, et al. Surgical gastrointestinal disorders during pregnancy. *Am J Surg.* 2007;193(2):223–32.

200

OVARIAN TORSION: TIPS TO MAKE THIS TOUGH DIAGNOSIS

KELLY M. MILKUS, MD

Ovarian torsion can be a challenging diagnosis to make. It is the fifth most common gynecologic emergency, comprising 2.7% of all gynecologic emergencies. It has subtle clinical features which are common in many diseases of the lower abdomen and pelvis. In addition, the rare incidence of this condition makes designing good clinical studies difficult, so evidence-based medicine is dependent on mostly retrospective and prospective observational studies. One review of ovarian torsion in the ED found that the diagnosis was missed almost half the time at the initial presentation.

Missed or delayed diagnosis of ovarian torsion can affect future fertility of the patient. Currently, the majority of patients undergo detorsion during laparoscopy or laparotomy, whereas in the past the majority of cases were treated with oophorectomy. Though conservative treatment has helped many women have preserved ovarian function, the more delayed the diagnosis the more likely the ovary is going to be necrotic and unsalvageable.

Multiple studies have shown that providers have low clinical suspicion for adnexal torsion. Ovarian torsion commonly does not present with sudden, severe, unilateral abdominal pain, as is classically described, so is often not considered in the differential diagnosis in women with abdominal pain. The diagnosis most likely to be mistaken for torsion is that of ovarian cyst or mass, appendicitis, tubo-ovarian abscess, or ectopic pregnancy.

While many patients will not have risk factors for ovarian torsion, there are several recognized risk factors associated with torsion that should raise clinical suspicion. The history of ovarian cysts, tubal ligation, ovarian hyperstimulation syndrome, polycystic ovarian syndrome, prior pelvic surgery, history of pelvic inflammatory disease (PID), and pregnancy are considered classic risk factors. About one quarter of patients with torsion are pregnant. The majority of patients with torsion are adult women of child-bearing age, though about 15% present after menopause and 15% present under the age of 20. Most cases present within 3 days of the onset of symptoms; however, women, presumed to have had intermittent torsion, have presented with chronic pelvic pain as much as 2 years later.

There are several features you will or will not see in torsion. Almost all torsion presents with abdominal pain. Most will present with lateralizing pain, but there are cases of contralateral pain, midline pain, flank pain, and epigastric pain. There may be a slight predominance of right-sided lesions. Nausea and vomiting are associated in many of the cases. Fever is not common in most patients. The presence of a palpable mass is highly variable, ranging from 40% to 80% in studies depending on the patient population. Most studies have shown that enlarged adnexae are almost always found in torsion. The range of ovarian measurements found in cases of torsion has been quite varied, from normal to thirty centimeters. However, studies have shown that 80% to 90% of torsed ovaries measured >5 cm.

Because the history and physical exam are so variable, imaging is essential to make the diagnosis. A pelvic ultrasound is typically the initial study. The presence of blood flow is variable in torsion and cannot be used to reliably exclude the diagnosis. Signs on pelvic ultrasound suggestive of torsion include an enlarged, edematous ovary and potentially, the presence of a cyst or mass that would predispose the ovary to torsion. CT and MRI can also be used to make the diagnosis. Features on CT and MRI suggestive of torsion again include enlargement and edema of the ovary, the presence of a mass, and deviation of the uterus to the side of the torsion.

The diagnosis of ovarian torsion requires a recognition of the risk factors, an appreciation of the variable presentation, and an understanding of the features seen on imaging.

SUGGESTED READINGS

Argenta PA, Yeagley TJ, Ott G, et al. Torsion of the uterine adnexa: Pathologic correlations and current management trends. *J Reprod Med*. 2000;45:831–836.

Houry D, Abbott JT. Ovarian torsion: A fifteen year review. *Ann Emerg Med*. 2001;38: 156–159.

Lee CH, Raman S, Sivanesaratnam V. Torsion of ovarian tumors: A clinicopathologic study. *Int J Gyn Obst*. 1989;28:21–25.

201

REMEMBER THAT ECLAMPSIA CAN OCCUR POSTPARTUM AND IN WOMEN WITH NO PRIOR DIAGNOSIS OF PREECLAMPSIA

JOHANNA C. MOORE, MD

The emergency physician is likely to be one of the first providers taking care of an actively seizing or postictal patient. Eclampsia is an uncommon but important cause of seizures that should always be considered in a woman of childbearing age getting first-time seizures. The underlying pathophysiology, treatment, and disposition of these patients are different than other seizure patients.

Hypertensive disorders occur in approximately 5% to 8% of pregnancies and contribute significantly to maternal and neonatal morbidity and mortality. Hypertensive disorders are, in fact, the second leading cause of maternal mortality in the United States.

Preeclampsia is traditionally defined as blood pressure ≥140 systolic and 90 diastolic with proteinuria in a previously normotensive female >20 weeks gestation. Proteinuria is defined as urinary excretion of >0.3 g protein in a 24-h specimen. This usually correlates with >30 mg/dL or >1+ reading on dipstick in a random urine specimen. Eclampsia is traditionally defined as new-onset seizures that cannot be attributed to other causes in a woman with preeclampsia.

In contrast to the definitions above, recent studies and reviews have illustrated that the diagnosis of preeclampsia is often not present in new-onset eclampsia. Hypertension or proteinuria is present in a majority of cases, ranging from 50% to 90%, but not all. Seizures can be the first manifestation of preeclampsia in up to 75% of cases. However, in retrospect, prodromal symptoms are present in a majority of these patients who initially present with a seizure. Most patients will describe having experienced headache with fewer patients describing nausea and vomiting, epigastric or right upper quadrant pain, or vision changes such as flashing lights, blurred vision, or scotoma. A minority of women have abnormal laboratory values such as elevated liver enzymes, elevated LDH, or thrombocytopenia, making the diagnosis more difficult.

Although in retrospect, a majority of patients who had prodromal symptoms prior to the onset of seizure did not think that their symptoms were worthy of seeking medical attention. More troubling is when the minority of patients did seek medical attention in the emergency department; preeclampsia was not considered as a diagnosis, even with concurrent hypertension. These findings suggest a need for emphasizing signs and symptoms of preeclampsia to patients in the antepartum and postpartum periods. It also calls for greater awareness on the part of the emergency physician to consider the diagnosis of preeclampsia in the pregnant and postpartum patient.

The overall incidence of eclampsia is declining. However, the incidence of postpartum eclampsia is relatively rising, that is, not declining as fast as antepartum and peripartum eclampsia. A British study done by Leitch et al. looking at 1,259 cases of eclampsia over a 60-year period documented a >90% decline in eclampsia with a relative increase in postpartum eclampsia. The incidence of postpartum eclampsia remained consistent in the last two decades of the study at 40% to 50% of all cases of eclampsia. Matthys et al. analyzed 3,988 cases of preeclampsia and discovered that 5.7% of them developed preeclampsia in the postpartum period. Of those, 15.9% also developed eclampsia. This study was also notable for the number of patients who were readmitted for hypertension or preeclampsia, with approximately 70% readmitted.

Of particular interest to the emergency provider is late postpartum eclampsia, or eclampsia occurring postpartum >48 h after delivery but <4 weeks after delivery. This entity is likely to present to the emergency department and may not be immediately apparent to the emergency provider, as the patient may not be able to provide a history and is not visibly gravid. The incidence of late postpartum eclampsia is also relatively increasing. In a review of 334 cases of eclampsia by Lubarsky et al., late postpartum eclampsia made up to 56% of their postpartum cases and 16% of all eclampsia cases. The timing of seizure presentation ranged from 3 to 24 days, and the mean was 6 days after delivery. Chames et al. found that one third of eclamptic patients they studied had postpartum eclampsia, 79% of whom had late postpartum eclampsia. These studies highlight that a significant percentage of patients with eclampsia will present to the ED after being discharged home with their babies. Most patients that present with late postpartum preeclampsia did not have elevated blood pressures during pregnancy.

Although there are traditional definitions of preeclampsia and eclampsia, it is important to remember that both occur as a spectrum of disease that is not fully understood. Eclampsia can occur in the absence of hypertension and proteinuria and in the postpartum period. The emergency provider must maintain a high index of suspicion in the postpartum period and also in pregnant women with seemingly benign or vague complaints.

SUGGESTED READINGS

Chames MC, Livingston JC, Ivester TS, et al. Late postpartum eclampsia: A preventable disease? *Am J Obstet Gynecol.* 2002;186:1174–1177.
Knight M, UKOSS. Eclampsia in the United Kingdom 2005. *BJOG.* 2007;114:1072–1078.
Leitch CR, Cameron AD, Walker JJ. The changing pattern of eclampsia of a 60 yr period. *BJOG.* 1997;104:917–922.
Lubarsky SL, Barton JR, Friedman SA, et al. Late postpartum eclampsia revisited. *Obstet Gynecol.* 1994;83:502–505.
Matthys LA, Coppage KH, Lambers DS, et al. Delayed postpartum preeclampsia: An experience of 151 cases. *Am J Obstet Gynecol.* 2004;190:1464–1466.
[No authors listed]. Report of the National High Blood Pressure Education Program Working Group on high blood pressure in pregnancy. *Am J Obstet Gynecol.* 2000;183:S1–S22.

202

DO NOT FOREGO A PELVIC ULTRASOUND IN PATIENTS WITH A CLINICAL SUSPICION FOR ECTOPIC PREGNANCY BUT A LOW β-HCG

JEREMY OLSEN, MD AND JOHN GULLETT, MD

Ectopic pregnancy (EP) is a critical diagnosis in the emergency department (ED), and yet it is still frequently misdiagnosed by emergency physicians. To complicate matters, the rate of occurrence per pregnancy is increasing. From 1970 to 1992, the EP rate nearly quadrupled climbing from 0.5% to 1.97%. The good news is that mortality has dropped by 90%; nevertheless, EP remains the leading cause of first-trimester pregnancy-related death and is implicated in up to 13% of all pregnancy-related deaths. This is a high-risk diagnosis that emergency physicians still frequently misdiagnose in the initial ED visit.

Unfortunately, a delay in EP diagnosis results in frequent patient morbidity and is one of the leading causes of malpractice lawsuits in emergency medicine. Therefore, it is essential that emergency physicians have a thorough understanding of the tools at their disposal to rule in or rule out this critical diagnosis. Serum β-hCG and pelvic ultrasound are useful for making this diagnosis, yet it is important to understand the proper use of these modalities as well as their limitations.

The serum β-hCG level is a measurement of the beta unit of human chorionic gonadotropin produced in pregnancy. Its measurement is standardized by the International Reference Preparation and it is measured in mIU/mL. This laboratory marker is useful in that it rises at a predictable rate in normal pregnancy. The serum level should increase by 1.5 to 2.0, or nearly double, every 48 until it reaches about 100,000 in which case the doubling rate slows down a bit. Ultimately, a peak of nearly 290,000 mIU/mL is reached usually around 9 to 12 weeks. An abnormally slow rise indicates an abnormal pregnancy, but a normal rise does not rule out an abnormality. Thus, single measurements of β-hCG are less useful; it is the pattern of increase that aids the clinician.

The first common misconception about diagnosing EP is that a very low β-hCG level rules out EP. Kaplan et al. in 1997 found that 40% of EPs had a serum β-hCG <1,000 mIU/mL. Furthermore, they found that this group had a fourfold higher relative risk for EP compared to those with a β-hCG level >1,000 mIU/mL. Also in 1997, Dart et al. found that over 50% of the EPs detected by ultrasound in their study had β-hCG levels below 500 mIU/mL. Even more striking is the finding of Counselman et al. in 1998 that 39% of the ruptured EPs in their study had β-hCG levels <1,000 mIU/mL.

A second misconception is that pelvic ultrasound is not beneficial in patients with a β-hCG level below 1,000 mIU/mL. A serum β-hCG level >1,000 mIU/mL is often described as the "discriminatory zone" in pelvic ultrasound for EP. This refers to the level above which an intrauterine pregnancy (IUP) should *always* be visualized by transvaginal ultrasonography. Therefore, a patient with a β-hCG level >1,000 mIU/mL and no IUP on ultrasound examination is presumed to have an EP.

However, a substantial number of EPs will be missed if the ultrasound exam is not done on patients with β-hCG levels below 1,000 mIU/mL. Counselman's study showed that 89% of the EPs with β-hCG level <1,000 mIU/mL had findings of EP on ultrasound that prompted obstetric consultation. Dart et al. found that 39% of EPs with β-hCG level <1,000 mIU/mL were detectable on ultrasound. Fleisher et al. found that there were suggestive or diagnostic findings in all of 50 patients studied with confirmed EP. There are numerous other studies confirming the benefit of pelvic sonography at any β-hCG level if suspicion for an EP is present. The abnormally slow rise of the serum β-hCG level in the setting of an EP means that there may be a visible EP or suggestive abnormality with a relatively low β-hCG.

The role of the discriminatory β-hCG level of 1,000 mIU/mL is now considered primarily for patients with indeterminant transvaginal ultrasounds. If a patient has an ultrasound that is indeterminant, a β-hCG level <1,000 mIU/mL, and is clinically stable and well appearing, then it is reasonable to discharge her with ectopic precautions and follow-up. If the serum β-hCG level is >1,000 mIU/mL, but the ultrasound is indeterminant, then an obstetric or gynecologic consult is warranted for the patient, and possibly an admission for observation. This may depend on the findings on ultrasound and the comfort level of the radiologist interpreting it. Bedside transvaginal ultrasound performed by an emergency physician has been well validated in the emergency medicine literature; however, for this discussion, we refer only to data from "formal" comprehensive transvaginal pelvic sonography performed and interpreted by radiology staff.

There is an abundance of data on these issues in both emergency medicine and obstetric or gynecologic literature, and certain things have been made clear. First, a low β-hCG level does not rule out EP and, in fact, may increase the patient's risk of having an EP. Second, pelvic ultrasound is beneficial at any β-hCG if EP is suspected.

SUGGESTED READINGS

Brennan DF. Ectopic pregnancy–part I: Clinical and laboratory diagnosis. *Acad Emerg Med*. 1995;2:1081–1089.

Counselman FL, Shaar GS, Heller RA, et al. Quantitative β-hCG levels less than 1000 mIU/ml in patients with ectopic pregnancy: Pelvic ultrasound still useful. *J Emerg Med*. 1998;16(5):699–703.

Dart RG, Kaplan B, Cox C. Transvaginal ultrasound in patients with low β-human chorionic gonadotropin values: How often is the study diagnostic? *Ann Emerg Med*. 1997;30: 135–140.

Fleisher A, Pennell R, Mckee M. Ectopic pregnancy: Features at transvaginal sonography. *Radiology*. 1990;174:375–387.

Fylstra DL. Tubal pregnancy: A review of current diagnosis and treatment. *Obstet Gynecol Surv*. 1999;54:138–146.

Kaplan BC, Dart RG, Moskos M, et al. Ectopic pregnancy: Prospective study with improved diagnostic accuracy. *Ann Emerg Med*. 1996;28:10–17.

Pisarska MD, Carson SA, Buster JE. Ectopic pregnancy. *Lancet*. 1998;351:1115–1120.

203

Perimortem Cesarean Section: The Clock Is Ticking

Francis J. O'Connell, MD

Cesarean sections date back to ancient civilization and were initially intended as a postmortem means of separating the fetus from the mother for burial purposes. The procedure was eventually adopted for the purpose of delivering a fetus from a moribund mother. The term "perimortem cesarean section" was introduced in a 1986 publication and used to describe cesarean sections performed during maternal cardiopulmonary resuscitation.

The primary goal in the resuscitation of the pregnant woman is to treat the mother, and thereby treat the fetus, and avoid emergent circumstances all together. However, pregnant patients present, on occasion, to emergency departments in extremis. In those circumstances, it is critical to understand the indications and the proper technique to perform a perimortem cesarean section which may be lifesaving for the fetus and beneficial for the mother.

Cardiovascular and respiratory physiologies in late pregnancy are different than that of nongravid and early pregnancy patients. Reduced venous return and distal aortic flow caused by aortocaval compression by the uterus occurs at 20 weeks gestation. A gravid uterus demands an increased amount of blood flow and causes a reduction in functional residual lung capacity. These factors are important in resuscitation in late pregnancy warranting timely control of the airway, movement of the uterus to a left lateral position (either by adjusting the position of the patient or manual displacement of the uterus), and the possibility of early cesarean delivery. All efforts should be made to position the patient in the appropriate position to facilitate cardiopulmonary resuscitation recognizing that the supine position is, by far, the most effective way to provide chest compressions.

The indications for performing a perimortem cesarean section are based on a small number (totaling hundreds) of reported cases in the medical literature. Recognizing that failures at perimortem cesarean sections may be underreported, there is currently no evidence to suggest that outcomes are worsened with perimortem cesarean section.

The most important factors to consider in performing a perimortem cesarean section are the timing of the procedure and the gestational age of the fetus. Based on retrospective data, the best outcomes (survival with no neurologic deficits) of perimortem cesarean section occurred within 5 min of maternal cardiac arrest. Therefore, the current recommendation is to perform a cesarean section if no pulse can be obtained at minute 4 of cardiopulmonary resuscitation. It should also be noted that successful delivery has occurred as late as 22 min beyond cardiac arrest, making cesarean section a viable option should patients present beyond the 5th min of cardiac arrest. Perimortem cesarean section should only be attempted on a fetus ≥24 weeks in gestational age. Should there be a question as to the dating of the pregnancy, gestational age may be approximated by measuring the distance from the pubic symphysis to the fundus in centimeters. A fundus that extends to the umbilicus may be approximated to 20 weeks gestation. Because time is critical in preparing for a cesarean section, performing an ultrasound for the purposes of dating is not recommended.

Perimortem cesarean sections are performed while resuscitation efforts are ongoing. If there is time to prepare for the arrival of a pregnant mother in extremis, securing the assistance and expertise of a neonatologist and obstetrician is recommended. Prior to starting the procedure, if time permits, the abdomen is prepped and a Foley catheter inserted to decompress the bladder. A traditional midline, vertical incision is then made starting just below the xiphoid process and extending to the pubic symphysis. The lower transverse (pfannenstiel) incision should not be used because it does not provide enough exposure to facilitate rapid fetal extraction. The rectus muscle layer is bluntly dissected due to its diastasis during late pregnancy with an incision made through the peritoneal layer. Once the uterus is exposed, any bowel or bladder that is visible is retracted out of the field. A small incision is made at the upper third of the uterus until amniotic fluid is reached. Using bandage scissors, with the other hand elevating the uterine wall from the fetus, the opening is continued inferiorly. Once the head is exposed, suctioning should be performed and the remainder of the body delivered with the cord clamped and cut as in the spontaneous vaginal delivery. The placenta is then delivered with the uterus wiped out and sutured back together in either single or double layer locked stitch with large absorbable suture. Because uterine bleeding may occur, watchful waiting in addition to the direct injection of oxytocin, carboprost, or methylergonovine into the myometrium is recommended before closing the other layers.

The major areas where errors may occur in perimortem cesarean section focus around identifying the appropriate situation where the procedure is indicated and acting in a timely fashion. Cesarean section should not be performed on protracted resuscitation efforts or in pregnancies dating <24 weeks. Ensuring that the appropriate people are notified and preparations made for a cesarean section when treating pregnant women in distress removes the element of surprise and reduces wasted time should the procedure be indicated.

SUGGESTED READINGS

Katz VL, Balderston K, DeFreest M. Perimortem cesarean delivery: Were our assumption correct? *Am J Obstet Gynecol.* 2005;192(6):1916–1920; discussions 1920–1911.

Katz VL, Dotters DJ, Droegemueller W. Perimortem cesarean delivery. *Obstet Gynecol.* 1986;68(4):571–576.

Lanoix R, Akkapeddi V, Goldfeder B. Perimortem cesarean section: Case reports and recommendations. *Acad Emerg Med.* 1995;2(12):1063–1067.

Mallampalli A, Guy E. Cardiac arrest in pregnancy and somatic support after brain death. *Crit Care Med.* 2005;33(10 Suppl):S325–S331.

Whitten M, Irvine LM. Postmortem and perimortem caesarean section: What are the indications? *J R Soc Med.* 2000;93(1):6–9.

Yeomans ER, Gilstrap LC. Physiologic changes in pregnancy and their impact on critical care. *Crit Care Med.* 2005;33(10 Suppl):S256–S258.

204

PELVIC INFLAMMATORY DISEASE IS A DIFFICULT DIAGNOSIS TO MAKE: KNOW THE CDC RECOMMENDATIONS

HEIDI F. WALZ, MD

Pelvic inflammatory disease (PID) afflicts over 1 million women per year in the United States. Of the 5 million patients who present to the emergency department (ED) each year with abdominal pain, approximately two thirds are women. The challenge for the emergency physician is to accurately determine which of these women have PID and to rule out other emergencies such as tuboovarian abscess (TOA), appendicitis, and ectopic pregnancy. PID is a very important diagnosis to make because the consequences of untreated PID are great: it is estimated that following untreated PID, the rate of ectopic pregnancy increases 12% to 15%, the rate of infertility is 12% to 50%, and up to 18% of women with even one episode of untreated PID will go on to develop chronic pelvic pain. Failure to diagnose PID is a common pitfall in the ED because there is no single historical, clinical, or laboratory finding that is both sensitive and specific for clinching the diagnosis. PID can be a subtle diagnosis with a varied presentation. The Centers for Disease Control (CDC) recommends empiric treatment if a sexually active young woman presents with lower abdominal or pelvic pain, cervical motion tenderness, or uterine or adnexal tenderness and no other cause for the pain is identified. Sounds relatively straight forward, until one thinks of a typical day in the ED and how many young women would fit the above description. Hence, a common emergency medicine pitfall is failure to assign the diagnosis of PID.

According to the CDC, additional signs and symptoms can increase the specificity of the diagnosis. This includes a temperature >101°F, abnormal or purulent cervical discharge, abundant white blood cells on wet mount, increased erythrocyte sedimentation rate, increased C reactive protein, or positive gonorrhea or Chlamydia testing. PID is rare without purulent cervical discharge, so look for white blood cells on wet mount obtained from the cervical os. The classic finding of cervical motion tenderness was found in only 20% of patients with laparoscopically diagnosed PID whereas abnormal uterine bleeding is found in up to one third of patients. The onset of pain is typically during or shortly after menses. Pain lasting longer than 2 weeks is less likely to be PID.

Remember that PID is a spectrum of disease, from endometritis and salpingitis to TOA and pelvic peritonitis. Between 10% and 18% of patients with PID also have a TOA. In general, these patients are more ill appearing with tenderness on exam. In these patients, an ultrasound to confirm or eliminate the diagnosis is essential. Patients with a TOA should be admitted for parenteral antibiotics. Appendicitis is another diagnosis that could be missed when diagnosing PID. Reviewing the aforementioned signs and symptoms of PID, many overlap with appendicitis. If a woman has bilateral abdominal tenderness, no migration of her pain, and no nausea and vomiting, she is more likely to have PID than appendicitis. If the diagnosis of appendicitis still cannot be eliminated, an abdominal CT or repeat examinations may be indicated. Ectopic pregnancy is yet another diagnosis not to be misinterpreted as PID. A pregnancy test is essential to rule out this diagnosis.

PID is often a difficult diagnosis to make because it rarely can be confirmed in the ED. Therefore, failure to assign the diagnosis of PID is a common pitfall in emergency medicine. The CDC definition is intentionally vague, because the risks of not treating PID are great. Prior to making the diagnosis, be sure to consider and rule out concomitant or alternative etiologies such as ectopic pregnancy, TOA, or appendicitis.

SUGGESTED READINGS

Blenning CE, Muench J, Judkins DZ, et al. Clinical inquires: Which tests are the most useful for diagnosing PID? *J Fam Pract*. 2007;56(3):216–220.

Eggert J, Sundquist K, van Vuuren C, et al. The clinical diagnosis of pelvic inflammatory disease—reuse of electronic medical record data from 189 patients visiting a Swedish university hospital emergency department. *BMC Womens Health*. 2006;6:16.

Morishita K, Gushimiyagi M. Clinical prediction rule to distinguish pelvic inflammatory disease from acute appendicitis in women of childbearing age. *Am J Emerg Med*. 2007;25:152–157.

Ness RB, Soper DE, Holley RL, et al. Effectiveness of inpatient and outpatient treatment strategies for women with pelvic inflammatory disease: Results from the Pelvic Inflammatory Disease Evaluation and Clinical Health (PEACH) Randomized Trial. *Am J Obstet Gynecol*. 2002;186(5):929–937.

[No author listed]. Sexually transmitted diseases treatment guidelines 2002. Centers for Disease Control and Prevention. *MMWR Recomm Rep*. 2002;51(RR-6):1–78.

Wiesenfeld HC, Hillier SL, Krohn MA, et al. Lower genital tract infection and endometritis: Insight into subclinical pelvic inflammatory disease. *Obstet Gynecol*. 2002;100(3):456–463.

205

Consider Pulmonary Embolism in Pregnancy and the Postpartum Period

Nathaniel L. Scott, MD

Pulmonary embolism (PE) is a common, life-threatening condition that is often difficult to diagnose. Pregnancy and the postpartum period are associated with wide-ranging anatomical, physiological, and hormonal changes which can confound the evaluation of many disease states, including PE. Data from the Center for Disease Control and Prevention gathered from 1991 to 1999 showed PE to be one of the leading causes of maternal mortality in the United States, outpacing pregnancy-induced hypertension, hemorrhage, and infection. The correct and expeditious diagnosis of PE in pregnant patients is a critical step in reducing mortality. Generally speaking, the reasons for failing to diagnose PE in pregnant and postpartum patients can be grouped as follows: (1) not recognizing pregnancy and postpartum period as risk factors, (2) incorrect interpretation of physical exam findings, and (3) misinterpretation of laboratory results.

It is necessary for the emergency physician to have a thorough knowledge of the risk factors for PE. Current algorithms for the diagnosis of PE often depend on appropriately risk-stratifying patients to direct additional testing. Unfortunately, pregnancy is usually an exclusion criterion in studies that determine risk factors for PE and, therefore, is absent in many clinical decision-making rules. Other studies specifically evaluating PE in pregnancy and the postpartum period have generated different estimates of risk. A study that included 285 women with venous thromboembolism (VTE) revealed a markedly increased risk for PE in the 3-month postpartum period (OR 34.4; 95% CI [13.3 to 88.5]). The risk for PE during pregnancy was less impressive (OR 2.3; 95% CI [1.0 to 5.2]), though the risk for VTE in pregnancy was significantly increased (OR 7.8, 95% CI [4.1 to 15.0]). In a different study of 105 cases, the 3-month postpartum period for PE had a relative risk of 15.0 (95% CI [5.13, 43.89]) compared to pregnancy. Furthermore, the incidence of PE has been observed to increase as pregnancy progresses. While many of these studies suffer from limited methodology, the data suggest that both the postpartum period and likely pregnancy confer a significant risk for PE. The consideration of pregnancy in women of childbearing age is dogmatic in the practice of emergency medicine; however, the possibility for recent childbirth is probably not as frequently assessed. It would be prudent to address the potential for recent childbirth in all women being evaluated for PE to avoid missing this risk factor.

While physical exam findings are generally not sensitive or specific in the evaluation of PE, the physical exam can be helpful to an extent. The presence or absence of dyspnea, tachypnea, pleuritic chest pain, tachycardia, rales with pulmonary auscultation, and unilateral lower extremity swelling can steer a clinician either toward or away from a diagnosis of PE. However, the interpretation of physical exam findings in pregnant patients can pose an even greater difficulty when evaluating a patient for PE. Normal pregnancy can produce tachycardia, tachypnea, dyspnea, and abnormal exam findings with pulmonary auscultation. Additionally, a number of conditions that can be confused with DVT are associated with pregnancy, including venous insufficiency, superficial venous thrombosis, and thrombophlebitis. Considering this overlap in exam findings between PE and pregnancy, it is important for the emergency physician not to erroneously attribute abnormal physical exam findings to normal pregnancy, when they could also suggest the presence of PE.

The serum D–dimer assay is an important tool in the workup of PE. It has been found to have a high negative predictive value in the evaluation of PE when a cutoff level of 500 ng/mL is used. Therefore, it is utilized in some clinical decision-making rules to rule out PE in patients in whom the clinical suspicion of PE is low. Pregnancy is known to increase the serum d-dimer level as the pregnancy progresses. A study of women with uncomplicated pregnancy found the mean serum d-dimer level to be 579 ng/mL (SD 363) in the first trimester, 832 ng/mL (SD 456) in the second trimester, 1,159 ng/mL (SD 573) in the third trimester, and 605 ng/mL (SD 433) postpartum. The commonly used cutoff of 500 ng/mL is probably not useful in pregnancy. At best, d-dimer results should be interpreted with caution in pregnancy, and some authors suggest not obtaining the test at all.

In summary, it is important that the postpartum period and pregnancy be correctly identified as risk factors for DVT and PE. Physical exam findings and d-dimer results should be interpreted cautiously. Current clinical decision-making rules have not been validated for pregnancy and the postpartum period. As with nonpregnant patients, when the clinical suspicion of PE is sufficient, additional testing should be performed. Computed tomography is both sensitive and specific for the evaluation of PE and results in less fetal radiation exposure than a V/Q scan.

SUGGESTED READINGS

Brown MD, Vance SJ, Klein JA. An emergency department guideline for the diagnosis of pulmonary embolism: An outcome study. *Acad Emerg Med*. 2005;12(1):20–25.

Chang J, Elam-Evans LD, Berg CJ, et al. Pregnancy-related mortality surveillance—United States, 1991–1999. *MMWR Surveill Summ*. 2003;52(2):1–8.

Chen MM, Coakley FV, Kaimal A, et al. Guidelines for computed tomography and magnetic resonance imaging use during pregnancy and lactation. *Obstet Gynecol*. 2008;112 (2 Pt 1):333–340.

Helt JA, Kobbervig CE, James AH, et al. Trends in the incidence of venous thromboembolism during pregnancy or postpartum: A 30-year population-based study. *Ann Intern Med*. 2005;142(10):697–706.

Kline JA, Williams GW, Hernandez-Nino J. D-dimer concentrations in normal pregnancy: New diagnostic thresholds are needed. *Clin Chem*. 2005;51(5):825–829.

Pomp ER, Lenselink AM, Rosendaal FR, et al. Pregnancy, the postpartum period and prothrombotic defects: Risk of venous thrombosis in the MEGA study. *J Thromb Hemost*. 2008;6(4):632–637.

206

DO NOT MISINTERPRET VITAL SIGNS IN THE PREGNANT PATIENT

MELISSA L. SHERMAN, MD

During pregnancy, women experience a myriad of physiologic changes, which can have important implications during their evaluation and management in the emergency department (ED). It is critical to consider the vital sign alterations which occur during pregnancy when treating this patient population. Some of these changes can both mask and mimic shock.

During a normal pregnancy, women will experience a 10 to 15 beat per min increase in resting heart rate. There is also a gradual increase in blood volume, which peaks at 32 to 34 weeks, to around 50% above normal. Cardiac output also increases by 30% to 50% before it plateaus at the end of the second trimester. Smooth muscle relaxation decreases the body's total peripheral vascular resistance. As a result, central venous pressure can drop to 4 mm Hg by the third trimester. Blood pressure, which starts to decline during the first trimester, climbs during the third trimester to near prepregnancy by the time of delivery.

As pregnancy progresses, some women become hypotensive when in the supine position, a condition long recognized as supine hypotensive syndrome. As the uterus enlarges, it compresses both the inferior vena cava and the lower portion of the aorta; therefore, the designation of aortocaval compression syndrome may be more accurate. This syndrome is a common complication of late pregnancy but has been reported as early as 16 weeks. While in the supine position, uterine compression on the inferior vena cava decreases preload causing cardiac output to diminish by up to 28%. This can lead to a drop in systolic blood pressure by up to 30 mm Hg. A wide spectrum of severity from asymptomatic, nonspecific complaints and minimal cardiovascular alterations to severe shock can result from aortocaval compression. It should be noted that a normal brachial arterial blood pressure in the mother does not exclude aortocaval compression with potential risk of uteroplacental hypoperfusion.

Awake and alert pregnant patients may naturally reposition themselves to avoid the symptoms of supine hypotension, but the patient with an altered mental status or on a backboard may be unable to do this. In these cases, it would be easy to misinterpret hypotension from aortocaval compression as a sign of shock. It is imperative for both the safety of the mother and fetus and the accuracy of collected vital signs that a pregnant woman beyond 16 to 20 weeks gestation be positioned in the left lateral decubitus position and avoid lying supine for any sustained length of time. When a backboard is indicated, it should be elevated to achieve an angle of 15 degrees by placing towels or blankets beneath the right side of the board. The significant increase in blood volume seen in pregnancy can delay clinical signs of maternal hypotension and blood loss. When true hypotension does occur, it should be considered an ominous sign prompting immediate intervention.

Even in the first trimester of pregnancy, vital signs can be deceiving. ED physicians should be aware that normal vital signs are a poor predictor of ruptured ectopic pregnancy. Early on, it was noted that hypotensive patients with ectopic pregnancy often did not mount a tachycardic response. Later studies showed that not only did they not become tachycardic, but they often remained normotensive. One study looking retrospectively at patients admitted for operative management of ectopic pregnancy showed that there was a poor correlation between vital signs and volume of hemoperitoneum. In this population, 20% of the patients found to have >1,500 mL of hemoperitoneum had normal vital signs. Understanding this phenomenon, others attempted to determine if a shock index, defined as the ratio of heart rate to systolic blood pressure (normal = 0.5 to 0.7), would be sensitive for identifying patients with ruptured ectopic pregnancies. Although more sensitive than heart rate or blood pressure alone, an elevated shock index was still only 75% sensitive. There is clear evidence that normal vital signs are a poor predictor of ruptured ectopic pregnancy and therefore should not be used in isolation to determine a patient's stability.

Be wary of a false sense of security with normal vital signs in the setting of trauma or ruptured ectopic pregnancy, as changes in blood pressure and pulse may not be seen until a blood loss of 1,500 to 2,000 mL has occurred. Special consideration of the physiologic changes of pregnancy is required to avoid the misinterpretation of vital signs in a pregnant patient.

- All pregnant patients beyond 16 to 20 weeks gestation should be positioned in the left lateral decubitus position to reduce the effect of aortocaval compression.

- Pregnant patients are likely to have a delayed hypotensive response to blood loss.

- Patients with ruptured ectopic pregnancies frequently have a normal blood pressure and heart rate despite significant hemorrhage.

SUGGESTED READINGS

Birkham RH, Gaeta TJ, Van Deusen SK, et al. The ability of traditional vital zigns and shock index to identify ruptured ectopic pregnancy. *Am J Obstet Gynecol.* 2003;189(5): 1293–1296.

Hick JL, Rodgerson JD, Heegaard WG, et al. Vital signs fail to correlate with hemoperitoneum from ruptured ectopic pregnancy. *Am J Emerg Med.* 2001;19(6):488–491.

Kinsella SM, Lohmann G. Supine hypotensive syndrome. *Obstet Gynecol.* 1994;83(5 Pt 1): 774–788.

Shah AJ, Kilcline BA. Trauma in pregnancy. *Emerg Med Clin North Am.* 2003;(21):615–629.

Snyder HS. Lack of a tachycardic response to hypotension with ruptured ectopic pregnancy. *Am J Emerg Med.* 1990;8(1):23–26.

207

ALWAYS MONITOR THIRD-TRIMESTER PREGNANT PATIENTS AFTER THEY HAVE SUSTAINED TRAUMA OF ANY SEVERITY

FRANK E. VILLAUME IV, MD

Pregnant patients presenting to the emergency department for evaluation after trauma pose unique challenges. Not only must we consider the anatomical and physiologic changes that occur during pregnancy, but we must now care for two patients rather than just one. It is important that we determine the status of the fetus early in our evaluation and initiate fetal monitoring as soon as possible in all women with viable gestations.

Among the most feared complications of trauma during pregnancy, and especially during the later stages, is placental abruption. At its most basic level, abruption is defined as bleeding into the deciduas basalis, separating the placenta from the uterus. This can be life threatening for both the mother and the fetus. Unfortunately, clinical signs of abruption, such as vaginal bleeding, abdominal pain, uterine contractions or tenderness, or amniotic fluid leakage, only have a sensitivity of about 50%. Although lab tests and imaging studies can assist in making the diagnosis, they are not sensitive enough to be solely relied upon. Hemorrhage and disseminated intravascular coagulation are both potential complications of abruption; however, the associated laboratory changes are generally late in the development of the disease. Due to low specificity, the use of the Kleihauer-Betke test to evaluate for fetomaternal hemorrhage has not shown utility for identifying abruption. Ultrasound, although useful in the ED to evaluate the status of the fetus, has been shown to have a very poor sensitivity for identifying abruption. At this point, fetal monitoring is considered the preferred test for detecting abruption.

Fetal heart tone evaluation represents an important and prognostic clinical "vital sign" for patients suffering trauma. Perhaps the most telling evidence illustrating the importance of fetal monitoring following trauma was a study which evaluated nearly 450 pregnant patients with viable pregnancies. This study showed that when fetal heart tones were absent, the fetus had no chance for survival, whereas simple detection of fetal heart tones in combination with a gestational age of 26 weeks or more indicated 75% survival of the fetus. The same study reported five infant deaths resulting from delayed recognition of fetal distress. 60% of these deaths were in mothers who had experienced mild to moderate injuries. In another study, where placental abruption complicated 3.5% of pregnant trauma victims, a fetal heart rate <110 bpm was shown to be a strong indicator of future fetal demise. More subtle abnormalities noted by continuous monitoring were observed in 24 patients. Seven underwent emergent c-section with maternal and fetal survival in all cases. These authors advocate for continuous fetal monitoring of all third-trimester trauma patients, claiming that good outcomes can be obtained if early fetal distress is identified and one proceeds to emergent cesarean section.

Management protocols for trauma in pregnancy are generally based on case reports and small series; however, there have been studies indicating the importance of monitoring across all degrees of trauma. One study looking at 514 pregnancies complicated by trauma showed that in the absence of symptoms of abruption, reassuring monitoring, defined as both fetal heart rate and uterine contraction monitoring, had a very high negative predictive value. These authors recommended that asymptomatic patients could safely be sent home with precautions and close follow-up after 4 h of reassuring monitoring. Although, in general, studies indicate that higher severity trauma has a stronger correlation with poor outcome of pregnancy, mild to moderate trauma warrants the careful attention that can be afforded by a period of monitoring. Of note, fetal monitoring does not have to be limited to the labor and delivery unit. If the patient is requiring ongoing evaluation and management for other injuries, continuous fetal monitoring can and should be instituted as early as possible in the ED. This may be facilitated with the assistance of labor and delivery nurses familiar with identifying more subtle signs of fetal distress.

An additional question is raised about the length of fetal monitoring, in particular, with regard to the delayed nature of some cases of placental abruption. Without the clinical symptoms that might indicate abruption (e.g., bleeding, uterine pain, contractions), the utility of monitoring beyond 4 to 6 h is by and large unnecessary. In summary, particular attention should be paid to women who have viable pregnancies and who sustain even mild abdominal trauma. These patients should all undergo at least 4 h of fetal monitoring to predict the course of fetal health and obstetrical management.

KEY POINTS

- Fetal heart tones are an important prognostic vital sign.
- Even relatively minor trauma warrants fetal monitoring for at least 4 h.
- Continuous fetal monitoring should be initiated as early as possible during the evaluation.

SUGGESTED READINGS

Baerga-Varela Y, Zietlow SP, Bannon MP, et al. Trauma in pregnancy. *Mayo Clin Proc.* 2000;75(12):1243–1248.

Connolly AM, Katz VL, Bash KL, et al. Trauma and pregnancy. *Am J Perinatol.* 1997;14(6): 331–336.

Cusick SS, Tibbles CD. Trauma in pregnancy. *Emerg Med Clin North Am.* 2007;25(3): 861–872.

Goodwin TM, Breen MT. Pregnancy outcome and fetomaternal hemorrhage after non-catastrophic trauma. *Am J Obstet Gynecol.* 1990;162(3):665–671.

208

BE PREPARED TO MANAGE POSTPARTUM HEMORRHAGE AT EVERY DELIVERY

EMILY E. VOGEL, MD

Postpartum hemorrhage (PPH) is a leading cause of pregnancy-related mortality in the United States, with an overall incidence of 4% to 8%. It is classically defined as blood loss of 500 mL or more; however, the American College of Obstetrics and Gynecology also includes in the definition a decrease in hematocrit of 10% or the need for transfusion after labor due to bleeding.

PPH can occur early (first 24 h) or late (between 24 h and 6 weeks after delivery). The former is more common, is associated with more blood loss and higher morbidity, and is most commonly due to uterine atony. The latter is most often due to retained placenta. The main risk factor for PPH due to uterine atony is overdistention (multiple gestations, polyhydramnios, and macrosomia). Precipitous labor, high parity, and hypertensive disorders are also associated with increased risk for PPH. Other causes of PPH include trauma (lacerations, hematomas, inversion, and rupture), accounting for 20%, tissue (retained placental tissue or abnormal placentation), accounting for 10%, and coagulopathies, accounting for 1%.

The best preventive strategy for PPH is active management of the third stage of labor, which decreases the risk of PPH by 68%. The most important step in active management is administering oxytocin (Pitocin), the first-line uterotonic drug, soon after the delivery of the placenta. Oxytocin should be administered at a dose of 10 U IM or 20 to 40 U in a liter of crystalloid, infused at 250 mL per h (or up to 500 mL over 10 min). Oxytocin has no contraindications and few side effects except for hypotension, which occurs much less commonly when administered by continuous infusion. Misoprostol (Cytotec), 1,000 μg per rectum, may be used when oxytocin is not available but can cause hyperpyrexia and is contraindicated in a woman with a prior C-section. Active mechanical uterine fundal massage should be performed after delivery of the placenta.

During the first few minutes that oxytocin is infusing, investigate other potential causes of hemorrhage, and resources should be mobilized in anticipation of the possible need for other interventions. If bleeding continues despite initial active management, the resuscitation phase should begin and, if possible, an obstetrical consultant should be involved emergently. The patient should have two large-bore intravenous (IV) lines and be placed on oxygen. Blood should be sent for a CBC, type and crossmatch, and coagulation studies. Patients may need transfusion of blood, fresh frozen plasma, and platelets.

A uterus that is not yet firm suggests uterine atony. Uterine massage should continue and additional uterotonic medications should be considered. Although there is not a clearly established algorithm for medical therapy with uterotonic drugs, if bleeding does not stop after oxytocin or misoprostol, there are two other well-studied alternative medications that can be given. Methylergonovine (Methergine) is an ergot alkyloid that is administered at 0.2 mg IM every 2 to 4 h but is contraindicated in hypertensive or preeclamptic patients. 15-methyl prostaglandin F2 (Hemabate) can be administered at 0.25 mg IM or intramyometrially every 15 to 90 min (maximum of eight doses), but it is contraindicated in patients with asthma or other active cardiac, pulmonary, renal, or hepatic disease. Side effects include nausea, vomiting, diarrhea, hypertension, headache, flushing, and hyperpyrexia. Hemabate has been shown to control PPH in 87% of patients but has more side effects than other uterotonics.

Postpartum bleeding with a uterus that is firm to palpation suggests an etiology other than atony. Retained placenta or delivery of a nonintact placenta occurs in <3% of vaginal deliveries. The management of retained placenta includes either manual extraction or injection of 20 mL of normal saline and 20 U of oxytocin directly into the umbilical vein. If a clear plane of separation between the placenta and the uterine wall cannot be identified during manual extraction, abnormal placentation, such as placenta accreta, should be suspected. The most common treatment for invasive placenta is hysterectomy.

The lower genital tract should be well visualized and explored from the cervix to the introitus. If a genital tract hematoma >3 cm is found, it may require I&D, irrigation, ligation of bleeding vessels, and a layered closure. Lacerations that are actively bleeding should also be repaired. Antibiotics should be given. At times, uterus inversion may be the cause of PPH. This must be rapidly identified and promptly replaced manually, ideally with analgesia. In these cases, the uterine fundus will not be palpable abdominally, but it also may not be easily visualized protruding from the introitus. The fundus should be replaced before attempts to remove any adherent placenta. If repositioning is unsuccessful, IV magnesium sulfate, terbutaline, nitroglycerine, or general anesthesia may be needed. When the uterus is in its normal position again, uterotonics should be given.

If medical therapies fail, surgical therapies, including uterine packing, arterial ligation, arterial embolization, uterine compression sutures, or hysterectomy, should be pursued.

SUGGESTED READINGS

Anderson JM, Etches D. Prevention and management of postpartum hemorrhage. *Am Fam Physician.* 2007;75(6):875–882.

Dildy GA. Postpartum hemorrhage: New management options. *Clin Obstet Gynecol.* 2002; 45(2):330–344.

McCormick ML, Sanghvi HCG, Kinzie B, et al. Preventing postpartum hemorrhage in low-resource settings. *Int J Gynecol Obstet.* 2002;77(3):267–275.

Sheiner E, Sarid L, Levy A, et al. Obstetric risk factors and outcome of pregnancies complicated with early postpartum hemorrhage: A population based study. *J Matern Fetal Neonatal Med.* 2005;18(3):149–154.

You WB, Zahn CM. Postpartum hemorrhage: Abnormally adherent placenta, uterine inversion, and puerperal hematomas. *Clin Obstet Gynecol.* 2006;49(1):184–197.

209

SIMPLE "RULES" OF PEDIATRIC RESUSCITATION

LAWRENCE A. DELUCA, JR, EDD, MD

An excellent veterinarian and highly skilled clinician taught me much about veterinary medicine that has had tremendous impact on my approach to pediatric care. In both disciplines, we often deal with patients who we have difficulty communicating with, who have concerned and occasionally neurotic parents or guardians, and whose size alone makes their care technically challenging. We can use the "Rules of the House of Dog" to help guide us in avoiding common pediatric resuscitation errors.

RULE 1: FIRST, DO NO HARM

Let children assume a position of comfort if at all possible! Children optimize their own airway and breathing. Forcing children to lie down increases their anxiety and their distress. Blow-by oxygen from mom or dad, although less consistent in delivery, is often better tolerated and can be more beneficial when the child will not (despite all efforts) tolerate an affixed mask.

Avoid creating iatrogenic resuscitation situations! Use tools such as the Broselow tape to help dose pediatric drugs and avoid accidental medication underdoses or overdoses. (See the "Medication Dosing Errors" section for more information on this topic.)

Planning and preparation for any pediatric resuscitation means knowing where your equipment is—your Broselow tape, your pediatric code kit, and how to find **the right size equipment** for the child you are treating. **Practice rarely performed procedures**—such as umbilical lines—whenever you get a chance in the simulation lab—it will pay off one day!

Take your own pulse first! Pediatric resuscitations are high-anxiety environments and emotionally charged situations for the parents, EMS, staff, and physicians.

RULE 2: YOU CAUSE MORE HARM BY NOT NOTICING THAN NOT KNOWING

Get as much history from the family and EMS as the situation allows! These people hold valuable clues that can help you figure out how the child got into this situation and how to get him or her out of it! A toxic ingestion is a perfect example that with a good history, you may have a treatment or antidote.

Have a reference to tell you the normal vital signs for the child's age! Trying to remember formulas or attempting to mentally calculate this information in a resuscitation situation is error prone and dangerous.

A fully clothed child is not an adequately examined child! Respiratory effort and the degree of distress cannot be adequately evaluated in small children without direct visualization of chest wall motion and signs of retractions. Trauma or suspected abuse also requires full exposure of the child to evaluate the extent of (potentially life-threatening) injuries.

Bradycardia and hypotension are ominous signs of impending arrest! Aggressively manage the ABCs to avoid these signs evolving in the first place! Blood pressure (BP) will be maintained until the point of near cardiovascular collapse. Do not wait for a dip in BP to begin fluid resuscitation.

Pay attention to the heart rate! Recognize that in small children, increasing heart rate (HR) rather than stroke volume is the primary means of increasing cardiac output. A dehydrated child may exhibit orthostatic HR changes in the absence of corresponding BP changes.

Resuscitation needs to be tailored to clinical endpoints! Tools such as the Broselow tape provide an estimate. Resolving tachycardia, adequate urinary output, and improved mental status are all good indicators of adequate resuscitation.

Keep the zebras in mind! Failure to diagnose can result in failure to treat, which can be fatal.

- **Ductal-dependant lesions** usually present in the 1st week of life with a child in severe *heart failure* with a *toxic appearance*. **Prostaglandins will be lifesaving!**
- **Sepsis requires prompt, broad-spectrum antibiotic therapy** *plus* **aggressive resuscitation!** Giving antibiotics without addressing volume issues will lead to worsening shock.
- **Stridor, drooling, and a toxic appearance suggest epiglottitis!** Are this child's immunizations up-to-date? Do not mistake this life-threatening condition for croup.
- **Abdominal pain and vomiting followed by an asymptomatic period could be iron toxicity or intussusception.** Both can lead to GI bleeding. You need a good history, too!

RULE 3: NEVER MAKE THE TREATMENT WORSE THAN THE DISEASE

Critically ill children may require aggressive and invasive management:

■ Use the intraosseous route (IO) after three failed IV attempts or 90 s have passed!

■ The primary cause of cardiac arrest in children is respiratory arrest—manage the airway aggressively and intubate early.

A less seriously ill child can often be managed more conservatively:

■ Use appropriate antiemetics and oral rehydration when the patient is alert and able to swallow.

■ Nasal continuous positive airway pressure (CPAP) can frequently help bronchiolitic infants avoid endotracheal intubation.

■ Blow-by oxygen might be better tolerated than a tight-fitting mask.

RULE 4: PAY ATTENTION!

The condition of critically ill children changes frequently! Once you have successfully resuscitated the patient and your presence is no longer required continuously at the bedside, you still need to go back and reassess often!

SUGGESTED READINGS

American Heart Association. 2005 American Heart Association (AHA) guidelines for cardiopulmonary resuscitation (CPR) and emergency cardiovascular care (ECC) of pediatric and neonatal patients: pediatric advanced life support. *Pediatrics*. 2006;117(5): e989–e1004.

Bellemare S, Hartling L, Wiebe N, et al. Oral rehydration versus intravenous therapy for treating dehydration due to gastroenteritis in children: A meta-analysis of randomised controlled trials. *BMC Med*. 2004;2:11.

Flomenbaum NE, Goldfrank LR, Hoffman RS, et al., eds. *Goldfrank's Toxicologic Emergencies*. 8th ed. New York, NY: McGraw-Hill; 2006.

Fuchs SM, Jaffe DM. Evaluation of the "tilt test" in children. *Ann Emerg Med*. 1987;16(4): 386–390.

Javouhey E, Barats A, Richard N, et al. Non-invasive ventilation as primary ventilatory support for infants with severe bronchiolitis. *Intensive Care Med*. 2008;34(9):1608–1614.

Nieman CT, Manacci CF, Super DM, et al. Use of the Broselow tape may result in the underresuscitation of children. *Acad Emerg Med*. 2006;13(10):1011–1019.

210

DO NOT FORGET THAT DRYING, WARMING, AND POSITIONING ARE AS IMPORTANT TO NEONATAL RESUSCITATION AS THE ABCs

CHARLES G. GILLESPIE, MD

Everyone knows that resuscitation begins with the ABCs. When it comes to neonatal resuscitation, the DWPs (drying, warming, and positioning) are as important to the algorithm as airway, breathing, and circulation. When performed promptly, these steps can promote spontaneous respiration and prevent hypothermia and unwanted metabolic derangements from occurring.

POINT 1: DWP STIMULATES SPONTANEOUS RESPIRATIONS

In utero, fetal respiration occurs via the placenta. Once the cord is clamped, the low-resistance placental circuit is eliminated, and blood is shunted to the newborn's lungs. Before gas exchange can occur, however, amniotic fluid must be displaced from the lungs. Suctioning the nares and oropharynx helps, though most is displaced with a vigorous cry. Infants cry in response to drying and gently flicking the soles of their feet. Crying promotes inspiration and distension of the alveoli, allowing oxygen exchange to occur. Gas exchange in turn relaxes the arterioles, further lowering the resistance of the lungs to blood flow. That is why DWP is the first block in the Neonatal Resuscitation Program (NRP) algorithm. Proper positioning is important for airway patency and to facilitate intubation, if warranted. Remember that persistent respiratory depression despite these measures is an indication of secondary apnea and the need for assisted ventilation.

POINT 2: DWP PREVENTS HYPOTHERMIA

Human survival depends on the body's ability to regulate temperature. In mature, healthy people, this is accomplished both consciously (e.g., changing the thermostat, adding/removing clothing, drinking liquids, etc.) and unconsciously (e.g., sweating and shivering). In utero, this is a passive process wherein the fetal environment is maintained one-half degree above maternal temperature. After delivery, the newborn is susceptible to heat loss via radiation, conduction, convection, and evaporative cooling. Newborns are not only incapable of taking conscious action to regulate temperature, but they are also limited in the unconscious mechanisms as well. In particular, premature (<30 weeks gestation) and low-birth weight (LBW; <1,500 g) infants are vulnerable to heat loss due to a greater body surface area-to-weight ratio, minimal fat stores, and thin skin that is prone to transdermal evaporative cooling. Although term infants have a limited capacity for nonshivering thermogenesis via the metabolism of brown fat, this response is diminished or absent in LBW infants. As heat generation increases metabolic demand, oxygen consumption, and utilization of glucose, neonates are susceptible to hypoxia, hypercarbia, hypoglycemia, and metabolic acidosis. Hypothermia can delay recovery from acidosis, setting up a vicious cycle. The best way to prevent this is by avoiding hypothermia from the moment of delivery.

One strategy for avoiding hypothermia is immediately placing the newborn under a radiant warmer following delivery. The infant should be promptly dried with warm linens, as radiant heat alone does not prevent evaporative heat loss. Replace the wet linens frequently to avoid further heat loss. Also, placing an infant cap on the baby may increase an infant's core body temperature. If you do not have a radiant warmer, place the newborn in direct skin-to-skin contact with the mother, covering both with dry linens. This technique has shown a significant reduction in hypothermia compared to the use of a radiant warmer alone. You may also crank up the temperature in the resuscitation area between 27°C and 31°C, although this may be uncomfortable for the adults. Be sure to check the infant's temperature regularly, with a goal axillary temperature between 36.5°C to 37.7°C. Avoid prolonged exposure of the infant during procedures (e.g., lines, tubes, imaging and nursing cares) whenever possible. Also, wrapping an LBW infant in food-grade plastic wrap (without predrying) has been shown to be an effective strategy for thermal stabilization and may decrease in-hospital mortality. Finally, positive-pressure ventilation can result in additional heat loss through conduction and insensible water loss. You may limit these losses by using warmed, humidified oxygen in line with the bag-mask ventilator.

In summary, DWPs are simple, proactive, preventative measures that may help you avoid some of the more aggressive interventions of the resuscitation algorithm. Suctioning the nares and oropharynx and vigorously drying may stimulate spontaneous respiration in the newborn. If this does not work, gentle heel flicking may do the trick. If not, consider secondary apnea and move down the algorithm to positive-pressure ventilation. To avoid hypothermia, place the newborn in a radiant warmer or in skin-to-skin contact with the mother or wrap LBW infants in plastic wrap without predrying. Monitor axillary temperature closely, avoid prolonged exposures, and use warmed, humidified oxygen during ventilation. Take these steps and you will avoid the pitfalls that occur from reflexively jumping to the ABC portion of the algorithm.

Suggested Readings

Behrman RE, Kliegman RM, Jenson HB, et al., eds. *Nelson Essentials of Pediatrics: Fetal and Neonatal Medicine.* 4th ed. New York, NY: Elsevier; 2002:203–204.

Bergman NJ, Linley LL, Fawcus SR. Randomized controlled trial of skin-to-skin contact from birth versus conventional incubator for physiological stabilization in 1200- to 2199 gram newborns. *Acta Paediatr.* 2004;93:779–785.

Braner DAV, ed. *Textbook of Neonatal Resuscitation.* 4th ed. Dallas, TX: American Heart Association; 2004:1–22.

Knobel R, Holditch-Davis D. Thermoregulation and heat loss prevention after birth and during neonatal intensive care unit stabilization of extremely low birth weight infants. *J Obstet Gynecol Neonatal Nurs.* 2007;36:280–287.

Roberts JR. *Use of a Stockinet Cap on Premature Infants After Delivery (dissertation).* Denton, TX: Texas Woman's University; 1981.

Vohra S, Grent G, Campbell V, et al. Effect of polyethylene occlusive skin wrapping on heat loss in very low birth weight infants at delivery: A randomized trial. *J Pediatr.* 1999;134: 547–551.

211

REMEMBER ... NOT ALL KIDS WITH WHEEZING HAVE ASTHMA

JAN M. SHOENBERGER, MD, FAAEM, FACEP

The patient who presents to the emergency department (ED) with wheezing is often presumed to have "asthma." This presumption often begins in the triage area before the physician sees the patient, and wheezing patients may even be triaged to a special area in the ED reserved for administering asthma treatment. But as every emergency physician knows, both adults and children who present with wheezing may have something other than asthma as a diagnosis.

"Wheezing" is a high-pitched adventitial sound heard on auscultation of the lungs. The characteristic high-pitched noise occurs during the rapid passage of air through airways that are narrowed but not yet at the point of closure. It most often occurs during the expiratory phase of breathing and is a nonspecific manifestation of airway obstruction. Children wheeze more often than adults because their bronchi are small to begin with, leading to higher peripheral airway resistance.

The most common cause of wheezing is, in fact, asthma. If the diagnosis is asthma, by definition, the wheezing and associated respiratory distress should respond to bronchodilator therapy. Although not usually necessary, the diagnosis can be confirmed in the pulmonary laboratory with a methacholine challenge test.

If asthma was initially suspected in a wheezing patient and standard therapies do not lead to clinical improvement, alternative diagnoses should be considered.

Alternative diagnoses in the wheezing patient are vast. Possibilities include

- Allergic reaction
- Congestive heart failure (CHF)
- Foreign body aspiration (especially if symptoms started suddenly)
- Gastroesophageal reflux disease (GERD)
- Infections: bronchiolitis, bronchitis, pneumonia, upper respiratory infection, croup
- Obstructive sleep apnea
- Pulmonary embolism
- Tumors/malignancy
- Vocal cord dysfunction

In pediatric patients, additional diagnoses to be considered include

- Bronchopulmonary dysplasia
- Congenital anomalies
- Cystic fibrosis
- Tracheo- or bronchomalacia
- Vascular rings

The time course of the disease may help the clinician narrow down the possibilities. If the onset is acute, foreign body aspiration, anaphylaxis, asthma, pneumonia, pulmonary embolism, CHF, or aspiration syndromes are in the differential diagnosis. If the onset is insidious, malignancies rise to the top of the list. CHF also may be slower in onset.

On physical examination, there may be more clues to the true diagnosis. Signs of cardiac disease, such as hepatic congestion and peripheral edema, may help to differentiate cardiac from pulmonary sources of wheezing. Auscultation of the heart is especially important; the presence of an S3 is one of the most specific signs of CHF. If unilateral wheezing is present, a localized cause, such as pneumonia, foreign body aspiration, pulmonary embolism, or a malignancy is more likely.

In the pediatric patient with wheezing, further history regarding timing should be obtained. A cough after eating in a wheezing child suggests GERD. A dry, unproductive cough that worsens at night could be GERD, allergies, or asthma. Obstructive sleep apnea should be considered in children whose coughing or wheezing awakens them at night and is associated with snoring. Sleep apnea in infants is usually a result of craniofacial abnormalities, but in older children, the main cause is adenotonsillar hypertrophy. Ask the parent if the wheezing improves or worsens with position. This may suggest tracheomalacia.

Chest radiography may be helpful in determining the etiology of wheezing. It will reveal whether the patient has cardiomegaly, pulmonary edema, or infiltrates suggestive of infection. If a foreign body is suspected, chest radiographs should be performed during inspiration and expiration or, in a child too young to cooperate, on both sides, in the decubitus position. These two views should be compared. If a mainstem bronchus is obstructed, the affected side will be hyperinflated and postobstructive changes may be seen such as atelectasis. Foreign body aspiration can occur anytime but is most common between 8 months and 4 years of age.

Testing for viral etiologies such as respiratory syncytial virus (RSV) may be helpful for making a specific diagnosis; however, testing should only be ordered if it will alter management. Spirometry may also be helpful in distinguishing etiologies. A low forced expiratory volume (FEV_1) with reversibility after administration of a bronchodilator or the ability to induce airflow restriction with provocative drug challenges indicates asthma. Flow-volume loop patterns can help diagnose other conditions, such as upper airway obstruction. There is also a role for computed tomography of the chest or neck in cases where airway compression is suspected. Bronchoscopy or endoscopy may also be helpful.

All emergency physicians know that "not all the wheezes are asthma"—it just helps to be reminded of the broad differential diagnosis every so often!

SUGGESTED READINGS

Holroyd HJ. Foreign body aspiration: Potential cause of cough and wheezing. *Pediatr Rev.* 1988;10(2):59–63.

Soto FJ, Guntupalli KK. All that wheezes is not asthma: Diagnosing the mimics. *Emergency Medicine.* November 2001. Available at: http://www.emedmag.com/html/pre/cov/covers/111501.asp

Swanson KL. Airway foreign bodies: What's new? *Semin Respir Crit Care Med.* 2004;25(4): 405–411.

Weiss LN. The diagnosis of wheezing in children. *Am Fam Physician.* 2008;77(8):1109–1114.

212

PEDIATRIC AIRWAYS ARE NOT JUST "LITTLE ADULT" AIRWAYS

RICHARD AMINI, MD

When assessing pediatric airways, one must first forget the adage that children are just small adults. The most common mistakes often stem from an adrenaline-induced mental block of basic differences in pediatric anatomy and physiology.

DO NOT FORGET THAT RESPIRATORY RESERVE IN PEDIATRIC PATIENTS IS MUCH MORE LIMITED THAN ADULTS

Anatomically, the thoracic cavities of pediatric patients have less intrinsic elasticity. Additionally, their intercostal muscles are not fully developed, and their diaphragm is shorter and more flattened, thereby decreasing its ability to pull down and further increase the negative force needed. These differences make their airways less capable of generating inspiratory force and more sensitive to fatigue.

Physiologically, having fewer Type I muscle fibers (the slow twitch red muscles lacking endurance), the child's respiratory drive is more fatigable than that of an adult. Their relatively smaller airway diameter increases resistance, while smaller alveolar size increases the likelihood of collapse. More importantly, children's basic metabolic rate is much greater than that of adults. This equates to increased oxygen metabolism/consumption which makes management of pediatric airway even more critical.

Decreased reserve, increased basal metabolic needs, and anatomical predisposition to collapse all help explain why 50% of pediatric deaths under 1 year of age are associated with respiratory failure. This also contributes to respiratory arrest as the leading cause of cardiac arrest in children.

When the patient's condition and the emergency physician's clinical acumen dictate that intubation is necessary, the understanding of basic pediatric anatomy and common mistakes will increase the success rate. Compared to the adult airway, children have a large tongue-to-mouth size ratio, anterocaudal laryngeal position, and a relatively large, inelastic epiglottis. Additionally, the narrowest portion of their airway is at the cricoid ring (more on that later). Finally, their large head-to-body surface area ratio anatomically creates passive flexion of the occiput which obstructs visualization of the vocal cords limiting the physician's ability to intubate.

DO NOT FORGET YOUR ANATOMY

Positioning the patient is vital to accessing the airway. Both in adult and pediatric patients, the key to a successful intubation is aligning the oral, laryngeal, and pharyngeal axes. Due to the pediatric patient's large occiput, the patient is in a passively flexed position. Placing a blanket under the shoulders helps overcome this and aligns the axes.

DO NOT FORGET TO SELECT THE CORRECTLY SIZED EQUIPMENT

Once the decision to intubate has been made, errors in choosing the best ET tube can be eliminated using length-based resuscitation tapes or the formula: ET tube size = Age/4 + 4. Remember that the pediatric airway is narrowest at the cricoid ring, which forms a natural anatomic seal around the ET tube. When choosing uncuffed versus cuffed tubes, the general recommendation is children <8 years of age require uncuffed tubes due to the anatomic seal. Children >8 years have larger, wider airways similar to adults, requiring a cuff.

DO NOT FORGET TO APPROPRIATELY PREOXYGENATE THE PEDIATRIC PATIENT

As discussed above, pediatric patients have an increased basic metabolic requirement and decreased residual capacity which forces them to consume oxygen at a higher rate and desaturate much faster than adults. Therefore, it is vital to maintain proper oxygenation prior to intubation. Remember that bag-mask ventilation is as effective in short-term oxygenation as intubation.

DO NOT FORGET TO BE GENTLE

Remember the pediatric airway is less rigid and more easily injured. Great care must be taken to avoid injuring the airway. Excessive force can create vocal cord spasms, airway swelling, lacerations, and permanent strictures. Using appropriate pediatric intubation supplies and a gentle hand will help avoid the need to reintubate which is the most common cause of airway injury.

DO NOT FORGET YOUR 9 PS OF RAPID SEQUENCE INTUBATION (RSI)

Remember to assess the

1) **Possibility** of success: consider the Mallampati classification, obstructions, neck mobility, etc.
2) **Preparation**: this goes without saying—have suction, oxygen, airway equipment, drugs, and monitoring equipment ready.
3) **Preoxygenate**: as previously mentioned, this is vital to success, especially in the pediatric patient whose oxygen demand is higher than that of an adult.
4) **Pretreatment**: keep in mind the adverse effects of inducing agents. Be cautious when dealing with increased ICP, increased intraocular pressure, potential bronchospasm, and possible bradycardia when using depolarizing neuromuscular blockade.
5) **Paralysis** with induction agents: chose the best agent.
6) **Protection**: while controversial, Sellick maneuver should be used.
7) **Positioning**: extremely important in children who may need a towel behind their shoulders to align the oral, laryngeal, and pharyngeal axes. (See above)
8) **Placement**: DO NOT MISS!
9) **Proof**: remember to check your work, assess placement by laryngoscopic observation of the endotracheal tube (ETT) passing through the vocal cords, and confirm with end-tidal CO_2. Auscultation of breath sounds, observation of symmetrical chest rise during ventilation, and condensation of the ETT tube also help. Remember to order an AP x-ray, and check the pulse oximetry.

Suggested Readings

Carpenter TC. Critical care. In: Hay WW, Levin MJ, Sondheimer JM, et al., eds. *Current Diagnosis and Treatment in Pediatrics*. 18th ed. New York, NY: McGraw-Hill; 2007.

Ganong WF. *Review of Medical Physiology*. 20th ed. New York, NY: McGraw-Hill; 2001.

Gausche M, Lewis RJ, Stratton SJ, et al. Effect of out-of-hospital pediatric endotracheal intubation on survival and neurological outcome: A controlled clinical trial. *JAMA*. 2000;283(6):783–790.

Gomes Cordeiro AM, Fernandes JC, Troster EJ. Possible risk factors associated with moderate or severe airway injuries in children who underwent endotracheal intubation. *Pediatr Crit Care Med*. 2004;5(4):364–368.

Hauda WE II. Pediatric cardiopulmonary resuscitation. In: Tintinalli JE, Kelen GD, Stapczynski JS, et al., eds. *Emergency Medicine: A Comprehensive Study Guide*. 65th ed. New York, NY: McGraw-Hill; 2003.

Hurford W. Orotracheal intubation outside the operating room: Anatomic considerations and techniques. *Respir Care*. 1999;44(6):615–626.

Mahadevan SV, Garmel GM. *An Introduction to Clinical Emergency Medicine*. 1st ed. New York, NY: Cambridge University Press; 2005.

Marx JA, Hockberger RS, Walls RM, eds. *Rosen's Emergency Medicine: Concepts and Clinical Practice*. 6th ed. Philadelphia, PA: Mosby; 2006.

213

DO NOT ASSUME THAT ALL STRIDOR IS CAUSED BY CROUP

JEREMY D. MEIER, MD

Stridor is defined as an abnormal, harsh noise caused by turbulent airflow through the upper airways. Stridor is NOT a diagnosis, it is a sign of an underlying disease. Stridor is not wheezing, which results from spasm or swelling of the small airways, nor is it stertor, which occurs from nasal or nasopharyngeal obstruction. Once you have heard stridor, you can identify it again. That is the easy part. Figuring out the cause and then knowing what to do about it is the challenge.

Evaluating a child with stridor is a true emergency that requires a rapid, systematic approach, in spite of any inner panic or palpitations you might be experiencing. When first hearing stridor, immediately assess the stability of the airway. A rapid clinical assessment can often make the difference between a lifesaving event and a fatal complication. A child in the classic tripod position, drooling, and unable to swallow secretions suggests an impending airway disaster; prepare for emergent endotracheal intubation, swallow your pride, and call for help (otolaryngology, pediatric surgery, etc.). This is one time that does not pay to go it alone.

If emergent intervention is not necessary, pull out your internist skills and obtain a complete history. The time of onset, alleviating or exacerbating factors, and the presence of persistent or intermittent complaints are all significant clues to the diagnosis. Common things are common. Croup, or laryngotracheobronchitis, is the most common cause of acute stridor in the pediatric population. However, too often when a stridulous child presents to the emergency department, he or she is given a diagnosis of croup, treated symptomatically with corticosteroids and nebulized epinephrine, and discharged home, only to return because the correct diagnosis was missed.

Bacterial tracheitis and epiglottitis are both serious, life-threatening infections that could be mistaken for croup. Symptoms of bacterial tracheitis include fevers and a toxic appearance, with little response to nebulized epinephrine. Initial treatment involves close airway monitoring and broad-spectrum antibiotics, typically a penicillinase-resistant penicillin and a third-generation cephalosporin. Although rare since the introduction of the HiB vaccine, patients with epiglottitis present with high fevers, drooling, and the sniffing position. With either of these diseases, management of the airway should be performed by the most experienced physician, and if possible in the operating room, by the otolaryngologist. Trying to be a hero in airway management without adequate experience or proper setup could lead to a disaster. This is one instance that should not draw the ire of the surgical consultant; just do not refer to the patient as a "kiddo" when calling the consult. You are running an emergency department not a daycare.

Croup often presents gradually, typically preceded by an upper respiratory infection, with symptoms worse at night or with agitation. If the onset is sudden, with a coughing or choking spell, you must rule out an airway foreign body. When an infant presents with stridor present for weeks or months, laryngomalacia is the likely culprit. This condition is caused by immature laryngeal structures leading to collapse within the airway and is usually worse when the child lies down or cries. A history of prolonged intubation or previous tracheostomy could suggest subglottic stenosis. Vocal cord paralysis should be considered in a child with a traumatic birth or prior neck surgery.

Differentiating inspiratory from expiratory stridor can help determine the site of obstruction. Inspiratory stridor typically occurs from a lesion above the glottis, while expiratory stridor suggests the location is intrathoracic. Biphasic stridor usually is caused by obstruction at the glottis or subglottis. Although the pitch and intensity can be clues to the severity of the obstruction, do not rely on this too heavily. Do not be fooled into a false sense of security if the stridor lessens in intensity. As the obstruction worsens, the stridor often becomes quiet, with minimal air flow. Needless to say, minimal air flow is not very good for your patient.

Direct examination of the airway, either performed fiberoptically at the bedside or in the operating room, can help make the diagnosis. Anteroposterior (AP) and lateral radiographic views of the neck are useful to assess the tonsils and adenoids, epiglottis, retropharynx, subglottis, and trachea. High-kilovoltage technique is preferred as this provides better views of the soft tissue. Radiographs can also potentially identify the presence of foreign bodies. Both AP and lateral views should be obtained, as instances have occurred where two or more coins were stacked upon each other, a fact obscured by a single AP view. A barium swallow is useful when vascular compression or gastroesophageal reflux is suspected.

Treatment for croup includes corticosteroids and nebulized epinephrine. While most children can be managed as outpatients, it is important to recognize admission criteria. Hospital admission is recommended in patients with any of the following: under 6 months of age, poor response to initial treatment, or inadequate oral intake (admission not necessarily mandated but certainly considered if the child's father is an attorney).

In summary, the differential diagnosis for stridor in children is extensive. When seeing a child with stridor, first ensure a stable or secure airway. Although croup is the most common cause of acute stridor, a complete history and physical examination are essential so that other less common diseases are not missed. Clinical acumen is essential, both in making the diagnosis and securing the airway when needed.

SUGGESTED READINGS

Bjornson CL, Johnson DW. Croup. *Lancet*. 2008;371:329–339.
Leung A, Cho H. Diagnosis of stridor in children. *Am Fam Physician*. 1999;60(8):2289–2296.
Savoy NB. Differentiating stridor in children at triage: It's not always croup. *J Emerg Nurs*. 2005;31:503–505.
Tunkel DE, Zalzal GH. Stridor in infants and children: Ambulatory evaluation and operative diagnosis. *Clin Pediatr*. 1992;31:48–55.

214

RECOGNIZE THE DIFFERENCES IN PEDIATRIC VERSUS ADULT BURN MANAGEMENT

ATANU BISWAS, MD, MSc

The time-dependent variables for all burn resuscitation formulas begin from the moment of injury not from the time the patient is seen in the emergency department. A common scenario is a burn patient being transferred from another hospital several hours after a burn and arriving in a severely underresuscitated or overresuscitated state. Calculations for the rate of fluid resuscitation should take the pre-ER resuscitative record into account and reflect the decreased or increased starting intravenous (IV) fluid rate.

Pediatric resuscitation protocols are based on the following formula (H is height [cm], W is weight [kg]):

$$BSA = (87 [H + W] - 2,600)/10,000$$

Pediatric resuscitation protocols are as follows:

- Shriners Burn Institute (Cincinnati)—4 mL/kg/percentage burn plus 1,500 mL/m² BSA
  - First 8 h—LR solution with 50 mEq sodium bicarbonate per liter
  - Second 8 h—LR solution
  - Third 8 h—LR solution plus 12.5 g of 25% albumin solution per liter
- Galveston Shriners Hospital—5,000 mL/m² TBSA burn plus 2,000 mL/m² BSA, using LR solution plus 12.5 g 25% albumin per liter plus D5W solution as needed for hypoglycemia

So what should you be thinking about when the burned child arrives to your ER? The first thing to remember is that there is no stone-cold right answer for resuscitation, but there are some important principles to be aware of. Regardless of the resuscitation formula or strategy used, initial presentation to the emergency department requires frequent adjustments based on your clinical judgment of volume status. Prehospital records of fluid therapy can offer objective clinical guidance to help you establish an appropriate fluid volume for resuscitation. It is important to keep in mind, however, that calculated volumes from all of the formulas should be viewed as estimates of the appropriate fluid volume. Strict adherence to a calculated number can lead to significant overresuscitation or underresuscitation if not correlated with the clinical context. An important point to remember is that overresuscitation is a major source of morbidity for burn patients and can result in increased pulmonary complications and escharotomies of the chest or extremities.

Two very important conceptual differences exist with regard to pediatric burn resuscitation. First, IV fluid resuscitations are usually required for patients with smaller burns (in the range of 10% to 20% vs. >20% for adults). Venous access in small children may be a difficult issue, and a saphenous vein cutdown or an interosseous line is an acceptable access site in the short term if no other peripheral sites are obtainable. Secondly, children have proportionally larger BSA than adults; TBSA burns must be estimated using pediatric modifications according to Lund-Browder tables (*Fig. 214.1*), which demonstrate the relatively larger head and smaller thigh. This results in higher weight-based calculations for resuscitation volume (~6 mL/kg/percentage burn) and has led some to advocate a BSA–based resuscitation in addition to the infusion of a maintenance requirement as described by the Galveston Shriners Hospital pediatric formula. Many other centers, however, simply use the Parkland formula with the addition of a maintenance rate. It is important to note that the Parkland formula can grossly underestimate volume requirements in patients with inhalational injury, electrical injury, or postescharotomy.

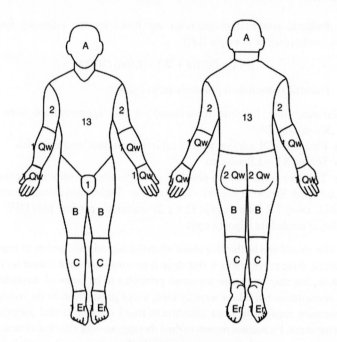

LUND-BROWDER CHART
Relative percentage of body surface area affected by growth

Age in years	0	1	5	10	15	Adult
A—head (back or front)	9 Qw	8 Qw	6 Qw	5 Qw	4 Qw	3 Qw
B—1 thigh (back or front)	2 Er	3 Qr	4	4 Qr	4 Qw	4 Er
C—1 leg (back or front)	2 Qw	2 Qw	2 Er	3	3 Qr	3 Qw

FIGURE 214.1. Lund-Browder tables.

Periodically increasing the fluid rate is better than giving frequent boluses of fluid for low urine output. Fluid boluses result in transient elevations in hydrostatic pressure gradients that further increase the shift of fluids to the interstitium and worsen the edema. However, you should not hesitate to administer a bolus as needed to patients early in the resuscitative period for hypotensive/hypovolemic shock. Also, the urge to maintain urine output at rates >2 to 4 mL/kg/h should be avoided. Fluid overload in the critical hours of early burn management leads to unnecessary edema and pulmonary dysfunction which subsequently can necessitate morbid escharotomies and prolonged ventilator requirements.

Recommended end points of resuscitation are also higher in children, with goal urine output closer to 2 to 4 mL/kg/h. Children approaching 50 kg are probably better served by adult resuscitation parameters of 1 to 2 mL/ kg/h urine output. Another concern with pediatric burn patients is the modest hepatic glycogen reserve, which can be quickly exhausted secondary to a relatively higher hypermetabolic state and sometimes require the change from Lactated Ringer solution to dextrose 5% in LR solution to prevent life-threatening hypoglycemia. For this reason, AccuChecks upon arrival to the ED and then every hour should be routine during this hypermetabolic state, especially for patients with larger burns. If you are having difficulty maintaining euglycemia with LR, then switching to D5LR is a wise choice.

Understanding the resuscitative differences of the pediatric population is the first step toward successful fluid management of a pediatric burn patient. In clinical practice, you should adopt a resuscitative protocol of choice and then know that you will have to titrate the resuscitative efforts based on sound clinical judgment. The most notable areas for improvement in the management of pediatric burns are in fluid resuscitation and airway control as reported by Gore et al. Historically, the main predictors of mortality from burn injury have been the extent of burn, age, presence of inhalational injury, and the worst base deficit in the first 24 h. As a mortal physician, you cannot change the age of the patient or the fact that inhalational injury or the burn even occurred. You can, however, affect the acid-base status of the patient by your fluid resuscitative efforts if you are adequately informed on resuscitative protocols for the pediatric population and are flexible enough to titrate the resuscitation based on clinical judgment. Lastly, transfer the patient to a pediatric burn hospital center sooner rather than later along with the appropriate documentation of your fluid management strategy.

SUGGESTED READINGS

Gore DC, Hawkins HK, Chinkes DL, et al. Assessment of adverse events in the demise of pediatric burn patients. *J Trauma*. 2007;63(4):814–818.

Merrell SW, Saffle JR, Sullivan JJ, et al. Fluid resuscitation in thermally injured children. *Am J Surg*. 1986;152(6):664–669.

O'Neill JA Jr. Fluid resuscitation in the burned child: A reappraisal. *J Pediatr Surg*. 1982;17(5):604–607.

Sheridan RL, Remensnyder JP, Schnitzer JJ, et al. Current expectations for survival in pediatric burns. *Arch Pediatr Adolesc Med*. 2000;154(3):245–249.

Wolfe SE, Rose JK, Desai MH, et al. Mortality determinants in massive pediatric burns. *Ann Surgery*. 1997;225(5):554–569.

Yowler CJ, Fratianne RB. Current status of burn resuscitation. *Clin Plast Surg*. 2000; 27(1):1–10.

215

DO NOT FORGET ABOUT THE SIMPLE, EASY-TO-FIX CAUSES OF IRRITABILITY IN INFANTS

SARAH CHRISTIAN-KOPP, MD

An irritable and inconsolable infant often strikes fear in many emergency physicians. We often begin a sepsis workup, leaving no body fluids unanalyzed and no chest free of imaging. While you *should* be conservative in the workup of an ill-appearing infant, there are a few conditions that have quick fixes and are of a more benign nature but may be easily missed if not specifically evaluated for on physical examination. These include hair tourniquets, corneal abrasions, bites and stings, and paraphimosis.

Hair tourniquets can be easily overlooked and, although rare, may result in morbidity if not treated in a timely manner. It occurs when a hair or other filament becomes wrapped tightly around an appendage. While all infants are susceptible, neonates are particularly prone, as postpartum women experience altered hormone levels resulting in the shedding of larger-than-normal volumes of hair in the months following delivery. The mittens and booties commonly worn early in life also provide a location for the formation of hair tourniquets. To avoid missing this condition, always inspect the genitals, all digits, and the uvula. If present, these regions may initially appear erythematous and edematous with a region of stricture and later may progress to necrosis. Upon careful inspection, the tourniquet may not be visible, and the use of a magnification device may be needed for visualization and is essential for removal of the object. Incision and hair removal cream have both been shown to be effective in the removal of the filament. Before proceeding toward any child's penis, clitoris, digit, or uvula with a scalpel, consider consulting the appropriate specialty if available and inform them of the planned procedure for removal.

An eye exam should also be conducted in an irritable infant in order to ensure there is no a corneal abrasion or foreign body. There may be no known history of ocular injury, and the eye may appear normal on gross examination. It is important to evaluate the eye as thoroughly as possible including the use of fluorescein. The use of topical anesthesia such as prilocaine as a carrier for the fluorescein will not only aid you in conducting the ocular exam (since even infants reflexively clamp an irritated eye shut) but will also give anecdotal confirmation of your suspicion when the irritability is alleviated by the topical analgesia. Also, consider dimming the lights in the room since infants are much more likely to open their eyes in dimmer light.

Insect, arachnid, and animal bites and stings may also be a source of irritability in an inconsolable infant. They may often lead to morbidity and have a significantly higher incidence in the pediatric than the adult population. Children are most often bitten by animals on the face, head, and neck; however, insect stings and bites may occur anywhere on the body. It is essential to do a quick yet thorough skin examination to evaluate for any regions of erythema, swelling, or bite/sting markings. Because the skin may appear normal, it is essential to remain alert for systemic signs of envenomation.

Conducting a genital exam on all irritable infants will prevent you from missing another easy fix: paraphimosis. Paraphimosis is the inability to retract the prepuce (foreskin) distally over the glans penis and is a true urologic emergency. The retracted foreskin serves as a ligature around the glans and prevents appropriate venous return leading to engorgement of the glans and compromised arterial blood flow. Prior to reduction, do not forget pain management via topical and/or parenteral routes. Since reduction will require lubrication, consider using topical viscous lidocaine at appropriate doses. The reduction maneuver includes using your thumb to apply gentle and steady pressure on the glans, while the other fingers are fixed proximal to the prepuce. Local ice, circumferential manual compression, or plastic wraps prior to this procedure help reduce the swelling to facilitate reduction. Success rates are generally high but may require more aggressive measures such as a dorsal slit procedure or even needle decompression. Although time is of the essence, one should consider consultation with urology prior to instrumentation. Following your successful reduction, do not discharge the patient until you verify that the patient is able to void spontaneously and that you have provided teaching on proper penile care and you have established urology follow-up.

TAKE HOME POINT

Always perform a thorough physical exam on any irritable infant, paying special attention to the eyes, skin, genitalia, extremities, and digits. You just may find a more benign source for the infant's irritability and avoid performing the septic infant workup.

SUGGESTED READINGS

Alverson B. A genital hair tourniquet in a 9-year-old girl. *Pediatr Emerg Care*. 2007;23(3): 169–170.

Amitai Y. Scorpion sting in children: A review of 51 cases. *Clin Pediatr*. 1985;24(3):136–140.

Harkness MJ. Corneal abrasion in infancy as a cause of inconsolable crying. *Pediatr Emerg Care*. 1989;December(4):242–244.

Hemmo-Lotem M, Barnea Y, Jinich-Aronowitz C, et al. Epidemiology of pediatric bite/ sting injuries: One-year study of a pediatric emergency department in Israel. *Scientific-WorldJournal*. 2006;6:653–660.

Rodriguez-Acosta A. Centipede envenomation in a newborn. *Rev Inst Med Trop Sao Paulo*. 2000;42(6):341–342.

Serour F, Gorenstein A. Treatment of the toe tourniquet syndrome in infants. *Pediatr Surg Int*. 2003;19(8):598–600.

Steele MT, Ma OJ, Nakase J, et al. Epidemiology of animal exposures presenting to emergency departments. *Acad Emerg Med*. 2007;14(5):398–403.

216

PEDIATRIC PROCEDURAL SEDATION: DO IT RIGHT (OR DO NOT DO IT!)

SARAH CHRISTIAN-KOPP, MD

Performing procedures on pediatric patients can often be rewarding. You become a hero to the parents if you are able to successfully extract a small object from the nose or ear. This is fine if the child holds still, but often, it is a bit more challenging and may require the use of sedation and monitoring.

In order to avoid any major errors in preparation for sedation and procedures, the "SOAPME" acronym should be utilized. This stands for suction, oxygen, airway, pharmacy, monitors, and equipment. You should always have suction catheters that are hooked up, already tested, and ready to go. An oxygen supply with the appropriately sized masks (bag-valve mask, nasal cannula, or simple face mask) should also be tested and pre-set up. "Appropriately sized" may mean that you need to secure access to adult airway equipment. There is nothing more fun than attempting an intubation on a 70-kg, 12-year-old "child" with a Miller 2 laryngoscope blade and a size 4 endotracheal tube!

Medications, including paralytics, sedatives, dissociatives, and analgesics, should be secured at the bedside. If you draw up medications prior to the procedure, make sure to label every syringe so you do not end up giving ketamine when you meant to give morphine. The initial doses should be drawn up and ready for administration as you begin, and additional doses should be available in the event of a prolonged procedure or an insufficient initial dose. Check, check, and triple check to ensure that you are giving the correct medication, in the right concentration, with the appropriate volume, and that your dosing calculations are correct. It is recommended to double check with the nurses as they often have more experience in dosing meds than you! Make sure the person administering the sedation medication is approved to do so according to hospital and state guidelines. In addition, reversal agents should be readily available. If using nitrous oxide, ensure your vacuum scavenger system is hooked up correctly or you will be taking a little journey down anesthesia lane!

Pulse oximetry and continuous cardiovascular monitoring should be in place and active prior, during, and after the procedure. Always have a pediatric crash cart and defibrillation directly available since as we all know—if you have it, you will not need it!

Always make sure you have a patent, functioning, nonpositional IV immediately prior to any procedure. There is nothing like discovering you have inadequate access when you are halfway through a reduction or complicated laceration repair. Also, find the location of a good, large, backup vein *prior* to the sedation in the event the primary line becomes nonfunctional during the sedation.

The importance of continuous cardiovascular and respiratory monitoring during procedures requiring procedural sedation cannot be understated. While most emergency physicians would agree with this statement, it is interesting to note that we often perform lumbar punctures on neonatal and infant patients in an unmonitored setting despite the risks of apnea. While we may assume that the lack of sedation or local anesthesia for this type of procedure lowers the importance of monitoring, it is essential in order to avoid deleterious events that may occur. During a lumbar puncture, the infant's malleable body is flexed to extremes. Do not forget, however, that hyperflexion of the pediatric neck can easily result in narrowing or occlusion of the airway and therefore recommend flexion at the shoulders rather than the neck. For all procedures, make sure that the patient's chest rise is visible and that no one is accidentally compressing the patient's chest or occluding the airway. If left unmonitored, this may not be noticed for some time, possibly even after an anoxic brain injury has occurred. The same precautions must be taken for any procedure where you are unable to continuously evaluate the patient for changes in level of consciousness, work of breathing, and overall general appearance. As a rule, if in doubt, place the patient on a monitor.

During procedures, the beeping sound of the pulse oximetry monitor may be frequent. It is important to differentiate between a low yet valid reading and an inadequate reading without error. First, assess the waveform of the pulse ox reading. If there is a poor waveform, the reading is inaccurate and the pulse ox needs to be adjusted or the monitor evaluated. If there is a good waveform, yet the pulse ox reading is low, assess whether monitored digit is cold. Vasoconstriction in the periphery may result in false low pulse ox readings. If the child appears well and there are no other cardiovascular or pulmonary abnormalities on the monitor, the extremity may be quickly warmed with the examiners hand or a heated towel for reevaluation. In addition, check for nail polish, synthetic nails, or a history of anemia all of which may lead to a low saturation. If the pulse ox reading remains low without explanation or the child appears hypoxic, proceed to airway management. Remember that low oxygen saturation is a *late* finding of respiratory compromise. Do not wait for your response to a low pulse ox reading! Conversely, you can get a false *elevated* pulse ox reading in patients exposed to carbon monoxide. If available, forehead sensors have been shown to provide better monitoring quality in the emergency setting. End-tidal CO_2 monitors should also be used when available since these will often be your most sensitive and most reliable indicators of apnea. Similar to pulse oximetry, an adequate wave form (implying an adequate sampling of exhaled gas) is required for reliable measurements.

Always plan ahead and be prepared for complications pediatric sedation. "SOAPME," redundant medication dosing calculations and labeling, age-appropriate equipment, oxygen and suction, and diligent observation are all required for successful outcomes of pediatric sedation.

SUGGESTED READINGS

American Academy of Pediatrics, American Academy of Pediatric Dentistry, Cote CJ, et al. Guidelines for the monitoring and management of pediatric patients during and after sedation for diagnostic and therapeutic procedures: An update. *Pediatrics*. 2006;118(6): 2587–2602.

American College of Emergency Physicians. Clinical Policy for procedural sedation and analgesia in the emergency department. *Ann Emerg Med*. 1998;31:663–677.

Glauser J. Documentation and standard forms for use during procedural sedation in the emergency department. In: Mace SE, Ducharme J, Murphy M, eds. *Pain Management and Sedation: Emergency Department Management*. New York, NY: McGraw Hill; 2006: 220–230.

Glauser J, Mace SE. Procedural sedation in the emergency department: Regulations as promulgated by the Joint Commission on Accreditation of Healthcare Organizations and establishment of procedural sedation policy within the emergency department. In: Mace SE, Ducharme J, Murphy M, eds. *Pain Management and Sedation: Emergency Department Management*. New York, NY: McGraw-Hill; 2006:15–21.

Godwin SA, Caro DA, Wolf SJ, et al. American College of Emergency Physicians Subcommittee (Writing Committee) on Procedural Sedation and Analgesia in the Emergency Department. Clinical Policy: Procedural sedation and analgesia in the emergency department. *Ann Emerg Med*. 2005;45:177–196.

Nuhr M, Hoerauf K, Joldzo A, et al. Forehead SpO_2 Monitoring compared to finger SpO_2 Recording in emergency transport. *Anaesthesia*. 2004;59(4):390–393.

217

INTUSSUSCEPTION IS A "CANNOT MISS" DIAGNOSIS ... KNOW HOW TO DIAGNOSE AND MANAGE THESE PATIENTS

SARAH CHRISTIAN-KOPP, MD

You have just walked into the emergency department ready for another winter shift full of patients with vomiting and diarrhea. Your colleague gives you one of the most feared lines in all of emergency medicine: "Do you remember that patient from yesterday?" Sadly, it is not an uncommon phenomenon when a patient, who was initially diagnosed with a "viral syndrome," now presents the following day with classic symptoms of an intussusception.

Intussusception is a "cannot miss" diagnosis, given the high incidence of mortality if left untreated. We all are probably guilty of disregarding this diagnosis when it does not present with the classical intussusception triad symptoms of abdominal pain, vomiting, and bloody stools. While this may be tempting, especially during "viral GI season," you must remain alert, as less than one third of cases of intussusception present with all three components. Approximately 75% of patients will have only two findings, and 13% will have only one or none, allowing it to masquerade as a more benign condition. We always look for the classic finding of bloody stools, but do not forget that this is a late finding and that the presentation may also include hematemesis. Also, remember that lethargy may be the only presenting sign of intussusception in infants and therefore should be considered when heading down the sepsis work-up pathway.

When obtaining a history for any child with GI complaints or lethargy, always ask about any recent viral illnesses. This may lead to enlarged Peyer patches that can function as a lead point for intussusception. Also, ask about a history of intussusception in siblings, which increases the risk about 15 to 20 times.

On physical exam, palpate for a sausagelike mass in the right upper quadrant, which is the actual intussusception, as well as a paucity of abdominal contents in the right lower quadrant, since everything is moved upward. This absence of bowel contents, known as Dance sign, is uncommon but pathognomonic for intussusception. If you have the slightest suspicion of an intussusception, obtain a three-view abdominal series. This series should include upright, lateral, and supine views. Look at the bowel gas pattern in the different positions. If there is air in the ascending colon on all three views, an intussusception is very unlikely. A series with air in the ascending colon on only one or zero views makes an intussusception much more likely. Make sure films allow for visualization of the entire colon and be sure to check for soft tissue masses, evidence of obstruction, free air, and obscuring of the liver margin. Remember, films can be normal in 30% of patients. If ultrasound, the preferred imaging of choice, is available, get one! Ultrasound is the least invasive and most commonly used diagnostic measure. Despite operator variability, ultrasound has been shown to have a sensitivity of 95% to 99% and a specificity of 88% to 98% for intussusception. Do not forget that most intussusceptions are ileocolic but may be ileoileal (particularly in patients with Henoch-Schonlein purpura), in which case, you may need to get a CT scan for better visualization.

A barium or air contrast enema is both diagnostic and therapeutic. If you have a choice, air contrast is the preferred method, since it allows for better colonic pressure control, and in the event of perforation, will not be deleterious if the air spills into the peritoneum. Be prepared for the less-than-ideal outcomes of perforation or failure, by ensuring that pediatric surgery has been informed of the impending procedure and remember to provide the patient with a fluid bolus (20 mL/kg), analgesics, IV access, and keep them NPO (nothing by mouth) status.

Do not discharge these children home once they are successfully reduced. There is a recurrence rate of 2% to 10% within the first 1 to 2 days, and therefore, they must be admitted for observation. If the child appears toxic, broad-spectrum antibiotic coverage with ampicillin, gentamicin, and either metronidazole or clindamycin should be started in the emergency department. Also, children over 2 years of age tend to have a lead point that initiated the intussusception. The pediatric surgery team should consider investigating this since a lead point may be as simple as mesenteric adenitis following viral gastroenteritis but could be as serious as a presenting complication of lymphoma.

To avoid mishaps in the management and diagnosis of intussusception, always remember that the majority of patients do not have the classic triad of symptoms. Get a three-view abdominal series to look for a paucity of gas in the ascending colon or, preferably, an ultrasound. An air contrast enema is the ideal choice as it is both diagnostic and therapeutic. Lastly, these kids are keepers, and admit them for observation.

SUGGESTED READINGS

Daneman A, Alton DJ, Ein S, et al. Perforation during attempted intussusception reduction in children-a comparison of perforation with barium and air. *Pediatr Radiol.* 1995;25(2):81–88.

Hadidi AT, El Shal N. Childhood intussusception: A comparative study of non-surgical management. *J Pediatr Surg.* 1999;34(2):304–307.

Kim YS, Ruh JH. Intussusception in infancy and childhood: Analysis of 385 cases. *Int Surg.* 989;74(2):114–118.

Marx J, Hockberger R, Walls R, et al., eds. Intussusception. In: *Rosen's Emergency Medicine. Concepts and Clinical Practice.* 6th ed. Philadelphia, PA: Saunders; 2006:2610–2612.

Meyer JS, Dangman BC, Duonomo C, et al. Air and liquid contrast agents in the management of intussusception: A controlled, randomized trial. *Radiology.* 1993;188(2):507–511.

Roskind CG, Ruzal-Shapiro CB, Dowd EK, et al. Test characteristics of the 3-view abdominal radiograph series in the diagnosis of intussusception. *Pediatr Emerg Care.* 2007;23(11): 785–789.

Tintinalli JE, Kelen GD, Stapczynski JS, et al., eds. Intussusception. In: *Emergency Medicine: A Comprehensive Study Guide.* 6th ed. New York, NY: McGraw-Hill; 2003:818–819.

218

Do not miss abdominal injuries after blunt trauma in the pediatric patient

Joseph J. DuBose, MD, FACS

The early and effective diagnosis of pediatric abdominal injuries remains one of the greatest challenges facing trauma providers. In the absence of clear operative indications (peritonitis, hypotension, and a positive focused abdominal sonography for trauma [FAST]), concerns over missed injuries continue to worry pediatricians, emergency physicians, and surgeons alike. Some retrospective studies estimate the incidence of missed injuries as high as 20%.

Several injury-related factors appear to be important and should raise the suspicion for intra-abdominal injuries. In retrospective reviews, mechanism of injury appears to be a particularly important factor. Patients with injury due to motor vehicle accident, falls of >10 ft, automobile hitting pedestrian, and assaults with loss of consciousness all warrant CT evaluation and intensive monitoring. If the event was unwitnessed, suspicion threshold for advanced imaging should, likewise, be low.

Physical examination of the abdomen remains the appropriate initial evaluation. Physical markings on the abdomen, particularly seat belt signs, significantly increase the likelihood of intra-abdominal injury and mandate evaluation with CT and intensive observation. Initial physical exam alone, however, does not possess adequate sensitivity to exclude significant intra-abdominal injury.

Several screening protocols utilizing laboratory evaluations have been proposed for use in detecting intra-abdominal injury. Based on existing data, however, laboratory evaluations are overly time-intensive tests that lack appropriate sensitivity to identify or exclude injury.

The use of ultrasound, in the form of the FAST exam, has become a routine practice for both adult and pediatric blunt abdominal trauma. While a useful screening tool if a positive exam is noted, the use of ultrasound in the pediatric population has been associated with disappointingly low sensitivity and questionable negative predictive value. Detection of free fluid alone has not proven a reliable indicator, as significant intra-abdominal injury is frequently present in the absence of free fluid. In fact, >40% of low-grade liver or spleen injuries and 11% of high-grade injuries would go undetected at FAST based on the absence of fluid. The sensitivity of FAST is also operator dependent and widely variable, with values ranging anywhere between 33% and 92.5% for detection of abdominal injury in children. Complete abdominal ultrasound, while providing a more comprehensive evaluation of the solid organs in addition to assessing for the presence of free fluid, also has a sensitivity of only between 65% and 71%.

Due to the limitations of physical exam and other imaging modalities, abdominal CT has seen increasing utilization in the trauma setting. This subsequent increase in CT use has also increased awareness regarding the radiation risk associated with these examinations. Although the assumptions, upon which some of these risk figures are published, are based largely on presumptive data, the risk of CT is, nevertheless, a real entity. All emergency physicians and surgeons should be well versed in these controversies. Involving trauma team members and the family in any discussion regarding the risk/benefit of CT is paramount. If CT use is deemed appropriate, then all efforts should be made to work with the radiologist to utilize radiation levels that are as low as reasonably achievable (ALARA) for the specific patient in question.

Until more reliable alternatives are developed, however, CT remains an integral part of the evaluation of the pediatric abdomen after trauma. Although CT has important limitations, including the inability to reliably diagnose hollow viscus injuries, the information obtained from appropriately performed CTs of the abdomen remains the gold standard for the diagnosis and triage of intra-abdominal injuries. If a CT is negative or inconclusive, and the mechanism of injury was significant, admission with serial exams and intensive observation should be undertaken.

In conclusion, the diagnosis of pediatric intra-abdominal injury remains a challenging task. Missed injuries are not uncommon and can be lethal. While the effective evaluation and treatment of these patients requires effective communication between emergency medicine physicians, surgeons, radiologists, and family decision makers, I strongly advise the judicious use of CT and admission for serial exams to prevent errors. Pediatrics colleagues, in particular, may be prone to advising parents that CT use is linked to cancer risk—politely remind them that cancer is a complication of trauma SURVIVORS and that while deciding not to use CT in appropriate settings may decrease cancer risk later in life, it will increase your risk of missing a lethal injury that may end that life much sooner.

SUGGESTED READINGS

Adamson WT, Hebra A, Thomas PB, et al. Serum amylase and lipase alone are not cost-effective screening methods for pediatric pancreatic trauma. *J Pediatr Surg.* 2003;38: 354–357.

Bixby SD, Callahan MJ, Taylor GA. Imaging in pediatric blunt abdominal trauma. *Semin Roentgenol.* 2008;43:72–82.

Bloom AI, Rivkind A, Zamir G, et al. Blunt injury of the small intestine and mesentery—the trauma surgeon's achilles heel? *Eur J Emerg Med.* 1996;3:85–91.

Chandler CF, Lane JS, Waxman KS. Seatbelt sign following blunt trauma is associated with increased incidence of abdominal injury. *Am Surg.* 1997;63:885–888.

Coley BD, Mutabagani KH, Martin LC, et al. Focused abdominal sonography for trauma (FAST) in children with blunt abdominal trauma. *J Trauma.* 2000;48:902–906.

Eppich WJ, Zonfrillo MR. Emergency department evaluation and management of blunt abdominal trauma in children. *Curr Opin Pediatr.* 2007;19:265–269.

Fenton SJ, Hansen KW, Meyers RL, et al. CT scan and the pediatric trauma patient: Are we overdoing it? *J Pediatr Surg.* 2004;39:1877–1881.

Holmes JF, Gladman A, Chang CH. Performance of abdominal ultrasonography in pediatric blunt trauma patients: A meta-analysis. *J Pediatr Surg.* 2007;42:1588–1594.

Krupnick AS, Teitelbaum DH, Geiger JD, et al. Use of abdominal ultrasonography to assess pediatric splenic trauma: Potential pitfalls in the diagnosis. *Ann Surg.* 1997;225:408–414.

Peery CL, Chendrasekhar A, Paradise NF, et al. Missed injuries in pediatric trauma. *Am Surg.* 1999;65:1067–1069.

Rice HE, Frush DP, Farmer D, et al. APSA Education Committee: Review of radiation risks from computed tomography: Essentials for the pediatric surgeon. *J Pediatr Surg.* 2007;42:603–607.

Salim A, Sangthong B, Martin M, et al. Whole body imaging in blunt multisystem trauma patients without obvious signs of injury: Results of a prospective study. *Arch Surg.* 2006;141:468–473; discussion 473–475.

Sievers EM, Murray JA, Chen D, et al. Abdominal computed tomography scan in pediatric blunt abdominal trauma. *Am Surg.* 1999;65:968–971.

Sokolove PE, Kuppermann N, Holmes JF. Association between the "seat belt sign" and intra-abdominal injury in children with blunt torso trauma. *Acad Emerg Med.* 2005;12:808–813.

Soyuncu S, Cete Y, Bozan H, et al. Accuracy of physical and ultrasonographic examinations by emergency physicians for the early diagnosis of intraabdominal haemorrhage in blunt abdominal trauma. *Injury.* 2007;38:564–569.

Velmahos GC, Tatevossian R, Demetriades D. The "seat belt mark" sign: A call for increased vigilance among physicians treating victims of motor vehicle accidents. *Am Surg.* 1999;65:181–185.

Venkatesh KR, McQuay N Jr. Outcomes of management in stable children with intra-abdominal free fluid without solid organ injury after blunt abdominal injury. *J Trauma.* 2007;62:216–220.

219

THE "SHOCKY" NEWBORN: THERE IS MORE TO CONSIDER THAN JUST SEPSIS

ANITA W. EISENHART, DO, FACOEP, FACEP
AND BRENNA K. YURSIK, MD, MPH

While sepsis is paramount in the differential when evaluating and managing the shocky newborn (1 to 4 weeks of age), there are other, less common, but just as life-threatening, diagnoses that need consideration by the emergency physician. Some of these problems include congenital adrenal hyperplasia (CAH) with acute salt wasting syndrome and cardiac ductal-dependent lesions, both of which can cause a shocky-appearing newborn.

CAH is a family of disorders, more than 90% of which are caused by a 21-hydroxylase deficiency. This form occurs in about 1:12,000 live births (1:300 in Yupik Eskimos of Alaska). While many American babies are routinely screened, some newborns with the disorder are undiagnosed, until they present to you in shock! There are several forms and presentations of CAH. However, the most important to recognize in the emergency department (ED) is acute salt-wasting syndrome. This newborn will present in the first month of life with progressively decreasing appetite and activity over hours to days. Other symptoms include irritability, weight loss, and vomiting. They are sometimes misdiagnosed with gastroenteritis or pyloric stenosis. Initial laboratory evaluation will include hyponatremia and hyperkalemia (the classic findings for adrenal crisis). Hypoglycemia is often seen in the stressed newborn, as they have increased metabolic demands, decreased carbohydrate intake, and an underutilized gluconeogenesis pathway with minimal glycogen stores. A metabolic acidosis and hemoconcentration from dehydration are also expected findings.

The initial resuscitation for the CAH baby with acute salt-wasting syndrome is supportive. Hypotension and electrolyte derangements will improve with intravenous or intraosseous isotonic sodium chloride boluses. Hypoglycemia should be treated with dextrose boluses as well as drips. Ultimately, you will need to administer glucocorticoids, which will additionally correct the electrolytes and halt the progression of salt wasting. Hydrocortisone is initially dosed as 1 to 2 mg/kg bolus. The major caveat here is the necessity for obtaining an extra serum sample for hormone testing before steroids are administered. Testing will include cortisol, aldosterone, and 17-hydroxyprogesterone levels. Again, serum for this testing must be obtained **prior** to the administration of any glucocorticoids, so as not to taint the results. Emergent pediatric endocrine and intensive care consultation with admission should follow stabilization efforts.

A second diagnosis to consider in the shocky newborn is a ductal-dependant cardiac lesion. These are the left heart lesions and include hypoplastic left heart, congenital aortic stenosis, interrupted aortic arch, and coarctation of the aorta. These babies present in cardiogenic shock as the ductus arteriosis closes, usually within the first few days of life. The typical history includes an uncomplicated delivery with a short well-baby nursery stay (often without a prenatal sonogram as these lesions are often diagnosed at that time). As the ductus arteriosis closes, the newborn will have less energy, decreased appetite, irritability, and increased sleep. This will develop over several hours and progress to symptoms of dehydration and poor perfusion secondary to cardiogenic shock.

They will present anywhere from pale and irritable to mottled, ashen gray, and obtunded. Tachycardia, tachypnea, and hypotension will all be noted as the baby decompensates and fails to perfuse from lack of left heart functional activity. Bedside glucose may be low from the increased metabolic demand of shock, decreased intake, and poor gluconeogenesis at this age. Initial resuscitation is supportive with airway, ventilation, and access. Fluids and pressors should be initiated and dextrose administered in the phase of hypoglycemia. The lifesaving maneuver in these children is to open up the ductus arteriosis so that the functioning right heart can resume circulatory support as systemic blood flow. This is done with prostaglandin (PGE_1). The dose is 0.05 to 0.1 $\mu g/kg/min$. Immediate consultation with pediatric intensive care and pediatric cardiology should ensue.

All shocky newborns, regardless of the ultimate diagnosis, should be evaluated for hypoglycemia (for reasons discussed above) and for sepsis. Blood and urine cultures must be obtained when possible and broad-spectrum antibiotics initiated as soon as intravenous or intraosseous access is established, regardless of the infant's temperature and white blood cell count. A lumbar puncture should not be performed until the baby is stabilized, as the tightly flexed position may prove dangerous for the already-decompensated patient. General principles of emergency stabilization should be employed, including establishing a reliable airway, ventilation, and circulatory support. Social support for the family is a high priority, and disposition should be arranged expeditiously to a pediatric intensive care unit (PICU).

SUGGESTED READINGS

American Academy of Pediatrics; Section on Endocrinology and Committee on Genetics. Technical report: Congenital adrenal hyperplasia. *Pediatrics*. 2000;106(6):1511–1518.

Cloherty JP, Stark AR, *Manual of Neonatal Care.* 4th ed. Philadelphia, PA: Lippincott-Raven; 1998.

Gerardi M. Neonatal emergencies. *Pediatric Emergency Medicine Reports.* 1996;1(12): 1–13.

Taeusch HW, Ballard RA, Gleason CA, et al., eds. *Avery's Diseases of the Newborn.* 7th ed. Philadelphia, PA: Saunders; 1998.

Wilson TA. *Congenital Adrenal Hyperplasia.* Updated April 2008. Available at: www.emedicine. com.

220

BE WARY OF MEDICATION DOSING ERRORS IN PEDIATRIC RESUSCITATION

LAWRENCE A. DeLuca, Jr, EdD, MD

Medication dosing errors in the pediatric emergency department setting are fairly common occurrences. Accurate dosing of medications and fluids is crucial to achieving a therapeutic effect while minimizing toxicity and side effects. Critical illness in both adults and children frequently requires weight- or body surface area–based dosing of medications. However, in the pediatric population, the smaller size of the patient can significantly worsen the impact of dosage errors.

Always look up the dosage! Aside from a few commonly used dosages that you likely already have committed to memory (15 mg/kg/dose of Tylenol, 20 mL/kg of isotonic crystalloid for boluses), use some sort of drug reference for pediatric dosing. Tools such as the Physician's Desk Reference or online resources such as www.rxlist.com can provide access to packaging inserts for most drugs.

Get as accurate an estimate of the child's weight as possible! Historically, in emergent situations, this has involved the use of tools such as the Broselow tape. However, there is evidence that a parent's weight estimate, if available, may be more accurate. The Broselow tape also may not accurately reflect weights in non-Caucasian populations. For example, the Broselow tape overestimates weight in Indian children by approximately 10%, and different tools may have different performance characteristics. Remember that the Broselow tape's weight estimates are just that—estimates! There is no "McBurger" edition that will provide corrections for obesity due to poor diet or sedentary lifestyle.

Be as explicit in your orders as possible—some medications come in multiple dosages! Perhaps the worst offender in this regard is epinephrine, available in both 1:1,000 and 1:10,000 dilutions, both of which are used in pediatric resuscitations. Selection of the wrong agent could result in severe under- or overdosing and could be fatal.

Use preprinted, weight-based tables for dosing rather than calculating dosages! In most emergency departments, this will be a Broselow tape or some other sort of dosing card. In some pediatric intensive care units, where daily weights are available on patients, dosages may be precalculated and posted in the room.

Titrate medications to clinical end points! Just as tools like the Broselow tape provide an estimate of body weight, drug dosages themselves provide an estimate of effect for an individual based upon a study cohort's response to a given dose of the drug. There will be considerable individual variability—especially in sedative medication in the pediatric population.

Use closed-loop communication during resuscitation! For example, the physician may give an order for "lidocaine 15 mg IV per the Broselow tape." The nurse or medic administering the medication should verify the dose and repeat back the order—"administered lidocaine 15 mg IV per the Broselow tape"—or request verification—"the suggested dosage range of lidocaine is 1 to 1.5 mg/kg. Do you still wish to administer 15 mg to this 10-kg child?"

Promote a respectful and congenial atmosphere! If colleagues are afraid to speak up, an obvious medication dosage error might go unchallenged.

Work with a pharmacist when possible! Full-time (but not part-time) clinical pharmacists have been shown (at least in the ICU setting) to reduce the rate of serious medication errors. If a clinical pharmacist is in-house, he or she should also attend any pediatric codes.

Use technology when available! Computer-based systems to reduce medication dosage errors have shown promise in adult care settings but have shown more modest gains in the pediatric environment. Improvements in technology may make these tools even more useful in the future.

Do not leave unlabeled syringes lying around! If you draw up a drug, label it immediately. Most drugs preparations are clear and can easily be confused with a flush, with potentially disastrous results.

THE BOTTOM LINE

Medication dosing errors are common! Attention to detail and use of resources such as clinical pharmacists, nurses, and dosage charts/calculators can help dramatically reduce the incidence of these errors and the resultant complications. The next time someone rankles you by questioning a dosage you have written—be sure to thank him or her! He or she may have helped avoid serious harm to your patient.

SUGGESTED READINGS

DuBois D, Baldwin S, King WD. Accuracy of weight estimation methods for children. *Pediatr Emerg Care*. 2007;23(4):227–230.

Kausha R, Bates DW, Abramson EL, et al. Unit-based clinical pharmacists' prevention of serious medication errors in pediatric inpatients. *Am J Health Syst Pharm*. 2008;65(13):1 254–1260.

Krieser D, Nguyen K, Kerr D, et al. Parental weight estimation of their child's weight is more accurate than other weight estimation methods for determining children's weight in an emergency department? *Emerg Med J*. 2007;24(11):756–759.

Lubitz DS, Seidel JS, Chameides L, et al. A rapid method for estimating weight and resuscitation drug dosages from length in the pediatric age group. *Ann Emerg Med*. 1988;17(6):576–581.

Physicians' desk reference: PDR. Oradel, NJ: Medical Economics Co. 2005.

Ramarajan N, Krishnamoorthi R, Strehlow M, et al. Internationalizing the Broselow tape: How reliable is weight estimation in Indian children. *Acad Emerg Med*. 2008;15(5):431–436.

Rinke ML, Moon M, Clark JS, et al. Prescribing errors in a pediatric emergency department. *Pediatr Emerg Care*. 2008;24(1):1–8.

Shamliyan TA, Duval S, Du J, et al. Just what the doctor ordered: Review of the evidence of the impact of computerized physician order entry system on medication errors. *Health Serv Res*. 2008;43(1 Pt 1):32–53.

Takata GS, Mason W, Taketomo C, et al. Development, testing, and findings of a pediatric-focused trigger tool to identify medication-related harm in US children's hospitals. *Pediatrics*. 2008;121(4):e927–e935.

221

DO NOT RELY SOLELY ON PATIENT APPEARANCE OR LABORATORY RESULTS WHEN DETERMINING THE DISPOSITION OF A FEBRILE NEONATE FROM THE EMERGENCY DEPARTMENT

STEPHANIE M. CASTRILLO, MD AND CONRAD J. CLEMENS, MD, MPH

Deciding the disposition of a febrile neonate is a common and often daunting task. This is particularly true when the neonate appears well, there are no pre- or perinatal risk factors, the neonate meets "low risk" criteria, and the parents are deemed reliable. Further confusion can ensue if the neonate is found to have a viral illness, such as respiratory syncytial virus (RSV). Despite attempts over the past few decades to develop guidelines, significant variability occurs in practice with regard to the workup and treatment of febrile neonates.

The term "neonate" has not been consistently used throughout the literature, which is essential, given that bacteremia is more than twice as frequent in the 1st month of life (7.4%) than it is in the 2nd month of life (3.1%), illustrating that 0 to 3 months of age is not a homogenous group, and therefore should not be treated like one. Strictly defined, a neonate is an infant ≤28 days old. In this age group, fever is defined as temperature of 100.4°F or 38.0°C measured rectally. Parental report of a fever should be treated similarly to a documented fever in the ED, even if, at the time of presentation, the neonate is afebrile.

When evaluating a febrile neonate, there are three well-known sets of criteria, including the "Boston Criteria," the "Philadelphia Criteria," and, probably the most widely used and recognized, the "Rochester Criteria." Each of these attempts to classify patients into high- and low-risk categories based on clinical appearance and laboratory results. *Table 221.1* summarizes the low-risk criteria for each.

However, when applying these criteria to neonates (<28 days old), a concerning picture emerges. Baker et al. (1993) found that when applying the Philadelphia criteria, 4.6% of neonates classified as low risk had serious bacterial infections (SBI). When applying the Rochester Criteria, Ferrera et al. (1997) found that 6% of neonates <29 days old had SBI, including one neonate who had two simultaneous infections, one of which was meningitis, thereby increasing the total number of SBI to four and proving that finding a single infectious etiology does not exclude the possibility of others. These findings demonstrate that although these criteria are fairly reliable at predicting SBI in neonates

TABLE 221.1	THREE CRITERIA FOR EVALUATING A FEBRILE NEONATE		
BOSTON CRITERIA	**PHILADELPHIA CRITERIA**	**ROCHESTER CRITERIA**
Well appearing	Well appearing	Well appearing
CSF: <10 WBC/hpf	CSF: <8 WBC/hpf, Negative Gram stain	
UA: <10 WBC/hpf, dipstick negative for leukocyte esterase	UA: <10 WBC/hpf, No/ few bacteria on spun urine specimen	UA: <10 WBC/hpf on spun urine sediment
Peripheral WBC <20,000/ mm^3	Peripheral WBC <15,000/ mm^3, band: neutrophil <0.2	Peripheral WBC <15,000/mm^3, normal absolute band counts (<1,500/mm^3)
Normal CXR (if indicated)	Normal CXR (if indicated)	
	Stool: negative for blood, few or no WBC (if indicated)	Stool: <5 WBC/hpf on smear (if indicated)

(the Rochester criteria were found to have a negative predictive value of 98.9%), they are not 100% sensitive and therefore should not be used as such.

Note a few reasons why the above mentioned criteria are less accurate in neonates:

1) *Well appearance*: Determining if an infant is well appearing relies on the experience of the physician with neonates.

2) *UA WBC count*: Urinalysis is often unreliable in neonates due to their decreased ability to concentrate urine. Marom et al. (2007) found the urinalysis to be normal in 12.9% of infants (<3 months old) with urinary tract infection (UTI).

Lastly, significant controversy surrounds the issue of managing neonates diagnosed with RSV, influenza, or other viral illnesses. Levine et al. (2004) found that although RSV-negative infants had a higher rate of SBI (12.5%), 7% of the RSV-positive infants had a bacterial superinfection. Therefore, a complete septic workup as well as administration of IV antibiotics and hospital admission is necessary even in febrile neonates with a confirmed viral diagnosis in the ED.

Although the most common cause of fever in neonates is of viral etiology and the majority of neonates with bacterial infection are found to have UTI/ pyelonephritis, the urgency of performing a complete septic workup, starting appropriate IV therapy (ampicillin 50 mg/kg q6h and cefotaxime 50 mg/kg q6h) and admitting the neonate for further observation and treatment, is due to the potentially devastating consequences of sepsis and meningitis, both of which are associated with high morbidity and possibly death. Therefore, no febrile neonate should ever be sent home from the ED because he or she appears well, is classified as "low risk" by any or all of the above mentioned criteria, is RSV positive, or his or her parents assure primary care physician (PCP) follow-up within 24 h.

SUGGESTED READINGS

Baker MD, Bell LM, Aner JR. Outpatient management without antibiotics of fever in selected infant. *N Engl J Med*. 1993;329(20):1437–1441.

Berman S. *Pediatric Decision Making*. 2nd ed. Philadelphia, PA: B.C Decker Inc.; 1991.

Ferrera PC, Bartfield JM, Snyder HS. Neonatal fever: Utility of the Rochester criteria in determining low risk for serious bacterial infections. *Am J Emerg Med*. 1997;15:299–302.

Jaskiewicz JA, McCarthy CA, Richardson AC, et al. Febrile infants at low risk for serious bacterial infection-an appraisal of the Rochester criteria and Implications for management. Febrile Infant Collaborative Study Group. *Pediatrics*. 1994;94(3):390–396.

Levine DA, Platt SL, Dayan PS, et al. Risk of serious bacterial infection in young febrile infants with respiratory syncytial virus infections. *Pediatrics*. 2004;113(6):1728–1734.

Marom R, Sakran W, Antonelli J, et al. Quick Identification of febrile neonates with low risk for serious bacterial infection: An observational study. *Arch Dis Child Fetal Neonatal Ed*. 2007;92(1):F15–F18.

Roberts KB. Young, febrile infants: A 30-year odyssey ends where it started. *JAMA*. 2004;291(10):1261–1262.

222

DO NOT RELY ON A URINALYSIS TO EXCLUDE URINARY TRACT INFECTION IN PATIENTS YOUNGER THAN 2 YEARS OLD

TYLER R. PEARCE, MD

Proper diagnosis and treatment of urinary tract infections (UTIs) in young children are essential to prevent life-threatening complications and long-term sequelae. The overall prevalence of UTI is 5% in all febrile children 3 to 24 months of age and is as high as 16% in white girls with a temperature >39°C. Unlike adults, children have few localizing symptoms of UTI and often present with fever, vomiting, and poor feeding. Pyelonephritis is more common than cystitis in young children and can lead to renal scarring, hypertension, and hasten end-stage renal disease. UTIs in children are also frequently associated with anatomic abnormalities of the GU tract, such as vesicoureteral reflux disease, which is detectable in as many as 30% to 40% of children 1 to 24 months old with febrile UTIs. Though the high risk of sepsis in children <3 months old with a febrile UTI is well known, remember that 5% of UTIs in those >3 months are also at risk for sepsis from concomitant bacteremia. Treatment of older infants and young children with suspected UTI is less uniform than for those <3 months of age. The American Academy of Pediatrics (AAP) recommends that catheterized urine cultures be sent of all children in whom UTI is suspected, but emergency physicians do not consistently follow this advice. One study indicated that emergency physicians only sent culture on 67% of urine samples of febrile children 3 to 36 months of age after urinalysis (UA) was obtained.

Diagnosis

One reason for this trend is over reliance on UA to diagnosis UTI in this age group. UA uses nitrite and leukocyte esterase as indicators to predict the likelihood of UTI, which are indirect measurements of pyuria and bacteriuria. In adults with urinary symptoms, the UA is an effective tool due to its high sensitivity, which is around 95%. This means that urinary dipstick is good at *ruling out* a UTI when negative, without the need of urine culture. However, both nitrite and leukocyte esterase require bacteria to incubate in the urine for at least 4 h in order for a detectable amount to be reached. This creates a dilemma in using the UA to diagnose UTI in younger children, since they do not hold their urine prior to the age of toilet training.

Consequently, the sensitivity of this test is significantly less in young children than in older children and adults. One study looked at the sensitivity of dipstick UA compared to urine culture and found that it was only 87.5% sensitive at detecting UTI in children 0 to 2 years of age but had a sensitivity of 100% in children 2 to 10 years of age. Another retrospective review of 37,450 children 0 to 2 years old demonstrated a sensitivity of 82% for detecting UTI by standard UA when compared to urine culture. The sensitivity did not differ when further broken down by age for the 0- to 2-year-old group. This means that both microscopic UA and urinary dipstick are much less sensitive at detecting UTIs in children <2 years old than in adults. Using UA alone, up to 18% of children with a UTI are missed!

A properly collected urine specimen must be sent for culture if UTI is suspected. Though a bag specimen may be used for UA if processed promptly, culture from a bag specimen is essentially useless. Studies have shown that as many as 85% of bagged urine specimens sent for culture are false positives and are only useful if negative. The AAP practice guidelines affirm that cultures must be obtained via suprapubic aspiration or catheterization in children 2 months to 2 years of age.

Bottom Line

A negative UA does not exclude a UTI in children <2 years old! The urine culture is diagnostic. Obtain urine specimens via SPA or urethral bladder catheterization in this age group and culture all urine specimens collected in the emergency department after initial UA. Do not obtain bagged specimens! Admit febrile neonates, dehydrated or toxic-appearing children to the hospital with parenteral antibiotics. If the patient is well enough to be discharged from the ED, begin antibiotics while awaiting urine culture if the UA is indicative of a UTI. If UA is negative, communicate positive culture results to patient's family or primary care physician and initiate antimicrobial therapy. If your emergency department does not have a reliable means to follow-up on urine cultures of discharged patients, establish one and make it work. The more serious clinical implications and less certain clinical diagnosis of UTI in this population require increased vigilance by the emergency physician.

SUGGESTED READINGS

[No authors listed]. Practice parameter: The diagnosis, treatment, and evaluation of the initial urinary tract infection in febrile infants and young children. American Academy of Pediatrics. Committee on Quality Improvement. Subcommittee on Urinary Tract Infection. *Pediatrics*. 1999;103(4 Pt 1):843–852.

Bachur R, Harper MB. Reliability of the urinalysis for predicting urinary tract infections in young febrile children. *Arch Pediatr Adolesc Med*. 2001;155(1):60–55.

Doley A, Nelligan M. Is a negative dipstick urinalysis good enough to exclude urinary tract infection in paediatric emergency department patients? *Emerg Med*. 2003;15(1):77–80.

Hoberman A, Charron M, Hickey RW, et al. Imaging studies after a first febrile urinary tract infection in young children. *N Engl J Med*. 2003;348(3):195–202.

Isaacman DJ, Kaminer K, Veligeti H, et al. Comparative practice patterns of emergency medicine physicians and pediatric emergency medicine physicians managing fever in young children. *Pediatrics*. 2001;108(2):354–358.

Pappas PG. Laboratory in the diagnosis and management of urinary tract infection. *Med Clin North Am*. 1991;75(2):313–325.

Shaikh N, Monroe NE, Bost JE, et al. Prevalence of urinary tract infection in childhood: A meta-analysis. *Pediatr Infect Dis J*. 2008;27(4):302–308.

Tobiansky R, Evans N. A randomized controlled trial of two methods for collection of sterile urine in neonates. *J Paediatr Child Health*. 1998;34(5):460–462.

223

NOT ALL EAR PAIN IS ACUTE OTITIS MEDIA … AND NOT ALL REQUIRE ANTIBIOTICS!

MICHAEL P. WILSON, MD, PhD AND GARY M. VILKE, MD

Acute otitis media (AOM) is a common cause of ear pain and is a prevalent infection in young children, with a majority of children receiving at least one diagnosis of AOM by their 7th year of life. According to the American Academy of Pediatrics, a diagnosis of AOM requires three criteria: rapid onset of symptoms

(<48 h), middle ear effusion or air-fluid level, and middle ear inflammation, which is generally indicated by erythema of the tympanic membrane. The otoscopic exam will note a bulging erythematous tympanic membrane, particularly when compared with the other "normal" ear. Features of the history or physical exam that suggest a diagnosis of otitis externa instead of AOM include pain upon traction of the pinna, a history of recent swimming, or erythema of the otic canal.

Often, AOM is difficult to confirm with certainty, since a crying infant will often have an angry-looking tympanic membrane (TM) that can be difficult to distinguish from infection. If the child is older than 2 years of age, or if diagnosis is uncertain in a child older than 6 months, a "wait and see" approach is appropriate, in which parents are given an antibiotic prescription and asked to wait to fill the prescription for approximately 2 days. Since many cases of uncomplicated and uncertain AOM get better on their own, a recent Cochrane review concluded that this option would reduce antibiotic use anywhere from 23% to 75%. Three studies reviewed by the Cochrane team, however, also showed that patient satisfaction was higher with traditional, immediate antibiotic approach. Remember that this option is only appropriate for children who do not appear ill, are not immunocompromised, do not have a perforated TM, and have not already failed an antibiotic trial.

However, not all ear pain is AOM. In fact, one study noted that 50% of adults with ear pain in a general medicine clinic have pain from another source that is referred to the ear. So, when should a more concerning cause of ear pain be suspected? Part of the diagnostic confusion comes from the fact that the ear receives inputs from multiple cranial nerves, and hence pain can be referred from almost any part of the head, including teeth, jaw, sinuses, throat, or neck. Case reports even document isolated ear pain from such distant sites as the chest in myocardial infarction, although this fortunately is a rarer cause.

The cardinal sign of referred ear pain is persistent pain with a normal ear exam. This should prompt a search for another source of the pain and to assess for the "must not miss" diagnoses. In these patients, look for a retraction in the superior pole of the tympanic membrane, which can be a subtle finding of a cholesteatoma. Ear pain in a diabetic or immunocompromised patient should prompt a careful search for granulation tissue in the otic canal, which may suggest malignant or necrotizing otitis externa. A history of dysphagia, odynophagia, weight loss, and neck masses may indicate that your patient has a head or neck malignancy, which can present with ear pain in over half of patients. You should examine the neck carefully and have a low threshold to image with a CT if any abnormal findings are noted, particularly if your patient is a heavy drinker or smoker, older than 50 years, or has multiple other medical problems. Finally, patients over 50 years of age with palpable pain over the area of the temporal artery along with the ear pain should have an erythrocyte sedimentation rate (ESR) drawn to assess for temporal arteritis.

So, what to do if your ear exam is, for some reason, equivocal or if the history does not clearly point you to a particular cause? Although there are few evidence-based studies to provide guidance, one must rule out the worse-case scenarios as above and assess for less critical diagnosis as well. Be sure to ask about hearing loss, which may be a sign of middle or inner ear disease, or sore throat, which can be a sign of pharyngitis. Examine the skin of the ear for cellulitis, which usually involves the earlobe, or relapsing polychondritis, which does not. Note any pain behind the ear, especially if your patient just recovered from AOM, as this can be a sign of mastoiditis. If this is normal, palpate the temporomandibular joint (TMJ) as the patient is chewing to evaluate for TMJ pain. Carefully feel along the gingiva and tap on the teeth with a tongue blade to identify dental caries or apical abscesses.

If your patient has any suspicious findings on your exam, is over 50 years, or has multiple medical problems, an early referral to an otolaryngologist may be appropriate. If your patient is otherwise young and healthy, you may consider a period of observation or empiric treatment with NSAIDS and close follow-up.

SUGGESTED READINGS

AAP Subcommittee on Management of Acute Otitis Media. Diagnosis and management of acute otitis media. *Pediatrics*. 2004;113(5):1451–1465.

Charlett SD, Coatesworth AP. Referred otalgia: A structured approach to diagnosis and treatment. *Int J Clin Pract*. 2007;61(6):1015–1021.

Ely JW, Hansen MR, Clark EC. Diagnosis of ear pain. *Am Fam Physician*. 2008;77(5): 621–628.

Kreiner M, Okeson JP, Michelis V, et al. Craniofacial pain as the sole symptom of cardiac ischemia: A prospective multicenter study. *J Am Dent Assoc*. 2007;138(1):74–79.

Pfaff JA, Moore GP. Otolaryngology. In: Marx JA, Hockberger RS, Walls RM, eds. *Rosen's Emergency Medicine: Concepts and Clinical Practice*. 6th ed. Philadelphia, PA: Mosby; 2006:1066–1078.

Sapira JD. *The Art and Science of Bedside Diagnosis*. 1st ed. Baltimore, MD: Urban & Schwarzenberg; 1990:209.

Shah RK, Blevins NK. Otalgia. *Otolaryngol Clin N Am*. 2003;36:1137–1151.

Spiro DM, Arnold DH. The concept and practice of a wait-and-see approach to acute otitis media. *Curr Opin Pediatr*. 2008;20:72–78.

Spurling GKP, Del Mar CB, Dooley L, et al. Delayed antibiotics for respiratory infections. *Cochrane Database Syst Rev*. 2007;(3):CD004417 [Review].

224

KNOW THE DIAGNOSTIC APPROACH TO PEDIATRIC ACUTE APPENDICITIS

EVAN S. GLAZER, MD, MPH

Pediatric appendicitis is very difficult to diagnose. Other etiologies for abdominal pain such as intussusception, inflammatory bowel disease, ulcer disease, and gall bladder disease need to be addressed based on age, history, and physical exam. A review of 25 studies by Bundy et al. (2007) (*Table 224.1*) found that patients under 12 years have a misdiagnosis rate between 28% and 57%.

The workup begins in the usual fashion—history and physical exam (*Table 224.2*). With preverbal children, this is especially difficult. I find that when the child is somewhat verbal (age >4 or 5), asking him or her questions directly is most useful. As usual, laboratory and other low-risk procedures (such as ultrasound) are performed next.

A 1-day history of abdominal pain is not useful. Furthermore, laboratory and radiologic changes may not have had happened at the time of presentation. Therefore, these patients should be observed in accordance with local practices of the ED, pediatric surgeon, and hospital pediatrician (i.e., observe with repeat exam and complete blood count (CBC)). A few days of worsening abdominal pain is much more typical of appendicitis (and other causes). Migratory pain is more reassuring of appendicitis. Nausea, vomiting, and fever clearly can be associated with many diseases, but pain first followed by nausea and vomiting

TABLE 224.1	LIKELIHOOD RATIOS FOR APPENDICITIS IN CHILDREN WITH ABDOMINAL PAIN
SIGNS AND SYMPTOMS OF PEDIATRIC APPENDICITIS	
SIGN OR SYMPTOM	**LIKELIHOOD RATIO (LR)**
Fever	3.4
Rebound tenderness	3
Pain migrating to RLQ	1.2
WBC <10 (1,000/mL)	0.22
CRP >24 (mg/L)	5.2

Notes: LR >1 is a positive correlation, while <1 is a negative correlation; All ratios are significant at $p < 0.05$.
RLQ, right lower abdominal quadrant; WBC, white blood cell count; CRP, C-reactive protein

---

TABLE 224.2	**EVIDENCE-BASED APPROACH**

HISTORY AND PHYSICAL EXAM: EVERYONE

<24-h duration → observe 24 to 48 h.

Pain from midabdominal to RLQ → suggests appendicitis.

Nausea/vomiting BEFORE any pain → suggests NOT appendicitis.

Family Hx doubles the rate of pathology-proven appendicitis.

High-grade fever → suggests appendicitis.

Worse RLQ, rebound, Rovsing sign, obturator sign → appendicitis.

INTERVENTIONS: ALMOST EVERYONE

IV Fluid Bolus → makes many feel better due to secondary dehydration.

Labs → WBC & CRP nonspecific but useful.

IMAGING: IF H&P NOT CLEAR

U/S → no ionizing radiation. Very operator and patient dependent.

CT → some surgeons prefer to be called prior to ionizing radiation, do not scan if <24 h of signs/symptoms→ high false-negative rate.

MRI → not ready for prime time… yet.

PEDIATRIC SURGEON

Consult when H&P, timeline, and labs all suggest acute appendicitis.

U/S is confirmatory for acute appendicitis.

CT clearly shows appendicitis.

---

followed by diarrhea is most often due to appendicitis rather than viral gastroenterovirus. In a randomized, placebo-controlled trial, morphine (low dose) was found to significantly reduce pain while there were no significant differences in rates of appendicitis, perforated appendicitis, missed appendicitis, or resolution of pain ($n = 108$).

After H&P, labs, and noninvasive imaging, we are left with three choices. They are (1) a clear diagnosis (i.e., gastroenterovirus or appendicitis), (2) the diagnosis is not clear, and radiologic imaging likely would be helpful, or (3) the diagnosis is not clear, but the patient clearly needs emergent intervention (i.e., frank peritonitis or hemodynamically unstable). Fortunately, situation (3) is rare but does require immediate intervention by the emergency physician, the pediatric surgeon, and possibly the pediatric intensivist. Situation (1) describes a common situation where a child may be sent home (i.e., likely gastroenterovirus with multiple recent sick contacts) or for a consult to the pediatric surgeon (i.e., appendicitis). Situation (2) brings up the issue of ionizing radiation.

Ultrasound is a safe alternative to CT scan, but it is slightly less accurate. In a study of pediatric and young adults, CT was significantly more accurate (94% vs. 89%, $p = 0.05$.) For those under 10 years of age however, there was only a trend toward significance.

Once a child has received antibiotics, it is difficult to distinguish improvement due to that intervention (and should undergo appendectomy for appendicitis) or if the child improved because of the natural history of some other disease (i.e., gastroenteritis). *Do not give antibiotics until it is decided that a patient has appendicitis and is going to the operating room* (or not). There are small cohorts of children who had antibiotics as their only treatment for acute appendicitis (planned interval appendectomy [IA] that never was performed). Of the 61 patients who did not have a planned IA, only 8% developed recurrent appendicitis. Although some would say then that IA is not required, the standard of care is to perform an IA.

On a final note, for everything we do, based on well-down studies, the median rupture rate is in the order of 36% in children while nearly 50% present atypically.

The kids do not read the textbook, but they do OK.

Suggested Readings

Bundy DG, Byerley JS, Liles EA, et al. Does this child have appendicitis? *JAMA*. 2007;298(4):438–451.

Green R, Bulloch B, Kabani A, et al. Early analgesia for children with acute abdominal pain. *Pediatrics*. 2005;116:978–983.

Moir C. Abdominal pain in infants and children. *Mayo Clin Proc*. 1996;71(10):984–989.

Morrow SE, Newman KD. Appendicitis. In: Ashcraft KW, Holcomb GW, Murphy JP, eds. *Pediatric Surgery*, 4th ed. New York, NY: Elsevier Inc.; 2005:577–585.

Puapong D, Lee SL, Haigh PI, et al. Routine interval appendectomy in children is not indicated. *J Pediatr Surg*. 2007;42(9):1500–1503.

Sivit CJ, Applegate KE, Stallion A, et al. Imaging evaluation of suspected appendicitis in a pediatric population: Effectiveness of sonography versus CT. *Am J Roentgenol*. 2000;175(4):977–980.

225

KNOW THE DIFFERENTIAL DIAGNOSIS AND PROPER WORKUP FOR THE LIMPING CHILD

NATHANIEL R. JOHNSON, MD, PhD

The limping child poses a significant diagnostic challenge for the emergency physician. The list of potential diagnoses is broad, and the etiology of the limp may be as benign as a bruise or as serious as cancer. Additionally, the potential morbidity and/or mortality that may result from a missed diagnosis such as nonaccidental trauma or septic arthritis are significant.

What follows is a brief review of some of the many causes of limping in a child and the important diagnoses that you, as a practitioner, do not want to miss.

TRAUMA

A history of trauma and a subsequent limp in a child should, obviously, raise concern for a fracture. While the mechanism of an injury and the location of pain are certainly important in accurately diagnosing the injury, so is the knowledge of some of the following basic principles.

First, it is important to understand that children break bones differently than do adults. In children, ligaments are relatively stronger than the bone or growth plate, and a mechanism that typically results in a ligamentous injury in the adult will more likely cause a fracture or physeal injury in a child. An example of this is femoral physeal separation instead of medial collateral ligament disruption in a knee injury. In addition, children have a more porous, immature bone structure than adults, which tends to prevent the extension of fracture lines. Compression and tension injuries are likely to result in buckle and greenstick fractures, respectively; so carefully inspect the entire cortex. This knowledge should direct how you evaluate for these injuries as well as encourage you to have a high index of suspicion for the presence of a fracture, even if not initially obvious on radiographs. If you are frequently diagnosing sprains in children with open physes, you are likely missing a number of nondisplaced fractures, especially Salter-Harris type I injuries!

Nonaccidental trauma should always be considered in the limping child as well. Abuse unfortunately occurs in some 1% of all children in the United States, and up to 40% to 50% of the fractures seen in abuse involve the femur or tibia—injuries that could present initially as a limp. Lesions suggestive of abuse on radiographs, including classic metaphyseal "corner" fractures or multiple fractures of differing ages, as well as injuries that do not match the reported mechanism should prompt further evaluation and the proper referrals.

Finally, a limping child with a history that suggests a repetitive source of injury—a high-school athlete, for example—should be evaluated for injuries resulting from chronic trauma. Osgood-Schlatter disease, shin splints, and stress fractures are just a few of these potential diagnoses.

Therefore, you must maintain a high degree of suspicion for fractures with the knowledge that children break bones differently than do adults, and always consider nonaccidental trauma as a potential cause of a child's limp.

INFECTION

An infectious process causing a child's limp may be superficial, such as cellulitis or small soft tissue abscess overlying a joint, or more invasive and serious, such as septic arthritis or osteomyelitis. Missing this diagnosis is a significant error given the serious potential morbidity that may result.

In general, children with osteomyelitis or a septic joint appear ill, and diagnostic studies such as erythrocyte sedimentation rate (ESR), C-reactive protein, blood cultures, and/or white blood cell (WBC) count tend to show significant abnormalities. Accurate and prompt diagnosis is imperative, with hospital admission, intravenous antibiotics, and possible surgical management when necessary. *Staphylococcus aureus* is frequently the offending organism, and one should initiate antibiotics with this in mind. MRI may be helpful to make the diagnosis of osteomyelitis as well.

Remember that transient synovitis of the hip, a self-resolving and ultimately benign process, should always be a diagnosis of exclusion. One source reports that a WBC count >12,000, along with fever >38.5°C, an ESR >40, and an inability to bear weight on the affected extremity may help distinguish toxic synovitis from septic arthritis—if all four are present, the chance of it being septic arthritis is 99%. Joint fluid aspirate will likely have elevated WBCs as well as elevated lactate.

The successful identification of other infectious causes of a limp—gono-coccal arthritis or arthritis in Lyme disease, for example—will be aided by findings on history and physical exam, as well as diagnostic testing.

The diagnosis of a septic arthritis or osteomyelitis should always be considered in a patient with sickle cell anemia presenting with an acute pain crisis involving a joint or long bone, especially near the physes.

TUMOR

Neoplasms, both benign and malignant, may present initially as a limp in a child. Tumors may be primary to the lower extremity—osteosarcoma, for example—or they may be disseminated—leukemias and lymphomas, for example. In fact, one study of pediatric leukemias suggests that more than 10% of children have a limp at initial presentation, just over 20% had some form of orthopedic functional impairment, and almost 6% had pathological fracture. Laboratory and radiographic studies may aid in making this diagnosis, though biopsy may ultimately be needed for a definitive diagnosis.

ABDOMEN AND SPINE

Pathology not localized to the lower extremities should also be considered in a limping child. Abdominal inflammation or infection, such as appendicitis, can cause gait abnormalities. One case report even describes the initial presentation of Crohn disease as limping in a child. The patient was later found to have a psoas abscess resulting from fistula formation.

Spinal pathologies including neoplasms, infections (osteomyelitis, discitis), and spondylolysis/spondylolisthesis may also present with limp and must be considered as well.

STRUCTURAL

Lastly, many assorted structural abnormalities—congenital and acquired, benign and potentially serious—can present as limping in a pediatric patient. These problems include limb-length discrepancies, hip dysplasia, Legg-Calve-Perthes disease (more common in boys, ages 2 to 10), and slipped capital femoral epiphysis (more common in adolescent males with elevated BMI). History, physical examination, imaging, and, again, maintaining a high degree of suspicion will aid in properly diagnosing these disorders.

A FEW FINAL THOUGHTS...

While many causes of limping in children are benign and self-limited (contusion, muscle or ligamentous strain, transient synovitis, etc.), many causes are not. These require prompt evaluation and intervention by the practitioner to prevent significant morbidity, and even mortality.

1) Always maintain a high degree of suspicion for fracture, recognize fracture patterns specific to pediatrics, and realize that a fracture may not always be seen initially on plain radiographs.
2) Always consider the possibility of nonaccidental trauma and recognize injury patterns pathognomonic for abuse.
3) Osteomyelitis and/or septic joint should always be high on a differential list and diagnosis and treatment initiated promptly.
4) Always consider other, potentially lethal, diagnoses—malignancy and intra-abdominal infection, for example. All that limps is not musculoskeletal.

SUGGESTED READINGS

Atkinson C, Morris SK, Ng V, et al. A child with fever, hip pain and limp. *CMAJ.* 2006;174(7):924.

Femino JD, Early SD, Skaggs DL. Current management of pediatric musculoskeletal infections and tumors. *Curr Opin Orthop.* 2002;13(6):419–423.

McMillan JA, Reigin RD, DeAngeles C, et al. *Oski's Pediatrics Principles and Practice.* 4th ed. Philadelphia, PA: Lippincott Williams & Wilkins; 2006.

Perez RH, Alonso Farto JC, Arias IA, et al. Small rounded B-cell lymphoma of bone presented by limp, with a positive multifocal 99mTc MDP bone scintigraphy pattern and a negative 99mTc HMPAO-labeled leukocytes study. *J Pediatr Hematol Oncol.* 2008;30(6):443–446.

Renshaw TS. The child who has a limp. *Pediatr Rev.* 1995;16(12):458–465.

Sinigaglia R, Gigante C, Bisinella G, et al. Musculoskeletal manifestations in pediatric acute leukemia. *J Pediatr Orthop.* 2008;28(1):20–28.

Wang CL, Wang SM, Yang YJ, et al. Septic arthritis in children: Relationship of causative pathogens, complications, and outcome. *J Microbiol Immunol Infect.* 2003;36(1):41–46.

226

KNOW THE CAUSES OF AND WORKUP FOR APPARENT LIFE-THREATENING EVENTS

LE N. LU, MD

Apparent life-threatening events (ALTEs) can provoke great anxiety and concern in caregivers and often generate significant discomfort regarding their management in the emergency department (ED). Since ALTE is not a diagnosis, but rather a collection of symptoms, the etiologies that must be considered are extensive. Most patients appear completely well upon arrival to the ED, making our job even more challenging. Often, out of uncertainty, we resign ourselves to simply admitting the patient and letting the pediatricians wade through the mess. While this may result in a valid disposition, it does the patient and our EM colleagues a disservice.

An ALTE is defined as "an episode that is frightening to the observer and that is characterized by some combination of apnea (centrally or occasionally obstructive), color change (usually cyanotic or pallid, but occasionally erythematous or plethoric), marked change in muscle tone (usually marked limpness), choking, and gagging." Many times, the caregivers relate that they feared that the child had died. This naturally generates an emotionally charged environment in which we are challenged to be both detective and consoler.

It is important to first differentiate between an ALTE and other clinical entities that may be similar in presentation. Neonates can have pauses in breathing (termed periodic breathing). This is a normal pattern of breathing that involves three or more respiratory pauses, between 3 and 20 s, without associated changes in color or heart rate. New parents engrossed by their newborn may become fixated on these apneic moments and present to your ED with great concern, which can be quickly abated. Conversely, *pathologic apnea* is a respiratory pause lasting 20 s or longer or that is associated with cyanosis, bradycardia, abrupt marked pallor, or hypotonia. This latter apnea necessitates further workup and admission to a monitored setting. The previous term "near-miss for sudden infant death syndrome (SIDS)" is no longer used as it implies a close relationship between ALTE and

SIDS, which has not been well established. This disconnection is substantiated by the fact that there has been a decrease in the incidence of SIDS with the "Back to Sleep" campaign, while there has been no change in the incidence of ALTEs.

Despite a standard definition for ALTE, diagnosis and patient management decisions remain elusive. Given the vast differential diagnosis, the evaluation can be overwhelming. While there is no standard minimal workup, there is also no maximal workup either. The most frequent identifiable causes of ALTE are digestive (~50%), neurological (~30%), respiratory (~20%), cardiovascular (~5%), metabolic and endocrine (<5%), and other problems, including child abuse. However, up to 50% of ALTEs have no identifiable etiology at first presentation. Unfortunately, even idiopathic ALTEs confer an appreciable risk for morbidity and mortality. Nearly 8% of admitted patients with ALTE require significant medical intervention during hospitalization, despite a negative ED workup. Therefore, it is often appropriate to admit these patients for observation.

So what, then, constitutes an appropriate evaluation in the ED? First and foremost, it is important to believe the caregivers. Avoid underestimating the significance of parental concern since most patients, even those with an occult pathology, are well appearing upon their evaluation in the ED. It is imperative to perform a thorough and detailed history and physical exam. In up to 70% of ALTE patients, the initial history and physical exam direct further workup. Be sure to take a detailed description of the surroundings and circumstances just before and during the ALTE. The history should include the position of the child during the event, whether the child was awake or asleep, events preceding the episode, and any interventions performed. Classifying the apnea as either obstructive or central may help further elucidate an etiology.

The dilemma then arises on evaluating the remaining 30% with inconclusive histories and physical exams. A reasonable initial ED evaluation includes obtaining a complete blood count (CBC), urinalysis and culture, electrocardiogram (arrhythmias, prolonged QT interval), chest radiography, blood sugar, and pulse oximetry. You can skip broad evaluations for systemic infections, metabolic diseases, and blood chemistry abnormalities, as they are not productive, unless directed by your H&P. If respiratory symptoms are present, obtain nasal swabs for respiratory syncytial virus (RSV) and pertussis. Although the risk of bacteremia or bacterial meningitis is very low (<1%), remember that any infant <1 month of age presenting with an ALTE or any child with recurrent ALTEs within a 24-h period warrants a full sepsis workup. In addition, consider metabolic causes in children <1 year old with a history of repeated ALTEs or previous infant deaths in the family. Better yet, let your pediatrician colleagues consider it during the inpatient evaluation. Three percent of ALTEs have been attributed to nonaccidental trauma, so a fundoscopic exam, skeletal surveys, and cranial imaging should be considered if the history is inconsistent or if a nonaccidental injury is suspected. Also, any family history of sudden death should raise several red flags.

Another potential pitfall is assuming that correlation implies causation. For example, although gastro esophageal reflux (GERD) is frequently present in infancy, its coexistence should not be attributed to causation. One study monitored infants with associated apnea and GERD, demonstrating that only 19% of apneic episodes documented by polysomnography were related to GERD documented by pH monitoring. In other words, be wary about diagnosing GERD and discharging infants without a more thorough workup, unless the caregiver gives a clear history of choking and then regurgitation (maybe even color change) immediately after feeding. When in doubt, admit the patient to a monitored setting. Consider an admission for ALTE as the equivalent of that soft-call chest pain-rule out patient: probably low yield, but too risky to send home.

SUGGESTED READINGS

Arad-Cohen N, Cohen A, Tirosh E. The relationship between gastroesophageal reflux and apnea in infants. *J Pediatr*. 2000;137:321–326.

Brand DA, Altman RL, Purtill K, et al. Yield of diagnostic testing in infants who have had an apparent life-threatening event. *Pediatrics*. 2005;115:885–893.

Brooks JG. Apparent life-threatening events. *Pediatr Rev*. 1996;17:257–259.

Claudius I, Keens T. Do all infants with apparent life-threatening events need to be admitted? *Pediatrics*. 2007;119:679–683.

Davies F, Gupta R. Apparent life threatening events in infants presenting to an emergency department. *Emerg Med J*. 2002;19:11–16.

De Piero AD, Teach SJ, Chamberlain JM. ED evaluation of infants after an apparent life-threatening event. *Am J Emerg Med*. 2004;22:83–86.

Gershan WM, Besch NS, Franciosi RA. A comparison of apparent life-threatening events before and after the back to sleep campaign. *WMJ*. 2002;101(1):39–45.

Kahn A. Recommended clinical evaluation of infants with an apparent life-threatening event. Consensus document of the European Society for the Study and Prevention of Infant Death, 2003. *Eur J Pediatr*. 2004;163:108–115.

McGovern MC, Smith MBH. Causes of apparent life threatening events in infants: A systematic review. *Arch Dis Child*. 2004;89:1043–1048.

National Institutes of Health. National Institutes of Health Consensus Development Conference on Infantile Apnea and Home Monitoring. *Pediatrics*. 1987;79:292–299.

Pitetti RD, Maffei F, Chang K, et al. Prevalence of retinal hemorrhages and child abuse in children who present with an apparent life-threatening event. *Pediatrics*. 2002;110:557–562.

Shah S, Sharieff GQ. An update on the approach to apparent life-threatening events. *Curr Opin Pediatr*. 2007;19:288–294.

227

KNOW HOW TO WORK UP A FEBRILE SEIZURE APPROPRIATELY

LE N. LU, MD

When a child has a fever and a seizure, do the age-appropriate workup for a fever and you will not go wrong!!!

Febrile seizures are common and usually benign, yet they require your vigilance to avoid mismanagement. About 2% to 5% of children 6 months to 5 years of age experience this type of seizure. We often breathe a sigh of relief when we diagnose a child with a febrile seizure, since the workup usually requires little more than consoling the caregivers. That holds true provided we have correctly diagnosed the condition and have not forgotten that the child had a fever that still requires investigation.

The appropriate workup is partially contingent upon the type of seizure. A "simple" febrile seizure is generalized, lasts <15 min, and occurs only once in a 24-h period in a febrile child 6 months to 5 years of age, without evidence of intracranial infection, severe metabolic disturbances, or known neurologic abnormalities. The latter criteria do not mandate laboratory investigation but do require that the patient return to his or her baseline. By contrast, "complex" febrile seizures are focal, last longer than 15 min, or recur within a 24-h period. While the "complex" entity may, in the end, have the same benign clinical course as the "simple" febrile seizure, it is too difficult to determine which patients have underlying pathology in the emergency department and, therefore, require a more conservative approach.

The management of febrile seizures is similar to that of other seizures (ABCs, benzodiazepines, phenytoin, and phenobarbital), but the evaluation is what often leads to trepidation. To help ease your uncertainty, remember two simple things: first, maintain a healthy respect for "complex" presentations and have a low threshold for a full sepsis workup, and second, any child with a febrile seizure requires an age-appropriate workup for the fever. Other than bedside glucose, routine labs and neuroimaging are not needed, unless they are part of the search for the source of the fever. Febrile seizures do not suggest a higher incidence of bacteremia than fever alone, so you can safely do the workup mandated by the fever. In other words, check the urine in an 8-month-old female, and look for herpangina in the 2-year-old refusing to eat.

Occasionally, this methodology needs to be altered. ACEP guidelines currently state that a lumbar puncture (LP) should be "strongly considered" in children <18 months old with febrile seizures plus any of the following features:

1) History of irritability, poor feeding, or lethargy
2) Abnormal mental status or appearance
3) Abnormal physical findings of meningitis
4) Complex seizures
5) Slow return from postictal state
6) Pretreatment with antibiotics

In the absence of these features, an LP can be deferred. But remember, a child on antibiotics the prior week for an ear infection does qualify for an LP! CTs prior to performing the LP are only needed for patients at risk of cerebral abscess (e.g., immunocompromised, focal findings, endocarditis) or showing signs of elevated intracranial pressure.

Keep in mind, many anxious parents reporting a seizure or "shaking all over" may actually be witnessing seizure mimics. These include gastroesophageal reflux (Sandifer syndrome), breathholding spells, cardiac dysrhythmias, benign myoclonus, infantile spasms, and acute dystonia. However, reports of focal shaking are, by definition, "complex" and warrant a more extensive workup. Remember, only epileptic seizures are followed by a postictal period.

Once you have made the diagnosis of simple febrile seizure and adequately evaluated the etiology of the fever, the final error to avoid is failing to provide appropriate information to console the family. Febrile seizures generally have a benign prognosis. While antiepileptic medication prophylaxis is effective in reducing the risk of recurrence, the potential toxicities outweigh the relatively minor risks and are not recommended. Also, prophylactic antipyretics do not need to be advocated for as they do not reduce the risk of recurrence. Febrile seizures recur 30% to 50% of the time, with risk factors including younger age (<12 months), lower temperatures (<40°C) at first presentation, shorter duration of fever (<24 h), and family history of febrile seizures. Despite high rates of recurrence, children with simple febrile seizures have only a slightly greater risk of developing epilepsy than the 1% risk in the general population. There is no evidence that recurrent simple febrile seizures produce structural central nervous system damage or lead to cognitive decline, learning problems, or premature death.

Since many may experience the recurrence of seizures, it is important to educate the family on how to manage the seizure while at home. Instruct families to always supervise their child during bathing. In the event of a seizure, the patient should be placed on his or her side on the floor, safely away from any furniture. Parents should avoid placing anything in the child's mouth: the patient will *not* swallow the tongue. Parents should also be instructed to time the seizure and observe for focal shaking. If two episodes occur in a 24-h period, they should return to the emergency department.

By properly diagnosing the condition, effectively treating the seizure, appropriately evaluating the fever, and providing adequate education to the family, you can provide excellent care for your littlest of patients, while working to avoid common pitfalls in the management of febrile seizures.

SUGGESTED READINGS

Armon K, Stephenson T, MacFaul R, et al. An evidence and consensus based guideline for the management of a child after a seizure. *Emerg Med J*. 2003;20:13–20.

Baumann RJ, Duffner PK. Treatment of children with simple febrile seizures: The AAP practice parameter. *Pediatr Neurol*. 2000;23:11–17.

Blumstein MD, Friedman MJ. Childhood seizures. *Emerg Med Clin N Am*. 2007;25:1061–1086.

Ellenberg JH, Nelson KB. Febrile seizures and later intellectual performance. *Arch Neurol*. 1978;35:17–21.

Friedman MJ, Sharieff GQ. Seizures in children. *Pediatr Clin N Am*. 2006;53:257–277.

[No author listed]. Practice parameter: Long-term treatment of the child with simple febrile seizures. American Academy of Pediatrics. Committee on Quality Improvement, Subcommittee on Febrile Seizures. *Pediatrics*. 1999;103(6 pt 1):1307–1309.

[No authors listed]. Practice parameter: The neurodiagnostic evaluation of the child with a first simple febrile seizure. American Academy of Pediatrics. Provisional Committee on Quality Improvement, Subcommittee on Febrile Seizures. *Pediatrics*. 1996;97(5):769–172.

Trainor JL, Hampers LC, Krug SE, et al. Children with first-time simple febrile seizures are at low risk of serious bacterial illness. *Acad Emerg Med*. 2001;8:781–787.

Van Esch A, Steensel-Moll V, Henriette A, et al. Antipyretic efficacy of ibuprofen and acetaminophen in children with febrile seizures. *Arch Pediatr Adolesc Med*. 1995;149:632–637.

van Stuijvenberg M, Derksen-Lubsen G, Steyerberg EW, et al. Randomized, controlled trial of ibuprofen syrup administered during febrile illnesses to prevent febrile seizure recurrences. *Pediatrics*. 1998;102(5):E51.

van Stuijvenberg M, Steyerberg EW, Derksen-Lubsen G, et al. Temperature, age, and recurrence of febrile seizure. *Arch Pediatr Adolesc Med*. 1998;152:1170–1175.

Warden CR, Zibulewsky J, Mace S, et al. Evaluation and management of febrile seizures in the out of hospital and emergency department settings. *Ann Emerg Med*. 2003;41:215–222.

228

PEDIATRIC HEAD TRAUMA: KNOW WHICH PATIENTS NEED A WORKUP ... AND WHICH PATIENTS DO NOT!

SARAH L. MILLER, MD

Our practice of emergency medicine will place us face to face with a vast array of illnesses and injuries. Pediatric head trauma will be encountered on nearly a daily basis. Traumatic brain injury resulting from blunt head trauma is the leading cause of morbidity and mortality among children and adolescents in the United States. Falls are the predominant mechanism for toddlers, whereas motor vehicle accidents cause the majority of head injuries in adolescence. Children's heads are uniquely at risk: infants and toddlers have proportionally larger heads causing them to fall head first whereas adolescents and teenagers often do not think with their heads and take ill-advised risks. While many incidents are truly accidents, up to 10% of head traumas in children are due to nonaccidental injuries.

The spectrum of injury will range from patients with decreased Glasgow Coma Score (GCS) to those running around your emergency department (ED). Yet, the goal of ED management is the same: diagnose primary head trauma and prevent secondary brain injury due to edema, hypotension, and hypoxia. The patient who arrives in a critical condition is often more straightforward in his or her management: Airway, Breathing, and Circulation! One important error to actively avoid is not maintaining adequate c-spine immobilization. A c-collar is reflexively placed on an adult with a head injury, but often it is forgotten in our younger patients by prehospital and ED providers. So, if it is not already on, be cautious and place an appropriately fitted c-collar.

While the critically ill patient is easily placed on an algorithmic path, the child who is opening every drawer in the exam room and running down the halls creates more misgivings about the appropriate management. With the knowledge that early exposure to radiation is placing our children at risk for the later development of oncologic processes, judicious use of imaging is important. As it is with every procedure or intervention we choose to order in the ED, our decision is based on a delicate risk–benefit ratio. Ordering a computed tomography (CT) for a patient with ominous signs and symptoms of altered mental status (GCS <13), focal neurologic exam, irritability, lethargy, or bulging fontanel is obviously appropriate as the risk-benefit ratio strongly favors imaging. The benefit may be less clear in a patient who is very active in the ED and the question of whether to obtain a CT or not is encountered. To help you answer this question, there are several concerning findings that should raise your suspicion and make you not as eager to rely solely on your physical exam.

Cranial CT scanning is indicated for

- Concerning mechanism
- Altered mental status or neurologic abnormalities on exam
- Known or suspected skull fracture, as skull fracture is strongly correlated with intracranial injury
- Hematoma in the parietal or temporal areas (associated with a higher incidence of intracranial injury)
- Vomiting >5 times or for >6 h after injury
- LOC >1 min
- Suspicion for abuse or a head injury with an inconsistent history

It is also important to not ignore your own "gut instinct." If a child has a concerning mechanism, but does not have any of the mentioned findings, or nonaccidental injury is suspected (implies that the reported mechanism cannot be believed), it may not be necessary to image the child's head. Multiple attempts have been made to quantify what constitutes a "concerning" mechanism. Definitions have been offered such as a fall >3 ft or a fall from a height that is greater than the height of a child (i.e., more than just a fall from standing). Mechanically, the degree of injury is a function of force per unit surface area justifying why a more significant mechanism can be seen when a child falls against the protruding end of furniture.

Observation is reasonable in cases of a normal exam, LOC <1 min, vomiting (<5 episodes) that is resolved, reported lethargy or irritability that is resolved on exam, and frontal scalp hematomas that are minor in nature. Typical observation strategies call for serial exams for up to 4 to 6 h after the trauma event. Admit patients of any age for observation when there is no reliable caregiver available or for the identification and management of persistent symptoms (e.g., headache, nausea, vomiting). Patients with an intracranial injury or basilar or displaced skull fracture require a neurosurgical consult as soon as possible. Also, do not forget a thorough cranial nerve exam for patients with basilar skull or temporal bone fractures since there is a potential for facial nerve injury and disruption of tympanic membrane or ossicles.

For those patients whom you have deemed safe to discharge home, clear anticipatory guidance through educating the caregiver is paramount. Caregivers must know to return immediately for reevaluation should the patient have any deterioration in mental status or neurologic function, worsening headache, or persistent vomiting. Routine follow-up with the primary care physician should be obtained within 48 h for the reevaluation of symptoms and injuries. Patients with concussion must be counseled on postconcussive syndrome: headaches, fatigue, dizziness, sleep disturbance, anxiety, depression, irritability, personality change, and problems with short-term memory. Concussive symptoms may persist for 7 to 10 days after an injury. Participation in sports can be resumed after being cleared by their pediatrician, generally after all concussive symptoms have resolved if there was no associated LOC or 2 weeks after symptom resolution in those patients who suffered LOC at the time of the injury.

While you are educating the patient and the guardian, this is also a great time to address injury prevention. Enforce that while this time the injuries were minor, if actions are not taken, the next time could be more severe. By discussing the appropriate use of car seats, seat belts, and helmets and reinforcing fall prevention and abstinence from drug and alcohol use, you may be preventing them from returning on your next shift.

SUGGESTED READINGS

Cook RS, Schweer L, Shebesta KF, et al. Mild traumatic brain injury in children: Just another bump on the head? *J Trauma Nurs.* 2006;13(2):58–65.

Da Dalt L, Marchi AG, Laudizi L, et al. Predictors of intracranial injuries in children after blunt head trauma. *Euro J Pediatr.* 2006;165:142–148.

Giza CC, Mink RB, Madinians A. Pediatric traumatic brain injury: Not just little adults. *Curr Opin Crit Care.* 2007;13(2):143–152.

Kirkwood MW, Yeates KO, Wilson PE. Pediatric sports-related concussion: A review of the clinical management of an oft-neglected population. *Pediatrics.* 2008;117(4):1359–1371.

Langlois JA, Rutland-Brown W, Thomas KE. *Traumatic Brain Injury in the United States.* Atlanta, GA: CDC, National Center for Injury Prevention and Control; January 2006.

Lee LK. Controversies in the sequelae of pediatric mild traumatic brain injury. *Pediatr Emerg Care.* 2007;23(8):580–586.

[No author listed]. Practice parameter: The management of concussion in sports (summary statement). Report of the Quality Standards Subcommittee. *Neurology.* 1997;48(3):581–585.

Schnadower D, Vazquez H, Lee J, et al. Controversies in the evaluation and management of minor blunt head trauma in children. *Curr Opin Pediatr.* 2007;19:258–264.

Thiessen ML, Woolridge DP. Pediatric minor closed head trauma. *Pediatr Clin North Am.* 2006;53:1–26.

229

FOCUS ON THE ABCs IN PATIENTS WITH CYANOTIC CONGENITAL HEART DISEASE

JARROD MOSIER, MD

Emergency Physicians are trained experts in all types of resuscitations. However, those involving the sick and crashing pediatric patient are the scenarios we most fear. Although we are trained to recognize and correct the threats to the "ABCs," commonly used therapies can be devastating to the crashing child with cyanotic congenital heart disease (CCHD). Anatomic variability and physiologic responses to therapies differ significantly from the adult patient, requiring us to be mindful when faced with sick children. Do not assume that all sick pediatric patients are septic. Consider the underlying physiology to avoid a potential disaster.

Initial history and evaluation should look for clues to CCHD. A common mistake is to assume that all CCHD patients are discovered either in utero or before discharge from the nursery. Prenatal ultrasound has only a 40% sensitivity of in utero diagnosis. Babies referred to a pediatric cardiologist for a murmur and/or abnormal pulse oximetry still miss nearly 25% of all CCHD lesions. Physical exam findings that demand the consideration of CCHD include feeding difficulties, abnormal height/weight, abnormal vital signs with or without fever, murmur, and diaphoresis. All critically sick infants should have blood pressure and pulse oximetry measured in the right upper and one lower extremity. A systolic blood pressure difference of 8 mm Hg or more, an O_2 sat < 95%, or >3% difference in O_2 saturation is significant. The earlier the age of presentation, the more likely the patient is to be in shock with a cyanotic lesion and/or ductal dependent lesion. Children who present later in infancy are more likely to present with congestive heart failure rather than shock.

Resuscitation requires careful consideration of the underlying physiologic process. Although older children and adults can increase contractility to improve stroke volume and cardiac output, infants lack such reserve. Rather, they use vascular resistance and heart rate to meet the increased demand. CCHD patients, especially those with single ventricle physiology, balance pulmonary vascular resistance (PVR) and systemic vascular resistance (SVR) to maintain cardiac output. SVR can be very high and thus maintain a normal blood pressure, but the infant can have no cardiac output if the central venous pressure or PVR is also high.

One method of differentiating sepsis from CCHD in the crashing infant is to provide a fluid challenge of 20 mL/kg bolus of crystalloid. This should improve a volume-depleted septic infant, whereas the CCHD patient may worsen from increased fluid overload of the lungs. Bedside or emergent formal echocardiographic evaluation of the heart and inferior vena cava (IVC) will help determine the specific lesion and guide the therapy.

Airway management can be the only procedure that improves both hemodynamics and gas exchange. CCHD infants decompensate from either increased or decreased pulmonary blood flow. Given their inability to increase contractility to overcome demand, manipulating PVR with intubation and mechanical ventilation can be lifesaving. Rapid sequence intubation drugs should be chosen carefully due to their side effects. If the underlying process is unknown, consider etomidate, fentanyl, succinylcholine, and rocuronium first due to their relatively neutral hemodynamic profile. Otherwise, choose your drugs based on the desired hemodynamic response. Ketamine will increase PA pressure and PVR while propofol, morphine, and benzodiazepines all decrease SVR and should be used only when afterload reduction is desired. Atropine may blunt the vagal response to intubation.

Intubation alone will increase PVR, while hypoventilation with decreased FiO_2 will augment this effect and drive blood flow downhill. Increased FiO_2 will relieve hypoxic vasoconstriction, improving pulmonary blood flow if desired, but will accelerate ductus arteriosus closure in ductal dependent lesions. Keep the O_2 sat 70% to 80% to maintain optimum pulmonary to systemic blood flow. Increasing the oxygen saturation will only increase pulmonary blood flow exponentially, increasing pulmonary edema. Add inhaled nitric oxide at 2 to 20 ppm to relieve pulmonary hypertension, decrease PVR, and increase oxygenation if unable to oxygenate despite full ventilator support. Prostaglandin (PGE1) infusion (0.5 to 0.2 μg/kg/min) should be given immediately for the infant <1 month old with cardiovascular collapse until ductus closure can be ruled out. PGE1 infusion requires close observation of side effects, including apnea and worsening hypotension.

While PVR is managed with intubation and ventilation, SVR is managed with vasoactive agents and fluids. Milrinone (50 to 75 μg/kg/min load and then 0.5 to 1 μg/kg/min), dobutamine (2 to 20 μg/kg/min), or nitroprusside (0.5 to 10 μg/kg/min) will be helpful to decrease SVR. Milrinone and dobutamine have the added benefit of inotropic effect. Vasopressors (e.g., levophed, dopamine, phenylephrine, vasopressin) should be used if increased SVR is required to increase the pulmonary blood flow and oxygenation. Do not overload the central circulation by administering too much crystalloid.

Awareness of the potential complications, proactive airway management, and manipulation of hemodynamics are critical skills required in the successful resuscitation of the crashing child with CCHD. While the principles of the ABCs are the same, critical differences exist that require attention. Consider the diagnosis and try to differentiate it from sepsis. Manage the airway with the appropriate medications and ventilator settings. Most importantly, manage the hemodynamic status with the appropriate balance of PVR, SVR, fluids, and oxygenation.

SUGGESTED READINGS

Abu-Harb M, Hey E, Wren C. Death in infancy from unrecognized congenital heart disease. *Arch Dis Child*. 1994;71:3–7.

Arlettaz R, Bauschatz AS, Monkhoff M, et al. The contribution of pulse oximetry to the early detection of congenital hear disease in newborns. *Eur J Pediatr*. 2006;165(2):94–98.

Carcillo J, Han K, Lin J, et al. Goal directed management of pediatric shock in the emergency department. *Clin Pediatr Emerg Med*. 2007;8(3):165–175.

Chew C, Stone S, Donath SM, et al. Impact of antenatal screening on the presentation of infants with congenital heart disease to a cardiology unit. *J Paediatr Child Health*. 2006;42(11):704–708.

Crapanzano M, Strong W, Newman I, et al. Calf blood pressure: Clinical implications and correlations with arm blood pressure in infants and young children. *Pediatrics*. 1996;97(2):220–224.

Mastropietro C, Tourner S, Sarnaik A. Emergency presentation of congenital heart disease in children. *Pediatr Emerg Med Practice*. 2008;5(5):1–32.

Park MK, Lee DH, Johnson GA. Oscillometric blood pressure in the arm, thigh, and calf in health children and those with aortic coactation. *Pediatrics*. 1993;91(4):761–765.

Photiadis J, Sinzobahamvya N, Fink C, et al. Optimal pulmonary to systemic blood flow ratio for best hemodynamic status and outcome early after Norwood operation. *Eur J Cardiothorac Surg*. 2006;29(4):551–556.

Woolridge D. Congenital heart disease in the pediatric emergency department. *Pediatr Emerg Med Reports*. 2002;7(8):81–92.

Yee L. Cardiac emergencies in the first year of life. *Emerg Med Clin N Am*. 2007;25:981–1008.

230

Do not fail to recognize or report child abuse or neglect

Kathleen O'Brien, MD

On a particularly busy evening shift, a 5-year-old previously healthy female is brought to the emergency department (ED) by her mother for an evaluation of abdominal pain. The child tells you that the pain is diffuse throughout her abdomen, dull in nature, and intermittent. She cannot identify any triggers for her pain. Her mother says that she has been complaining of intermittent abdominal pain daily for the last 3 weeks. There has been no nausea, vomiting, fever, dysuria, hematuria, or change in bowel habits. She has no past medical history and is up-to-date with her immunizations. She is in kindergarten and had previously enjoyed school but recently does not want to go because of her pain. She lives at home with mom, infant sister, and mom's boyfriend. On exam, she is well appearing and in no acute distress. Her vital signs are unremarkable. Her abdomen is mildly tender to deep palpation, poorly localized. There is no guarding or rebound, bowel sounds are normal, and there is no significant right lower quadrant (RLQ) tenderness. The remainder of the physical exam is unremarkable. Complete blood count (CBC), comprehensive metabolic panel, and urinalysis are all within normal limits. Serial abdominal exams during the ED stay are unchanged.

Your suspicion for serious intra-abdominal pathology is very low. Before sending the child home with strict follow-up instructions for ongoing abdominal pain, a thought dawns on you. Could the child's ongoing pain be a physical manifestation of underlying emotional distress? What would cause a 5-year-old girl significant emotional distress? You reevaluate the child and speak with her mother privately. After thorough questioning, her mother begins to cry and admits that she is terrified that her new live-in boyfriend may be sexually abusing her daughter. Child Protective Services (CPS) is notified immediately.

More than 3 million cases of child abuse and neglect are reported annually in the United States. Thirty-five percent of these are cases of physical abuse, 15% are cases of sexual abuse, and the remaining 50% are cases of neglect. Infants aged 0 to 4 are at the greatest risk of abuse. It has been estimated that one in four girls and one in eight boys will be sexually abused before the age of 18. The overwhelming majority of abuse cases occur within the family or by a perpetrator well known to the child.

Children may be fearful or ashamed of disclosing abuse. A child's emotional distress may manifest as a common physical complaint, such as headache or abdominal pain. Your suspicion for abuse should be extremely high in children with vague symptoms or chronic pain and in children with numerous or extensive medical evaluations that repeatedly reveal no etiology for the pain. Research indicates that chronic abdominal pain in children has two age peaks: age 4 to 6 years and 7 to 12 years. It has been suggested that girls more frequently develop chronic abdominal pain than do boys, but the topic remains controversial. Little research exists regarding the direct association between sexual abuse and the development of chronic abdominal pain; however, one small ($n = 72$) case–control study showed that abused children report more functional disorders than controls. Another prospective study showed that abused boys versus nonabused boys report a similar frequency of functional disorders, but there is a significantly longer duration of symptoms in the boys who had been abused.

As physicians, we may be the only individuals able to broach the difficult subject of abuse with caregivers. Despite our own discomfort with discussing the possibility of abuse with caregivers, it is our medical obligation to explore every possible explanation for our patient's symptoms, including abuse and neglect. It is also our obligation to report any suspicion of abuse or neglect to CPS. Reassure the caregiver that the well-being of the child is our top priority and for that reason we must involve CPS. Be sure that the caregiver understands that by calling CPS, we are not accusing him or her of abuse but feel that the situation merits further exploration. Sadly, there are >1,500 child abuse deaths annually. What can we do about this devastating number? Always consider abuse or neglect in your pediatric differential diagnosis and should you even suspect the slightest chance of abuse, involve CPS immediately. While discharging a child home without addressing a suspicion of abuse may cost you your medical license, this negligence might cost the child much, much more!

SUGGESTED READINGS

Administration for Children and Families. Available at: http://www.acf.hhs.gov

Apley J, Naish N. Recurrent abdominal pains: A field survey of 1,000 school children. *Arch Dis Child*. 1958;33(168):165–170.

Berger MY, Cieteling MJ, Benninga MA. Chronic abdominal pain in children. *Br Med J*. 2007;334(7601):997–1002.

Centers of Disease Control and Prevention. Available at: http://www.cdc.gov/mmwr.

Childhelp: The prevention and treatment of child abuse. Available at: http://www.childhelp.org/resources/learning-center/statistics.

Guthrie E, Thompson D. ABC of psychological medicine. Abdominal pain and functional gastrointestinal disorders. *Br Med J*. 2002;325:701–703.

Price L, Maddocks A, Davies S, et al. Somatic and psychological problems in a cohort of sexually abused boys. A six year follow-up case-control study. *Arch Dis Child*. 2002;86:164–167.

Rimsza ME, Berg RA. Sexual abuse: Somatic and emotional reactions. *Child Abuse Neg*. 1988;12:201–208.

231

UNDERSTAND THE PROPER MANAGEMENT OF PEDIATRIC SUBMERSION INJURIES

ERIKA DEE SCHROEDER, MD, MPH

When you're drowning, you don't say 'I would be incredibly pleased if someone would have the foresight to notice me drowning and come and help me,' you just scream.

—John Lennon

It is important to understand some potential pitfalls when it comes to the management of pediatric submersion injuries. Presentation of near-drowning patients can range from a child who is acting tired to one who is in cardiopulmonary arrest. As you are trying to maintain, or regain, control in your emergency department (ED), do not fall into the trap of being less than diligent with a patient following a submersion injury.

Drowning, defined as a death that occurs within 24 h of a submersion event, is the *second leading cause of death* in children aged 1 to 14. Victims of submersion injury tend to fall into one of four practical categories: asymptomatic, symptomatic, in cardiopulmonary arrest, or dead. While those who appear sick or have obvious symptoms will easily attract your attention, it is imperative that you remain vigilant with all near-drowning patients as even well-appearing patients can acutely decompensate. This conservative caution needs to be especially heeded when directing prehospital care. All submersion victims need to be transported to a hospital unless they have obviously been dead for a long time. Unless there is clear evidence against associated trauma (eye witness), remind EMS providers to place a c-collar preventatively. If a patient arrives to your facility without a c-collar, applying one must be part of your primary survey prior to moving the patient.

As it is with many clinical scenarios in emergency medicine, determining the management of a well-appearing patient in whom there is the chance of an occult life-threatening condition is one of the unique challenges of our job. While the patient who comes in playful after a near-drowning experience may appear well enough to be quickly discharged home, you must resist the urge to move the meat in this situation, despite how anxious the patient and family may be to leave the ED. As the nursing staff members roll their eyes at you for occupying one of the valuable beds with a "well child," remind everyone that, unfortunately, these patients have the propensity to decompensate and it is imperative to observe near-drowning victims for *at least 6 h*. As you ignore the staff's deep and audible sigh, ask that someone obtain an ECG for you to evaluate, as swimming can trigger long QT syndrome and other arrhythmias.

Patients who are symptomatic, but not critically ill, following a submersion event can have a variety of symptoms, including anxiety, respiratory distress, and altered mental status. Patients with respiratory symptoms should be placed on oxygen via facemask, monitored using pulse oximetry, and checked on frequently. BiPAP/CPAP is useful in awake, cooperative patients. Be particularly wary of the patient with abnormal vital signs. Unless the patients resolve all of their symptoms and have normal vitals, keep them in the ED for prolonged observation or admit them for observation overnight.

Manage critically ill patients as you would in any other situation, but pay particular attention to the hypothermic patient. Do not be the doctor to prematurely declare a 3-year-old child dead. Children who are submerged in cold water can develop apnea, bradycardia, and vasoconstriction that allow them to survive prolonged submersion with minimal neurological effects. Thus, the old adage "patients are not dead until they are warm and dead" holds especially true with pediatric cold-water drowning.

That being said, it is extremely difficult to decide when to end the resuscitation of a near-drowning patient. Patients who are in asystole upon presentation to the ED have a uniformly poor outcome. Unfortunately, no laboratory values have been found to reliably predict death in the pediatric drowning victim. PRISM, the pediatric risk of mortality score, has been validated for use in EDs and can be useful in discussions with parents if resuscitation efforts become futile.

During your resuscitative measures, it is also necessary to investigate the etiology of the submersion event. Seizures, hypoglycemia, and syncope can all be the cause of a near-drowning episode. Your chances of a good outcome will be improved by determining that the patient is hypoglycemic and needs dextrose as part of the resuscitation. It is also essential to entertain nonaccidental trauma (NAT) and neglect as possible etiologies of the event. This is particularly true if there has been a delay in obtaining care, histories do not match, or there are any signs of a struggle. If there is significant concern for NAT, admit the patient regardless of clinical condition.

Near drowning is also an area where your guidance and advice can help prevent a future, more significant event. Approximately 80% of deaths due to drowning are deemed preventable. Just as you would recommend that a child wear a helmet while riding a bike or be appropriately restrained in a car, it is part of your job to help educate parents during this opportunity while they are likely to be listening more astutely. Often, common-sense advice can save lives (i.e., do not leave your kid alone in the bathtub and do not expect that the toddler is safe because he or she is in the tub with the older siblings). Installation of fences around private pools and the use of personal floatation devices have been found to be extremely effective as well. Lastly, encourage families to learn CPR as bystander resuscitation significantly improves neurological outcome following a submersion injury.

SUGGESTED READINGS

Ackerman MJ, Tester DJ, Porter CJ. Swimming, a gene-specific arrhythmogenic trigger for inherited long QT syndrome. *Mayo Clin Poc.* 1999;74(11):1088–1094.

Kyriacou DN, Arcinue EL, Peek C, et al. Effect of immediate resuscitation on children with submersion injury. *Pediatrics.* 1994;94(2):137–142.

Pollack MM, Ruttimann UE, Getson PR. Pediatric risk of mortality (PRISM) score. *Crit Care Med.* 1988;16(11):1110–1116.

Spack L, Gedeit R, Splaingard M, et al. Failure of aggressive therapy to alter outcome in pediatric near-drowning. *Pediatr Emerg Care.* 1997;13(2):98–102.

Welcome to WISQARS™. Centers for Disease Control and Prevention. Available at: http://www.cdc.gov/ncipc/wisqars. Accessed August 13, 2008.

Wollenck G. Cold water submersion and cardiac arrest in treatment of severe hypothermia with cardiopulmonary bypass. *Resuscitation.* 2002;52(3):255–263.

Zuckerman GB, Gregory PM, Santos-Damiani SM. Predictors of death and neurologic impairment in pediatric submersion injuries. *Arch Pediatr Adolesc Med.* 1998;152(2):134–140.

232

NEVER MISS A CASE OF KAWASAKI DISEASE

SARAH K. SOMMERKAMP, MD

A 5-year-old child presents to the emergency department (ED) with a fever. She is diagnosed with a viral illness and discharged. The next time she is in the ED, she is in cardiac arrest. On autopsy, multiple coronary artery aneurysms (CAAs) are observed. How could you have avoided this tragedy? The only way to avoid this error is to entertain Kawasaki disease (KD) on your differential of fever.

KD is difficult to diagnose and can have disastrous consequences if the diagnosis is missed. Emergency physicians are at a disadvantage as they will likely only have a single chance to make the diagnosis and may only see a select few of the symptoms during the single ED visit. Certainly you are familiar with making significant decisions with limited information. What may be less familiar is the set of clinical criteria that KD is based on.

Symptoms of KD include a high fever for at least 5 days, combined with four or more of the following:

1) Conjunctival injection, usually bilateral and nonpurulent
2) Cervical lymphadenopathy >1.5 cm

3) Oral mucosal changes or strawberry tongue
4) Polymorphous rash and/or swelling of the hands and feet with late desquamation
5) No other diagnosis that can explain these symptoms.

The variation in symptom presentation, with symptoms being apparent at different times, increases the difficulty of successful diagnosis and demands that you be wary. Not all fevers are due to benign viral illnesses. Ask the caregiver whether any of the criteria were present recently, but now resolved. If clinical criteria are met, then treatment should begin expeditiously.

And just when you thought that you had figured out KD, along comes incomplete KD. Incomplete KD occurs when the patient does not have all the requisite symptoms to meet the criteria for diagnosis of KD yet still has the risk of developing the deadly CAAs. It seems incredibly unfair to have to make a diagnosis of a condition that has significant morbidity and mortality when all of the criteria for that condition are not even present. It is the job you choose, though.

Suspect incomplete KD in any patient with fever and any two of the aforementioned criteria. The trick now is to determine who has incomplete KD and who has a viral illness leading to a fever, rash, and red eyes. In an effort to limit unnecessary treatment, but prevent missing the entity, laboratory studies should be performed looking for systemic inflammatory response. There is no single lab test that will diagnose KD, but there are characteristic abnormalities: elevations in erythrocyte sedimentation rate (ESR) and c-reactive protein (CRP), platelets, white blood cell count (WBCs), aspartate transaminase (AST), and alanine transaminase (ALT), along with normochromic normocytic anemia, hyponatremia, and sterile pyuria, are common and can aid in confirming initial diagnosis. If you diagnose incomplete KD, treat it as aggressively as you would the complete version.

If your labs do not clearly substantiate your diagnosis, but you are still concerned, then you have the unique opportunity to order an echo from the ED. Echocardiography may show evidence of the presence of CAAs and should be performed within the first few days of diagnosis. A patient presenting with incomplete KD should have an echo earlier, even while in the ED, as the presence of CAA can confirm KD and must lead to immediate treatment. If the echo is normal, realize that CAAs may have not yet developed and know that the patient needs a repeated echo within a few days.

Once you have made the diagnosis, then there is only one more error to avoid—not starting appropriate treatment quickly. Current initial treatment of KD includes intravenous immunoglobulin (IVIG) and high-dose aspirin. Give the IVIG as a single infusion of 2 g/kg initial dose over 8 to 12 h to decrease the incidence of CAA. High-dose aspirin, 80 to 100 mg/kg/day divided into four doses, is used for its antiplatelet effects. These therapies should be ordered while the patient is in the ED and started as soon as possible which, depending on your hospital dynamics, may still be in your ED. If the initial treatment does not lead to the resolution of symptoms, a second dose of IVIG may be required at a later time.

Ideally, IVIG and aspirin treatment should be administered as soon as possible but at least within the first 7 to 10 days of symptom onset as delayed treatment leads to higher risk of CAA. Treatment of incomplete KD should be started within the same timeframe. Also be aware that IVIG dosing constitutes a fairly large-volume challenge requiring caution in the patient with cardiac dysfunction. Other treatments, including steroids, plasmapheresis, TNF inhibition, and cyclophosphamide, have been used for refractory disease but are more controversial since they yield mixed results. None of these treatments should be used instead of, or delay, the administration of IVIG and aspirin combination. Hopefully your hospital is efficient enough so that you do not have to manage refractory KD, but it could be possible.

It is essential that you, the emergency physician, know about KD since the consequences of missing the diagnosis are severe. With appropriate and prompt treatment, significant decreases in CAA formation have been shown. By knowing and utilizing the clinical criteria, while acknowledging the existence of incomplete disease, at-risk children will be identified and appropriately managed by you.

SUGGESTED READINGS

Belay ED, Maddox RA, Holman RC, et al. Kawasaki syndrome and risk factors for coronary artery abnormalities. *Pediatr Infect Dis J.* 2006;25(3):245–249.

Celik U, Alhan E, Arabaci F. Incomplete Kawasaki disease: A pediatric diagnostic conflict. *Anatdolu Kardiyol Derg.* 2007;7(3):343–344.

Freeman AF, Shulman ST. Kawasaki disease: Summary of the American Heart Association guidelines. *Am Fam Physician.* 2006;74(7):1141–1148.

Furusho K, Kamiya T, Nakano H, et al. High-dose intravenous gammaglobulin for Kawasaki disease. *Lancet.* 1984;2(8411):1055–1058.

Inoue Y, Okada Y, Shinohara M, et al. A multicenter prospective randomized trial of corticosteroids in primary therapy for Kawasaki disease. *J Pediatr.* 2006;149(3):336–341.

Juan CC, Hwang B, Lee PC, et al. The clinical manifestations and risk factors of a delayed diagnosis of Kawasaki disease. *J Chin Med Assoc.* 2007;70(9):374–379.

Kato H. Cardiovascular complications in Kawasaki Disease: Coronary artery lumen and long-term consequences. *Progress Pediatr Cardiol.* 2004;19(2):137–145.

Wolff AE, Hansen KE, Zakowski L. Acute Kawasaki disease: Not just for kids. *J Gen Intern Med.* 2007;22(5):681–684.

233

BEWARE THE COMPLICATIONS IN MANAGING DIABETIC KETOACIDOSIS, ESPECIALLY CEREBRAL EDEMA

BRYAN C. THIBODEAU, MD

Over the past two decades, cerebral edema in diabetic ketoacidosis (CEDKA) has remained a serious life-threatening condition in the pediatric diabetes population whose incidence has not changed despite advances in management protocols. CEDKA is traditionally thought of as a disease of childhood, with 95% of cases occurring in those under 20 years old, 33% under 5 years of age, and 67% of cases diagnosed in those with new-onset diabetic ketoacidosis (DKA). Worldwide literature reports an incidence of 0.7% to 1.0% per episode of childhood DKA, with a mortality range of 21% to 27%, and 21% to 35% having long-term neurologic sequelae. The greatest risk of mortality is associated with DKA at first presentation, those with a long history of symptoms prior to presentation, and anyone within the first 24 h from the onset of therapy. As an emergency medicine physician, it is imperative that you know how to recognize and manage a patient with CEDKA.

There is no consensus over the mechanism of or the predisposing risk factors for developing CEDKA. This reflects the poor understanding of the underlying nature of the metabolic derangements in DKA and the effects of the treatments. There are several common risk factors that you need to be aware of, including elevated BUN, low serum CO_2, sodium bicarbonate administration, the rate and type of fluid administered, and the rapid fall of glucose without equivalent rise of serum sodium. Whether these are individual risk factors or rather signs of severe disease is unclear.

So that you can hold your own with the ICU team when you call to admit the patient, a brief review of the pathophysiology is useful. In patients with DKA, profound dehydration results in reduced plasma volume, which is aggravated by low serum CO_2 (from acidosis, ketosis, and hyperventilation), and leads to cerebral vasoconstriction and cerebral ischemia, hypoxia, and increased capillary permeability. This increased permeability represents a vasogenic insult, which permits the movement of free water across the barrier. Additionally, the brain protects itself from the hyperosmolar state by producing idiogenic osmoles from cerebral metabolic breakdown products. According to this mechanism, a DKA patient who is aggressively hydrated and whose serum osmolality is quickly normalized will experience a relative elevation in brain cell osmolality, which will allow for the influx of free water into its cells; that is, a cellular osmotic insult. While the pathophysiology is fun to ponder, in the end, it is imperative to remember the importance of judiciously administering isotonic fluids and closely monitoring the change in glucose and sodium in pediatric DKA so as not to aggravate this osmotic effect.

Being aware of the risk of CEDKA is the first step, but being able to detect it is equally important. The diagnosis of CEDKA is based on **clinical signs and symptoms**, which usually occur as the metabolic parameters of DKA are resolving. In the ED, you will need to be aware of how the classic CEDKA patient will present. The presentation commonly begins with signs and symptoms of neurologic deterioration, worsening coma and loss of consciousness, fixed or dilated pupils, and eventual respiratory arrest. This typically progresses over a range of 4 to 12 h after the onset of DKA therapy, possibly while the patient is still in your ED.

Though currently a standardized set of clinical criteria to diagnose symptomatic CEDKA does not exist, there is a clinical model that is extremely useful for early detection. Their retrospective chart study produced a protocol that detects CEDKA early with 92% sensitivity and 96% specificity. Their findings, summarized in *Table 233.1*, are based on definable signs and symptoms of neurologic collapse and are tiered according to diagnostic, major, and minor criteria.

TABLE 233.1	MUIR DIAGNOSTIC CRITERIA

DIAGNOSTIC CRITERIA

- Abnormal motor or verbal response to pain
- Decorticate/decerebrate posturing
- Cranial nerve palsy (especially CNs 3, 4, 6)
- Abnormal neurogenic respiratory pattern (grunting, tachypnea, Cheyne Stokes, apneusis)

MAJOR CRITERIA

- Altered mentation/fluctuating level of consciousness (LOC)
- Sustained heart decelerations (>20 bpm decline) not due to improved intravascular volume or sleep-state
- Age-inappropriate incontinence

MINOR CRITERIA

- Vomiting
- Headache (HA)
- Lethargy or not easily aroused
- DBP >90 mm Hg
- Age <5 y

While it is known that cerebral edema can be present in patients subclinically, it is also important to realize that initial CT results are negative in up to 40% of cases of CEDKA in the acute stage. Remember that the diagnosis is clinical. If your suspicion is high, do not delay treatment for a head CT which may not reliably direct your management.

After overcoming the first hurdle of diagnosing CEDKA and avoiding the pitfall of overreliance on neuroimaging, the next error to avoid is not being aggressive enough with treating it. Your initial reflex should be to turn off your intravenous (IV) fluids immediately. The treatment of CEDKA often feels contrary to your management of the DKA; however, the brain is swelling and that will compromise your ABCs in short course. After the fluids are stopped, you have several agents available to you to treat CEDKA. Your first option is IV mannitol at a dose of 0.2 to 0.5 g/kg, with a maximum dose of 1 g/kg/dose. It produces an osmotic diuresis and reduces plasma viscosity, thus improving cerebral blood flow and tissue oxygen delivery. An alternative to mannitol is hypertonic saline, which works similarly to mannitol in its osmotic diuretic effect, with the additional advantage that it prevents or mitigates hyponatremia and hypovolemia.

Unfortunately, some patients will deteriorate despite your best efforts and will require intubation. If this occurs, aim to ventilate the patient at the estimated baseline pCO_2 when he or she was symptomatic just prior to intubation. Hyperventilation and rapidly lowering arterial $paCO_2$ worsen cerebral vasoconstriction and produce blood-brain barrier ischemia, leading to a vasogenic-type injury. For the acidotic patient, resist the urge to administer sodium bicarbonate as it results in hypoxia and paradoxical CSF acidosis and worsening cerebral vasoconstriction.

The management of pediatric DKA and its feared complication of CEDKA highlights several potential pitfalls and errors that we need to be aware of, so that we can actively take steps to avoid them. Anticipating the development of CEDKA and knowing a plan of care prior to its onset will hopefully benefit our patients and make our time in the pediatric emergency department less stressful.

SUGGESTED READINGS

Dunger DB, Edge JA. Predicting cerebral edema during diabetic ketoacidosis. *N Engl J Med*. 2001;322(4):302–303.

Edge JA. Cerebral oedema during treatment of diabetic ketoacidosis: Are we any nearer finding a cause? *Diabetes Metab Res Rev*. 2000;16:316–324.

Glaser NS, Wootton-Gorges SL, Marcin JP, et al. Mechanisms of cerebral edema in children with diabetic ketoacidosis. *J Pediatr*. 2004;145:164–171.

Inward CD, Chambers TL. Fluid management in diabetic ketoacidosis. *Arch Dis Child*. 2002;86:443–445.

Lawrence SE, Cummings EA, Gaboury I, et al. Population-based study of incidence and risk factors for cerebral edema in pediatric diabetic ketoacidosis. *J Pediatr*. 2005;146:688–692.

Levin DL. Cerebral edema in diabetic ketoacidosis. *Pediatr Crit Care Med*. 2008;9(3):320–329.

Muir AB, Quisling RG, Yang MCK, et al. Cerebral edema in childhood diabetic ketoacidosis. *Diabetes Care*. 2004;27(7):1541–1546.

234

DO NOT MISS (OR MISMANAGE) THE PEDIATRIC DIARRHEAL ILLNESS THAT IS MORE THAN JUST DIARRHEA

CHAD VISCUSI, MD

Diarrhea is one of the more common reasons children seek emergency department (ED) care in the United States, representing 15% to 20% of all pediatric ED visits in some series. Acute infectious enteritis or colitis can be quite troublesome to the emergency physician and even more so to the patient, particularly when the diarrhea is bloody. *Escherichia coli* is one pathogen that deserves special attention because of its association with the single most frequent cause of acute renal failure in previously healthy children in the United States, the hemolytic uremic syndrome (HUS). Approximately 90% of HUS in the United States is associated with a diarrheal illness, and most of these cases are caused by Shiga toxin–producing strains of *E. coli* (STEC), particularly the O157:H7 subtype.

The triad of microangiopathic hemolytic anemia, thrombocytopenia, and renal insufficiency is vitally important for the emergency physician to recognize, especially in children <4 years of age with a recent diarrheal illness. The shrewd physician will identify the symptoms of lethargy and decreased urine output in a well-hydrated child and also the subtle signs of pallor (look at the conjunctiva) and edema (often periorbital upon awakening). These early signs and symptoms occur between 2 and 14 days after the onset of diarrhea and obligate us to perform a CBC with smear, chemistry panel with BUN and creatinine, and urinalysis. Remember that thrombocytopenia (<150,000/mm^3) presenting within 7 days of a diarrheal prodrome is an early sign of impending HUS and may precede the anemia and renal failure. Sending a stool culture to evaluate for STEC is also a nice touch, and one that is sure to impress your colleagues on higher hospital floors.

The treatment of HUS, once established, is mainly supportive and may require dialysis in children with oliguria or anuria. Since there is currently no cure for HUS, prevention is of vital importance. Early isotonic volume expansion and maintenance fluid before HUS takes hold may decrease the risk of progression to dialysis-dependent oligoanuric renal failure. Therefore, isotonic saline should be judiciously administered parenterally early in its course to children presenting with bloody diarrhea possibly caused by STEC.

Limited studies show little, if any, clinical benefit from antidiarrheal agents. With unacceptably high rates of lethargy, ileus, respiratory depression, coma, and death, the current consensus is that these agents should not be used in the treatment of young children with diarrhea, especially if it is inflammatory or bloody.

The role of empiric antibiotics in the treatment of infectious enteritis or colitis in children is somewhat controversial. A few situations exist where antibiotic treatment has been found to be useful. Evidence- and consensus-based guidelines recommend the treatment of confirmed invasive *Salmonella typhi*, *Shigella*, *Giardia*, and amebiasis.

However, the predominant cause of diarrheal illness in developed countries is a viral or self-limited bacterial infection which is not shortened by empiric antibiotic agents. Furthermore, a small but well-done prospective cohort study of 71 children <10 years old published by Wong et al. in 2000 demonstrated an increased risk of HUS in children with *E. coli* O157:H7 who were treated with antibiotics (RR = 17.3/OR = 14.25). The proposed mechanism by which this might occur is an increased release or induced production of the Shiga toxin in the presence of trimethoprim-sulfamethoxazole, quinolones, or β-lactams. In August of 2002, a meta-analysis of nine studies conducted by Safarm et al. failed to show any higher risk of HUS with antibiotic administration.

Critics of the Safdar study cite that due to heterogeneity of the included studies, it was not possible to control for the choice of drug, timing, or duration of therapy or specific infecting strain of STEC. In vitro studies have shown that different strains respond differently in their production of Shiga toxin in response to different antibiotics, particularly when dosing results in subinhibitory drug concentration. A well-controlled randomized study is surely needed, but until then, do not try to be different than your pediatric colleagues. As empiric antibiotics have shown no significant clinical benefit in the treatment of inflammatory or bloody diarrhea and have been linked in some studies to precipitating or worsening HUS in children, they should still be avoided in young children <8 years old, unless of course you want to get yourself and your patient into an even bloodier mess.

SUGGESTED READINGS

Ake JA, Jelacic S, Ciol MA, et al. Relative nephroprotection during *Escherichia coli* O157:H7 infections: Association with intravenous volume expansion. *Pediatrics*. 2005;115: e673–e680.

Armon K, Stephenson T, MacFaul R, et al. An evidence and consensus based guideline for acute diarrhea management. *Arch Dis Child*. 2001;85:132–142.

Fiorino EK, Rafaelli RM. Hemolytic-uremic syndrome. *Pediatr Rev*. 2006;27(10):398–399.

King CK, Glass R, Bresee JS, et al. Managing acute gastroenteritis among children: Oral rehydration, maintenance, and nutritional therapy. *MMWR Recomm Rep*. 2003;52(RR-16): 1–16. Available at: www.cdc.gov/mmwr/PDF/RR/RR5216.pdf.

[No authors listed]. Practice parameter: The management of acute gastroenteritis in young children.American Academy of Pediatrics, Provisional Committee on Quality Improvement, Subcommittee on Acute Gastroenteritis. *Pediatrics*. 1996;97(3):424–435.

Safdar N, Said A, Gangnon RE, et al. Risk of hemolytic uremic syndrome after antibiotic treatment of *Escherichia coli* O157:H7 enteritis: A meta-analysis. *JAMA*. 2002;288(8): 996–1001.

Wong CS, Srdjan J, Habeeb RL, et al. The risk of hemolytic-uremic syndrome after antibiotic treatment of *Escherichia coli* O157:H7 infections. *N Eng J Med*. 2000;342:1930–1936.

235

DO NOT LET ATHLETES WITH CONCUSSIONS RETURN TO PLAY TOO EARLY

ANNA L. WATERBROOK, MD

Concussions, minor traumatic brain injuries, are common in sports and represent approximately 5% to 10% of all high school and collegiate sport-related injuries. The management of these patients can be frustrating because there is not much evidence in the literature to guide us. Returning athletes to their sports too early can lead to prolonged or worsening concussive symptoms, postconcussive syndrome, or even the controversial, but dreaded, "second-impact syndrome," which is rare, but often rapid and fatal, cerebral edema sustained after a second concussion. Conversely, we do not want to keep them out longer than necessary because this may lead to depression, feelings of isolation, sleep disturbances, or deconditioning.

The 2nd International Symposium on Concussion in Sport held in Prague in November 2004 provides us the most up-to-date information and recommendations for providing care to athletes with concussions, including sideline assessments and help with return-to-play decisions. In addition, it recommends that old grading scales for concussions be abandoned and replaced with the distinction between simple and complex concussions. Simple concussions, by definition, completely resolve within 7 to 10 days, while complex concussions last longer. Concussion severity can only be determined in retrospect, after all concussion symptoms have cleared, the neurologic examination is normal, and cognitive functions have returned to baseline.

When a player sustains an acute injury on the field, evaluation and management should begin immediately. The sideline assessment of a potentially concussed athlete should include the medical provider's general impression and the patient's orientation, immediate and delayed memory, concentration, and game situation responsibilities. Orientation questions to person, place, and time have been shown to be inaccurate in the evaluation of concussed patients. Thus, different orientation questions, including the name of the venue, the opponent, and the quarter or period of the game, should be used. This strategy works great because playing the game requires answering these questions correctly. It is also important to examine cranial nerves, sensation, strength, and the vestibular system. Balance testing is an integral part of performance and should be tested with tandem gait, finger-to-nose, Romberg, and rapid alternating movements. Even if a thorough assessment of the athlete is normal, he or she must be removed from play for 15 min and reassessed. If the athlete is asymptomatic both cognitively and physically, and serial physical exams are normal, he or she should be tested with exertion on the sidelines. Have him or her perform five push-ups, five sit-ups, and a 40-yard sprint. If testing is normal and he or she remains asymptomatic, the athlete may be allowed to return to play. However, if she or he shows ANY signs or symptoms of a concussion, the player should not be allowed to return to play the same day. The player should not be left alone, and regular monitoring for deterioration is essential over the initial few hours following the injury. A player should never return to play while symptomatic. "When in doubt, sit them out!"

The majority of concussions will resolve spontaneously over several days, and these athletes will usually be able to proceed rapidly through a stepwise return-to-play strategy. During this period of recovery in the first few days following an injury, it is important to emphasize to the athlete that physical AND cognitive rest is required. Activities that require concentration and attention may exacerbate the symptoms and, as a result, delay recovery. The return to play following a concussion should be gradual and follow a medically supervised stepwise process and includes

1) No activity and complete rest until fully asymptomatic
2) Light aerobic exercise such as walking or stationary cycling, without resistance training
3) Sport-specific exercise (e.g., skating in hockey, running in soccer), with progressive addition of resistance training
4) Noncontact training drills
5) Full-contact training after medical clearance
6) Game play

With this stepwise progression, the athlete should continue to proceed to the next level if asymptomatic at the current level. If any concussive symptoms occur, such as headache, dizziness, or feeling "foggy," the patient should drop back to the previous asymptomatic level and try to progress again after 24 h. Because more research is needed to better understand the physiologic changes sustained by children with head trauma, younger athletes should be treated more conservatively than adults. In cases of complex concussion, the rehabilitation will be more prolonged and return-to-play advice will be more circumspect. In particularly difficult cases, physicians with specific expertise in the management of such injuries, such as neurologists, should be consulted.

In summary, the management of concussed athletes is complex. Every brain injury is unique, even in the same athlete. However, there are a few simple rules to use with every athlete who may have a concussion to keep them safe and healthy—always have a consistent approach; never allow a symptomatic athlete to return to play; and always allow the brain adequate rest to fully recover after an injury.

SUGGESTED READINGS

Gessel LM, Fields SK, Collins CL, et al. Concussions among United States high school and collegiate athletes. *J Athl Train*. 2007;42(4):495–503.

McCrory P, Johnston K, Meeuwisse W, et al. Summary and agreement statement of the 2nd International Conference on Concussion in Sport, Prague 2004. *Clin J Sport Med*. 2005;15(2):48–55.

Maddocks DL, Dicker GD, Saling MM. The assessment of orientation following concussion in athletes. *Clin J Sport Med*. 1995;5:32–35.

[No authors listed]. Guidelines for assessment and management of sport-related concussion. Canadian Academy of Sports Medicine concussion Committee. *Clin J Sport Med*. 2000;10(3):209–211.

236

DO NOT MISS A PEDIATRIC THORACIC INJURY IN BLUNT TRAUMA

BRENNA K. YURSIK, MD, MPH AND ANITA W. EISENHART, DO, FACOEP, FACEP

Pediatric thoracic injuries, while not very common, can result in devastating outcomes if overlooked. Children with isolated chest trauma carry a 4% to 12% mortality rate and in a multiple-injured child, death is ten times more likely if chest trauma is present. While performing your pediatric trauma evaluation, look for predictors of thoracic injury which include tachypnea, abnormal thoracic and chest auscultation findings, low systolic blood pressure (SBP), and presence of a femur fracture. Be mindful that there may be no evidence of thoracic injury due to rib cage pliability in young children. Focus your exam to look for crackles, diminished breath sounds, crepitus over the chest wall, and external marks indicating trauma. Adequate oxygenation in a pediatric patient does not always ensure sufficient ventilation; it is important to rely on auscultatory and other physical findings rather than just the pulse oximetry.

Blunt trauma accounts for 83% of thoracic injuries in children which can result in rib fractures and pulmonary contusions (50%), pneumothorax (20%), and hemothorax (10%). Children and infants are anatomically protected against blunt thoracic cage trauma because of the compliance of the rib cage, but this protection may also mask complex thoracic injuries. Children with multiple rib fractures must be admitted for observation to exclude associated injuries since this can be a marker of serious injury with the mortality rate exceeding 40%.

Signs and symptoms of pneumothorax include external evidence of chest trauma, tachypnea, respiratory distress, hypoxemia, and chest pain. Remember that diminished breath sounds may not be appreciated in children with a pneumothorax due to the wide transmission of breath sounds in the chest and upper abdomen. The mobile pediatric mediastinum favors the development of rapid ventilatory and circulatory collapse in the presence of a tension pneumothorax. Signs are similar to a pneumothoarx but are often more severe, such as a shift in the point of maximal impact (PMI) and mediastinum resulting in tracheal deviation and distention of neck veins. Depending on the age of the child, do not rely solely on these signs since children often have short necks and compliant soft tissue structures. Definitive treatment is a chest tube, but needle thoracostomy may be necessary as a temporizing measure. If you have a patient with a pneumothorax who is intubated, make sure you have performed a tube thoracostomy **prior** to mechanical ventilation. Also, do not forget to check a chest radiograph to confirm your chest tube placement. If intubation is not required, and the pneumothorax is <20% (not under tension), the child may be observed while being treated with 100% oxygen and reassessed by repeat-interval chest radiographs.

Hemothorax is most often associated with severe impact. Listen for decreased breath sounds and check for dullness to percussion on the affected side. It may present with signs of hypovolemic shock, so remember to check for a hemothorax in shocky children. It is difficult to quantify the degree of bleeding on plain radiographs without an upright film. A hemothorax can hold about 40% of a child's blood. Treat with a chest tube, fluid replacement, and transfusion, using an autotransfuser if possible. Remember that the initial hemoglobin is unreliable for estimating the amount of acute blood loss.

The compliance of the pediatric rib cage makes the patient susceptible to pulmonary contusion even without external signs of trauma. A child with major thoracic injuries may appear normal at first glance. Injury to the capillary membranes allows collection of blood in the interstitial spaces, resulting in hypoxia and respiratory distress; if the bleeding is severe enough, oxygenation and ventilation are impaired. The initial chest radiograph may not show classic findings of pulmonary consolidation, and blood gas evaluation may be normal in the early stages of the injury. Do not assume that a child with a normal chest x-ray and ABG (arterial blood gas) result has no injury. Evidence of pulmonary contusion usually appears on the chest radiograph within 6 h of the injury and appears like an opacified lung segment. If a child has unexplained respiratory distress after blunt trauma, a CT might be helpful, as it is somewhat more sensitive for the presence of a pulmonary contusion. Suspicion of pulmonary contusion should be raised by the mechanism of injury or by the presence of hypoxemia or rib fractures. Significant force is necessary to cause a pulmonary contusion, so be suspicious for additional injuries. Treatment includes oxygen, pain control, and monitoring in an ICU. Most resolve, but in rare cases, pulmonary contusion can be associated with the development of ARDS.

Other less common but important injuries in pediatric blunt trauma scenarios include blunt cardiac injury (most commonly myocardial contusion), commotio cordis, flail chest, rupture of the thoracic aorta, and injury of the tracheobronchial tree.

It is important to have a high index of suspicion for thoracic injuries in children. Children may present differently from adults or may appear well and have normal labs and imaging. This can lead a physician down the wrong path unless there is a healthy suspicion for thoracic injury based on the mechanism of injury and the often subtle findings on physical exam.

SUGGESTED READINGS

Allen GS, Cox CS. Pulmonary contusion in children: Diagnosis and management. *South Med J.* 1998;91:1099–1106.

American College of Surgeons. *Advanced Trauma Life Support (ATLS) for Doctors Student Course Manual.* 6th ed. Chicago, IL: American College of Surgeons; 1997.

Baum VC. Cardiac trauma in children. *Pediatrc Anesth.* 2002;12(2):110–117.

Bauman MH, Sahn SA. Tension pneumothorax: Diagnostic and therapeutic pitfalls. *Crit Care Med.* 1993;21(2):177–179.

Bender TM, Oh KS, Medina JL, et al. Pediatric chest trauma. *J Thorac Imaging.* 1987; 2(3):60–67.

Bonadio WA, Hellmich T. Post-traumatic pulmonary contusion in children. *Ann Emerg Med.* 1989;18(10):1050–1052.

Furnival RA, Woodward GA, Schunk JE. Delayed diagnosis of injury in pediatric trauma. *Pediatrics.* 1996;98(1):56–62.

Genc A, Ozcan C, Erdener A, et al. Management of pneumothorax in children. *J Cardiovas Surg.* 1998;39:849–851.

Grisoni ER, Volsko TA. Thoracic injuries in children. *Respir Care Clin North Am.* 2001; 7:25–38.

Holmes JF, Sokolove PE, Brant WE, et al. A clinical decision rule for identifying children with thoracic injuries after blunt torso trauma. *Ann of Emerg Med.* 2002;39:492–499.

Hormuth D, Cefali D, Rouse T, et al. Traumatic disruption of the thoracic aorta in children. *Arch Surg.* 1999;134:759–763.

Lateef F. Commotio cordis an underappreciated cause of sudden death in atheletes. *Sports Med.* 2000;30(4):301–308.

Meller JL, Little AG, Shermeta DW. Thoracic trauma in children. *Pediatrics.* 1984;74(5): 813–819.

Peclet MH, Newman KD, Eichelberger MR, et al. Thoracic trauma in children: An indicator of increased mortality. *J Pediatr Surg.* 1990;25(9):961–965.

Slimane MA, Becmeur F, Aubert D, et al. Tracheobronchial ruptures from blunt thoracic trauma in children. *J Pediatr Surg.* 1999;34(12):1847–1850.

237

NEVER MISS A CASE OF SPINAL CORD INJURY WITHOUT RADIOGRAPHIC ABNORMALITY (SCIWORA)

BRENNA K. YURSIK, MD, MPH AND ANITA W. EISENHART, DO, FACOEP, FACEP

Despite advances in imaging, diagnosis of spinal cord injury without radiographic abnormality (SCIWORA) can be difficult, and missing one is a frightening thought for an emergency physician. The incidence is 18% to 38% of all pediatric spinal injuries. The most common overall mechanism of injury is motor vehicle collision (MVC), which ranks highest for infants. Falls are most common for children between 2 and 9 years old, and sports for those between 10 and 14 years old. The most common injury level is the occiput to C4, but complete lesions of the cord are associated more frequently with lower c-spine injuries. Predictors of mortality include a younger age, MVC-related mechanism, C1 dislocations, and closed head injury.

The flexibility and elasticity of the pediatric vertebral column are more than that of the spinal cord, so a distraction injury can cause cord traction or ischemia without anatomic defects. SCIWORA has been found in 25% to 50% of patients with spinal cord injuries (SCI) under the age of 8. The anatomic features of the c-spine approach adult patterns at 8 to 10 years of age, but injury patterns identical to those of adults are often not fully manifested until the age 15 years, once again proving children are NOT little adults. Some of these features in children are proportionally larger heads, more elastic ligaments, less calcified cartilaginous structures, different orientation of bones and joints, and underdeveloped neck musculature.

Over 50% of children with SCIWORA have a delayed onset of paralysis, up to 4 days. Significant head, neck, or back trauma and any trauma associated with speed, height, MVC, or falls are suspicious for SCI. The presence of paralysis, paresthesia, ptosis, or priapism, even if transient, should result in an assumption of SCI until established otherwise by a neurosurgeon.

Only 2.5% of the patients in the NEXUS study were 8 years old or younger. Fear and agitation may make the NEXUS criteria difficult to apply in children. Until more conclusive pediatric studies are done, c-spine imaging in children should be included for the following criteria: moderate- to high-risk head or neck injury, multiple trauma, signs or symptoms of spine injury, altered mental status or focal neurologic findings, and a distracting, painful injury with possible mechanism for SCI.

If a child has none of the above findings and is awake, alert, and cooperative, the c-collar may be removed for further examination. This is one of those times when skill at establishing a rapport with a child is very helpful. If there is no neck tenderness, allow gentle, active range of motion of the neck. Children with spinal injury often limit their neck motion due to pain to protect the area of injury, so never passively move the neck. In this scenario, the patient knows better than the physician. If there is neck tenderness or limitation of movement due to pain, replace the collar and order radiographic exams. Otherwise, the c-spine can be cleared clinically.

Your radiographic orders should include a cross-table lateral view of the c-spine, an AP view, and a Water view to visualize the odontoid. With these three views, the sensitivity for detecting cervical fractures is 93%, and the specificity is 91%. The negative predictive value of these three views is 99%. The role of flexion-extension films is controversial, and they should not be done if there are neurologic signs or symptoms of injury.

A common mistake in reading pediatric cervical spine films occurs when one confuses pseudosubluxation and true subluxation. To determine the difference, use the posterior cervical line or the spinolaminar line. If the spinolaminar line, drawn from the anterior cortical margin of the spinous process of C1 through the anterior cortical margin of C3, crosses the anterior cortical margin of the spinous process of C2 or is off by <2 mm and no fractures are visualized, the patient has pseudosubluxation at that level. The predental space should not exceed 4 to 5 mm in children under 10 years, and the prevertebral soft tissue space should not be greater than normal. The four cervical radiographic lines should be evaluated, and the atlanto-occipital alignment should be assessed for dislocation in this region.

If the child has had any paresthesias, numbness, or weakness or if there is any doubt about the plain films, do not hesitate to order a CT. Even if all imaging is negative, there is still a possibility of SCIWORA. If the CT is negative and diagnosis is being considered, order an MRI. In light of all the evidence of complications of high-dose radiation from a CT, one may wonder if going straight to an MRI evaluation of a child is more beneficial. After all, if the patient has a neurologic deficit and a negative CT, we order an MRI. Conversely, if the CT is positive with a deficit, the neurosurgeon *still* wants an MRI. However, MRIs are not perfect, and it is difficult or impossible to sedate a child from the ED, with a possible spine injury, for a lengthy MRI study. This issue should be discussed in advance with the consulting neurosurgeon and based upon your facilities resources.

MRI studies have demonstrated five classes of post-SCIWORA cord findings: complete transaction, major hemorrhage, minor hemorrhage, edema only, and normal. These findings are highly predictive of outcome. Again, MRIs are not perfect. In one small study, the predominant neurological presentation of

SCIWORA was a mild, partial syndrome that resolved within 72 h, but the MRI revealed abnormalities only in patients who had complete neurological deficits. MRI may lack the sensitivity to demonstrate abnormalities associated with partial or temporary nerurological deficits of SCIWORA, even when those deficits persist beyond 72 h.

Treatment may require steroids but discuss this volatile topic with a neurosurgeon prior to use. Give supplemental oxygen and ventilatory assistance if required and remember that hypotension can be secondary to spinal shock. If a SCIWORA is strongly considered, perform radiographic imaging, utilize a neurosurgical consultation, admit for observation, and continue c-spine immobilization.

SUGGESTED READINGS

Brown RL, Brunn MA, Garcia VF. Cervical spine injuries in children: A review of 103 patients treated consecutively at a level 1 pediatric trauma center. *J Pediatr Surg*. 2001;36; 1107–1114.

Cattell HS, Filtzer DL. Pseudosubluxation and other normal variations in the cervical spine in children. *J Bone Joint Surg Am*. 1965;47(7):1295–1309.

Chen LS, Blaw ME. Acute central cervical cord syndrome caused by minor trauma. *J Pediatr*. 1986;108(1):96–97.

Cirak B, Ziegfeld S, Knights VM, et al. Spinal injuries in children. *J Pediatr Surg*. 2004; 39(4):607–612.

Dare AO, Dias MS, Li V. Magnetic resonance imaging correlation in pediatric spinal cord injury without radiographic abnormality. *J Neurosurg*. 2002;97(1 Suppl):33–39.

Hadley MN, Zabramski JM, Browner CM, et al. Pediatric spinal trauma: Review of 122 cases of spinal cord and vertebral column injuries. *J Neurosurg*. 1988;68(1):18–24.

Hill SA, Miller CA, Kosnik EJ, et al. Pediatric neck injures: A clinical study. *J Neurosurg*. 1984;60(4):700–706.

Hoffman JR, Mower WR, Wolfson AB, et al. Validity of a set of clinical criteria to rule out injury to the cervical spine in patients with blunt trauma. *N Engl J Med*. 2000;343(2):94–96.

Jaffe DM, Binns H, Radowski, NA, et al. Developing a clinical algorithm for early management of cervical spine injury in child trauma victims. *Ann Emerg Med*. 1987;16:270–276.

Kokoska ER, Keller MS, Rallo MC, et al. Characteristics of pediatric cervical spine injuries. *J Pediatr Surg*. 2001;36:100–105.

Pang D. Spinal cord injury without radiographic abnormality in children, 2 decades later. *Neurosurgery*. 2004;55(6):1325–1342; discussions 1342–1343.

Pang D, Wilberger JE. Spinal cord injury without radiographic abnormalities in children. *J Neurosurg*. 1982;57(1):114–129.

238

ANESTHESIA FOR FRACTURE REDUCTION: KNOW YOUR OPTIONS

JESSE H. KIM, MD

Emergency departments (EDs) frequently treat a wide range of orthopedic fractures. Emergency physicians are commonly presented with the challenge of providing adequate analgesia and/or sedation to patients undergoing orthopedic and wound care maneuvers. Fracture reduction is one of the most painful procedures commonly performed in EDs, and patients expect the ED to provide adequate pain relief. The challenge lies in the fact that many different anesthetic methods exist with an array of possible pitfalls and complications unique to each.

Arguably, the most well-documented anesthesia associated with fracture management in the medical literature centers around reduction of the distal radius fracture in adults. In that setting, many options are available. The hematoma block is provided by injecting a local anesthetic directly into the fracture site. Intravenous regional anesthesia (IVRA), also commonly known as Bier block, involves IV infusion of a local anesthetic into the arm after exsanguination using a pneumatic tourniquet. Regional nerve blocks can be provided in the elbow or, more distinctively, in the brachial plexus, with or without catheter implantation. Procedural sedation, often vaguely called "conscious sedation" in older literature, may be provided with an IV sedative. In some cases, outside of the ED, the patient may go through general anesthesia with orotracheal or oropharyngeal intubation in the operating room.

Hematoma block is perhaps the simplest and quickest anesthesia and has gained wide acceptance in EDs. A survey of 54 UK accident and emergency (A&E) departments in 1989 showed that for reduction of Colles fracture (distal radial fracture), general anesthesia was used in 44% of patients, Bier block in 33%, IV sedation in 13%, and hematoma block in just 7%. A later 1994 survey of 86 UK A&E departments showed the use of Bier block in 33%, hematoma block in 33%, general anesthesia in 24%, and IV sedation in 7% of patients.

Thus, the use of hematoma block increased substantially in the ED, which appears to be a safe and cost-effective option.

The hematoma block provided significantly better pain control than moderate procedural sedation in a study of 67 patients in India where pentazocine and diazepam IV were compared to a hematoma block with xylocaine in Colles fracture reduction. A recent pediatric study comparing hematoma block with 2.5 mg/kg lidocaine plus nitrous oxide to ketamine/midazolam regimen for forearm fracture reduction found that patients and parents both reported less pain with the hematoma block.

Rare but potential complications from injection into the hematoma include compartment syndrome, infection, vascular infiltration, or local anesthetic toxicity. One case of altered mental status and seizure after hematoma injection of 5 mg/kg lidocaine was reported, presumably from inadvertent IV administration. Manufacturer recommendation for the total amount of infiltrated plain lidocaine is a maximum of 5 mg/kg (or 7 mg/kg with epinephrine). However, for hematoma blocks, a dosage of 2.5 mg/kg is typically effective and results in safe plasma lidocaine levels far below toxic levels. Proper location of the block also should be confirmed by aspiration of the blood in the hematoma. Slow infusion of lidocaine at multiple sites of the hematoma by repositioning the needle may allow more effective dissemination within the hematoma. This serves to help prevent inadvertent injection of the total dose of lidocaine intravascularly.

Bier block, or IVRA, is more resource consuming in general. Regular blood pressure cuffs are not appropriate for use as an upper extremity tourniquet due to the risk of rupture or leakage; a reliable pneumatic tourniquet and IV access are mandatory to achieve optimal results. Compared to the hematoma block, however, a Cochrane database review of the literature found that all trials included in the review showed significantly less pain during fracture manipulation in patients receiving IVRA. However, an evidence review from the Cochrane group showed insufficient evidence to confirm overall clinical superiority of IVRA over hematoma block.

Given the direct IV administration of lidocaine in Bier block, safety is more of a concern than in the hematoma block. Bier block was originally introduced with 3-mg/kg lidocaine dose, to be used principally in the operating room. However, given the risk of serious toxicity, Farrell et al. experimented "mini-dose Bier block" in 105 ED patients using 1.5 mg/kg lidocaine, which resulted in a 95% success rate in attaining pain levels of minimum to none. The lidocaine should also be diluted to 0.5% solution, and 20 to 30 min of inflation should be allowed before deflation of pneumatic cuff to prevent sudden increase in systemic lidocaine concentration. Bupivacaine use in IVRA is highly controversial due to sporadic reports of severe and fatal complications and should generally be avoided.

In an overall comparison of IVRA, hematoma block, procedural sedation, nerve block, and general anesthesia in adult distal radial fractures, a Cochrane review found insufficient evidence to establish relative effectiveness, except that IVRA seemed to provide better analgesia than a hematoma block and, perhaps, resulted in less need for remanipulation. In one systemic review of pediatric fracture reductions, data were again lacking to make direct comparison between the different forms of anesthesia. However, ketamine-midazolam combination was associated with less adverse events than other parenteral drug combinations and was more effective than propofol.

Knowing the various options of anesthesia in fracture reduction as well as the unique associated complications with each, combined with experience and clinical judgment in individual patients, should help anticipate and avoid common errors in fracture reduction anesthesia.

SUGGESTED READINGS

Dorf E, Kuntz AF, Kelsey J, et al. Lidocaine-induced altered mental status and seizure after hematoma block. *J Emerg Med*. 2006;31:251–253.

Farrell RG, Swanson SL, Walter JR. Safe and effective IV regional anesthesia for use in the emergency department. *Ann Emerg Med*. 1985;14:239–243.

Handoll HHG, Madhok R, Dodds C. Anaesthesia for treating distal radial fractures in adults. *Cochrane Database Syst Rev*. 2002;(3):CD003320 [Review].

Hunter JB, Scott MJL, Harries SA. Methods of anaesthesia used for reduction of Colles' fractures. *Br Med J*. 1989;299:1316–1317.

Kalso E, Rosenberg PH. Bupivacaine and intravenous regional anaesthesia: A matter of controversy. *Ann Chir Gynaeco*. 1984;73(3):190–196.

Kendall JM, Allen PE, McCabe SE. A tide of change in the management of an old fracture? *J of Accid Emerg Med*. 1995;12(3):187–188.

Luhmann JD, Schootman M, Luhmann SJ, et al. A randomized comparison of nitrous oxide plus hematoma block versus ketamine plus midazolam for emergency department forearm fracture reduction in children. *Pediatrics*. 2006;118:e1078–e1086.

Meining RP, Quick A, Lobmeyer L. Plasma lidocaine levels following hematoma block for distal radial fractures. *J Orthop Trauma*. 1989;3:187–191.

Migita RT, Klein EJ, Garrison MM. Sedation and analgesia for pediatric fracture reduction in the emergency department: A systemic review. *Arch Pediatr Adolesc Med*. 2006;160:46–51.

Roberts JR. Intravenous regional anesthesia. In: Roberts H, ed. *Clinical Procedures in Emergency Medicine*. 4th ed. Philadelphia, PA: Saunders; 2004:591–595.

Singh GK, Manglik RK, Lakhtakia PK, et al. Analgesia for the reduction of Colles fracture. A comparison of hematoma block and intravenous sedation. *Online J Curr Clin Trials*. 1992 October 1; Doc No 23:[3614 words; 43 paragraphs].

Younge D. Haematoma block for fractures of the wrist: A cause of compartment syndrome. *J Hand Surg*. 1989;14:194–195.

239

BE FAMILIAR WITH INTRAOSSEOUS ACCESS IN THE EMERGENCY DEPARTMENT

MATTHEW J. LEVY, DO, MSc

Obtaining rapid vascular access in the critically ill or injured patient is a key step in the initial resuscitative efforts. However, in critically ill patients, vascular collapse often occurs and results in the inability to secure peripheral intravenous (IV) lines, posing a major challenge for the resuscitation team. While central venous access serves an important role in these patients, the chaotic first moments of the resuscitation of these patients place both the provider and the patient at risk for iatrogenic and untoward effects of central venous access attempts. Furthermore, even in the most skilled hands, obtaining central access can take minutes during a time where seconds count. Intraosseous infusion (IOI) is an ideal alternate route for providing vascular access to administer fluids, blood products, and medications.

Intraosseous (IO) access is not a new method of access by any means. Prior to the advent of plastic IV catheters, IO was shown to be an effective route of administration of medications and fluids. IOI has been shown by radionucleotide technique to deliver fluids as rapidly as IV techniques.

The basic indication for IOI is the need for emergent vascular access when conventional methods have failed. IOI is recommended in Advanced Cardiac Life Support, Advanced Trauma Life Support, and Pediatric Advanced Life Support treatment protocols as alternative means of vascular access in the event that IV cannulation is delayed or not feasible. The American Heart Association recommends the use of IOI in patients under 6 years of age in need of vascular access who have had two failed IV attempts or where >2 min have elapsed at attempting IV access. The Eastern Association of Surgeons of Trauma recommends the use of IO access in adult trauma patients requiring vascular access in which IV access is unobtainable or has failed two attempts. The only accepted absolute contraindication to IOI is a fracture of the bone near the access site. Some authors feel that osteogenesis imperfecta and osteoporosis should also be considered absolute contraindications. Relative contraindications to IOI include cellulitis over the insertion site and inferior vena caval injury.

Complications of IOI are rare and outweighed by the benefits of immediate vascular access. Fluid extravasation is the most common complication, can occur from a misplaced needle, from multiple attempts in the same bone, or from movement of the needle enlarging the penetration site, and may precipitate compartment syndrome. Osteomyelitis is a rare complication, occurring in 0.6% of cases, and occurs most frequently with prolonged needle placement, preexisting bacteremia, and the use of hypertonic fluids. Rarely, fractures at the insertion site, compartment syndrome, fat emboli, cellulitis, and local abscess have occurred.

Any standard IV fluid, including blood products, may be administered through the IO needle. All drugs that can be administered via the IV route can be administered by IOI. It is not necessary to adjust drug dosages based on the IOI insertion site. Although fluids may infuse by gravity, flow rates of 10 mL per min by gravity can be increased to 41 mL per min by using pressurized bags. Blood aspirated from the IOI site may be used for certain laboratory analyses including hemoglobin, hematocrit, and chemistries. Note that some authors have reported discrepancies between potassium and glucose levels from bone marrow when compared to serum.

There are several anatomic sites for IOI placement. The most common location of IOI is the proximal tibia. The distal tibia is an acceptable alternate placement site. To avoid the saphenous vein, the distal tibia may be entered 1 to 2 cm superior to the medial malleolus. Other documented sites for IO placement include the proximal humerus, sternum, and distal tibia. Many commercial devices, such as drills and spring-loaded devices, exist to facilitate IO placement. These devices use some form of mechanical advantage to penetrate the bone cortex. Regardless of the device, the fundamental concept remains the same. Familiarization with the device used at your institution is highly recommended.

When placing an IO device, the patient's extremity should be restrained and a towel roll placed under the knee (for the proximal tibia site). The area should be cleaned and draped using a sterile technique (chlorhexidine). A local anesthetic is recommended in the conscious patient (1% lidocaine injected subcutaneously and over the periosteum). The IO needle is inserted through the skin and subcutaneous tissues until the bone is felt. If using a manual IO needle, the needle is then inserted into the bone using a twisting motion until a loss of resistance or "pop" is felt, indicating entry into the marrow. The trocar is removed from the needle and proper placement is verified. Proper IO placement in the marrow canal can be confirmed by three methods. First, the needle should stand on its own without support. Second, after unscrewing the inner trocar from the needle, bone marrow should be able to be aspirated through the needle. Third, a 5- to 10-mL saline bolus injection should enter with little resistance and without evidence of extravasation; this can be confirmed by carefully observing the calf area for acute swelling or discoloration. To minimize the possibility of extravasation, only one IO attempt should be made in each bone.

In summary, IOI serves as an ideal, fast, and easy method to perform a procedure that enables the resuscitation team to obtain rapid vascular access in the critically ill or injured patient with vascular collapse. Many commercial devices such as drills and spring-loaded devices exist to facilitate IO placement. Any medication, IV fluid, or blood product that can be given through a peripheral IV can be given through an IO. The most common complication of an IO is fluid extravasation, and the IO site requires close monitoring for evidence of extravasation.

SUGGESTED READINGS

American College of Surgeons, eds. *ATLS, Advanced Trauma Life Support for Doctors, Student Manual*. Chicago, IL: American College of Surgeons; 1997:12, 97.

Cameron JL, Fontanarosa PB, Passalaqua AM. A comparative study of peripheral to central circulation delivery times between intraosseous and intravenous injection using radionucleotide technique in normovolemic and hypovolemic canines. *J Emerg Med*. 1989;7: 123–127.

Chameides L, Hazinski MF, eds. Intraosseous cannulation. In: *Textbook of Pediatric Advanced Life Support*. Dallas, TX: American Association of Pediatrics–American Heart Association; 1994:5–6.

Cotton BA, Jerome R, Collier BR, et al. Guidelines for prehospital fluid resuscitation in the injured patient. *Trauma*. 2009;67(2):389–402.

Fiser DH. Intraosseous infusion. *N Engl J Med*. 1990;322:1579–1581.

Hurren JS. Can blood taken from intraosseous cannulations be used for blood analysis? *Burns*. 2000;26:727–730.

Kanter RK, Zimmerman JJ, Strauss RH, et al. Pediatric emergency intravenous access: Evaluation of a protocol. *Am J Dis Child*. 1986;140:132–134.

LaRocco BG, Wang HE. Intraosseous infusion. *Prehosp Emerg Care*. 2003;7(2):280–285.

Miner WF, Corneli HM, Bolte RG, et al. Prehospital use of intraosseous infusion by paramedics. *Pediatr Emerg Care*. 1989;5(1):5–7.

Orlowski JP, Julius CJ, Petras RE, et al. The safety of intraosseous infusions: Risks of fat and bone marrow emboli to the lung. *Ann Emerg Med*. 1989;18:1062–1067.

Rosetti V, Thompson BM, Aprahamian C, et al. Difficulty and delay in intravascular access in pediatric arrests. *Ann Emerg Med*. 1984;13(5):406.

Shoor PM, Berryhill RE, Benumof JL. Intraosseous infusion: Pressure—flow relationships and pharmacokinetics. *J Trauma*. 1979;19:772–774.

Vidal R, Kissoon N, Gayle M. Compartment syndrome following intraosseous infusion. *Pediatrics*. 1993;91:1201–1202.

240

CONSIDER THE INTRA-ARTICULAR SALINE LOAD FOR OPEN KNEE INJURIES

SUSAN MARIE PETERSON, MD

Knee injuries are regularly seen in the emergency department with common mechanisms such as motor vehicle accidents, contact sports, and falls from a height. Knee injuries commonly involve the ligaments (anterior cruciate ligament, posterior cruciate ligament, and the medial and lateral collateral ligaments) and cartilage (medial and lateral menisci) but can include fractures of the patella, distal femoral condyles, or proximal tibial plateau. MRI is typically used to diagnose injury to the ligaments or cartilage, but often radiographs are done first to rule out fracture. Decision rules have been created to help guide clinicians to decide when to obtain imaging. In particular, the Pittsburg decision rules indicate that a knee should be radiographed if blunt trauma has been sustained and the patient is younger than 12, older than 50, or unable to bear weight for four consecutive steps. Using these rules, 99% specificity and 60% sensitivity can be achieved.

While radiographs are useful, they give limited indication of the degree of disruption of the synovial membrane. If penetration of the synovial membrane occurs, aggressive intervention with antibiotics, exploration, and irrigation is necessary as a result of contamination of the joint. Open capsular injuries can have severe consequences for the patient, including infections and long-term limitations to mobility, making an accurate diagnosis critical. Confirmation of synovial membrane compromise is often done using the intra–articular saline load test. In this procedure, the knee is draped and prepared in a sterile fashion with the patient in the supine position with the knee relaxed (contraction of the quadriceps muscles can limit the patellofemoral joint space). A local anesthetic may be used in the skin just lateral or medial to the patella (anterior approaches may be used but are associated with higher rates of inaccuracy and meniscal injury). A 20- to 22-gauge needle is inserted in the soft tissue between the femur and the patella when using the lateral approach and just under the middle of the patella when using the medial approach. The needle is then advanced into the lateral or medial patellar facet, and the location of the needle in the bursa can be confirmed by aspirating a small amount of joint fluid. The needle is then secured, and sterile saline is injected into the joint until the joint is distended. The joint is then inspected for extravasation of fluid at rest and with passive movement. Sterile methylene blue may be used in place of sterile saline to make the extravasation of fluid more obvious. In patients with a methylene blue allergy, a fluorescein solution may be used alternatively. Patients with a positive test should be started on antibiotics immediately, and orthopedists should be consulted for exploration and irrigation.

Intra–articular saline load test is indicated with an obvious soft tissue injury and periarticular fracture, a visible joint capsule, or a laceration in proximity to the capsule. However, it should be noted that false negatives are possible with small open defects in the synovial membrane causing only a slow leakage of fluid. False negatives are also possible if there is an insufficient amount of dye injected, not allowing for the extravasation of fluid. A 2007 study by Keese et al. found that an injection of 50 mL of fluid had a sensitivity of 46% while the injection of 194 mL of saline achieved a sensitivity of 95%. Injecting sufficient quantities of dye is crucial for the test to be diagnostically valuable but may be painful to the patient, and sufficient analgesics should be used.

While the injection of saline or methylene blue is useful, it may not always be necessary. Open fractures with obvious joint involvement, intra-articular air, or foreign bodies on plain radiographs do not necessitate saline injection. In these cases, radiographs are highly suggestive of open injuries, and joint exploration and irrigation are already indicated. Further diagnostic workup with saline injection is likely to cause pain to the patient without offering any further diagnostic utility.

In summary, knee injuries are commonly seen in the emergency department but an open capsule injury should not be missed as it may have severe consequences for the patient, including long-term mobility limitations and infections. Intra-articular saline load test can be a useful diagnostic tool and is indicated with an obvious soft tissue injury and periarticular fracture, a visible joint capsule, or a laceration in proximity to the capsule. However, false negatives are possible with insufficient dye injection and small open defects. Saline injection is not indicated in cases of open fractures with obvious joint involvement, intra-articular air, or foreign bodies on radiograph as these are by themselves indications for exploration and irrigation.

SUGGESTED READINGS

Bauer SJ, Hollander JE, Fuchs SH, et al. A clinical decision rule in the evaluation of acute knee injuries. *J Emerg Med*. 1995;13:611–615.

Keese GR, Boody AR, Wongworawat MD, et al. The accuracy of the saline load test in the diagnosis of traumatic knee arthrotomies. *J Orthop Trauma*. 2007;21(7):442–443.

Patazakis MJ, Dorr LD, Ivler D, et al. The early management of open injuries: A prospective study of one hundred and forty patients. *J Bone Joint Surg Am*. 1975;57(8):1065–1670.

Tornetta P III, Boes MT, Schepsis AA, et al. How effective is a saline arthrogram for wounds around the knee? *Clin Orthop Relat Res*. 2008;466(2):432–435.

241

CONSIDER TREPHINATION INSTEAD OF NAIL PLATE REMOVAL FOR MOST SUBUNGUAL HEMATOMAS

SAMIT DESAI, MD

One of the oldest documented surgical procedures is trephination. The word trephination most likely comes from a Greek word meaning auger or borer. There is some evidence that the practice of cranial trephination dates back nearly 7,000 years. It is a procedure that has been relatively pervasive in a number of cultures throughout history. Trephination refers to the process of drilling a hole through the cranium but can also refer to creating a hole in a toenail or fingernail. In the case of a subungual hematoma, trephination is used for the evacuation of blood or serosanguineous material from underneath the nail plate using any one of a number of techniques. Increasingly, it is supplanting the traditional removal of the nail plate for a subungual hematoma.

A subungual hematoma is an accumulation of blood between the nail plate and the nail bed. Its presence is due to a traumatic event and represents an injury to the capillaries within the underlying nail bed. Associated injuries include a fracture of the distal phalanx, nail bed laceration, surrounding damage to the soft tissue (nail fold, eponychium) nail plate fracture, and nail plate avulsion.

The management of subungual hematomas has long served as a source of controversy. Traditional management of a subungual hematoma without an associated nail avulsion or surrounding soft tissue damage included nail removal for all hematomas that constituted >25% of the nail bed. Others recommend nail plate removal for hematomas >50%. However, there are a number of studies suggesting that trephination alone is sufficient irrespective of the percentage of nail bed involvement.

When a nail plate fracture or avulsion is present, there is little debate that the nail must be removed. Similarly, nail plate removal is advocated with severe damage to the surrounding soft tissue, such as nail folds and the eponychium. Controversy arises when the nail plate remains affixed to the bed and a hematoma is >25% to 50% of the nail bed. In one prospective, observational study, trephination alone for those patients with subungual hematomas demonstrated no adverse outcomes of infection, osteomyelitis, or nail deformity. Of note, 76% of patients had hematomas that were >50% of the nail bed and 38% had an underlying distal phalanx fracture. Yet another randomized, controlled trial came to the similar conclusion that trephination is an appropriate intervention with no untoward consequences.

There are several methods of trephination. The first involves using a pre-sterilized needle, generally an 18-gauge needle, but any appropriate sized needle can be used that takes into account the size of the nail. The needle is rotated slowly back and forth with gentle downward pressure until there is a release of fluid. In some cases, several holes can be created to relieve the pressure and drain the fluid. A second method is to use a heated straightened sterilized paperclip to burn a hole through the nail until the hematoma can be expressed. This method has its detractors due to the possibility of coagulation of the hematoma as well as the potential to add carbon particles. A third method favored by many authors is to use a high-temperature electrocautery, but this also has the disadvantage of potentially causing a heat-induced coagulation preventing complete expression of the hematoma. A tool was recently introduced in the literature that employs a technology that creates microcuts in the nail. It has an advantage of using electrical signals to terminate the cutting process once the nail is penetrated, thereby avoiding nail bed injury. The mesoscission handheld device contains two small electric motors that create small cuts in the nail with a 400-μm diameter tissue. There are only a few studies attesting to the effectiveness of this tool.

Trephination represents a relatively painless and conservative strategy in the treatment of a subungual hematoma. Several methods are available to perform a nail trephination. In appropriate circumstances, there is good evidence to suggest that the time-honored removal of the nail plate may no longer be necessary.

SUGGESTED READINGS

Bowman SH. Subungal hematoma evacuation. In: Reichmann E, Simon R. *Emergency Medicine Procedures.* New York, NY: McGraw-Hill; 2003.

Ciocon D, Gowrishankar TR, Herndon T, et al. How low should you go: Novel device for nail trephination. *Dermatol Surg.* 2006;32(6):828–833.

Roser SE, Gellman H. Comparison of nail bed repair versus nail trephination for subungual hematomas in children. *J Hand Surg Am.* 1999;24(6):1166–1170.

Seaberg DC, Angelos WJ, Paris PM. Treatment of subungual hematomas with nail trephination: A prospective study. *Am J Emerg Med.* 1991;9(3):209–210.

Simon RR, Wolgin M. Subungal hematoma: Association with occult laceration requiring repair. *Am J Emerg Med.* 1987;5(4):302–304.

Tintinalli JE, Kelen GD, Stapczynski JS, et al., eds. *Emergency Medicine: A Comprehensive Study Guide.* 6th ed. New York, NY: McGraw-Hill; 2003.

242

CORNEAL FOREIGN BODY REMOVAL IN THE EMERGENCY DEPARTMENT: KNOW "WHEN," AND KNOW "HOW"

BRYAN S. LEE, MD, JD

Patients who present to the emergency department (ED) with a foreign body sensation in their eye are not uncommon. Although there are many different causes of a foreign body sensation, one common cause is a corneal foreign body (CFB). Fortunately, in most cases, the CFB removal is a straightforward procedure that can be done with a slit lamp.

The emergency physician should assess the patient's subjective visual symptoms and consider whether the patient may have a potentially more serious injury, such as an open–globe or an intraocular foreign body. Typical symptoms of a CFB are nonspecific, such as a gritty or sandy sensation, pain, tearing, and redness.

The history should be focused on the mechanism of injury, the size and composition of the CFB, and its speed when it struck the eye. The physician should ask whether the patient was wearing eye protection and whether the CFB hit the eye directly or obliquely. The time to presentation also is important because metallic objects rust rapidly. Doctors should not neglect a possible injury to the other eye and past ophthalmic history. A good occupational history often confirms that many patients have had multiple CFBs in the past. A CT scan is not warranted routinely, but the circumstances of the case may dictate otherwise.

The examination should begin with checking visual acuity prior to CFB removal. If the patient is uncooperative because of extreme pain, a drop of an anesthetic may facilitate examination. Under no circumstances should a patient be allowed to leave with a topical anesthetic because of the risk of neurotrophic ulceration and perforation. The physician should ensure that both the pupils are round, symmetric, and reactive. Any irregularity or peaking of the pupil is concerning for an open–globe injury.

A systematic slit lamp exam begins with a lid examination followed by a search for a conjunctival foreign body, laceration, or open globe. The exam must include the upper and lower fornices. The upper lid should be everted by having the patient look down, pulling on the eyelashes, and flipping the tarsus over the handle of a cotton tip. A pattern of linear corneal abrasions is highly suspicious for a forniceal foreign body.

The physician should apply fluorescein and look at the cornea under the cobalt blue light of the slit lamp; CFBs are usually easily visible. Switching back to white light, the physician can narrow the slit beam and estimate the depth of penetration as a percentage of corneal thickness. Also, the size and shape of the CFB, its location relative to the visual axis, and the presence of a rust ring should be noted. A hazy infiltrate around the CFB is common and is usually sterile if the CFB is metallic but is more concerning for infection if the CFB is vegetable matter. Deep, multiple, or infected CFBs often merit ophthalmologic consultation.

The examiner should check the anterior chamber for a hyphema or intraocular foreign body and look for iris tears or defects. Doctors should ensure that the pupil remains round and reactive under high magnification and evaluate the lens for any evidence of trauma.

The key to CFB removal is patient positioning and cooperation. The physician should give more topical anesthetic prior to the procedure. Many physicians also give a preprocedure drop of an antibiotic such as a fourth-generation fluoroquinolone. It is important to explain to the patient the need for concentration and communication if the patient feels the urge to make any sudden movements. Both the emergency physician and the patient should sit at the slit lamp as comfortably as possible, with the patient anchored on the chin rest and pushed against the forehead bar. Before proceeding, the doctor should give the patient as small and specific a fixation target as possible and make sure that the patient has both eyes open.

An extremely shallow CFB may sometimes be removable with irrigation. Some use a moistened cotton tip, but this is discouraged because it often pushes the CFB deeper into the cornea. A corneal burr may have the same effect if used initially. Instead, a 27- or 30-gauge needle attached to a tuberculin syringe is the instrument of choice. Doctors should hold the syringe so that the bevel of the needle faces toward them and make sure that their hands are well anchored on the slit lamp or the patient's face.

The beam should be broad and the slit lamp set at 10× magnification. The physician should locate the needle tip in the field of view and then move it toward the patient bevel-up. Ideally, the hollow end will be able to slip under the CFB and flick it out in one piece, but CFBs sometimes break up, necessitating multiple passes. Having a moistened cotton tip ready to collect freed CFBs from the ocular surface is a good idea because the patient's blinking may move the CFB to the fornix otherwise.

The goal is complete removal of the CFB because residual material often causes irritation and inflammation. However, a rust ring may be difficult to remove entirely, and at that point, use of the Alger burr is helpful. Deep or central rust may be left to migrate more superficially for safer removal by an ophthalmologist at a later time.

After removal, treatment for several days with bacitracin ointment qid helps prevent superinfections. Lens wearers and patients with vegetable matter eye exposure should have a fourth-generation fluoroquinolone qid as well. Contact lens wearers should resist putting anything in their eyes until they have completely healed. A patient with a small, superficial, completely removed CFB may not need follow-up, but someone with a large or central defect or any concern for infection should receive close outpatient ophthalmology follow-up.

CFBs are commonly encountered in the ED. With a good history and physical examination, judicious use of topical anesthetic and antibiotics, and the proper use of a slit lamp, most CFBs can be safely removed. As is true for all ED patients, close follow-up and clear discharge instructions are essential.

SUGGESTED READING

Babineau MR, Sanchez LD. Ophthalmologic procedures in the emergency department. *Emerg Med Clin North Am.* 2008;26(1):17–34.

243

CRICOTHYROTOMY: STABILIZE THAT LARYNX

ARJUN S. CHANMUGAM, MD, MBA

All emergency physicians need to have expertise in certain procedures. These procedures include those lifesaving techniques that can be instituted quickly and efficiently. Some of these procedures are infrequently performed which can pose some difficulty for the clinician. Fortunately, there are reference books, Web sites, and journals that serve as a resource to help the practitioners perform their duties. However, there can be variations in the description of the performance of the procedure. In the case of cricothyrotomy, there are some elements of the procedure that are either omitted or underemphasized in different references.

Cricothyrotomy is a case in point. This procedure is one of the most valued critical procedures in medicine because it allows physicians a reliable way to establish a definitive airway. The problem with the procedure is that for most physicians, it is not performed very often. Thankfully, most patients do not require the procedure. When it is necessary, cricothyrotomy may be the only intervention that can preserve life.

Although the procedure is fairly straightforward, there are descriptions of the procedure that vary slightly on Web sites and textbooks. In some cases, the references themselves can be misleading or lack emphasis on key elements. In the case of cricothyrotomy, the procedure is straightforward, but there is one step that is often underemphasized in references.

One critical element to the performance of cricothyrotomy is the stabilization of the larynx and/or the cricothyroid cartilage with the nondominant hand (or by some other equivalent means). It is particularly important to stabilize the area if the patient continues to move or is attempting to breathe. Even if the patient is not moving or attempting to breathe, stabilizing the thyroid and/or cricothyroid cartilage during the incision and tube insertion process will facilitate the procedure. In fact, it could be a key factor in the success of the procedure as it can help ensure proper incision and tube placement and prevent the scourge of the failed cricothyrotomy—creation of false lumens. Such reasoning is consistent with the basic surgical principle to ensure that the field is stable before commencing an invasive intervention.

A common complication in the performance of cricothyrotomy occurs after the initial skin incision. For various reasons, the exact location of the membrane can become somewhat obscured after the initial incision. Having an exact idea of the location of the elusive cricothyroid membrane can be facilitated by having a firm hold on the lateral aspects of the larynx or the inferior portion of the thyroid cartilage or cricoid cartilage with the nondominant hand. This allows for a tactile determination to aid in visual confirmation. A firm stabilizing grip can help prevent loss of landmarks or obscuring of key features. Without the stabilization accorded by the nondominant hand, incision pressure or other forces could disrupt the operator's sense of where the midline of the cricothyroid membrane lies.

Interestingly, there are multiple references that make minimal, if any, mention for the need to stabilize the larynx and/or cricothyroid membrane with the nondominant hand (or by some other means). The importance of stabilizing the membrane before insertion is underemphasized in these references but could be critically important for success with the procedure.

SUGGESTED READINGS

Cricothyrotomy. From Wikipedia, the free encyclopedia. Available at: http://en.wikipedia.org/wiki/Cricothyrotomy#Procedure.

Dilational cricothyrotomy. From Maquet/Drägermedical. Available at: http://www.aic.cuhk.edu.hk/web8/dilational_cricothyrotomy.htm.

Helm M, Gries A, Mutzbauer T. Surgical approach in difficult airway management. *Best Pract Res Clin Anaesthesiol.* 2005;19(4):623–640.

Schober P, Hegemann MC, Schwarte LA, et al. Emergency cricothyrotomy—a comparative study of different techniques in human cadavers. *Resuscitation.* 2009;80(2):204–209 [Epub 2008 December 5].

Stone KC, Humphries RL, eds. *Current Diagnosis and Treatment Emergency Medicine.* 6th ed. New York, NY: McGraw-Hill; 1992.

Tintinalli JE, Kelen GD, Stapczynski JS, et al., eds. *Emergency Medicine: A Comprehensive Study Guide.* 65th ed. New York, NY: McGraw-Hill; 2003.

244

DO NOT ASSUME THAT NEEDLE DECOMPRESSION OF A TENSION PNEUMOTHORAX IS 100% RELIABLE AND EFFECTIVE

JULIANNA JUNG, MD, FACEP

Medical students are often taught that needle decompression is an essential first-line treatment for tension pneumothorax. Indeed, it is a potentially lifesaving procedure that every physician should know how to do. Many physicians who are confronted with tension pneumothoraces, particularly those that occur in the context of medical disease or mechanical ventilation, will have limited or no experience with tube thoracostomy. In these cases, the use of needle decompression can stabilize the patient until surgical backup is available. However, is needle decompression the best immediate treatment for tension pneumothorax? Is tube thoracostomy superior? Which procedure should be considered the standard of care for emergency physicians, who are skilled in both?

The evidence on this topic is quite limited. There are no randomized controlled trials that evaluate outcomes of patients with tension pneumothorax who undergo needle decompression compared to those who undergo tube thoracostomy. However, the trauma literature suggests that there are significant failure rates associated with needle decompression and limited clinical benefits to patients undergoing this procedure.

One major argument against needle decompression is that the needle or catheter may not reach the pleural space and effectively achieve pleural drainage. Indeed, a recent study showed that the mean chest wall thickness at the second intercostal space, where needle decompression is performed, is 3.5 cm, and 9% to 19% of men and 24% to 35% of women have a chest wall thickness of >4.5 cm. Given that a standard 16- to 18-g angiocath is only 4.77 cm long, it is possible that this commonly used device would not be long enough to reach the pleural space of many patients, particularly women.

Another argument against needle decompression is the possibility of needle or catheter malposition. Training physicians are taught to listen for the "whoosh" of air escaping from the pleural space or to aspirate air using a syringe—either of these findings is said to confirm the presence of pneumothorax. However, a short catheter lodged in the subcutaneous tissue will not return air, giving a false-negative result. Even a catheter of sufficient length can be misdirected into the subcutaneous tissue, also producing a false-negative result. The use of longer needles has its drawbacks; they can increase the risk of injury to the lung or heart. With a long needle, or even any needle that is long enough, placement of that needle within the lung parenchyma can produce a false-positive result—aspiration of air from the lung parenchyma itself in the absence of a pneumothorax. Needle decompression attempts can even create a pneumothorax or hemothorax where none was present before!

Tube thoracostomy is not without its own complications—malposition has been reported in up to 20% of patients, and associated morbidity can be significant. However, this procedure is felt to be more reliable, and complications more apparent, compared to needle decompression. In the ED setting, where physicians are skilled in tube thoracostomy and able to perform this procedure rapidly, it seems that the utility of needle decompression is limited at best. Possibilities for complications and misinterpretation of results abound, with all the attendant risk of delayed diagnosis and inappropriate management of an already unstable patient.

It should be emphasized that virtually all of the literature on the management of tension pneumothorax pertains to trauma patients. Tension pneumothorax in medical patients is reported but rare, and there are little or no data regarding its management. For physicians with limited experience in tube thoracostomy, needle decompression may be the only means of temporizing an unstable patient until help arrives, and outcomes in these patients may be different than in trauma patients. Additionally, for stable patients with spontaneous pneumothoraces, needle thoracostomy shows significant promise as a definitive treatment.

The bottom line: Immediate chest tube placement is preferable to needle decompression for unstable patients with tension pneumothorax, but as a treatment of last resort, needle decompression remains an essential skill for all physicians.

SUGGESTED READINGS

Cullinane DC, Morris JA Jr, Bass JG, et al. Needle thoracostomy may not be indicated in the trauma patient. *Injury.* 2001;32(10):749–752.

Fitzgerald M, Mackenzie CF, Marasco S, et al. Pleural decompression and drainage during trauma reception and resuscitation. *Injury.* 2008;39(1):9–20.

Zengerink I, Brink PR, Laupland KB, et al. Needle thoracostomy in the treatment of a tension pneumothorax in trauma patients: What size needle? *J Trauma.* 2008;64(1):111–114.

245

DO NOT BE LAZY ... USE MAXIMAL BARRIER PROTECTION WHEN PERFORMING INVASIVE PROCEDURES IN THE EMERGENCY DEPARTMENT

SUSAN MARIE PETERSON, MD

Catheter placement has become a necessity in the treatment of the majority of patients seen in the emergency department, including peripheral intravenous (IV) catheters, midline catheters, arterial catheters, and central venous catheters. However, catheter-related bloodstream infections (CRBSIs) are common and can have a high associated morbidity and mortality. On average, there are 250,000 CRBSIs per year in the United States, with an estimated mortality rate of 12% to 25% and an average increased health care cost of $35,000 to $54,000. The high financial costs and significant health consequences of these infections make prevention critical.

The current rate of CRBSI is unacceptably high. A systemic review done in 2006 of 200 prospective trials found that peripheral IVs, the most commonly placed catheters, have an infection rate of 0.5 per 1,000 IVD-days or 0.1%, midline catheters have a 0.4% infection rate, and arterial catheters have a 0.8% infection rate. Noncuffed, nonmedicated central venous catheters had a significantly higher infection rate of 4.4%.

While these numbers are staggering, they may be understated because the diagnosis of these infections is complex. Confirmation of a CRBSI requires standardized techniques to determine the colonization of the catheter and subsequent isolation of the same organism from the bloodstream. These studies are time consuming and may not always be conclusive.

Numerous preventative methods have been proposed, but one of the most obvious interventions has been the use of maximal barrier precautions. A 1994 study by Raad et al. found that the use of maximal sterile precautions, including sterile gloves, long-sleeved sterile gown, mask, cap, and large sterile sheet drape, when inserting a central venous catheter significantly decreased infection rates when compared with standard precautions of sterile gloves and a small drape. Infection rates were shown to decrease from a rate of 0.5/1,000 catheter days to 0.08/1,000 catheter days.

The effectiveness of this intervention was combined with further intervention in a 2007 study in the *NEJM*. This study found that the implementation of five evidence-based procedures, in addition to improved oversight and communication techniques, reduced infection rates by 66%. These procedures included maximal barrier techniques during insertion of the catheter, hand washing, use of chlorhexidine for skin preparation, avoiding the femoral site if possible, and removal of unnecessary catheters.

While these studies were primarily done in the setting of the insertion of central venous catheters and subsequently confirmed by other observational and prospective studies, full barrier precautions were recommended in a 2000 Annals of Internal Medicine review article for all types of venous and arterial catheter insertion. The CDC recommends that maximal barrier precautions be taken when introducing an arterial or central catheter but states that clean gloves may be used for the insertion of peripheral and midline catheters provided the access site is not touched after the application of a skin antiseptic.

In summary, CRBSI is a significant cause of nosocomial morbidity and mortality and has an annual cost of an estimated 2.3 billion dollars. Infection rates are lowest for the most commonly placed vascular catheters, the peripheral IV, with a rate of 0.1% and highest for central venous catheters with a rate of 4.4%. Maximal barrier methods, including sterile gloves, long-sleeved sterile gown, mask, cap, and large sterile sheet drape, have been shown repeatedly to significantly decrease the rate of infection when compared to the use of sterile gloves and a sterile drape alone. The CDC recommends the use of maximal barrier precautions for the placement of both arterial and central venous catheters. For peripheral and midline catheters, the CDC states that clean gloves alone can appropriately prevent an infection during placement provided the insertion site is not manipulated after the application of a skin antiseptic.

SUGGESTED READINGS

Maki DG, Kluger DM, Crnich CJ. The risk of bloodstream infection in adults with different intravascular devices: A systematic review of 200 published prospective studies. *Mayo Clinic Proc.* 2006;81(9):1151–1152.

Mermel LA. Prevention of intravascular catheter-related infections. *Ann Intern Med.* 2000;132:391–402.

O'Grady NP, Alexander M, Dellinger EP. Guidelines for the prevention of intravascular catheter-related infections: Centers for Disease Control and Prevention. *MMWR Recomm Rep.* 2002;51(44–10):1–29.

Pronovost P, Needham D, Berenholtz S, et al. An intervention to decrease catheter-related bloodstream infections in the ICU. *N Engl J Med.* 2006;355(26):2725–2732.

Raad II, Hohn DC, Gilbreath J, et al. Prevention of central venous catheter-related infections by using maximal sterile barrier precautions during insertion. *Infect Control Hosp Epidemiol.* 1994;15:231–238.

246

KNOW HOW TO INTERPRET LUMBAR PUNCTURE RESULTS PROPERLY

JIM YEN, MD

The most common indications for lumbar puncture (LP) in the emergency department (ED) are for diagnosing central nervous system (CNS) infections and ruling out subarachnoid hemorrhage (SAH). LPs are also useful for identifying elevated intracranial pressure (ICP) in a number of conditions. Most errors in the interpretation of LP results are in the setting of a traumatic LP. It is important for the emergency physician not to dismiss grossly elevated red blood cell (RBC) counts or disproportionately abnormal white blood cell (WBC) counts as due to a "traumatic tap." In the setting of possible SAH, it is also important to assess the CSF for the presence or absence of xanthochromia.

If the LP can be performed in the lateral recumbent position, then one should measure the opening pressure. This piece of information requires only an extra minute to obtain and can aid in the diagnosis. Opening pressures can be abnormally elevated in SAH, CNS infection, and cerebral venous sinus thrombosis or abnormally low in intracranial hypotension. Normal opening pressures range from 5 to 20 cm H_2O (which correspond to the marks on the

LP kit manometer) and up to 25 cm H_2O in obese patients. Values outside this range suggest CSF pathology. Pressures should be measured with the patient lying slightly extended in the lateral recumbent position because they can be artificially elevated while patients are sitting upright or in extreme flexion.

Traumatic LP occurs in 9% to 13% of LPs performed in the ED. CSF is normally acellular; however, in the setting of an LP, the presence of five RBCs or WBCs is accepted as normal in adults. In the traumatic LP, CSF contains elevated RBCs and WBCs due to incidental trauma to a capillary or venule. The interpretation of traumatic taps can lead to the false-positive diagnosis of SAH or meningitis; however, the more serious clinical error is to assume that an elevated RBC or WBC count in a true case of SAH or meningitis is due only to trauma.

Several methods have been described to differentiate between traumatic LPs and true CNS pathology. The first and last CSF collection tubes should be analyzed for cell count, and if the last tube is normal, then this is generally accepted as adequate for excluding SAH. Several studies have looked at the absolute and percentage decrease in RBC count between the first and the last tubes. Beyond a normal RBC count in the last tube, no clear numbers or trends have been identified that can rule out SAH with absolute certainty.

Even with an RBC count of zero or close to zero in the CSF, patients may still have an SAH that can be detected with LP by the presence of xanthochromia. Xanthochromia is a pink or yellow discoloration of CSF caused by the lysis of RBCs and breakdown of hemoglobin. Typically, xanthochromia begins to appear 2 to 4 h after RBCs enter the CSF and may persist for weeks. Therefore, in the setting of an acellular LP result, one should also check the CSF for the presence of xanthochromia as evidence of SAH.

In the setting of a traumatic LP, one may also be tempted to dismiss abnormally elevated WBCs. The ratio of WBCs to RBCs in a traumatic LP depends on their ratio in the blood:

$$\frac{\text{WBC in CSF}}{\text{RBC in CSF}} = \frac{\text{WBC in blood}}{\text{RBC in blood}}$$

In patients with normal peripheral blood, it is acceptable to subtract one WBC per 1,000 RBCs in a traumatic tap. Any disproportionate elevation of WBCs must be considered evidence for CNS infections. It is also important to note that immunocompromised patients may have normal WBC counts in CSF despite a serious infection. If CNS infections are suspected in these patients, they should be treated with antimicrobial therapy and admitted for follow-up of their CSF culture results.

The bottom line for interpreting LP results is as follows: Use the opening pressure, xanthochromia, and the history and physical examination to diagnose

CNS pathology in the setting of normal CSF cell counts. Treat and admit immunocompromised patients for suspected CNS infections regardless of the cell count. Check that the RBC elevations clear to normal in the last tube and that WBC elevations adhere to an expected ratio before dismissing them. Think twice before assuming that elevated cell counts are only due to a "traumatic tap"!

SUGGESTED READINGS

Shah KH, Edlow JA. Distinguishing traumatic lumbar puncture from true subarachnoid hemorrhage. *J Emerg Med*. 2002;23:67–74.

Shah KH, Richard KM, Nicholas S, et al. Incidence of traumatic lumbar puncture. *Acad Emerg Med*. 2003;10:151–154.

Whiteley W, Al-Shahi R, Warlow CP, et al. CSF opening pressure: Reference interval and the effect of body mass index. *Neurology*. 2006;67(9):1690–1691.

247

KNOW HOW TO PERFORM A LATERAL CANTHOTOMY AND CANTHOLYSIS

ESTHER I. CHANG, MD

The orbital socket is a fixed space bounded by a bone, with the globe sitting anteriorly within that space. In the setting of trauma, bleeding from vessels behind the globe can cause a retrobulbar hemorrhage which pushes the globe forward. While the eye is able to displace forward to some degree, its movement anteriorly is restricted by the medial and lateral canthal tendons, which insert onto the orbital rim.

When the globe can no longer move forward, an orbital compartment syndrome results. Compression of the retinal artery and the optic nerve results in acute optic neuropathy as well as retinal ischemia, which, within hours, can result in permanent vision loss. As the veins are compressed, the intraocular pressure within the globe rises acutely, which in itself can cause permanent vision loss if left untreated for hours.

Every emergency physician should be able to firstly accurately determine whether a lateral canthotomy is indicated and secondly to perform an emergent lateral canthotomy and cantholysis in that setting.

Firstly, is a lateral canthotomy indicated? Certainly not for every retrobulbar bleed! While a CT scan of the orbits can confirm the presence of retrobulbar blood, the indication for a lateral canthotomy is a clinical one. The affected eye should be proptotic, bulging forward more so than the contralateral eye, with tight eyelids. Extraocular movements can be restricted. The intraocular pressure should be elevated, as measured with a tonopen or Schiotz tonometer. Normal intraocular pressures are <21 mm Hg but are usually elevated to the forties or above in this setting. If the measurement of intraocular pressure is absolutely not possible, palpation of the globe through a closed lid should reveal greater resistance to retropulsion on the affected side. Of note, palpation is contraindicated in the case of an open-globe injury.

Signs of acute optic nerve damage should also be present. There should be an afferent pupillary defect on the affected side using the swinging flashlight test. The affected pupil will dilate rather than constrict as the light shines back and forth due to damage of the afferent fibers of cranial nerve II. Many other causes of trauma can cause pupillary abnormalities; the whole clinical picture must be kept in mind.

The patient may report an acute decrease in vision or eye pain, though these findings can be less reliable in the acute setting. If normal visual acuity is reliably measured, of course, acute damage is unlikely. It should also be noted that a lateral canthotomy is rarely indicated in the setting of a concurrent orbital fracture, as the fracture itself decompresses the orbital space.

Should a lateral canthotomy be indicated—there is proptosis, elevated intraocular pressure, an afferent pupillary defect, or decreased vision—then do not wait to refer the patient, but do the canthotomy yourself:

1) Inject 2% lidocaine with epinephrine into the lateral canthal area, pointing the needle away from the eye.
2) Place a hemostat horizontally at the lateral canthus and clamp for 1 min to reduce bleeding.
3) Place a blunt-tipped pair of scissors (e.g., Wescott or Stevens) across the lateral canthus and incise the canthus full thickness. This step provides exposure to the canthal tendons and does *not*, in itself, decompress the orbit.
4) Grasp the lower eyelid at the inner edge of the incised canthus with toothed forceps. Pulling the eyelid away from the face, place the scissors in an open position just beneath the skin with the tips pointing against the orbital bone and slightly down toward the nose, and begin cutting to sever the inferior lateral canthal tendon. Sometimes the tendon itself can be visualized, but the key is to *keep cutting* until the eyelid releases completely away from the globe and the globe itself moves forward. Once released, the lower eyelid should retract medially; if not, keep cutting!
5) Hold pressure over the orbital bone, as the area will tend to bleed.
6) Wait 15 min; the results of a successful cantholysis are usually evident within that period of time. Remeasure the intraocular pressure, which should decrease. Often, the vision begins to improve as well.

The most common mistake is not cutting deeply enough. Make sure that you not only have incised not only skin and soft tissue, which in themselves do not decompress the orbit, but also have cut through the tendon itself and seen the eyelid retract and the globe come forward.

Of note, incising the superior lateral canthal tendon is typically avoided as it has not been shown to significantly decrease intraorbital pressure in cadaver studies and carries with it the additional danger of incising the lacrimal gland.

After successfully carrying out the cantholysis, refer the patient as necessary to an ophthalmologist for further evaluation. And congratulations! You have just saved someone's vision.

SUGGESTED READINGS

Carrim ZI, Anderson IW, Kyle PM. Traumatic orbital compartment syndrome: Importance of prompt recognition and management. *Eur J Emerg Med.* 2007;14(3):174–176.

Ehlers JP, Shah CP. *The Wills Eye Manual.* 5th ed. Philadelphia, PA: Lippincott Williams & Wilkins; 2008.

McInnes G, Howes DW. Lateral canthotomy and cantholysis: A simple, vision-saving procedure. *CJEM.* 2002;4(1):49–52.

248

KNOW HOW TO PERFORM A LUMBAR PUNCTURE PROPERLY

JIM YEN, MD

In general, lumbar puncture (LP) is a very safe procedure with rare complications. However, there are several things that should be checked prior to performing an LP to avoid adverse outcomes such as spinal hematoma, post-LP meningitis, or cerebral herniation. These include measuring coagulation parameters and platelet counts in patients with suspected coagulopathy, considering the diagnosis of epidural abscess, assessing the patient for altered mental status or any neurologic deficits, acquiring head computed tomography (CT) in patients at risk for herniation, and recognizing the signs of increased intracranial pressure (ICP) on head CT. In patients who are clinically deteriorating with clear evidence of meningitis or cerebral herniation, aggressive treatment should precede a diagnostic workup.

Several studies have reported serious bleeding with spinal cord compression in patients on anticoagulation therapy. Some medical texts recommend arbitrary cutoffs of international normalized ratio (INR) <1.5 and platelets >50,000 to 75,000 as safe levels to proceed with an LP; however, no data are available regarding the incidence of adverse outcomes in patients with low platelet counts or elevated INR. Nonetheless, thrombocytopenia and coagulopathy have been considered a relative contraindication to LP. When the LP is an essential part of the workup, plasma or platelets can be infused to mitigate the risk of complications.

A second relative contraindication to LP is the patient with suspected spinal epidural abscess. An LP performed through infected skin or an abscess can introduce organisms into the subarachnoid space, thereby inducing meningitis. Before performing an LP, patients should be assessed for red flags that would suggest the possibility of epidural abscess. These include back pain, fever, intravenous drug abuse, leg weakness, dermatomal numbness, and bladder or bowel dysfunction. If suspected, MRI is indicated.

Cerebral herniation is the most severe complication of LP secondary to brain lesions or edema causing increased supratentorial pressure relative to infratentorial pressure after an LP. There is some controversy regarding the causal role of an LP because cerebral herniation also occurs in severe acute bacterial meningitis and intracranial hemorrhage even when an LP is not done. Furthermore, elevated ICP by itself does not predict cerebral herniation. This is most evident in patients with idiopathic intracranial hypertension, for whom treatment includes therapeutic LP to lower the elevated ICP. It is important to differentiate these patients clinically into two groups: those who are well appearing and will be sent home if the LP is normal and those who are ill appearing and will be admitted regardless of the LP results. For ill-appearing and clinically deteriorating patients, the benefits of immediate LP are limited, and therefore management of meningitis (steroids and antimicrobials) or cerebral herniation (mannitol and hyperventilation) should be initiated immediately, while diagnostic workup (head CT and LP) is delayed until the patient becomes more stable. In patients who are well appearing and have no risk factors for intracranial lesions, edema, or cerebral herniation, diagnostic LP can be performed without a head CT. Patients with risk factors for abnormal head CT findings can be identified by the following features on history and physical exam: altered mental status, focal neurological deficits, papilledema, seizure in the past week, history of CNS disease, immunocompromise, and age >60. These patients should undergo a head CT before an LP.

Another pitfall for emergency physicians is failure to recognize signs on head CT that may make an LP dangerous. These include a lateral shift of midline structures, loss of suprachiasmatic basilar cisterns, obliteration or shift of the fourth ventricle, and obliteration of the superior cerebellar and quadrigeminal plate cisterns with sparing of the ambient cisterns. Even then, the head CT is not 100% sensitive for predicting the risk of cerebral herniation. Cerebral herniation has occurred soon after an LP in patients with a normal head CT.

What is the bottom line? Before performing the LP, consider coagulopathy, paraspinous infection, and herniation risk. For stable patients with risk factors for intracranial lesions or edema, check the head CT and be able to identify the head CT contraindications to LP. Clinically deteriorating patients with clear evidence of meningitis or cerebral herniation should be treated with immediate and aggressive therapy first—the CT and LP can wait!

SUGGESTED READINGS

Gower DJ, Baker AL, Bell WO, et al. Contraindications to lumbar puncture as defined by computed cranial tomography. *J Neurol Neurosurg Psychiatr.* 1987;50(8):1071–1074.

Hasbun R, Abrahams J, Jeleel J, et al. Computed tomography of the head before lumbar puncture in adults with suspected meningitis. *N Engl J Med.* 2001;345(24):1727–1733.

Joffe AR. Lumbar puncture and brain herniation in acute bacterial meningitis: A review. *J Intensive Care Med.* 2007;22(4):194–207.

Reihsaus E, Waldbaur H, Seeling W. Spinal epidural abscess: A meta-analysis of 915 patients. *Neurosurg Rev.* 2000;23(4):175–204; discussion 205.

Rennick G, Shann F, de Campo J. Cerebral herniation during bacterial meningitis in children. *Br Med J.* 1993;306(6883):953–955.

Ruff RL, Dougherty JH Jr. Complications of lumbar puncture followed by anticoagulation. *Stroke.* 1981;12(6):879–881.

Silverman RS, Kwiatkowski T, Bernstein S, et al. Safety of lumbar puncture in patients with hemophilia. *Ann Emerg Med.* 1993;22(11):1739–1742.

249

KNOW HOW TO PERFORM AN ESCHAROTOMY

MELISSA W. COSTELLO, MD, FACEP

Escharotomy is a specific procedure that has been a staple in the treatment of severe burns since Pruitt published his original paper in 1968. The burned tissue, in a deep second- or third-degree burn, rapidly loses elasticity and will become constricting as fluid resuscitation is initiated and tissue edema begins. Escharotomy is used to release the pressure in extremity, abdomen, chest, and/ or neck compartments after a circumferential or nearly circumferential burn. The progressive tissue swelling beneath the burn eschar will begin to compromise venous flow, then capillary and lymphatic flow, and ultimately arterial flow. As perfusion becomes more and more compromised, the resulting cell death and tissue necrosis will increase the edema of the tissues, creating a self-perpetuating process that can be stopped only by the release of the pressure on the tissues. The edema in the chest, neck, and abdomen can compress critical structures (tracheal and vessels) and restrict chest and abdominal excursion necessary for adequate oxygenation.

Despite the physiology of this process being well-known and dogmatically taught to surgeons, burn specialists, and emergency physicians, a review of the literature shows that burn patients need escharotomies more often, more aggressively, and far sooner than they are being performed. One of the multiple studies of this issue looked at the adequacy of limb escharotomies in burn patients transferred to a major burn center and found that 44% had inadequate limb escharotomies with an average compartment pressure of >50 mm Hg. Additionally, as the measurement of bladder pressure and the recognition of abdominal compartment syndrome have become more standard in the trauma literature, the burn community is adopting this assessment technique to assess the need for abdominal escharotomy.

Burd et al. did a thorough review of the topic of escharotomy along with a clinical review of 5 years of patients admitted to their burn intensive care unit published in Burns in 1996. Based on this review and clinical data, they have advocated a total change in the way that escharotomy is taught. They argue that escharotomy should no longer be taught as a singular procedure but as a process of decompression and reassessment that is repeated throughout the initial management of a severely burned patient. The constrictive eschar is only a part of the process causing loss of perfusion. Particularly in patients with thermal burns, electrical burns, or a combination of burns and trauma, muscle damage and edema can result in elevated compartment pressures requiring not only the skin or eschar release of escharotomy but also the compartmental release of fasciotomy.

In Burd's clinical group, the authors make a point to emphasize that while many of the patients had the traditional signs of adequate perfusion of hands and feet, the eschar and edema from the burns had compressed the forearm and leg compartments to the point that the patients required emergent decompression escharotomy and fasciotomy. Despite the absence of the traditionally taught clinical signs of compartment syndrome (pain, pallor, paresthesia, pressure, and pulselessness), it is important to remember that these are often signs that appear late in the course, particularly pulselessness. The authors discuss the fact that in burns, far too much attention has been paid to the periphery (hands and feet) and far less to the compartments which can develop critically elevated pressures long before pulses are lost.

Early, aggressive management of severe burns should include the basics of securing airway, breathing, and circulation. After these steps are complete, the attention of the provider should turn to fluid resuscitation and the adequate assessment of the extremity, chest, abdominal, and neck compartments. Early escharotomy, with or without fasciotomy, can be potentially limb saving, preventing permanent nerve damage, muscle necrosis, and, ultimately, amputation. Additionally, preventing muscle necrosis by early fasciotomy can eliminate a large culture medium of dead muscle that is a prime source for hospital-acquired and bloodstream infections which are now no longer reimbursed by several payment entities.

The specific technique of escharotomy is beyond the scope of this chapter, and there are several very good, comprehensive descriptions available online and in various textbooks and articles about burn management. Interestingly, very little has changed since the original diagrams published by Pruitt. Burd's review did, however, recommend a more chevron-shaped escharotomy of the lower chest in order to more adequately separate the chest and the abdominal compartments and advocates for limb escharotomies in locations that facilitate the easy conversion to fasciotomy should the need arise. Compartment pressure monitoring should become a more routine part of burn management with the recognition that compartment pressures of >30 mm Hg for 8 h have been shown in the orthopedic literature to result in permanent nerve dysfunction and pressures of >50 mm Hg will result in cellular death.

In summary, escharotomy should be viewed as part of an ongoing serial evaluation of the patient with severe burns. Recognition of the tendency to perform this procedure too late and too conservatively is important to give providers, particularly in rural, outlying hospitals, the necessary push to perform escharotomy or, at minimum, measure compartment pressures and Doppler pulses on extremities. Elevated pressures or any diminishing of the Doppler flow should prompt immediate decompression.

SUGGESTED READINGS

Bethel CA, Krisanda TJ. Emergency escharotomy. In: Roberts JR, Hedges JR, eds. *Clinical Procedures in Emergency Medicine*. 4th ed. Philadelphia, PA: Elsevier; 2004:769–771.

Brown RL. The adequacy of limb escharotomies-fasciotomies after referral to a major burn center. *J Trauma*. 1994;37(6):916–920.

Burd A, Noronha FV, Ahmed K, et al. Decompression not escharotomy in acute burns. *Burns*. 2006;32:284–292.

Demling R, DeSanti L. Initial management of the burn patient. BurnSurgery.org. Available at: http://www.burnsurgery.org/Modules/initial_mgmt/index_initial_mgmt.htm. Accessed January 20, 2009.

Pruitt BA, Dowling JA, Moncreif JA. Escharotomy in early burns care. *Arch Surg*. 1968;96:502–507.

250

KNOW THE POTENTIAL COMPLICATIONS OF CLOSED TUBE THORACOSTOMY

EVELINE A. HITTI, MD

Tube thoracostomy can be a lifesaving intervention for patients presenting with pneumothoraces, effusions, and hemothoraces. It is, however, associated with significant morbidity and mortality. Chan et al. demonstrated that chest tube insertion in the emergency department can be done as safely and as effectively as in the operating room. This requires a solid understanding of the complications of the procedure, pitfalls of insertion, high-risk patient characteristics, and indications for surgical backup.

Reported mortality rate of closed tube thoracostomy ranges from 0.4% to 3.4%. The complication rate for chest tube insertion ranges from 6% to 38%. Failure rates and nonresolution of the effusion or pneumothorax, however, account for much of the high rates. A study of complications of tube thoracostomy performed in the emergency department for thoracic trauma, spontaneous pneumothoraces, and iatrogenic pneumothoraces had an overall complication prevalence rate of 37.2% with only 1.7% being major complications (potentially life threatening, requiring corrective surgery and administration of blood products or intravenous antibiotics to manage the complication). Immediate complications accounted for 26% with the majority involving minor complications secondary to misplaced thoracostomy tube. The prevalence of delayed complications was 16.5%, the majority of which were minor complications related to failure of drainage and 0.8% was due to major complications involving empyema development.

Complications of pneumothorax can be early or late. Empyema is the most common late complication with a prevalence that varies between 0.8% and 2.8%. Other complications include hemorrhage from an injury to the internal mammary artery, intercostal vessels, or central vessels. Visceral organ injury is another well-documented early major complication with lacerations to the liver, spleen, and lung being most common followed by rare heart injury. Diaphragmatic and esophageal perforation and death from vagal nerve irritation have also been reported. Finally, re-expansion pulmonary edema (REPO) is an uncommon but potentially life-threatening complication with reported incidence of 1% to 14%.

Some complications of chest tube insertion are related to technical factors. The use of the trocar, more common in the past, is associated with a higher risk of organ injury. An alternative to the trocar is blunt dissection followed by insertion of finger with 360-degree rotation to sweep away adhesions and ensure correct position. This method combined with inspection for diaphragmatic injury in trauma situations is aimed at reducing the risk of inadvertent organ injury. Insertion of the tube at the T4 interspace with careful posterosuperior positioning when using the lateral approach can also avoid inadvertent abdominal organ injuries.

Conformity with universal precautions and sterile technique is essential to reducing the risk of infection and empyema. The role of prophylactic antibiotics is controversial with some studies showing no benefit and others demonstrating a small difference in infection rates in patients receiving antibiotics.

Bleeding from the intercostal vessels is best avoided by dissecting into the pleural space superior to the rib. Insertion of chest tubes in the second intercostal space midclavicular line may reduce the risk of organ injury but has been associated with major bleeding usually from an injury to the internal mammary artery.

Risk factors for developing REPO include the presence of a large pneumothorax, collapse of the affected lung for >3 days, and negative pleural pressure suction of >20 cm H_2O. Slow, gradual evacuation of pneumothoraces and avoiding extreme negative intrapleural pressures are thus suggested.

There are little data on inherent patient characteristics that are associated with higher complication rates. Pleural adhesions, however, have been reported as the cause of major complications including lung injury. Trauma leading to diaphragmatic injury is a documented risk factor for transabdominal placement of chest tubes. A high index of suspicion for diaphragmatic injury should be maintained in patients presenting with trauma to the upper abdomen and lower thorax. Perforation of the heart has been reported in patients with cardiomegaly. Any coagulopathy, whether hereditary or medication related, increases the risk of bleeding. Surgical backup should be considered when performing tube thoracostomy in all of these high-risk patients.

Tube thoracostomy is an important skill set in the emergency department. Adhering to sterile technique, blunt dissection with finger sweep, and careful adherence to recommended landmarks are important to ensure safe placement. Patients with pleural adhesions, underlying coagulopathy, cardiomegaly, or history of trauma are at high risk for complications, and surgical backup should be considered in these settings when tube thoracostomy is indicated.

SUGGESTED READINGS

Beng S, Mahadevan M. An uncommon life-threatening complication after chest tube drainage of pneumothorax in the ED. *Am J Emerg Med.* 2004;22:615–619.

Chan L, Reilly K, Henderson C, et al. Complication rates of tube thoracostomy. *Am J Emerg Med.* 1997;15:368–370.

Deneuville M. Morbidity of percutaneous tube thoracostomy in trauma patients. *Eur J Cardiothoracic Surg.* 2002;22:673–678.

Fitzgerald M, Mackenzie C, Marasco S, et al. Pleural decompression and drainage during trauma reception and resuscitation. *Injury.* 2008;39:9–20.

Kerger H, Blaettner T, Froehlich C, et al. Perforation of the left atrium by a chest tube in a patient with cardiomegaly: Management of a rare, but life-threatening complication. *Resuscitation.* 2007;74:178–182.

Kitami A, Suzuki T, Suzuki S, et al. Bilateral pneumothorax accompanied by mild deficiency type hemophilia: A report of a case. *Surg Today.* 2003;33:861–863.

Millikan J, Moore E, Steiner E, et al. Complications of tube thoracostomy for acute trauma. *Am J Surg.* 1980;140:738–741.

Rawlins R, Brown K, Carr C, et al. Life threatening haemorrhage after anterior needle aspiration of pneumothoraces: A role for lateral needle aspiration in emergency decompression of spontaneous pneumothorax. *Emerg Med J.* 2003;20:383–384.

Sethuraman K, Duong D, Mehta S, et al. Complications of tube thoracostomy placement in the emergency department. *J Emerg Med.* 2008 Dec 19 [Epub ahead of print].

251

KNOW WHEN A HEAD CT IS NEEDED BEFORE THE LUMBAR PUNCTURE ... AND WHEN IT IS NOT

SUSAN MARIE PETERSON, MD

The lumbar puncture (LP) is a commonly performed procedure in the emergency department. However, the feared complication of neurological decompensation and cerebral herniation following the procedure has increased the request for computed axial tomography (CT) scans prior to the procedure. In the current environment of competing priorities of heightened patient safety verses utilization and cost reduction, what role does the CT scan have prior to performing the LP?

Contraindications to the LP include unequal pressure between the supratentorial and infratentorial compartments and includes a shifting of intracranial contents (as is found in cases with a midline shift). Most of these situations can be inferred from CT findings. In cases with a suspected diagnosis of subarachnoid hemorrhage (SAH), CT scan is considered by some to be the gold standard (sensitivity 90% to 93%, specificity not calculated) and is often followed by a LP (sensitivity 93%, specificity 95%) to capture the remaining undiagnosed positive patients. The LP procedure is considered safe in patients with a normal level of consciousness, who have no focal deficits or papilledema, although no rigorous studies have been pursued for this purpose. However, in patients with a suspected diagnosis such as meningitis where a CT scan is not considered the gold standard for diagnosis, is it safe to perform the LP without a CT scan?

Numerous studies have tried to address this issue. A 2001 study in the *New England Journal of Medicine* looked at 301 patients with suspected meningitis. Two hundred and thirty-five patients received a head CT of which 24% (56 patients total) were found to have abnormalities. They evaluated the clinical features of these 56 patients including age >60 years, known CNS lesions, seizure within 1 week of presentation, and immunocompetency. They compiled neurological similarities between these patients including abnormal level of consciousness, inability to answer two consecutive questions, and focal neurological deficits. None of these clinical or neurological features were present in 96/235 patients scanned, and 93/96 had normal CT scans giving these clinical features a negative predictive value of these features of 97%. While the presence of neurological deficits is a good indicator of space-occupying lesions, it is important to know the sensitivity of this parameter. A 2006 study out of the United Kingdom found that the neurological exam alone has a sensitivity of 0.72% and a negative predictive value of 0.85% for space-occupying lesions. These two studies suggest that clinical features and a negative neurologic exam can appropriately rule out the need for a CT scan in many patients.

While the neurological exam and clinical features may be sufficient to determine the safety of the LP for many patients, the CT scan alone may have limitations. A 2007 review looking at LP and brain herniation found that while a CT can be invaluable for indicating midline shift, obliteration of suprachiasmatic and basil cisterns, obliteration of the fourth ventricle, and obliteration of the superior cerebellar plate cisterns, there have notably been four case reports and three case series where the patients had normal CT scans with subsequent herniation following LP. These reports indicate the inadequate correlation between CT scan and elevated intracranial pressure (ICP) and highlight that CT alone is not sufficient. Similarly, there are nine case reports and three case series of patients with clinical signs of elevated ICP with herniation subsequent to LP. All patients in this series were noted to have altered levels of consciousness that got precipitously worse following LP, three had a seizure within 24 h, one had decerebrate posturing, and one had a dilated pupil. For this reason, a thorough neurological exam looking for clinical signs of elevated ICP is always indicated, which includes a search for papilledema, posturing, dilated pupils, diminished levels of consciousness (Glasgow Coma Scale (GCS) < 12), focal deficits, and recent seizure.

In summary, a CT scan is indicated in cases of suspected SAH prior to the LP as the diagnosis of SAH can often be made without the LP. If the CT is negative for blood or other signs of increased ICP, and the patient has no other contraindications, then it is reasonable to perform an LP if the index of suspicion is high enough. A CT scan is indicated in patients with suspected bacterial meningitis prior to performing an LP when the patient is older than 60 years, there is a known CNS lesion, the patient has had a seizure within 1 week of presentation, or the patient is immuncompromised. A CT is also indicated if there are focal findings on the neurological exam, if elevated ICP is suspected by physical exam, or if the patient has an altered level of consciousness (GCS < 12). A CT scan cannot replace the neurological exam and physicians must use their best clinical judgment when ordering these imaging studies keeping in mind the acute clinical risks, cost, and radiation exposure.

SUGGESTED READINGS

Byyny R, Mower W, Shum N, et al. Sensitivity of noncontrast cranial computed tomography for the emergency department diagnosis of subarachnoid hemorrhage. *Ann Emerg Med.* 2008;51(16):697–703.

Dupont SA, Wijdicks EF, Manno EM, et al. Thunderclap headache and normal computed tomographic results: Value of cerebrospinal fluid analysis. *Mayo Clin Proc.* 2008;83(12):1326–1331.

Greig PR, Goroszeniuk D. Role of computed tomography before lumbar puncture: A survey of clinical practice. *Postgrad Med J.* 2006;82(965):162–165.

Hasbun R, Abrahams J, Jekel J, et al. Computed tomography of the head before lumbar puncture in adults with suspected meningitis. *N Engl J Med.* 2001 Dec;345(24):1727–1733.

Joffe AR. Lumbar puncture and brain herniation in acute bacterial meningitis: A review. *J Intensive Care Med.* 2007;22(4):194–207.

252

KNOW WHEN A LARGE-VOLUME PARACENTESIS IS INDICATED IN THE EMERGENCY DEPARTMENT

CYRUS SHAHPAR, MD, MPH

PARACENTESIS

Paracentesis, or needle drainage of fluid from the abdominal cavity, is a procedure often performed in the emergency department (ED). This procedure is typically classified into two types, diagnostic and therapeutic. Diagnostic paracentesis typically involves removal of a small volume of fluid in order to determine the etiology or nature of the fluid removed. It can be used to determine transudative versus exudative ascites and the presence of malignancy or to diagnose bacterial peritonitis. This method of paracentesis encompasses the majority of those carried out in EDs. Therapeutic paracentesis, however, is less frequently performed in the ED. It involves the removal of large amounts of ascitic fluid (usually >4 L) to relieve abdominal pain or pressure or assuage

Table 252.1	**WSACS Definitions**
Intra-abdominal pressure (IAP)	IAP is the steady-state pressure concealed within the abdominal cavity expressed in mm Hg and measured at end-expiration in the complete supine position.
Abdominal perfusion pressure (APP)	APP = MAP − IAP MAP = Mean arterial pressure
Intra-abdominal hypertension (IAH)	IAH is a sustained or repeated pathological elevation in IAP ≥ 12 mm Hg.
Abdominal compartment syndrome (ACS)	ACS is a sustained IAP > 20 mm Hg (with or without an APP < 60 mm Hg) that is associated with new organ dysfunction/failure
Primary ACS	Primary ACS is a condition associated with injury or disease in the abdominopelvic region
Secondary ACS	Secondary ACS refers to conditions that do not originate from the abdominopelvic region

respiratory distress that may be secondary to ascites. Despite its infrequent usage, it should be cautiously considered a viable emergency procedure when indicated.

Indications for Emergent Therapeutic Paracentesis

Large-volume paracentesis should be considered in a patient whose ascites is causing severe pain or damage to intra-abdominal or extra-abdominal organs. This scenario is characterized by abdominal compartment syndrome (ACS), a disease process more commonly associated with the critical care setting.

Abdominal Compartment Syndrome

ACS and its associated terminology have recently been described by the World Society of the Abdominal Compartment Syndrome (WSACS) (*Table 252.1*). This expert panel defined ACS as a combination of elevated intra-abdominal pressure (IAP) with associated new organ dysfunction. This is similar to a more common ED disease process, hypertensive emergency. As with hypertensive emergency and blood pressure, there is no agreed upon strict threshold for the magnitude of IAP which defines the disease. Rather, given the variation amongst patients, ACS can present at various levels of IAP.

Etiology and Pathophysiology of ACS

There are both primary and secondary causes of ACS (*Table 252.1*). Primary causes include those related to intra-abdominal injury or disease. This includes

TABLE 252.2	**RISK FACTORS FOR IAH/ACS**
Decreased abdominal wall compliance	Acute respiratory failure Abdominal surgery with 1 degree closure Major trauma/burns Prone positioning
Increased intraluminal contents	Gastroparesis Ileus Colonic pseudo-obstruction
Increased abdominal contents	Hemoperitoneum/pneumoperitoneum Ascites/liver dysfunction
Capillary leak/fluid resuscitation	Acidosis Hypotension Hypothermia Poly transfusion (>10 U/24 h) Coagulopathy Massive fluid resuscitation (>5 L/24 h) Oliguria Sepsis Major trauma/burns

abdominal trauma, ascites, pancreatitis, and other processes. Secondary ACS arises outside the abdominopelvic area and includes massive fluid resuscitation and tension pneumothorax. Each disease may contribute to the development of intra-abdominal hypertension (IAH) and ACS by a number of mechanisms, which generally include decreased abdominal wall compliance, increased intraluminal contents, increased abdominal contents, and capillary lead/fluid resuscitation. In the ED, one may identify those at risk for ACS by considering the pathophysiology of the disease (*Table 252.2*).

DIAGNOSIS AND MONITORING

IAP is most commonly measured using intravesical pressure, a method which can easily be performed in the ED. A standardized method of measuring bladder pressure has been described by Cheatham et al. An elevation in IAH can affect nearly every organ system, which can lead to the development of ACS. IAH decreases cardiac output by reducing venous return and impairing cardiac function. This can lead to an increase in central venous pressure which may misguide fluid resuscitation. IAH can also decrease vital capacity and lung compliance, which may lead to increase airway pressures, barotrauma, hypoxemia, and hypercarbia. Renal impairment is often seen in IAH, secondary to decreased renal plasma flow which can lease to a decline in urine output and renal failure. Similarly, IAH reduces splanchnic blood flow which may lead to increased bacterial translocation in the gut. Lastly, increases in IAP have also been shown to be associated with increases in intracerebral pressure (ICP), which may lead to cerebral hypoperfusion. ED providers must be aware of the effects of IAH in order to properly diagnose and treat the disease.

TREATMENT

Surgical abdominal decompression is the definitive treatment for ACS. Large-volume paracentesis in the ED, however, is a recommended treatment in the emergent setting. In management guidelines published by WSACS, the authors identified nine studies which found that paracentesis was effective for treatment of IAH/ACS. These studies encompassed a variety of patients, including pediatric, medical, burn, and trauma patients. In one such study, Latenser et al. compared percutaneous decompression with decompressive laparotomy in burn patients (>40% total body surface area). In this study, five of nine patients who developed IAH (defined as IAP ≥25 mm Hg) were successfully treated with percutaneous decompression, while four progressed to ACS requiring decompressive laparotomy. Inhalational injury and burn area of >80% total body surface area appeared to predict failure of percutaneous decompression. Overall, the WSACS guidelines state that percutaneous catheter decompression should be considered in patients, with intraperitoneal fluid, abscess, or blood, who demonstrate symptomatic IAH or ACS (grade 2C recommendation).

ULTRASOUND GUIDANCE

When available, routine bedside ultrasonography prior to every ED paracentesis is advised. In a study of 100 ED patients with suspected ascites, Nazeer et al. found that procedure success rates were 95% in the ultrasound-assisted group and 61% in the traditional (nonultrasound assisted) group. As with other ED procedures, ultrasound has been shown to improve safety and efficacy.

SUMMARY

Large-volume paracentesis is indicated in the ED in the patient whose ascites is causing severe pain, respiratory distress, or new organ dysfunction. This is true in the case of ACS, where paracentesis has been shown to help prevent associated multisystem failure and avert the imminent need for surgical decompression.

SUGGESTED READINGS

Cheatham ML, Malbrain ML, Kirkpatrick A, et al. Results from the International Conference of Experts on Intra-abdominal Hypertension and Abdominal Compartment Syndrome. II. Recommendations. *Intensive Care Med.* 2007;33(6):951–962.

Harrison SE, Smith JE, Lambert AW, et al. Abdominal compartment syndrome: An emergency department perspective. *Emerg Med J.* 2008;25(3):128–132.

Latenser BA, Kowal-Vern A, Kimball D, et al. A pilot study comparing percutaneous decompression with decompressive laparotomy for acute abdominal compartment syndrome in thermal injury. *J Burn Care Rehabil.* 2002;23:190–195.

Ma O, Mateer J, Blaivas M. *Emergency Ultrasound.* 2nd ed. New York, NY: McGraw-Hill; 2008.

Malbrain ML, Cheatham ML, Kirkpatrick A, et al. Results from the International Conference of Experts on Intra-abdominal Hypertension and Abdominal Compartment Syndrome. I. Definitions. *Intensive Care Med*. 2006;32:1722–1732.

Nazeer SR, Dewbre H, Miller AH. Ultrasound-assisted paracentesis performed by emergency physicians vs the traditional technique: A prospective, randomized study. *Am J Emerg Med*. 2005;23(3):363–367.

253

KNOW WHEN TO CONSIDER AWAKE ENDOTRACHEAL INTUBATION

JULIANNA JUNG, MD, FACEP

Rapid sequence intubation (RSI) is the mainstay of emergency airway management. This technique involves administration of an anesthesia induction agent followed by a paralytic agent in order to facilitate endotracheal intubation. While RSI is generally safe and effective, it can be fraught with peril for patients with difficult airways. Induction of deep sedation and paralysis leads to loss of airway protective reflexes and apnea. If the airway is difficult and intubation cannot be achieved, mask ventilation may be adequate to maintain oxygenation until spontaneous respiration resumes. However, if the patient cannot be effectively oxygenated using mask ventilation, a true airway emergency develops, often requiring the establishment of a surgical airway.

Anticipating the potentially difficult airway is of paramount importance. A wide variety of patient factors may lead to difficult intubation, including abnormal facial anatomy, obesity, late pregnancy, impaired mouth opening, impaired cervical mobility, and pharyngeal/laryngeal abnormalities. Factors contributing to difficult mask ventilation include age >55 years, obesity, lack of teeth, presence of beard, and a history of snoring. Classification schemes like the Mallampati score have also been used to predict airway difficulty. Unfortunately, no single test adequately predicts airway difficulties. There are more complex scoring systems which show greater promise; however, these may be difficult to employ in the ED setting, where airway management tends to be urgent or emergent and there is little time for assessment prior to intubation. One large meta-analysis of all rapid bedside tests showed that Mallampati class III or IV combined with thyromental distance >6 cm yielded the best discriminative power of available tests, though sensitivity was still poor.

While prediction of difficult intubation is challenging, it is nonetheless crucial. When a difficulty airway is anticipated, the EM physicians must modify their approach to airway management to optimize patient safety. This means assessing the urgency of intubation, choosing the safest possible intubation plan, and being prepared to manage a failed airway. When intubation is needed but it is not an urgent priority, it is prudent to involve consultants experienced in difficult airway management prior to attempting intubation. However, when intubation is needed emergently, the EM physician must proceed unaided. In either case, when a difficult airway is anticipated, there is a general consensus that awake intubation is the first-line technique for establishing an airway.

Awake intubation avoids the use of deep sedatives and paralytics, thereby allowing the patient to maintain airway protection and continue breathing throughout the procedure. However, "awake" is something of a misnomer, as virtually all patients require some degree of sedation or anxiolysis in order to tolerate the procedure. The nasotracheal route is preferred over the orotracheal route in the awake patient, as it is better tolerated and requires less cooperation. Topical anesthesia is recommended, using a "spray as you go" technique. Most anesthesiologists use fiberoptic guidance for awake nasal intubation. However, fiberoptic bronchoscopes are not universally available in EDs, and many EM physicians are not facile with their use. For this reason, EM physicians may need to rely on blind nasotracheal intubation for patients they do not wish to paralyze. This technique is particularly useful for patients with short or immobile necks, limited mouth opening, and oral injuries. Apnea is the only absolute contraindication, as spontaneous respiration is required to abduct the vocal chords and advance the tube into the trachea. Midface trauma, basilar skull fractures, and coagulopathy are relative contraindications.

Orotracheal intubation can also be performed in awake patients, although this as well as nasotracheal intubation is not tolerated, as laryngoscopy stimulates the gag reflex. However, intubation has been successfully performed without use of medications in obtunded patients and in those receiving moderate pharmacologic sedation. A major risk of this technique, and also of awake nasal intubation, is simply failure. Data on overall success rates of various techniques are lacking, and every clinical scenario is different. In general, failed intubation is less lethal in awake patients, as they will continue breathing on their own and maintain some degree of pharyngeal tone. In some cases, it may be possible to support the patient with supplemental oxygen or mask ventilation while arranging appropriate backup maneuvers and personnel. However, if intubation is urgently needed to treat respiratory failure or if sedation drugs lead to loss of airway protection, an alternate plan to rapidly secure the airway is needed.

In addition to failed awake intubation in patients who are known or suspected to have difficult airways, unanticipated difficult airways will inevitably be encountered in clinical practice. There are many options available for difficult airway management, and it is not possible to detail all of them here. Essential techniques for every EM physician include placement of laryngeal mask airway (LMA), use of multiple sizes and types of laryngoscope blades, use of gum elastic bougie, and, failing all else, surgical cricothyrotomy. Use of intubating LMA, placement of esophageal-tracheal combitube, fiberoptic bronchoscopy, and video laryngoscopy are other techniques to consider. Every EM physician must be prepared to manage difficult airways, both anticipated and not.

In short, predicting a difficult airway is problematic. When a patient is suspected to have a difficult airway, it is prudent to avoid RSI. Awake intubation is the preferred option for these patients, and fiberoptic nasal intubation is optimal, though blind nasal intubation is also possible. EM physicians must be skilled in difficult airway management in order to manage the airways of patients for whom awake intubation is unsuccessful and those who prove unexpectedly difficult to intubate.

SUGGESTED READINGS

Lavery GG, McCloskey BV. The difficult airway in adult critical care. *Crit Care Med.* 2008;36(7):2163–2173.

McGill JW, Clinton JE. Tracheal intubation. In: Roberts JR, Hedges JR, eds. *Clinical Procedures in Emergency Medicine*. Philadelphia, PA: WB Saunders; 1998:15–44.

Shigs T, Wajima Z, Inoue T, et al. Predicting difficult intubation in apparently normal patients: A meta-analysis of bedside screening test performance. *Anesthesiology*. 2005;103(2): 429–437.

254

LEARN HOW TO DIAGNOSE LOWER EXTREMITY DEEP VENOUS THROMBOSIS WITH BEDSIDE EMERGENCY DEPARTMENT ULTRASOUND

BEATRICE HOFFMANN, MD, PhD, RDMS

Deep venous thrombosis (DVT) of the lower extremity is a common medical problem. If DVTs remain undetected, they carry a high morbidity and mortality. Physical exam alone for detecting or excluding DVT has a poor diagnostic accuracy. As a result, many physicians often utilize clinical prediction rules to determine which patient has low, moderate, or high probability for DVT and initiate the appropriate diagnostic tests and treatment accordingly. In the ED setting, if patients are deemed to require diagnostic imaging of the venous system, compression ultrasonography has become the imaging modality of choice for diagnosing acute lower extremity DVT. This modality has largely replaced more invasive imaging tests such as venous contrast and radionuclide venography.

The classic approach for the sonographic exam for suspected lower extremity DVT is whole-leg compression ultrasound. This allows for the evaluation of all the deep veins from the groin to the ankle using a compression technique. In recent years, more advanced methods combine compression sonography with sophisticated Doppler techniques. Such a combination results in a very high negative predictive value (NPV) for lower extremity DVT ($\geq 99\%$). The downside is that it requires high operator skill and sophisticated equipment. Hence, the availability of comprehensive whole-leg venous Duplex compression ultrasound for patients presenting with symptoms suggestive of DVT can be very limited, especially for patients presenting after hours. This can result in diagnostic delay and unnecessary anticoagulation prophylaxis. Also, despite the high operator skill and equipment, the efficiency at detecting isolated calf DVT is not always adequate. This is particularly true for patients with challenging exam conditions and often requires follow-up examinations for persisting symptoms or limited initial exams.

In recent years, serial two-point venous compression ultrasound has emerged as an alternative to comprehensive whole-leg venous sonography for the diagnosis of acute lower extremity DVT. This ultrasound exam is restricted to compression sonography of the common femoral vein at the groin and the popliteal vein at the knee fossa. Such a technique completely abandons the evaluation of the deep subpopliteal and calf veins. It requires less sophisticated ultrasound equipment and even novice operators to show a steep learning curve, making this a more accessible test for the general patient population. However, if used alone, there is a need for repeat testing of patients with an initial negative exam. This repeat exam is usually performed within 1 week of first presentation in order to detect formerly concealed calf DVTs, which have progressed to proximal DVTs. Proximal DVTs have a higher morbidity and mortality and require anticoagulation.

Because repeat sonographic testing for patients with initial negative two-point ultrasound is a major limitation and an inconvenient approach, other diagnostic approaches have been evaluated. New evidence suggests that in patients with suspected DVT, the combination of a single negative D-dimer test and a single negative two-point compression ultrasound can rule out DVT with a degree of certainty and efficiency. These findings are equivalent to comprehensive whole-leg venous ultrasound, making repeat sonographic evaluations for this patient group less of a requirement. The D-dimer test utilized in this approach is a blood test detecting fibrin degradation products after a blood clot is degraded by fibrinolysis. It is important to note that a variety of commercial D-dimer assays are available. These assays have a range of sensitivities and NPVs for detecting DVT. When used alone, tests with lower sensitivity have only limited diagnostic value. It is important that the clinician becomes familiar with the specific type of D-dimer test utilized by the laboratory and its limitations in clinical practice. However, newer studies have shown that a negative D-dimer test result, including those from assays with lower sensitivity, combined with a negative two-point compression ultrasound is highly accurate at excluding DVT.

In summary, DVTs can be challenging to diagnose. Although whole-leg compression ultrasound serves as a comprehensive examination, the two-point compression ultrasound in combination with a d-dimer can be a reasonable alternative as a diagnostic strategy.

SUGGESTED READINGS

Anderson DR, Wells PS, Stiell I, et al. Thrombosis in the emergency department: Use of a clinical diagnosis model to safely avoid the need for urgent radiological investigation. *Arch Intern Med*. 1999;159(5):477–482.

Blaivas M. Ultrasound in the detection of venous thromboembolism. *Crit Care Med*. 2007;35(5 Suppl):S224–234.

Blaivas M, Lambert M, Harwood R, et al. Lower extremity doppler for deep venous thrombosis: Can emergency physicians be accurate and fast? *Acad Emerg Med*. 2000;7:120–126.

Bernardi E, Camporese G, Büller HR, et al. Serial 2-point ultrasonography plus D-dimer vs whole-leg color-coded Doppler ultrasonography for diagnosing suspected symptomatic deep vein thrombosis: A randomized controlled trial. *JAMA*. 2008;300(14):1653–1659.

Elias A, Mallard L, Elias M, et al. A single complete ultrasound investigation of the venous network for diagnostic management of patients with a clinically suspected first episode of deep vein thrombosis of the lower limbs. *Thromb Haemost*. 2003;89:221–227.

Frederick MG, Hertzber BS, Kliewer MA, et al. Can the US examination for lower extremity deep venous thrombosis be abbreviated? A prospective study of 755 examinations. *Radiology*. 1996;199:45–47.

Hamper UM, DeJong MR, Scoutt LM. Ultrasound evaluation of the lower extremity veins. *Radiol Clin North Am*. 2007;45(3):525–547.

Heijboer H, Büller HR, Lensing AW, et al. A comparison of real-time compression ultrasonography with impedance plethysmography for the diagnosis of deep-vein thrombosis in symptomatic outpatients. *N Engl J Med*. 1993;329(19):1365–1369.

Hirsh J, Bates SM. Prognosis in acute pulmonary embolism. *Lancet*. 1999;353(9162):1375–1376.

Jacobson AF. Diagnosis of deep venous thrombosis: A review of radiologic, radionuclide, and non-imaging methods. *Q J Nucl Med*. 2001;45(4):324–333.

Kearon C, Ginsberg JS, Douketis J, et al. A randomized trial of diagnostic strategies after normal proximal vein ultrasonography for suspected deep venous thrombosis: D-dimer testing compared with repeated ultrasonography. *Ann Intern Med*. 2005;142(7):490–496.

Landefeld CS. Noninvasive diagnosis of deep vein thrombosis. *JAMA*. 2008;300(14):1696–1697.

Michiels JJ, Gadisseur A, van der Planken M, et al. Different accuracies of rapid enzyme-linked immunosorbent, turbidimetric, and agglutination D-dimer assays for thrombosis exclusion: Impact on diagnostic work-ups of outpatients with suspected deep vein thrombosis and pulmonary embolism. *Semin Thromb Hemost*. 2006;32(7):678–693.

Prandoni P, Lensing AW, Prins MR. Long-term outcomes after deep venous thrombosis of the lower extremities. *Vasc Med*. 1998;3(1):57–60.

Righini M. Is it worth diagnosing and treating distal deep vein thrombosis? No. *J Thromb Haemost*. 2007;5(Suppl 1):55–59.

Scarvelis D, Wells PS. Diagnosis and treatment of deep-vein thrombosis. *CMAJ*. 2006;175(9):1087–1092.

Schellong SM, Schwarz T, Halbritter K, et al. Complete compression ultrasonography of the leg veins as a single test for the diagnosis of deep vein thrombosis. *Thromb Haemost*. 2003;89:228–234.

Stevens SM, Elliott G, Chan KJ, et al. Withholding anticoagulation after a negative result on duplex ultrasonography for suspected symptomatic deep vein thrombosis. *Ann Intern Med*. 2004;140:985–1001.

Useche JN, de Castro AM, Galvis GE, et al. Use of US in the evaluation of patients with symptoms of deep venous thrombosis of the lower extremities. *Radiographics*. 2008;28(6): 1785–1797.

Wells PS, Anderson DR, Bormanis J, et al. Value of assessment of pretest probability of deep-vein thrombosis in clinical management. *Lancet*. 1997;350(9094):1795–1798.

Wells PS, Owen C, Doucette S, et al. Does this patient have deep vein thrombosis? *JAMA*. 2006;295(2):199–207.

255

Learn how to perform ultrasound-guided peripheral intravenous access

Jesse H. Kim, MD

Use of ultrasound (US) has gained great acceptance in the medical community for central venous catheter (CVC) cannulation. In fact, Agency for Healthcare Research and Quality has reported that real-time US guidance for CVC insertion, with or without Doppler assistance, improves catheter insertion success rates, reduces the number of venipuncture attempts prior to successful placement, and reduces the number of complications associated with catheter insertion. In some emergency departments (EDs), US is now being used for guiding peripheral intravenous (IV) access in those patient populations (e.g., IV drug users, dialysis patients, obese patients, etc.) who have failed IV access attempts by traditional landmark and palpation approach. It avoids the complexities and some of the major complications associated with the central lines in patients not deemed to require such level of IV access.

US-guided peripheral IV insertion in EDs first generated great interest in the literature after a report from Keyes et al. in 1999. In that report of 100 patients who failed two attempts at IV placement by landmark and palpation approach, 91% of patients were successfully able to be cannulated in brachial or basilic veins using a 7.5-MHz US probe, with only 2% risk of arterial puncture. In the study, deep brachial vein was identified simply as the compressible vascular structure adjacent to the pulsatile and noncompressible deep brachial artery. Basilic vein was also identified, without mention of Doppler assistance, simply as the more superficial compressible vascular structure radial to the deep brachial vessels. The study involved attending physicians or senior ED residents who had a brief US training session.

In 2005, Costantino et al. reaffirmed the successful nature of US-guided peripheral IV insertion by allocating 39 patients on odd days to US-guided insertion and 21 patients on even days to traditional cannulation method. Their report stated that the US-guided IV insertion took less time overall (13 vs. 30 min), took less time to successful cannulation from first puncture (4 vs. 15 min), required less repeat punctures (1.7 vs. 3.7 punctures), and resulted in greater patient satisfaction. Overall success rates of cannulation after three attempts were 97% in the US arm compared to dismal 33% in the traditional method arm.

The US-guided peripheral IV placement is not without its fault. The deep locations of the brachial veins compared to the superficial veins, as well as the proximity of the biceps muscle and tendon to the IV site, make it more prone to dislodgement of the short IV catheters. Keyes et al. noted 8% frequency of line infiltration or line falling out within 1 h of cannulation. This led to the recommendation that longer than normal IV catheters be used and that a central line be considered if long-term IV access is desired. The concept of longer IV catheters achieving longer duration of uncomplicated cannulation was addressed by Mills et al. who used a 15-cm 16-gauge catheter for deep brachial or basilic vein cannulation with US guidance on 25 ED patients. In their study, 92% of patients were successfully cannulated, and all catheters remained in place until IV access was no longer required, with a median duration of access of 26 h.

Although praised for its efficiency and success rates, some studies have questioned the validity of previous study results. Stein et al. did a randomized study involving 59 patients comparing US-guided peripheral IV access to the traditional method on patients who failed two IV access attempts by nursing staff. In their study, there was no difference in the median number of attempts before successful cannulation in each group, and the median time to cannulation was longer in US group (39 min) compared to the non-US group (13 min). However, in this study, there were three times more obese patients in the US group compared to the non-US group. Also, the US machine could be used only by the attendings, while the peripheral IV without US guidance could be placed by either the residents or attendings, introducing potentially different providers with different levels of training systematically to each arm. Another study of US-guided upper extremity peripheral IV placements in 35 adult patients by Certified Registered Nurse Anesthetists (CRNAs) also did not show any significant differences in time to successful cannulation or number of attempts compared to the traditional approach. However, patients were enrolled not after failed attempts but based on subjective history of difficult IV access in the past or if the provider identified them as having a potential difficulty with IV access.

US-guided peripheral IV access is a viable and excellent option for selected, but not all, ED patients. Ideally, these are the patients who have failed traditional IV access attempts multiple times and who require small number of blood samples or short-term, temporary IV access. Longer catheters may be more stable and last longer compared to standard catheters, and the procedure can be done by providers with relatively simple training. Following these principles, some of the common errors, such as inappropriate selection of patients or using standard-length catheters that may be too short for the deep veins of obese patients, may be avoided.

Suggested Readings

Aponte H, Acosta S, Rigamonti D, et al. The use of ultrasound for placement of intravenous catheters. *AANA J*. 2007;75:212–216.

Costantino TG, Parikh AK, Satz WA, et al. Ultrasonography-guided peripheral intravenous access versus traditional approaches in patients with difficult intravenous access. *Ann Emerg Med*. 2005;46:456–461.

Keyes LE, Frazee BW, Snoey ER, et al. Ultrasound-guided brachial and basilic vein cannulation in emergency department patients with difficult intravenous access. *Ann Emerg Med*. 1999;34:711–714.

Mills CN, Liebmann O, Stone MB, et al. Ultrasonographically guided insertion of a 15-cm catheter into the deep brachial or basilic vein in patients with difficult intravenous access. *Ann Emerg Med*. 2007;50:68–72.

Rothschild JM. Ultrasound guidance of central vein catheterization: Making healthcare safer: A critical analysis of patient safety practices [Agency for Healthcare Research and Quality Web site]. Publication No. 01-E058. Available at: http://www.ahrq.gov/clinic/ptsafety. Accessed January 25, 2009.

Stein J, George B, River G, et al. Ultrasonographically guided peripheral intravenous cannulation in emergency department patients with difficult intravenous access: A randomized trial. *Ann Emerg Med*. 2009;54(1):33–40 [Epub September 27, 2008].

256

Minimize the Risk of Infection When Placing Central Lines

Susan Marie Peterson, MD

Central venous lines, including the access to the subclavian, internal jugular, and femoral veins, are a common necessity in the emergency room and in the intensive care unit setting. In the emergency setting, these lines are required when peripheral IV access cannot be gained, but blood, rehydration, or medication must be given intravenously. In the intensive care unit, these lines are often placed in order to deliver long-term IV antibiotics, parenteral nutrition, pain medications, chemotherapy, dialysis, or frequent blood draws.

Catheters are considered to be colonized when >1,000 colony-forming units (CFUs) can be quantitatively cultured from the tip segment. Local infection is indicated by colonization and clinical symptoms such as purulence or significant erythema. Catheter-related bacteremic systemic infection is defined as positive blood cultures with clinical evidence of the catheter site as a source of infection.

An estimated 5 million central lines are placed every year. While many of these lines are placed in the emergency department, the infection rate data are available primarily from the intensive care unit. On average, 48% of patients in the intensive care unit have a central line with a 4% infection rate associated with these lines. Of those with infections, there is a 14-day increase in the length of stay, a $25,000 increase in cost per infection, and an 18% increase in the mortality rate. This accounts for 250,000 infections per year and nearly 45,000 deaths annually. These are often preventable causes of nosocomial morbidity and mortality, and it is important to be aware of the factors that increase risks.

Evidence-based strategies to decrease central line infections include hand hygiene, maximizing sterile barriers, using chlorhexidine for skin asepsis, and removing unnecessary lines.

Catheters impregnated with antiseptic or antibacterial agents such as chlorhexidine/silver sulfadiazine or minocycline/rifampin have shown to decrease costs as well as the incidence of infection and death. Hypersensitivity does not appear to be a factor; however, there is a concern that these catheters may increase the incidence of resistant organisms, and ongoing surveillance is required.

Factors directly associated with an increased risk of infection include neutropenia, prolonged duration of catheterization, prolonged hospitalization prior to catheterization, total parenteral nutrition, heavy microbial colonization at the insertion site or catheter hub, prematurity, excessive manipulation, moisture under the dressing, and reduced nurse:patient ratio.

An ongoing debate exists as to whether the anatomical site of the central venous line contributes to a patient's risk for infection. A 2005 study in critical care medicine done in 2,000 patients found that a femoral line was an independent risk factor for catheter-related blood stream infections (CR-BSI). However, a study done in the same year and published in the same journal with 657 patients found no clinically or statistically significant differences in infection and colonization for subclavian lines, internal jugular lines, and femoral lines. A subsequent trial conducted in 2008 and published in *Journal of American Medical Association* with 750 patients found that jugular venous access did not reduce the risk of infection when compared with femoral access. Because of the conflicting data, a multicenter trial is underway beginning in 2009 entitled the Central Line Emergency Access Registry (CLEAR), which will attempt to identify complication rates based on factors including the anatomical site, level of training, and use of ultrasound guidance.

In summary, central venous lines are commonly required in the emergency department. However, in the long term, this form of access can be associated with high rates of infection, high costs of care, and a high mortality rate associated with infection. Known risk factors include prolonged insertion, colonization, poor management of the line, and neutropenia. Known factors that decrease risk of infection include hand hygiene, maximum barrier techniques, aseptic skin cleansing, removal of unnecessary lines, and the use of catheter impregnated with antibacterial agents. Recent evidence suggests that the site of line insertion is not a factor in central venous line infection rates, and studies are ongoing.

SUGGESTED READINGS

Alonso-Echanove J, Edwards JR, Richards MJ, et al. Effect of nurse staffing and antimicrobial-impregnated central venous catheters on the risk for bloodstream infections in intensive care units. *Infect Control Hosp Epidemiol*. 2003;24:916–925.

Berenholtz SM, Pronovost PJ, Lipsett PA, et al. Eliminating catheter-related bloodstream infections in the intensive care unit. *Crit Care Med*. 2004;32:2014–2020.

Centers for Disease Control and Prevention (CDC). Reduction in central line-associated bloodstream infections among patients in intensive care units—Pennsylvania, April 2001-March 2005. *MMWR Morb Mortal Wkly Rep*. 2005;54(40):1013–1016.

Deshpande KS, Hatem C, Ulrich HL, et al. The incidence of infectious complications of central venous catheters at the subclavian, internal jugular, and femoral sites in an intensive care unit population. *Crit Care Med*. 2005;33(1):13–20; discussion 234–235.

Lorente L, Henry C, Martin MM, et al. Central venous catheter-related infection in a prospective and observational study of 2,595 catheters. *Crit Care*. 2005;9(6):631–635.

McGee DC, Gould MK. Preventing complications of central venous catheterization. *N Engl J Med*. 2003;348:1123–1133.

Mermel LA. Infections caused by intravascular devices. In: Pffeifer JA, ed. *APIC Text of Infection Control and Epidemiology*. 2nd ed. St. Louis, MO: Mosby; 2000:30–38.

O'Grady NP, Alexander M, Dellinger EP, et al. Guidelines for the prevention of intravascular catheter-related infections: Centers for Disease Control and Prevention. *MMWR Recomm Rep*. 2002;51(RR-10):1–29.

Parienti JJ, Thirion M, Mégarbane B, et al. Femoral vs jugular venous catheterization and risk of nosocomial events in adults requiring acute renal replacement therapy: A randomized controlled trial. *JAMA*. 2008;299(20):2413–2422.

Raad II, Bodey GP. Infectious complications of indwelling vascular catheters. *Clin Infect Dis*. 1992;15:197–208.

Sherertz RJ, Heard SO, Raad II. Diagnosis of triple-lumen catheter infection: Comparison of roll plate, sonication, and flushing methodologies. *J Clin Microbiol*. 1997;35:641–646.

Soufir L, Timsit JF, Mahe C, et al. Attributable morbidity and mortality of catheter-related septicemia in critically ill patients: A matched, risk-adjusted, cohort study. *Infect Control Hosp Epidemiol*. 1999;20:396–401.

Veenstra DL, Saint S, Sullivan SD. Cost-effectiveness of antiseptic-impregnated central venous catheters for the prevention of catheter-related bloodstream infection. *JAMA*. 1999;282:554–560.

257

Not all shoulder dislocations require procedural sedation for reduction

Emilie J. B. Calvello, MD, MPH

Shoulder dislocations are a common reason for presentation to the emergency department (ED) and account for approximately 50% of all joint dislocations. Of all dislocations from the glenohumeral joint, anterior dislocations are by far the most common accounting for 95% to 97% of cases. Anterior dislocations consist of four different anatomic variants: subcoracoid (the most common), subglenoid, subclavicular, and intrathoracic (very rare). Diagnosis is made by history (mechanism of injury, history of previous dislocation), physical exam (arm in slight abduction and external rotation with loss of the rounded contour of the shoulder and palpable humeral head), and radiographs.

Once the diagnosis is made, the physician should consider analgesia and sedation in a stepwise fashion ranging from least to most risk to the patient. Certain features of the history are associated with an increased need for analgesia and/or procedural sedation. Those are time of injury >24 h, associated fractures, and recurrent dislocations. There are a number of techniques in the literature that are reported to have little need for any analgesic agent at all, although the physician should consider each patient's needs individually. The Oza method (direct humeral head manipulation) has been reported in a small case series to require no analgesia or sedation. Other methods shown to require little to no analgesia include external rotations, scapular manipulation, or Milch technique, all of which do not require a substantial amount of traction.

For those patients who require analgesia but in whom systemic narcotics or procedural sedation is not desired, the use of lidocaine in a variety of methods has been described. Perhaps the simplest and best described in the ED setting is the use of intra-articular lidocaine (IAL). In this technique, 20 mL of 1% lidocaine is placed in the glenoid fossa either under ultrasound guidance or using external landmarks (lateral approach, 1 cm inferior to the acromion process). The needle is advanced medially and inferiorly to a depth of 2 to 3 cm. After administration of lidocaine, reduction attempts should be delayed 15 to 20 min while adequate analgesia is achieved. A recent review of all available randomized controlled trials comparing IAL and procedural sedation showed that reduction rates were the same, while the complication rate and ED length of stay were much higher in the sedation group. The time since injury is an important variable as this technique is more likely to fail if the patient presents >6 h after injury.

Ultrasound guided brachial plexus blocks have also been described in the literature as obviating the need for procedural sedation or large doses of narcotics. In particular, the use of ultrasound-guided interscalene brachial plexus block has been reported to be effective in decreasing the need for other analgesia or sedation. However, this technique has not been fully validated in the hands of more unexperienced clinicians and should be approached with caution secondary to possibility of unintended effects (pneumothorax, phrenic nerve paralysis, intra-arterial injection, total spinal block, and high epidural block).

In summary, there are a number of validated methods which avert the need for procedural sedation in the patient who presents with a simple anterior shoulder dislocation. Utilization of these methods will put the patient at decreased risk of complications and decrease the all important ED length of stay.

SUGGESTED READINGS

Blaivas M, Lydon M. Ultrasound guided interscalene block for shoulder dislocation reduction in the ED. *Am J Emerg Med*. 2006;24(3):293–296.

Fitch R, Kuhn J. Intraarticular lidocaine versus intravenous procedural sedation with narcotics and benzodiazepines for reduction of the dislocated shoulder: A systematic review. *Acad Emerg Med*. 2008;15:703–708.

Howell S, Serafini M. Ultrasound-guided interscalene block: More than meets the eye. *Am J Emerg Med*. 2008;26(5):627–628.

Kosnik J, Shamsa F, Raphael E, et al. Anesthetic methods for reduction of acute shoulder dislocations: A prospective randomized study comparing intraarticular lidocaine with intravenous analgesia and sedation. *Am J Emerg Med*. 1999;17(6):566–570.

Kroner K, Lind T, Jensen T. The epidemiology of shoulder dislocations. *Arch Orthop Trauma Surg*. 1989;108(5):288–290.

O'Connor DR, Schwarze D, Fragomen AT, et al. Painless reduction of acute anterior shoulder dislocations without anesthesia. *Orthopedics*. 2006;29(6):528–532.

Oza M. Direct humeral head manipulation (Oza maneuver) for anterior shoulder dislocation. *Ann Emerg Med*. 2004;44(3):282.

Wen DY. Current concepts in the treatment of anterior shoulder dislocations. *Am J Emerg Med*. 1999;17(4):401–407 [Review].

258

PARACENTESIS IN THE EMERGENCY DEPARTMENT: KNOW THE INDICATIONS AND TECHNIQUE

SHANNON B. PUTMAN, MD

Ascites, the pathological accumulation of free flowing fluid in the abdomen and pelvis, is due to cirrhosis >80% of the time. It is the most common complication of decompensated liver disease. Ascites develops in approximately 50% of patients within 10 years of the diagnosis of compensated cirrhosis, as compared with only 25% of patients who develop variceal bleeding. The development of ascites is a poor prognostic indicator, with 50% of patients surviving 2 years from the time of diagnosis.

The other causes of ascites include malignancy, congestive heart failure, tuberculosis, renal failure, and pancreatic disease. The diagnosis of ascites in the emergency department is based on history (identifying risk factors and symptoms of cirrhosis), physical examination, and imaging, typically ultrasonography. The accuracy of the physical exam in diagnosing ascites varies based on the amount of fluid present, the technique used, and patient body habitus. A focused physical exam should include inspection for bulging flanks, percussion for flank dullness, assessment of shifting dullness, and a test for a fluid wave. Only 10% of patients without flank dullness have ascites on ultrasound examination, making it a useful negative predictor. However, it takes roughly 1,500 mL of ascites for dullness to be appreciated; therefore, it is not a sensitive test and smaller volumes may be missed. Ultrasound is the imaging study of choice when diagnosing a patient with ascites and can detect fluid as minimal as 100 mL. It can be done without intravenous access and does not expose patients to radiation or contrast risks. Additionally, it can "mark" pockets of ascitic fluid safe for paracentesis, identify portal hypertension and splenomegaly, access liver size, and confirm portal vein patency.

Once the diagnosis of ascites is confirmed, who should undergo paracentesis? General consensus recommends paracentesis be performed on patients with new-onset ascites, patients admitted to the hospital, and those with clinical deterioration, including fever, abdominal pain, encephalopathy, and signs of infection. Paracentesis is both helpful at narrowing the differential diagnosis of the cause of ascites as well as identifying patients with spontaneous bacterial peritonitis (SBP). Peritonitis is a frequent and often fatal complication of ascites with a prevalence of 8% to 27% and a mortality rate of 48% to 57%. Cell count with a manual differential, sent to the lab in a purple top tube containing ethylenediaminetetraacetic acid [EDTA], is the most useful test to identify patients at high risk for SBP. Any patients with >250/mm³ polymorphonuclear cells should be empirically treated for peritonitis. Ascitic fluid (at least 10 mL) should also be directly innoculated into blood culture bottles in order to assist in the antibiotic treatment of patients with SBP.

Other routine tests that should be sent on ascitic fluid include albumin and total protein. Calculating the serum-to-ascites albumin gradient (SAAG) is useful for identifying the presence of portal hypertension and is obtained by subtracting the ascitic fluid albumin from the serum albumin. A SAAG of >1.1 identifies portal hypertension with 97% accuracy and is seen, for example, in patients with cirrhosis, fulminant hepatic failure, Budd-Chiari syndrome, and portal vein thrombosis. A SAAG of <1.1 indicates an exudative process as the cause of ascites and can be seen with peritoneal carcinomatosis, tuberculous peritonitis, pancreatic ascites, and nephrotic syndrome. Ascitic total protein may provide additional information, and in the past, values >2.5 to 3 g/dL have identified patients with an exudative process, while lower values indicate a transudative process. Although the SAAG is more specific at determining the presence of portal hypertension and has replaced the classification of transudate versus exudative process, ascitic total protein of <1 g/dL identifies patients at high risk for the development of SBP. Patients with a low ascitic total protein should be considered for primary prophylaxis against SBP.

Is paracentesis a safe procedure? Generally, paracentesis is thought to be safe with minimal risks of serious complications despite the coagulopathy present in many patients with cirrhosis. A prospective study of 229 abdominal paracenteses performed on 125 patients found only a single patient requiring transfusion for an abdominal wall hematoma (0.9% of paracenteses) and only two minor complications with non–transfusion-requiring hematomas (0.9% of paracenteses). In this series, there were no cases of procedure-related bacterial peritonitis or death. Another study of 1,100 paracenteses in 628 patients found no need for transfusion despite an INR as high as 8.7 and platelets as low as 19,000, supporting the practice guidelines of the American Association for the Study of Liver Diseases which states that routine correction of the prothrombin time or thrombocytopenia is not required before performing paracentesis. One review of 4,729 paracenteses found that rates of severe hemorrhage and death were estimated to be 0.19 and 0.016, respectively. Most cases of bleeding in this series occurred in patients with severe cirrhosis and some degree of renal failure. Another review found that the incidence of death in a variety of studies ranged from 0% to 16.9% (within 48 h of procedure) with a majority of studies finding an overall incidence of death to be <2%. Overall, paracentesis is considered safe in most patients with coagulopathy, with the exception of those with evidence of disseminated intravascular coagulation who are at higher risk for bleeding-related complications. Special caution should be given to those with hepatorenal syndrome, recent abdominal surgery, or severe intestinal distention. Given these data, it should be concluded that paracentesis is a safe procedure for most patients whose benefits of ruling out SBP and evaluating for portal hypertension far outweigh the risk of bleeding complications.

Patients with ascites are not unusual in the emergency department and should be evaluated thoroughly for the presence of peritonitis given the high mortality of a missed diagnosis. Bedside paracentesis is a quick procedure, taking only minutes of the physician's time and with minimal risk to the patient. Ascitic fluid should routinely be sent for cell count, albumin, total protein, and culture in order to optimize the care of the patient with ascites.

SUGGESTED READINGS

Bhuva M, Ganger D, Jensen D. Spontaneous bacterial peritonitis: An update on evaluation, managment, and prevention. *Am J Med*. 1994;97:169–174.

Grabau CM, Crao SF, Hoff LK, et al. Performance standards for therapeutic abdominal paracentesis. *Hepatology*. 2004;40:484–488.

Inadomi J, Cello JP, Koch J. Ultrasonographic determination of ascitic fluid. *Hepatology*. 1996;24(3):549–551.

Pache I, Bilodeau M. Severe haemmorrhage following abdominal paracentesis for ascites in patients with liver disease. *Aliment Pharmacol Ther*. 2005;21:525–529.

Runyon BA. Paracentesis of ascitic fluid: A safe procedure. *Arch Intern Med*. 1986;146(11): 2259–2261.

Runyon BA. Care of patients with ascites. *N Engl J Med*. 1994;330:337–342.

Runyon BA, Montano AA, Akriviadis EA, et al. The serum-ascites albumin gradient is superior to the exudate-transudate concept in the differential diagnosis of ascites. *Ann Intern Med*. 1992;117(3):215–220.

Williams JW, Simel DL. Does this patient have ascites. *JAMA*. 1992;267:2645–2648.

Wong CL, Holroyd-Leduc J, Thorpe KE, et al. Does this patient have bacterial peritonitis or portal hypertension? How do I perform a paracentesis and analyze the results? *JAMA*. 2008;299(10):1166–1178.

259

PIGTAIL CATHETERS: KNOW THE INDICATIONS AND PITFALLS

EVELINE A. HITTI, MD

Chest tubes have historically been the standard intervention for the treatment of substantial pneumothoraces and pleural effusions. Chest tube insertion, however, requires patient hospitalization, is painful, and is associated with significant morbidity and mortality. With growing interest in minimally invasive therapies to reduce cost as well as pain associated with procedures, the use of small-bore pigtail catheters as an alternative to chest tubes is increasing. Understanding the advantages, indications, and limitations of pigtail catheters is important to using them safely and effectively in the emergency department.

Pigtail catheters are small catheters (usually smaller than 14F) inserted either anteriorly at the midclavicular line in the second intercostal space or laterally at the anterior axillary line in the 4th or 5th intercostal space using Seldinger technique. The appeal of pigtail catheters is multifold: they are easier and less traumatic to insert than traditional chest tubes, select patients can be discharged home with these attached to a Heimlich valve, and they offer more patient mobility than chest tubes. These advantages translate to significant reduction in pain with activities of daily living as well as substantial increases in cost savings.

The safety profile of pigtail catheters compares favorably to that of traditional chest tubes. Injury of the spleen, liver, diaphragm, and heart and infection are the major complications of traditional chest tubes. Visceral organ injury is rarely seen with pigtail catheters. A historical comparison of empyema rates suggests comparable rates for pigtail catheters and chest tubes.

Multiple retrospective studies have evaluated the use of pigtail catheters in both primary and secondary spontaneous pneumothorax. These studies have demonstrated no statistically significant difference in the length of hospital stay, success rate, recurrence rate, or complication of patients treated with pigtail catheters compared to those treated with chest tubes. Thus, they offer a safe and effective alternative to chest tubes in this population.

Iatrogenic pneumothoraces that are symptomatic or large require pleural air drainage. This can be done safely and effectively with pigtail catheters. Furthermore, patients with iatrogenic pneumothoraces who require drainage with pigtail catheters and show no progression on repeat 4-h chest radiograph can be managed safely as outpatients at a cost saving.

The use of pigtail catheters in the treatment of effusions has been looked at in multiple retrospective studies. Patients with malignant pleural effusions treated with pigtail catheters had similar recurrence and complication rates as those reported for patients treated with large-bore catheters. However, given the high failure rate of pigtail catheters placed for empyemas (80%), their use in this setting is not advocated.

There are no studies that have investigated the safety and efficacy of pigtail catheters in trauma patients. Given the high incidence of hemothorax in patients with chest trauma, failure of small-bore catheters secondary to blockage is of concern in this setting and, as such, not recommended.

Though the safety of pigtail catheters has been well established, there are functional complications that have been reported with their use. Displacement of pigtail catheters is common with one study reporting a 21% displacement with 13% of patients requiring repeat pleural procedures. The second most common complication is tube blockage (9%) mainly in patients treated for effusions. The use of pigtail catheters to drain empyemas is associated with the highest blockage rate.

Pigtail catheters are safe and effective alternatives to chest tubes for treatment of spontaneous and iatrogenic pneuomothoraces as well as malignant effusions requiring drainage. Their use is not recommended for traumatic pneumothoraces or empyemas, as tube blockage is a concern in these conditions. Though pigtail catheters are gaining widespread acceptance as a way to improve pain control and reduce costs, tube dislodgement is a common complication that must be considered.

SUGGESTED READINGS

Argall J, Desmond J, Mackway-Jones K. Seldinger technique chest drains and complication rate. *Emerg Med J*. 2003;20:169–170.

Davies HE, Merchant S, McGown A. A study of the complication of small bore "Seldinger" intercostal chest drains. *Respirology*. 2008;13(4):603–607.

Dernevik L, Roberts D, Hamraz B, et al. Management of pneumothorax with a mini-drain in ambulatory and hospitalized patients. *Scand Cardiovasc J*. 2003;37:172–176.

Horsley A, Jones L, White J, et al. Efficacy and complications of small-bore, wire-guided chest drains. *Chest*. 2006;130(6):1857–1863.

Liu C, Hang L, Chen W, et al. Pigtail tube drainage in the treatment of spontaneous pneumothorax. *Am J Emerg Med*. 2003;21:241–244.

Pancione L. The treatment of iatrogenic pneumothorax with small-gauge catheters. The author's personal experience in 30 cases. *Radiol Med*. 2000;100:42–47.

Tsai W, Chen W, Lee J, et al. Pigtail catheters vs large-bore chest tubes for management of secondary spontaneous pneumothoraces in adults. *Am J Emerg Med*. 2006;24:795–800.

260

PROCEDURAL SEDATION: KNOW YOUR OPTIONS

JESSE H. KIM, MD

In the emergency departments (EDs), emergency physicians play a central role in providing sedation and analgesia to patients in need of procedures. In turn, patients have a high expectation for their pain to be relieved. In fact, in a survey, patients reported that their expectation was that their pain be relieved at least by 72% when in the ED.

Procedural sedation and analgesia (PSA) is on a continuum from minimal sedation to general anesthesia. Many different procedural sedation methods exist. Detailed analysis of PSA is beyond the scope of this chapter, but we will examine some of the commonly used agents along with the potentially useful and commonly discussed issues.

Midazolam is a commonly used agent, often combined with fentanyl for analgesia. It may be given by various routes, including intravenously (IV), intramuscularly (IM), or orally. IV is the preferred route in general, secondary to the delayed onset of action and erratic absorption by oral and IM routes. In pediatric dental procedures, intranasal (IN) midazolam at 0.3 mg/kg showed three times faster onset of action compared to oral route while demonstrating no significant difference in overall behavior and vital signs. In adults, 1 or 2 mg of IN midazolam resulted in 97% success rate in MRI completion in claustrophobic patients, while oral midazolam resulted in only 50% success in one randomized study. Thus, it seems that IN midazolam may be a viable option for painless procedures requiring minimal sedation or when avoiding invasive administration of medication.

Methohexital is a rapid-acting barbiturate and may be used for sedation in painless procedures. In a prospective study of 100 pediatric population, 95% efficacy for successful completion of computed tomography (CT) scanning was achieved with 25 mg/kg methohexital given rectally with a mean time to sedation of 8.2 min. Although six patients had brief desaturation, all recovered completely without a need for endotracheal intubation. In another study of 50 pediatric patients, methohexital 10 mg/kg IM achieved 92% success rate for CT scanning with a mean onset of 3.3 min.

Ketamine is another very popular agent for procedural sedation. It is a dissociative agent that is also a potent analgesic. "Emergence reaction" or "emergence phenomena" described as emergence anxiety, nightmares, hallucinations, and delirium have been reported, and Chudnofsky et al. tested the hypothesis that midazolam 0.07 mg/kg IV added to ketamine may result in fewer emergence reactions. In their study of 70 adult patients, 7% had mild emergence reactions without any hallucinations or delirium noted when midazolam was added. However, no comparison group was present in the study. In a pediatric randomized, blinded, controlled study of 266 patients, addition of midazolam 0.1 mg/kg IV did not result in any difference in emergence phenomena compared to ketamine alone. In yet another randomized study of 104 pediatric patients, addition of IV midazolam in 0.05- to 2-mg/kg dosages did not affect recovery agitation and had no measurable beneficial effect compared to ketamine alone.

Laryngospasm is a potential side effect of ketamine. However, both the incidence and magnitude of the side effects are very low in general. Laryngospasm was reported in 1.4% of 1,022 pediatric patients receiving IM ketamine, and in a pooled-data analysis of 11,589 pediatric ketamine administrations among 97 published reports, laryngospasm necessitating intubation occurred in only 0.017% of cases. Ketamine can also cause increased salivary and tracheobronchial secretions, and atropine 0.01 mg/kg or glycopyrrolate 0.005 mg/kg has been used to prevent the bronchorrhea as noted in the literature. However, it is known that ketamine has been successfully and extensively used without these adjunctive agents as well.

Etomidate is an agent that has gained wide acceptance in the rapid sequence intubation and also in procedural sedation. Etomidate has shown to frequently induce deep sedation. In a retrospective study of 150 procedures by Vinson and Bradbury, moderate sedation was achieved in 32%, while 68% of patients achieved deep sedation with mean dose of 0.2 mg/kg etomidate. Etomidate is frequently used as a monoagent during procedural sedation, and literature data are sparse overall in terms of adding an analgesic. In the absence of clear literature data, it may be reasonable to use adjunctive analgesic agent in cases of relatively prolonged and painful procedures. This area clearly needs further investigation.

Propofol is another widely accepted agent in ED procedural sedation. It is both safe and effective in both adult and pediatric populations. It has been used successfully both with adjunctive analgesia (fentanyl) with 31% rate of transient oxygen desaturation and without analgesia with 11.6% rate of transient desaturation in painful ED procedures in pediatric population. In a study of bone marrow aspiration, the use of propofol plus remifentanil resulted in significantly shorter recovery ($p < 0.001$) and less total use of propofol ($p < 0.001$) compared to propofol alone, although transient respiratory depression was higher and satisfaction scores were similar. It is, thus, reasonable, as with etomidate, to add adjunctive analgesia in cases of relatively prolonged and painful procedures although further investigation in this area for risk-benefit is needed. Even though propofol is relatively new to emergency medicine practice, recent cost-effectiveness analysis has shown that propofol is more cost saving in the ED compared to midazolam due to its shorter recovery time.

Overall, many methods exist for ED PSA, and likely many more will appear. Knowing and being comfortable with the various methods and relative idiosyncrasy of different methods, as well as solid experience and individualized clinical judgment, will help us anticipate and avoid common errors.

SUGGESTED READINGS

Bahn EL, Holt KR. Procedural sedation and analgesia: A review and new concepts. *Emerg Med Clin North Am*. 2005;23:503–517.

Chudnofsky CR, Weber JE, Stoyanoff PJ, et al. A combination of midazolam and ketamine for procedural sedation and analgesia in adult emergency department patients. *Acad Emerg Med*. 2000;7:228–235.

Falk J, Zed PJ. Etomidate for procedural sedation in the emergency department. *Ann Pharmacother*. 2004;38:1272–1277.

Fosnocht DE, Heaps ND, Swanson ER. Patient expectations for pain relief in the ED. *Am J Emerg Med*. 2004;22:286–288.

Godambe SA, Elliot V, Matheny D, et al. Comparison of propofol/fentanyl versus ketamine/midazolam for brief orthopedic procedural sedation in a pediatric emergency department. *Pediatrics*. 2003;112:116–123.

Green SM. Research advances in procedural sedation and analgesia. *Ann Emerg Med.* 2007;49:31–36.

Green SM, Johnson NE. Ketamine sedation for pediatric procedures: Part 2, Reviews and implications. *Ann Emerg Med.* 1990;19:1033–1046.

Green SM, Rothrock SG, Lynch EL, et al. Intramuscular ketamine for pediatric sedation in the emergency department: Safety profile in 1,022 cases. *Ann Emerg Med.* 1998;31: 688–697.

Havel CJ Jr, Strait RT, Hennes H. A clinical trial of propofol vs midazolam for procedural sedation in a pediatric emergency department. *Acad Emerg Med.* 1999;6:989–997.

Hohl CM, Nosyk B, Sadatsafavi M, et al. A cost-effectiveness analysis of propofol versus midazolam for procedural sedation in the emergency department. *Acad Emerg Med.* 2008;15:32–39.

Keidan I, Berkenstadt H, Sidi A, et al. Propofol/remifentanil versus propofol alone for bone marrow aspiration in paediatric haemato-oncological patients. *Paediatr Anaesth.* 2001;11:297–301.

Lee-Kim SJ, Fadavi S, Punwani I, et al. Nasal versus oral midazolam sedation for pediatric dental patients. *J Dent Child.* 2004;71:126–130.

Mace SE, Barata IA, Cravero JP, et al. Clinical Policy: Evidence-based approach to pharmacologic agents used in pediatric sedation and analgesia in the emergency department. *Ann Emerg Med.* 2004;44:342–377.

Pomeranz ES, Chudnofsky CR, Deegan TJ, et al. Rectal methohexital sedation for computed tomography imaging of stable pediatric emergency department patients. *Pediatrics.* 2000;105:1110–1114.

Sherwin TS, Green SM, Khan A, et al. Does adjunctive midazolam reduce recovery agitation after ketamine sedation for pediatric procedures? A randomized, double-blind, placebo-controlled trial. *Ann Emerg Med.* 2000;35:229–238.

Tschirch FT, Göpfert K, Fröhlich JM, et al. Low-dose intranasal versus oral midazolam for routine body MRI of claustrophobic patients. *Eur Radiol.* 2007;17:1403–1410.

Varner PD, Ebert JP, McKay RD, et al. Methohexital sedation of children undergoing CT scan. *Anesth Analg.* 1985;64:643–645.

Vinson DR, Bradbury DR. Etomidate for procedural sedation in emergency medicine. *Ann Emerg Med.* 2002;30:592–598.

Wathen JE, Roback MG, Mackenzie T, et al. Does midazolam alter the clinical effects of intravenous ketamine sedation in children? A double-blind, randomized, controlled, emergency department trial. *Ann Emerg Med.* 2000;36:579–588.

261

THE INTRAVENOUS CATHETER: IS BIGGER BETTER?

MICHAEL E. NOTTIDGE, MD, MPH

One of the first and crucial steps in the resuscitation of the trauma patient is establishment of intravenous (IV) access and administration of an appropriate amount of fluid. A widely held notion is that central venous catheters (i.e., central lines) are necessary for adequate resuscitation of the critically ill or

TABLE 261.1	VENOUS CATHETER DIMENSIONS	
	CATHETER SIZE	**CATHETER LENGTH**
Peripheral venous catheters	14–22 ga	4–7 cm
Central venous catheters	16–30 ga	8–15 cm
	7–7.5 Fr[a]	15–25 cm[a]

[a]Dimensions for double- and triple-lumen catheters.

trauma patient. This notion rests on the belief that more fluid can be delivered faster through the central venous catheter, which typically will have a larger internal diameter than a standard peripheral venous catheter (*Table 261.1*). As such, a lot of time and effort is spent in securing central venous access in critically ill or trauma patients. But is bigger always better when it comes to venous catheters?

It seems intuitive that IV infusion into the central circulation is more effective than that done through a peripheral vein.

However, flow dynamics suggest that the flow through a catheter depends on several independent factors based on the Hagen-Poiseuille equation:

$$\text{Flow rate} = \Delta P \, (r^4 / 8 \, \mu L)$$

where

ΔP is the applied pressure or pressure gradient
r is the radius of the catheter
μ is the viscosity of the fluid
L is the length of the catheter

According to the above equation, the flow rate increases greatly with even small increases in the radius of the catheter. However, the flow rate decreases with any increases in length. This becomes important when considering catheters because the average central line is two to three times as long as the average peripheral catheter. For the same lumen diameter, the flow through the catheters can be expected to be significantly slower, depending on its length.

This has been demonstrated in several studies. Mateer et al. in an in vitro study comparing flow rates through different peripheral and central venous catheters and tubing showed higher flow rates for shorter catheters with the diameter held constant (*Figs. 261.1* and *261.2*). In a combined in vitro and in vivo study using dogs, Aeder et al. showed a 50% increase in flow rates for 2-in. versus 8-in. venous catheters.

An important point of note is that in addition to catheter size, the size of the connected tubing also significantly affects flow rates. In one article, it was

Infusion Time by Catheter Size

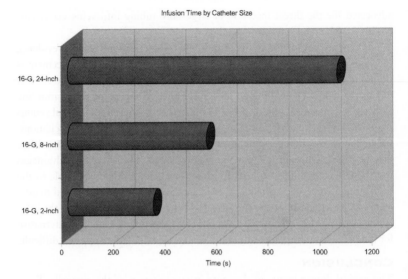

FIGURE 261.1. Infusion time by catheter size.

Catheter Infusion Rates (In Vitro)

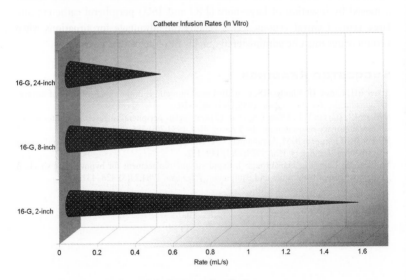

FIGURE 261.2. Catheter infusion rates (in vitro).

advocated for the direct insertion of large-bore tubing into veins via venous cutdown without an interposing catheter!

There are advantages to the central line catheterization. There is evidence to suggest that the main advantage of central over peripheral line placement is the rapid achievement of effective central drug concentrations in the context of cardiac arrest. Depending on its site, another advantage of the central line catheter is that central venous pressure can be easily monitored. Central venous pressures are particularly useful in guiding fluid therapy during resuscitations. Finally, in cases when peripheral venous cannulation is difficult, a central line may be the only option in obtaining venous access. The latter two advantages may be less compelling as there are now alternative methods available to the well-trained emergency provider. For instance, ultrasound can be used to estimate intravascular volume noninvasively with a quick examination of the inferior vena cava. Also, the intraosseous catheter is becoming a suitable alternative for fluid resuscitation, especially when venous catheterization appears difficult.

CONCLUSION

The critical determinants of flow rate in resuscitation of the critically ill are diameter and length of the venous catheter. Optimal flow rates are readily achieved by insertion of large-bore (14G and 16G) peripheral catheters into large veins. Central venous access retains the advantage for situations when certain drugs must be administered quickly into the central circulation.

SUGGESTED READINGS

Aeder MI, Crowe JP, Rhodes RS, et al. Technical limitations in the rapid infusion of intravenous fluids. *Ann Emerg Med*. 1985;14(4):307–310.

Hedges JR, Barsan WB, Doan LA, et al. Central versus peripheral intravenous routes in cardiopulmonary resuscitation. *Am J Emerg Med*. 1984;2(5):385–390.

Mateer JR, Thompson BM, Aprahamian C, et al. Rapid fluid resuscitation with central venous catheters. *Ann Emerg Med*. 1983;12(3):149–152.

Millikan JS, Cain TL, Hansbrough J. Rapid volume replacement for hypovolemic shock: A comparison of techniques and equipment. *J Trauma*. 1984;24(5):428–431.

262

TREATMENT OF PNEUMOTHORAX: CONSIDER PERFORMING NEEDLE ASPIRATION

EVELINE A. HITTI, MD

Needle aspiration is an underutilized intervention for patients presenting to the emergency department with pneumothoraces. Compared to closed tube thoracostomy, the advantages of needle aspiration include reduced hospital admission rates, lower length of stay, and reduced pain. The success rate of needle aspiration ranges from 68% to 75% with a safety profile that compares favorably to closed tube thoracostomy. Thus, needle aspiration can be an effective and safe first-line treatment of pneumothoraces in select patients presenting to the emergency department.

Needle aspiration of pneumothoraces involves manual evacuation of air from the pleural space. An over-the-needle catheter, usually 16 guage, is placed anteriorly in the second intercostal midclavicular space with the patient in a semisupine (45 degrees) position. Alternatively, the needle can be placed laterally along the anterior axillary line in the fourth or fifth intercostal space. After the pleural space is entered, the needle is withdrawn and the catheter is connected to a three-way stopcock and a 60-mL syringe. Manual aspiration of the air is performed until no more air can be aspirated. The catheter is then removed. This is generally a safe procedure with few complications. However, when performed in the second intercostal space midclavicular line, hemorrhage from injury to the internal mammary artery can occur. This is a serious complication often requiring surgical intervention.

Although the American College of Chest Physicians 2001 consensus guidelines for treatment of primary spontaneous pneumothorax found the use of simple aspiration to be rarely appropriate, the British Thoracic Society (BTS) 2003 guidelines recommend simple aspiration as the first step in the management of any primary spontaneous pneumothorax requiring pleural drainage (breathless or rim of air >2 cm on chest radiograph). A second aspiration attempt is reasonable if the patient remains symptomatic after the first aspiration and <2.5 L are aspirated on first attempt. If simple aspiration is successful, the guidelines support patient discharge after a brief period of observation. The BTS approach is supported by multiple randomized studies that have compared needle aspiration for primary spontaneous pneumothoraces to tube thoracostomy. In patients with clinically significant pneumothoraces requiring drainage, needle aspiration has been shown to reduce need for admission, reduce hospitalization rate, and reduce amount of analgesia required for pain control as well as number of days lost from work. Failure rates of the two groups are comparable, as is the 1-year recurrence rate. The RR of 2-year recurrence rate is 1.23 for needle aspiration compared to tube thoracostomy. Some studies have shown that higher failure rates are associated with age >50 and large pneumothoraces (>40%) and thus advocate chest tube placement in these patients. Patients with recurrent primary spontaneous pneumothorax should also be treated with chest tubes as more definitive therapy with pleurodesis or video-assisted thorascopic surgery may be indicated in this setting.

Although the success rate of needle aspiration for secondary spontaneous pneumothorax (33% to 67%) is lower than with primary spontaneous pneumothorax (59% to 83%), the BTS guidelines still recommend simple needle aspiration for small secondary pneumothoraces (visible rim between lung margin and chest wall <2 cm) in patients <50 years old who are not breathless. However, contrary to primary pneumothorax, patients successfully treated with needle aspiration should not be discharged but rather admitted for a 24-h observation period to ensure no recurrence.

Emergency department physicians are often faced with managing iatrogenic pneumothoraces complicating either an emergency department intervention or an ambulatory surgical intervention with delayed presentation. The use of needle aspiration as a first-line therapy in treating iatrogenic pneumothoraces that require intervention is successful in up to 89% of cases. In patients with iatrogenic pneumothoraces who require mechanical ventilation, have underlying chronic obstructive pulmonary disease (COPD), or have >670 mL of air aspirated, a chest tube should be considered as failure rates are high.

Simple needle aspiration is advocated in the treatment of traumatic pneumothoraces only as a first step in decompressing a tension pneumothorax. Otherwise, there is no role for simple needle aspiration in this population as the rate of hemothorax requiring closed tube thoracostomy is high.

Needle aspiration can be a safe and effective intervention for patients with pneumothoraces. It can reduce hospitalization rates and length of hospital stay and improve patient comfort. Its use should be strongly considered as first-line intervention in patients presenting with primary spontaneous pneumothorax or iatrogenic pneumothorax requiring pleural air evacuation. It may be attempted in young, asymptomatic patients with secondary spontaneous pneumothoraces who require drainage. Failure rates are higher in this population and admission is required to observe for recurrence. Needle aspiration has no role in traumatic pneumothorax management beyond initial decompression of a tension pneumothorax when present.

SUGGESTED READINGS

Chan S. The role of simple aspiration in the management of primary spontaneous pneumothorax. *J Emerg Med*. 2008;34:131–138.

Henry M, Arnold T, Harvey J. BTS guidelines for the management of spontaneous pneumothorax. *Thorax*. 2003;58:ii39–ii52.

Rawlins R, Brown K, Carr C, et al. Life threatening haemorrhage after anterior needle aspiration of pneumothoraces: A role for lateral needle aspiration in emergency decompression of spontaneous pneumothorax. *Emerg Med J.* 2003;20:383–384.

Yamagami T, Kato T, Hirota T, et al. Usefulness and limitation of manual aspiration immediately after pneumothorax complicating interventional radiological procedures with the transthoracic approach. *Cardiovasc Interven Radiol.* 2006;29:1027–1033.

Zehtabchi S, Rios C. Management of emergency department patients with primary spontaneous pneumothorax: Needle aspiration or tube thoracostomy? *Ann Emerg Med.* 2008;51: 91–100.

263

USE THE OPTIMAL POSITION WHEN PERFORMING A LUMBAR PUNCTURE

SUSAN MARIE PETERSON, MD AND JULIANNA JUNG, MD, FACEP

The lumbar puncture (LP) is a commonly performed procedure in the emergency department. The analysis of the cerebrospinal fluid (CSF) obtained using this procedure allows the clinician to test for life-threatening diseases such as meningitis and subarachnoid hemorrhage. LP is a relatively safe procedure but can lead to complications, including superficial hematoma and postprocedure headache or backache, as well as rare but serious and potentially life-threatening complications such as infection, epidural hematoma, and cerebral herniation.

It is possible to minimize complications and increase success rates of the procedure with appropriate positioning of the patient. Typically, the patient is positioned in either the lateral decubitus position or the upright sitting position. To perform the procedure in the decubitus position, the patient is asked to lie on his side with neck flexed and knees drawn toward the chest in order to maximize the interlaminar spaces. To perform the procedure in the upright sitting position, the patient is seated upright, leaning forward with arms on a tray or Mayo stand. The feet may also be supported in order to increase lumbar flexion and maximize the interlaminar spaces.

There is no evidence that either technique is more likely to result in success than the other. Given the paucity of evidence on this subject, practitioners should use the technique with which they feel most comfortable. However, each technique has potential advantages and disadvantages that must be considered.

Many practitioners feel that the sitting position makes anatomic markers easier to palpate. While this cannot be proven, it has been clearly demonstrated that this position optimizes the interlaminar spaces. A 2004 study used ultrasound to examine the space between the lumbar spinous processes in three positions: lateral decubitus, sitting upright with feet unsupported, and sitting upright with feet supported. They found that patients sitting upright with feet supported had significantly greater interspinous distances compared to patients in the other groups. Another study compared L-spine radiographs of patients with hips at 90 degrees (as in the upright sitting position) versus those of patients with hips more fully flexed (as in the feet supported position). This study found that the width of the L2-3, L3-4, and L4-5 spaces increased by 7%, 11%, and 21%, respectively, when hips were placed in the flexed position.

While the sitting position does indeed maximize interlaminar distances, particularly with feet supported, it has never been shown to yield superior success rates. This position does have significant disadvantages. Patients who are very ill may not be able to tolerate sitting up. Furthermore, it does not allow the clinician to reliably measure opening pressure. Studies have shown that for every 10 degrees of head elevation, intracranial pressures (ICP) decreases by 1 mm Hg on average. Opening pressure can provide critical clinical and diagnostic information, thus not being able to measure it in the sitting up position is a significant disadvantage. Additionally, some studies have suggested that this position may increase the incidence of post-LP headache. Post-LP headache is thought to be due to persistent leak of CSF from the LP site, causing intracranial hypotension and traction on intracranial structures. Symptoms can be mild or severe prompting revisits to the emergency department. A 1988 controlled study found no correlation between position and post-LP headache. However, subsequent studies found that the upright position causes increased CSF pressure and flow, which may increase the incidence and severity of post-LP headache. Also, the upright sitting position is often used after attempts in the lateral decubitus position have failed, resulting in multiple puncture attempts and dural damage, which is a known risk factor for post-LP headache.

While the standard positions allow for a successful procedure in the majority of cases, some patients may have anatomical limitations that these positions cannot overcome. A 2003 study found that the interlaminar spaces decrease in both height and width with advancing age, potentially making LP more difficult in older patients. Conditions such as ankylosing spondylitis, osteoarthritis of the spine, and prior spinal surgery can further complicate the procedure. In these situations, the paramedian approach may be useful. In this technique, the patient is placed in the lateral decubitus position, and the needle is introduced 1 cm lateral to the midline of the L4-5 interspace. The needle is advanced perpendicular to the skin until the bone is contacted, at which time it is withdrawn 1 cm and redirected at a 15-degree angle medially and cephalad and advanced until CSF is elicited. The major benefit of this approach is that it does not require flexion of the hips or spine, which is useful in patients with limited range of motion. However, this approach is rarely used in the emergency department, and limited experience with this technique may decrease success rates.

In summary, LP can be successfully performed in a variety of positions, and no data clearly support the use of one position over another. The seated position optimizes interlaminar distances, particularly with feet flexed. However, the decubitus position allows for easy and accurate measurement of ICP and may reduce the risk of post-LP headache, though literature evidence is contradictory. Patients with impaired range of motion may benefit from the paramedian approach. Practitioners should use the techniques with which they are comfortable and are most likely to achieve success if they become facile with multiple techniques.

SUGGESTED READINGS

Adams RD, Maurice V, Ropper AH. *Principles of Neurology*. 6th ed. New York, NY: McGraw-Hill; 1997:13–14.

Ahmed SV, Jayawama C, Jude E. Post Lumbar puncture headache: Diagnosis and management. *Postgrad Med J*. 2006;82:713–716.

Boon JM, Abrahams PH, Meiring JH, et al. Lumbar puncture: Anatomical review of a clinical skill. *Clin Anat*. 2004;17:544–553.

Boon JM, Prinsloo E, Raath RP. A paramedian approach for epidural block: An anatomic and radiologic description. *Reg Anesth Pain Med*. 2003;28(3):221–227.

Brocker RJ. Technique to avoid spinal-tap headache. *JAMA*. 1958;168:261–263.

Cook TM. Combined spinal-epidural techniques. *Anaesthesia*. 2000;55:42–64.

Fisher A, Lupu L, Gurevitz B, et al. Hip flexion and lumbar puncture: A radiologic study. *Anaesthesia*. 2001;56(3):262–266.

Frank RL. Lumbar puncture and post-dural puncture headache. *J Emerg Med*. 2008;35(2):149–157.

Lee SJ, Lin YY, Hsu CW, et al. Intraventricular hematoma, subarachnoid hematoma and spinal epidural hematoma caused by lumbar puncture: An unusual complication. *Am J Med Sci*. 2009;337(2):143–145.

Mericq O, Colombani A, Eychenne B, et al. Paramedian lumbar puncture for spinal anesthesia in the elderly. *Cah Anesthesiol*. 1985;33:685–687.

Norris MC, Grieco WM, Borkowski M, et al. Complications of labor analgesia: Epidural versus combined spinal epidural techniques. *Anesth Analg*. 1994;79:529–537.

Rabinowitz A, Bourdet B, Minville V, et al. The paramedian technique: A superior initial approach to continuous spinal anesthesia in the elderly. *Anesth Analg*. 2007;105(6):1855–1857.

Rosner MJ, Coley IB. Cerebral perfusion pressure, intracranial pressure, and head elevation. *J Neurosurg*. 1986;65(5):636–641.

Sandoval M, Shestak W, Sturmann K, et al. Optimal patient position for lumbar puncture, measured by ultrasonography. *Emerg Radiol*. 2004;10(4):179–181.

Vilming ST, Schrader H, Monstad I. Post-lumbar puncture headache: The significance of body posture: A controlled study of 300 patients. *Cephalgia*. 1988;8:75–78.

264

USE BEDSIDE ULTRASOUND FOR THE DETECTION OF PNEUMOTHORAX

BEATRICE HOFFMANN, MD, PhD, RDMS

Bedside lung ultrasound including an evaluation for pneumothorax became an emergency ultrasound core application in 2008 and is now part of the scope of practice for emergency physicians. Sonography for pneumothorax is carried out in association with the Extended Focused Assessment with Sonography for Trauma, or E-FAST, protocol. The exam is also performed in patients suspected of having a partial or complete lung collapse from nontraumatic causes. Its increasing use by emergency physicians and physicians of other nonradiology specialties can be largely attributed to the fact that it can detect pneumothorax with higher sensitivities than portable or supine chest x-ray.

The evaluation for pneumothorax using sonography relies on the assessment of a cluster of sonographic features, mainly ultrasound artifacts, thereby ruling pneumothorax in or out with high accuracy when compared to computed tomography as the gold standard technique. An initial step is an assessment of lung sliding. The presence of lung sliding virtually excludes pneumothorax, with a reported negative predictive value of 100%. By contrast, pneumothorax abolishes lung sliding, and documentation of such a finding predicts a positive diagnosis with sensitivity and specificity in the general population reaching 95% and 91%, respectively. However, in the critically ill, the specificity can drop considerably (≤60%), as a variety of pulmonary diseases can present without this sonographic feature, especially in patients requiring mechanical ventilation. It is thus important to recognize that the absence of lung sliding is not specific to pneumothorax and can occur with other lung pathologies including right main stem intubation and atelectasis, severe pulmonary fibrosis, or pleural inflammatory changes.

The efficiency of ultrasound in the evaluation of pneumothorax can be significantly improved with an assessment for comet-tail artifacts and lung point sign. Comet-tail artifacts arise from the visceral pleura and represent an inflated lung adherent to the chest wall. They may be absent in normal lung ultrasound, but similar to lung sliding, their presence practically excludes pneumothorax. The absence of both lung sliding and comet-tail artifact resulted in an increased sensitivity and negative predictive value of 100% and a specificity of 96.5%.

Another sonographic attribute of pneumothorax is the lung point sign, representing the lead point of the collapsed lung. When detected, it is 100%

specific and has a sensitivity of 66% in the overall study population. The sensitivity decreases, however, with the increasing size of pneumothoraces.

Further evidence for the accuracy of ultrasonographic pneumothorax detection is derived from two studies evaluating the performance of imaging modalities in patients presenting with small pneumothoraces. Ultrasound not only outperformed bedside chest x-ray and detected 79% to 83% of occult pneumothoraces, the investigators concluded that it was an alternative to computed tomography in the emergency or critical care setting with only slightly lower accuracies.

Overall, ultrasound seems to be a powerful bedside tool in the diagnosis of pneumothorax. It can be performed faster than radiography, with a higher efficiency than bedside chest x-ray, and has proven to be a relatively quickly acquired skill among physicians previously unacquainted with the technique. The highest accuracies in the detection of pneumothorax with bedside ultrasound are achieved by evaluating the presence of several sonographic features simultaneously, such as lung sliding, comet-tail artifacts, and lung point sign, and, of course, by putting these findings into clinical context.

SUGGESTED READINGS

Blaivas M, Lyon M, Duggal S. A prospective comparison of supine chest radiography and bedside ultrasound for the diagnosis of traumatic pneumothorax. *Acad Emerg Med*. 2005;12(9):844–849.

Chan SS. Emergency bedside ultrasound to detect pneumothorax. *Acad Emerg Med*. 2003;10(1):91–94.

Dulchavsky SA, Schwarz KL, Kirkpatrick AW, et al. Prospective evaluation of thoracic ultrasound in the detection of pneumothorax. *J Trauma*. 2001;50:201–205.

Kirkpatrick AW, Sirois M, Laupland KB, et al. Hand-held thoracic sonography for detecting post-traumatic pneumothoraces: The Extended Focused Assessment with Sonography for Trauma (EFAST). *J Trauma*. 2004;57(2):288–295.

Knudtson JL, Dort JM, Helmer SD, et al. Surgeon-performed ultrasound for pneumothorax in the trauma suite. *J Trauma*. 2004;56(3):527–530.

Lichtenstein DA. Ultrasound in the management of thoracic disease. *Crit Care Med*. 2007;35(5):S250–S261.

Lichtenstein DA, Menu Y. A bedside ultrasound sign ruling out pneumothorax in the critically ill. Lung sliding. *Chest*. 1995;108(5):1345–1348.

Lichtenstein D, Mezière G, Biderman P, et al. The "lung point": An ultrasound sign specific to pneumothorax. *Intensive Care Med*. 2000;26(10):1434–1440.

Lichtenstein DA, Mezière G, Lascols N, et al. Ultrasound diagnosis of occult pneumothorax. *Crit Care Med*. 2005;33(6):1231–1238.

Reissig A, Kroegel C. Accuracy of transthoracic sonography in excluding post-interventional pneumothorax and hydropneumothorax: Comparison to chest radiography. *Eur J Radiol*. 2005;53(3):463–470.

Soldati G, Testa A, Sher S, et al. Occult traumatic pneumothorax: Diagnostic accuracy of lung ultrasonography in the emergency department. *Chest*. 2008;133(1):204–211.

Tayal V, ed. *ACEP Policy Statement: Emergency Ultrasound Guidelines 2008*. Dallas, TX: American College of Emergency Physicians; 2008. Available at: http://www.acep.org/workarea/downloadasset.aspx?id = 32878

Volpicelli G. Significance of comet tail artifacts at lung ultrasound. *Am J Emerg Med*. 2007;25:981–982.

265

USE CAUTION WHEN STOPPING A CODE DUE TO CARDIAC STANDSTILL ON BEDSIDE ECHO

JOHN GULLETT, MD

Since the 1980s, bedside echocardiography has been used to assess cardiac activity in the setting of a cardiopulmonary arrest or "code" situation. As in all emergency ultrasound applications, the tool is only as good as the operator's knowledge of its uses and limitations. Fortunately, bedside echocardiography can be quite straightforward in answering focused "yes or no" questions with direct visualization that can guide therapy with greater accuracy.

Bedside ultrasound, or in this case echocardiography, can provide pivotal information to the emergency physician (EP) who is treating a critical or arresting patient. Among the multiple causes of pulseless electrical activity (PEA), emergency ultrasound has been studied in diagnosing hypovolemia, tamponade, massive PE, pneumothorax, and cardiogenic shock from MI (cardiac standstill, low ejection fraction, and myocardial dyskinesia). Kaul et al. in 1994 found that echocardiography correctly distinguished cardiogenic from noncardiogenic shock in 86% of their cases. Furthermore, EPs at the bedside have been shown to accurately estimate left ventricular (LV) function, particularly when there is severe dysfunction. Some interesting studies have shown that it is a common misstep to rely on palpable pulses alone when conducting a code. Additionally, studies have shown that relying on palpable pulses is an unreliable estimation of blood pressure and hemodynamics, as is commonly done in codes.

Transthoracic cardiac ultrasound is an invaluable tool in code situations for making informed management decisions. When treating a cardiac arrest, one of the most challenging decisions for the EP is to decide at what point further resuscitative efforts are futile and should be stopped. An important study by Blaivas et al. in 2001 found that, in 169 arrests, cardiac standstill, essentially directly visualized asystole, was 100% predictive of death in the emergency department regardless of initial electrical rhythm. The compelling data have indicated that it is reasonable to cease efforts when cardiac standstill is visualized on bedside transthoracic echocardiography (TTE). Indeed, many EPs now cease efforts in a code when cardiac standstill is visualized with ultrasound.

There are difficulties in acquiring quality images of the heart in a code setting. Chest compressions physically impair the exam, and pauses in CPR are the only opportunity to quickly acquire an image. Unfortunately, this often prolongs the pause in CPR by several seconds, which can be problematic.

The American Heart Association (AHA) emphasizes more consistent CPR with fewer and shorter pulse checks during resuscitation. Furthermore, obese patients and patients with COPD frequently yield a poor image quality. These factors, in addition to the hectic environment of a code, make TTE a potentially challenging ultrasound application.

A recent case series, also by Blaivas, demonstrates the limitations of TTE in comparison with transesophageal echocardiography (TEE) in cardiac arrests. He describes six codes in which the initial TTE was poor in quality and/or incorrect in its assessment. In one case, cardiac standstill was diagnosed on TTE, but subsequent TEE revealed myocardial contractions, a low ejection fraction, and a measurable carotid pulse wave Doppler. A second patient was also diagnosed with cardiac standstill on TTE, but the subsequent transesophageal view revealed organized but very bradycardic contractions due to hyperkalemia. Among the other examples was a case of ventricular fibrillation unappreciated on TTE.

This is a small series and larger studies using TEE are necessary, but nonetheless, this provocative series suggests that the transthoracic approach in the chaotic setting of a code can be misleading. The accuracy of the code TTE is likely decreased in the presence of suboptimal body habitus, COPD, the rushed and logistically awkward environment of a code, and inexperienced operators. The TEE is advantageous in that it provides superior cardiac images, can be placed during CPR and left in place as a constant visual cardiac monitor, and even provides a means of measuring carotid flow. TEE, however, is currently unavailable to most EPs.

The lesson we can learn from Blaivas's case series is that while TTE may be greatly useful in codes, it has limitations. This is not to discourage its use; in fact, the AHA strongly encourages the use of ultrasound in its ACLS guidelines. As always, the EP needs to understand the role and limitations of his or her tools, especially when using bedside ultrasonography for medical management decisions. If a TTE is questionable, indeterminant, or the operator is uncomfortable with it, one should use caution in making management decisions based on the findings. For instance, if a clinician feels that the patient has had several advantageous factors in his or her resuscitation (constant good quality CPR, brief downtime, few comorbidities, etc.), it may be reasonable to consider continuing resuscitative efforts despite cardiac standstill seen on TTE. It is important to remember that TTE and all bedside ultrasound are only as good as the image quality and the interpreters' comfort level.

SUGGESTED READINGS

Blaivas M. Transesophageal echocardiography during cardiopulmonary arrest in the emergency department. *Resuscitation.* 2008;78:135–140.
Blaivas M, Fox JC. Outcome in cardiac arrest patients found to have cardiac standstill on the bedside emergency department echocardiogram. *Acad Emerg Med.* 2001;8:616–621.

Deakin CD, Low JL. Accuracy of the advanced trauma life support guidelines for predicting systolic blood pressure using carotid, femoral, and radial pulses: Observational study. *Br Med J.* 2000;321(7262):673–674.

Kaul S, Stratienko AA, Pollock SG, et al. Value of two-dimensional echocardiography for determining the basis of hemodynamic compromise in critically ill patients: A prospective study. *Echocardiography.* 1994;7:598–606.

Moore CL, Rose GA, Tayal VS, et al. Determination of left ventricular function by emergency physician echocardiography of hypotensive patients. *Acad Emerg Med.* 2002;9:186–193.

Randazzo MR, Snoey ER, Levitt MA, et al. Accuracy of emergency physician assessment of left ventricular ejection fraction and central venous pressure using echocardiography. *Acad Emerg Med.* 2003;10:973–977.

266

USE THE RIGHT DOSE OF VECURONIUM FOR RAPID SEQUENCE INDUCTION

JESSE H. KIM, MD

The proper management of the airway is one of the most important priorities for any emergency physician. The range of management techniques varies from noninvasive support to endotracheal intubation all the way to surgical intervention, the cricothyrotomy. One of the critical management issues when supporting a patient who is in severe respiratory distress is the use of pharmacological adjuncts, especially the paralytic agents. Perhaps the most widely used paralytics are the depolarizing agents. Equally effective and with a slightly different risk-benefit profile are the nondepolarizing agents. In this chapter, vecuronium is profiled as a medication that may be an excellent option for a variety of clinical situations in which endotracheal intubation is being considered.

As with any medication, there is variability in the response that individuals will have to vecuronium. Vecuronium is a classic nondepolarizing agent that works by interfering with the binding of acetylcholine to its receptors. The onset is fairly quick, about 60 s. The duration of its effect is reported to be 30 to 40 min. The ED_{95} (95% effective dose for paralysis) dose of vecuronium is 0.049 mg/kg based on available data. The traditional, typical paralytic dose of vecuronium used clinically is twice the amount of ED_{95}, which comes to about 0.1 mg/kg.

One of the most common preintubation procedures is the rapid sequence induction (RSI), which allows for expeditious endotracheal intubation. The principal difference between the RSI technique and more controlled intubations is that in RSI, there is a minimal amount of time between induction agent administration and paralytic agent administration. RSI's initial intention was to prevent aspiration in patients who may have a full stomach. RSI is now often performed in situations of severe respiratory distress and trauma settings or in any situation when the patient is assumed to have a full stomach. In the ED, there are many situations that require rapid onset of neuromuscular blocking agent for the most efficient intubating conditions for definitive airway control. At the same time, there is concern that too much dose of a paralytic agent may result in prolonged paralysis time.

Although effective for complete paralysis in most populations, the typical paralytic dose of vecuronium ($2\times ED_{95}$) may not be the most optimal dose for RSI. In fact, in his book Emergency Airway Management, Ron Walls specifically recommends 0.15 mg/kg ($3\times ED_{95}$) for vecuronium as intubation dose.

The literature supporting this concept of higher multiples of ED_{95} resulting in faster onset time comes from a comparison of various ED_{95} doses of vecuronium being tested in adductor pollicis muscle paralysis time in train-of-four tests in patients undergoing surgery. In that study, up to $8\times ED_{95}$ doses (0.4 mg/kg) of vecuronium were used for comparison. At $3\times ED_{95}$ (0.15 mg/kg), the shortest onset time was achieved, after which there was no significant drop in onset time. This study did not specifically look at intubating conditions at various ED_{95} doses, but it has compelling data supporting the optimal dose for the fastest onset time of intubation conditions of 0.15 mg/kg.

Vecuronium has a relatively short period of duration. After RSI, paralytic agents are often used for patient comfort and sedation. In the ED setting, the very indications of RSI are usually of a serious nature that requires good deal of medical or surgical work. The potential side effect of a slightly increased neuromuscular paralytic time with $3\times ED_{95}$ dose of vecuronium may be overshadowed by the benefit of complete paralysis in the shortest period of time as compared to the standard paralytic dose of $2\times ED_{95}$. Thus, if vecuronium is to be used as an RSI drug, it is reasonable to use 0.15 mg/kg vecuronium dose as standard ED intubation dose, instead of typical 0.1 mg/kg ($2\times ED_{95}$) paralytic dose.

SUGGESTED READINGS

Casson WR, Jones RM. Vecuronium induced neuromuscular blockade: The effect of increasing dose on speed of onset. *Anaesthesia*. 1986;41(4):354–357.

Kopman AF, Khan NA, Neuman GG. Precurarization and priming: A theoretical analysis of safety and timing. *Anesth Analg*. 2001;93(5):1253–1256.

Walls RM, Luten RC, Murphy MF, et al., eds. *Manual of Emergency Airway Management.* 2nd ed. Philadelphia, PA: Lippincott Williams & Wilkins; 2004.

267

USE THE SUPRACLAVICULAR APPROACH TO CENTRAL LINES

JAE LEE, MD

Many providers shun the supraclavicular (SpC) catheter placement. This is largely due to a number of misconceptions rooted in neither logic nor literature. Often erroneously attributed to Yoffa but actually initially described by Aubinac in 1952, the SpC line has withstood the test of time. It has recently enjoyed a resurgence of popularity supported by a wealth of literature examining over 13,000 placements. These data suggest that the SpC is a safe and efficient option in a variety of clinical settings and situations.

The anatomic advantages of this approach are many. Landmarks for the SpC approach tend to be surprisingly reliable in a broad spectrum of patients ranging from neonates to the elderly and cachectic to the morbidly obese. The target of cannulation is the confluence of the internal jugular (IJ) and subclavian vein and forms the "IJ-Subclavian Sling" which makes for a large and attractive target. The relatively superficial location (typically 1 to 3 cm deep to the surface) makes for a site that is frequently visualized by ultrasound and is reasonably compressible. Prepping the IJ or infraclavicular (IC) site simultaneously with the SpC site conveniently allows for a rapid "back-up" approach for those instances where initial cannulation attempts prove difficult.

The insertion of SpC lines may be performed in a variety of challenging scenarios, including the upright patient and the patient undergoing active chest compressions with minimal interruption. An elegantly designed study shows higher SpC cannulation rates than even femoral vein (FV) access during cardiac arrest. A growing body of literature supports the SpC approach for fast, reliable access for emergency transvenous pacing.

Complications can be conveniently divided into those related to insertion and those related to intravascular indwelling. Overall rates of insertion failure, spanning an extensive review of the literature, are 12% for IJ approach and 12% to 20% for the IC approach versus 3.2% for SpC. Pneumothorax rates are always of significant concern in all of the upper extremity central catheter placement techniques. The most comprehensive reviews reveal rates of 1% (IJ) to 1.5% (IC) versus 0.3% (SpC). Malposition rates of the various upper extremity catheter techniques range from 5% (IJ) to 15% (IC) versus 0.3% (SpC). Arterial puncture rates are reported at 6% (IJ) to 2% (IC) versus 1% (SpC).

The indwelling complications most widely encountered are thrombosis and infection. Occlusive thrombosis rates are most commonly reported as 0% to 1% (IJ), 1% to 2% (IC), and 6% to 30% (FV). Occlusive rates are unavailable for SpC but overall thrombosis (occlusive and nonocclusive) rates are reported at 5%. A vast minority of thromboses are actually occlusive, which are likely to yield occlusion rates similar to IJ and IC. Infection rates resulting in systemic sepsis thought to be catheter related are reported as 4% (IJ) to 2.5% (IC) to 3.5% (FV). Current data for SpC infection risk are limited and rather speculative but theoretically favorable.

A number of slightly differing placement techniques have been described. In this author's experience, the most favorable results are obtained by initiating needle entry 2 cm lateral to the clavicular head of the sternocleidomastoid muscle and 2 cm posterior to the clavicle. The needle is then advanced directly in the coronal plane toward the contralateral nipple. The "Sling" is typically encountered in 1 to 3 cm.

Clearly, the placement of central venous catheters is a complex issue with a significant number of variables. The goal is to produce the best short-term and long-term outcomes for an individual patient given a particular clinical scenario, resources, and operator ability. An SpC approach is by no means a "one size fits all" solution but compares quite favorably to other techniques and merits serious consideration under a variety of circumstances.

SUGGESTED READINGS

Aubinac R. L'injection intraveineuse sous-claviculaire. *Presse Med.* 1952;60:1456–1457.

Cunningham SC, Gallmeier E. Supraclavicular approach for central venous catheterization: "Safer, simpler, speedier". *J Am Coll Surg.* 2007;205(3):514–517.

Dronen S. Subclavian vein catheterization during cardiopulmonary resuscitation: A prospective comparision of the supraclavicular and infraclavicular percutaneous approaches. *JAMA.* 1982;247(23):3227–3230.

Emerman CL, Bellon EM, Lukens TW, et al. A prospective study of femoral versus subclavian vein catheterization during cardiac arrest. *Ann Emerg Med.* 1990;19:26–30.

Kusminsky R. Complications of central venous catheterization. *J Am Coll Surg.* 2007;204: 681–696.

Laczika K, Thalhammer F, Locker G, et al. Safe and efficient emergency transvenous ventricular pacing via the right supraclavicular route. *Anesth Analg.* 2000;90(4):784–789.

Malatinský J, Faybik M, Sámel M, et al. Surgical, infectious and thromboembolic complications of central venous catheterization. *Resuscitation.* 1983;10(4):271–281.

Marino PL. *The ICU Book.* 3rd ed. Philadelphia, PA: Lippincott Williams & Wilkins, 2007;117.

Merrer J, De Jonghe B, Lefrant JY, et al. Complications of femoral and subclavian venous catheterization in critically ill patients: A randomized controlled trial. *JAMA.* 2001;286: 700–707.

Trottier SJ, Veremakis C, O'Brien J, et al. Femoral deep vein thrombosis associated with central venous catheterization; results from a prospective, randomized trial. *Crit Care Med.* 1995;23:52–59.

Yoffa D. Supraclavicular subclavian venepuncture and catheterization. *Lancet.* 1965;2: 614–617.

268

USE VERTICAL INCISION IN EMERGENCY CRICOTHYROTOMIES

JULIANNA JUNG, MD, FACEP AND SAMIUR R. KHANDKER, MD

Airway management is the single most important skill of the emergency physician, and maintenance of a patent airway supersedes all other clinical considerations in the management of an unstable patient. Preparation and training in difficult airway management are crucial but problematic: the stakes are astronomical, but opportunities to practice are rare. Complete airway obstruction in a patient who cannot be intubated or noninvasively ventilated is the ultimate airway emergency, requiring rapid establishment of a surgical airway. Cricothyrotomy is the procedure of choice in this situation, and it is a procedure with which few physicians are truly comfortable. The standard or open technique is the most commonly used, though other techniques have been described and used quite successfully.

The first step in a successful cricothyrotomy is understanding the anatomy. The prominent thyroid cartilage is identified first. Palpating caudally, the first indentation encountered will be the cricothyroid membrane. The membrane is roughly 0.5 to 1 cm high and 3 cm wide and is relatively avascular. However, the anterior jugulars lie just lateral to the membrane on either side, and there is substantial risk of serious bleeding if these vessels are transected. For this reason, when performing standard open cricothyrotomy, a *vertical* incision is recommended—this approach will minimize the risk of venous injury.

Another benefit of a vertical skin incision in open cricothyrotomy is the ability to easily extend cephalad or caudad in the event that the original incision fails to expose the cricothyroid membrane. As noted before, the membrane is only 0.5 to 1 cm high, and it may be difficult to palpate in obese patients or those with abnormal neck anatomy. It is therefore quite easy to make an initial incision that is too high or too low, and a vertical orientation allows rapid correction of this error.

That being said, it is must be emphasized that the incision through the membrane itself is always horizontal. The cricothyroid artery traverses the superior aspect of the membrane, and the highly vascular thyroid artery lies just inferior to the membrane. It would be easy to injure these structures with a vertical incision through the membrane. The membrane itself is wider than it is high, and a vertical incision could also injure the laryngeal cartilages.

After the cricoid membrane is incised, a tracheal hook held by an assistant is placed in the cephalad aspect of the incision, followed by the introduction of a dilator and ultimately the endotracheal tube.

There are no data regarding outcomes of various incision techniques in open cricothyrotomy. These recommendations are based solely on the anatomy. Alternate techniques for cricothyrotomy have been described, notably the rapid four-step technique (RFST) and the wire-guided technique. The RFST uses a horizontal stab incision through the skin and membrane, followed by the introduction of the tracheal hook in the caudad aspect of the incision. This technique has been associated with higher rates of soft tissue damage compared to the standard open technique in one study. The wire-guided technique uses a needle to puncture the skin and membrane followed by the introduction of a guidewire. A stab incision is then made through the skin and membrane, and a cannula is advanced over the wire into the trachea. A recent study showed that this technique took longer and was associated with more complications compared to the standard open technique.

The bottom line is that there are several emergency cricothyrotomy techniques, but the old-fashioned open technique remains as good as, or better than, the alternatives. Using a vertical skin incision, followed by a horizontal membrane incision, is important to the success and low complication rate of this procedure.

Equipment

- Skin sterilization material (betadine or chlorhexidine)
- Face mask, gown, cap, sterile gloves
- No. 11 scalpel
- Hemostat or Kelly clamp
- Sterile gauze sponges
- Tracheostomy tube
- Bag-valve-mask unit with 100% oxygen source
- Tape

Technique

1) Place the patient supine with a rolled towel under the shoulders and neck in hyperextension (if no C-spine injury suspected)
2) Ensure proper sterile preparation of the entire neck as well as sterile garb
3) Stabilize and apply slight downward traction to the cricoid cartilage with the thumb and index finger of the nondominant hand
4) Using a number 11 scalpel, make a 1.5-cm vertical incision along the midline of the cricothyroid membrane, avoiding lateral vessels

5) Cut through the skin and subcutaneous tissue, exposing the cricothyroid membrane

6) Use the scalpel to make a transverse puncture through the cricothyroid membrane into the airway lumen

7) Dilate the opening with a hemostat or Kelly clamp

8) Insert the tracheostomy tube into the opening inferiorly and inflate the cuff

9) Connect the bag-valve-mask to the tube and ventilate with 100% oxygen

10) Tape the tracheostomy tube into place

SUGGESTED READINGS

Brofeldt BT, Panacek EA, Richards JR. An easy cricothyrotomy approach: The rapid four step technique. *Acad Emerg Med.* 1996;3(11):1060–1063.

Chang RS, Hamilton RJ, Carter WA. Declining rate of cricothyrotomy in trauma patients with an emergency medicine residency: Implications for skills training. *Acad Emerg Med.* 1998;5(3):247–251.

Davis DP, Bramwell KJ, Vilke GM, et al. Cricothyrotomy technique: Standard versus the rapid four-step technique. *J Emerg Med.* 1999;17(1):17–21.

DiGiacomo C, Neshat KK, Angus LD, et al. Emergency cricothyrotomy. *Mil Med.* 2003;168(7):541–544.

Friedman Z, You-Ten KE, Bould MD, et al. Teaching lifesaving procedures: The impact of model fidelity on acquistion and transfer of cricothyrotomy skills to performance on cadavers. *Anesth Analg.* 2008;107(5):1663–1669.

Liess BD, Scheidt TD, Templer JW. The difficult airway. *Otolaryngol Clin N Am.* 2008; 41(3):567–580.

McGill J, Clinton JE, Ruiz E. Cricothyrotomy in the emergency department. *Ann Emerg Med.* 1982;11(7):361–364.

Narrod JA, Moore EE, Rosen P. Emergency cricothyrostomy: Technique and anatomical considerations. *J Emerg Med.* 1985;2:443–446.

Nicholls SE, Sweeney TW, Ferre RM, et al. Bedside sonography by emergency physicians for the rapid identification of landmarks relevant to cricothyrotomy. *Am J of Emerg Med.* 2008;26(8):852–856.

Partin WR. Emergency procedures. In: Stone CK, Humphries RL, eds. *Current Diagnosis & Treatment: Emergency Medicine.* 6th ed. New York: McGraw-Hill, 2008.

Schillaci CR, Iacovoni VF, Conte RS. Transtracheal aspiration complicated by fatal endotracheal hemorrhage. *N Engl J Med.* 1976;295(9):488–490.

Schober P, Hegemann MC, Schwarte LA, et al. Emergency cricothyrotomy: A comparative study of different techniques in human cadavers. *Resuscitation.* 2009;80(2):204–209 [Epub 2008 Dec 5].

Spaite DW, Joseph M. Prehospital cricothyrotomy: An investigation of indications, technique, complications, and patient outcome. *Ann Emerg Med.* 1990;19(3):279–285.

Vanner R. Emergency cricothyrotomy. *Curr Anaesth Crit Care.* 2001;12(4):238–243.

269

NEVER ASSUME THAT ACUTE DELIRIUM IS CAUSED BY PREEXISTING PSYCHIATRIC DISEASE

MARY LOUISE MARTIN, MD AND
JORGE A. FERNANDEZ, MD, FAAEM, FACEP

Caring for the acutely psychotic patient can be a challenge even for the most experienced emergency physician. These patients frequently compromise the safety of the medical staff and require extensive time and resources. It is a normal human countertransference behavior to want to hurry these patients out of the department. Emergency physicians should be mindful of the potential to misdiagnose their patients when these feelings occur. Otherwise, transfer to a facility not fully equipped to deal with complex medical conditions could occur, and any necessary diagnostic and therapeutic interventions would be delayed. Therefore, it is best to be extra diligent in completing a thorough medical and psychiatric evaluation of all psychotic patients in the emergency department.

Acute psychosis can be the presenting symptom in an extensive array of disease processes. For example, there are a multitude of case reports in the literature focusing on the misdiagnosis of psychiatric diseases in cases of hypoglycemia, meningoencephalitis, and subarachnoid hemorrhage.

Risk factors for an underlying organic cause of psychosis include (a) abnormal vital signs, (b) predominance of visual hallucinations, (c) lethargy or clouded sensorium, (d) disorientation, (e) memory loss, (f) acute change from baseline functional status, (g) age >40 years without a history of previous psychiatric diagnosis, and (h) coexisting medical diagnoses. If timing is sudden and reaches maximal severity acutely, a nonpsychiatric etiology should be highly suspected. A negative family history of psychiatric illness and documentation of a high level of functioning immediately prior to presentation also make a psychiatric diagnosis less likely. Other discrete clues that may indicate an organic cause include (a) extreme emotional lability, (b) a history of recent illness (even minor), (c) intermittent periods of lucidity with absence of symptoms, and (d) minimal response to antipsychotic medications. In the absence of a previous history, the diagnosis of functional or nonorganic psychosis is a diagnosis of exclusion and should never be made in the emergency department setting without an extensive barrage of medical tests.

When evaluating someone with acute psychosis, the extensive differential diagnosis of toxic, traumatic, infectious, metabolic, structural, and nutritional causes should be sought for and treated. All patients must receive a complete history and physical examination. The history can be difficult and, when possible, should utilize all resources available including family, caregivers, medical records, and prehospital personnel. Every effort should be made to establish the patient's baseline level of functioning. A screening mental status examination should be performed in all cases by applying the mnemonic, "OH-MAT": orientation, hallucinations, memory, affect, and thought. The physical examination should search for evidence of toxidromes, trauma, infection, and neurological deficits.

In patients with a known psychiatric disease who present acutely agitated and who are noted to display characteristic behaviors, the history and physical examination are all that are necessary for medical clearance. In those with an established diagnosis of psychiatric illness, but who exhibit an atypical or extreme change from baseline as well as anyone without a known psychiatric history, further evaluation and testing are required. Many psychiatric facilities require a baseline CBC, electrolyte panel, BUN, creatinine, urinalysis, blood alcohol level, and urine drug screen prior to admission. More extensive laboratory testing can be used to evaluate for metabolic derangements, nutritional deficiencies, and toxic substances. Neuroimaging may be necessary to locate structural or traumatic etiologies and should be considered as a screening tool in all cases of new-onset psychosis. All possible organic causes of psychosis should be reasonably excluded prior to transfer to a psychiatric facility. Therefore, under most circumstances, patients are admitted to a medical facility to undergo extensive evaluation prior to transfer.

The evaluation of the patient with acute psychosis is a challenge. The important points to note include (a) acute psychosis can be the primary symptom for a large number of medical emergencies; (b) a new diagnosis of psychiatric illness can only be made after an extensive evaluation for nonpsychiatric causes has been completed; (c) acute changes in a person's psychiatric symptoms may indicate a concomitant medical condition. By conducting a thorough medical clearance evaluation with these points in mind, emergency physicians should avoid the pitfall of discharging patients inappropriately to a psychiatric facility.

SUGGESTED READINGS

Binder RL, McNeil DE. Contemporary practices in managing acutely violent patients in 20 psychiatric emergency rooms. *Psychiatr Serv*. 1999;50(12):1553–1554.

Morris RJ, Chandran KN, Newcombe RL. Psychiatric presentation of aneurysmal subarachnoid haemorrhge. *ANZ J Surg*. 2001;71(1):69–70.

Richards CF, Gurr DE. Psychiatric emergencies: Psychosis. *Emerg Med Clin North Am*. 2000;18(2):253–262.

Shefrin A, Puddester D, Greenham S, et al. What investigations are ordered in patients with first-episode psychosis? *Jefferson J Psychiatry*. 2006;20(1):4–12. Available at: jdc.jefferson. edu/jeffjpsychiatry.

Xavier M, Correa B, Coromina M, et al. Sudden psychotic episode probably due to meningoenchephalitis and Chlamydia pneumoniae acute infection. *Clin Pract Epidemiol Ment Health*. 2005;1:15.

270

THINK TWICE BEFORE DIAGNOSING "ANXIETY" IN THE EMERGENCY DEPARTMENT

ROXANNA SADRI, MD

Anxiety is defined as "a feeling of apprehension, fear, nervousness, or dread accompanied by restlessness or tension." Anxiety disorders include general-ized anxiety disorder (GAD), panic disorder, obsessive-compulsive disorder, specific phobias, posttraumatic stress disorder, and substance-induced anxiety. As the lifetime prevalence of GAD is approximately 3%, panic disorder up to 3.5%, and specific phobias up to 13%, many of these patients will present to the emergency department (ED) with anxiety either as their chief complaint or as a comorbid condition. In addition, anxiety may present with physical symptoms, and organic diseases may present with anxiety as the chief complaint or one of the main symptoms. Making the distinction between a primary anxiety disorder and an underlying organic disease is often difficult and may be a fateful error in the ED setting.

It is not unusual for the clinician to become easily frustrated with an anx-ious patient and thus cut short interactions. Moreover, an acute exacerbation of a patient's anxiety may be a result of an acute exacerbation of one of his or her underlying medical conditions. One should not make the diagnosis of anxiety until other life-threatening medical conditions have been ruled out; in the ED, anxiety must be a diagnosis of exclusion.

Multiple papers have been published addressing the misdiagnosis of paroxysmal supraventricular tachycardia as anxiety or panic disorder. Other cardiac diseases, such as myocardial infarction and mitral valve prolapse, can also present similarly to a panic attack. Multiple pulmonary diseases can also be confused with panic, such as acute exacerbations of chronic obstructive pul-monary disease, acute asthma attacks, spontaneous pneumothorax, pneumonia, and tuberculosis. Endocrine disorders that are commonly associated with the presentation of anxiety are pheochromocytoma, hyperthyroidism and hypothyroidism, hypoparathyroidism, hypoglycemia, and hyperadrenocortisonism. Strong associations have been shown in a variety of neurologic disorders, including epilepsy, myasthenia gravis, and transient ischemic attacks.

In some cases, anxiety disorders may be closely intertwined with underlying medical conditions. For example, 50% of patients with irritable bowel syndrome have a concurrent diagnosis or depression or anxiety. In fibromyalgia, symptoms such as muscle pain and stiffness have been known to be exacerbated by anxiety. In asthma, it can occur either way: an asthma exacerbation can cause an anxiety attack, or anxiety can precipitate an asthma attack. Anxiety can also cause hypertension (white coat syndrome). Patients with mental illness (including depression and anxiety) are also at a higher risk for other comorbid medical diseases.

In the ED setting, a complete review of systems, at a minimum, is necessary to screen for organic pathology. Laboratory tests that may be useful in individual cases include a complete blood count, serum chemistry panel, urine and serum toxicologies, and thyroid function tests. More extensive testing may be indicated to look for underlying cardiac, neurologic, or endocrine pathology. If there is a high suspicion for an organic cause of symptoms, particularly of cardiac or neurologic origin, hospital admission is sometimes necessary. Finally, patients with suspected psychiatric disease should be screened for suicidal and homicidal behaviors.

Once the diagnosis of anxiety has been made, there are several approaches to treatment. In cases of acute, severe anxiety, benzodiazepines are most effective. While benzodiazepines were once commonly prescribed in chronic anxiety disorders, selective serotonin receptor inhibitors (SSRIs) are now the treatment of choice. Although the initiation of SSRIs in the ED is generally not recommended, it is important to refer these patients to either their primary care provider or a psychiatrist who can advise them on various therapeutic options. Proven, effective therapeutic modalities that can be safely recommended to all patients include stress reduction techniques such as daily exercise, improved sleep habits, cognitive behavioral therapy, meditation, and biofeedback.

SUGGESTED READINGS

Aydin IO, Uluşahin A. Depression, anxiety comorbidity, and disability in tuberculosis and chronic obstructive pulmonary disease patients: Applicability of GHQ-12. *Gen Hosp Psychiatry*. 2001;23(2):77–83.

Emery EJ, Szymanski HV. Psychological symptoms preceding diagnosed myasthenia gravis. *Psychosomatics*. 1981;22(11):993–995.

Lessmeier TJ, Gamperling D, Johnson-Liddon V, et al. Unrecognized paroxysmal supraventricular tachycardia: Potential for misdiagnosis as panic disorder. *Arch Intern Med*. 1997;157(5):537–543.

McCrank E, Schurmans K, Lefcoe D. Paroxysmal supraventricular tachycardia misdiagnosed as panic disorder. *Arch Intern Med.* 1998;158(3):297.

Paradis CM, Friedman S, Lazar RM, et al. Anxiety disorders in a neuromuscular clinic. *Am J Psychiatry.* 1993;150:1102–1104.

271

USE CHEMICAL OR PHYSICAL RESTRAINTS JUDICIOUSLY

MARY LOUISE MARTIN, MD AND JORGE A. FERNANDEZ, MD, FAAEM, FACEP

When patients present in an agitated and combative state, they pose a threat to the safety of the staff and themselves. Both physical and chemical restraints may be necessary. However, the use of restraint devices carries with it many legal, ethical, and medical concerns. The use of restraints is the subject of recent policies by both The Joint Commission on Accreditation of Healthcare Organizations and Centers for Medicare and Medicaid Services. In addition, practitioners are also accountable for their own institutional policies. The liability associated with an injury to a patient or others resulting from lack of restraints is generally greater than the liability associated with their use. As long as physicians adhere to these guidelines and act with their patients' best interest in mind, the risk of liability will be low.

The American College of Emergency Physicians policy on restraints states that "restraints should be individualized and afford as much dignity to the patient as the situation allows." Other less restrictive attempts at de-escalation should be exhausted first. Restraints should never be placed punitively or for convenience. Ideally, the treating physician should not be involved in the placement of restraints. A team of at least five appropriately trained staff members with a leader who gives orders is recommended. Once a decision has been made to restrain a patient, it should be completed despite a sudden change in behavior and attempts for negotiation. Seclusion generally should be avoided in most circumstances.

Improperly applied restraints have multiple risks, including direct injury to limbs from excessive pressure, aspiration, and sudden death. Positioning the patient in the lateral decubitus position or with the head of the bed raised may decrease the risk of aspiration.

The most feared adverse event associated with restraint use is sudden death. Over the last 10 years, 142 deaths secondary to restraint use have been reported, with 26% of these occurring in children. Catecholamine excess, from toxic or endogenous mechanisms, is frequently associated with these fatal events. Factors associated with sudden death include (a) violent and prolonged struggling, (b) cocaine or stimulant intoxication, (c) comorbid medical disease, and (d) morbid obesity. The prone and hobbled positions should be avoided, as these are associated with an increased risk of sudden death. Patients under the influence of alcohol or illicit substances should be continuously monitored because of the increased risks of asphyxiation and aspiration. Chest restraints should be used with extreme caution as they can restrict chest expansion leading to asphyxiation. Any patient with acutely diminished struggling or decreased rate of breathing should be immediately assessed, as this may indicate impending cardiopulmonary arrest.

The U.S. Department of Health and Human Services rules and regulations mandate that physicians must evaluate their patients, face to face, within 1 h of the application of restraints. The physician is required to document each of the following: (a) the immediate situation, (b) the patient's response to intervention, (c) the patient's medical and behavioral conditions, and (d) a determination of the need for continued restraint or seclusion. Physicians must also evaluate the continued need for restraints and renew orders at 4-h intervals for adults (>18 years old), 2-h intervals for adolescents (9 to 17 years old), and 1-h intervals for children (<9 years old). Most institutions recommend that these patients be under continuous, direct observation by an appropriately trained staff member.

Patients who continue to struggle after being placed in physical restraints require a chemical restraint in order to prevent self-induced injury and rhabdomyolysis. Benzodiazepines and neuroleptics are the most widely used drugs for the treatment of acute agitation. Life-threatening adverse effects of the most commonly used medications include respiratory depression, prolonged QT syndrome, and neuroleptic malignant syndrome. A medication history, if available, may identify contraindications prior to the choice of agent(s). For example, benzodiazepines are more likely to result in respiratory failure in the alcohol-intoxicated patient. Patients already taking medications with QT prolonging properties, however, are at increased risk for life-threatening dysrhythmias with the use of neuroleptics. Dosages should always be the lowest possible and titrated as necessary. As with a physical restraint, continuous monitoring for adverse reactions is indicated. Furthermore, frequent repositioning of the patient may be necessary in order to prevent pressure sores, thrombosis, and nerve injury.

SUGGESTED READINGS

Centers for Medicare & Medicaid (CMS), DHHS. Medicare and Medicaid programs; hospital conditions of participation: Patient rights. Final rule. *Fed Regist.* 2006;71(236): 71377–71428.

Sorrentino A. Chemical restraints for the agitated, violent, or psychotic. *Curr Opin Pediatr.* 2004;16(2):201–205.

Stratton SJ, Rogers C, Brickett K, et al. Factors associated with sudden death of individuals requiring restraint for excited delirium. *Am J Emerg Med.* 2001;19(3):187–191.

272

Sedate patients with delirium or dementia with care

Samuel N. Melton, MD and Jorge A. Fernandez, MD, FAAEM, FACEP

Sedative and pain medications are among the most common medications prescribed by emergency physicians. Rather than apply a one-size-fits-all approach, it is far safer to tailor the use of these agents to the underlying condition. This is one of many reasons why establishing the cause for acutely altered mental status quickly is a high priority for the emergency physician.

The differential diagnosis for altered mental status is exhaustive and beyond the scope of this chapter; however, it can be useful when choosing a sedative to subcategorize altered mental status into hyperactive and hypoactive delirium. Hyperactive, or "agitated," delirium is more often seen in young patients and may be associated with sympathomimetic or anticholinergic toxidromes, as well as sedative withdrawal (e.g., alcohol withdrawal). In these cases, benzodiazepines are frequently required for sedation. Hypoactive delirium is more often seen in elderly patients, carries a worse prognosis, and should provoke an investigation for underlying infection; ischemia; and metabolic, endocrine, pharmacologic, and neurologic causes. Even patients with hypoactive delirium may require sedation; however, the choice of agents and doses will likely be less aggressive than in hyperactive delirium. Regardless of the presentation, altered mental status requires a diligent attempt by the emergency physician to illicit history from family, caretakers, EMS personnel, and other sources to evaluate the timing and associated factors contributing to the illness.

The greatest pitfall in the sedation of patients with altered mental status is to simply sedate the patient without considering emergent etiologies for altered mental status. The patient is often framed as a "psych" patient who is merely "crazy." If a patient has escalated to the point that the nurse is requesting sedation, the physician should come to the bedside to assess the patient if possible. Important etiologies for agitation such as hypoxia, hypoglycemia, and pain should immediately be ruled out or treated if present. If the diagnosis is unclear and the patient is violent or too agitated to assess, hospital security should be notified to assist with restraining the patient so that medications may be administered safely. An appropriate initial choice for sedation in an acutely agitated or violent adult is haloperidol either alone or in combination with lorazepam. Doses should start modestly and be repeated until the patient is calm enough to allow safe assessment and definitive management. Haloperidol is contraindicated in cases of prolonged QT/torsade de pointes or if neuroleptic malignant syndrome is suspected.

Another common error is to administer sedative medication when analgesic medication is indicated. Oligoanalgesia (inadequate pain treatment) is well documented in the emergency setting, and it can be more difficult to identify pain in the pediatric and geriatric populations. Federal guidelines now mandate assessment and treatment of pain whenever possible and have encouraged adoption of pain as the "fifth" vital sign. Regardless, an ethical approach to patient care requires us to relieve pain. Physical examination in an altered elderly patient should include palpation and inspection to assess for pain. In demented or chronically ill patients, particularly those who have difficulty communicating, a trial of short-acting analgesics such as fentanyl may be indicated to see if agitation is relieved with analgesia prior to initiating sedation. As with all medications, the risk of respiratory and cardiac suppression must be balanced with benefits, and advanced airway management should be available if needed.

Management of the demented patient in the emergency department is particularly difficult and prone to error. First and foremost, the diagnosis of dementia should be a diagnosis of exclusion in the emergency department and should never be used to explain an acute worsening in mental status. There is no ideal medication for the sedation of the agitated demented patient. Until recently, some authors recommended low-dose antipsychotics such as haloperidol, risperidone, and olanzapine for neuropsychiatric manifestations of dementia. The FDA's latest recommendations state, however, that "antipsychotics are not indicated for the treatment of dementia-related psychosis." They cite this due to two studies showing an increase in mortality (of unclear etiology). Sedation with low-dose benzodiazepines and antihistamines may be effective and are likely the best initial choice; however, they may also cause paradoxical disinhibition and worsening agitation. As always, the possibility of an underlying pain complaint should be addressed.

SUGGESTED READINGS

Ayalon L, Gum AM, Feliciano L, et al. Effectiveness of nonpharmacological interventions for the management of neuropsychiatric symptoms in patients with dementia: A systematic review. *Arch Intern Med*. 2006;166:2182–2188.

Lukens TW, Wolf SJ, Edlow JA, et al. Clinical policy: Critical issues in the diagnosis and management of the adult psychiatric patient in the emergency department. *Ann Emerg Med*. 2006;47(1):79–99.

Phillips DM. JCAHO pain management standards are unveiled. *JAMA*. 2000;284(4): 428–429.

U.S. Food and Drug Administration Center for Drug Evaluation and Research Website. Available at: http://www.fda.gov/cder/drug/InfoSheets/HCP/antipsychotics_conventional.htm. Accessed July 11, 2008.

273

NEVER DIAGNOSE MALINGERING OR FACTITIOUS DISORDER UNTIL YOU HAVE RULED OUT ORGANIC DISEASE

ROXANNA SADRI, MD

Factitious disorder and malingering are similar conditions; they both involve the intentional feigning of symptoms for an incentive. While malingering involves an external incentive, such as gaining disability status or getting out of jail, the incentive of factitious disorder is only to assume the sick role. Munchausen syndrome, the chronic form of factitious disorder, can be concurrent in approximately 10% to 20% of patients with factitious disorder. Malingering is not classified as a psychiatric disorder, whereas factitious disorder does respond to psychiatric treatment.

There are multiple potential errors made by emergency physicians who suspect malingering or factitious disorder. The most important error is the failure to recognize true organic disease as the cause of the patient's symptoms. Particular patient groups, such as those incarcerated or those seeking workers' compensation, are often erroneously assumed to be malingering. Symptoms commonly attributed to malingering, such as hyperalgesia (pain out of proportion to findings), hypoesthesia, and allodynia, may all be seen in life-threatening and painful conditions including necrotizing fasciitis, mesenteric ischemia, discitis, trigeminal neuralgia, endometriosis, or reflex sympathetic dystrophy.

If factitious disorder and malingering are not considered, patients may receive tests, treatments, and surgical procedures that are unnecessary and potentially harmful. Moreover, patients may not receive the psychiatric care required to prevent future iatrogenesis. Munchausen syndrome is most common in middle-aged individuals who are estranged from their families. While Munchausen's is considered a psychiatric illness, Munchausen's by proxy is child abuse. If not recognized and reported, there is a significant risk of morbidity and mortality to the child.

Confrontation of patients with either factitious disorder or malingering is inadvisable in the emergency department. It is possible that a person with factitious disorder may escalate his or her behavior to try to "prove" that he or she has an organic illness. This type of self-harm can cause significant patient morbidity or mortality. Confronting a malingering patient, on the other hand, can be potentially dangerous to the physician or ED staff. It is important in suspected cases to not directly accuse the patient of lying; instead, allow the patient every opportunity to "save face." There is a potential for malingerers to become violent when directly confronted or not given what they are seeking, so it is vital for the physician to remain cautious and vigilant. Actions that may deter violence in the ED include the presence of visible law enforcement personnel, keeping sharps or other potential weapons out of patient rooms, constant mindfulness of escape routes, and maintaining a passive posture and empathy toward these patients.

Patients with suspected factitious disorder and malingering should be advised about the lack of evidence of any emergent medical condition, and the need for primary care should be emphasized. Patients with suspected factitious disorder or Munchausen's should also be referred to a psychiatrist. Emergency physicians can safely tell these patients that chronic pain responds best to a multidisciplinary approach that may include psychiatric care in order to teach effective coping skills and reduction of associated stress and anxiety.

SUGGESTED READINGS

Folks DG, Freeman AM III. Munchausen's syndrome and other factitious illness. *Psychiatr Clin North Am*. 1985;8:263–278.
Thompson JW, LeBourgeois HW, Black FW. Malingering. In: Simon R, Gold L, eds. *Textbook of Forensic Psychiatry*. Washington, DC: American Psychiatric Publishing; 2004.

274

CHECK THE QT INTERVAL PRIOR TO ADMINISTRATION OF ANTIPSYCHOTICS WHENEVER POSSIBLE

DIEGO ABDELNUR, MD AND JORGE A. FERNANDEZ, MD, FAAEM, FACEP

Prolongation of the QT interval is a potentially life-threatening side effect of many medications, including commonly administered neuroleptics. Haloperidol and droperidol are first-line agents in the treatment of agitated and combative patients. However, the U.S. Food and Drug Administration (FDA) has recently issued warnings regarding the use of these medications, despite the lack of strong supporting evidence. Droperidol, in particular, was issued a "black box" warning in 2001, effectively limiting its use in many EDs.

Unfortunately, obtaining a baseline ECG may be difficult in acutely agitated patients until they are adequately sedated. The QT interval is measured from the start of the QRS deflection to the end of the T wave on the surface ECG. Modern ECG machines also calculate a corrected QT interval (QTc), which takes into account the patient's heart rate. Although there is no consensus concerning the upper limit of normal for the QTc, a value >450 ms is considered prolonged, with values >500 ms causing particular concern. The most serious consequence of a prolonged QTc is the type of ventricular tachycardia known as torsade de pointes (TdP). This ventricular tachycardia can quickly degenerate into ventricular fibrillation if there is no intervention.

Both haloperidol and droperidol are butyrophenones, neuroleptic medications that are extremely useful in treating acute agitation due to their rapid onset, clinical efficacy, and mild side-effect profile when compared with sedative-hypnotics such as the benzodiazepines. Commonly used both intramuscularly (IM) and intravenously (IV), recent literature has called into question the "off-label" IV use of these medications for acute agitation due to the measurable increase in prolonging the QTc. A study of six different antipsychotics by Harrigan et al. (2004) showed that haloperidol increased the QTc by 4 to 6 ms, whereas thioridazine caused the longest QTc prolongation of 35 ms. Another study found that there was no significant difference among droperidol, ondansetron, and normal saline in causing QTc prolongation. Furthermore, the relationship between QTc prolongation and resulting TdP is not always linear. For example, some drugs prolong the QTc beyond 500 ms yet rarely cause TdP, while other drugs that prolong the QTc only minimally have stronger associations with TdP. Roden et al. (2004) identified certain risk factors that seem to predispose a patient to developing TdP. These include female sex, hypokalemia, hypomagnesemia, rapid infusion of QT prolonging drugs, congestive heart failure, bradycardia, baseline QT prolongation, and recent conversion from atrial fibrillation. High-risk patients in the ED therefore include females, alcoholics, and patients with obvious cardiac disease. Regardless of the presence of these risk factors, there is often no better choice of sedative than haloperidol or droperidol. Newer atypical antipsychotics often have a higher risk of QTc prolongation than the butyrophenones. Furthermore, benzodiazepines have a significantly higher risk of respiratory or circulatory compromise in patients with underlying alcoholism or severe congestive heart failure, respectively.

Despite the fact that there are little data to suggest that haloperidol is safer when given IM instead of IV, the FDA currently recommends the use of IM injections of haloperidol (in 5-mg increments) with no need for continuous cardiac monitoring. If an emergency physician is faced with an agitated patient who is not amenable to cardiac monitoring, doses of haloperidol in 5-mg IM increments can be given with little fear of causing TdP. If more rapid sedation is desired using IV haloperidol, a baseline ECG and continuous cardiac monitoring are recommended. It is noteworthy that there have been only 28 case reports of haloperidol causing TdP, despite the hundreds of thousands of patients who have safely received the drug in emergency departments around the world.

Delaying sedation of agitated patients places both the patient and the hospital staff at increased risk of injury and resulting liability. These concerns dwarf the exceedingly small risk of TdP associated with haloperidol and droperidol. Nonetheless, an awareness of the recent FDA warnings and risk factors for TdP will help to steer the practitioner away from the liability that can be associated with using these drugs.

SUGGESTED READINGS

Charbit B, Albaladejo P, Funck-Brentano C, et al. Prolongation of QTc interval after postoperative nausea and vomiting treatment by droperidol or ondansetron. *Anesthesiology*. 2005;102(6):1094–1100.

Harrigan EP, Miceli JJ, Anziano R, et al. A randomized evaluation of the effects of six antipsychotic agents on QTc, in the absence and presence of metabolic inhibition. *J Clin Psychopharmacol*. 2004;24(1):62–69.

Roden DM. Drug-induced prolongation of the QT interval. *N Engl J Med*. 2004;350: 2618–2621.

Zept B. Drug induced prolongation of the QT interval. *Am J Family Prac*. 2005;71(1):284.

275

BEWARE SUICIDAL IDEATION OR BEHAVIOR

MARY LOUISE MARTIN, MD AND JORGE A. FERNANDEZ, MD, FAAEM, FACEP

Emergency physicians must identify any patient at immediate risk of successful suicide. Unfortunately, suicidal behavior can sometimes be difficult for physicians to recognize. Frequently, patients at highest risk of successful suicide do not directly state their intention to a physician. Furthermore, occult and silent suicide attempts may be intentionally misleading.

Studies have shown that patients, immediately prior to attempting suicide, may present to the emergency department with vague complaints. In fact, these vague presentations may be subtle cries for help. Emergency physicians should be mindful in these situations to screen for depressive symptoms and, if positively identified, to directly query patients regarding suicidal ideation.

Occult suicidal behavior is defined as a suicide attempt that appears accidental. Examples include motor vehicle accidents involving a single driver or pedestrian, an unexplained fall from a height, medication or drug overdose, lacerations involving the wrist, or risky behavior such as Russian roulette. There is also a phenomenon known as "suicide by cop." This occurs when an individual provokes a police officer in order to receive a fatal gunshot wound. Occult suicide is a consideration when the events and circumstances surrounding a patient's injury are questionable.

Silent or passive suicidal behavior is described as nonviolent behavior with the intent of death. Passive suicidal behavior is more common in the elderly or chronically ill; these patients often present with complications associated with medical noncompliance. Other examples of passive suicide include self-starvation or continuing to drink or smoke, in the setting of cirrhosis or emphysema, respectively.

Emergency physicians should screen all patients presenting with any of the above presentations for suicidal ideation and risk. The investigation should be undertaken in a nonthreatening but direct manner. It is important to elicit from the patient: the events surrounding the perceived attempt (concentrating on clues to the intent), a mental health history, a substance abuse history, and social support. At sometime during the evaluation, the patient should be asked directly if the event was indeed a suicide attempt. Obviously, there is room for interpretation when attributing suicide intent with some of the behaviors listed above.

If suicidal ideation is identified by the emergency physician, the patient's plans and risks should be evaluated. Risk factors associated with successful suicide include (a) male sex, (b) adolescent or elderly age, (c) previous suicide attempt, (d) prior severe depression, (e) chronic illness, (f) a family history of suicide, (g) recent loss, (h) lack of social support, and (i) substance abuse.

Emergency physicians should become proficient at identifying and documenting suicidal behaviors, attempts, and risks. Mislabeling a suicide attempt as an accident may have fatal consequences. In suspected cases, particularly those with multiple risk factors for successful suicide, psychiatric consultation should be obtained.

SUGGESTED READINGS

Alesopoulos GS, Bruce ML, Hull J, et al. Clinical determinants of suicidal ideation and behavior in geriatric depression. *Arch Gen Pyschiatry*. 1999;56(11):1048–1053.

Cochrane-Brink KA, Lofchy JS, Sakinofsky I. Clinical rating scales in suicide risk assessment. *Gen Hosp Psychiatry*. 2000;22(6):445–451.

Garrison CZ, McKeown RE, Valois RF, et al. Aggression, substance use, and suicidal behaviors in high school students. *Am J Public Health*. 1993;83(2):179–184.

Hirschfeld RM, Russell JM. Assessment and treatment of suicidal patients. *N Engl J Med*. 1997;337:910–915.

Ho TP. The suicide risk of discharged psychiatric patients. *J Clin Psychiatry*. 2003;64(6):702–707.

Hutson RH, Anglin D, Yarbrough J, et al. Suicide by cop. *Ann Emerg Med*. 1998;32(6):665–669.

Maris RW. Suicide. *Lancet*. 2002;360(9329):319–326.

276

DO NOT FORGET TO ADMINISTER STEROIDS IN PATIENTS WITH ACUTE ASTHMA EXACERBATIONS

EDUARDO BORQUEZ, MD

Steroids are a cornerstone in the treatment of both chronic and acute exacerbations of asthma. Although opinions vary as to which patients should receive systemic and inhaled preparations of steroids, the National Asthma Education and Prevention Program (NAEPP) has explicit recommendations and guidelines for their use.

In acute exacerbations, systemic steroids are recommended for treating moderate to severe exacerbations or in patients who do not completely respond to inhaled β-agonists. Additionally, they should be considered in patients with a recent history of an exacerbation and prolonged symptoms or for those already on steroids. In patients with acute symptoms, systemic steroids have been shown to decrease hospital admissions and return visits to the emergency department (ED).

It has been shown that asthmatics receive steroids 77% of the time when they present to the ED. What is important to remember is that the majority of patients presenting to the ED will have more than just a "mild exacerbation." Mild exacerbations, by definition, are those that are "usually treated in the home, have prompt relief with short-acting β-agonists, and have dyspnea only on exertion," according to the NAEPP.

Relatively recently, inhaled corticosteroids (ICS) have been employed in the treatment of asthma. Inhaled corticosteroids have the advantage of being delivered directly into the airway, causing fewer systemic side effects. The NAEPP recommends the use of ICS, as they have been shown to reduce exacerbations, relapse rates, ED visits, admissions, and mortality. The NAEPP recommends that patients who have "persistent asthma" be treated with ICS. This implies that only those patients classified as having "intermittent asthma" should *not* receive ICS. To determine whether a patient has persistent asthma, remember the "rules of two." These are

- more than two uses of quick-relief inhalers (β-agonists) per week
- more than two nighttime awakenings per month due to asthma
- more than 2 days with symptoms per week

Just over half of those (55%) presenting to the ED will be classified as having mild to severe persistent asthma according to the rules above. Consequently, there has been an increasing call to action to increase the percentage of patients discharged from the ED with ICS. Despite this call, it has been observed that ICS are given upon discharge from the ED to <25% of patients. Many emergency physicians are resistant to prescribing ICS because they believe that the classification of asthma as intermittent or persistent is better determined by the primary care provider. Additionally, many have concerns that they will not be monitoring the patient for side effects from chronic ICS. However, from a practical standpoint, it has been observed that patients frequently do not get ICS at follow-up. If patients are not discharged from the ED with an ICS, less than half (42%) with an exacerbation will receive ICS from their primary care providers at follow-up. Moreover, ICS have a relatively safe side effect profile, especially compared with the systemic steroids routinely prescribed from the ED in short bursts.

In conclusion, systemic corticosteroids should be used as a mainstay therapy for the patient presenting with acute exacerbations of moderate to severe asthma. Inhaled corticosteroids should be given when discharging a patient whom the emergency physician believes is suffering from persistent asthma, regardless of severity and independent from the classification of the acute exacerbation. Adding ICS to the discharge regimen of persistent asthmatics will not only improve the patient's health but also decrease the number of bounce-backs!

SUGGESTED READINGS

Camargo CA, Clark S. Emergency department management of acute asthma between 1996–2001: Potential impact of the 1997 NAEPP guidelines. *J Allergy Clin Immunol.* 2002;109(1):S156.

Cydulka R, Tamayo-Sarver JH, Wolf C, et al. Inadequate follow-up controller medications among patients with asthma who visit the emergency department. *Ann Emerg Med.* 2005;46(4):316–322.

Kwok MY, Walsh-Kelly CM, Gorelick MH, et al. National Asthma Education and Prevention Program severity classification as a measure of disease burden in children with acute asthma. *Pediatrics.* 2006;177(4):S71–S77.

National Asthma Education and Prevention Program (NAEPP). *Expert Panel Report 3: Guidelines For The Diagnosis and Management of Asthma.* Bethesda, MD: National Institutes of Health; National Heart, Lung, and Blood Institute; 2007. Publication No. 07–4051.

Ornato J. Treatment strategies for reducing asthma-related Emergency Department visits. *J Emerg Med.* 2007;32(1):27–39.

Singer AJ, Camargo C, Lampell M, et al. A call for expanding the role of the emergency physician in the care of patients with asthma. *Ann Emerg Med.* 2005;45:295–298.

277

CONSIDER CRYPTOGENIC ORGANIZING PNEUMONIA AS A CAUSE OF PERSISTENT PULMONARY INFILTRATES

SHANNON B. PUTMAN, MD

The diagnosis of cryptogenic organizing pneumonia (COP), previously referred to as bronchiolitis obliterans with organizing pneumonia (BOOP), is based on specific histopathological criteria found in the appropriate clinical setting. It is a disease with clinical features of pneumonia (fever, malaise, and productive cough) rather than those of a primary airway disorder, such as asthma or emphysema. Organizing pneumonia can be seen as a primary idiopathic disorder in a previously healthy person or as a secondary reaction to a number of different lung pathogens or toxins. It has been associated with various drugs, including cocaine, amiodarone, bleomycin, and sulfasalazine, as well as with infections, including human immunodeficiency virus, adenovirus, and mycoplasma.

COP can also be a pulmonary manifestation of a systemic disease, such as with myelodysplastic syndrome, ulcerative colitis, and with a number of different connective tissue diseases. The diagnosis is made by biopsy, and important pathological features include evidence of immature granulation tissue. Inflammation of the distal airspaces can also be present, including the bronchioles, alveolar ducts, and alveoli. Changes appear temporally uniform and underlying lung architecture is preserved. The distribution is patchy and always involves the alveolar space. Pertinent negative findings include the absence of interstitial fibrosis, granulomas, or microabscesses. There is no evidence of vasculitic involvement in organizing pneumonia, nor should there be a prominent infiltration of neutrophils or eosinophils. The pathogenesis of these findings is poorly understood.

The incidence and prevalence of cryptogenic organizing pneumonia are unknown but are likely not rare and were reported to be six to seven patients per 100,000 cumulative hospital admissions at one university hospital. Men and women are affected equally, and although the diagnosis has been made in patients from ages 20 to 70 years, it is most common in the fifth and sixth decades of life. Unlike many pulmonary processes, tobacco abuse is not thought to be a risk factor. COP has a subacute presentation with the majority of patients reporting symptoms for <2 months prior to seeking medical care. This is in contrast to patients ultimately diagnosed with idiopathic pulmonary fibrosis who may be symptomatic for up to 18 months prior to presentation. COP shares features with community-acquired pneumonia with 50% of patients reporting fever, malaise, fatigue, and cough at symptom onset. The most common symptoms at presentation are progressive dry cough (56% to 88% of patients), dyspnea with exertion (50% to 88%), and weight loss of >10 lb (63% to 75%). Three quarters of patients will have inspiratory rales on physical exam, while wheezing is rare. One quarter of patients will have a normal physical exam.

The classic radiographic manifestations of COP are bilateral diffuse air-space opacities with normal lung volumes, seen in up to two thirds of patients. Peripheral distribution of infiltrates, similar to that associated with chronic eosinophilic pneumonia, is common. Patchy migratory infiltrates can be seen in 50% of cases and allow a narrowing of the differential diagnosis to include COP and eosinophilic pulmonary syndromes including Churg-Strauss vasculitis, drug hypersensitivity, parasitic infection, and allergic bronchopulmonary aspergillosis. Unusual radiographic findings include unilateral disease, honeycombing, pleural effusions, cavities, and hyperinflation. Computed tomography (CT) scan may reveal a more extensive disease than expected based on plain radiograph findings. Patchy consolidation may range from minimal to diffuse involving all lung zones and is more likely to be found both peripherally and in the lower lobes. High-resolution CT may also show ground glass infiltrates, bronchial wall thickening, and bronchiole dilation. CT scan may be useful for guiding the site of lung biopsy by localizing the radiographically most abnormal tissue. Laboratory studies are nonspecific with the most common abnormalities being an elevated total white blood cell count, erythrocyte sedimentation rate (ESR), and C-reactive protein (CRP). Pulmonary function studies most often show a mild to moderate restrictive ventilatory defect with reduced lung volumes and an impaired gas transfer defect with decreased diffusing capacity for carbon monoxide (DLCO). Obstructive lung defects (FEV1/FVC of <70% of predictive value) are seen in <20% of patients, most of whom have a history of tobacco abuse.

When a patient fitting the clinical syndrome of subacute respiratory insufficiency presents with systemic symptoms, the differential diagnosis is broad. In addition to, community-acquired pneumonia, other entities like COP, sarcoidosis, amyloidosis, pulmonary manifestations of connective tissue disease, hypersensitivity pneumonitis, one of the eosinophilic pulmonary syndromes, and malignancy should be considered. Clinically and radiographically, COP may be most similar to eosinophilic pneumonia, but patients with the later frequently have wheezing on exam and peripheral eosinophilia. It is worth noting that other forms of bronchiolitis, including obliterative bronchiolitis (OB), can easily be distinguished from COP by the predominance of obstructive physiology with expiratory wheezing on exam, hyperlucent lung fields on radiographic images, and obstructive changes on pulmonary function studies. Confusion over nomenclature and the erroneous interchange of the terms BOOP and OB among practitioners led to the more recent recommendation to focus on the pneumonia-like illness associated with COP.

Open lung biopsy is the preferred procedure of choice to confirm the diagnosis in patients with the appropriate clinical spectrum. Spontaneous resolution is rare, and most patients require an extensive course of glucocorticoid therapy. Generally, therapy is initiated with 1 mg/kg of prednisone up to a maximum of 100 mg daily for 1 to 3 months. Prednisone may then be tapered slowly over the next 6 months in patients who remain stable.

From an emergency medicine standpoint, most patients ultimately diagnosed with COP will be empirically treated for community-acquired pneumonia on presentation. Careful consideration of the returning patient with pneumonia-like illness and persistent infiltrates on serial chest radiographs should include concern for antibiotic failure, patient noncompliance, and an alternative diagnosis. COP should be on one's differential diagnosis and, if suspected, should lead to hospital admission for diagnostic biopsy and treatment with steroids.

SUGGESTED READINGS

Alasaly K, Muller N, Ostrow D, et al. Cryptogenic organizing pneumonia: A report of 25 cases and a review of the literature. *Medicine*. 1995;74(4):201–211.

Arakawa H, Kururihara Y, Niimi H, et al. Bronchiolitis obliterans with organizing pneumonia versus chronic eosinophilic pneumonia: High resolution ct findings in 81 patients. *Am J Roentgenol*. 2001;176:1053–1058.

Bartter T, Irwin R, Nash G, et al. Idiopathic bronchiolitis obliterans organizing pneumonia with periperhal infiltrates on chest roentgenogram. *Arch Intern Med*. 1989;149:273–279.

Cordier JF. Cryptogenic organizing pneumonia. *Eur Respir J*. 2006;28:422–446.

Epler GR. Bronchiolitis obliterans organizing pneumonia. *Arch Intern Med*. 2001;161:158–165.

Epler G, Colby T, McLoud T, et al. Bronchiolitis obliterans organizing pneumonia. *N Eng J Med*. 1985;312:152–158.

Wright L, King TE Jr. Cryptogenic organizing pneumonia (idiopathic bronchiolitis obliterans organizing pneumonia): An update. *Clin Pul Med*. 1997;4(3):152–158.

278

CONSIDER VENOUS THROMBOEMBOLISM MORE HIGHLY IN PATIENTS WITH HIV

CYRUS SHAHPAR, MD, MPH

VENOUS THROMBOEMBOLISM

Venous thromboembolism (VTE) is a leading cause of morbidity and mortality in the United States, with more than 200,000 cases annually. Of these cases, 30% die within 30 days, one fifth suffer sudden death due to pulmonary embolism (PE), and about 30% develop recurrent VTE within 10 years.

TABLE 278.1	RISK FACTORS FOR VTE
ACQUIRED RISK FACTORS	
Strong risk factors (odds ratio > 10)	Fracture (hip or leg)
	Hip or knee replacement
	Major general surgery
	Major trauma
	Spinal cord injury
Moderate risk factors (odds ratio 2–9)	Arthroscopic knee surgery
	Central venous lines
	Chemotherapy
	Congestive heart or respiratory failure
	Hormone replacement therapy
	Malignancy
	Oral contraceptive therapy
	Paralytic stroke
	Pregnancy, postpartum
	Previous VTE
	Thrombophilia
Weak risk factors (odds ratio <2)	Bed rest >3 days
	Immobility due to sitting
	Increasing age
	Laparoscopic surgery
	Obesity
	Pregnancy, antepartum
	Varicose veins
Inherited risk factors for VTE	Factor V Leiden mutation
	Prothrombin gene mutation
	Protein S deficiency
	Protein C deficiency
	AT deficiency
	Dysfibrinogenemia
	Increased factor VIII coagulant activity

Source: Anderson FA Jr, Spencer FA. Risk factors for venous thromboembolism. *Circulation*. 2003;107(23 Suppl 1):I9–I16.

Emergency physicians are adept at identifying major and minor risk factors for PE (*Table 278.1*). These include both acquired and inherited factors with varying levels of risk. Despite the substantial burden of disease, however, one risk factor for VTE that is often overlooked is the presence of human immunodeficiency virus (HIV) infection.

HIV INFECTION AND VTE

HIV infection is a common chronic disease in the United States, and by the end of 2003, over 1 million persons in the United States were living with HIV/AIDS, with 24% to 27% undiagnosed and unaware of their HIV infection.

In recent years, several studies have examined whether HIV is an independent risk factor for VTE (specifically deep vein thrombosis [DVT] and PE), and the results of these studies imply that there is a moderate association between the two disease entities.

In a systematic review of the literature from 1986 to 2004, Klein et al. (2005) identified 10 relevant epidemiological studies that investigated the risk of venous thrombotic disease and HIV. After reviewing these largely retrospective studies, the authors concluded that the overall risk of DVT in patients with HIV infection may be roughly estimated to be twofold to tenfold higher in comparison with a healthy population of comparable age. This implies that HIV infection is a moderate risk factor for VTE, similar to oral contraceptive therapy, pregnancy, and malignancy, conditions that are commonly screened for when VTE is suspected.

COAGULATION SYSTEM ABNORMALITIES

Several studies have examined the various hemostatic changes that may explain the relationship between VTE and HIV. These changes can be summarized as an increase in procoagulant factors such as endothelial TF expression and thrombogenic properties of microparticles, which are upregulated in HIV patients. Studies have also shown that HIV-infected patients have decreased levels of certain anticoagulant factors, including lower levels of antithrombin (AT), protein C, and protein S. These factors have also been associated with an increased risk of DVT. Overall, it is likely that HIV infection represents a hypercoaguable state that increases the risk of VTE.

POTENTIAL CONFOUNDERS

Age. Among patients with HIV infection, the traditional direct relationship between the age and the risk of VTE may not be valid. In a large study examining the relationship between HIV and VTE, Matta et al. (2008) examined data from the National Hospital Discharge Survey from 1990 through 2005. In this study, among 2,429,000 patients older than 18 years hospitalized with HIV infection, the relative risks compared with all hospitalized non-HIV patients of PE, DVT, and VTE were 0.91, 1.26, and 1.21. Of note, the risk for PE among those aged 30 to 49 was greater than in the rest of the population, with relative risks of 1.23, 1.72, and 1.65, respectively. Similarly, Copur et al. (2002) found that in a retrospective study of 362 HIV-positive patients from 1998 to 1999, HIV-positive patients under the age of 50 were at increased risk for VTE compared with non–HIV-positive individuals. It is not clear why this relationship is seen, and further investigation by controlled studies is needed.

Low CD4 Count. Low CD4 count has been found to be an independent risk factor for VTE. In a study of 160 patients with HIV and VTE, Ahonkhai et al. (2008) found that those with a CD4 count <500 had three times the risk of

VTE as those with higher CD4 counts. In their review of 10 studies, Klein et al. (2005) found two studies that showed higher risks for VTE among patients with AIDS or CD4 count <200. The authors surmise that this relationship is likely due to active ongoing triggering of the immune system by both HIV infection and superimposed infections.

Highly Active Antiretroviral Therapy (HAART). Treatment with HAART, especially protease inhibitors, has been linked to an increased risk of venous thrombosis. In a large prospective study of more than 42,900 patients, Sullivan et al. (2000) found a heightened risk of venous thrombosis among HIV patients on the protease inhibitor indinavir. Subsequent studies, however, have failed to confirm this association. Recent evidence suggests that this association is likely small and clinically insignificant.

SUMMARY

VTE and HIV are common entities in the emergency department. Recent evidence has shown that there is a clear association between HIV infection and the risk of VTE. While traditional decision rules for assessing VTE risk are extremely valuable in patient management, they clearly do not reflect all risk factors for VTE. More specifically, health care providers should consider HIV as a significant risk factor when assessing a patient's pretest probability for VTE. This may be even more important in middle-aged HIV-positive patients or in those with low CD4 counts.

SUGGESTED READINGS

Ahonkhai AA, Gebo KA, Streiff MB, et al. Venous thromboembolism in patients with HIV/AIDS: A case-control study. *J Acquir Immune Defic Syndr*. 2008;48(3):310–314.

Anderson FA Jr, Spencer FA. Risk factors for venous thromboembolism. *Circulation*. 2003;107(23 Suppl 1):I9–I16.

Copur AS, Smith PR, Gomez V, et al. HIV infection is a risk factor for venous thromboembolism. *AIDS Patient Care STDS*. 2002;16(5):205–209.

Glynn M, Rhodes P. Estimated HIV prevalence in the United States at the end of 2003. *National HIV Prevention Conference*. June 2005, Atlanta [Abstract 595].

Heit JA. Venous thromboembolism epidemiology: Implications for prevention and management. *Semin Thromb Hemost*. 2002;28(Suppl 2):3–13.

Klein SK, Slim EJ, de Kruif MD, et al. Is chronic HIV infection associated with venous thrombotic disease? A systematic review. *Neth J Med*. 2005;63(4):129–136.

Matta F, Yaekoub AY, Stein PD. Human immunodeficiency virus infection and risk of venous thromboembolism. *Am J Med Sci*. 2008;336(5):402–406.

Sullivan PS, Dworkin MS, Jones JL, et al. Epidemiology of thrombosis in HIV-infected individuals. The Adult/Adolescent Spectrum of HIV Disease Project. *AIDS*. 2000;14:321–324.

279

CROUP IS COMMON ... SO KNOW IT WELL!

MELISSA W. COSTELLO, MD, FACEP

Croup, also known as laryngotracheitis or laryngotracheobronchitis, is the most common upper respiratory obstruction in childhood and the most common cause for stridor in febrile children. It is an illness of young children with most cases occurring between 6 months and 6 years of age. The peak incidence occurs at age 2 (24 to 36 months), although cases of croup have been reported up to 12 to 15 years of age. Most cases occur during the late fall, winter, and early spring. Most often, croup has a viral cause with parainfluenza type 1 accounting for about 50% of cases and parainfluenza type 1, 2, and 3 combining for nearly 80% of all cases. Other causative agents include influenza A and B, adenoviruses, respiratory syncitial virus, and rhinovirus. Other rare causes include herpes simplex, *Mycoplasma pneumoniae*, and measles.

Clinically, croup is characterized by hoarseness, fever, and a distinctive "seal-like" barking cough which may or may not be accompanied by stridor. Generally, the stridor is inspiratory and is perceived to worsen at night. Given this, it is not surprising that most emergency department (ED) visits for croup occur between 10 PM and 4 AM and account for nearly 15% of clinic and ED visits for pediatric respiratory infections. Most children will have had a 1- to 2-day prodrome of mild fever and upper respiratory symptoms prior to the onset of the characteristic cough. The majority of croup is self-limiting. Only 2% to 5% of children require hospitalization and fewer than 2% of those hospitalized require endotracheal intubation (EI). Overall mortality is difficult to determine, but it is likely to be exceptionally low given that one study showed only 0.5% mortality among intubated patients (who are already only 2% of the 2% to 5% that are admitted).

Differential diagnosis of croup should include bacterial tracheitis, epiglottitis, peritonsillar or retropharyngeal abscess, diphtheria, foreign body aspiration, hereditary angioedema, subglottic stenosis, vascular ring, and right-sided aortic arch. The first five of these conditions will often present with a more toxic-appearing child and a slightly different clinical picture whereas the latter five will usually be afebrile and present with stridor unresponsive to standard croup treatment.

The pathophysiology of the stridor and cough associated with croup is narrowing of the subglottic airway due to edema of the mucosal tissues. The subglottic airway at the level of the cricoid ring is already the narrowest portion of the pediatric airway. Edema here, combined with the baseline pliability of the pediatric trachea, can generate significant inspiratory stridor during the negative pressure of inspiration and the seal-like bark during the forced expiration of coughing. The classification of the severity of croup and therapeutic goals are aimed at evaluation, mitigation, and serial observation of these symptoms and the degree of respiratory compromise present. Several scoring systems have been developed over the years to help classify croup patients, with the two most commonly cited ones being the Westley score and the Alberta Clinical Practice Guidelines. The Westley score evaluates a patient by assessing five factors and assigning a point value (*Table 279.1*). The scores are added and <3 indicates mild disease, 3 to 6 being moderate and >6 being severe. Unfortunately, while the system has been tested in multiple studies for reliability, no large prospective validation has been done either to correlate the scoring system with outcomes or to reliably guide ED treatment and disposition. The Alberta Clinical Practice Guidelines Working Group developed a grading system released in July 2003 (revised July 2008) which classifies croup patients based on clinical presentation into one of four categories: mild, moderate, severe, or impending respiratory failure. Each of these categories is accompanied by a clinical description that closely correlates with the Westley scoring system. In the Canadian trials of this classification system, 85% of children presenting to the ED were classified as mild and <1% were classified as severe or impending respiratory failure.

Laboratory and radiographic evaluations are likely to add little to a diagnosis of croup. Lateral and anterior-posterior (AP) soft tissue neck radiographs will often show classic "steepling" or cone shaped narrowing of the subglottic trachea and will help rule out other diseases (particularly epiglottitis). Generally, radiographs should be performed only if there is a doubt about the clinical diagnosis and only if they can be done without significant agitation of the child. Labs will generally be normal and can be avoided when there is a clear clinical picture of croup.

The mainstay of croup treatment is corticosteroids with the addition of nebulized racemic epinephrine in children with moderate to severe disease. The typical child with mild to moderate croup will present with a normal oxygen

TABLE 279.1	WESTLEY SCORING SYSTEM EVALUATES A PATIENT BY ASSESSING FIVE FACTORS AND A POINT VALUE

Inspiratory stridor: None=0, with agitation=1, at rest=2;

Retractions: mild=1, moderate=2, severe=3;

Air entry: normal=0, mild decrease=1, marked decrease=2;

Cyanosis: none=0, with agitation=4, at rest=5;

Level of consciousness: normal=0, depressed=5.

saturation and minimal distress when quiet. Antipyretics should be given for fever, and efforts to minimize agitation of the child are essential. A single dose of dexamethasone should be given (0.3 mg/kg) intramuscular, intravenous, or orally in all children with croup. The administration of dexamethasone has shown benefit in clinical studies of even the mildest cases. Studies have looked at dexamethasone dosing ranges from 0.15 to 0.6 mg/kg and have found that there is little difference in clinical effect from 0.3 to 0.6 mg/kg. Minimal effect is lost by decreasing the dose to 0.15 mg/kg, but the dose increase to 0.3 mg/kg does allow for some rounding and the inevitable loss of medication in oral administration routes. In multiple studies, oral and parenteral routes have been found to be dose and onset equivalent. The key management step is the administration of steroids early in the clinical course.

Steroids should be given in the first hour with an expected onset of 30 to 120 min and peak effect at 2 h. Dexamethasone has a long half-life (54 h), and thus a single dose is usually adequate for croup, providing the edema reduction and anti-inflammatory effects desired through the remainder of the disease course. Comparison studies of the standard dexamethasone to the alternatives—oral prednisolone and inhaled budesonide—have shown good efficacy for croup. The prednisolone group had a slightly higher bounce back rate (likely due to the shorter half-life of the drug). The budesonide group did nearly as well as the dexamethasone group but several authors point out that nebulized budesonide is prohibitively expensive for most departments, especially in the face of an arguably more effective, vastly cheaper alternative. However, budesonide may be useful in cases of severe respiratory distress prohibiting oral intake or with cases of vomiting.

Nebulized racemic epinephrine (0.05 mL/kg of 2.25% solution—max 0.5 mL) should be given to children who present with moderate to severe disease characterized by stridor at rest or respiratory distress. The onset of effect is usually about 10 min, with the peak effect at approximately 60 min. Continuous nebulization should be avoided (case reports of ventricular tachycardia and myocardial infarction), and any child who receives racemic epinephrine should be observed in the ED for at least 3 h prior to discharge. Standard cardiac epinephrine (1:1,000) can be substituted for racemic epinephrine if needed at a dose of 0.5 mL/kg (max 5 mL).

Other treatment modalities in the management of croup are mostly reserved for severe disease and for those children with impending respiratory failure. These include heliox, which can improve air movement in severely constricted airway. The definite management is endotracheal intubation (EI). EI should be approached with the added diligence, preparation (bedside needle cricothyroidotomy or pediatric tracheostomy equipment), and personnel that accompany a pediatric difficult airway scenario given the degree of *subglottic* narrowing that is expected in severe disease. Antibiotics are not indicated in the management of viral croup.

Disposition, much like the diagnosis, should be guided by the clinical picture. Children should ideally be observed until 4 h after the initial dose of steroids or 3 h after the last inhaled racemic epinephrine treatment, whichever is longer. The patient should be tolerating oral fluids, have no findings consistent with dehydration, and an oxygen saturation >90%. The caretaker should be able to reasonably recognize worsening symptoms and have the ability to return to the ED easily. Children with severe distress, those who receive multiple racemic epinephrine treatments, and those with unpredictable social situations should be admitted either to the appropriate pediatric service or to short-term observation.

Croup can be a profoundly disturbing disease for patients, parents, and providers. With a knowledge of the disease process and prognosis, the astute provider should be able to institute an appropriate management plan that adequately prepares parents for the likely outcomes.

SUGGESTED READINGS

Cordle R. Viral croup. In: Tintinalli JE, Kelen GD, Stapczynski JS, eds. *Emergency Medicine: A Comprehensive Study Guide*. 6th ed. New York, NY: McGraw-Hill; 2004:851–854.

Guideline for the diagnosis and management of croup. Alberta, ON, Canada: Alberta Medical Association, 2008. Available at: http://www.topalbertadoctors.org/cpgs/croup.html. Accessed January 20, 2009.

Manno M. Viral croup. In: Marx J, Hockberger R, Walls R, eds. *Rosen's Emergency Medicine: Concepts and Clinical Practice*. 5th ed. St. Louis, MO: Mosby; 2002:2251–2253.

Muniz A, Molodow RE, Defendi GL. Croup. *eMedicine*. Available at: http://emedicine.medscape.com/article/962972-print. Accessed January 20, 2009.

Steele DW. Croup. In: Rosen P, Barkin RM, Hayden SR, et al., eds. *The 5 Minute Emergency Medicine Consult*. 3rd ed. Philadelphia, PA: Lippincott Williams & Wilkins; 1999:270–271.

Vernacchio L, Mitchell AA, Marchetti F, et al. Oral dexamethasone for mild croup. *N Engl J Med*. 2004;351:2768–2769.

280

DO NOT WITHHOLD OXYGEN FROM A HYPOXIC PATIENT WITH CHRONIC OBSTRUCTIVE PULMONARY DISEASE

MELISSA W. COSTELLO, MD, FACEP

There are few myths more pervasive in the world of medicine than the one about patients with chronic obstructive pulmonary disease (COPD) who should not get "too much oxygen." Years of dogma have taught that giving extra oxygen to these patients is dangerous. The reason given is that oxygen will interfere with the patient's hypoxic drive ultimately exacerbating hypercarbia, resulting in apnea and death. This belief is particularly entrenched in the prehospital environment where it often makes an appearance in textbooks, treatment protocols, and therapeutic pathways as stern warnings about apnea in COPD patients who are receiving supplemental oxygen.

While there are certainly data and studies that show a link between increasing supplemental oxygen and an increase in $PaCO_2$, this reality often leads to a potentially tragic miscalculation on the part of medical personnel to decrease the amount of oxygen given to a sick or failing patient. Dr John Hoyt summarized this nicely in his editorial in *Critical Care Medicine* (1997) "Key organs such as the heart and brain, are not at all forgiving of insufficient supplies of oxygen ... withholding or delivering inadequate doses of oxygen to meet the metabolic needs of the patient in respiratory failure ... is generally fatal for the patient and a treatment tragedy for the misinformed physician." A careful examination of the respiratory physiology and the pathophysiology of COPD will reveal that the elevation of $PaCO_2$ is both transient and essentially unrelated to depression of the hypoxic drive.

Lee and Read postulated as early as 1967 that increasing oxygen above a PaO_2 of 60 torr would cause a rise in $PaCO_2$ due to an increase in pulmonary dead space. Their study looked at COPD patients in stable condition and showed that the dead space increased by $\geq 6\%$ when the patients were breathing 100% oxygen. The mechanism described suggested reversal of the pulmonary vasoconstriction that is well documented to be present in a chronic hypoxic state. The alveolar vasculature is very adept at constricting during hypoxic states ($PaO_2 < 60$ torr) to shunt blood to the best ventilated areas of the lung. When the PaO_2 is allowed (or supplemented) to rise above this threshold, the hypoxic pulmonary vasoconstriction is released, and this creates an increased blood flow to poorly ventilated areas of the lung. This creates a V/Q mismatch, resulting in a rise in $PaCO_2$.

Crossley et al. did an elegant study of this theory in 1997 when they examined a small population of known CO_2-retaining COPD patients whose medical condition had stabilized after a period of mechanical ventilation. These patients were spontaneously breathing on the ventilator, were not hypoxic, and had varying levels of supplemental oxygen. All had a documented paO_2 of >60 torr prior to entry into the study. These patients then had their FiO_2 increased from baseline (0.3 to 0.4) to 0.7 for 20 min and the $PaCO_2$ was remeasured. The study showed that, in the absence of baseline alveolar hypoxia, there was no significant change in $PaCO_2$, dead space or respiratory drive.

The ability of a patient to increase his or her minute volume in response to the transient increase in $PaCO_2$ that results from supplemental oxygen–induced pulmonary vasodilatation may be significantly compromised during a severe acute respiratory distress event. This becomes the true issue in the "retainers" that are often seen in the emergency department. Truly it is unrelated to the supplemental oxygen and much more related to the impending respiratory failure. Several well-performed studies have shown that patients who are not stressed to their absolute physiologic maximum minute volume are capable of rebounding from the $PaCO_2$ bump with an increase in minute volume. The solution for the acute respiratory distressed group is, and always has been, invasive or noninvasive mechanical ventilation. For the latter, the solution is certainly NOT deprivation of needed oxygen but a bit of patience and restraint on the part of the treating physician.

Withholding oxygen from a hypoxic COPD patient is never a good idea. Careful monitoring and judicious use of noninvasive or invasive mechanical ventilatory support should be the prime consideration in the patient with severe acute respiratory distress.

SUGGESTED READINGS

Crossley DJ, McGuire GP, Barrow PM, et al. Influence of inspired oxygen concentration on deadspace, respiratory drive, and $PaCO_2$ in intubated patients with chronic obstructive pulmonary disease. *Crit Care Med.* 1997;25(9):1522–1526.

Hoyt JW. Debunking myths of chronic obstructive lung disease. *Crit Care Med.* 1997;25(9): 1450–1451.

Lee J, Read J. Effect of oxygen breathing on distribution of blood flow in chronic obstructive lung disease. *Am Rev Respir Dis.* 1967;96:1173–1180.

Whitnack J. The death of the hypoxic drive theory. *Speech to 22nd Annual Tahoe Odyssey Conference.* Available at: http://home.pacbell.net/whitnack/the_death_of_the_hypoxic_drive_theory.htm. Accessed November 17, 2008.

281

DO NOT ASSUME THAT A NORMAL OXYGEN SATURATION ALWAYS MEANS THAT THE PATIENT IS OXYGENATING OR VENTILATING ADEQUATELY

EMILIE J. B. CALVELLO, MD, MPH

Vital signs are one of the most important objective data elements in the emergency physicians' armamentarium. In addition to the standard five vital signs, blood pressure, heart rate, temperature, respiratory rate, and mental status, two other measures are commonly thought of as vital signs as well. Increasingly, blood glucose and pulse oximetry are reported with the other triage vital signs, although arguably pulse oximetry will have a more universal application.

In the current era of emergency medicine, oxygen saturation is used in variety of situations, especially in patients who may be in a hypoxic state. Given the importance that pulse oximetry plays in monitoring patients, physicians need to have a clear understanding of the principles behind its function and its limitations.

The functionality of pulse oximetry is based on a basic law of physics, the Beer-Lambert law. Simply stated, the Beer-Lambert law states that the absorption of a wavelength of light by a solute is proportional to the solute concentration. In human tissue, deoxyhemoglobin absorbs light in the red spectrum at 600 to 750 nm, whereas oxyhemoglobin absorbs light in the infrared spectrum at 850 to 1,000 nm. Current pulse oximeter probes emit two frequencies, 660 and 940 nm. The relative absorptions of the two wavelengths are measured and used via a computerized algorithm to estimate saturation.

The first common misconception applied to the interpretation of pulse oximetry is that normal oxygen saturation reflects adequate ventilation. If patients are placed on supplemental oxygen, detection of significant alveolar hypoventilation may be further delayed as the oxygen prevents hypoxemia. Capnography or blood gas analysis (arterial or venous) to directly measure $PaCO_2$ should be considered in situations where inadequate alveolar ventilation may occur, such as procedural sedation.

The acute clinician should be aware of two abnormal hemoglobin states that can significantly alter the interpretation of pulse oximetry: carboxyhemoglobin and methemoglobin. Carboxyhemoglobin and oxyhemoglobin both absorb light at 660 nm which leads to errors in the summation calculations. This can lead to the clinical scenario where substantial concentrations of carboxyhemoglobin may be present with adequate saturations. Carboxyhemoglobin concentration must be assessed with co-oximetry from an arterial blood gas. Newer generation pulse oximeters now exist, which have the capacity to measure carboxyhemoglobin concentrations. Methemoglobin absorbs light both at 660 and 940 nm. The summation calculation produces a saturation that tends toward 80% to 85% independent of the true concentration of oxyhemoglobin. Notably, this will produce the clinical scenario of persistent saturations of 85% despite administration of 100% oxygen. Blood gas analysis with co-oximetry will reveal both the concentration of methemoglobin if present and the saturation of dissolved oxygen in the blood which will be higher than that measured by pulse oximetry.

In conclusion, pulse oximetry has become an important measurement—as valuable as a vital sign should be. It is an indispensible tool to care for the critically ill patient. Understanding the basic concepts of function allows better appreciation for the scenarios in which the oxygen saturation is unreliable in detecting clinically significant illness.

SUGGESTED READINGS

Ayas N, Bergstrom LR, Schwab TR, et al. Unrecognized severe postoperative hypercapnea: A case of apnic oxygenation. *Mayo Clin Proc.* 1998;73:51.

Barker SJ, Curry J, Redford D, et al. Measurement of carboxyhemoglobin and methemoglobin by pulse oximetry: A human volunteer study. *Anesthesiology*. 2006;105:892.

Barker SJ, Tremper KK. The effect of carbon monoxide inhalation on pulse oximetry and transcutaneous PO2. *Anesthesiology*. 1987;66:677.

Barker SJ, Tremper KK, Hyatt J. Effects of methemoglobinemia on pulse oximetry and mixed venous oximetry. *Anesthesiology*. 1989;70:112.

Fu ES, Downs JB, Schwiger JW, et al. Supplemental oxygen impairs detection of hypoventilation by pulse oximetry. *Chest*. 2004;126:1552.

Grace RF. Pulse oximetry: Gold standard or false sense of security? *Med J Aust*. 1994;160:638.

Hampson NB. Pulse oximetry in severe carbon monoxide poisoning. *Chest*. 1998;114:1036.

Jubran A. Pulse oximetry. *Intensive Care Med*. 2004;30:2017.

Wright RO, Lewander WJ, Woolf AD. Methemoglobinemia: Etiology, pharmacology and clinical management. *Ann Emerg Med*. 1999;34:646.

282

DO NOT ASSUME THAT SUCCINYLCHOLINE IS THE PARALYTIC OF CHOICE FOR ALL ADULTS UNDERGOING RAPID-SEQUENCE INTUBATION

JOHN W. BURGER, MD

Succinylcholine (SCh) is a popular drug widely used by emergency physicians. With its rapid onset and relatively short duration of action, SCh appears to be the perfect choice of paralytic for an adult patient undergoing rapid-sequence intubation (RSI). While this is indeed true for many patients encountered in the acute setting, there are several conditions in which the side effects of administering this particular drug can be deleterious or even fatal to the patient and therefore must be avoided.

HYPERKALEMIA

Perhaps the most important side effect of SCh is hyperkalemia. When SCh binds to the postsynaptic acetylcholine receptor found at the motor end plate of the neuromuscular junction, sodium enters the cells in exchange for potassium. For most adults, this rise in potassium occurs 3 to 5 min after administration of IV SCh and corresponds to 0.5 to 1.0 mEq/L increase in serum potassium concentration. The transient increase, lasting anywhere from 5 to 10 min, can be clinically significant in certain patients. Those individuals with rhabdomyolysis, preexisting hyperkalemia, or disease states that cause up-regulation of postjunctional acetylcholine receptors are at greatest risk.

Up-regulation produces isoforms of the acetylcholine receptor that are expressed beyond the neuromuscular junction throughout the muscle membrane. With more receptors available, more potassium will enter the bloodstream leading to an increase in serum potassium levels that can result in cardiac dysrhythmias and eventual cardiac arrest.

Conditions that up–regulate acetylcholine receptors include

1) Myopathies (muscular dystrophy)
2) Denervation diseases (Guillain-Barre syndrome, multiple sclerosis)
3) Disuse atrophy (prolonged immobilization)
4) Botulism/tetanus
5) Traumatic injuries (burn injuries, crush injuries)

For acutely injured patients, the greatest risk of hyperkalemia typically occurs 7 to 10 days after the initial injury. However, it is suggested that SCh be avoided in patients with burn or crush injuries >48 to 72 h old because the exact onset of up–regulation is highly variable.

SCh is not contraindicated in patients with myasthenia gravis. Even though myasthenia is a disease involving the neuromuscular junction, patients are not at risk for developing hyperkalemia. In fact, these patients are often resistant to SCh and require doses up to 2 mg/kg to achieve adequate paralysis.

Despite its association with chronic hyperkalemia, renal failure does not constitute an absolute contraindication to single-dose SCh use. Studies have shown that a single dose of SCh does not result in a significantly larger increase in serum potassium levels when compared to individuals without renal disease. It is important to note that SCh should be avoided in renal failure patients already exhibiting EKG changes suggestive of elevated serum potassium.

MALIGNANT HYPERTHERMIA
Patients with a personal or family history of malignant hyperthermia should not receive SCh. SCh can precipitate the acute onset of malignant hyperthermia, a potentially fatal hypermetabolic disorder.

TRISMUS
0.001% to 0.1% of all patients experience masseter muscle spasms after receiving SCh. This increase in muscle tone can be severe enough to interfere with direct laryngoscopy and even prevent adequate oxygenation with a bag-valve mask. Nondepolarizing neuromuscular blocking agents can be used to relax the spasm, but other airway rescue techniques may need to be employed. Though rare, trismus can be a harbinger of impending malignant hyperthermia and must be taken seriously.

FASCICULATIONS
The fasciculations caused by SCh may elevate both intracranial and intraocular pressure. The transient increase in intraocular pressure has the potential to exacerbate eye injuries, though several studies suggest that SCh is indeed safe in patients with open globe trauma.

BRADYCARDIA

SCh can also have side effects beyond the neuromuscular junction. Since it resembles two joined acetylcholine molecules, it has the ability to bind to any cholinergic receptor throughout the sympathetic and parasympathetic nervous systems. The most common cardiovascular side effect is bradycardia caused by sinus node sensitization from succinylmonocholine, a metabolite of SCh.

PROLONGED PARALYSIS

Typically, paralysis from SCh lasts <10 min. However, some patients will experience prolonged neuromuscular blockade. This is usually due to high dosages or abnormal metabolism. SCh is metabolized by an enzyme produced in the liver called pseudocholinesterase. The length of the blockade depends on extent of the enzymatic activity. One out of every fifty patients will have a heterozygous pseudocholinesterase deficiency. For most patients with a deficient enzyme, paralysis lasts 20 to 30 min. Keep in mind that several medications can also cause decreased enzymatic activity.

KEY POINTS

SCh use is absolutely contraindicated in patients with a personal or family history of malignant hyperthermia, pre-existing hyperkalemia with EKG changes, or disorders that up-regulate acetylcholine receptors. SCh causes fasciculations that may lead to increased intracranial pressure and increased intraocular pressure. Some patients experience trismus after administration of SCH that can make airway protection extremely challenging. Because of its similarity to acetylcholine, SCh can also act beyond the neuromuscular junction. Lastly, it is important to recognize that neuromuscular blockade can persist significantly longer than anticipated in patients with inherited or acquired variations in pseudocholinesterase activity.

SUGGESTED READINGS

Allen G, Rosenberg H. Malignant hyperthermia susceptibility in adult patients with masseter muscle rigidity. *Can J Anesthesia*. 1990;37:31–35.

Bauer S, Orio K, Adams B. Succinylcholine induced masseter spasm during rapid sequence intubation may require a surgical airway: Care report. *Emerg Med J*. 2005;22:456–458.

Chakravarty E. Cardiac arrest due to succinylcholine-induced hyperkalemia in a patient with wound botulism. *J Clin Anesth*. 2000;12:80–82.

Gill M, Graeme K, Guenterberg K. Masseter spasms after succinylcholine administration. *J Emerg Med*. 2005;29:167–171.

Gronert G. Cardiac arrest after succinylcholine: Mortality greater with rhabdomyolysis than receptor upregulation. *Anesthesiology*. 2001;94:523–529.

Levitan R. Safety of succinylcholine in myasthenia gravis. *Ann Emerg Med*. 2005;45:225–226.

Maiorana A, Roach RB Jr. Heterozygous pseudocholinesterase deficiency: A case report and review of the literature. *J Oral Maxillofac Surg*. 2003;61:845–847.

Martyn JAJ. Succinylcholine hyperkalemia after burns. *Anesthesiology*. 1999;91:321–322.

Martyn J, Richtsfeld M. Succinylcholine-induced hyperkalemia in acquired pathologic states: Etiologic factors and molecular mechanisms. *Anethesiology*. 2006;104:158–169.

Morgan G, Mikhail M, Murray M. *Clinical Anesthiology*. 4th ed. Los Angeles, CA : McGraw Hill; 2005.

Thapa S, Brull S. Succinylcholine-induced hyperkalemia in patients with renal failure: An old question revisited. *Anesth Analg*. 2000;91:237–241.

Vachon C, Warner D, Bacon D. Succinylcholine and the open globe. Tracing the teaching. *Anesthesiology*. 2003;99:220–223.

Yasuda I, Hirano T, Amaha K. Chronotropic effects of succinylcholine and succinylmonocholine on the sinoatrial node. *Anesthesiology*. 1982;57:289–292.

Zink B, Snyder H, Raccio-Robak N. Lack of a hyperkalemic response in emergency department patients receiving succinylcholine. *Acad Emerg Med*. 1995;2:974–978.

283

USE OF TERBUTALINE AND EPINEPHRINE IN ACUTE MANAGEMENT OF ASTHMA

JESSE H. KIM, MD

The myth that subcutaneous or intravenous (IV) terbutaline or epinephrine adds additional benefit over that of albuterol in severely bronchoconstricted asthmatics is extremely prevalent. Often, these systemic therapies are administered by emergency medical services (EMS) and continued in IV drip fashion over continuous albuterol nebulization therapy in in-patient settings. Perhaps the biggest rationale comes from providers who believe that the severely decreased airflow limits delivery of nebulized albuterol to the airways. However, although plausible, the evidence supporting benefit from this common treatment rationale is sparse at best. The following are five pieces of literature which illustrate this point.

- Adding an IV terbutaline drip on pediatric asthma patients already on continuous albuterol neb did not improve any outcome in a randomized study done in a pediatric emergency department (ED).

- Comparison of out-of-hospital use of single-dose albuterol nebulization (2.5 mg) versus subcutaneous terbutaline (0.25 mg) in COPD and asthma exacerbations did not show a significant difference in respiratory severity scores (measured by EMS personnel), peak flow rate, or hospital admission frequencies upon ED presentation. However, subjective scores by patients did show significant improvement in the albuterol arm ($p < 0.05$).

- Subcutaneous use of epinephrine before albuterol nebulization did not provide any significant improvement in clinical scores, peak flow, or respiratory rate in pediatric asthma patients in the ED (mean age 8.9 years) at 20 min and 2 h after treatment.

- A Cochrane review of 15 randomized controlled trials in the literature involving 584 patients compared IV β_2-agonists versus placebo, inhaled β_2-agonists, or other standard of care. The conclusions did not find any conferred advantage of IV β_2-agonist therapy over inhalation in severe acute asthma patients presenting to EDs.

- Systemic β_2-agonist therapy is not only an unproven treatment, but there is some evidence that it may be harmful. An in-patient study of severely asthmatic patients in Boston Children's Hospital showed that patients who were on IV isoproterenol therapy were significantly more likely to suffer from cardiac ischemia as measured by cardiac enzymes, CK-MB values and EKG abnormalities when compared to patients who were not on an isoproterenol infusion.

The latest National Heart, Lung and Blood Institute 2007 Asthma guideline states that IV β_2-agonits remain largely unproven treatments and that insufficient evidence exists to make recommendations regarding their routine use in the ED. Given the sparse literature support and possible systemic side effects, inhalation bronchodilator therapy should remain the treatment of choice over systemic β_2-agonists, including subcutaneous or IV terbutaline or epinephrine.

SUGGESTED READINGS

Bogie AL, Towne D, Luckett PM, et al. Comparison of intravenous terbutaline versus normal saline in pediatric patients on continuous high-dose nebulized albuterol for status asthmaticus. *Pediatr Emerg Care*. 2007;23(6):355–361.

Kornberg AE, Zuckerman S, Welliver JR, et al. Effect of injected long-acting epinephrine in addition to aerosolized albuterol in the treatment of acute asthma in children. *Pediatric Emerg Care*. 1991;7(1):1–3.

Maguire JF, O'Rourke PP, Colan SD, et al. Cardiotoxicity during treatment of severe childhood asthma. *Pediatrics*. 1991;88(6):1180–1186.

National Heart Lung and Blood Institute (NHLBI), National Asthma Education Prevention Program (NAEPP). Expert panel report 3. Guidelines for the diagnosis and management of asthma: full report; 2007.

Travers A, Jones AP, Kelly K, et al. Intravenous beta2-agonists for acute asthma in the emergency department. *Cochrane Database Syst Rev*. 2001;(2):CD002988.

Zehner WJ Jr, Scott JM, Iannolo PM, et al. Terbutaline vs albuterol for out-of-hospital respiratory distress: Randomized, double-blind trial. *Acad Emerg Med*. 1995;2(8):686–691.

284

Do not exclude pneumonia simply based on a "negative" chest x-ray

Mustapha Saheed, MD

Pneumonia is one of the leading causes of death in the world. Together with influenza, pneumonia accounts for over 60,000 deaths a year making it the eighth leading cause of death in the United States (2005 data). Early diagnosis and proper treatment are critical to the prevention of additional morbidity and mortality. Early treatment has become a public health priority so much so that the Agency for Health Care Research and Quality has made empiric antibiotic treatment for community-acquired bacterial pneumonia an emergency department performance measure. Given the importance of early diagnosis and treatment, the question of how best to diagnose pneumonia should be examined. In particular, how reliable is the chest x-ray in making a diagnosis?

The diagnosis of pneumonia is based on the combination of a clinically appropriate history, physical exam, and a positive imaging study. Multiple studies have attempted to identify clinical features that provide sufficient diagnostic certainty to subvert the need for imaging. Unfortunately, the data consistently show that clinical judgment alone cannot be used to identify pneumonia or distinguish it from other respiratory pathology. Accordingly, the reference gold standard for the diagnosis of pneumonia is by radiograph. However, while the x-ray, as a result of its wide availability, relatively low cost, and easy deployment, has become a ubiquitous diagnostic adjunct, it is not without limitations.

Certainly, as with all imaging modalities, there is interobserver variability in radiographic interpretations. Albaum et al. (1996), in a prospective multi-center study, evaluated the agreement between two radiologists' assessments of chest radiographs of over 282 patients and showed that there was only fair agreement ($\kappa = 0.37$, 95% CI 0.22 to 0.52) on the presence or absence of an infiltrate. And when descriptive aspects of the x-rays between the two radiologists were compared, like the classification of an infiltrate as lobar or the presence of air bronchograms, the agreement further declined! ($\kappa = 0.09$, 95% CI 0.04 to 0.22; and $\kappa = 0.01$, 95% CI -0.13 to 0.15, respectively). Other studies corroborate the poor reliability in the radiologic classifications of pneumonia morphology. Moreover, several studies show that despite traditional teaching, radiographic findings are poorly predictive of causative agents in lower respiratory infections.

Chest x-rays may altogether "miss" the diagnosis of lower respiratory infections. In a study by Syrjala et al. (1998), 47 patients with signs and symptoms concerning for possible pneumonia were evaluated by chest x-ray and high-resolution CT scan. All 18 cases of pneumonia recognized radiographically were identified on CT scan, but an additional 8 cases were also visualized on CT—suggesting a possible x-ray miss rate of 31%. Certainly, there is ambiguity about the import of the cases identified only by CT scan. There were no supplemental data presented to convincingly show that the CT-identified cases likely represent pneumonia. Furthermore, without clinical course and outcomes data, the clinical significance of the cases is debatable.

In a series of 2,706 patients, Basi et al. (2004) reviewed the clinical course of patients admitted with the clinical diagnosis of pneumonia and managed by a predefined clinical treatment pathway. Of the sample studied, 30% had negative initial radiographs for pneumonia. These patients tended to be older, had a higher initial pneumonia severity index score, and were more likely to have positive blood or sputum cultures for microbes other than Streptococcal pneumonia. The study revealed that both patient populations, with and without roentgenography-confirmed pneumonia, had significant similarities including presenting pulmonary symptoms, rates of positive sputum cultures and bacteremia, general laboratory test results, and in-hospital mortality. The authors acknowledge the inherent controversy in defining a cohort of "pneumonia" patients with negative radiographs, especially as a positive radiographic study is the reference standard for diagnosis. However, they conclude that these patients likely represent a population with a clinically significant lower respiratory illness.

Notably, Basi et al. (2004) also discovered that 7% of patients, who presented with initial negative x-ray for pneumonia, developed radiographic findings consistent with pneumonia within 72 h of admission. This finding, while certainly lower than the 31% possible miss rate found by Syrjala et al. (1998), suggests that the chest x-ray may have a much lower sensitivity than typically accepted for a "gold standard" test.

There is already a consensus that immunocompromised patients may require more sophisticated imaging and laboratory diagnostic tests for diagnosis of pneumonia. Approximately 10% of these symptomatic patients may have normal radiographs. To be sure, there are subsets of immunocompromised patients who have a higher rate of false-negative radiographs. For example, in one series of 93 patients with HIV and microbiologically confirmed *Pneumocystis carinii* pneumonia (PCP), 39% had initial x-rays interpreted as normal. Neutropenic patients also represent another subpopulation that may present with initially negative radiographs. In a study of febrile patients who had bone marrow transplant, the sensitivity of the chest x-ray was only 46%. As such, the recommendations for immunocompromised patients generally encourage clinicians to consider more sophisticated imaging modalities as appropriate.

Radiographs are clearly important diagnostic adjuncts in the diagnosis of pneumonia. However, we should be cautious in our overreliance on radiographic imaging and pursue further testing as appropriate in patients with negative x-rays but concerning clinical presentation for pneumonia.

SUGGESTED READINGS

Albaum MN, Hill LC, Murphy M, et al. Interobserver reliability of the chest radiograph in community-acquired pneumonia. *Chest.* 1996;110(2):343–350.

Barloon TJ, Galvin JR, Mori M, et al. High-resolution ultrafast chest CT in the clinical management of febrile bone marrow transplant patients with normal or nonspecific chest roentgenograms. *Chest.* 1991;99:928–933.

Basi SK, Marrie TJ, Huang JQ, et al. Patients admitted to hospital with suspected pneumonia and normal chest radiographs: Epidemiology, microbiology, and outcomes. *Am J Med.* 2004;117(5):305–311.

Boersma WG, Daniels JM, Löwenberg A, et al. Reliability of radiographic findings and the relation to etiologic agents in community-acquired pneumonia. *Respir Med.* 2006;100(5):926–932.

Bruns AH, Oosterheert JJ, Prokop M, et al. Patterns of resolution of chest radiograph abnormalities in adults hospitalized with severe community-acquired pneumonia. *Clin Infect Dis.* 2007;45(8):983–991.

Dalhoff K. Worldwide guidelines for respiratory tract infections: Community-acquired pneumonia. *Int J Antimicrob Agents.* 2001;18(Suppl 1):S39–S44.

Dawson N, Speroff T, Siciliano C, et al. Comparison of physician judgment and decision aids for ordering chest radiographs for pneumonia in outpatients. *Ann Emerg Med.* 1991;20(11):1215–1219.

DeLorenzo U, Huang CT, Maguire OP, et al. Roentgenographic patterns of Pneumocystis carinii pneumonia in 104 patients with AIDS. *Chest.* 1987;91:323–327.

Gruden JF, Huang L, Turner J, et al. High-resolution CT in the evaluation of clinically suspected Pneumocystis carinii pneumonia in AIDS patients with normal, equivocal, or nonspecific radiographic findings. *Am J Roentgenol.* 1997;169(4):967–975.

Gulati M, Kaur R, Jha V, et al. High-resolution CT in renal transplant patients with suspected pulmonary infections. *Acta Radiol.* 2000;41(3):237–241.

Heussel CP, Kauczor HU, Ullmann AJ. Pneumonia in neutropenic patients. *Eur Radiol.* 2004;14(2):256–271.

Hopstaken RM, Muris JW, Knottnerus JA, et al. Contributions of symptoms, signs, erythrocyte sedimentation rate, and C-reactive protein to a diagnosis of pneumonia in acute lower respiratory tract infection. *Br J Gen Pract.* 2003;53(490):358–364.

Hopstaken RM, Stobberingh EE, Knottnerus JA, et al. Clinical items not helpful in differentiating viral from bacterial lower respiratory tract infections in general practice. *J Clin Epidemiol.* 2005;58(2):175–183.

Hopstaken RM, Witbraad T, Engelshoven JM, et al. Inter-observer variation in the interpretation of chest radiographs for pneumonia in community-acquired lower respiratory tract infections. *Clin Radiol.* 2004;59:743–752.

Katz DS, Leung AN. Radiology of pneumonia. *Clin Chest Med.* 1999;20(3):549–562.

Kennedy CA, Goetz MB. Atypical roentgenographic manifestations of Pneumocystis carinii pneumonia. *Arch Intern Med.* 1992;152:1390–1398.

Macfarlane JT, Miller AC, Roderick Smith WH, et al. Comparative radiographic features of community acquired Legionnaires' disease, pneumococcal pneumonia, mycoplasma pneumonia, and psittacosis. *Thorax.* 1984;39(1):28–33.

Mandell LA, Bartlett JG, Dowell SF. Update of practice guidelines for the management of community-acquired pneumonia in immunocompetent adults: Infectious Diseases Society of America. *Clin Infect Dis.* 2003;37(11):1405–1433.

Margolis P, Gadomski A. The rational clinical examination: Does this infant have pneumonia? *JAMA.* 1998;279(4):308–313.

Melbye H, Dale K. Interobserver variability in the radiographic diagnosis of adult outpatient pneumonia. *Acta Radiol.* 1992;33:79–81.

Nambu A, Saito A, Araki T, et al. Chlamydia pneumoniae: Comparison with findings of Mycoplasma pneumoniae and Streptococcus pneumoniae at thin-section CT. *Radiology.* 2006;238(1):330–338.

Niederman MS, Mandell LA, Anzueto A, et al. American Thoracic Society Guidelines for the management of adults with community-acquired pneumonia: Diagnosis, assessment of severity, antimicrobial therapy, and prevention. *Am J Respir Crit Care Med.* 2001;163(7):1730–1754.

Opravil M, Marincek B, Fuchs WA, et al. Shortcomings of chest radiography in detecting Pneumocystis carinii pneumonia. *J Acquir Immune Defic Syndr.* 1994;7:39–45.

Shreeniwas R, Schulman LL, Berkmen YM, et al. Opportunistic bronchopulmonary infections after lung transplantation: Clinical and radiographic findings. *Radiology.* 1996;200: 349–356.

Singal BM, Hedges JR, Radack KL. Decision rules and clinical prediction of pneumonia: evaluation of low-yield criteria. *Ann Emerg Med.* 1989;18(1):13–20.

Syrjälä H, Broas M, Suramo I, et al. High-resolution computed tomography for the diagnosis of community-acquired pneumonia. *Clin Infect Dis.* 1998;27(2):358–363.

Tew J, Calenoff L, Berlin BS. Bacterial or nosocomial pneumonia: accuracy of radiographic diagnosis. *Radiology.* 1977;124:607–612.

Washington L, Palacio D. Imaging of bacterial pulmonary infection in the immunocompetent patient. *Semin Roentgenol.* 2007;42(2):122–145.

Weber C, Maas R, Steiner P, et al. Importance of digital thoracic radiography in the diagnosis of pulmonary infiltrates in patients with bone marrow transplantation during aplasia. *Fortschr Röntgenstr.* 1999;171:294–301.

Wipf JE, Lipsky BA, Hirschmann JV, et al. Diagnosing pneumonia by physical examination: relevant or relic? *Arch Intern Med.* 1999;159(10):1082–1087.

285

DO NOT EXCLUDE PULMONARY EMBOLUS SIMPLY BASED ON A NEGATIVE CHEST COMPUTED TOMOGRAPHY

JULIANNA JUNG, MD, FACEP

Computed tomography (CT) of the chest has become the most commonly used initial test in the evaluation of patients with suspected pulmonary embolus (PE). There are good reasons for this: chest CT is fast, convenient, and allows simultaneous evaluation of alternative diagnoses. Many physicians use chest CT as their sole test for PE and consider PE to be ruled out on the basis of a negative CT, regardless of the pretest probability of the diagnosis. However, the sensitivity of chest CT is not adequate to exclude the diagnosis of PE in high-risk patients, and it is by no means clear that using CT as a sole test for PE is a safe or appropriate practice.

In the PIOPED II study, overall sensitivity of multidetector-row chest CT for the diagnosis of PE was 83%—this means that CT missed the diagnosis of PE in 17% of cases. The overall positive predictive value (PPV) of chest CT was 86%—this means that 14% of CT scans showing PE proved to be false positive. On first glance, this might shake one's faith in CT. However, when CT (like any test) is interpreted in the context of clinical pretest probability, these numbers make a lot more sense. Indeed, in PIOPED II, the predictive value of CT varied dramatically when clinical assessment of pretest probability was taken into account.

For patients with low clinical probability of PE, a negative chest CT had negative predictive value (NPV) of 97%, but a positive chest CT had a PPV of only 58%. As one may expect, patients who were judged clinically *unlikely* to have PE had a very *low* rate of false-negative studies—if the doctor thought the patient did not have a PE and the scan did not show a PE, then there was almost never a PE. On the other hand, among this group there was a very *high* rate of false-positive studies—if the doctor thought the patient did not have a PE but the scan showed a PE, the scan was often wrong.

By contrast, for patients with high clinical probability of PE, a negative chest CT had an NPV of only 60%, while a positive CT had a PPV of 96%. In this case, patients who were judged *likely* to have a PE had a very *high* rate of false-negative studies—if the doctor really thought there was a PE but the scan did not show one, the scan was often wrong. *In fact, the scan was wrong 40% of the time in this study—a really dangerous error level for such a deadly diagnosis.* This is why CT alone is not adequate to rule out PE in high probability patients—it is just not sensitive enough.

So, what to do? The PIOPED II investigators have offered clear recommendations. First and foremost, *determine pretest probability of PE in each and every patient in whom the diagnosis is considered.* This study used the Wells criteria, but others are available, and experienced clinicians get similar results with "empirical assessment" (i.e., good old-fashioned gestalt). Pretest probability determines how all studies for PE are to be interpreted.

For low or moderate probability patients, D-dimer testing is sufficient, provided the quantitative ELISA assay is used. If this test is negative, the workup is over. However, for patients with positive d-dimers and those with high clinical probability, further workup is needed. Note that D-dimer testing has no role in the assessment of high probability patients.

Chest CT is the first-line test after the d-dimer for these patients. The numbers cited above refer specifically to CT angiography (CTA) of the pulmonary vessels—if CT venography (CTV) of the inferior vena cava (IVC) and pelvic/leg veins is added, the diagnostic accuracy of the test increases. For high probability patients, the NPV of a negative CTA-CTV is 82%, compared to only 60% for CTA alone. However, CTV is not universally available, and the

PIOPED II group recommends CTA and CTA-CTV interchangeably in their algorithms. CTV substantially increases radiation exposure for the patient, and it is probably a good idea to use this test judiciously and avoid it altogether in women of childbearing age.

For low probability patients, a negative CT can be considered adequate to rule out PE. However, a positive CT is problematic: with a 42% false-positive rate in this group, treating every positive scan would lead to lot of unnecessary anticoagulation. The location of the PE becomes important for these patients, as the PPV of CT varies according to where the PE is seen—97% for main or lobar arteries, 68% for segmental vessels, and 25% for subsegmental vessels. Therefore, for low probability patients, all main or lobar PEs should be treated, but further workup is recommended for segmental or subsegmental PEs. This may take the form of repeat CT, CTV (if only CTA done initially), ultrasound, ventilation/perfusion scan, or pulmonary angiography.

For intermediate probability patients, a negative CT can also be considered adequate to rule out PE, though the NPV is lower in this group compared to the low probability group (89% vs. 96%). For this reason, CTV or ultrasound are considered optional if there is a lingering concern despite a negative chest CT. For this group, all positive CT scans should be treated with anticoagulation, given the higher pretest risk.

For high probability patients, a negative CT is *not* considered adequate to rule out PE! Again, the NPV of a negative chest CT is only 60%, meaning that CT misses 40% of patients with PE in this group. It is therefore recommended that these patients undergo additional testing using the options listed above and that they be anticoagulated pending the results of these tests. For practical purposes in the ED, it is probably prudent to admit these patients for this purpose.

The bottom line is to know your pretest probability and interpret your chest CT accordingly. A negative CT alone does *not* rule out a PE.

SUGGESTED READINGS

Stein PD, Fowler SE, Goodman LR, et al. Multidetector computed tomography for acute pulmonary embolism. *N Engl J Med*. 2006;354(22):2317–2327.

Stein PD, Woodard PK, Weg JG, et al. Diagnostic pathways in acute pulmonary embolism: Recommendations of the PIOPED II investigators. *Radiology*. 2007;242(1):15–21.

286

Do not exclude tuberculosis simply based on a "negative" chest x-ray

Mustapha Saheed, MD

Tuberculosis (TB) is one of the most frequent infectious causes of death worldwide. Over 8 million people develop active TB, with another 2 million people succumbing to the infection yearly. While TB infection rates have generally decreased in the industrialized world, migration patterns from endemic areas may be causing an increase in parts of the developed world. The advancing antibiotic resistance patterns and relatively high communicability further make the identification, quarantine, and treatment of this infection a priority. Unfortunately, early identification can be somewhat difficult as symptoms of TB infection are nonspecific, and diagnostic testing is relatively complicated. The chest x-ray has historically been a central part of the diagnostic algorithm. However, despite "common misconceptions," radiography has multiple limitations in the diagnosis of TB.

Mycobacterium TB is an intracellular organism with well-developed defenses against host immunity. After initial exposure to bacteria in respiratory droplets, immunocompetent individuals respond with a cell-mediated phagocytic response. Unfortunately, this response is generally unsuccessful as mycobacterium TB can survive intracellularly in the macrophage. The bacteria replicates rapidly, invading local tissues and lymph nodes. Over the next 2 to 4 weeks, the host reacts with a T-cell mediated humoral response, a fact that is exploited diagnostically by the tuberculin skin test. With the advent of specific immunity, most immunocompetent individuals will be now able to halt the bacterial expansion and eventually clear the infection. However, after the primary infection, 5% of exposed individuals will continue to develop a progressive primary infection. Others will develop latent TB that is characterized by noninfectious foci that lies dormant until, for unclear reasons, the immune system fails, and the infection reactivates. Of those with primary TB, 5% to 10% develop reactivation TB.

During primary TB infection, the x-ray findings are varied. Unlike the classically described upper lung zone infection in reactivation TB, primary TB tends to appear more as an infiltrative process with a mild predilection for the lower lobes. Additionally, 10% to 20% of patients may present with a solitary cavitary infiltrate or multiple macronodular infiltrates, and 10% may only have a pleural effusion.

Reactivation TB typically involves the upper lung zone. Notably, the posterior and apical segments of the right upper lobe, apical posterior left upper lobe, and superior segments of the lower lobes are involved in the descending order of frequency. Initially, there is fibronodular involvement, which progresses to larger nodules as lesions coalesce and generally results in cavitary lesions that can vary in size and often have necrotic cores.

However, despite the distinctly described x-ray findings, distinguishing between primary versus reactivation TB or progressive primary TB on radiologic features is unreliable. Geng et al. (2005), in a retrospective review of 456 patients who were culture positive for TB, found that the time of disease acquisition and clinical progression did not accurately predict radiographic abnormalities

Moreover, TB patients often have variable radiographic presentation, sometimes with no distinctive features from other causes of community-acquired pneumonia. van Cleef et al. (2005) evaluated 993 patients with suspected TB based on symptomatology. The patients received three sputum smears and cultures and a chest x-ray. Notably, 46 of the 226 patients with culture-positive sputum had chest x-rays interpreted as "pathology but not TB," or "no pathology," suggesting a 20% radiographic miss rate. Their data demonstrate the difficulty of excluding the diagnosis of TB based on isolated radiographic findings and emphasize the variability in radiographic presentation.

Furthermore, there is already considerable evidence showing that x-ray findings are poorly predictive of the pneumonia etiology. In a series of 162 patients with pneumonia of known etiology as confirmed by sputum cultures, blood cultures, and serological tests, Boersma et al. (2006) found no relationship between general radiographic features and causative agents.

The limitations of the x-ray are not clearly circumvented by the use of computed tomography (CT). Certainly, the CT is more sophisticated, allowing for three-dimensional modeling of the lung parenchyma. However, its sensitivity must be balanced—with the need to minimize overtreatment, the greater cost, and the increased radiation exposure. In a study evaluating pulmonary infections in patients with AIDS, Kang et al. (1996) showed that the CT scan has an increased sensitivity of 96% to 90% over chest radiography. The authors conclude that the modest improvement with CT imaging makes it more useful for targeted testing as opposed to screening. Generally, CT scans are recommended for immunocompromised patients or patients with high suspicion for infection as they are more likely to have atypical or negative radiographs on presentation.

Imaging studies, especially the standard chest x-ray, are still a central part of the diagnostic algorithm for TB. When used in the appropriate clinical context and in conjunction with other diagnostic tools including the tuberculin skin test, the radiograph helps to identify patients with active TB infection. However, in patients with a moderate to high pretest likelihood of the disease, the variability in radiographic presentation and the difficulty in predicting etiologic agents from radiographic findings preclude the isolated use of the chest x-ray to rule out the diagnosis of TB.

SUGGESTED READINGS

Baum GL, Crapo JD. *Baum's Textbook of Pulmonary Diseases*. 7th ed. Philadelphia, PA: Lippincott Williams & Wilkins; 2004.

Boersma WG, Daniels JM, Löwenberg A, et al. Reliability of radiographic findings and the relation to etiologic agents in community-acquired pneumonia. *Respir Med*. 2006;100(5): 926–932.

Bruns AH, Oosterheert JJ, Prokop M, et al. Patterns of resolution of chest radiograph abnormalities in adults hospitalized with severe community-acquired pneumonia. *Clin Infect Dis*. 2007;45(8):983–991.

Campbell IA, Bah-Sow O. Pulmonary tuberculosis: Diagnosis and treatment. *Br Med J* 2006; 332(7551):1194–1197.

Cecil RL, Goldman L, Bennett JC. *Cecil Textbook of Medicine*. 19th ed. Philadelphia, PA: W.B. Saunders; 1992.

Centers for Disease Control. Trends in tuberculosis—United States, 2005, *MMWR Morb Mortal Wkly Rep*. 2006;55:305–308.

Geng E, Kreiswirth B, Burzynski J, et al. Clinical and radiographic correlates of primary and reactivation tuberculosis: A molecular epidemiology study. *JAMA*. 2005;293(22): 2740–2745.

Janzen DL, Padley SP, Adler BD, et al. Acute pulmonary complications in immunocompromised non-AIDS patients: Comparison of diagnostic accuracy of CT and chest radiography. *Clin Radiol*. 1993;47(3):159–165.

Jones BE, Ryu R, Yang Z, et al. Chest radiographic findings in patients with tuberculosis with recent or remote infection. *Am J Respir Crit Care Med*. 1997;156(4 pt 1):1270–1273.

Kang EY, Staples CA, McGuinness G, et al. Detection and differential diagnosis of pulmonary infections and tumors in patients with AIDS: Value of chest radiography versus CT. *Am J Roentgenol*. 1996;166(1):15–19.

Kunimoto D, Long R. Tuberculosis: Still overlooked as a cause of community-acquired pneumonia–how not to miss it. *Respir Care Clin N Am*. 2005;11(1):25–34. Review.

Lee KS, Im JG. CT in adults with tuberculosis of the chest: Characteristic findings and role in management. *Am J Roentgenol*. 1995;164(6):1361–1367.

Lee KS, Song KS, Lim TH, et al. Adult-onset pulmonary tuberculosis: Findings on chest radiographs and CT scans. *Am J Roentgenol*. 1993;160(4):753–758.

Lee MP, Chan JW, Ng KK, et al. Clinical manifestations of tuberculosis in HIV-infected patients. *Respirology*. 2000;5(4):423–426.

Liam CK, Pang YK, Poosparajah S. Pulmonary tuberculosis presenting as community-acquired pneumonia. *Respirology*. 2006;11(6):786–792.

Macfarlane JT, Miller AC, Roderick Smith WH, et al. Comparative radiographic features of community acquired Legionnaires' disease, pneumococcal pneumonia, mycoplasma pneumonia, and psittacosis. *Thorax*. 1984;39(1):28–33.

McAdams HP, Erasmus J, Winter JA. Radiologic manifestations of pulmonary tuberculosis. *Radiol Clin N Am*. 1995;33(4):655–678.

van Cleeff MR, Kivihya-Ndugga LE, Meme H, et al. The role and performance of chest X-ray for the diagnosis of tuberculosis: A cost-effectiveness analysis in Nairobi, Kenya. *BMC Infect Dis*. 2005;5:111.

Washington L, Palacio D. Imaging of bacterial pulmonary infection in the immunocompetent patient. *Semin Roentgenol*. 2007;42(2):122–145.

WHO. Framework for effective tuberculosis control. WHO/TB/94.179, Geneva: WHO; 1994.

287

DO NOT RELY ON ARTERIAL BLOOD GAS MEASUREMENTS TO MANAGE PATIENTS WITH ASTHMA

EMILIE J. B. CALVELLO, MD, MPH

Asthma prevalence in the United States is 4% to 5% of the population. Intimate knowledge of the management of acute asthma exacerbations is a necessity for the emergency physician. The National Heart, Blood and Lung Institute Expert Panel Report 3 published new guidelines for the diagnosis and management of asthma in 2007. *Figure 287.1* shows the panel's summary recommendations for emergency department (ED) care. To briefly review, ED presentations are broken down into mild-moderate (peak expiratory flow [PEF] > 40%), severe (PEF < 40%), and life-threatening presentations which must be managed immediately with endotracheal intubation. Clinical findings can help practitioners identify severe asthma attacks; however, the more objective measurements of peak flow can aid in severe asthma diagnosis with the added benefit of being able to monitor the patient's response to treatment. For those severe asthmatics not requiring emergent airway control, aggressive early management includes corticosteroids and short-acting β-agonists plus ipratropium over the first hour of presentation. Mild-moderate exacerbations should also receive short-acting β-agonists and steroids but do not necessitate the need for ipratropium.

Arterial blood gases (ABGs) are not recommended in the general management of asthma patients. Considerations for relative hypercapnia may be inferred by simple peak flow which obviates the need for routine blood gas analysis. In addition, hypercapnia or acidosis only takes place when the PEF is <25% the predicted norm in the absence of other respiratory depressant medication. Therefore, the guidelines now state that ABGs are recommended only in patients who have PEF <25% after initial therapy, persistent dyspnea, or suspicion for hypoventilation secondary to respiratory fatigue. Of course, ABGs may be required in a patient in severe distress who cannot produce a PEF, however, that the patient will likely require aggressive intervention requiring ventilatory control regardless of the amount of hypercarbia.

In addition, the venous blood gas (VBG) has proven its role as a useful screening tool in asthma for hypercarbia in the ED setting. The risks of the ABG include pain, thrombosis, bleeding, infection, and compressive neuropathies which further strengthen the case for screening VBG. A pCO_2 of >45 is associated with relative hypercarbia in the asthmatic. Remember that patients

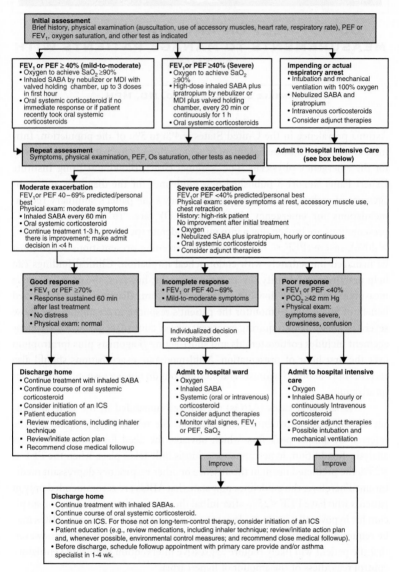

FIGURE 287.1. Management of asthma exacerbations: ED and hospital-based care. (From National Heart, Lung, and Blood Institute, National Institutes of Health. National Asthma Education and Prevention Program. Expert Panel Report 3 [EPR-3]: Guidelines for the Diagnosis and Management of Asthma – Summary Report 2007. Washington DC: USDHHS; 2007.)

with asthma may present with a variety of blood gas measurement ranging from respiratory alkalosis through "normalization" of $PaCO_2$ to a respiratory acidosis. Given the increased ventilatory stimulation, a normal or mildly elevated $PaCO_2$ indicates significant airway obstruction that may progress to ventilatory failure.

In summary, the common presentation of asthma in the ED requires strict attention to physical exam and assessment of response to initial aggressive therapy monitored by serial peak flow measurements. The use of blood gas analysis should only be reserved for a subset of patients, and in general, VBG sampling may be an adequate screening tool to evaluate for hypercarbia.

SUGGESTED READINGS

Kelly AM, Kyle E, McAlpine R. Venous pCO(2) and pH can be used to screen for significant hypercarbia in emergency patients with acute respiratory disease. *J Emerg Med.* 2002a;22(1):15–19.

Kelsen SG, Kelsen DP, FLeeger BF, et al. Emergency room assessment and treatment of patients with acute asthma: Adequacy of the conventional approach. *Am J Med.* 1978;64:622–628.

Mannino DM, Homa DM, Akinbami LJ, et al. Surveillance for asthma: United States, 1980–1999. *MMWR Surveill Summ.* 2002;51(SS1):1–14.

Martin TG, Elebaas RM, Pingleton SH. Use of peak expiratory flow rates to eliminate unnecessary arterial blood gases in acute asthma. *Ann Emerg Med.* 1982;11(2):70–73.

McFadden ER Jr, Lyons HA. Arterial-blood gas tension in asthma. *N Engl J Med.* 1968;278:1027–1032.

National Heart, Lung, and Blood Institute, National Institutes of Health. National Asthma Education and Prevention Program. Expert Panel Report 3 (EPR-3): Guidelines for the Diagnosis and Management of Asthma - Summary Report 2007. Washington DC: USDHHS; 2007.

288

FIGHT THE URGE TO PRESCRIBE ANTIBIOTICS IN ACUTE, UNCOMPLICATED BRONCHITIS

DREW L. FULLER, MD, MPH, FACEP

Acute bronchitis is a common presentation in most emergency departments. It is important to define acute bronchitis in both adult and pediatric populations and to distinguish such cases from acute exacerbations of chronic bronchitis, pneumonia, bronchiolitis, pertussis, or asthma. Acute bronchitis is a clinical term implying the self-limited inflammation of the large airways. It is typically an acute respiratory infection that is manifested by cough and, at times, sputum production that usually lasts for no more than 3 weeks. Occasionally, cough may persist for 4 or more weeks. Uncomplicated acute bronchitis is characterized as being afebrile, with symptoms lasting from 5 to 21 days, and no exposure to pertussis or influenza.

Because of its frequency as well as patient expectation and provider complacency, antibiotics are frequently used for the treatment of acute bronchitis. This is a common error in emergency medicine and primary care. The routine use of antibiotics is not indicated for acute bronchitis. Several reports have shown that up to 65% to 80% of patients inappropriately receive antibiotics for this condition. Inappropriate use is even higher in the elderly and smokers with reports of up to 90% of patients being prescribed antibiotics.

Viruses are usually the cause of acute bronchitis. Respiratory viruses such as influenza A and B, parainfluenza, rhinoviruses, respiratory syncytial virus (RSV), coronavirus, and adenoviruses are often cited as causative agents. While bacteria causing community-acquired pneumonia are occasionally cultured in patients with bronchitis, there is little evidence to support their invasiveness as a cause of symptoms. *Bordetella pertussis, Mycoplasma pneumoniae*, and *Chlamydia pneumoniae* are also rarely implicated but typically have different clinical profiles.

The presence of purulent mucous, which is secondary to epithelial sloughing, and inflammatory cells, is reported by approximately 50% of patients, and it does not change the treatment.

Multiple randomized controlled trials (RCTs), meta-analyses, and a Cochrane Review have all demonstrated that the routine use of antibiotics is not indicated in acute bronchitis. The only benefit, if any, was for an improvement in symptoms by hours. This is generally believed to not be worth the risk in light of the fact that adverse reactions secondary to antibiotics have been reported to be as high as 20% (RR1.22) in these populations.

While it is clear that the use of antibiotics in acute uncomplicated bronchitis is not indicated, other proposed therapies such as bronchodilators, antitussives, mucolytics, and inhaled corticosteroids are worth mentioning. Inhaled β-agonists are not routinely recommended. There is some suggestion that their use may be helpful if there are baseline obstructive symptoms or wheezing; however, the results from multiple RCTs are mixed and the benefit, even with obstruction, is not well supported. Antitussive use is also mixed. Although no clinical trials support the use of antitussives, expert consensus in the 2006 American College of Chest Physicians (ACCP) gave it a grade C recommendation stating, "Antitussive agents are occasionally useful and can be offered for short-term symptomatic relief of coughing." Mucolytics are universally not recommended for use according to the 2006 ACCP guidelines. Inhaled corticosteroid use is also mixed. While there are no clinical trials that support their use and in general, they are not routinely recommended, expert opinion based on clinical practice suggests that the use of mucolytics may be helpful for cough persisting longer than 3 weeks.

In summary, the routine use of antibiotics is not indicated for uncomplicated acute bronchitis.

SUGGESTED READINGS

Braman S. Chronic cough due to acute bronchitis: ACCP evidence-based clinical practice guideline. *Chest*. 2006;129:95–103.

Bent S. Antibiotics in acute bronchitis: A meta-analysis. *Am J Med*. 1999;107:62–67.

Fahey T, Smucny J, Becker L, et al. Antibiotics for acute bronchitis. *Cochrane Database Syst Rev*. 2004;(4):CD000245; doi: 10.1002/14651858.CD000245.pub2.

Gonzales R, Sande MA. Uncomplicated acute bronchitis. *Ann Intern Med*. 2000;133: 981–991.

Linder J, Sim I. Antibiotic treatment of acute bronchitis in smokers. *J Gen Intern Med*. 2002;17:230–234.

Macfarlane J, Holmes W, Gard P, et al. Prospective study of the incidence, aetiology and outcome of adult lower respiratory tract illness in the community. *Thorax*. 2001;56:109–114.

Oeffinger K, Snell L, Foster B, et al. Treatment of acute bronchitis in adults: A national survey of family physicians. *J Fam Pract*. 1998;46:469–475.

Wenzel RP, Fowler AA. Acute bronchitis. *N Eng J Med*. 2006;355:2125–2130.

289

KNOW HOW TO PROPERLY USE A D-DIMER IN THE EVALUATION OF PULMONARY EMBOLISM

JESSE H. KIM, MD

The diagnosis of venous thromboembolism (VTE) has been a challenge for many decades. VTE actually represents two related disease entities, deep venous thrombosis (DVT) and pulmonary embolism (PE). Both occur as a result of thrombus formation. In the case of DVT, red blood cells, fibrin and, to a lesser extent, platelets and leukocytes form a thrombotic mass within an intact vein usually deep within the lower extremity. The cause is not always known, but vascular injury is often considered an inciting culprit. PE results when a thrombus fragment travels and becomes lodged within the pulmonary arteries. More than 70% of all pulmonary emboli originate in the pelvis and deep veins of the lower extremities. There are other areas where thrombosis occurs, including the superior vena cava, upper extremity veins, and the right heart chambers, but they are less common. Making a diagnosis of DVT or PE often relied on complicated testing until recently.

There has been tremendous research in biomarkers for VTE and their role as a diagnostic tool. This has led to the development of the assay for d-dimer, which is a fibrin degradation product, a small protein fragment that results when a thrombus undergoes fibronolysis. The advantages to a serum test are obvious, ease of use, lower cost compared to invasive imaging, and relatively fast lab result time. However, under the surface, there exist far-reaching complexities and problems associated with the sole reliance on D-dimer testing.

First, many variations of D-dimer testing methods exist. Also, equipment from diagnostic lab companies for validation of screening for VTE varies. Some tests, such as ELISA quantitative D-dimers and turbidimetric D-dimer assays, have proven to have high sensitivities, measuring 94% and 93%, respectively, in meta-analysis. Some assays have proven to have lower sensitivity, including Simplify D-dimer assay with reported 80.6% sensitivity. Also, assays differ in their clinical validation data, with some assays having been validated over and over while other types of assays have only scantly appeared in the literature.

As with any assay, D-dimer assays' negative predictive value (NPV) in screening for VTE rests on the pretest probability of the patient being tested. The original extended Wells criteria resulted in PE probability of 3%, 28%, and 78% for low, moderate, and high risks, respectively. The simplified Wells rule resulted in 1.3%, 16.2%, and 40.6% for low, moderate, and high risks, respectively (Wells, 2001). A study of the Geneva rule in assessing pretest probability resulted in 10%, 38%, and 81% pretest probability of PE in low, moderate, and high risks, respectively. Another prediction rule published by Kline also found 13.3% pretest probability of PE and 42.1% in "nonhigh" and "high" categories. When a nonstructured clinical gestalt was used, actual PE probabilities of 9%, 30%, and 68% were obtained when physicians initially categorized the risk as low, moderate, and high, respectively.

The NPV of any given test varies tremendously with the sensitivity of the test being utilized and the prevalence of disease. Given the relatively high sensitivity of some D-dimer assays and low prevalence of PE in low-risk patients, whether by structured rules or by clinical gestalt, d-dimer can be very useful in screening out PE in low-risk patients. Indeed, NPV of 99.5% (CI, 99.1% to 100%) was achieved for PE in Wells low-risk criteria patients with negative d-dimers in Wells (2001) study. In that study, the NPV of D-dimer assay dropped to 88.5% (CI, 69.9% to 97.6%) in high-risk patients.

In summary, given the varying test sensitivities and PE prevalence in different populations, the d-dimer by itself should not be used indiscriminately to rule out PE in any and all populations. The exact type of D-dimer assay being utilized, its sensitivity, and its validation in published literature data need to be known. In addition, the estimated pretest probability of PE, whether by clinical gestalt or by structured clinical scoring systems, should be considered when utilizing the d-dimer in the screening of PE.

SUGGESTED READINGS

Begelman, SM. Venous thromboembolism. In: Cleveland Clinic Center for Continuing Education, eds. *Disease Management*. Available at: http://www.clevelandclinicmeded.com/medicalpubs/diseasemanagement/cardiology/venous-thromboembolism/.

Brown MD, Lau J, Nelson RD, et al. Turbidimetric d-dimer test in the diagnosis of pulmonary embolism: A meta-analysis. *Clin Chem.* 2003;49:1846–1853.

Brown MD, Rowe BH, Reeves MJ, et al. The accuracy of the enzyme-linked immunoabsorbent assay d-dimer test in the diagnosis of pulmonary embolism: A meta-analysis. *Ann Emerg Med.* 2002;40:133–144.

Browse NL, Thomas ML. Source of non-lethal pulmonary emboli. *Lancet.* 1974;1(7851): 258–259.

Kline JA, Nelson AD, Jackson RE, et al. Criteria for the safe use of d-dimer testing in emergency department patients with suspected pulmonary embolism: A multicenter US study. *Ann Emerg Med.* 2002;39:144–152.

Kline JA, Runyon MS, Webb WB, et al. Prospective study of the diagnostic accuracy of the simplify d-dimer assay for pulmonary embolism in emergency department patients. *Chest.* 2006;129:1417–1423.

The PIOPED investigators. Value of the ventilation/perfusion scan in acute pulmonary embolism: Results of the Prospective Investigation of Pulmonary Embolism Diagnosis (PIOPED). *JAMA.* 1990;263:2753–2759.

Wells PS, Anderson D, Rodger M, et al. Excluding pulmonary embolism at the bedside with suspected pulmonary embolism presenting to the emergency department by using a simple clinical model and D-dimer. *Ann Intern Med.* 2001;135:98–107.

Wells PS, Ginsberg JS, Anderson D, et al. Use of a clinical model for safe management of patients with suspected pulmonary embolism. *Ann Intern Med.* 1998;129:997–1005.

Wicki J, Perneger TV, Junod AF, et al. Assessing clinical probability of pulmonary embolism in emergency ward. *Arch Intern Med.* 2001;161:92–97.

290

KNOW THE BASICS OF MANAGING PULMONARY HYPERTENSION IN THE EMERGENCY DEPARTMENT

RANDOLPH N. BROWN, MD

EPIDEMIOLOGY

The incidence of primary pulmonary hypertension has been estimated at 2 cases per million. It is a disease associated with early mortality. Women are affected approximately twice as often as men in adulthood; however, no gender predilection is present in childhood. Most patients are diagnosed in the third or fourth decade of life, with an average of 2.5 years from the onset of symptoms to diagnosis. While primary pulmonary hypertension is relatively uncommon, secondary causes of pulmonary hypertension occur more frequently. Numerous causes of secondary pulmonary hypertension exist, many of which are routinely seen in the emergency department (ED). These causes include COPD and pulmonary emboli. Although most pulmonary emboli completely resolve, approximately 2% of patients with chronic pulmonary emboli may develop pulmonary hypertension.

PATHOPHYSIOLOGY

The pulmonary vasculature is a high-capacity (high distensibility) low-resistance system. Therefore, it is able to tolerate significant rises in pulmonary blood flow with a relatively inconsequential rise in overall pressure. Hence, pulmonary hypertension results from an increase in pulmonary vascular resistance rather than an increase in pulmonary blood flow. When pulmonary vascular resistance is increased, pulmonary alveolar gas exchange is impaired, which causes an increase in pulmonary arterial pressure. When the pulmonary pressure is normal (pulmonary artery pressure <30 mm Hg and mean pressure <20 mm Hg), normal right ventricle output only requires minimal contractile force. In addition, the right ventricle is able to compensate for acute increases in pulmonary pressure generating systolic blood pressure of up to 50 mm Hg without resultant right heart failure. However, when the progression of pulmonary hypertension is more insidious, right ventricle hypertrophy occurs, which may result in right heart failure. The right heart failure that results from pulmonary hypertension may subsequently cause left heart failure. This occurs because the elevated pressure in the right ventricle causes bowing of the interventricular septum which causes a decrease in left ventricle size, compliance, and stroke volume.

DIAGNOSIS

The diagnosis of pulmonary hypertension can be difficult. Echocardiography and the measurement of the right ventricle systolic pressure (RVSP) can provide some indication that pulmonary hypertension exists. Echocardiography is not definitive, but findings of RVSP ≥ 35 mm Hg, especially when accompanied by evidence of right heart pressure overload such as right atrial enlargement, right ventricular enlargement, hypertrophy, or dysfunction, should suggest pulmonary hypertension. The definitive diagnosis of pulmonary hypertension requires a right heart cardiac catheterization, which is beyond the scope of the ED.

While primary pulmonary hypertension is relatively rare, there are many illnesses that cause secondary pulmonary hypertension (*Table 290.1*). Many of these diseases are encountered quite routinely in the ED. These include pulmonary emboli, COPD, sleep apnea, HIV, and cocaine (as well as crack cocaine) use. Regardless of the etiology of pulmonary hypertension, the signs and symptoms are unchanged. These include progressive shortness of breath with activity and fatigue. Hoarseness may occur due to compression of the recurrent laryngeal nerve between the aorta and the dilated pulmonary artery (Ortner syndrome). Progression of the disease causes angina-like chest pain, presyncope, and exertional syncope as a result of decreased myocardial perfusion and left ventricular failure, respectively. A physical exam may reveal an increased jugular venous pressure and reduced carotid pulse. Auscultation of the heart frequently reveals an increased pulmonary component of the second heart sound, a third or fourth heart sound,

---

TABLE 290.1   CAUSES OF PULMONARY HYPERTENSION

Pulmonary artery abnormalities

- Pulmonary embolic disease
- Parenchymal lung disease (COPD, pulmonary fibrosis, etc.)
- Toxic (crack cocaine, L-tryptophan, etc.)
- HIV associated
- Vasculitides (systemic lupus, systemic sclerosis, etc.)
- Primary pulmonary hypertension

Reactive pulmonary vasoconstriction

- Hypoxia (e.g., high altitude)
- Acidosis
- Hypoventilation syndromes (e.g., sleep apnea, neuromuscular disorders)
- Sickle cell (mechanism not well understood)

Elevated pulmonary venous pressure

- Left ventricular failure
- Mitral stenosis
- Mitral regurgitation
- Pulmonary venous thrombosis

Structural heart disease

- Atrial and ventricular septal defects
- Patent ductus arteriosus
- Peripheral arteriovenous shunts

---

or murmurs of tricuspid regurgitation, mitral stenosis, or mitral regurgitation. Chest x-ray usually reveals large pulmonary arteries with clear lung fields. EKG generally shows right axis deviation and right ventricular hypertrophy. Chest CT scan may be valuable in diagnosing some secondary causes of pulmonary hypertension. CT may reveal pulmonary emboli, fibrosis, and bullous emphysema.

TREATMENT

The treatment of pulmonary hypertension regardless of etiology remains the same for the emergency physician. ABCs (airway, breathing, and circulation) remain paramount in all patients, especially for the patient presenting in respiratory distress. This mantra of emergency medicine is indeed essential in the case of both primary and secondary pulmonary hypertension. The institution of supplemental oxygen in patients with pulmonary hypertension may decrease pulmonary pressures and thus improve right ventricular function. This occurs due to a blunting of the hypoxia-induced pulmonary vasoconstriction.

Once the ABCs are stabilized, the emergency physician should then embark on the quest of diagnosing the source of secondary pulmonary hypertension. The classic treatment of pulmonary hypertension includes oxygen, diuretics, and digoxin. However, in some patients with secondary pulmonary hypertension, fluid management may be difficult, because the patient may present with hypovolemia compounding secondary pulmonary hypertension. In such cases, as in the sickle cell patient in vasoocclusive crisis who also suffers from pulmonary hypertension, very gentle fluid administration may be in order as opposed to diuresis. The treatment of secondary pulmonary hypertension is aimed at treating the underlying cause. Hence, obtaining a thorough history and physical exam is very essential. If the patient is incapacitated, obtaining a history from family members and EMS personnel is necessary. In emergency medicine, while the history obtained must be thorough, emphasis should be placed on obtaining a history about imminent life-threatening conditions. For patients with secondary pulmonary hypertension, questions regarding pulmonary emboli risk factors, COPD, and structural heart disease should be explored.

Regarding the treatment of primary pulmonary hypertension, the emergency physician should be aware of the pathophysiology of this disease. This is because given the potential of vascular thrombosis in these patients, many of them are on prescribed chronic anticoagulation therapy. Hence, obtaining a history regarding adherence to treatment and last prothrombin time must be elicited. In addition, a review of the patient's medication regimen may reveal chronic vasodilator therapy, namely, calcium channel blockers, inhaled nitric oxide, phosphodiester inhibitor blocker, and/or continuous intravenous infusion of epoprostenol (prostacyclin). Eliciting this history may imply that the patient responds to or improves with vasodilator therapy. Unfortunately in patients with progressive disease, lung transplantation or heart-lung transplantation may be necessary. In a posttransplantation patient, the emergency physician must work in close consultation with pulmonary medicine and transplant surgery. Nonetheless, the principles previously mentioned for the patient in respiratory distress still pertain.

Pulmonary hypertension is an insidious disease with an early mortality. The principles of management are not overly complex but they must be addressed, which include supplemental oxygen, judicious diuresis when appropriate, and treatment of the underlying disease in secondary pulmonary hypertension. In primary pulmonary hypertension, the treatment must involve a careful review of recent anticoagulation therapy and consideration of the various vasodilator therapies.

SUGGESTED READINGS

Benedict N, Seybert A, Mathier MA. Evidence-based pharmacologic management of pulmonary arterial hypertension. *Clin Ther*. 2007;29(10):2134–2153.

Leuchte HH, Schwaiblmair M, Baumgartner RA, et al. Hemodynamic response to sildenafil, nitric oxide, and iloprost in primary pulmonary hypertension. *Chest*. 2004;125:580–586.

Lykouras D, Sampsonas F, Kaparianos A, et al. Pulmonary arterial hypertension: Need to treat. *Inflamm Allergy Drug Targets*. 2008;7(4):260–269.

Vichinsky EP. Pulmonary hypertension in sickle cell disease. *N Engl J Med*. 2004;350(9): 857–859.

291

KNOW THE CAUSES AND MANAGEMENT OF HEMOPTYSIS WELL

SHANNON B. PUTMAN, MD

Hemoptysis, coughing up of blood from the lower respiratory tract, can range from scant blood-streaked sputum to frank blood in large volumes. Massive hemoptysis refers to life-threatening amounts of blood loss ranging from 100 to 600 mL over a 24-h period. In the emergency department, it is critical to quickly identify whether your patient qualifies as having massive hemoptysis both because it may be a sign of a serious underlying illness and because the bleeding itself may be life threatening due to aspiration and asphyxiation. Although only 5% of patients with hemoptysis qualify as being massive, it carries a mortality rate of up to 80%. The management of hemoptysis is complex due to a broad differential diagnosis with bleeding capable of being localized to the airway, the pulmonary parenchyma, or the pulmonary vasculature. Further, bleeding may be unpredictable, and there is no consensus regarding the optimal management in a patient presenting with hemoptysis.

One of the most important initial triage steps in evaluating a patient with hemoptysis is confirming that the blood is coming from the lower airway (below the vocal cords) and not the upper airway or gastrointestinal tract. This may be difficult, if not impossible, in the emergency setting, sometimes requiring both gastroenterology and otolaryngology evaluations. Although blood from the lungs can be swallowed and gastrointestinal blood can be aspirated, generally the presence of an alkaline pH, foamy appearance, and the presence of pus are most suggestive of lungs as being the source of bleeding.

Pulmonary arteries and bronchial arteries make up the arterial vasculature of the lungs. The pulmonary arteries deliver the majority of right-sided cardiac output at low pressure during the delivery of blood to the pulmonary capillary bed for oxygenation. The bronchial arteries, on the other hand, are under much higher pressure but receive much less of the cardiac output. Each lung typically has one or two bronchial arteries, arising from either the aorta or the intercostal arteries. They function to provide nutrients and oxygen to the airways, visceral pleura, and mediastinum. Although the bronchial arteries carry much less blood through the lungs, they are more likely to be the source of hemoptysis due to their systemic pressure and location along the airways, the most common site of bleeding.

The most common causes of hemoptysis from the airway include the "three B's"—bronchitis, bronchiectasis, and bronchogenic carcinoma. Other causes include metastatic lung disease, Kaposi sarcoma, foreign body, trauma, and fistulas between the aorta and the airway. Thoracic aortic aneurysms, in particular, may be associated with life-threatening fistulas with the left bronchopulmonary tree. Dieulafoy lesion, a subepithelial bronchial artery traversing the bronchial mucosa, may be a rare cause of hemoptysis. Pulmonary parenchymal diseases associated with bleeding include infections, autoimmune diseases, coagulopathies, and iatrogenic injuries during a procedure. Infections that are most likely to be associated with hemoptysis include tuberculosis, lung abscess, and aspergilloma. Inflammatory or autoimmune diseases typically associated with pulmonary hemorrhage include Goodpasture syndrome, Wegener granulomatosis, lupus pneumonitis, and pulmonary hemosiderosis. Other less common causes of hemoptysis from the parenchyma are cocaine-induced hemorrhage and catamenial hemoptysis secondary to intrathoracic endometriosis. Pulmonary vascular lesions associated with hemoptysis include pulmonary embolism, pulmonary arteriovenous malformations, and elevated pulmonary capillary pressure seen with severe left ventricular dysfunction. Up to one third of patients have no identifiable bleeding site despite extensive workup. Generally, the prognosis is good for this group of patients, but one series found that 7 out of 115 patients were diagnosed with lung cancer over a mean follow-up of 6.6 years. Other studies have identified a higher percentage of these patients with Dieulafoy lesion, ultimately identified during emergency surgery for massive hemoptysis.

When a patient presents to the emergency department for an evaluation of hemoptysis, a detailed history and physical exam can help narrow the differential diagnosis. Information about chronicity, associated symptoms, and disease risk factors are key elements in the history. Pulse oximetry and arterial blood gas analysis give important information regarding oxygenation. A complete blood count, coagulation profile, renal function, and urinalysis also supply valuable information about the severity of bleeding and the identification of associated illnesses, such as coagulopathy, thrombocytopenia, and pulmonary renal syndromes. A type and screen should be done for patients with large amounts of blood loss who may need transfusion.

One of the most valuable initial studies is a chest radiograph, allowing the visualization of any underlying lung pathology, such as a mass or an infection. Sputum analysis for Gram stain and cytology can be useful, particularly in patients with abnormal chest films. High-resolution chest CT and flexible bronchoscopy are very important in the evaluation of a patient with hemoptysis and a normal chest film. Although the likelihood of identifying a lung cancer by bronchoscopy in the setting of a normal chest film is <5%, its yield may be higher in patients at risk for lung cancer. This includes men older than 40 years of age with a history of smoking more than 40 packs a year and a history of hemoptysis for more than 1 week.

Flexible bronchoscopy performed within 48 h of presentation is more likely to identify either active bleeding or the site of bleeding as compared with delayed bronchoscopy. High-resolution chest CT is most useful in evaluating patients at lower risk for malignancy and is particularly useful for identifying bronchiectasis, arteriovenous malformation, pulmonary embolism, and atypical infections such as aspergilloma. Chest CT may not detect subtle mucosal lesions seen with bronchitis and Kaposi sarcoma. Patients without concerning risk factors, normal labs, a normal chest radiograph, and minimal amounts of hemoptysis may be empirically treated for bronchitis and followed up closely to monitor for resolution.

The acute management of patients with massive hemoptysis includes airway protection, adequate ventilation, and maintenance of cardiovascular function. Patients with severe dyspnea, poor gas exchange, rapid blood loss, and hemodynamic compromise should be intubated urgently with a large-bore endotracheal tube. Protection of the nonbleeding lung is critical as contamination of blood can block the airway with clot or fill the alveoli, preventing adequate gas exchange. If the location of bleeding is identified, placing the patient in the lateral decubitus position with the bleeding lung in a dependent position may be useful. For patients with rapid blood loss who are at risk for exsanguination, a double-lumen endotracheal tube can be placed to allow for selective intubation of either the right or the left main stem bronchus in order to adequately ventilate the nonbleeding lung and block the flow of blood from the bleeding side. Bronchoscopy may be used acutely both to identify the site of hemorrhage and to slow or stop the bleeding with balloon tamponade, application of topical epinephrine, or iced saline lavage. None of these methods have been tested in controlled trials, and results are dependent on local expertise. Another option for patients with ongoing bleeding is arteriographic embolization which successfully stops the bleeding 85% of the time. Unfortunately, rebleeding may occur in 10% to 20% of patients over the next 6 to 12 months due to incomplete embolization, revascularization, or recanalization. Patients with uncontrolled bleeding unresponsive to less invasive procedures should be considered for surgical intervention. Surgical mortality for patients with massive hemoptysis requiring emergent surgery is up to 20%. Relative contraindications for surgery include severe underlying lung disease (including cystic fibrosis, multiple arteriovenous malformations, diffuse bronchiectasis, and severe emphysema), active tuberculosis, and diffuse alveolar hemorrhage.

In summary, patients presenting with hemoptysis should quickly be triaged as having massive or nonmassive bleeding. A broad differential should be entertained and adequate oxygenation should be maintained at all times. For both massive and nonmassive bleeding, the airway is the most common site with the most common causes being bronchitis, bronchiectasis, and bronchogenic carcinoma.

SUGGESTED READINGS

Adelman M, Haponi EF, Bleecker ER, et al. Cryptogenic hemoptysis: Clinical features, bronchoscopic findings, and natural history in 67 patients. *Ann Intern Med.* 1985;102:829.

Cahill BC, Ingbar DH. Massive hemoptysis: Assessment and management. *Clin Chest Med.* 1994;15:147.

Heimer D, Bar-ziv J, Scharf SM. Fiberoptic bronchoscopy in patients with hemoptysis and nonlocalizing chest roentgenograms. *Arch Intern Med.* 1985;145:1427.

Herth F, Ernst A, Becker HD. Long-term outcome and lung cancer incidence in patients with hemoptysis of unknown origin. *Chest.* 2001;120:1592.

Johnston H, Reisz G. Changing spectrum of hemoptysis: Underlying causes in 148 patients undergoing diagnostic flexible bronchoscopy. *Arch Intern Med.* 1989;149:1666.

Lederle FA, Nichol KL, Parenti CM. Bronchoscopy to evaluate hemoptysis in older men with nonsuspicious chest roentgenograms. *Chest.* 1989;95:1043.

Savale L, Parrott A, Khalil A, et al. Cryptogenic hemoptysis: From a benign to a life-threatening pathologic vascular lesion. *Am J Respir Crit Care Med.* 2007;175:1181.

Swanson KL, Johnson CM, Praash UB, et al. Bronchial artery embolization: Experience with 54 patients. *Chest.* 2002;121:789.

292

KNOW WHEN YOU NEED TO TAPER STEROIDS ... AND WHEN YOU DO NOT NEED TO

MUSTAPHA SAHEED, MD

In 1898, Sir William Osler successfully employed adrenal cell extracts in the treatment of a patient with Addison disease. Fifty years later, the first synthetic steroids were created. Since then, our understanding of the role of steroids in the regulation of multiple body systems has expanded, as well as its use in the management of different pathological processes. This rapid growth in the clinical utility of steroid therapy has also been associated with the discovery of varied harmful side effects.

Specifically, the constellation of adverse findings is collectively termed Cushing syndrome, which includes classically described features such as central obesity, buffalo hump, moon facies, extremity wasting, and abdominal striae. Fortuitously, many of these symptoms resolve with the cessation of steroid therapy. However, the abrupt cessation of steroid therapy may also result in significant adverse effects, the most severe being the precipitation of adrenal crises. These adverse effects are broadly caused by three general processes: worsening of underlying disease process, steroid withdrawal syndrome, or adrenal insufficiency.

Clearly, when steroid therapy is terminated, there may be a risk of recurrence of chronic underlying process. While it may seem intuitive, some processes treated by steroids may present initially with vague nonspecific signs or symptoms. As such, clinicians should have a high index of suspicion and must be aware of subtle signs that may indicate a worsening underlying pathological process and the possible need for early diagnostic testing.

Steroid withdrawal syndrome is a rare diagnosis that may result from the abrupt cessation of steroids. The disease is characterized by multiple vague symptoms including "weakness, fatigue, nausea, arthralgias, and dizziness" that are often initially attributed to adrenal insufficiency or crises. However, these patients, on testing, have normal hypothalamic–pituitary–adrenal (HPA) axis function. As such, the symptomatology represents a distinct clinical entity from adrenal-mediated pathology.

The etiology of steroid withdrawal syndrome is unclear but is postulated to be related to cytokine release and possibly a proinflammatory state. It has been observed that nonsteroidal anti-inflammatory agents may provide some relief from symptoms. Moreover, the use of a very slow taper may be required to prevent recurrent symptoms. And while there is no clear literature to guide the specific taper regimen, clinical experience suggests that the taper must be completed in a manner that reduces steroid therapy without eliciting clinical symptoms.

Adrenal insufficiency is most commonly associated with the abrupt cessation of steroid therapy. The HPA axis is responsible for the steady-state regulation of endogenous steroids production. The system employs complex feedback mechanisms to maintain adequate steroid production. Exogenous steroids suppress the endogenous production from the adrenal glands through interactions with the pituitary-hypothalamic axis. Furthermore, this complex interaction may also result in adrenal gland atrophy. Adrenal crisis, a life-threatening illness of severe systemic steroid deficiency generally precipitated by stressors, is more likely to occur in patients with HPA axis suppression that directly involves the adrenal gland.

Notably, even patients with short-term usage of exogenous steroids, as little as 20 to 30 mg of prednisone or equivalency daily for >5 days, may have HPA axis suppression and adrenal insufficiency. Common symptoms of adrenal insufficiency include weakness and fatigability, anorexia, nausea, vomiting, and orthostatic hypotension. Additionally, some patients may have subclinical adrenal insufficiency. These patients have adrenal insufficiency by ACTH testing but are asymptomatic. Some of these patients may respond to stressors such as surgery or infection, with adrenal crises, and may represent a clinical challenge for the unsuspecting provider.

On the other hand, while short courses of steroid therapy may have some effect on the HPA axis, clinically significant axis suppression rarely occurs in steroid treatments for <1 to 2 weeks. Patients receiving these short bursts generally do not develop significant adrenal insufficiency or have catastrophic response to stressors and tend to have a rapid rebound in the HPA axis within 2 to 5 days. Furthermore, the considerable clinical experience and data, especially in the treatment of asthmatic patients, reinforce the principle that short courses (<1 to 2 weeks) of steroid therapy are low risk for clinically significant adrenal suppression.

In patients who do receive a longer steroid regimen, it is appropriate to taper their steroid regimen slowly to reduce the risk of adrenal suppression. Also, patients who receive multiple steroid bursts, without an appropriate rebound of the HPA axis in between, may also require a taper. However, there is a paucity of data defining the optimal method for the taper. Generally, steroids are tapered until there is a reduction to replacement physiologic doses (around 5 mg per day) from supratherapeutic anti-inflammatory doses. If the patient remains asymptomatic, the taper can then be continued until cessation. Patients should be advised that they may become symptomatic after stressful physiologic events and may require further steroid therapy for up to 1 year after the taper is completed.

In short, while steroid therapy has provided a potent tool in the treatment of multiple disease processes, there are significant side effects. Notably, concern about steroid cessation and associated complications—including adrenal insufficiency—may have contributed to the belief that steroid therapy should always be tapered. However, patients receiving <1 to 2 week course of steroid generally do not require a taper. As many patients are on chronic steroids and/ or receive repetitive steroid doses for chronic conditions, clinicians should continue to have a high index of suspicion for adrenal suppression and associated complications in these patients.

SUGGESTED READINGS

Cydulka RK, Emerman CL. A pilot study of steroid therapy after emergency department treatment of acute asthma: Is a taper needed? *J Emerg Med*. 1998;16(1):15–19.

Jones AM, Munavvar M, Vail A, et al. Prospective, placebo-controlled trial of 5 vs 10 days of oral prednisolone in acute adult asthma. *Respir Med*. 2002;96(11):950–954.

Karan RS, Pandhi P, Behera D, et al. A comparison of non-tapering vs. tapering prednisolone in acute exacerbation of asthma involving use of the low-dose ACTH test. *Int J Clin Pharmacol Ther*. 2002;40(6):256–262.

Krasner A. Glucocorticoid-induced adrenal insufficiency. *JAMA*. 1999;282:671–676.

Kountz DS, Clark CL. Safely withdrawing patients from chronic glucocorticoid therapy. *Am Fam Physician*. 1997;55:521–525.

Lederle FA, Pluhar RE, Joseph AM, et al. Tapering of corticosteroid therapy following exacerbation of asthma. A randomized, double-blind, placebo-controlled trial. *Arch Intern Med*. 1987;147(12):2201–2203.

Marx JA, Hockberger RS, Walls RM, eds. *Rosen's Emergency Medicine: Concepts and Clinical Practice.*, 6th ed. St. Louis, MO: Mosby Inc.; 2006.

Streck WF, Lockwood DH. Pituitary adrenal recovery following short-term suppression with corticosteroids. *Am J Med*. 1979;66:910–914.

Torrey SP. Recognition and management of adrenal emergencies. *Emerg Med Clin N Am*. 2005;23(3):687–702, viii.

Welbourn RB. The emergence of endocrinology. *Gesnerus*. 1992;(49 pt 2):137–150.

293

PNEUMOTHORAX: TO TUBE OR NOT TO TUBE

EVELINE A. HITTI, MD

There are few randomized clinical trials evaluating the different treatment modalities for pneumothoraces. Given the lack of comprehensive studies, optimal management strategies are still evolving. Pneumothoraces can be classified as spontaneous, traumatic, or iatrogenic. The physiology depends on the underlying cause as do the surgical management options and reoccurrence prognosis. Regardless of the underlying cause, the central initial management decision in the emergency department (ED) is the same: should a chest tube be placed? Closed-tube thoracostomy carries the risk of organ injury, infection, empyema, and extended hospitalization. Thus, understanding the indications for closed-tube thoracostomy is essential to the management of patients presenting to the ED with a pneumothorax.

Spontaneous pneumothorax occurs in individuals without any preceding trauma or injury and affects >20,000 patients per year in the United States. This type of pneumothorax is further subdivided into primary spontaneous, when there is no known underlying lung disease, and secondary spontaneous, when there is underlying parenchymal disease. In 2001, the American College of Chest Surgeons developed practice guidelines for the management of spontaneous pneumothorax based on existing evidence as well as expert opinion which was thought to be necessary given the lack of high-quality randomized clinical studies. In these guidelines, the key elements were pneumothorax size and patient clinical stability. The size was classified as small or large with small being any pneumothorax with an apex-to-cupola distance <3 cm. Clinical stability was defined as the presence of respiratory rate <24 breaths per min, heart rate >60 and < 120 beats per min, room air oxygen saturation >90%, and a patient's ability to speak in whole sentences between breaths. Any patient not fulfilling the definition of stable was classified as clinically unstable. There was "very good consensus" on placing chest tubes in any patient who was either clinically unstable or who had a large pneumothorax irrespective of clinical stability.

Traumatic pneumothoraces are those caused by either blunt or penetrating chest trauma resulting in alveolar rupture. Up to 20% of patients with chest trauma or multitrauma have an associated hemothorax. Traumatic pneumothoraces should, in general, be treated with large-bore (28°F to 36°F) chest tube placement with few exceptions. There is some evidence that small pneumothoraces in hemodynamically stable patients may be observed. In addition, occult pneumothoraces detected on CT scanning but not on initial screening chest radiograph may be treated by observation alone. The need for mechanical ventilation, however, precludes this option even in the presence of occult pneumothorax as it is associated with 38% progression of pneumothorax necessitating chest tube placement with more severe complications than immediate closed-tube thoracostomy. In these cases, as well as in cases with an associated hemothorax, a large-bore chest tube should be placed.

Iatrogenic pneumothorax generally occurs as a complication of inadvertent transthoracic needle biopsy. This type of pneumothorax is usually preceded by central venous catheter insertion, thoracentesis, transbronchial lung biopsy, pleural biopsy, or positive-pressure ventilation. Here again, large, symptomatic iatrogenic pneumothoraces and the need for mechanical ventilation are indications for closed-tube thoracostomy. Small and asymptomatic iatrogenic pneumothoraces may be treated conservatively with observation for progression. An exception to this is patients who have underlying emphysema. The significantly greater need for chest tubes after sustaining iatrogenic pneumothoraces in this population supports the placement of drainage catheter over observation in emphysematous patients.

No matter what the underlying etiology, any patient with tension pneumothorax—that is, complete collapse of the lung with disruption of venous return—requires immediate chest tube placement. Furthermore, any patient presenting with simultaneous bilateral pneumothoraces, regardless of the underlying cause, requires chest tube placement because of the high risk of progression to tension pneumothorax.

Patients often present to the ED with spontaneous, traumatic, or iatrogenic pneumothorax. Understanding the indication for closed-tube thoracostomy in treating these patients is essential as this procedure carries significant morbidity and mortality risks. These indications include any large pneumothorax, any clinically unstable patient regardless of pneumothorax size, tension pneumothorax, bilateral simultaneous pneumothorax, any pneumothorax with associated hemothorax, any patient requiring ventilator support, and any iatrogenic pneumothorax in a patient with underlying emphysema.

SUGGESTED READINGS

Baumann M. Pneumothorax. *Semin Respir Crit Care Med.* 2001;22(6):647–655.

Baumann M, Strange C, Light R, et al. Management of spontaneous pneumothorax. *Chest.* 2001;119:590–602.

Enderson B, Abdalla R, Frame S, et al. Tube thoracostomy for occult pneumothorax: A prospective randomized study of its use. *J Trauma.* 1993;35:726–730.

Jenner R, Sen A. Chest drains in traumatic occult pneumothorax. *Emerg Med J.* 2006;23: 138–139.

Millikan S, Moore E, Steiner E, et al. Complications of tube thoracostomy for acute trauma. *Am J Surg.* 1980;140:738–741.

Noppen M, Keukeleire T. Pneumothorax. *Respiration.* 2008;76(2):121–127.

Sayar A, Turna A, Metin M, et al. Simultaneous bilateral pneumothorax report of 12 cases and review of the literature. *Acata Chir Belg.* 2004;104:572–576.

Symington L, McGugan E. BET1: Is a chest drain necessary in stable patients with traumatic pneumothorax? *Emerg Med J.* 2008;25:439–440.

294

REMEMBER THAT ALL THAT WHEEZES IS NOT NECESSARILY ASTHMA (OR CHRONIC OBSTRUCTIVE PULMONARY DISEASE)

MELISSA W. COSTELLO, MD, FACEP

Asthma and chronic obstructive pulmonary disease (COPD) are commonly encountered in the emergency department (ED). Both conditions are a frequent cause of wheezing in the ED and can lull physicians into believing that all wheezing is attributed to these two conditions. It is important for the clinician to remember that there are literally dozens of causes of wheezing. In the most general of terms, wheezing can result from anything that causes narrowing of the small airways: injury, infection, inflammation, and irritation. Rather than simply generating a laundry list of the important differential diagnoses for wheezing, this section will review the important history and physical exam elements to differentiate the symptoms of asthma and COPD from the other, less common causes.

AGE

The age of the patient can be an important factor in the determination of the underlying cause of wheezing. Consider newborns and infants; they can develop wheezing from things such as recurrent aspiration during feeding, respiratory syncytial virus (RSV) bronchiolitis, and congenital heart defects. These causes are much less common in older children and adults. Although asthma has become the most common chronic disease of childhood in the industrialized world, children can wheeze from other conditions such as foreign body aspiration, known or previously undiagnosed cystic fibrosis, and reflux disease. For adults, while asthma and COPD certainly head the list of wheezing causes, other causes such as masses, interstitial lung diseases, and cardiac problems can also present with wheezing.

HISTORY

A thorough history should include questions about onset, duration, and timing (i.e., symptoms that only occur in the morning, only at work or school, etc.), progression or changes, sick contacts or other exposures (smoke, allergens, new medications, chemicals, etc.), family history, and psychosocial stressors. This level of detailed history taking is often much more realistic in the primary care setting rather than in a busy ED or in managing a patient in extremis. In the ED, this history is often covered in a quick "Is this the same as it always has been?" format. When the answer is "yes," the physician can continue down an abbreviated algorithm. When the answer is either "no" or "I've never had this before," this should give the emergency physician (EP) a pause, and a much more detailed history is warranted.

PHYSICAL EXAM

It goes without saying that a wheezing patient should have a lung exam. Close attention should be paid to asymmetric findings, particularly in children or whenever the patient has a fever. The clinician should be careful to discriminate between wheezing and other respiratory sounds such as rales (small clicking, bubbling, or rattling sounds in the lung), rhonchi (resemble snoring, occur when air movement is blocked or becomes rough through the large airways), and stridor (wheeze-like sound heard on exhalation, usually due to an obstruction of airflow in the upper airway). The distressed patient with quiet lungs should be of particular concern as this indicates a reduction of airflow to <20% of normal; in other words, so little air is moving that no sound can be generated. A patient who appears to have some respiratory compromise but quiet lung fields is at high risk and should be very closely monitored with the consideration of impending respiratory failure.

The cardiovascular exam should be performed with an eye and ear tuned to detect extra heart sounds or murmurs, muffled heart sounds, jugular venous distention, or peripheral edema in order to not miss the signs and symptoms of new or progressing congestive heart failure causing cardiac asthma. Such a careful examination should not be relegated to adults, because a similar cardiac asthma presentation can occur in infants with congenital defects. The remainder of the general physical exam can be performed quickly with attention paid to the presence or absence of rashes, neck swelling or masses, clubbing digits, and extremity tenderness or swelling.

LAB/RADIOLOGY

Very little is added to the diagnosis of wheezing with the addition of lab testing. Arterial or venous blood gas (ABG or VBG) can help to guide the management of the fatiguing or failing patient but do very little to contribute to narrowing a differential for the wheezing patient. Additionally, most experienced EPs make decisions regarding ventilatory assistance in wheezing patients on a purely clinical basis and forgo blood gases in the initial management phase. Although ABGs/VBGs may be useful in the longitudinal evaluation, in the acute setting, they offer only minor diagnostic support. A complete blood count will help confirm a clinical exam that points to anemia. Leukocytosis, a common finding, can point to infection or simply can be the result of stress demargination or steroid response and thus tends to offer little diagnostic help. Although other lab tests, cardiac enzyme profiles, and B-naturetic peptide levels may help to confirm a diagnosis of cardiac asthma or respiratory failure, these tests should certainly not be ordered on every wheezing patient. Radiography can help direct the physician's workup, particularly in a first-time wheezer. In children with asymmetric clinical findings, unilateral hyperinflation or infiltrate can be very helpful in pointing to a foreign body aspiration or pneumonia. In adults, a chest radiograph (with or without soft tissue neck radiographs, depending on the clinical picture) can help in the diagnosis of congestive failure, infiltrates, pneumothorax, or large compressive mass. Thus, the chest roentgenogram can help guide the next steps in management. Electrocardiogram (ECG) may also give the EP clues when the clinical picture points to cardiac disease or pulmonary embolism as a cause of wheezing with the caveat that the answer rarely lies in the ECG alone.

In summary, wheezing is a symptom that most EPs will see on a daily basis, and the majority will often be due to the two most common causes: asthma and COPD. A methodical approach to those patients who fall outside the "typical asthma/COPD flare" group will prevent missed diagnoses and allow the EP to more quickly guide the clinical care of these patients. Asking patients if their symptoms are new or different can be helpful in determining the etiology of the wheezing. All that wheezes is not asthma (or COPD) (*Table 294.1*).

TABLE 294.1	BRIEF DIFFERENTIAL DIAGNOSIS FOR WHEEZING
Pediatric	Asthma, bronchiolitis, bronchopulmonary dysplasia, recurrent aspiration, infection, reflux disease, congenital heart disease, foreign body aspiration, cystic fibrosis, tracheoesophageal fistula, sinusitis, immotile cilia, mediastinal mass
Adults	Asthma, COPD, chronic bronchitis, angioedema, foreign body, extrinsic compression of the airways (thyroid, tumors, hematoma, abscess), vocal cord dysfunction, chemical irritants, medication reaction, pneumonia, pulmonary edema, carcinoid syndrome, pulmonary embolism, tracheomalacia, postlobectomy bronchial torsion, interstitial lung disease

SUGGESTED READINGS

Bent T. Wheezing. In: *The 10-Minute Diagnosis Manual: Symptoms and Signs in the Time-Limited Encounter.* Philadelphia, PA: Lippincott Williams & Wilkins; 2000. Available at: http://www.wrongdiagnosis.com/w/wheezing/book-diseases-10b.htm. Accessed November 2008.

Epstein SK. Wheezing. In: Rosen P, Barkin RM, Hayden SR, et al., eds. *Rosen and Barkin's 5 Minute Emergency Medicine Consult.* Philadelphia, PA: Lippincott Williams & Wilkins; 2007.

Kreiger BP. When wheezing may not mean asthma. Other common and uncommon causes to consider. *Postgrad Med.* 2002;112(2):101–111.

[No author noted]. Wheeze. Available at http://en.wikipedia.org/wiki/Wheeze. Accessed November 2008.

295

UNDERSTAND PROPER VENTILATORY MANAGEMENT IN PATIENTS WITH ASTHMA

TINA M. LATIMER, MD, MPH

Acute asthma exacerbations are on the rise. As the prevalence of asthma increases in the general population, so does the risk of an emergency medicine (EM) physician being faced with an asthmatic needing emergency airway management. With 10% of individuals admitted for asthma needing to go to the ICU and 2% of those admitted requiring intubation, airway management and ventilator management are essential competencies in EM. Fraught with pitfalls that can lead to worsening respiratory status, ventilator-induced lung injury, and even death, this chapter focuses on reducing the complications of severe gas trapping.

Asthma produces a combination of bronchoconstriction, airway edema, and mucous plugging. The airway resistance that these processes produce creates both an inward and an outward flow problem that disrupts the ventilation that occurs during normal spontaneous negative-pressure breathing. The end product of the disruption in ventilation is gas trapping. Gas trapping occurs when ventilatory flow cannot overcome the frictional resistance in the airways needed to empty to the alveoli. Coupled with an asthmatic's inability to fully exhale before the next breath (low expiratory flow rates mandate longer expiratory time), hyperinflation of the lungs ensues. This leads the lungs and chest wall to operate on the suboptimal portion of the pressure-volume curve and an increase in auto-positive end-expiratory pressure (PEEP).

The decision to intervene with noninvasive or invasive mechanical ventilation is made after medical therapy (oxygen, inhaled beta agonists, inhaled ipratropium bromide, steroids, IV magnesium sulfate, etc.) has been optimized. A physician should consider noninvasive positive-pressure ventilation in the setting of acute hypercapnic and hypoxemic insufficiency. Noninvasive positive-pressure ventilation uses a nasal or face mask to deliver mechanical breaths without airway invasion. While there are only two prospective, randomized studies using noninvasive positive-pressure ventilation in asthma, both show improved lung function and reduced need for hospitalization. All other prospective, randomized studies done in patients with COPD collectively show a reduced need for endotracheal intubation, reduced in-hospital mortality rates, and improved long-term survival. Nonetheless, there are clinical cases where invasive ventilation via intubation is the only appropriate next step in managing an asthmatic's worsening respiratory failure.

Multiple prospective studies have demonstrated that early failed response to noninvasive positive-pressure ventilation is predictive of the need for intubation and invasive mechanical ventilation. A prospective study that included 1,033 patients with COPD exacerbation found the following to predict the risk of failure >70% on admission:

- A Glasgow Coma Score < 11
- A pH < 7.25
- A respiratory rate ≥ 30 bpm

Even with strong predictors of failure of noninvasive positive-pressure ventilation, there has been no study that shows any single objective value (pH, pCO_2, PaO_2, etc.) that indicates the need for mechanical ventilation. Ultimately, the decision to intubate is a clinical one. Intubation decisions should be based on a patient's lack of improvement, including increased fatigue, decreasing mental status, and hemodynamic status.

Once the decision is made to intubate, optimizing mechanical ventilation is necessary to help reverse the gas trapping that has occurred during the acute asthma exacerbation. Without proper ventilation, gas trapping continues and leads to lung hyperinflation and barotrauma known as ventilator-induced lung injury. Hypotension and refractory respiratory acidosis can also result if the ventilator is not used properly. The most effective way to reduce the worsening effects of lung hyperinflation is to reduce minute ventilation. Minute ventilation is the product of tidal volume and respiratory rate per minute (MV = TV × RR). Minute volume can be reduced a number of ways, including

- *Decrease of tidal volume:* Use tidal volume of 6 mL/kg predicted body weight and can increase to 8 to 10 mL/kg as long as plateau pressure remains <30 cm H_2O. If plateau pressure is >30 cm H_2O at 6 mL/kg, decrease the tidal volume to 4 to 5 mL/kg.

- *Decrease of respiratory rate*: A rate of 6 to 8 breaths per min allows longer expiration times and reduces alveolar overdistention.
- *Shortened inspiratory time*: It allows longer expiratory time to correct hyperinflation. Evidence of this working is a reduction in plateau pressure.

Adjusting these variables reduces minute ventilation, decreases hyperinflation, and leads to alveolar hypoventilation and hypercapnia. This permissive hypercapnic ventilation results in a well-tolerated acidosis. While there is no evidence that points to what the exact safe level of hypercapnia is, a pH ≥ 7.2 or $PaCO_2$ < 90 mm Hg is used as a parameter during ventilator management. Excess CO_2 production should be limited by controlling fever and pain and by providing adequate sedation. It should be noted that the resulting alveolar hypoventilation and decrease in minute ventilation have the potential for lowering serum oxygenation. For this reason, supplemental oxygenation should be used.

Just as important as reduced minute ventilation is the reduction of expiratory flow resistance. Use the largest endotracheal tube appropriate for the patient to minimize airflow resistance. Bronchodilators should be added to the ventilatory circuit to help reduce airway constriction. Steroid therapy will decrease the inflammatory component of asthma and help reduce airway edema. Suctioning will help to reduce airway secretions. Lastly, PEEP of 5 to 10 cm H_2O should be employed to help splint airways open by counteracting the auto-PEEP that occurs with dynamic hyperinflation.

SUGGESTED READINGS

The Acute Respiratory Distress Syndrome Network. Ventilation with lower tidal volumes as compared with traditional tidal volumes for acute lung injury and the acute respiratory distress syndrome. *N Eng J Med*. 2000;342(18):1301–1308.

Amato M, Barbas C, Medeiros D, et al. Effect of a protective-ventilation strategy on mortality in the acute respiratory distress syndrome. *N Engl J Med*. 1998;338(6):347–354.

Anton A, Guell R, Gomez J, et al. Predicting the result of noninvasive ventilation in severe acute exacerbations of patients with chronic airflow limitation. *Chest*. 2000;117(3): 828–833.

Antonelli M, Conti G, Rocco M, et al. A comparison of non-invasive positive pressure ventilation and conventional mechanical ventilation in patients with acute respiratory failure. *N Engl J Med*. 1998;339:429–435.

Antonelli M, Conti G, Moro M, et al. Predictors of failure of noninvasive positive pressure ventilation in patients with acute hypoxemic respiratory failure: A multi-center study. *Intensive Care Med*. 2001;27(11):1718–1728.

Bellomo R, McLaughlin P, Tai E, et al. Asthma requiring mechanical ventilation. A low morbidity approach. *Chest*. 1994;105:891–896.

Bott J, Carroll MP, Conway JH, et al. Randomized, control trial of nasal ventilation in acute ventilatory failure due to chronic obstructive pulmonary disease. *Lancet*. 1993;341: 1555–1557.

Brochard L, Mancebo J, Wysocki M, et al. Non-invasive ventilation for acute exacerbations of chronic obstructive pulmonary disease. *N Eng J Med*. 1995;333:817–822.

Caramez M, Borges J, Mauro R. Paradoxical responses to positive end-expiratory pressure in patients with airway obstruction during controlled ventilation. *Crit Care Med*. 2005;33(7):1519–1528.

Confalonieri M, Garuti G, Cattaruzza M, et al. A chart of failure risk for noninvasive ventilation in severe acute exacerbations of patients with chronic obstructive disease. *Eur Respir J.* 2005;25(2)348–355.

Darioli R, Perret C. Mechanical controlled hypoventilation in status asthmaticus. *Am Rev Respir Dis.* 1984;129:385–387.

Keenan S, Sinuff T, Cook D, et al. Which patients with acute exacerbation of chronic obstructive pulmonary disease benefit from noninvasive positive-pressure ventilation? A systematic review of the literature. *Ann Intern Med.* 2003;138(11):861–870.

Kondili E, Prinianakis G, Georgopoulos D. Patient-ventilator interaction. *Br J Anaesth.* 2003;91(1):106–119.

Kramer N, Meyer TJ, Meharg J, et al. Randomized, prospective trial of non-invasive positive pressure ventilation in acute respiratory failure. *Am J Respir Crit Care Med.* 1995;151: 1799–1806.

Levy BD, Kitch B, Fanta CH. Medical and ventilatory management of status asthmaticus. *Intensive Care Med.* 1998;24:105–117.

Martin T, Hovis J, Costantino J, et al. A randomized, prospective evaluation of non-invasive ventilation of acute respiratory failure. *Am J Resp Crit Care Med.* 2000;161:807–813.

Meduri G, Cook T, Turner R, et al. Noninvasive positive pressure ventilation in status asthmaticus. *Chest.* 1996;110(3):767–774.

Pendergraft T, Sanford R, Beasley R, et al. Rates and characteristics of intensive care unit admissions and intubations among asthma-related hospitalizations. *Ann Allergy Asthma Immunol.* 2004;93:29–35.

Phua J, Kong K, Lee K, et al. Noninvasive ventilation in hypercapnic acute respiratory failure due to chronic obstructive pulmonary disease vs. other conditions: Effectiveness and predictors of failure. *Intensive Care Med.* 2005;31(4):533–539.

Rana S, Jenad H, Gay P, et al. Failure of noninvasive ventilation in patients with acute lung injury: Observational cohort study. *Crit Care.* 2006;10(3):R79.

Tobin M, Jubran A, Laghi F. Patient-ventilatory interaction. *Am J Respir Crit Care Med.* 2001;163(5):1059–1063.

296

USE ANTIBIOTICS WISELY IN PATIENTS WITH CHRONIC OBSTRUCTIVE PULMONARY DISEASE

DREW L. FULLER, MD, MPH, FACEP

Chronic obstructive pulmonary disease (COPD) is a common entity in most emergency departments (EDs). It is a disease with a relatively high mortality and is often cited as the sixth leading cause of death worldwide and a leading cause of death in the United States. The economic impact due to the cost of treatment and lost productivity is staggering and reported to exceed 42 billion dollars in the United States alone. Understanding the pathophysiology and the interventions available in the ED may be helpful in the efficient management of the patient with COPD.

COPD is a condition associated with air flow narrowing and, unlike asthma, is only partially reversible. Airflow obstruction is attributed to either chronic bronchitis or emphysema. Chronic bronchitis is associated with a chronic cough and excessive mucus secretions. Emphysema is characterized by the destruction of the bronchial walls without fibrosis and abnormal enlargement of the distal air spaces. Most patients will have features of both disorders. One of the characteristics of this disease is that it is a disorder marked by inflammation, both airway and systemically. COPD is associated with significant comorbidities. In fact, many of the deaths attributed to COPD are due to extrapulmonary comorbid conditions and have been associated with a host of systemic markers of inflammation.

COPD exacerbations have been defined by the Global Initiative for Chronic Obstructive Lung Disease (GOLD) as a change in baseline dyspnea, cough, and/or sputum beyond day-to-day variations and acute in onset, which warrants a change in regular medication in the patient with COPD. Lung inflammation and infection are the underlying mechanisms behind COPD that respond to bacterial or viral involvement or environmental pollution. Most clinical guidelines recommend bronchodilators to reduce hyperinflation, steroids to reduce lung inflammation, and the judicious use of noninvasive positive-pressure ventilation as well as antibiotics to treat potential pathogens.

Antibiotics are commonly used in the ED for the treatment of COPD. The antibiotics that are used most often are the oral Beta lactams and the tetracycline derivatives. In a recent literature review, B. Quon et al. found only five studies that showed that antibiotics reduced treatment failures as compared to placebo. In this case, treatment failure was defined as requiring additional antibiotics within the first 7 days or unchanged or deteriorated symptoms within 21 days. Overall, Quon found that antibiotics significantly reduced treatment failures when they were administered to patients who were hospitalized but not when they were used in ambulatory patients.

Overall, antibiotics should not be prescribed for all COPD exacerbations. While the definition of exacerbation in the literature is inconsistent, most studies list common factors such as dyspnea, increased sputum production, and sputum purulence. Benefit has only been shown for patients with significant exacerbations requiring hospitalization and has been consistently demonstrated by multicenter randomized controlled trials over the past 40 years, as well as multiple meta-analyses and a Cochrane Review. In these populations, antibiotics reduced treatment failure by up to 46% and in-hospital mortality by 78%. Patients with the features of increased sputum and purulence have been shown to benefit the most.

Outpatients with mild or type 3 exacerbations, defined as having only one of the three common symptoms of dyspnea, increased sputum, or sputum purulence, did not show a benefit from empiric antibiotics. Although COPD is a disease that is characterized by both an airway and a systemic inflammatory state, the routine use of antibiotics is not suggested. A more judicious application of antibiotics is recommended. The current data support antibiotics for patients with significant COPD exacerbation who are likely to be hospitalized.

SUGGESTED READINGS

El Moussaoui R, Roede BM, Speelman P, et al. Short-course antibiotic treatment in acute exacerbations of chronic bronchitis and COPD: A meta-analysis of double-blind studies. *Thorax.* 2008;63;415–422.

Puhan MA, Volenweider D, Latshang T, et al. Exacerbations of chronic obstructive pulmonary disease: When are antibiotics indicated? A systematic review. *Respir Res.* 2007;8:30.

Quon Bs, Gan WQ, Sin DD. Contemporary management of acute exacerbations of COPD: A systematic review and meta-analysis. *Chest.* 2008;133;756–766.

Ram F, Rodriguez RR, Granados NA, et al. Antibiotics for exacerbations of chronic obstructive pulmonary disease. *Cochrane Database Syst Rev.* 2006;(2): CD004403; doi: 10.1002/14651858. CD004403. pub2.

297

VENTILATION/PERFUSION VERSUS COMPUTED TOMOGRAPHY FOR PULMONARY THROMBOEMBOLISM IN PREGNANCY

MICHAEL E. NOTTIDGE, MD, MPH

Pulmonary thromboembolism (PE) is an extremely common manifestation of venous thrombosis and is often difficult to diagnose. It has a high morbidity and mortality and, by some estimates, is one of the leading causes of unexpected death in all age groups, including pregnant patients. PE is estimated to occur in approximately 1 in every 7,000 pregnancies. It remains a leading cause of maternal morbidity and mortality in the United States, in some series accounting for up to one fifth of all maternal deaths. The diagnosis in pregnancy is even more complex than in other populations. It presents a challenge for most emergency physicians because of not only the consequences the undiagnosed disease has to the mother and to the fetus but also the risk that the diagnostic modalities have for the fetus.

The difficulty in diagnosing PE in pregnancy rests on its varied presentations. The initial clinical features of PE are practically indistinguishable from normal changes and symptoms in pregnancy. Historically, most diagnoses of PE were made postmortem, because of the difficulty in making the diagnosis. Whereas prediction rules have been shown to improve accuracy, the diagnosis in pregnancy has hinged on either helical computed tomographic pulmonary angiography (CTPA) or ventilation/perfusion (V/Q) scintigraphy. For the emergency physician, making the decision to subject a pregnant patient to radiation of any kind is difficult and is likely to cause consternation among the treatment team.

The diagnostic dilemma that a potential PE raises has to be counterbalanced by the potential damage to the fetus caused by testing. A helpful reminder is that the risks of undiagnosed PE far outweigh the potential risks of radiation to the fetus. Nevertheless, the principle of avoiding ionizing radiation of any type during pregnancy has to be honored. Because of these counterbalancing issues, there is a great deal of controversy over the safest way to diagnose a PE in pregnancy.

Interestingly, a widely held notion is that V/Q scintigraphy administers less radiation and is therefore safer for the fetus than CTPA. This was borne out in a recent survey of 163 UK physicians, in which only about half indicated the impression that V/Q scans give a higher fetal dose of radiation than CTPA.

Ionizing radiation dose (i.e., amount absorbed by tissue) is usually measured in the conventional unit of rad or the SI unit of Gray (Gy)—1 Gy equals 100 rad. On the other hand, the biological risk of exposure to radiation is measured in the conventional units of rem or SI units of sievert (Sv)—1 Sv equals 100 rem.

On average, CT angiography gives a higher total radiation dose to the mother than does V/Q scintigraphy (14 mSv vs. 2.2 mSv). Furthermore, the usual convention for pregnant patients is to do perfusion-only scintigraphy with no ventilation study in order to minimize radiation exposure. The usual expected doses are shown in *Table 297.1*.

On the other hand, the actual dose to the fetus is higher even with perfusion-only scintigraphy than with CTPA (640 to 800 μGy vs. 3 to 131 μGy). By some estimates, perfusion scintigraphy gives the fetus at least five times the radiation dose as CTPA through all trimesters of pregnancy.

Overall, the risk of diagnostic imaging to the fetus is considerably small and can be considered in the broad categories of teratogenesis, carcinogenesis, and toxic effects. The teratogenetic effects of the ionizing radiation include death, congenital anomalies, growth and mental retardation, intellectual impairment, and microcephaly. These effects are not known to occur below a dose of 50 mGy

TABLE 297.1	DIAGNOSTIC EXAM AND RADIATION DOSES TO MOTHER AND FETUS		
	V/Q SCAN (MGY)	Q-ONLY SCAN (MGY)	CT SCAN (MGY)
Mother	0.9–1.8	0.9	14
Fetus	0.9–1.8	0.9	0.14

and are most severe with earlier gestational exposure. Radiation-induced cancer risk is increased with fetal irradiation in utero. Although the risk is thought to persist through all stages of pregnancy, the precise type and incidence of cancer remain unclear.

The major potentially toxic consideration in CTPA is the use of iodinated contrast agents which can cross the placenta. This can cause depression of thyroid function in the fetus. However, this is thought to be less of a factor unless the maternal thyroid function is also abnormal. The duration of exposure is also thought to be limited. There is, however, a lack of systematic research into this question. The standard practice in the United States is to have thyroid function tests in the first week of life, and this is especially important for cases of prenatal maternal contrast exposure.

CONCLUSION

CTPA is an overall safer test for the diagnosis of pulmonary emboli in pregnancy than V/Q or Q-only scanning. CTPA also has the added advantage of defining the pulmonary anatomy and identifying other pathologies. V/Q scans, however, deliver a lower radiation dose to the maternal mammary glands than older CT modalities and pose a lower risk of malignancy for pregnant women undergoing diagnostic studies for PE.

SUGGESTED READINGS

ACOG Committee Opinion. Number 299, September 2004 (replaces No. 158, September 1995). Guidelines for diagnostic imaging during pregnancy. *Obstet Gynecol.* 2004;104(3): 647–651.

Berg CJ, Chang J, Callaghan WM, et al. Pregnancy-related mortality in the United States, 1991–1997. *Obstet Gynecol.* 2003;101(2):289–296.

Chang J, Elam-Evans LD, Berg CJ, et al. Pregnancy-related mortality surveillance—United States, 1991–1999. *MMWR Surveill Summ.* 2003;52(2):1–8.

De Santis M, Di Gianantonio E, Straface G, et al. Ionizing radiations in pregnancy and teratogenesis: A review of literature. *Reprod Toxicol.* 2005;20(3):323–329.

Groves AM, Yates SJ, Win T, et al. CT pulmonary angiography versus ventilation-perfusion scintigraphy in pregnancy: Implications from a UK survey of doctors' knowledge of radiation exposure. *Radiology.* 2006;240(3):765–770.

Huda W. When a pregnant patient has a suspected pulmonary embolism, what are the typical embryo doses from a chest CT and a ventilation/perfusion study? *Pediatr Radiol.* 2005; 35(4):452–453.

Le Gal G, Righini M, Roy PM, et al. Prediction of pulmonary embolism in the emergency department: The revised Geneva score. *Ann Intern Med.* 2006;144(3):165–171.

Patel SJ, Reede DL, Katz DS, et al. Imaging the pregnant patient for nonobstetric conditions: Algorithms and radiation dose considerations. *Radiographics.* 2007;27(6):1705–1722.

Simpson EL, Lawrenson RA, Nightingale AL, et al. Venous thromboembolism in pregnancy and the puerperium: Incidence and additional risk factors from a London perinatal database. *BJOG.* 2001;108(1):56–60.

Streffer C, Shore R, Konermann G, et al. Biological effects after prenatal irradiation (embryo and fetus). A report of the International Commission on Radiological Protection. *Ann ICRP.* 2003;33(1–2):5–206.

Webb JA, Thomsen HS, Morcos SK. The use of iodinated and gadolinium contrast media during pregnancy and lactation. *Eur Radiol.* 2005;15(6):1234–1240.

Wells PS, Anderson DR, Rodger M, et al. Excluding pulmonary embolism at the bedside without diagnostic imaging: Management of patients with suspected pulmonary embolism presenting to the emergency department by using a simple clinical model and d-dimer. *Ann Intern Med*. 2001;135(2):98–107.

Winer-Muram HT, Boone JM, Brown HL, et al. Pulmonary embolism in pregnant patients: Fetal radiation dose with helical CT. *Radiology*. 2002;224(2):487–492.

RESUSCITATION

298

REMEMBER TO INITIATE THERAPEUTIC HYPOTHERMIA FOR POST-CARDIAC ARREST PATIENTS

ERIN E. WILKES, MD

In late 2002, the International Liaison Committee on Resuscitation (ILCOR) incorporated the following into their recommendations:

- Unconscious adult patients with spontaneous circulation after out-of-hospital cardiac arrest should be cooled to 32°C to 34°C for 12 to 24 h if the initial rhythm was ventricular fibrillation (VF)
- Such cooling may also be beneficial for other rhythms or in-hospital cardiac arrest

Since that time, many hospitals have instituted protocols to comply with these recommendations. However, cooling measures are still far from universally instituted in the emergency department (ED), even in the first group of patients described in the ILCOR guidelines. Failure to initiate therapy in the ED can delay the time to reach the recommended goal temperature and potentially reduce the benefit of this important therapy.

ILCOR recommendations, and similar ones from the American Heart Association, were based off of two prospective randomized trials published in 2002. Both studies identified a highly specific patient population in which mild hypothermia might be beneficial to mitigate the severe brain damage usually sustained during cardiac arrest. The idea was to reduce cerebral oxygen consumption as well as other potentially harmful chemical and physical processes initiated subsequent to a prolonged period of cerebral ischemia. These processes can persist for some hours postresuscitation and include destructive enzymatic reactions, free radical production, increased oxygen demand in low flow areas, intracellular acidosis, biosynthesis, and the use of neurotransmitters. Both trials demonstrated a significant improvement in neurological outcome and mortality.

Strict criteria should be outlined in identifying the patient population that is proven to benefit from this therapy. There should be a presumed cardiac origin of the arrest, and the initial acceptable rhythms on the monitor include only VF or pulseless ventricular tachycardia (VT). Patients who arrest secondary to traumatic brain injury, cerebrovascular accident, respiratory causes, have a terminal illness or preexisting coagulopathy, or demonstrate other rhythms on the monitor have not been sufficiently studied to warrant this treatment. Furthermore, these trials were only validated for patients who experienced an out-of-hospital, witnessed arrest, regained spontaneous circulation within 60 min of collapse, and remained comatose after resuscitation. Arrest after the arrival of emergency personnel on the scene was not studied nor was the pediatric or pregnant patient population.

Several methods, both active and passive, can be applied to achieve the desired therapeutic temperature range of 32°C to 34°C. Cooling blankets, ice packs to the groin, axillae, and neck, wet towels, fanning, application of a cooling helmet, and infusion of IV saline cooled to 4°C are all common methods. Target time to desired temperature should be approximately 4 to 16 h and maintained for 12 to 24 h. Measures should be undertaken to monitor temperature, prevent shivering, prevent cardiac dysrhythmias, and prevent infection. Other therapeutic interventions aimed at treating the underlying cause of the arrest, including thrombolytic therapy, heparinization, and percutaneous coronary intervention (PCI), need not be delayed. Once the therapy is completed, patients may be actively or passively rewarmed with normothermia restored in 6 to 12 h. The above details varied slightly between the two core studies and have not been further refined since that time. However, despite this variability, both studies showed similar outcomes.

The use of hypothermia to mitigate brain damage during periods of ischemia was pioneered in the 1950s in a study that looked at the use of moderate hypothermia. Practice was not altered at the time because the adverse effects on rates of infection, coagulopathy, and dysrhythmias seemed to outweigh the benefits. Recent studies with the use of mild hypothermia seem to strike a more appropriate balance in favor of the therapy, with sepsis being the most problematic of the complications.

Postarrest hypothermia is an exciting and rapidly expanding branch of resuscitation research with many smaller animal and human studies showing potential benefit for a wider range of patients. But for the time being, its effectiveness in patients with witnessed out-of-hospital arrest who remain unconscious after successful cardiopulmonary resuscitation is supported by literature and should be initiated in the ED.

SUGGESTED READINGS

Bernard SA, Gray TW, Buist MD, et al. Treament of comatose survivors of out-of-hospital cardiac arrest with induced hypothermia. *N Engl J Med*. 2002;346:557–563.

Hypothermia after Cardiac Arrest Study Group. Mild therapeutic hypothermia to improve the neurolgoic outcome after cardiac arrest. *N Engl J Med*. 2002;346(8):549–556.

Nolan JP, Morley PT, Hoek TL, et al. Therapeutic hypothermia after cardiac arrest: An advisory statement by the Advancement Life Support Task Force of the International Liaison Committee on Resuscitation. *Resuscitation.* 2003;57(3):231–235.

Wolfrum S, Pierau C, Radke PW, et al. Mild therapeutic hypothermia in patients after out-of-hospital cardiac arrest due to acute ST-segment elevation myocardial infarction undergoing immediate percutaneous coronary intervention. *Crit Care Med.* 2008; 36(6):1780–1786.

299

ALLOW FAMILIES THE OPPORTUNITY TO BE PRESENT DURING THE RESUSCITATION OF A LOVED ONE

JAN M. SHOENBERGER, MD, FAAEM, FACEP

In the past decade, it became more common for emergency department physicians and nurses to allow families into the clinical area to witness the resuscitation of their family member. However, there are still physicians and nurses who object to this practice and do not extend an invitation to family members to witness the care of their loved ones.

There are four main arguments against allowing family members to witness the resuscitation. The primary objection is the fear that it will be too traumatic for them. It is believed that an already emotionally stressed family is not prepared to handle the additional stress of witnessing CPR, electrical shocks, and artificial ventilation of their loved one. Another argument is that the patient has the right to confidentiality, even when unconscious. The third argument is that the presence of family will influence the resuscitation team. It is believed that family members may impede the resuscitation effort by either physically being in the way or distracting the team members through the emotional distress that the family member is experiencing. The fourth significant concern is a medicolegal one. If a procedure, such as securing the airway, is difficult or complicated by aspiration, the family at the bedside may be more likely to initiate legal proceedings. Although this has not been shown to be true, it is still a perception of many care providers.

Research on this topic has yielded interesting results. In one study of family members who witnessed resuscitations, there was no long-lasting psychological stress related to their experiences on follow-up interviews. Family members also felt satisfied with their decision to remain with their loved one during the resuscitation efforts. Another study found that over 90% of family members present for a resuscitation of a relative would do so again if faced with that decision in the future. In the case of children, a 1999 study that surveyed parents found that approximately 80% of parents expressed a desire to be present during their child's resuscitation.

The argument against the breach of an unconscious patient's right to confidentiality is primarily an ethical one, and there has never been a lawsuit to determine precedent. Emergency departments routinely call family members of unconscious patients to inform them of the patient's presence in the department. This would also be considered a breach of confidentiality. When a patient is rendered unconscious by illness or accident, we often go to family members to obtain valuable medical information or to aid in decision making. This is widely accepted. Moreover, it is likely that approaching family members to consider the option of witnessing the resuscitation will become more accepted as it becomes more commonplace in our practice.

In 2005, the European Resuscitation Council and the American Heart Association (AHA) endorsed the concept of allowing family members to witness resuscitations. The AHA states the following in its 2005 guidelines:

in the absence of data documenting harm and in light of data suggesting it may be helpful, offering select family members the opportunity to be present during a resuscitation seems reasonable and desirable

To ensure a successful experience for the team members as well as family members, several steps should be taken. These are as follows:

- Family members should be carefully screened and asked about their willingness to participate. Relatives who are overly emotional, intoxicated, or unsure/unwilling should not be allowed into the resuscitation.
- The family members should be briefed prior to entering the resuscitation area. This should be done either by a physician or by a nurse, and the language used should be simple layperson terms so that they can understand.
- Continual assistance should be available to support the family member throughout the experience. A nurse trained in this subject should be standing next to the family member and answer questions and explain the actions of the team.

SUGGESTED READINGS

Baskett PJF, Steen PA, Bossaert L. European Resuscitation Council Guidelines for Resuscitation 2005. Section 8. The ethics of resuscitation and end-of-life decisions. *Resuscitation.* 2005;67S1:S171–S180.

Boie ET, Moore GP, Brummett C, et al. Do parents want to be present during invasive procedures performed on their children in the emergency department? A survey of 400 parents. *Ann Emerg Med.* 1999;34(1):70–74.

Doyle CJ, Post H, Burney RE. Family participation during resuscitation: An option. *Ann Emerg Med.* 99;16(6);673–675.

ECC Committee, Subcommittees and Task Forces of the American Heart Association. 2005 American Heart Association Guidelines for Cardiopulmonary Resuscitation and Emergency Cardiovascular Care. *Circulation*. 2005;112(24 Suppl):IV1–203.

Robinson SM, Mackenzie-Ross S, Campbell Hewson GL, et al. Psychological effect of witnessed resuscitation on bereaved relatives. *Lancet*. 1998;352(9128):614–617.

300

BE WILLING TO DISCUSS END-OF-LIFE WISHES AND DO-NOT-ATTEMPT-RESUSCITATION ORDERS IN THE EMERGENCY DEPARTMENT

STEVEN NAZARIO, MD

Many patients present to the emergency department (ED) without advance directives. While some people may have some cursory understanding of what it means to be kept alive "on machines" or what CPR is, most have neither decided what they would do in just such a circumstance nor have they selected a health care surrogate. In addition, patients often have unrealistic expectations about what medical treatment in advanced disease can accomplish. For example, recent literature indicates that the lay public has the expectation that most individuals undergoing CPR will be successfully resuscitated. It is important to address the realistic outcomes of such interventions.

The onus falls on the emergency physician to provide guidance to the patient and the family in their understanding of what a do–not–attempt-resuscitation (DNAR; also often referred to as "DNR") order means, to assess their wishes for their end-of-life care, and to comply with those directives. Some ED providers believe that it is not their role to discuss the DNAR issues. If not addressed by the patient's primary doctor beforehand, they would elect to leave this issue to the admitting physician. However, to do so suspends a patient's right to autonomy while they are in the ED. With most EDs in the country experiencing rising volumes, ED providers may also feel that they do not have enough time for DNAR discussions. The pressures of attending to the next patient and of clearing out the ED must not prejudice the patient who is at or near the end of life. Our care for these patients requires allotting the time necessary to make informed decisions. If the patient needed additional time with us to secure vascular access, would we not spend that time with them?

For moribund patients, one must inquire above advance directives. In patients who appear to have decisional capacity, ask about their understanding of their illness and the future of their condition. Ask if they would like a friend or family member with them while you interview them. Answers to these questions will give you a sense of how they are approaching the prospect of death. Often patients are still uncertain about these decisions. Allow for a break should the session prove too intense.

Broad statements like "Do you want us to do everything?" simply will not convey the meaning that you intend. Ask what specific procedures they want applied. Explain that you wish to know how to respond if and when their condition worsens. Clarify what is meant by intubation and CPR. Often, patients and their families feel that a DNAR order is equivalent to abandoning care altogether; assure them that a DNAR order will not stop the treatment of their symptoms or pain. At times, patients may question your motives. Be transparent in your answers, avoid vague language, and assure them that you want them to have control over their treatment should they become incapacitated.

Be attuned to disagreements or sources of discord between family members. Ask who will be the surrogate should the patient become incapacitated and have them involved in the discussions about end-of-life issues, if possible. If the patient's decision-making capacity is in question, then speaking with the family is vitally important. In the absence of a legal surrogate, each state has delineated a hierarchy among family members for obtaining consent.

Providers may feel that they do not have enough information to approach a DNAR discussion. A good faith effort should be applied to acquire information from the medical record, prior hospitalizations, or primary care doctor as to end-of-life decisions. Moribund patients who arrive in the ED with DNARs already in place can be a special source of frustration. Why would someone call 911 if there is a DNAR order? However, it is common for family caregivers to become distressed as they watch a loved one enter the dying process. They may be unsure whether the presentation is a symptom, a new illness, or a natural death. Moreover, patients are entitled to change their DNAR preferences. We must strive to respect patient autonomy, even if it is at odds with our own values.

SUGGESTED READINGS

American College of Emergency Physicians. Practice resources: "Do not attempt resuscitate" orders in the out-of-hospital setting. ACEP, October 2003. Available at: http://www.acep.org/practres.aspx?id = 30108

American College of Emergency Physicians. Practice resources: Code of ethics for emergency physicians. ACDP, October 2001. Available at: http://www.acep.org/practres.aspx?id = 29144

Emanuel LL, Quest T, eds. *Education in Palliative and End-of-Life Care for Emergency Medicine (EPEC-EM) Curriculum*, 2008.

Fox E, Siegler M. Redefining the emergency physician's role in do-not-resuscitate decision-making, *Am J Med*. 1992;92(2):125–128.

301

KNOW YOUR RESUSCITATION EQUIPMENT

THOMAS M. MAILHOT, MD, FAAEM

Emergency physicians (EPs) are experts in resuscitation, acting quickly upon limited data to stabilize patients. Given the time-critical nature of resuscitation, the EP cannot afford to divert his or her full attention to waste precious moments attempting to understand the resuscitation equipment. This issue is complicated by the fact that many EPs work in more than one ED. Each ED is variable with respect to how the resuscitation areas are stocked, so the EP should take the time to understand what equipment exists in each location. This same advice holds true if the EP is responsible for running codes outside of the ED (e.g., on the wards or in intensive care areas).

AIRWAY/BREATHING

All EDs will have standard airway tools: Macintosh/Miller blades and endotracheal tubes of various sizes. But if this fails, what backup airway options are available? Depending on the ED, the backup airway of choice may be a laryngeal mask airway, an esophageal obturator device (e.g., Combitube), a gum elastic bougie, or a no. 11 blade to perform a cricothyrotomy. In many EDs, a wide variety of backup airway options may exist. But if one is not familiar with the function of any of these items, they cease to be options and become distractions, or even worse, impediments. They might as well not exist and would be better off being removed from the cart. A thorough familiarity with two or three airway options (including a surgical option—cricothyrotomy—as one of them) is far superior to a cursory knowledge of multiple options.

The first time you set up a tracheostomy tube should not be when you are performing a cricothyrotomy. Tracheostomy kits have three essential parts: an outer cannula, an inner cannula, and an obturator. The obturator has no lumen and serves to guide the placement of the tracheostomy tube upon insertion. The obturator is inserted into the outer cannula before it is inserted into the trachea. The obturator is then removed and the inner cannula is inserted in its place.

Percutaneous transtracheal jet ventilation, the ventilation of the lungs by intermittent bursts of oxygen through a needle or cannula in the cricothyroid membrane, is the surgical airway of choice for children under 10 years of age. Jet ventilation is extremely rare, and although simple to perform, its rarity leads to an unfamiliarity that causes delays. A large (14 gauge or larger) catheter must be used, along with high-pressure tubing to prevent kinking or collapse. This tubing should be secured to the catheter via an adapter: this can be a 3–0 endotracheal tube adapter, if necessary. A high-pressure oxygen source is needed, with recommended pressures of 30 mm Hg for children aged 5 to 12 (less for children under 5 years old). Ventilation is accomplished via a one-way valve, allowing for a 1:3 inspiratory-to-expiratory ratio. Both oral and nasal airways should be placed to ensure adequate exhalation and to prevent barotrauma.

Understanding how to connect and troubleshoot the suction equipment can make the difference between a successful intubation and converting to a surgical airway. One should not wait until blood or secretions obscure a clear view of the vocal cords to figure out how to dial up the force of suction.

CIRCULATION

When the 400-lb patient goes into cardiac arrest in the ED, what options exist for intravenous access? There may be a central line with nearly impossible-to-palpate landmarks. In some EDs, an ultrasound machine may be available to identify a central vein for cannulation. In other facilities, an intraosseous line may be the best option. Understanding what technology is available will allow quicker and more decisive action to be taken.

Faced with a massive GI bleed, the EP may need to place a gastroesophageal balloon device such as a Sengstaken-Blakemore or Linton tube. Each device has slightly different specifications, but generally, these devices consist of a gastric balloon ± an esophageal balloon. The typical volume inflated in the gastric balloon is 450 to 500 mL of air, while the esophageal balloon takes just enough air to stop bleeding (normally a much smaller volume). The pressure from the esophageal balloon should not exceed 45 mm Hg. A small amount of traction must be exerted on the device (usually equivalent to the weight of a 1-L bag of saline) to tamponade varices at the gastroesophageal junction.

SUGGESTED READINGS

Mace SE. Cricothyrotomy and translaryngeal jet ventilation. In: Roberts JR, Hedges JR, eds. *Clinical Procedures in Emergency Medicine.* 3rd ed. Philadelphia, PA: W. B. Saunders; 1998:57–74.

Panacek E. Balloon Tamponade of gastroesophageal varices. In: Roberts JR, Hedges JR, eds. *Clinical Procedures in Emergency Medicine.* 3rd ed. Philadelphia, PA: W. B. Saunders; 1998:713–718.

Vissers RJ, Bair AE. Surgical airway techniques. In: Walls RM, Murphy MF, eds. *Manual of Emergency Airway Management.* 3rd ed. Philadelphia, PA: Lippincott Williams & Wilkins; 2008:193–220.

302

ABANDON THE USE OF HIGH-DOSE EPINEPHRINE

TONY PEDUTO, MD

High-dose epinephrine (HDE) should not be used during resuscitation of either adult or pediatric patients in cardiac arrest. HDE has been shown in multiple well-designed, randomized, double-blind controlled trials to not improve outcome when compared to standard-dose epinephrine (SDE). Moreover, its use may raise resource stewardship and ethical issues.

Current American Heart Association guidelines recommend epinephrine IV (SDE), at a dose of 1 mg for adults and 0.01 mg/kg for pediatric patients, for the treatment of ventricular fibrillation, pulseless electrical activity (PEA), and asystole. There is no consensus on the exact dose of HDE, although various studies have used doses of 2 to 15 mg, in either fixed or escalating dosage regimens. Early animal research had found improved survival with the use of HDE as compared with SDE. However, a recent meta-analysis by Vandycke et al. of all large, well-designed human studies does not demonstrate improved outcomes in adults using HDE. Perondi et al. recently published a large, well-designed trial in pediatric patients that not only showed a lack of superiority of HDE to SDE but also suggested worse outcomes in the HDE group.

While no studies have shown improved functional outcomes (and few demonstrate a trend toward increased survival to hospital discharge), studies do show improved rates of return of spontaneous circulation (ROSC) with HDE. This disconnect speaks to the favorable cardiac (but not necessarily neurologic) resuscitative qualities of epinephrine as it is utilized in cardiac arrest. Patients who would otherwise have died are "resuscitated" to either a persistent vegetative state or a state of profound neurological disability requiring total care. Even those who do not survive to hospital discharge require days to months of futile ICU care prior to their death. Recent studies suggest that cardiac arrest patients with ROSC using HDE do quite poorly from a functional standpoint compared to those treated with SDE. Even if critical care beds were not a scarce resource, HDE significantly increases the chance of patients, families, and the medical team being forced into the dilemma of when to suspend futile care.

One can easily lose sight of the "big picture" if one focuses only upon the emergency department (ED) course. What may initially be perceived as an "amazing save" by the ED team may in reality become a prolonged death. No studies have demonstrated improved neurological or functional outcomes with the use of HDE, and a recent well-designed study by Behringer et al. suggests that increasing cumulative doses of epinephrine are associated with worsening neurological outcome. This raises profound ethical questions of futility: are families being given false hope? is the patient's death being prolonged? does this prolongation of death increase suffering?

The best evidence available at this time suggests that HDE should not be used as a "rescue therapy" when SDE fails. Failure of SDE indicates nonsurvivable cardiac arrest. HDE does not improve functional patient outcome; it leads to increased utilization of scarce resources, increases health care costs, prolongs death, and probably leads to increased suffering of both patients and families.

SUGGESTED READINGS

Behringer W, Kittler H, Sterz F, et al. Cumulative epinephrine dose during cardiopulmonary resuscitation and neurologic outcome. *Ann Intern Med.* 1998;129(6):450–456.

Cummins RO, Hazinski MF. The next chapter in the high-dose epinephrine story: Unfavorable neurologic outcomes? *Ann Intern Med.* 1998;129(6):501–502.

Gueugniaud PY, Mils P, Goldstein P, et al. A comparison of repeated high doses and repeated standard doses of epinephrine for cardiac arrest outside the hospital. *N Engl J Med.* 1998;339(22):1595–1601.

Perondi MB, Reis AG, Paiva EF, et al. A comparison of high-dose and standard-dose epinephrine in children with cardiac arrest. *N Engl J Med.* 2004;350(17):1722–1730.

Vandycke C, Martens P. High dose versus standard dose epinephrine in cardiac arrest: Ameta-analysis. *Resuscitation.* 2000;45(3):161–166.

303

BE EXTRA CAREFUL WITH MEDICATION DOSAGES DURING PEDIATRIC RESUSCITATION

THOMAS M. MAILHOT, MD, FAAEM

Pediatric resuscitations are very stressful events for most emergency physicians (EPs). Aside from the emotional issues surrounding ill or injured children, many EPs feel less comfortable with pediatric dosing than with adult dosing. Having a strong command of pediatric dosing can considerably lessen the anxiety associated with pediatric resuscitations.

Pediatric dosing is weight based, and the Broselow tape has been shown to be fairly reliable in estimating pediatric weights. Use the Broselow tape if you have one available. If it is missing, even 1 min spent looking for it can jeopardize the resuscitation. Therefore, every EP must know how to approximate pediatric weight based on age. One method uses the formula: weight in kilograms = 10 + (age × 2). Thus, a 4–year-old child weighs approximately 18 kg. A simpler approach that avoids any calculation at all is to remember that at ages 1, 3, 5, 7, and 9, the average child weighs approximately 10, 15, 20, 25, and 30 kg, respectively.

Medications that might be needed in an emergency situation must be familiar to the EP, including drugs needed to address issues of airway, breathing, circulation, neurological disability, and exposure. This is no time to be thumbing through the pharmacopeia or placing a call to the pharmacist. Moreover, in a stressful situation, it can be extremely difficult to perform even basic calculations. Thus, if there is any advanced warning that an unstable child is arriving in your ED, calculate doses in advance. All doses below are for intravenous (IV) administration unless otherwise indicated.

AIRWAY

Rapid sequence intubation drugs consist of induction agents and paralytics. Induction is typically accomplished with etomidate (0.3 mg/kg). Other options include ketamine (1 to 2 mg/kg) and propofol (2 mg/kg). Succinylcholine (2 mg/kg in infants, 1.5 mg/kg in children) or rocuronium (0.6 to 1.2 mg/kg) are frequently used paralytics. Although controversy now surrounds its routine use, atropine (0.02 mg/kg, minimum dose 0.1 mg) should be given prior to succinylcholine in children <8 years old in order to blunt the vagal response that young children typically experience with succinylcholine and intubation.

Endotracheal tubes (ETTs) are sized according to the formula (age/4) + 4. A simple way of estimating the ETT size is by using the width of the patient's small finger as an estimate of the inner diameter that the ETT should have. Because cuffed tubes are now more routine in children, one can err on a tube one-half size smaller when making the estimate.

Laryngoscope blades' sizes are estimated according to age as well, with a size 0 (Miller or Macintosh) being appropriate for preterm infants and neonates, size 1 for ages 0 to 1, size 2 for ages 2 to 10, and a size 3 for ages >10 years.

BREATHING

Asthmatic patients can be given albuterol (0.5 mg/kg/nebulization treatment). Magnesium (25 to 50 mg/kg IV) and epinephrine (0.01 mg/kg of 1:1,000 solution intramuscularly) can also be given.

Once a pediatric patient is intubated, ventilator settings that are weight appropriate should be chosen. Tidal volumes of 6 to 8 mL/kg are usually adequate, and a respiratory rate that is age appropriate should be selected. A normal respiratory rate in a neonate is 30 to 60 bpm, in a young child, 20 to 40, and in an older child, 15 to 25.

CIRCULATION

In a code situation, epinephrine (0.01 mg/kg) is given IV or via an intraosseous line in a 1:10,000 concentration. Atropine (0.02 mg/kg) has a minimum dose of 0.1 mg because below this dose, paradoxical bradycardia can be seen. Adenosine (0.1 mg/kg) is given as a rapid push, doubling the dose if ineffective. For cardioversion, use doses of 0.5 J/kg initially and double if ineffective. Defibrillation should be attempted at 1 J/kg initially before being doubled as needed.

Fluid administration is also weight based. Normal saline and lactated Ringer solution are given as 20 mL/kg boluses. Packed red blood cells are given in 10 mL/kg increments.

DISABILITY

In the seizing child, the proper dose for benzodiazepines (diazepam, lorazepam, and midazolam) is 0.05 to 0.1 mg/kg. Phenobarbital (10 to 20 mg/kg) and fosphenytoin (10 to 20 phenytoin equivalents/kg) may also be needed. Phenobarbital is preferred after benzodiazepines in neonates.

If cerebral herniation is suspected, mannitol (0.25–1g/kg) may be needed.

EXPOSURE

Children who are poisoned may need emergent treatment, including calcium chloride (20 mg/kg or 0.2 mL/kg of 10% solution), sodium bicarbonate (1 mEq/kg; use 4.2% solution in neonates, 8.4% in children), and naloxone (0.1 mg/kg). Dextrose (0.5 to 1 g/kg) should not be given in high concentrations to pediatric patients for fear of inducing hyperosmolarity, which may result in morbidity. Whereas in adults 1 to 2 mL/kg of D50W may be appropriate, children should be given either D25W (2 to 4 mL/kg; infants and children) or D10W (5 to 10 mL/kg; neonates). Glucagon (0.02 mg/kg intramuscularly) may be needed if no IV access can be obtained.

A thorough knowledge of pediatric dosing will help avoid errors in medication administration and allow for a greater comfort level in conducting pediatric resuscitation.

SUGGESTED READINGS

Black K, Barnett P, Wolfe R, et al. Are methods used to estimate weight in children accurate? *Emerg Med (Fremantle)*. 2002;14(2):160–165.

Ralston M, Hazinski MF, Arno L, et al., eds. *PALS Provider Manual*. Dallas, TX: American Heart Association; 2007.

304

BEWARE THAT AMIODARONE PRODUCES QT PROLONGATION

TONY PEDUTO, MD

A prolonged QT interval (QTc > 0.44 s) on ECG increases the risk of torsade de pointes (TdP), a potentially fatal dysrhythmia. Amiodarone administration prolongs the QT interval and can lead to TdP in patients whose QT is already prolonged. Recognizing that a patient has, or is at risk for, a prolonged QT interval should prompt the physician to avoid amiodarone in the resuscitation of the patient with a wide-complex tachydysrhythmia or cardiac arrest.

Out-of-hospital cardiac arrest patients arrive in the ED with little or no available history. Nonetheless, any patient with a known history of a congenital long QT syndrome or a history of TdP should be considered to have a prolonged QT until proven otherwise. This is sometimes found on a "medical alert" bracelet or by patient/family report. Many drugs are also known to prolong the QT interval, and TdP should be considered as the precipitating event in all cardiac arrest patients known to be taking such a drug. Important classes of drugs that prolong the QT interval include many antidysrhythmics, antipsychotics, antidepressants, antibiotics, antimalarials, antifungals, and antihistamines.

Additional risk factors for TdP include hypomagnesemia (e.g., alcoholic patients), hypokalemia (e.g., a patient who arrests immediately following hemodialysis), hypocalcemia (e.g., recent parathyroid resection), bradycardia (absolute lengthening of QT), hypothyroidism, congestive heart failure (CHF), left ventricular hypertrophy (LVH), recent cardioversion, digoxin therapy, and a history of ventricular arrhythmia. Finally, the presence of T-wave alternans on ECG has been described as a risk factor for TdP.

Amiodarone is recommended by the American Heart Association Advanced Cardiac Life Support (ACLS) guidelines as a treatment option for wide-complex dysrhythmias and ventricular fibrillation that is refractory to electrical cardioversion. Yet, administering amiodarone to patients with a prolonged QT interval places the patient at high risk for refractory TdP, which can degenerate to ventricular fibrillation. Lidocaine does not prolong the QT interval and thus is the antidysrhythmic of choice in these patients. By using lidocaine in those patients at risk for, or known to have, a prolonged QT interval, the physician can avoid induction of iatrogenic TdP.

In the event that TdP occurs following administration of amiodarone, the infusion should be stopped immediately and IV magnesium should be given. Other electrolyte disturbances (e.g., hypokalemia and hypocalcemia), whether known or suspected, should immediately be treated. If TdP is persistent, or if bradycardia occurs, pacing can be initiated and titrated to effect (most patients will respond if paced above 70 bpm). If electrical pacing fails, overdrive pacing can be initiated with isoproterenol or atropine. The goal of overdrive pacing is to induce tachycardia, which in turn shortens the myocardial refractory period (the QT interval), reducing the risk and recurrence of TdP. The bile acid sequestrant cholestyramine can be also given orally or by nasogastric tube to speed amiodarone elimination, as it undergoes enterohepatic circulation.

Amiodarone is only one option in the treatment of ventricular dysrhythmias. Even during the "adrenaline-charged" setting of a cardiac arrest, attention to all available information is important and may lead to different therapeutic options such as magnesium, lidocaine, or electrical cardioversion.

Suggested Readings

Dorian P, Cass D, Schwartz B, et al. Amiodarone as compared with lidocaine for shock-resistant ventricular fibrillation. *N Engl J Med*. 2002;346(12):884–890.

Foley P, Kalra P, Andrews N. Amiodarone—avoid the danger of torsades de pointes. *Resuscitation*. 2008;76(1):137–141.

Kudenchuk PJ, Cobb LA, Copass MK, et al. Amiodarone for resuscitation after out-of-hospital cardiac arrest due to ventricular fibrillation. *N Engl J Med*. 1999;341(12):871–878.

Trohman RG, Sahu J. Drug-induced torsade de pointes. *Circulation*. 1999;99(16):E7.

Yap YG, Camm AJ. Drug induced QT prolongation and torsades de pointes. *Heart*. 2003; 89(11):1363–1372.

305

REMEMBER TO SYNCHRONIZE CARDIOVERSION IN PATIENTS WITH PULSES

THOMAS M. MAILHOT, MD, FAAEM

Electricity has been used to treat cardiac dysrhythmias since 1962, when Lown et al. described its use. Since then, electricity has taken on an important role in advanced cardiac life support (ACLS). When applying this technology, however, the emergency physician must avoid common errors relating to the use of the "sync" mode.

The R-on-T phenomenon occurs when a cardiac depolarization (i.e., a QRS complex) begins during ventricular repolarization (i.e., a T wave). This can result in polymorphic ventricular tachycardia (VT) or ventricular fibrillation (VF). In order to avoid this dreaded complication, synchronized cardioversion should be used whenever indicated. Synchronized cardioversion times, or synchronizes, the delivery of a shock to occur with the QRS complex, thus avoiding a shock during the relative refractory period of the cardiac cycle.

Synchronized cardioversion is indicated for the treatment of unstable tachy-dysrhythmias. These include certain atrial dysrhythmias (paroxysmal supraventricular tachycardia, atrial fibrillation, atrial flutter) as well as monomorphic VT. Synchronized cardioversion is *not* indicated in the treatment of VF or polymorphic VT. These rhythms require high-dose unsynchronized shock (i.e., defibrillation).

Unsynchronized cardioversion, or defibrillation, delivers electricity without regard to position in the cardiac cycle. Rhythms amenable to defibrillation include VF and pulseless VT. In addition, because it is very difficult to achieve reliable synchronization with polymorphic VT, the American Heart Association recommends using defibrillation rather than synchronized cardioversion for polymorphic VT.

When using the unsynchronized or defibrillating mode, a low-energy shock is more likely to result in VF or asystole than a high-energy shock. Because of this, low-energy shocks should never be used in the unsynchronized mode. When using a monophasic defibrillator, use 360 J. For the newer biphasic defibrillators, use the recommended device-specific dose. If no dose is recommended, use 200 J.

Take care when using an automated external defibrillator (AED), as these devices are not programmed to deliver synchronized shocks. AEDs are designed for patients without signs of life. AEDs will thus recommend an unsynchronized (defibrillating) shock for monomorphic VT, which could transform your patient from unstable to pulseless.

It is also an error to attempt synchronized defibrillation on a patient without pulses. Pushing the "sync" button on the defibrillator will essentially prevent a shock from being delivered until a QRS complex is identified. Since QRS complexes are unidentifiable in VF, a long delay to defibrillation can occur, or it may not occur at all. Because it is estimated that each minute without CPR results in a 7% to 10% decrease in survival, it is crucial that as little time as possible be wasted when preparing to deliver an electrical countershock. If the synchronization button has been selected in error, simply pushing the button again will shut the function off in most machines. When the synchronization function has been selected, a light on the "sync" button goes on.

Equipment is constantly being replaced in hospitals, due both to wear and tear as well as to technological advances. Familiarity with the location and the use of the "sync" function to select synchronized cardioversion rather than defibrillation can make the difference between a successful cardioversion and an unfortunate (and preventable) degeneration into a more malignant dysrhythmia through the R-on-T phenomenon.

What is the bottom line when it comes to synchronization? If the patient has pulses, perform synchronized cardioversion. If the patient is pulseless, defibrillate. The exception occurs in patients with polymorphic VT, who should receive defibrillation rather than synchronized cardioversion.

SUGGESTED READINGS

ECC Committee, Subcommittees and Task Forces of the American Heart Association. 2005 American Heart Association guidelines for cardiopulmonary resuscitation and emergency cardiovascular care. *Circulation*. 2005; 112(24 Suppl): IV1–203 [Epub Nov 28, 2005].

Lown B, Amarasingham R, Neuman J. New method for terminating cardiac arrhythmias. Use of synchronized capacitor discharge. *JAMA*. 1986;256(5):621–627.

Xavier LC, Memon A. Synchronized cardioversion of unstable supraventricular tachycardia resulting in ventricular fibrillation. *Ann Emerg Med*. 2004;44(2):178–180.

306

CONSIDER THE POTENTIAL CAUSES OF PULSELESS ELECTRICAL ACTIVITY AND TREAT ACCORDINGLY

TONY PEDUTO, MD

Pulseless electrical activity (PEA) is defined as organized cardiac electrical activity in the absence of a palpable pulse. It results when the myocardium is unable to generate sufficient force to sustain perfusion. Over the past few decades, the incidence of PEA as the presenting rhythm in cardiac arrest has increased, while the incidence of ventricular fibrillation has decreased. This relative increase in PEA may be a result of successful implementation of pre-hospital basic life support (BLS) and defibrillation programs.

PEA is an extreme form of shock, one where end-organ perfusion ceases entirely. Its causes can be categorized as cardiogenic (pump failure, which has multiple causes), obstructive (cardiac tamponade, tension pneumothorax, massive pulmonary embolus), hypovolemic (including massive hemorrhage), and distributive (profound vasodilatation, generally secondary to sepsis or drug overdose). The American Heart Association classifies the various causes of PEA into a useful mnemonic: "The H's and T's". The H's include (1) hypoxia, (2) hypovolemia, (3) hydrogen ion/acidosis, (4) hyperkalemia or hypokalemia, (5) hypoglycemia, and (6) hypothermia; the T's are (1) toxins, (2) tamponade, (3) tension pneumothorax, (4) thrombosis (coronary), and (5) thrombosis (pulmonary).

Virkkunen et al. recently demonstrated that we have a tendency to severely overestimate acute coronary syndrome as the etiology of PEA while discounting other common causes. Emergency physicians should neither assume that PEA is caused by massive pump failure nor rely upon epinephrine alone to reverse the underlying condition.

Once PEA is identified, a rapid, systematic assessment must be performed. Any available history should be obtained from available sources such as paramedics or bystanders. Attention should be paid to preceding events, recent trauma, medications, or drug paraphernalia on the scene. The physical examination should include a rapid search for airway obstruction, unequal breath sounds, jugular venous distension, shunts, indwelling catheters, unilateral or bilateral leg swelling, or any abnormal odor that would indicate ketoacidosis or toxin ingestion. All orifices should be examined for bleeding; a core temperature should also be obtained.

Treating the cause of PEA requires empiric treatment prior to definitive diagnosis. In addition to basic BLS, a normal saline bolus should be administered routinely, as should epinephrine and dextrose. Needle decompression and thoracostomy are required in cases of suspected pneumothorax. Narcan should be administered intravenously to all patients with suspected opioid overdose. Calcium chloride and sodium bicarbonate should be administered intravenously in any suspected renal failure patient, with the exception of patients who are known to be hypokalemic. Cases of suspected massive myocardial infarction or pulmonary embolism should receive systemic fibrinolytics. Pericardiocentesis should be performed in all cases of suspected cardiac tamponade. While emergency interventions are made on the basis of likelihood of a given pathology, they are often tantamount to "educated guesswork" and can only be confirmed by a positive response to treatment.

Bedside ultrasound (US) has revolutionized the accurate identification of causes of PEA. In 2005, Niendorff et al. validated the use of bedside US by non-expert sonographers to identify severe hypovolemia, tension pneumothorax, cardiac tamponade, and massive pulmonary embolus in cardiac arrest. Since 2005, numerous protocols for use of bedside US in cardiac arrest have been proposed. Furthermore, numerous studies have recently evaluated the use of point-of-care (POC) testing in critically ill patients in order to rapidly identify electrolyte and acid-base derangements at the bedside. Nevertheless, the successful resuscitation of coding patients with suspected electrolyte abnormalities should never be delayed for POC test results. Notably, abnormal POC test results could potentially increase liability, if the electrolyte abnormality documented is not adequately treated prior to the cessation of resuscitative efforts.

Failure to identify and rapidly treat the cause of PEA results in inevitable death. Emergency physicians are experts at resuscitation, which includes correctly diagnosing and treating all causes of PEA.

SUGGESTED READINGS

American Heart Association. *ACLS Provider Manual*. Dallas, TX: American Heart Association; 2006:62.

Breitkreutz R, Walcher F, Seeger FH, et al. Focused echocardiographic evaluation in resuscitation management: Concept of an advanced life support-conformed algorithm. *Crit Care Med*. 2007;35(5 Suppl):S150–S161.

Kost GJ, Vu HT, Inn M, et al. Multicenter study of whole-blood creatinine, total carbon dioxide content, and chemistry profiling for laboratory and point-of-care testing in critical care in the United States. *Crit Care Med*. 2000;28(7):2379–2389.

Niendorff DF, Rassias AJ, Palac R, et al. Rapid cardiac ultrasound of inpatients suffering PEA arrest performed by nonexpert sonographers. *Resuscitation*. 2005;67(1):81–87.

O'Beirne P, Robotis DA, Rosenthal L. Pulseless electrical activity. eMedicine.com, May 11, 2009. Available at: http://www.emedicine.com/med/topic2963.htm

Parish DC, Dinesh Chandra KM, Dane FC. Success changes the problem: Why ventricular fibrillation is declining, why pulseless electrical activity is emerging, and what to do about it. *Resuscitation*. 2003;58(1):31–35.

Virkkunen I, Paasio L, Ryynänen S, et al. Pulseless electrical activity and unsuccessful out-of-hospital resuscitation: What is the cause of death? *Resuscitation*. 2008;77(2): 207–210 [Epub Feb 4, 2008].

307

MINIMIZE INTERRUPTIONS IN CHEST COMPRESSIONS WHILE MANAGING PATIENTS IN CARDIAC ARREST

TONY PEDUTO, MD AND JORGE A. FERNANDEZ, MD,
FAAEM, FACEP

Failure to perform continuous chest compressions during cardiac arrest increases the likelihood of death or poor neurologic outcome. Multiple well-designed clinical trials have shown improved outcomes with early and high-quality chest compressions. Interrupting chest compressions during cardiac arrest resuscitation for any reason degrades the quality of resuscitation and places the patient's recovery in jeopardy.

American Heart Association (AHA) and European Resuscitation Council (ERC) guidelines for cardiopulmonary resuscitation (CPR) have been updated recently to emphasize the primary importance of high-quality, uninterrupted chest compressions during cardiac arrest. The trend has been to simplify existing protocols and to place more emphasis on the "basics" of resuscitation. This emphasis on Basic Life Support (BLS) measures follows data suggesting that the addition of Advanced Life Support (ALS) to BLS-based emergency medical services (EMS) systems does not improve outcome in out-of-hospital cardiac arrest. To date, the only links in the AHA's "Chain of Survival" that have improved patient outcomes in large prospective studies are (1) early CPR and (2) early defibrillation. Recent data drive home the necessity of high-quality uninterrupted chest compressions by making the striking suggestion that epinephrine, the prototypical ALS drug, is indeed useless without good quality CPR. Another recent study documented 100% return of spontaneous circulation (ROSC) in animals receiving >80 compressions per min compared with 10% ROSC in animals receiving <80 compressions per min during the first 3 min of CPR.

The most common reasons for interruption of chest compressions during CPR are (1) ventilation maneuvers, (2) rhythm analysis, (3) pulse checks, (4) shock delivery, and (5) human error. Researchers refer to interrupted chest compressions as "no flow time"; circulatory standstill causes cessation of myocardial and cerebral oxygen delivery. Recent AHA and ERC modifications include (1) initiation of CPR before ventilation, (2) increased compression to ventilation (C:V) ratio from 15:2 to 30:2, (3) reducing shock delivery to one attempt at any given time, and (4) resumption of CPR immediately following shock for 2 min without pausing for pulse checks or rhythm analysis. These modified guidelines have been shown to reduce "no-flow time" by 50%.

Recently, a modified BLS protocol called "cardiocerebral resuscitation" has been shown to even further improve neurologic outcomes in cardiac arrest. This technique goes beyond current recommendations in emphasizing the importance of chest compressions over ventilation. In a large study published in 2008, after instituting the cardiocerebral resuscitation protocol, survival to hospital discharge increased from 20% to 47% and neurologically intact survival increased from 15% to 39%.

Research is currently focusing on even more ways to minimize interruption of chest compressions. Berger et al. have recently published a study demonstrating the technology to acquire rhythm analysis without interrupting compressions. Lloyd et al. have recently demonstrated the safety of defibrillation *during* chest compressions. Eliminating interruptions in CPR for rhythm analysis and defibrillation may improve patient outcomes even further.

In summary, high-quality uninterrupted chest compressions are the foundation of BLS protcols; ALS protocols will fail unless they are accompanied by high-quality BLS measures. Interruptions in chest compressions should be minimized or avoided entirely in order to maintain circulation.

SUGGESTED READINGS

Berger RD, Palazzolo J, Halperin H. Rhythm discrimination during uninterrupted CPR using motion artifact reduction system. *Resuscitation*. 2007;75(1):145–152 [Epub Apr 30, 2007].

Hostler D, Rittenberger JC, Roth R, et al. Increased chest compression to ventilation ratio improves delivery of CPR. *Resuscitation*. 2007;74(3):446–52 [Epub Mar 23, 2007].

Jäntti H, Kuisma M, Uusaro A. The effects of changes to the ERC resuscitation guidelines on no flow time and cardiopulmonary resuscitation quality: A randomised controlled study on manikins. *Resuscitation*. 2007;75(2):338–344 [Epub Jul 12, 2007].

Kellum MJ, Kennedy KW, Barney R, et al. Cardiocerebral resuscitation improves neurologically intact survival of patients with out-of-hospital cardiac arrest. *Ann Emerg Med*. 2008;52(3):244–252 [Epub Mar 286, 2008].

Kellum MJ, Kennedy KW, Ewy GA. Cardiocerebral resuscitation improves survival of patients with out-of-hospital cardiac arrest. *Am J Med*. 2006;119(4):335–340.

Lloyd MS, Heeke B, Walter PF, et al. Hands-on defibrillation: An analysis of electrical current flow through rescuers in direct contact with patients during biphasic external defibrillation. *Circulation*. 2008;117(19):2510–2514 [Epub May 5, 2008].

Pytte M, Kramer–Johansen J, Eilevstjønn J, et al. Haemodynamic effects of adrenaline (epinephrine) depend on chest compression quality during cardiopulmonary resuscitation in pigs. *Resuscitation*. 2006;71(3):369–378 [Epub Oct 4, 2006].

Stiell IG, Wells GA, Field B, et al. Advanced cardiac life support in out-of-hospital cardiac arrest. *N Engl J Med*. 2004;351(7):647–656.

Yannopoulos D, Aufderheide T. Acute management of sudden cardiac death in adults based upon the new CPR guidelines. *Europace*. 2007;9(1):2–9.

Yu T, Weil MH, Tang W, et al. Adverse outcomes of interrupted precordial compression during automated defibrillation. *Circulation*. 2002;106(3):368–372.

308

DO NOT RELY ON ABNORMAL VITAL SIGNS AND TREMOR TO DIAGNOSE ALCOHOL WITHDRAWAL

JONATHAN S. ANDERSON, MD

Alcohol-related complaints make up a large percentage of today's emergency department visits. Rough estimates suggest that every year there are around half a million episodes of withdrawal requiring pharmacologic treatment in the United States. Dangerous withdrawal occurs more often in patients with heavier drinking histories, but there is a large degree of unexplained individual variation. Withdrawal syndromes can occur while the patient is still intoxicated (from a laboratory standing). Some authors report withdrawal in patients with serum alcohol levels still two to four times above the legal driving limit. All emergency physicians are familiar with the classic picture of an alcoholic after a day or two of sober living, who arrives anxious, tremulous, and hypertensive. However, alcohol withdrawal is a spectrum of disease with multiple, and potentially vague, presentations.

Alcohol withdrawal can be divided into four separate syndromes: minor withdrawal symptoms (or alcoholic tremulousness), alcoholic hallucinations, withdrawal seizures (or rum fits), and delirium tremens (DT). These syndromes can overlap, but often patients present with the key features of just one syndrome.

Alcoholic tremulousness is perhaps the most common form of withdrawal, and also the most easily recognized. It presents a collection of signs and symptoms including tachycardia, hypertension, diaphoresis, anxiety, tremor, insomnia, agitation, and GI upset. In general, the patient is agitated but otherwise has a normal mental status. Classically, the symptoms occur between 6 and 48 h after the last drink. A patient with tolerance may still have an elevated serum alcohol level. There are reports of cases of this type of withdrawal as far as 7 days out from the last drink.

Alcoholic hallucinations are generally visual but can be auditory or tactile. They occur within 12 and 24 h of abstinence and resolve within 48 h. They are often confused with DT; alcoholic hallucinations are not associated with a delirium or otherwise clouded sensorium. They are discrete and specific hallucinations. These hallucinations can occur with no other signs or symptoms, including normal vital signs.

Withdrawal seizures are classically single, generalized tonic-clonic seizures that occur in patients with long alcohol abuse histories within 2 days of the last drink. They can occur as early as 2 h from the last drink and, like alcoholic hallucinations, can occur without the classic signs of tremor and altered vital signs preceding the seizure.

DT is a constellation of symptoms that occur in about 5% of alcohol withdrawal cases. There is a significant risk of morbidity and mortality when dealing with DT. The presentation generally includes disorientation and delirium, hallucinations, tachycardia and hypertension, fever, and diaphoresis. Typically, they occur 2 to 4 days after the last drink and can last up to a week. Risk factors include prior DT, older age, and greater drinking history.

Thankfully, the treatment of all four withdrawal syndromes involves the same class of drugs: benzodiazepines. The pathophysiology of alcohol withdrawal is not fully understood, but we do know that reduced neurotransmission in gamma-aminobutyric acid (GABA) pathways likely causes a number of symptoms and probably triggers the seizures that can be part of alcohol withdrawal. It is likely that the GABA activity of benzodiazepines is the reason for their protective effects. Not surprisingly, benzodiazepines offer a huge benefit versus placebo treatment. Authors differ over their choice of agent, but many agree that the long-acting benzodiazepines such as diazepam and chlordiazepoxide offer easier dosing and a smoother withdrawal. Patients with hepatic dysfunction may benefit from using lorazepam. Regardless of the choice of a drug, symptom-triggered therapy is superior to a fixed schedule of dosing.

Alcohol withdrawal includes a spectrum of signs and symptoms from minor to life threatening. The classic picture of alcoholic tremor or DT is fairly easy to recognize. However, remember that a patient with a single seizure or with simple visual hallucinations could also be in alcohol withdrawal without manifesting the classic symptoms of tremor and tachycardia. Keeping an open mind is the key to successful diagnosis and treatment.

Suggested Readings

Etherington JM. Emergency management of acute alcohol problems. Part 1: uncomplicated withdrawal. *Can Fam Physician*. 1996;42:2186–2190.

Kosten TR, O'Connor PG. Management of drug and alcohol withdrawal. *N Engl J Med*. 2003;348(18):1786–1795.

Ntais C, Pakos E, Kyzas P, et al. Benzodiazepines for alcohol withdrawal. *Cochrane Database Syst Rev*. 2005;(3):CD0050063.

Schuckit MA, Tipp JE, Reich T, et al. The histories of withdrawal convulsions and delirium tremens in 1648 alcohol dependent subjects. *Addiction*. 1995;90(10):1335–1347.

309

DO NOT RELY ON THE PRESENCE OF TACHYCARDIA TO CONFIRM ANTICHOLINERGIC SYNDROME

EDWARD KIMLIN, MD

Anticholinergic syndrome can occur after the ingestion of several over-the-counter preparations, prescription pharmaceuticals, illegal drugs, and naturally occurring substances, including antihistamines, tricyclic antidepressants, scopolamine, heroin, atropine, and jimson weed. While tachycardia is a classic, early, and particularly reliable manifestation of anticholinergic toxicity, its absence certainly does not exclude anticholinergic syndrome.

Anticholinergic poisoning produces a wide variety of signs and symptoms due to the broad distribution of acetylcholine receptors throughout the human body, including the central nervous system (CNS) and peripheral organs. Toxicologists frequently make the distinction between the central anticholinergic syndrome, which is the alteration of mental status due to CNS muscarinic blockade, and the peripheral anticholinergic syndrome, which is the byproduct of the antagonism of muscarinic receptors outside the CNS.

Central muscarinic antagonism produces a variety of neuropsychiatric manifestations, including anxiety, agitation, dysarthria, confusion, disorientation, visual hallucinations, bizarre behavior, delirium, psychosis (typically in the form of paranoia), coma, and seizures. Central anticholinergic toxicity frequently exhibits a characteristic pattern of mumbling speech, agitation that is redirectable to appropriate response to questioning, and the observation that the patient picks at invisible objects.

Alternatively, peripheral anticholinergic toxicity refers to the constellation of signs and symptoms observed following the antagonism of peripheral nervous system muscarinic receptors. One of the earliest and most frequently identified hallmarks of peripheral anticholinergic toxicity is tachycardia, which is due to decreased vagal tone on the atrioventricular node, and, in some ingestions, the inhibition of synaptic norepinephrine uptake (Thanacoody et al.). Other common signs of peripheral anticholinergic poisoning include antimuscarinic anhidrosis with secondary anhidrotic hyperthermia and compensatory peripheral vasodilatation (e.g., "dry as a bone," "hot as a hare," and "red as a beet"), antimuscarinic nonreactive mydriasis (e.g., "blind as a bat"), antimuscarinic gastrointestinal disturbances, and antimuscarinic urinary retention (e.g., "full as a flask").

Although the central and peripheral components of the anticholinergic syndrome typically occur concomitantly, the central phenomenon can occur with minimal or no peripheral signs. Thus, reliance on peripheral anticholinergic findings can often mislead the clinician. One common mistake involves inflexibly grouping anticholinergic poisoning with tachycardia. Due to the wide variety of agents that cause anticholinergic toxicity, the broad distribution of acetylcholine receptors throughout the body, and the discrepancy between central and peripheral manifestations, the lack of tachycardia does not exclude an anticholinergic toxidrome. For example, tricyclic antidepressants can cause atrioventricular block, thereby preventing anticholinergic tachycardia. Moreover, diphenhydramine poisonings tend to favor central rather than peripheral symptoms, resulting in a bizarre behavior in the absence of tachycardia.

The take-home lesson: while tachycardia is a classic, early, and common manifestation of anticholinergic toxicity, its absence certainly does not rule out anticholinergic toxicity and must be weighed against the preponderance of clinical evidence in making the diagnosis.

SUGGESTED READINGS

Köppel C, Ibe K, Tenczer J. Clinical symptomatology of diphenhydramine overdose: An evaluation of 136 cases in 1982 to 1985. *J Toxicol Clin Toxicol.* 1987;25(1–2):53–70.

Pragst F, Herre S, Bakdash A. Poisonings with diphenhydramine: A survey of 68 clinical and 55 death cases. *Forensic Sci Int.* 2006;161(2–3):189–197.

Schonwald S. *Medical Toxicology: A Synopsis and Study Guide.* Philadelphia, PA: Lippincott Williams & Wilkins; 2001:893.

Su M, Goldman M. *Anticholinergic Poisoning.* UpToDate. 2007

Thanacoody HK, Thomas SH. Tricyclic antidepressant poisoning: Cardiovascular toxicity. *Toxicol Rev.* 2005;24(3):205–214 [Review].

310

CONSIDER β-BLOCKER OR CALCIUM CHANNEL BLOCKER TOXICITY IN THE PATIENT WITH UNEXPLAINED BRADYCARDIA OR HYPOTENSION

LAURA BURKE, MD

Toxic ingestion of β-blockers (BBs) and calcium channel blockers (CCBs) may cause bradycardia, dysrhythmias, hypotension, and even cardiogenic shock. Both agents interfere with calcium entry into myocardial cells, inhibiting myocyte contractility, action potential generation in pacemaker cells, and vascular smooth muscle tone. Central nervous system affects such as altered mental status, seizures, or coma may be seen, especially in the setting of ingestion of lipophilic BBs with membrane-stabilizing activity (carvedilol, propranolol, labetalol, and metoprolol). It is crucial to consider medication toxicity in these patients and to promptly institute treatment to reverse the hemodynamic instability.

A number of ECG abnormalities may be seen in BB and CCB toxicity; bradycardia and first-degree atrioventricular block are most common. QRS prolongation may be present when BBs that block sodium channels (propranolol) are ingested. Sotalol ingestion may cause QT prolongation and ventricular dysrhythmias.

Atropine may reverse hypotension and bradycardia but generally has a limited role. Sodium bicarbonate may improve the acidemia that potentiates CCB toxicity as well as the QRS widening commonly seen with sotalol and BBs with sodium channel activity. Transcutaneous or transvenous pacing may be necessary for heart block or persistent bradycardia with poor perfusion. Gastric decontamination and activated charcoal are of greatest benefit within 2 h of ingestion or following the ingestion of sustained-release preparations.

The administration of intravenous calcium may overcome the receptor antagonism by CCBs and improve negative inotropy in BB overdose. One suggested dosing regimen is the administration of a 0.6 mL/kg of 10% calcium gluconate bolus over 5 to 10 min followed by a continuous infusion (0.6 to 1.5 mL/kg/h) of calcium gluconate.

Glucagon increases myocyte cAMP independently of β-adrenergic receptors and has been shown in case studies and animal models to improve heart rate and contractility in the setting of both BB and CCB toxicities. The suggested dose is a 3 to 5 mg or 50 to 150 μg/kg bolus repeated in 3 to 5 min and followed by an infusion at 0.05 to 0.10 mg/kg/h titrated to heart rate and blood pressure. Vasopressors may be required in high doses to support heart rate and blood pressure, although controversy exists over which agent is superior.

The administration of both insulin and dextrose has also been reported to treat CCB and BB overdoses. The administration of insulin is thought to promote the utilization of carbohydrate by myocardial cells, improving cardiac metabolism and function. No standard dosing regimen has been defined, but one review suggests an insulin bolus of 1 U/kg followed by a continuous infusion of 0.5 U/kg/h. In the absence of severe hyperglycemia, a concomitant dextrose regimen of a 25-g bolus followed by a continuous infusion of 0.5 g/kg/h is suggested. Serum glucose should be monitored every 30 min to 1 h and the medications titrated to the heart rate and blood pressure.

Nonpharmacologic treatments of CCB and BB toxicities including aortic balloon pump and extracorporeal membrane oxygenation (ECMO) have been reported in severe, refractory cases of CCB and BB toxicities. No CCBs are amenable to dialysis, but selected BBs (atenolol, nadolol, and sotalol) may be dialyzed in cases of severe toxicity.

All patients with evidence of hemodynamic instability following a BB or CCB overdose should be admitted to an intensive care unit for monitoring. One retrospective study of children with CCB ingestion recommended an observation period of 3 h in asymptomatic children following an ingestion of immediate-release preparation and 14 h for extended-release preparations. Studies of adults have suggested that symptoms typically develop within 4 to 6 h of BB overdose, but there is no general duration of observation for ingestion of either class of drug in adults or children. Patients who have ingested sotalol, extended-release preparations, or other medications or substances should be observed for an extended period.

In summary, it is crucial to consider BB and CCB toxicities in a patient with bradycardia, hypotension, cardiogenic shock, or altered mental status. Pitfalls to avoid include failure to evaluate for coingestants, to treat concomitant metabolic abnormalities, or to observe for a sufficient period of time.

SUGGESTED READINGS

Bailey B. Glucagon in beta-blocker and calcium channel blocker overdoses: A systematic review. *J Toxicol Clin Toxicol*. 2003;41:595–602.

Belson MG, Gorman SE, Sullivan K, et al. Calcium channel blocker ingestions in children. *Am J Emerg Med*. 2000;18:81–86.

Kerns W II. Management of beta-adrenergic blocker and calcium channel antagonist toxicity. *Emerg Med Clin North Am*. 2007;25:309–331.

Love JN, Enlow B, Howell, JM. Electrocardiographic changes associated with beta-blocker toxicity. *Ann Emerg Med*. 2002;40:603–610.

Love JN, Howell JM, Litovitz TL, et al. Acute beta blocker overdose: Factors associated with the development of cardiovascular morbidity. *J Toxicol Clin Toxicol*. 2000;38(3):275–281.

Ramoska EA, Spiller HA, Winter M, et al. A one-year evaluation of calcium channel blocker overdoses: Toxicity and treatment. *Ann Emerg Med*. 1993;22:196–200.

311

BE WARY OF DRUG-DRUG INTERACTIONS WHEN TREATING COCAINE-INTOXICATED PATIENTS

JON B. COLE, MD

Cocaine is a complex pharmacological agent, with significant drug–drug interactions. When treating intoxicated patients, careful consideration of your pharmacologic therapy will lead to optimal care of the patient. Cocaine has a complex mechanism of action. It blocks the reuptake of biogenic amines, especially dopamine, norepinephrine, and epinephrine, and increases excitatory amino acid concentrations in the brain. Cocaine also blocks sodium channels in myocardial tissue and is classified as a Vaughn-Williams type I(A) antidysrhythmic agent. The original medicinal use of cocaine was as a local anesthetic. Subsequent local anesthetics, such as procaine, were developed to mimic the sodium channel–blocking capabilities of cocaine.

The metabolism of cocaine is complex. Approximately half of a dose of cocaine is hydrolyzed to form benzoylecognine (BE), a potent vasoconstrictor and the most common metabolite screened for on a urine drug screen. Plasma cholinesterase (PChE) is also involved in the metabolism of cocaine and converts active cocaine to a minimally active metabolite. Lastly, smoked cocaine produces a unique metabolite from the pyrolysis of the drug called anhydro-ecognine methyl ester (AEME) that is a direct muscarinic (M_2) agonist. This particular property of smoked cocaine may be the underlying cause of asthma exacerbation commonly seen with smoked cocaine.

Because patients intoxicated on cocaine often require intubation, it is important to consider the potential interactions of drugs used during rapid sequence intubation. The use of succinylcholine as a paralytic is relatively contraindicated. Cocaine intoxication is associated with an increased incidence of rhabdomyolysis. Hyperkalemia, from rhabdomyolysis and its subsequent life-threatening arrhythmias, may be exacerbated by succinylcholine's depolarizing properties. Both succinylcholine and a significant portion of cocaine are metabolized by PChE, which can prolong both cocaine intoxication and the effects of succinylcholine. The use of a nondepolarizing agent such as rocuronium would avoid these potential complications.

Cocaine is a documented arrhythmogenic agent. This is partially due to its sodium channel–blocking properties, which manifest as prolongation of the QRS intervals and can lead to Brugada pattern changes as well. Cocaine also blocks potassium channels, leading to an increase in the QTc interval which can progress to torsades de pointes. Additionally, as a sympathomimetic agent, cocaine will increase ventricular irritability and lower the threshold for ventricular fibrillation. Other class IA antidysrhythmics, such as procainamide, should be avoided because they may exacerbate the effects of cocaine and slow its metabolism. Both lidocaine and sodium bicarbonate have been used safely in patients with cocaine intoxication and wide-complex tachycardias. Other than antiarrhythmic selection, there is no deviation in the treatment of cocaine-associated arrhythmias.

Patients intoxicated on cocaine commonly present with agitation. If cocaine intoxication is known or strongly suspected, the use of butyrophenones (e.g., haloperidol) and phenothiazines (e.g., promethazine) is relatively contraindicated. Animal models demonstrate increased toxicity (lowered seizure threshold) and increased lethality. Both agents also prolong the QTc interval. The optimal sedative medications in the cocaine-intoxicated patient are parenteral benzodiazepines. Midazolam and diazepam are preferable to lorazepam, as they have a more rapid onset and are thus more titratable.

Perhaps the greatest area of controversy in cocaine-associated drug interactions involves the concomitant use of β-blockers (BBs). In theory, the use of BBs with cocaine leads to unopposed α-adrenergic stimulation causing increased systemic arterial pressure and coronary vasospasm. This was substantiated by Lange et al. in a study where they performed a randomized double-blind placebo controlled trial in which patients undergoing cardiac catheterization received cocaine and either saline or propranolol. Patients receiving propranolol had a significant decrease in coronary artery diameter and no significant decrease in arterial pressure. A similar study was performed with labetalol given its unique α-blocking properties. This study revealed a reduction in mean arterial pressure, but persistent coronary vasospasm. This is not unanticipated when considering that labetalol has β to alpha blockade ratios of 3:1, when taken orally, and 7:1, when taken intravenously.

By contrast, there is evidence that BBs may actually be beneficial. In a retrospective cohort study of 363 patients admitted with positive urine cocaine tests, BBs were associated with a statistically significant reduction in the incidence of myocardial infarction (MI). The incidence of death was also much lower in the BB group.

Controversy continues; however, it is probably still wise to recommend avoiding the use of BBs in the cocaine-intoxicated patient in the ED. Hypertensive crisis should be treated with sodium nitroprusside. If this is inadequate, IV phentolamine (a short-acting alpha blocker), dosed at 1 to 2.5 mg IV to titration, can be used. If a BB must be used acutely to lower blood pressure, esmolol would be a prudent choice given its extremely short half-life of 9 min.

Currently, sodium nitroprusside should still be considered the first-line therapy for treating a hypertensive crisis in cocaine-intoxicated patients. If this is inadequate, IV phentolamine can be added. If a BB must be used, esmolol would be a prudent choice given its extremely short half-life.

KEY POINTS

- Succinylcholine is relatively contraindicated.
- Lidocaine and sodium bicarbonate are good antiarrhythmic choices.
- Benzodiazepines are the agent of choice for agitation and chest pain.
- Concomitant use of BBs is strongly discouraged. Hypertensive crisis should be treated with sodium nitroprusside and, if necessary, phentolamine. If a BB must be used, esmolol would be the ideal choice.

SUGGESTED READINGS

Boehrer JB, Moliterno DJ, Willard JE, et al. Influence of labetalol on cocaine-induced coronary vasoconstriction in humans. *Am J Med.* 1993;94(6):608–610.

Counselman FL, McLaughlin EW, Kardon EM, et al. Creatine phosphokinase elevation in patients presenting to the emergency department with cocaine-related complaints. *Am J Emerg Med.* 1997;15(3):221–223.

Dattilo PB, Hailpern SM, Fearon K, et al. Beta-blockers are associated with reduced risk of myocardial infarction after cocaine use. *Ann Emerg Med.* 2008;51(2):117–125.

Lange RA, Cigarroa RG, Flores ED, et al. Potentiation of cocaine-induced coronary vasoconstriction by beta-adrenergic blockade. *Ann Intern Med.* 1990;112(12):897–903.

Page RL II, Utz KJ, Wolfel EE. Should beta-blockers be used in the treatment of cocaine-associated acute coronary syndrome? *Ann Pharmacother.* 2007;41(12):2008–2013.

312

IN SUSPECTED TRICYCLIC ANTIDEPRESSANT OVERDOSE, START SODIUM BICARBONATE AS SOON AS THE QRS DURATION IS OVER 100 MS

ANDREA DUGAS, MD

Tricyclic antidepressant (TCA) overdoses can proceed quickly to a fatal arrhythmia within minutes to hours after presentation. Due to the urgent nature of this toxicity, drug levels are often unavailable and are not used to guide emergency treatment. Conversely, electrocardiography (ECG) can be performed quickly and repeated throughout the hospital course as the clinical picture changes.

Due to the lack of laboratory data in an acute setting, the suspicion of TCA toxicity comes from clinical diagnosis and associated EKG changes. In cases of fatal TCA overdose, the most common initial symptoms in serious toxicity include coma, tachycardia, hypotension, respiratory depression, and seizures. Other signs of TCA toxicity include mental status changes and typical anticholinergic effects such as dry mouth, flushing, dilated pupils, urinary retention, hyperthermia, and tachycardia. Mental status can vary from agitation, confusion, or hallucinations to sedation, coma, and seizures.

Cardiac toxicity is the most common cause of death and usually develops <3 to 6 h from the time of presentation. Sinus tachycardia is the earliest and most common arrhythmia but does not predict toxicity as it is often from the anticholinergic properties of these drugs. Cardiac toxicity is associated with ventricular dysrhythmias, heart block, bradyarrhythmias, tachyarrhythmias, and asystole.

TCAs cause cardiac toxicity via blockade of the fast-acting sodium channels, which prolongs the QRS complex. This prolongation can be increased by concurrent acidosis caused by the medication itself, hypotension, and seizures. The other ECG finding associated with TCA toxicity is right axis deviation of the terminal 40 ms of the QRS complex. Seen as a terminal R wave in aVR, or a terminal S wave in I or aVL, a terminal QRS axis between 130 and 270 degrees is a sensitive and specific indicator of TCA toxicity.

A major prospective study showed that no patient with a QRS duration of <100 ms developed seizures or ventricular dysrhythmias. For patients with a QRS duration above 100 ms, the incidence of seizures was 34% and that of ventricular dysrhythmias was 14%. Ventricular dysrhythmias were only seen in patients whose QRS duration was longer than 160 ms, and that same group had a 50% incidence of seizures. The risk of toxicity appropriately decreased with the normalization of the QRS interval.

Signs of cardiac toxicity appear early in the course of a TCA overdose. Over 80% of cases have reached their maximum QRS duration by the time of presentation, and the remainder will reach it within 3 h. QRS widening can develop rapidly, so serial ECGs must be checked frequently, especially if the patient is showing other signs of toxicity, such as mental status changes. Half of in-hospital fatalities from TCA overdose develop toxicity within the first hour.

The treatment of TCA overdoses focuses initially on resuscitation, decontamination if appropriate, and using sodium bicarbonate to preserve cardiac function and prevent seizures. Sodium bicarbonate works by a number of mechanisms. It increases the serum sodium concentration, corrects the acidosis, and decreases the serum concentration of TCAs by increasing protein binding. Sodium bicarbonate is indicated for ventricular dysrhythmias, refractory hypotension, marked acidosis, cardiac arrest, and ECG changes, including a QRS duration of >100 ms or a terminal right axis deviation of >120 degrees. If a patient has a previously documented QRS duration longer than 100 ms, sodium bicarbonate treatment can be deferred until the QRS duration increases from its previous length. Recommended treatment includes starting with an IV bolus of 50 mEq of sodium bicarbonate and repeating it as necessary with a target serum pH of 7.45 to 7.55.

Hypotension is a common manifestation in TCA overdoses, and initial treatment includes correction of acidosis and dehydration using sodium bicarbonate and intravenous fluids. In the persistently hypotensive patient, the choice of a vasopressor remains unclear. Numerous agents have been suggested for TCA overdose, including norepinephrine, dopamine, isoproterenol, and glucagon. Concern over the use of dopamine, which relies on presynaptic norepinephrine stores possibly depleted by the mechanism of TCAs, has not been conclusively shown. Studies in humans with direct comparison are limited, and the choice of a vasopressor remains controversial.

TCA toxicity is both rapid and fatal demanding swift diagnosis and treatment. ECG changes assist with both diagnosis and directing treatment, so they should be attained early and often in patients with an appropriate clinical suspicion. QRS prolongation beyond 100 ms occurs quickly and is associated with severe toxicity. Early sodium bicarbonate therapy for a QRS >100 ms can reverse the prolongation and prevent seizures and ventricular dysrhythmias.

SUGGESTED READINGS

Boehnert MT, Lovejoy FH. Value of the QRS duration versus the serum drug level in predicting seizures and ventricular arrhythmias after an acute overdose of tricyclic antidepressants. *N Engl J Med.* 1985;313:474–479.

Callaham M, Kassel D. Epidemiology of fatal tricyclic antidepressant ingestion: Implications for management. *Ann Emerg Med.* 1985;14:1–9.

Haddad LM, Shannon MW, Winchester JF. *Clinical Management of Poisoning and Drug Overdose.* 3rd ed. Philadelphia, PA: W.B. Saunders Company; 1998.

Liebelt EL, Ulrich A, Francis PD, et al. Serial electrocardiogram changes in the acute tricyclic antidepressant overdoses. *Crit Care Med.* 1997;25:1721–1726.

Niemann JT, Bessen HA, Rothstein RJ, et al. Electrocardiographic criteria for tricyclic antidepressant cardiotoxicity. *Am J Cardiol.* 1986;57:1154–1159.

313

DIGIBIND IS YOUR FRIEND ... DO NOT LET IT BECOME YOUR ENEMY

RUSSELL BERGER, MD

Digoxin toxicity occurs in 20% of people treated with the drug. Recognizing and treating this toxicity is an important part of emergency practice.

Acute digoxin toxicity is characterized by profound nausea, vomiting, bradycardia, hyperkalemia, and ECG changes. Initially, ischemic appearing T-wave inversions may be present. These T-wave changes are then frequently followed by QT interval shortening. Later ECG changes include scooping of the ST segment and an increase in the amplitude of the U wave. Accelerated junctional rhythms and bidirectional ventricular tachycardias are relatively specific for cardiac glycoside toxicity, and their presence should suggest this condition until proven otherwise.

Digoxin levels may be elevated due to intrinsic host conditions or iatrogenically. Renal insufficiency, for example, impairs digoxin clearance. Dehydration, too, carries the risk of artificially concentrating digoxin levels, potentiating toxicity. Patients who, for example, have received antibiotics, particularly macrolides, may be at increased risk for toxicity as these agents deplete gut flora responsible for partial breakdown of digoxin.

In addition, agents such as quinidine and procainamide, part of the family of IA antidysrhythmics, depress AV nodal conduction and exacerbate digoxin toxicity.

Hypokalemia, hypercalcemia, and hypomagnesemia predispose to increased sensitivity to digoxin and, when present, may exacerbate toxicity. Underlying cardiac disease, ischemia, cardiomyopathy, and conduction disturbances play a role in sensitizing patients to the toxic effects of digoxin.

In acute intoxications, digoxin is effectively adsorbed by activated charcoal if ingestion has occurred within 6 to 8 h. Associated bradycardia responds to atropine. Hemodialysis and hemoperfusion have no role in the treatment of digoxin toxicity.

As emergency doctors, we are fortunate to have digibind. Digibind is indicated for the treatment of digoxin overdose when there is hemodynamic instability, life-threatening arrhythmias, severe bradycardia, plasma potassium concentrations above 5 mEq/L, plasma digoxin concentrations above 10 ng/mL, ingestion of >10 mg of digoxin in adults and >4 mg in children, or in the presence of a digoxin toxic rhythm in the setting of an elevated dig level.

Digibind works by binding molecules of digoxin, making these molecules unavailable for binding with their receptors. There are no contraindications to digibind administration. However, anaphylactic and hypersensitivity reactions have been reported.

After the administration of digibind, one may expect clinical improvement within 30 min. Roughly 5 to 10 vials of digibind should be empirically administered to a patient in overdose. Those individuals who rely on digoxin for its inotropic support may develop cardiogenic shock when receiving this agent.

As digitalis toxicity may produce significant electrolyte disturbance and acid-base changes, patients should be monitored in an intensive care unit. Serial EKGs, vital sign checks, and chemistries should be obtained. Digoxin levels should be checked every 3 to 4 h after an acute ingestion.

When digibind is administered, the measured serum level of digoxin may be markedly elevated prompting grave concerns. This is a reflection of the immunoassay used to determine the serum digoxin and not a reflection of bioavailable digoxin. The immunoassay measures both bound and unbound digoxin, and therefore serum digoxin levels will appear markedly elevated as a function of the measurement of digibind-digoxin adducts.

Still another consideration associated with digibind administration is significant alterations in potassium levels associated with its use. As digibind captures digoxin, poisoned Na/K ATPases recover function. As a result, this transporter works to bring serum potassium back into affected cells. In a patient with normal renal function, this period of elevated serum potassium is met with an increased renal excretion of potassium. Thus, when the Na/K ATPase is reactivated, the patient may rapidly become hypokalemic.

Digoxin has held a long place in treating heart disease, but its therapeutic window is very narrow. Toxicity is common, and complications can be lethal. As emergency physicians, we must be prepared to recognize and effectively address digoxin toxicity. Digibind is a highly effective agent for digoxin toxicity, but it is easy to get into a situation where your patient's potassium bottoms out, particularly in patients with normal renal function. The bottom line is keep an eye on your patient's potassium level and do not be deceived by apparently elevated levels of digoxin in the face of digibind administration.

SUGGESTED READINGS

Goldfrank LR, Flomenbaum NE, Lewin NA, et al., eds. *Goldfrank's Toxicologic Emergencies.* 8th ed. New York, NY: McGraw Hill; 2006.

Greenberg MI. Digibind, an important antidote, if used properly. *Emerg Med News.* 2002;24(2):18, 21–22. Available at: http://www.em-news.com/pt/re/emmednews/fulltext.00132981–200202000–00015.htm;jsessionid = LwLDWG7PpGjTV7wTyKyqXY hkvdr62Ph21s4jq421dpSMRcgdx4Ws!2126095447!181195629!8091!-1.

Nuhad I. Digitalis poisoning. UpToDate.com. Jan 23, 2008. Available at: http://www.uptodate.com/home/index.html.

Schreiber D. Digitalis toxicity. eMedicine.com. Jan 3, 2006. Available at: http://www.emedicine.com/EMERG/topic137.htm.

Tintinalli JE, Kelen GD, Stapczynski JS, et al., eds. *Emergency Medicine: A Comprehensive Study Guide.* 5th ed. New York, NY: McGraw-Hill; 2003.

Wolfson AB, Hendey GW, Hendry PL, et al., eds. *Harwood Nuss' Clinical Practice of Emergency Medicine.* Philadelphia, PA: Lippincott Williams & Wilkins; 2005.

314

BEWARE OF CARDIAC COMPLICATIONS WITH INTRAVENOUS ADMINISTRATION OF PHENYTOIN AND FOSPHENYTOIN

RUSSELL BERGER, MD

Phenytoin works by blocking voltage-sensitive and frequency-dependent sodium channels in neurons. It was discovered in the early 1900s but found clinical use in 1938 as an antiepileptic.

Dilantin is approved for the management of generalized tonic-clonic (grand mal) and complex partial seizures. It is also used in the prevention of seizures following head trauma. It is not indicated for usage in treating absence seizures. Its role is limited for toxin-induced seizures and alcohol withdrawal seizures.

Dilantin interacts strongly with hepatic enzymes and, therefore, has marked effects on the metabolism of commonly prescribed drugs. These effects may serve to potentiate toxicity or diminish effectiveness on a drug-to-drug basis. Therefore, care must be taken when prescribing this medication in the setting of polypharmacy.

Initial signs of dilantin toxicity are nystagmus, decreased consciousness, lethargy, ataxia, and dysarthria. This may progress to coma and apnea in a large overdose. Paradoxical seizure activity may be noted.

Important local skin toxicity has been noted with IV phenytoin administration. Complications after intravenous infusion have included skin and soft tissue necrosis that, in severe cases, has resulted in death. A delayed bluish discoloration characterized by redness, swelling, vesicle formation, and tissue ischemia, termed purple glove syndrome, has been described. In addition, hirsutism, gingival hyperplasia, hypocalcemia, DIC, hepatitis, pseudolymphoma, and Stevens-Johnson syndrome are among the more notable toxicities linked to this agent. Of particular note, significant cardiovascular toxicity has also been described.

One of the more concerning complications of dilantin use is that rapid IV administration at a rate higher than 50 mg per min is linked to hypotension and arrhythmias. These complications are believed to be secondary to the diluent, propylene glycol.

These effects may be more pronounced in patients over the age of 50 with known atherosclerotic cardiovascular disease.

In a recent study of 200 patients loaded with IV dilantin, seven patients had cardiovascular complications. However, when the IV infusion rate was slowed or temporarily stopped, cardiovascular complications resolved in each case.

One alternative to IV dilantin that has been touted for its safety is fosphenytoin, a parenterally administered prodrug of phenytoin. It may be loaded more rapidly than phenytoin and requires no intravenous filter.

However, fosphenytoin may be prohibitively expensive and may have some of the same rate-related cardiac toxicity as phenytoin. A recent study identified 29 applicable reports of adverse cardiac events likely related to fosphenytoin infusion, including 10 cardiac deaths. Adverse effects in patients receiving IV fosphenytoin relative to the incidence in patients receiving IV phenytoin have not been systematically evaluated to date. In addition, although IV fosphenytoin loading is faster, from an adverse-drug event perspective, no advantage of IV fosphenytoin over IV phenytoin is apparent.

Studies have shown that oral phenytoin is the most cost-effective loading method in most settings. IV phenytoin, while easier to load than its oral equivalent, is more expensive and riskier than oral loading. However, the use of the IV formulation is associated with more rapid ED discharges.

Dilantin is an agent that has significant side effects and a complex pharmacologic profile with a proclivity for multiple drug interactions. Perhaps its most concerning potential side effect is its ability to produce cardiac instability when improperly administered. The notion that fosphenytoin should replace phenytoin administration because of a safer cardiovascular profile has not been established. When using the IV formulation instead of a PO formulation, use it with care and monitor your patient's hemodynamics closely.

SUGGESTED READINGS

Adams BD, Buckley NH, Kim JY, et al. Fosphenytoin may cause hemodynamically unstable bradydysrhythmias. *J Emerg Med.* 2006;30(1):75–79.

Donovan PJ, Cline D. Phenytoin administration by constant intravenous infusion: Selective rates of administration. *Ann Emerg Med.* 1991;20(2):139–142.

Earnest MP, Marx JA, Drury LR. Complications of intravenous phenytoin for acute treatment of seizures: Recommendations for usage. *JAMA.* 1983;249(6):762–765.

Holliday SM, Benfield P, Plosker GL. Fosphenytoin: Pharmacoeconomic implications of therapy. *Pharmacoeconomics.* 1998;14(6):685–690.

Swadron SP, Rudis MI, Azimian K, et al. A comparison of phenytoin-loading techniques in the emergency department. *Acad Emerg Med.* 2004;11(3):244–252.

315

DO NOT RELY UPON THE PRESENCE OF AN ANION GAP ACIDOSIS OR AN ELEVATED OSMOL GAP TO DIAGNOSE TOXIC ALCOHOL INGESTION

FIONA M. GARLICH, MD

The most commonly encountered toxic alcohols are methanol and ethylene glycol. Both are eliminated through successive hepatic metabolism by alcohol dehydrogenase (ADH) and aldehyde dehydrogenase (ALDH), with the eventual formation of acid byproducts that cause significant end-organ toxicity.

Methanol, a common component of windshield washer fluid, model airplane fuel, and camp stove fuel, is metabolized to formaldehyde and then formic acid, which exerts its toxic effects primarily by inhibiting oxidative phosphorylation in retinal and optic nerve cells. This results in visual impairment (the classic "snowfield blindness") with occasional progression to permanent blindness, coma, and death. The lethal dose of pure methanol is approximately 1 g/kg, with windshield washer fluid containing a methanol concentration of 30% to 40%. Fatalities have been reported with ingestions as low as 30 mL.

Ethylene glycol, the primary component of antifreeze, is successively metabolized by ADH and ALDH to eventually form oxalic acid. This acid complexes with calcium and can precipitate as crystals in the renal tubules, causing acute tubular necrosis and renal failure. Oxalate crystals can also cause significant damage to the brain, liver, vasculature, and pericardium. In cases of severe poisoning, clinically significant hypocalcemia can occur. The lethal dose of ethylene glycol is 100 mL, or 1 to 1.5 mg/kg in adults.

The hallmarks of methanol and ethylene glycol ingestions are elevated anion gap acidosis and elevated osmol gap. Methanol and ethylene glycol are both osmotically active substances that will contribute to the difference between measured and calculated serum osmols (using the formula 2Na + BUN/2.8 + glucose/18 + ethanol/4.6). As the alcohols are metabolized to their acidic byproducts, the concentration of the osmotically active alcohols decreases and an anion gap acidosis develops. However, this anion gap elevation becomes evident only when significant metabolism of the parent alcohol compounds has occurred. This may take 3 to 8 h in the case of ethylene glycol toxicity or up to 24 h after methanol ingestion. Additionally, when concomitant ethanol ingestion has occurred, the inhibition of ADH results in a delay in toxic acid formation and therefore a delay in the onset of acidosis.

These successive changes in alcohol concentration, osmol gap, and anion gap create several pitfalls in the diagnosis of clinically significant toxic alcohol poisoning. This comes into play primarily in two common clinical scenarios: the early presenter and the late presenter. In the hours after a toxic alcohol ingestion, there will be a high serum concentration of ethylene glycol or methanol, and thus an elevated osmol gap; however, acidosis will not yet be present because acid metabolites have not yet been formed. Given the difficulty in obtaining routine quantitative serum levels (this lab is often a "send-out" with a multiday turnaround time), an elevated osmol gap in the right clinical scenario might be the only clue to toxicity. Furthermore, coingestion with ethanol can prolong the period when an elevated osmol gap may be the only laboratory abnormality. Therefore, when recent toxic alcohol exposure is expected, the presence of a high osmol gap, even in the absence of acidosis, should prompt the clinician to initiate an early inhibition of ADH with fomepizole or ethanol to prevent further metabolite formation.

The other clinical scenario that may challenge the emergency clinician is that of the late presenter. A patient who presents many hours to days after a potentially toxic ingestion has already undergone full metabolism of the parent compound to toxic acids. Therefore, the osmol gap has closed, but a large anion gap acidosis should exist. Symptoms may vary, signs of intoxication may be absent, and the patient may already display evidence of end-organ damage. At this point, hemodialysis should be prioritized to remove toxic acids. Indications for hemodialysis in ethylene glycol toxicity include significant metabolic acidosis, renal dysfunction, and serum levels >25 to 50 mg/dL. For methanol toxicity, indications include significant metabolic acidosis, any ocular findings, a serum level >20 mg/dL, and a history of ingesting more than 30 mL (0.4 mg/kg).

In summary, it is crucial to remember that both an anion gap acidosis and an elevated osmol gap will not occur simultaneously in many cases of significant toxic alcohol ingestion. The time of ingestion and the presence of ethanol must be carefully considered.

- In the patient with significantly altered mental status and presumed ingestion, obtain a serum ethanol level and calculate the osmol gap early on.
- In the early presenter, an elevated osmol gap may be present without an anion gap acidosis. Ethanol, if present, will delay the formation of acidosis. If suspicion is high, treat with an ADH blocker such as fomepizole before the anion gap widens.
- In the late presenter, the anion gap is elevated but the osmol gap has closed. Treatment at this point is hemodialysis.

SUGGESTED READINGS

Brent J, McMartin K, Phillips S, et al. Fomepizole for the treatment of ethylene glycol poisoning: Methylpyrazole for Toxic Alcohols Study Group. *N Engl J Med.* 1999;340(11): 832–838.

Mycyk MB, Aks SE. A visual schematic for clarifying the temporal relationship between the anion and osmol gaps in toxic alcohol poisoning. *Am J Emerg Med.* 2003;21(4):333–335.

Trummel J, Fored M, Austin P. Ingestion of an unknown alcohol. *Ann Emerg Med.* 1996;27: 368–374.

Wiener SW. Toxic alcohols. In: Flomenbaum NE, Goldfrank LR, Hoffman RS, et al., eds. *Goldfrank's Toxicologic Emergencies.* 8th ed. New York, NY: McGraw-Hill Professional Publishing; 2006:1447–1459.

316

REMEMBER TO MAINTAIN MODERATE ALKALEMIA IN PATIENTS SUFFERING FROM ACETYL SALICYLIC ACID TOXICITY

JOHN E. JESUS, MD

Salicylates have been a mainstay analgesic, antipyretic, and anti-inflammatory agent for centuries. Their medicinal properties were first harvested from the bark of the willow tree (Salix alba vulgaris), and in the later part of the 19th century, the derivative, acetyl salicylic acid (ASA, also known as Aspirin), was made commercially available by the company named Bayer. Today, salicylate derivatives may also be found in a variety of products including PeptoBismol, Arthropan, and oil of wintergreen among others. Though the use of ASA declined because of its association with Reye syndrome and the presence of safer alternatives, it is still widely available and commonly prescribed as an antiplatelet therapy for those with cardiovascular and cerebrovascular diseases. Since 2000, analgesics have consistently ranked first among the substances responsible for the largest number of deaths, and of those deaths, aspirin, alone or in combination, was responsible for approximately 12.6% of them.

Acid-base disturbances and CNS abnormalities reflect the more important underlying mechanisms of salicylate toxicity, which produces a well-described set of signs and symptoms including nausea, vomiting, tachypnea, hyperpyrexia, tinnitus, agitation, psychosis, confusion, and coma. Single ingestions of <150 mg/dL are unlikely to result in significant toxicity, while ingestions >500 mg/dL are considered potentially lethal. Salicylate toxicity produces two primary acid-base disorders. Directly and indirectly, salicylates stimulate the medulla respiratory center and increase its sensitivity to pH and carbon dioxide partial pressure PCO_2. In response, the depth and frequency of respiration increase, producing a primary respiratory alkalosis. This change is compensated for by the exchange of intracellular hydrogen ions for extracellular cations and the urinary excretion of bicarbonate. As salicylate toxicity increases, a primary metabolic acidosis results from the buildup of lactate and other organic acids caused by the inhibition of the Krebs cycle as well as the uncoupling of cellular oxidative phosphorylation increasing the body's metabolic rate and temperature. Though the exact mechanism of cerebral dysfunction is unknown, it is associated with increased capillary permeability and cerebral edema.

Salicylates are metabolized in the liver and excreted by the kidneys. At therapeutic levels, salicylate metabolism by hepatic conjugation and subsequent excretion follows first-order kinetics and is directly proportional to the amount of salicylate ingested. Levels of salicylate >30 mg/dL, however, saturate hepatic metabolic pathways and follow zero-order kinetics; further increases in elimination are defined by independent urinary excretion of free salicylate, the degree to which is dependent on urinary pH.

The management of ASA toxicity revolves around the prevention of salicylate penetration into tissues and further facilitating elimination by urinary excretion. Important to these strategies is the principle of ion trapping. Because ASA has a low pK_a (3.5), there exists only a small proportion of nonionized salicylate. It is this form, however, that is able to penetrate into cell membranes and across the blood-brain barrier. With progressive acidemia, an increasing proportion of salicylate exists in the nonionized form. Alkalinizing the serum maintains salicylate in its ionized conformation, trapping it in the intravascular space. This technique also alkalinizes the urine inhibiting salicylate reabsorbed in the proximal tubule, thereby enhancing its excretion.

Gastric decontamination with activated charcoal is generally effective only within the 1st hour of ingestion unless a bezoar has formed or the ingested ASA is enteric coated.

Errors in the management of acute ASA toxicity occur when medical personnel fail to recognize the need for moderate alkalemia or attempt to produce an alkalemia inappropriately. The goal of alkalinization is to achieve and maintain a serum pH of 7.5 (not to exceed 7.55) and a urine pH of 8.0. When salicylate levels exceed 100 mg/dL, bicarbonate should be used in combination with hemodialysis as an initial bridge through dialysis set up time and as a definitive treatment. Although there are other methods to alkalinize urine, they should be avoided. For example, acetazolamide is contraindicated as it alkalinizes the urine at the expense of acidifying the serum.

In severe ASA toxicity, coma and signs of impending respiratory failure may necessitate intubation. Sedation and airway management, however, have resulted in patient deaths. The respiratory alkalosis produced by salicylate-induced tachypnea compensates for the ASA-induced metabolic acidosis. Neglecting to set appropriately high minute ventilation may exacerbate a patient's acidemia. Furthermore, hyperventilation should only be used in combination with sodium bicarbonate therapy.

A proportion of ASA exposures, especially those that are intentional, occur in the setting of coingestion with other agents. ASA and sedative hypnotic agents are particularly lethal combinations because of the sedative hypnotic–induced respiratory depression. Not only does this effect mask the classic sign of tachypnea, which may lead to misdiagnosis, it also blunts the initial respiratory alkalosis, making those patients more vulnerable to acidemia.

The bottom line in the management of an acute ASA toxic patient: use sodium bicarbonate to achieve a moderate alkalemia of a pH of 7.5 and a urine pH of 8.0, avoid intubation if at all possible, and be aware of potential co-ingestions.

SUGGESTED READINGS

Almond G. Salicylates. In: Viccellio P, Bana T, Ament J, et al., eds. *Emergency Toxicology.* 2nd ed. Philadelphia, PA: Lippincott-Raven Publishers; 1998:553.

Berk WA, Anderson JC. Salicylate-associated asystole: Report of two cases. *Am J Med.* 1989;86(4):505–506.

Flomenbaum N. Salicylates. In: Flomenbaum NE, Goldfrank LR, Hoffman RS, et al., eds. *Goldfrank's Toxicologic Emergencies.* 8th ed. New York, NY: McGraw-Hill Professional Publishing; 2006.

Higgins RM, Connolly JO, Hendry BM. Alkalinization and hemodialysis in severe salicylate poisoning: Comparison of elimination techniques in the same patient. *Clin Nephrol.* 1998;50(3):178–183.

Kerr F, Krenzelok E. Salicylates. In: Shannon M, Borron S, Burns M, eds. *Haddad and Winchester's Clinical Management of Poisoning and Drug Overdose.* 4th ed. Philadelphia, PA: Saunders; 2007:846.

317

Acute Lithium Intoxication Is More Dangerous in Individuals Already Taking Lithium Than in Those Who Are Lithium Naïve

Cheri N. M. Weaver, MD

Lithium is widely used in the treatment of depressive and manic disorders. It is particularly useful in the management of bipolar disease and has become a mainstay of the treatment of this disorder. However, this medication has a narrow therapeutic window mandating that its administration and dosing be closely monitored. Emergency medicine physicians routinely manage patients presenting with a chief complaint of an acute ingestion of a chemical. Acute ingestions often incite a higher level of anxiety in treating physicians as compared to a patient who accidentally took an extra pill of a routinely prescribed medication. With lithium, however, the latter of the two aforementioned patients is at greatest risk of complications from his or her ingestion if not treated aggressively.

The exact mechanism through which lithium works to treat psychiatric disorders is unknown. Much investigation into the topic has suggested that the cation may alter electrolyte, ion, or neurotransmitter transport or may work intracellularly to modify second messenger actions. Lithium absorption is quick, with most of the ingested dose being absorbed into the body within 6 to 8 h. Initially, the drug distributes through the circulatory plasma volume. It typically reaches a peak serum concentration 2 to 4 h after ingestion. At a slower rate, the drug enters the intracellular compartments of the body. Lithium clearance is managed exclusively by renal filtration and urinary excretion with a plasma half-life nearing 20 h. With its volume of distribution and tissue penetration, it can be difficult to dose lithium appropriately to keep serum concentrations in the therapeutic window. While adverse side effects of lithium therapy have been noted to occur while serum levels are within the therapeutic window, the incidence of adverse side effects increases significantly when the serum lithium concentration rises beyond this level.

Three distinct classifications of lithium poisoning have been recognized: acute, acute-on-therapeutic, and chronic. Acute poisoning occurs in the lithium-naïve individual. Serum lithium levels in this group of patients will be acutely elevated. However, as the drug redistributes throughout the body tissues, the serum level falls. Thus, without intervention, the body is exposed to elevated lithium levels for a relatively short amount of time. Acute-on-therapeutic poisoning occurs when an individual currently on a maintenance regimen ingests additional amounts of lithium. Serum levels of lithium rise acutely in this subgroup as well. However, unlike the acutely poisoned group, tissue penetration has already occurred, so less tissue redistribution can occur. Thus, without intervention, serum levels of lithium will remain elevated. In the chronically poisoned group, no additional ingestion of lithium occurs. Rather, this subgroup develops toxic levels of the drug while on maintenance therapy. Serum lithium levels rise due to a decrease in the renal function. This leads to a decrease in the renal excretion of lithium and thus, a prolonged half-life of the drug.

Although data vary regarding correlation of serum lithium levels and ultimate severity of lithium poisoning, there is a general consensus that as the serum levels of lithium rises so does the severity of the symptomatology of the intoxication. Mild symptoms, generally associated with lithium levels no higher than 3.5 mEq/L, include gastrointestinal upset, tremors, and fascicular twitching. While more severe symptoms, associated with serum lithium levels over 3.5 mEq/L, include cardiac arrhythmia, stupor, coma, and seizure. However, this "lithium level" approach does not account for the different categories of lithium poisoning.

In 2007, Waring et al. reviewed all events of lithium ingestion reported to the Scottish Poison Information Bureau between 2000 and 2005. In the paper, each category of lithium poisoning—acute, acute-on-therapeutic, and chronic—was evaluated. Each of the three categories of lithium poisoning had a similar distribution of serum lithium levels. However, the evaluation of poisoning severity was much higher in the later two groups. Thus, suggesting a lithium level that causes mild symptoms in an acutely poisoned patient may have devastating effects in a chronically poisoned patient. Furthermore, one could surmise based on the pharmacokinetics of lithium that the acute-on-therapeutic and chronically poisoned patients have a prolonged exposure time to the elevated levels of lithium as compared to the acute ingestion group and thus more severe symptoms.

Treatment for lithium poisoning, as with the majority of intoxications, has supportive care and hydration as its mainstay of therapy. Activated charcoal is of no benefit in lithium ingestion. Hemodialysis, however, is remarkably effective in removing lithium from the body. As an emergency medicine physician, one must remember to involve both the toxicology and renal services early in the care of any patient with a lithium poisoning. In a patient chronically on lithium, even slight elevations in his or her serum lithium levels can have devastating effects on both renal and neurologic functions.

SUGGESTED READINGS

Okusa MD, Crystal LJ. Clinical manifestations and management of acute lithium intoxication. *Am J Med.* 1994;97(4):383–389.

Potter W, Hollister L. Antipsychotic agents and lithium. In: Katzung B, ed. *Basic and Clinical Pharmacology*. New York, NY: McGraw-Hill; 2001:478–497.

Timmer RT, Sands JM. Lithium intoxication. *J Am Soc Nephrol*. 1999;10(3):666–674.

Waring WS, Laing WJ, Good AM, et al. Pattern of lithium exposure predicts poisoning severity: Evaluation of referrals to a regional poisons unit. *QJM*. 2007;100(5):271–276.

318

TREATING AN OPIOID OVERDOSE: KNOW WHEN IT IS TIME TO START THE NALOXONE DRIP

ALDEN LANDRY, MD

Patients who present to the emergency department due to an opioid overdose often present with bradycardia, respiratory depression, altered mental status, and in some cases, cardiopulmonary arrest. Quickly identifying that opioids are the cause of an arrest or near arrest is imperative in treating these patients properly. Some physical exam findings to suggest an opioid overdose include miotic (constricted) pupils, decreased bowel sounds, respiratory depression, hypotension, bradycardia, and crackles indicating pulmonary edema. Skin findings such as track marks or abscesses which indicate skin popping are also helpful in identifying a potential opioid overdose.

When treating patients with respiratory depression or arrest suspicious for opioid overdose, treatment with naloxone can temporarily reverse the opioids. Naloxone works on a signaling level by competitively binding to the mu receptors. It is a short-acting opioid antagonist and can be given via various routes with intravenous being the best. Naloxone, when taken orally, must go through hepatic metabolism to be converted to an active form. Naloxone can also be given subcutaneously, intramuscularly, or via the endotracheal tube, but using such routes results in slower absorption and unpredictable duration making the drug difficult to titrate.

The time of onset of naloxone is approximately 1 min and lasts 20 to 60 min. Unfortunately, the half-life of naloxone is shorter than that of heroin or other common opioids of abuse (*Table 318.1*). When patients in the emergency department are brought in with suspected opioid overdose and are treated with naloxone, either prior to arrival by EMS or while in the emergency department, it is imperative to watch these patients closely as the naloxone may wear off and the underlying opioid overdose will reappear. These patients must then be retreated with the medication.

TABLE 318.1	HALF-LIFE OF COMMON OPIOIDS OF ABUSE
DRUG[a]	HALF LIFE
Heroin	15–30 min
Morphine	2–3 h
Fentanyl	3–12 h
Oxycodone	3–4.5 h
Hydrocodone	3–4.5 h
Methadone	24–36 h
Meperidine	3–5 h
Codeine	2.5–3 h

[a]opiates are converted to morphine thus prolonging the symptoms.

The goal when using naloxone is not to restore the patient to a normal mental status; instead, it is to maintain adequate ventilation. Measuring the carbon dioxide level via capnometry, watching for hypoxia, and measuring the ventilatory efforts are all ways to ensure adequate ventilation. An arbitrary number of 12 breaths per min is often sited as a goal when resuscitating opioid overdoses.

Physicians must decide whether to bolus or to start a naloxone drip in patients with opioid overdose. Giving a bolus is easy to do but does carry some risks. Patients given repeated boluses of naloxone can suffer from opioid withdrawal, apnea, seizures, and fatal arrhythmias. Signs and symptoms of opioid withdrawal include vomiting, diarrhea, agitation, piloerection, lacrimation, and yawning. Another concern about naloxone administration is the cardiovascular effects. Large boluses are associated with hypotension, especially if a patient has also ingested medications affecting blood pressure, but this should respond to an IV fluid bolus. If hypotension persists, consider starting vasopressor therapy.

When deciding to start a naloxone drip, the appropriate dose can be calculated by giving a patient two thirds of the initial loading dose to reverse an opioid overdose as a drip over an hour will supply adequate naloxone to maintain a respiratory rate of 12. If a patient develops signs and symptoms of opioid withdrawal, the drip can be stopped. If the patient develops respiratory depression during the infusion, then the patient should be treated with one half of the initial bolus, and then, the rate of the drip should also be increased by one half.

Close observation is essential when treating a patient with an opioid overdose. Given that naloxone has a shorter half-life (2 to 3 h) of most opioids, opioid-related symptoms can recur. If intoxication is so severe that it will require a naloxone drip, then inpatient management is strongly recommended.

SUGGESTED READINGS

Chamberlain JM, Klein BL. A comprehensive review of naloxone for the emergency physician. *Am J Emerg Med*. 1994;12(6):650–660.

Goldfrank L, Weisman RS, Errick JK, et al. A dosing nomogram for continuous infusion intravenous naloxone. *Ann Emerg Med*. 1986;15(5):566–570.

Osterwalder JJ. Naloxone–for intoxications with intravenous heroin and heroin mixtures–harmless or hazardous? A prospective clinical study. *J Toxicol Clin Toxicol*. 1996;34(4):409–416.

319

DO NOT DISCONTINUE *N*-ACETYLCYSTEINE IF ANAPHYLACTOID SYMPTOMS DEVELOP

LINDSAY ROBERTS, MD

N-acetylcysteine (NAC) has turned acetaminophen overdose into an extremely treatable entity. Acetaminophen hepatotoxicity begins at approximately 8 h postoverdose when nontoxic metabolism is overwhelmed and the processing of acetaminophen to the toxic NAPQI predominates. NAC replenishes nontoxic pathways, detoxifies NAPQI, and provides direct cellular protection. Whenever possible, it is of utmost importance to start NAC within 8 h of overdose, before hepatocellular damage has already occurred.

NAC is manufactured in both oral and IV formulations. Although both have proven efficacy, controversy exists over which should be used first line, as discussed by Prescott (2005). Nausea and vomiting are the most common side effects of oral NAC. This is not a surprise given oral NAC's barely palatable taste (despite dilution in cola) and relatively large dosing requirement (the loading dose for a 70-kg patient is about 220 oz, which is two thirds of a soda can prior to dilution). Although seemingly benign, nausea and vomiting are significant concerns as they may prevent adequate delivery of NAC, especially in the most at-risk population: patients who have already developed gastrointestinal side effects from the acetaminophen overdose. Thus, although oral NAC is safe, it can be complicated to use. If a patient vomits within an hour of the NAC dose, it needs to be repeated. If the patient begins drinking the NAC loading dose within but approaching the 8-h time window and subsequently vomits, the 8-h window is violated. Due to such concerns, many toxicologists recommend IV NAC as the first-line treatment of choice. Additionally, only IV NAC is recommended for use in patients who have already developed liver failure.

Approximately 15% of IV NAC use results in an "anaphylactoid" type reaction. Most of these reactions are mild with flushing and urticaria predominating, though angioedema, bronchospasm, and hypotension can occur. These side effects are believed to be dose related and most often occur during the 15-min loading dose infusion (the highest infusion rate). For this reason, many experts give the NAC loading dose over an hour instead of the originally recommended 15 min.

Guidelines published by Bailey and McGuigan (1998) provide instructions on how to treat the common side effects of IV NAC. Flushing is a benign side effect and most often does not require any treatment. Mild urticaria can be treated with diphenhydramine and NAC can be continued without a pause. However, severe urticaria may require that NAC be stopped temporarily, until resolution (which should occur within an hour). Respiratory symptoms and angioedema require diphenhydramine and additional symptomatic treatment such as albuterol, as well as holding the NAC infusion until the symptoms resolve (again, usually within an hour). In severe cases where the angioedema or respiratory symptoms do not improve significantly, one can consider transitioning to oral NAC. The bottom line is that IV NAC should not be completely discontinued unless a life-threatening reaction (unresolving bronchospasm) has developed or unless lab data support its discontinuation.

Asthmatics are reported by Schmidt and Dahloff (2001) to be at greater risk for anaphylactoid reactions, particularly bronchospasm due to NAC. Though extremely rare, there is a case report by Appleboam et al. (2002) of a death associated with NAC use in a severe asthmatic. Due to this higher frequency of side effects, it would be reasonable to start with oral NAC as first-line treatment in asthmatics. If the patient cannot tolerate oral NAC due to nausea or vomiting, IV NAC can be used: it is not contraindicated. However, it may be prudent to consider pretreatment in these patients with diphenhydramine and/ or albuterol.

Recent studies by Schmidt and Dalhoff (2001), as well as Waring et al. (2008), have found a trend toward fewer anaphylactoid reactions in those with higher acetaminophen concentrations. Additionally, oral NAC does not reach serum concentrations as high as IV NAC and does not cause anaphylactoid reactions. Taken together, the data imply that "free" or "unused" NAC serum concentration may be the culprit in the anaphylactoid side effects of IV NAC. Perhaps, future NAC dosing will consider acetaminophen level in addition to the current weight-based dosing.

PEARLS

- Negative APAP levels drawn BEFORE 4 h postingestion can be used to rule out toxicity. However, NAC treatment should be based on a 4-h level and the Matthew-Rumack Nomogram.

- For overdoses of unknown timing, start IV NAC immediately (do NOT wait for lab results). Send an APAP level and an AST: if the AST is elevated or if the APAP is >10, continue treatment.
- Oral NAC may be given IV if the IV formulation of NAC is not available.
- NAC is a pregnancy category B drug. The risks of fetal APAP overdose outweigh the risks of using NAC.

SUGGESTED READINGS

Appleboam AV, Dargan PI, Knighton J. Fatal anaphylactoid reaction to N-acetylcysteine: caution in patients with asthma. *Emerg Med J*. 2002;19(6):594–595.

Bailey B, McGuigan MA. Management of anaphylactoid reactions to intravenous N-acetylcysteine. *Ann Emerg Med*. 1998;31(6):710–715.

Hendrickson RG, Bizovi KE. Acetaminophen. In: Goldfrank LR, Flomenbaum NE, Lewin NA, et al., eds. *Goldfrank's Toxicologic Emergencies*. 8th ed. New York, NY: McGraw Hill; 2006: 523–543.

Howland MA. N-acetylcysteine. In: Goldfrank LR, Flomenbaum NE, Lewin NA, et al., eds. *Goldfrank's Toxicologic Emergencies*. 8th ed. New York, NY: McGraw Hill; 2006:544–547.

Prescott L. Oral or intravenous N-acetylcysteine for acetaminophen poisoning. *Ann of Emerg Med*. 2005;45(4):409–412.

Schmidt LE, Dalhoff, K. Risk factors in the development of adverse reactions to N-acetylcysteine in patients with paracetamol poisoning. *Br J Clin Pharmacol*. 2001;51(1):87–91.

Waring WS, Stephen AF, Robinson ED, et al. Lower incidence of anaphylactoid reactions to N-acetylcysteine in patients with high acetaminophen concentrations after overdose. *Clin Toxicol (Phila)*. 2008;46(6):496–500.

320

KNOW THE BASICS OF ELECTRICITY TO UNDERSTAND THE INJURY PATTERNS

MATTHEW J. LEVY, DO, MSc

INTRODUCTION

The widespread use of electricity in modern society has caused a large number of electrical injuries and deaths. The first known death from modern electrocution occurred in 1881 when Samuel W. Smith fell onto a generator outside a saloon. Shortly thereafter, an entrepreneurial dentist commercialized death by electrocution by the invention of the Electric Chair. Electrocution is defined as death caused by electricity. An electrical injury is tissue damage resulting from the flow of electrical current through tissue. Electrical burns are cutaneous injuries and necrosis resulting from electrical current flow through the skin. An electric shock is a sudden response caused by a body part coming in contact with an electric current.

BACKGROUND

Each year, over 17,000 victims of electrical injuries are treated in emergency departments. The true incidence of electrical injuries is likely much higher, as many incidents are underreported, while others are hidden by associated blunt trauma such as falls from a height. Three unique populations are at risk for electrical injury, each evenly accounting for approximately 20% to 25% of electrical injuries. Toddlers who sustain electrical injuries from household electrical sockets and cords constitute the first group. The second group is adolescents who engage in dangerous behaviors around electrical power lines. The third population is those that work with electricity for a living. The annual incidence of death amongst U.S. electrical workers is approximately 1 per 10,000.

TYPES OF ELECTRICITY

Electricity is the flow of charged particles between positive and negative terminals. Voltage (V) describes the potential difference between these terminals. Electricity is commonly thought of as either high voltage or low voltage. Standard household voltage is 110 V, and the third rail in a subway is 600 V. Power lines in U.S. residential areas are typically 7,620 V. Discrepancy exists in the medical literature as to what actual voltage should be considered high voltage. Some authors suggest 600 V while traditional literature states 1,000 V. For the purposes of management of electrical injuries, any voltage >600 V should be considered high voltage, as evidence states that the risk for serious and fatal electrical injury increases significantly with voltages above 600 V. Although high voltage is more dangerous, low voltage sources account for about half of all electrical injuries and deaths since the general population has much greater access to them.

Electrical current, commonly referred to as amperage, describes the volume-charged particles that are flowing. Electrical current exists in two forms: DC (direct current) and AC (alternating current). The DC describes that the continuous flow of electrons is principally used in medical devices and those with batteries. Lightening is also a form of DC. AC has a periodic reversal in the direction of current flow and is found in the electricity supplied to homes and businesses. AC is more dangerous to the human body but is the most efficient means to transmit current long distances. Power supplies or "transformers" are devices that convert AC to DC power or vice versa.

A conductor is any item through which electricity can flow. When energized, the human body can be a conductor and this often results in some degree of electrical injury. An insulator does not allow the flow of electrical current.

Resistance describes the impedance to flow caused by energy loss through a conductor. Most of the body's resistance is concentrated in the skin. The thicker the skin, the greater its resistance; likewise, the skin's resistance decreases when broken (for example, punctured or scraped) or when wet.

FLOW OF ELECTRICITY THROUGH THE HUMAN BODY

Regardless of the type of electrical current, electricity will flow through a person if his or her body completes a circuit. Completing a circuit requires a positive voltage terminal, contact point with the body (including entry and exit points), and a negative terminal. For example, a person who inadvertently grasps an energized metal ladder with his or her left hand while his or her left foot is on the ground will have current flow from his or her left hand to the ground. Electrical current will not necessarily flow through his or her head or unaffected arm.

A common misconception often described in the medical literature is that electricity will flow exclusively through the body in the "path of least resistance." This implies that electricity is flowing through one tissue type and assumes that the body is a single tissue (like a big copper wire). However, electricity may flow through different tissues at the same time. Some tissues are better conductors than others. Bone, for example, has a high resistance, while vessels and nervous tissue have considerably lower resistance, yet all are vulnerable to the effects of electricity. The degree of damage sustained to these tissues is related to the type of tissue and resistance and cross-sectional area of a given tissue.

Electricity affects the body in three primary ways. Direct contact results in tissue damage altering the membrane potentials of cells resulting in muscle tetany, seizures, and arrhythmias. When AC current flows through the arm, flexor tetany of the fingers and forearm overpowers that of the extensor's, and the hand may grasp the conductor tighter, leading to an extended exposure. Conversion of electrical to thermal energy results in burns, tissue destruction, and coagulation necrosis. Blunt trauma is sustained from falls, violent muscle contraction, or other mechanical injury. Contact with high-voltage AC and DC tends to cause a single violent skeletal muscle contraction, leading to the person appearing to "be thrown" from the voltage source, and produce mechanical trauma. Other forceful muscle contractions can cause fractures and joint dislocations, especially dislocations of the shoulder.

MANAGEMENT OF THE PATIENT WHO IS POST ELECTRICAL INJURY

Safety of the rescuers is a primary consideration in regard to electrical injuries. Countless cases exist where well-meaning Good Samaritans or unaware professional rescuers become patients themselves when exposed to the same electrical source that initially injured the primary patient. A common misconception is that a downed power line is safe to be around as long as it is not directly touched. Some power lines may conduct tens of thousands of volts and may energize a considerable area of the ground it is touching. A safe rule of thumb is to stay at least 30 ft away from any downed power line.

The initial management of a patient following electrical injury is no different than that of the trauma patient. Advanced cardiac life support medications and interventions should be performed as indicated. If burns are present, wound care should be performed, with attention to removing constricting items such as rings and detailed historical factors such as the voltage, current, duration of time exposed, secondary injuries such as falls and whether the patient was wet or dry is crucial to determining the type and duration of electrical current exposure. Laboratory analysis of serum electrolytes, renal function, and creatine kinase levels, along with urinalysis, to detect evidence of myoglobinuria should be performed.

Patients having contact with over 600 V should be admitted for observation, even in the absence of apparent injury. Any patient with an abnormal physical exam, laboratory finding, or symptoms concerning for systemic injury should be admitted. It is commonly thought that these patients require telemetry monitoring; however, routine cardiac monitoring is not required unless the initial ECG is abnormal. Adults with electrical injury caused by household voltage (110 to 220 V) have minimal risk for delayed arrhythmias. Asymptomatic patients who sustain a household electrical shock can be discharged home if they have a normal ECG on presentation and normal examination findings. Children with only hand wounds from electrical outlet injuries and no evidence of cardiac or neurologic involvement can be discharged with local wound care, provided that the assessment of the child's home supervision ensures adequate supervision and safety.

SUGGESTED READINGS

Fish RM. Electric injury: Part II. Specific injuries. *J Emerg Med.* 2000;18:27.
Fish RM. Electric injury: Part III. Monitoring indications, the pregnant patient, and lightning. *J Emerg Med.* 2000;18:181–187.
Ore T, Casini V. Electrical fatalities among US construction workers. *J Occup Environ Med.* 1996;38:587–592.
Tintinalli JE, Kelen GD, Stapczynski JS, eds. *Emergency Medicine: A Comprehensive Study Guide.* 6th ed. New York, NY: McGraw-Hill Professional; 2003: ch 201.

321

CONDUCTIVE ENERGY WEAPONS (TASER): AN INCREASING CAUSE OF INJURY—YOU BETTER KNOW HOW TO TREAT!

MATTHEW J. LEVY, DO, MSc

Emergency physicians have to be prepared to manage all types of patients, including those who may be victims of many different weapons. Perhaps one of the more controversial weapons is the TASER. This device was first introduced in 1969, modified in 1974, and modified again in 1990s. It gained notoriety in 1991 when it was reportedly used in the Rodney King episode. The modern incarnation involves two electrodes that are released forcibly by nitrogen charges and are connected to a wire that allows an electrical charge to be transmitted to the victim. In addition, the device can discharge its electrical charge by direct contact with a subject.

TASERs are a form of conducted electrical weapon that induce transient incapacitation by inducing involuntary muscle contractions. This weapon is often used by law enforcement personnel against individuals who exhibit dangerous or threatening behaviors and who fail to comply with the instructions of a police officer. Given that background, for all TASER victims, it is essential that the emergency physicians consider underlying medical and psychiatric conditions that may have contributed to the behavior, in addition to the injuries associated with TASER use.

Devices such as the TASER use a compressed nitrogen gas canister to propel two barb-tipped probes about 21 ft at a velocity less than a firearm or paintball gun. The probes are attached to the device by thin wires. The best way to think of a barb is to consider it as a straight no. 8 fishhook. The length of the barb is 4 mm and the length of the shaft is 9.5 mm. The weapon delivers up to 50,000 V through the probes, pulsating rapidly for up to 5 s. It delivers electrical impulses of approximately 1.76 J (26 W) per pulse. The average current of the widely used TASER model ×26 is 2.1 mAmps, well below the threshold for ventricular fibrillation of 50 to 100 mAmps, but enough to be remarkably uncomfortable and transiently disabling.

The TASER's barbs do not penetrate deeply and therefore pose little risk for penetrating the lungs, heart, or bowel. However, there are certain parts of the body that are vulnerable. Barbs that inadvertently penetrate the eyes, major vasculature, or genitalia need close attention and should be evaluated and treated as necessary. Barbs embedded elsewhere on the body can be removed easily. The first step is to stabilize the skin surrounding the puncture site. The second step is to grasp the probe with either a gloved hand or a clamp and pull away from the puncture site with purposeful consistent traction. In some cases, a directly applied traction on the probe is sufficient to dislodge the probe, but in many cases, the barb provides sufficient resistance to the extraction effort. Once removed, the TASER barbs should be considered evidence and turned over to law enforcement personnel as dictated by local policy.

If direct and purposeful traction fails to dislodge the probe, a small incision may be necessary. One method is to anesthetize the area around the wound and then incise down to the base of the barb using a no. 11 scalpel. The skin can be stabilized by using an open clamp around the barb, then removing the probe by applying steady, inline traction. There is no need to advance the end of the barb through the skin as with other fishhooks. The wound should be managed as any other wound with appropriate wound cleansing, irrigation as needed, appropriate wound care, dressing, and tetanus vaccination review.

Every patient who is a victim of trauma should be carefully evaluated, including assessments for airway, breathing, and circulation. In many cases, TASER barb removal forms the basis of the emergency physician's management if there are no other medical issues. To this point, it is unnecessary to obtain an electrocardiogram routinely in patients subjected to a TASER discharge, provided there are no signs or symptoms of other medical conditions. One condition that must be considered is excited delirium. Patients who remain agitated and combative after being subjected to a TASER should be assessed carefully for "Excited Delirium"; a condition associated with in-custody deaths following TASER use. Excited Delirium is an ill defined syndrome presenting as agitation, tachycardia, hyperthermia, metabolic acidosis, and sudden death. This condition is seen frequently in association with cocaine and stimulant use.

TABLE 321.1	CONCERNING ELEMENTS OF THE TASER VICTIMS EXAMINATION

- Persistent, abnormal vital signs, including hyperthermia
- History or physical findings consistent with amphetamine or hallucinogenic drug use
- Cardiac history
- Altered level of consciousness or aggressive, violent behavior including resistance to evaluation
- Evidence of hyperthermia
- Abnormal, subjective complaints, including chest pain, shortness of breath, nausea or headaches

Historical factors associated with Excited Delirium include a history of schizophrenia, psychosis or mania, previous similar presentation(s), history of illicit substance abuse, ethanol use. Physical findings in Excited Delirium include seeming superhuman strength; imperviousness to pain, including injuries sustained during violent outbursts; bizarre, purposeless and violent behavior; hyperactivity; paranoia; tachycardia; very hot skin; profuse sweating or skin extremely dry for level of exertion.

One of the most controversial aspects about the use of the TASER are deaths that have been associated with its use. The majority of deaths associated with TASER discharge occur minutes to hours after TASER application. There is little scientific evidence implicating a causal relationship between TASER use and death. Clinical studies indicate that the risk of cardiac harm to subjects from a TASER is very low. Patients showing signs of Excited Delirium who were exposed to multiple TASER discharges are at an increased risk for sudden in-custody death compared to those subjected to a single TASER discharge.

In summary, TASER victims presenting to an Emergency Department do well with careful removal of the probes followed by good wound care. If the probes enter a delicate region, including the eye or genitals, additional resources may be necessary. If any of the elements listed in *Table 321.1* are noted, close and careful evaluation and monitoring is warranted. There is an association of TASER injury and death that needs to explored more in the literature. In most cases, TASER probe removal is a straightforward procedure without much complication.

SUGGESTED READINGS

Lutes M. Focus on: Management of TASER injuries. *ACEP News*. May 2006.
Manojlovic D, Hall C, Laur D, et al. Technical Report TR-01–2006 Review of Conducted Energy Devices. Canadian Association of Chiefs of Police. August 22,2005. Canadian Police Research Centre (CPRC) Ottawa, ON K1A 0R6.
Vilke G, Sloane C, Levine S, et al. Does the TASER Cause Electrical Changes in 12-Lead EKG Monitoring of Human Subjects. Society for Academic Emergency Medicine, 2007 Meeting.

322

KNOW WHEN INTUBATION CAN MAKE A TRAUMA PATIENT ACUTELY WORSE

JONATHAN C. BERGER, MD AND ELLIOTT R. HAUT, MD, FACS

In the trauma bay, airway evaluation is a critical first step in the treatment of every injured patient. In patients without a secure or stable airway, endotracheal intubation can be a lifesaving procedure. In general, once an injury requiring definitive airway control is identified, endotracheal intubation should not be delayed. However, in the trauma patient who can protect his or her airway, premature endotracheal intubation can result in serious consequences. There are instances in which endotracheal intubation can lead to rapid clinical deterioration, rather than the improvement the clinician was hoping for when deciding to intubate a patient. Three mechanisms by which this deterioration can occur are commonly encountered: (a) causing air embolism in a patient with penetrating chest trauma, (b) converting a simple pneumothorax into a tension pneumothorax with positive-pressure ventilation, and (c) precipitating cardiopulmonary collapse in a patient in hemorrhagic shock who relies on sympathetic tone to maintain blood pressure. The following scenarios will illustrate these points.

CAUSING AIR EMBOLISM IN A PATIENT WITH PENETRATING CHEST TRAUMA

A young man presents to the trauma bay shortly after sustaining a gunshot wound to the chest. He has decreased breath sounds on the left side but his blood pressure is stable at 110/60 and his pulse is 110. He is alert and oriented and has oxygen saturations of 95%. A chest tube is placed which immediately dumps 1 L of blood, prompting a plan for thoracotomy in the operating room by the trauma surgeon who is coming to the hospital. The emergency medicine physician decides to expedite his care and electively intubates the patient before his transport to the operating room. While waiting for surgical intervention, the patient decompensates into cardiac arrest and dies. The postmortem examination shows air emboli in the coronary arteries and the cerebral circulation.

This patient sustained a fatal air embolism from an unrecognized fistula between the bronchial tree and a branch of the pulmonary vein. Hypovolemic patients with penetrating injuries that cause direct communication between the airways and the pulmonary veins are at particularly high risk. As a consequence of positive-pressure ventilation, air can be transmitted from the airway to the relatively low-pressure pulmonary venous system, potentially introducing air directly to the left heart and the systemic circulation. Immediate consequences include myocardial infarction, stroke, mesenteric ischemia, and other end-organ infarctions.

This condition is best prevented by thoughtful consideration of the risks and benefits of intubating a patient with penetrating chest trauma. One should consider whether positive-pressure ventilation is truly indicated in any patient with penetrating chest trauma who can protect his or her airway and maintain arterial oxygen saturation. In patients going to surgery for thoracotomy, the time delay between intubation and surgical control of the lung injury should be minimized by intubating in the operating room immediately before thoracotomy, if possible. In addition, fluid resuscitation to fill the venous system can also help prevent this deadly problem. Unfortunately, once air embolism occurs, it is very difficult to treat. If the clinician suspects an air embolus, 100% inspired oxygen therapy should be instituted. The patient should be placed in Trendelenburg position (head down) and the left decubitus position in an effort to trap the embolus in the ventricle. Aspiration of air can be attempted, although this maneuver is rarely successful.

CONVERSION FROM A SIMPLE TO A TENSION PNEUMOTHORAX WITH POSITIVE-PRESSURE VENTILATION

A patient presents to the trauma bay with blunt trauma (i.e., motor vehicle collision). The patient has a dislocated hip which requires immediate reduction. Breath sounds are present, and he is hemodynamically stable; however, an initial chest x-ray shows a small right-sided pneumothorax with multiple rib fractures. The physician performs endotracheal intubation to allow adequate sedation for joint reduction. After a few minutes, the patient is hypotensive, tachycardic, and difficult to ventilate due to elevated airway pressures. On physical examination, he has jugular venous distension, no breath sounds on the right side, and his trachea is deviated to the left. Prompt diagnosis and treatment of a tension pneumothorax save his life.

This trauma patient presented with a simple pneumothorax. Without any other concomitant injury, this may not have needed aggressive treatment. However, by submitting him to intubation and positive-pressure ventilation, his simple pneumothorax was converted to a life-threatening tension pneumothorax. With each delivered positive-pressure breath, air is pushed into the pleural space through the lung injury. This situation ultimately results in tension pneumothorax physiology manifested by decreased venous return to the heart and increased airway pressures. Treatment of a tension pneumothorax is prompt decompression of the pleural space by needle decompression followed by tube thoracostomy.

PRECIPITATING CARDIOPULMONARY COLLAPSE IN A PATIENT IN HEMORRHAGIC SHOCK WHO RELIES ON SYMPATHETIC TONE TO MAINTAIN BLOOD PRESSURE

A middle-aged woman is the unbelted driver in a high-speed motor vehicle collision. In the trauma bay, her breath sounds are equal bilaterally, and she is alert with a Glasgow Coma Scale Score of 15. However, she is hypotensive (blood pressure 85/50 mm Hg) and tachycardic (pulse 150 beats per min). She has bruising over her left-upper quadrant, abdominal tenderness, and a positive abdominal FAST ultrasound exam (Focused Abdominal Sonogram for Trauma). The on-call trauma surgeons will be taking her for urgent laparotomy upon their arrival to the hospital. A well-meaning resident decides to intubate the patient to expedite her surgery. Upon the administration of etomidate, she becomes more hypotensive and deteriorates to cardiopulmonary arrest.

This patient suffered a high-grade splenic rupture with intra-abdominal bleeding and presents in class IV hemorrhagic shock. Her blood pressure is maintained mainly by endogenous catecholamines and high sympathetic tone resulting in peripheral vasoconstriction. In a profoundly hypovolemic patient, even a small loss in sympathetic drive associated with sedation can result in a catastrophic fall in blood pressure. In a patient such as this one who has a stable airway but will likely need operative management, it may be safer to intubate this patient in the operating room when the surgical procedure to control hemorrhage is imminent. Adequate IV access should be obtained in this type of patient, with packed red blood cells available, if possible. A planned "hypotensive resuscitation" can be employed; however, the pitfall of removing the sympathetic stimulation should be considered before any sedation is given.

SUGGESTED READING

Haut ER. Evaluation and acute resuscitation of the trauma patient. In: Evans SRT, ed. *Surgical Pitfalls: Prevention and Management*. Philadelphia, PA: Saunders; 2009:757–771.

323

KNOW THE ZONES OF THE NECK AND THE APPROPRIATE WORKUP FOR PENETRATING INJURIES IN EACH ZONE

BENJAMIN BRASLOW, MD

The management of injuries to the neck that penetrate the platysma is dependent upon the anatomic level of an injury. Anatomically, the anterior neck (between the left and the right sternocleidomastoid muscles) is divided into threes zones. Zone I, the lowest, extends from the clavicles up to the level of the cricothyroid membrane and includes the thoracic outlet vasculature, trachea, esophagus, thoracic duct, and major cervical nerve trunks. Zone III, the most cephalad area, lies between the angle of the mandible and the skull base. It contains the pharynx, jugular veins, vertebral arteries, and distal internal carotid arteries. Zone II, between zones I and III, contains parts of all major vascular and hollow viscus organs of the neck. Because of the density of vital structures in this zone, multiple injuries are common and mortality, particularly for major vascular injuries, may reach 50%. Obtaining proximal surgical control of a vascular injury in zone I often requires a technically difficult and large operation such as median sternotomy, clavicle resection, and/or anterolateral thoracotomy. Similarly difficult, distal control in zone III might necessitate the disarticulation of the mandible or resection of the base of the skull. Only in zone II can proximal and distal control of a vascular injury readily be obtained with a relatively simple incision along the anterior border of the sternocleidomastoid muscle (or via a transverse collar incision for bilateral exposure) and minor soft tissue dissection.

For patients with "hard" signs of significant vascular and/or aerodigestive injuries, operative management is indicated regardless of the zone of an injury. The "hard" signs include active hemorrhage, expanding hematoma, audible bruit, pulse deficit, massive subcutaneous emphysema, stridor, respiratory distress, and/or hemiparesis.

Controversy arises over the management of the patient with penetrating neck trauma with only "soft" signs of an injury, such as dysphagia, voice change, hemoptysis, or a wide mediastinum on chest x-ray evaluation. Traditionally, unless such a patient had profound hemodynamic instability, a selective management approach (often including angiography, esophagoscopy, and bronchoscopy) has been advocated for both zone I and zone III because of the difficulty in examining and operatively exposing these areas. The management of similar patients with zone II injuries, however, has evolved from an era of mandatory surgical exploration, which led to many nontherapeutic explorations, to an era of more selective management based on both civilian and military clinical experience and new imaging modalities. Recent data have shown that <25% of gunshot wounds to the neck and only 10% of stab wounds to the neck require a therapeutic operation.

A careful physical exam is mandatory and is the most efficient first step in evaluating the neck with respect to a penetrating injury. The Advanced Trauma Life Support guidelines to this exam provide a systematic approach to identifying major vascular, aerodigestive, and neurologic signs and symptoms that would mandate immediate intervention. For hemodynamically stable patients with penetrating neck injury (with or without "soft" signs), regardless of zone, helical computed tomographic angiography (CTA) has emerged as the initial diagnostic test of choice. Not only is it extremely sensitive and specific for identifying a significant vascular injury, but it is also excellent for identifying or ruling out an aerodigestive tract injury and spinal injuries. As the speed and resolution of this modality continue to improve, many suggest that it could supplant all other more invasive modalities and serve as a "one stop shop" to evaluate asymptomatic patients for selective operative management.

If a CTA demonstrates that the trajectory is remote from vital structures, the need for additional invasive studies can be eliminated. Helical CTA is limited, however, by artifacts due to a metal (i.e., bullets), which may obscure arterial segments mandating conventional catheter-based angiography with digital subtraction capabilities. An arterial injury identified on CTA warrants either open operative repair or formal angiography with endovascular intervention (i.e., stent, embolization).

Trajectory on CTA concerning for aerodigestive injury warrants further evaluation. Either contrast esophagography or esophagoscopy (flexible and/or rigid) can be used to rule out an esophageal perforation that requires operative repair with acceptable sensitivities and specificities. Combining the two modalities, however, results in nearly 100% sensitivity and specificity. Special attention must be devoted to visualizing the proximal 3 to 5 cm of the cervical esophagus immediately inferior to the cricopharyngeal constrictor as this area can be easily missed during scope insertion and withdrawal. A diagnostic workup of pharyngeal or esophageal injuries should be expeditious because morbidity increases if repair is delayed by more than 24 h.

Concerns for laryngeal and/or tracheal injuries on CT scan or physical exam mandate further evaluation. Direct laryngoscopy is the modality of choice for identifying a suspected laryngeal injury while fiberoptic bronchoscopy should be utilized to detect a suspected tracheal or proximal bronchial injury. A secured airway is recommended before undertaking further workup of a suspected airway injury. For patients requiring urgent airway management, the oral endotracheal approach by an experienced practitioner will often be the first option.

Emergency surgical airway (cricothyroidotomy) should be a mandatory skill as it will be the lifesaving backup procedure for most failed intubation scenarios.

Although frequently performed, immobilization of the cervical spine is unnecessary in patients with penetrating neck trauma unless there is an overt neurologic deficit, unless an adequate physical examination cannot be performed (e.g., unconscious victim), or for patients with concomitant blunt trauma. Neurologic deficits from penetrating assault usually are established and final at the time of presentation. Cervical immobilization devices can obscure critical physical examination findings, leading to missed injuries with potential life-threatening consequences.

SUGGESTED READINGS

Asensio JA, Trunkey DD, eds. *Current Therapy of Trauma and Surgical Critical Care*. St. Louis, MO: Mosby; 2008:197–202.

Schermer CR, Boffard KD. Penetrating neck trauma. In: Peitzman AB, Rhodes M, Schwab CW, eds. *The Trauma Manual: Trauma and Acute Care Surgery*. 3rd ed. Philadelphia, PA: Lippincott Williams & Wilkins; 2007:197–203.

Tisherman SA, Bokhari F, Collier B, et al. Clinical practice guidelines: Penetrating zone II neck trauma. *J Trauma*. 2008;64(5):1392–1405.

Weireter LJ, Britt LD. Penetrating neck injuries: Diagnosis and selective management. In: Asensio JA, Trunkey DD, eds. *Current Therapy of Trauma and Surgical Critical care*. 1st ed. St. Louis, MO: Mosby;2008:197-202.

324

KNOW WHEN AND HOW TO DO A RESUSCITATIVE THORACOTOMY

J. BRACKEN BURNS JR, DO AND ANDREW J. KERWIN, MD

A resuscitative thoracotomy is a high-adrenaline, high-stress situation that can produce dramatic results. Overall, survival is about 4% to 12% for patients requiring resuscitative thoracotomy when considering all patients who present in extremis and have the procedure. More importantly, more than 90% of survivors have normal neurologic functions following resuscitative thoracotomy.

Survival is determined by the type and mechanism of injury, location of major injury, and the presence of signs of life before the procedure is performed. A resuscitative thoracotomy following blunt trauma has about 1% survival compared to about 10% survival following penetrating trauma. In penetrating trauma, because of the higher energy of gunshot wounds, patients who suffer stab wounds typically have better survival than those who suffer gunshot wounds. Survival following stab wounds is around 15%, while it is about 5% for gunshot wounds. Patients with cardiac injuries will have the best survival rate (19.4%) when the location of major injury is analyzed as an outcome variable. Finally, patients with signs of life in the field have a survival that exceeds 10% while those with no signs of life in the field only have about a 1% survival rate.

In order to have a chance at a successful outcome (survival with normal neurologic function), the procedure must be done for appropriate indications. Indications for a resuscitative thoracotomy include patients with penetrating injuries who lose signs of life either just prior to arrival or in the trauma center. Patients who lose signs of life in the trauma center following blunt trauma may be candidates for resuscitative thoracotomy in selected cases. Patients who have no signs of life in the field are not candidates for resuscitative thoracotomy, regardless of the mechanism of injury.

As with any major trauma patient, a coordinated effort at resuscitation is key to success. The algorithm outlined by Advanced Trauma Life Support is one safe way to approach the resuscitation of these patients. Many resuscitative efforts must be initiated simultaneously to the actual thoracotomy. All patients should be orotracheally intubated. At the same time as the resuscitative thoracotomy is taking place, an effort should be made to evaluate the right hemithorax by finger thoracostomy or chest tube placement. Ensuring the safety of hospital personnel is of paramount importance.

The procedure for resuscitative thoracotomy involves a left anterior-lateral thoracotomy. The patient should be supine with the arms extended. Someone should quickly prep and drape the chest while the surgeon and assistant gown and glove themselves to ensure sterility as well as personnel protection.

The incision should be made in the fourth intercostal space. This usually corresponds to the nipple in a male patient. In a female patient, lift the breast and the incision is made in the inframammary crease at the same anatomic level. The incision is curved to follow the path of the rib and should extend from the sternal border to the midaxillary line.

The initial incision should be made with a number-10 scalpel blade and carried down to the intercostal muscles. This should take two or three quick strokes of the scalpel blade to get to this level. At this point, Mayo scissors are used to incise the intercostal muscles above the rib and enter the chest. The pleura should be incised along the length of the incision. A rib spreader should now be inserted with the handle down toward the table. This is an important point to remember as it is easy to insert the rib spreader backward during this chaotic time. If this is done incorrectly, you will not be able to easily extend the incision across the sternum and enter the right chest should the need arise.

Once inside the chest cavity, the first move is to evacuate all of the blood in the chest to help identify the site of bleeding. This is a very dramatic point in the procedure as you are likely to encounter a majority of the patient's blood volume in the chest. The lung can be mobilized by dividing the inferior pulmonary ligament. Next, the pericardium should be grasped, tented, and incised with scissors in a parallel fashion to the phrenic nerve. It is important to identify the phrenic nerve when opening the pericardium to prevent an injury. The opening of the pericardium will allow for the evaluation of tamponade and facilitate open cardiac massage. Small cardiac injuries can be repaired with sutures or staples or can have a Foley catheter inserted into the hole as a temporizing measure to allow for continued resuscitation and transport to the operating room. In the case of a massively bleeding lung, consideration should be given to twisting the lung 180 degrees around the hilum to temporarily halt blood flow to the lung.

Next, attention is turned to cross clamping of the descending thoracic aorta. In order to successfully cross clamp the aorta, several things should be considered as the aorta is generally flat and easily confused with the thoracic esophagus. Anatomically, the aorta is the first structure anterior to the spine. An orogastric tube must be placed as soon as the airway is secured, which may aid in the differentiation between the aorta and the esophagus. Successful cross clamping can only be accomplished safely if the parietal pleura is opened by finger or scissor dissection. If there is difficulty in doing this maneuver, the thoracic aorta can be compressed against the thoracic spine with a finger while resuscitation is continued. Ongoing resuscitation may begin to restore some of the intravascular volume and facilitate easier dissection of the aorta.

Patients who survive initial resuscitative efforts should be transferred immediately to the operating room for the definitive management of their injuries.

SUGGESTED READINGS

American College of Surgeons. *ATLS Advanced Trauma Life Support Program for Doctors: Student Course Manual*. 7th ed. Chicago IL: American College of Surgeons; 2004:108.

Branney SW, Moore EE, Feldhaus KM, et al. Critical analysis of two decades of experience with postinjury emergency department thoracotomy in a regional trauma center. *J Trauma*. 1998;45:87–94.

Cothren CC, Moore EE. Emergency department thoracotomy for the critically injured patient: Objectives, indications, and outcomes. *World J Emerg Surg*. 2006;1:4.

Hirshberg A, Mattox KL, eds. *Top Knife: The Art and Craft of Trauma Surgery*. Shropshire, UK: TFM Publishing Ltd; 2005:157–168.

Rhee PM, Acosta J, Bridgeman A, et al. Survival after emergency department thoracotomy: Review of published data from the past 25 years. *J Am Coll Surg*. 2000;190:288–298.

325

UNDERSTAND THE BASICS OF GUNSHOT WOUND TREATMENT

KATHERINE W. KHALIFEH, MD AND ELLIOTT R. HAUT, MD, FACS

When patients come to the trauma bay following a gunshot wound (GSW), adrenaline is high. Understanding some basic principles of gunshot evaluation and management is imperative. Always start with the ABCs (airway, breathing, and circulation) of trauma just as in every other case. GSW victims may have impressive or deforming injuries that should not distract experienced practitioners from the basics of trauma care. Delay in attention to these fundamental tenants of acute care management can worsen injuries and cause long-term sequela. While bleeding from GSWs can be excessive, most hemorrhage can be controlled by direct pressure, allowing time for a more thorough exam so that other subtle but possibly devastating injuries are not missed. Blind clamping of vascular bleeding should be avoided, as it may worsen injuries and cause a more extensive surgery to be necessary. Tourniquets have come back in favor for exsanguinating extremity injuries and can be lifesaving in these instances.

Basic "gunshot wound math" tells us that the number of bullets (often identified on x-ray or palpation) plus the number of holes must be an even number. Every gunshot entrance wound must have an accompanying exit wound or a retained bullet. An odd number requires further physical and/or radiologic examination and evaluation. Common places to miss a wound are in the hair lines, axillae, groins, rolls of fat, mouth, ear, nose, and anus. In addition, cervical collars, blood pressure cuffs, EKG leads, and Zoll pads have been known to cover GSWs. Complete radiography is mandatory, but never assumed. Retained bullets are often missed if the soft tissue of a patient is not included on an otherwise acceptable chest x-ray. Bullets can be missed in a similar fashion in the abdomen, which is not routinely imaged in trauma even when the chest and pelvis are. Because retained bullets are often missed on plain film x-rays, CT scans may be helpful. Ask patients if they have been shot before. Some patients may have retained bullets from prior trauma, but this should never be assumed.

For patients with GSW injury, the often-quoted mantra is "trajectory determination equals injury identification." This is often straightforward, especially in the case of a single GSW. In the patient with multiple holes and/ or retained bullets, this can sometimes be more challenging. Once the trajectory is determined, the correct course of action based upon the likely injury must be undertaken. This may include simple maneuvers such as further physical examination (i.e., an arterial pulse index in penetrating injury of the extremity), diagnostic imaging (i.e., CT scan), or ultrasound examination (i.e., FAST exam of the pericardium). Other trajectories may necessitate immediate operative intervention or a diagnostic and/or therapeutic conventional arteriogram for a solid organ or vascular injury. In some cases, patients can be safely discharged from the emergency department.

GSWs to the chest always need rapid evaluation. Patients who are hypotensive or are in respiratory distress need rapid tube thoracostomy. However, in those patients who are stable, a rapid upright chest x-ray will help determine the injuries and the need for a chest tube. When placing an urgent (as opposed to emergent) chest tube, antibiotics, sedation, and sterile techniques should be used as long as time allows. Injuries below the nipple line are at risk of intra-abdominal or diaphragm injury since the location of the diaphragm is variable during the respiratory cycle. Injuries in the left thoracoabdominal region warrant surgical exploration (often diagnostic laparoscopy) to rule out a diaphragm injury, a risk for future diaphragmatic hernias.

Hemodynamic stability alone does not exclude a significant injury in an abdominal GSW patient. Clinical peritonitis mandates a trip to the operating room and is often the first sign of significant intra-abdominal injury. Delaying transfer to the operating room can lead to the need for more extensive surgery, higher rates of abdominal sepsis, and death. Femoral intravenous (IV) access should be avoided in patients with abdominal GSWs if possible. Major venous injuries will often not allow volume resuscitation via femoral access. Large-bore peripheral antecubital IV lines or central internal jugular or subclavian access is preferred.

Most civilian GSWs are from low-velocity weapons that cause injuries primarily in the direct path of the bullet with limited surrounding damage. The exception to this is a shotgun wound. At close range, shotguns are high-velocity weapons, which cause damage in a large cavitary area with significant tissue devitalization and loss. In general, most close-range shotgun wounds need operative exploration, debridement, and removal of the various parts of the shotgun shell (i.e., casing, wadding). At longer distance, shotguns have more low-velocity type injuries but cause these injuries over a large area as the bullet shot is dispersed over a larger area.

There are certain commonly asked questions from patients and/or family members of GSW victims. Inform patients if they have retained bullets. Bullets are generally left in place because retrieval can cause more harm than leaving the bullet in place. Bullets are not known to cause lead poisoning. In general, they do not migrate. Delayed infection is uncommon. Patients will need to know about retained bullets for future CT/MRI scanning. Retained bullets will not set off airport security and other metal detectors. Patients should be informed that they had a tetanus shot (which providers should ensure happens) and they are currently up-to-date.

SUGGESTED READINGS

Gestring ML, Gestring BJ. Gunshot injury: Overview of ballistics, wounding, and clinical management principles. In: Flint L, Meredith JW, Schwab CW, et al., eds. *Trauma: Contemporary Principles and Therapy*. Philadelphia, PA: Lippincott Williams & Wilkins; 2008:111–119.

Haut ER. Evaluation and acute resuscitation of the trauma patient. In: Evans SRT, ed. *Surgical Pitfalls: Prevention and Management*. Philadelphia, PA: Saunders; 2009:757–771.

326

CHECK FOR THUMB LAXITY TO AVOID MISSING THE DIAGNOSIS OF "GAMEKEEPER'S THUMB"

LISA FORT, MD

BACKGROUND

Gamekeeper's thumb is an injury to the ulnar collateral ligament (UCL) of the metacarpophalangeal (MCP) joint of the thumb. It was named historically for Scottish gamekeepers who sustained the injury while grasping various wild games between their thumb and index finger to kill the animal by stretching and hyperextending the neck. The injury was frequently a result of repetitive motion and developed over time as a chronic process. More recently, acute injuries of the UCL have been described as "skier's thumb," where the injury often occurs due to a sports injury such as falling with a ski pole attached to the hand causing lateral stress or valgus stress on the joint and the UCL ligament. The injury can occur many other ways in other sports, falls, as a result of an arthritic process, or in grasping injuries. Ultimately, the severity of the injury can range from partial tear of the UCL to a gamekeeper's fracture, a complete avulsion of the base of the medial proximal phalanx of the thumb. The diagnosis is easily missed in the emergency department without a high index of suspicion in thumb injuries and requires proper testing and diagnostic maneuvers. There is significant morbidity with a delayed diagnosis because future functionality of the hand can be affected.

ANATOMY

The UCL is a structure that plays a major role in the stability of the first MCP joint. Its two components are the accessory collateral ligament, which is most important in extensor stability, and the proper collateral ligament, which stabilizes the MCP joint during flexion. The origin of the UCL is at the metacarpal head and it inserts at the medial base of the proximal phalanx of the thumb. The UCL is covered superficially by the adductor aponeurosis, which occasionally becomes lodged between the UCL and its insertion site after an injury takes place. This complication, known as a Stener lesion, prevents the ruptured UCL from reattaching to its insertion point and healing.

DIAGNOSIS

An initial history should assess whether an acute injury took place. If an injury is present, details such as the mechanism of injury (specifically position of the thumb), the pattern and type of pain, presence of Stener lesion, and grasp weakness are important to elicit.

As with any bilateral structures, physical examination can be initiated with a comparison of the affected and the unaffected thumb. The unaffected thumb can be examined first and before radiographs are obtained to look for range of motion, stability of the joint under valgus stress, and stability under valgus stress in extension and 30 degrees of flexion. The initial examination of the injured thumb should focus on areas of swelling, tenderness, and ecchymosis as well as gentle palpation for specific areas of nodularity or swelling, gross deformities, or displacement. Before manipulation of the joint is attempted, however, three views of the thumb joint should be obtained.

Stress testing should not be performed if a fracture is present. The patient should be placed in a functional splint and given prompt orthopedic follow-up for further treatment. If no fracture is present, the patient can be further evaluated with stress testing. The thumb should be anesthetized with approximately 3 mL of 1% lidocaine prior to stress testing and injected directly into the MCP joint. If this anesthesia is inadequate, a metacarpal or digital block should be considered. Stress testing is best performed with additional radiography. Valgus stress on the thumb is applied both with the thumb extended as well as flexed to 30 degrees. If there is >40 degrees of radial deviation in extension or 20 degrees in flexion, the joint is unstable. 15 degrees more laxity than the uninjured thumb also indicates laxity. Finally, if there is >3 mm of volar subluxation of the phalanx relative to the first metacarpal on plain film, consider UCL instability (*Table 326.1*).

MANAGEMENT

Injuries of the MCP joint should be treated with immobilization. Ulnar or radial deviation can place further stress on the joint and will prevent adequate healing. Plaster casting and thumb spica splints have been used historically, but a prospective randomized study by Sollerman et al. (1991) demonstrated that functional splinting was much preferred by patients with no difference in outcome between the modalities after either surgical or nonsurgical treatment.

Instability of the MCP joint, Stener lesions, and gamekeeper's fracture are indications for urgent orthopedics follow-up, preferably within 24 h of

TABLE 326.1	SIGNS OF THUMB INSTABILITY WITH VALGUS STRESS APPLIED

>40 degrees radial deviation with thumb in 30-degree extension

>20 degrees radial deviation with thumb in 30-degree flexion

≥15 degrees more laxity compared to uninjured thumb

≥3 mm volar subluxation of phalanx relative to metacarpal

presentation. Best outcomes are associated with surgical repair within the first week after injury. Surgical repair is necessary for all complete tears of the UCL, and repair within the first 3 weeks after injury shows decreased incidence of weakness and pain within the joint. Small, nondisplaced fractures and partial tears of the UCL with no associated joint instability are less urgent and may be conservatively managed with thumb spica splinting for 4 to 6 weeks. However, close orthopedics follow-up is prudent in these patients within the first few days after injury so that they may be followed up over time by the appropriate specialist.

SUGGESTED READINGS

Heyman P. Injuries to the ulnar collateral ligament of the thumb metacarpophalangeal joint. *J Am Acad Orthop Surg*. 1997;5(4):224–229.

Husband JB, McPherson SA. Bony skier's thumb injuries. *Clin Orthop Relat Res*. 1996;327: 79–84.

Peterson JJ, Bancroft LW. Injuries of the fingers and thumb in the athlete. *Clin Sports Med*. 2006;25(3):527–542, vii–viii.

327

USE ABDOMINAL COMPUTED TOMOGRAPHY SCANNING LIBERALLY BASED ON MECHANISM OR IN UNEVALUABLE PATIENTS TO RULE OUT BLUNT ABDOMINAL TRAUMA

JACQUELINE GARONZIK-WANG, MD AND
ELLIOTT R. HAUT, MD, FACS

Modern helical CT scanners have made astounding changes in all fields of medicine, with trauma surgery being no exception. The liberal use of CT scanning can lead to earlier diagnosis and subsequent treatment of an occult injury. In addition, abdominal CT scans can rule out intra-abdominal pathology in a patient who might otherwise have to be admitted overnight for serial examinations and monitoring. While an alert, oriented, nonintoxicated person may immediately show signs and symptoms that can aid in the diagnosis of an abdominal injury, many trauma patients are intoxicated or have had a significant head injury, making their physical exam unreliable.

The liberal use of abdominal CT scan in trauma patients often allows for early diagnosis and treatment of an injury that may have otherwise gone unnoticed or taken longer to diagnose. An abdominal CT scan often finds pathology that is not suspected based on the patients' mechanism of injury or presentation. In a study by Deunk et al., abdominal CT scan revealed unexpected diagnoses in 40% of patients and these findings resulted in a change in treatment plan in 16% of the patients. Other studies have shown similarly high numbers of patients with unexpected findings resulting in a change in management plans in large numbers of injured patients. Earlier detection of unsuspected abdominal pathology can lead to quicker surgical intervention which may prevent unnecessary complications, decreasing morbidity and hospital stay. Early CT scan may also identify patients who will benefit from catheter-based interventions (i.e., invasive angiographic embolization for solid organ or pelvic fracture–related bleeding).

CT scans can also save money by reliably ruling out an abdominal injury, preventing costly admissions and helping to decrease the ever-rising strain and demand on busy, overburdened emergency departments and trauma centers. Livingston et al. performed a multi-institutional prospective study at four level I trauma centers which demonstrated that "the negative predictive power of an abdominal CT scan based on the preliminary reading ... was 99.63%." Their study suggests that patients suspected of having blunt abdominal trauma with a negative scan did not need to be admitted or undergo prolonged observation.

Intoxication or altered level of consciousness often makes physical examination unreliable making these two types of trauma patients ideal candidates for abdominal CT scan. Patients with blunt traumatic brain injury or those whose mental status is altered from drugs or alcohol are frequently encountered in the trauma bay. They may suffer an injury to their chest, abdomen, and extremities but lack the ability to communicate where they hurt, and they often harbor an occult injury. A negative CT scan in a patient such as this may allow safe early disposition from the emergency department directly to an inpatient surgical floor for the management of other injuries.

While the argument has been made to liberally use CT scans in trauma patients, we agree that not every patient needs a CT scan. Some patients should be immediately taken to the operating room without obtaining a CT scan. Any patient with hypotension and a positive FAST exam and/or peritonitis should be taken directly to the operating room. While CT can be a useful tool, no patient should ever die on the scanner table. It is important that every provider treating trauma patients be able to quickly determine which patient needs emergent surgery and which patients are stable enough to undergo a more thorough workup.

Some factors that weigh against routine abdominal CT scanning include cost as well as the small possible risks of intravenous (IV) contrast and long-term cancer development from the added radiation. Although the radiologist charges may be quite high, the actual costs may be very small. In a hospital that already has the CT scan machine and a technologist to run it, the only incremental cost may be the actual bottle of IV contrast. However, many would argue that the costs are outweighed by the amount saved by avoiding costly admissions and earlier diagnosis of occult injury, therefore preventing later complications and morbidity. There is also a risk associated with IV contrast and with the amount of radiation delivered with routine scanning. However, there are no studies that have determined if the benefits outweigh the risks associated with radiation and IV contrast. Trauma care providers must be cognizant of these factors and consider them for each individual patient.

SUGGESTED READINGS

Deunk J, Dekker HM, Brink M, et al. The value of indicated computed tomography scan of the chest and abdomen in addition to the conventional radiologic work-up for blunt trauma patients. *J Trauma*. 2007;63:757–763.

Huber-Wagner S, Lefering R, Qvick LM, et al. Effect of whole-body CT during trauma resuscitation on survival: A retrospective, multicentre study. *Lancet*. 2009;373(9674): 1455–1461.

Livingston DH, Lavery RF, Passannante MR, et al. Admission or observation is not necessary after a negative abdominal computed tomographic scan in patients with suspected blunt abdominal trauma: Results of a prospective, multi-institutional trial. *J Trauma*. 1998;44:273–282.

Salim A, Sangthon B, Martin M, et al. Whole body imaging in blunt multisystem trauma patients without obvious signs of injury. *Arch Surg*. 2006;141:468–475.

Self ML, Blake A, Whitley M, et al. The benefit of routine thoracic, abdominal, and pelvic computed tomograpy to evaluate trauma patients with closed head injuries. *Am J Surg*. 2003;186:609–614.

328

INTUBATE EARLY FOR PATIENTS WITH TRAUMATIC BRAIN INJURY

SARAH E. GREER, MD, MPH AND RAJAN GUPTA, MD, FACS, FCCP

Patients who arrive in the trauma bay are assessed during the primary trauma survey with the Glasgow coma scale (GCS) to quantify the extent of neurologic disability. Patients with a GCS score of 8 or less are considered to have a severe traumatic brain injury (TBI) and require immediate intubation for airway protection. Agitation or combativeness in patients with any GCS score should be assumed to be secondary to hypoxia or TBI until proven otherwise, and early intubation for these patients should be considered.

Primary brain injury occurs at the time of the initial traumatic event and includes focal lesions such as parenchymal contusions; intracranial hemorrhages such as epidural, subdural, or subarachnoid hematomas; as well as diffuse axonal injury. Secondary injury occurs as a result of hypoperfusion or inadequate oxygen delivery following the initial traumatic event and often leads to worse outcomes in TBI patients. Two of the most common causes of secondary brain injury are hypoxia and hypotension and are both associated with significant increases in morbidity and mortality. Avoiding these events is essential in the management of TBI in order to prevent further damage to brain tissue. Early intubation and control of respiratory physiology can minimize both the duration and the extent of hypoxia. Preliminary studies examining brain tissue oxygenation in the penumbra of the injury suggest that a more liberal use of inspired oxygen to achieve higher arterial partial pressures may improve oxygen delivery to injured brain tissue and improve outcomes. Patients with TBI need an aggressive euvolemic resuscitation to prevent systemic hypotension. The autoregulatory mechanisms that maintain cerebral blood flow may be disrupted in TBI, and standard TBI management of maintaining intracranial pressures (ICP) <20 mm Hg and cerebral perfusion pressures (CPP) >60 mm Hg should be instituted. The use of crystalloids appears to be safer than certain colloids such as albumin for fluid resuscitation in the setting of TBI. More recently, studies examining the use of hypertonic saline for resuscitation suggest improved management of ICP, CPP, and brain tissue oxygenation.

Early recognition of TBI is paramount. Many patients with TBI have associated injuries involving multiple systems and are often subject to hypoxia and hypotension. Early intubation and aggressive euvolemic resuscitation are critical in the prevention of secondary injury and the reduction of morbidity and mortality associated with TBI.

SUGGESTED READINGS

Bratton SL, Chestnut RM, Ghajar J, et al. Intracranial pressure thresholds. *J Neurotrauma*. 2007;24(1):S55–S58.

Bratton SL, Chestnut RM, Ghajar J, et al. Cerebral perfusion thresholds. *J Neurotrauma*. 2007;24(1):S59–S64.

Chestnut RM, Marshall LF, Klauber MR, et al. The role of secondary brain injury in determining outcome from severe head injury. *J Trauma*. 1993;34:216–222.

Gracias VH, Guillamondegui OD, Stiefel MF, et al. Cerebral cortical oxygenation: A pilot study. *J Trauma*. 2004;56:469–474.

Jacob M, Chappell D, Bilotta F, et al. Saline or albumin for fluid resuscitation in traumatic brain injury. *N Engl J Med*. 2007;357:874–884.

Pascual JL, Maloney-Wilensky E, Reilly PM, et al. Resuscitation of hypotensive head-injured patients: Is hypertonic saline the answer? *Am Surg*. 2008;74:253–259.

Stiefel MF, Spiotta A, Gracias VH, et al. Reduced mortality rate in patients with severe traumatic brain injury treated with brain tissue oxygen monitoring. *J Neurosurg*. 2005;103: 805–811.

329

KNOW THE APPROPRIATE INDICATIONS FOR EMERGENT ANGIOGRAPHY IN PATIENTS WITH PENETRATING EXTREMITY INJURIES

SARAH E. GREER, MD, MPH AND RAJAN GUPTA, MD, FACS, FCCP

Peripheral vascular injury may be limb and/or life threatening, and delays in diagnosis or treatment can have devastating consequences. Prolonged ischemia lasting >6 h often leads to irreversible damage. These injuries are more commonly seen in penetrating trauma. Different types of vascular injuries commonly encountered are contusions or intimal flaps resulting in spasm and/or thrombosis, laceration or transection resulting in frank hemorrhage or hematoma, and pseudoaneurysm formation leading to delayed rupture. Clinical manifestations of hemorrhage or distal ischemia may be readily apparent but often are occult.

When a trauma patient presents with penetrating injury to the extremity, immediate evaluation for vascular injury is paramount. The presence of hard signs on the initial physical exam is a reliable indicator of vascular injury. Hard signs include external hemorrhage, expanding pulsatile hematoma, absent distal pulses, palpable thrill, audible bruit, and distal ischemia (pain, pallor, paralysis, paresthesia, and poikilothermia). Frykberg demonstrated the reliability of hard signs on physical exam to have a 100% positive predictive value (PPV) of vascular injury. Patients with hard signs of vascular injury do not routinely require angiography and should be taken directly to the operating room for surgical intervention. In patients at risk for peripheral vascular injury at multiple levels in the same extremity, angiography may help identify the level and/or prioritize the management of multiple vascular injuries. Ideally, these studies should be performed in the operating room to facilitate rapid intervention.

When no hard sign is present in a patient with penetrating extremity trauma, physical exam alone is not adequate to rule out vascular injury. The patient should be examined for soft signs of vascular injury including history of hemorrhage, nonpulsatile hematoma that is not expanding, injury in proximity to major vessels (fractures or missile trajectories), diminished peripheral pulses, and peripheral nerve deficit. The presence of these soft signs can suggest vascular injury; however, they are not 100% predictive. In addition, the lack of any physical signs and the presence of normal pulses also do not exclude vascular injury. Further evaluation with arterial pressure indices (APIs) is warranted. The API is performed by taking the blood pressure in both injured legs by using a Doppler and determining the ratio of the affected to the noninjured leg. Lynch compared API's with the gold standard of angiography and demonstrated a 99% negative predictive value (NPV) for APIs >0.90. Arterial injury can be reliably excluded in patients with APIs >0.90. In patients with APIs <0.90, further evaluation using angiography is required. The use of arterial duplex instead of angiography has been described; however, the sensitivity and specificity of duplex compared to the gold standard of angiography have not been confirmed. Additionally, clinical utility is limited—as duplex requires advanced expertise in ultrasound technology as well as equipment that is often not readily available at the bedside in emergent settings, especially during evening and night time hours. More recently, CT angiography has emerged as a potential diagnostic option. Data are still preliminary, and although it may be an adequate diagnostic tool, it lacks the potential therapeutic benefits of standard angiography.

In penetrating extremity trauma, rapid evaluation and intervention to restore perfusion as quickly as possible are vitally important to minimize tissue ischemia, reperfusion injury, and subsequent complications such as rhabdomyolysis. Angiography is an important tool in this evaluation process when used for appropriate indications. It should not delay rapid intervention in limb- or life-threatening injury. A useful algorithm for evaluation of penetrating extremity trauma can be found on the Web site of the Eastern Association for the Surgery of Trauma (www.east.org).

SUGGESTED READINGS

Frykberg ER, Dennis JW, Bishop K, et al. The reliability of physical examination in the evaluation of penetrating extremity trauma for vascular injury: Results at one year. *J Trauma*. 1991;31:502–511.

Lynch K, Johansen K. Can doppler measurements replace exclusion arteriography in the diagnosis of occult extremity arterial trauma? *Ann Surg.* 1991;214:737–741.

Modrall JG, Weaver FA, Yellin AE. Diagnosis and management of penetrating vascular trauma and the injured extremity. *Emerg Med Clin North Am.* 1988;16:129–144.

330

KNOW THE BASICS OF COMPUTED TOMOGRAPHY INTERPRETATION FOR PATIENTS WITH TRAUMATIC BRAIN INJURY

MICHAEL D. GROSSMAN, MD, FACS

CT scanning has high utility in patients with suspected traumatic brain injury (TBI). Sensitivity is above 90% though this figure is problematic as accurate determination of sensitivity depends upon definition of the traumatic lesion visualized and the timing of the study with respect to injury. In general, large lesions producing mass effect will be diagnosed, and CT remains the gold standard imaging modality for acute traumatic injury. All scans are "noncontrast," meaning no intravenous contrast as this will mask small hemorrhages. Magnetic resonance imaging (MRI) may help further characterize TBI injuries or be beneficial when the diagnosis is in doubt, but it has no role in the acute phase of trauma care. In general, hemodynamically unstable trauma patients should NOT be taken to CT for neuroimaging. When operative intervention is required to stabilize and treat patients, it should be done first.

Traumatic intracranial hemorrhages (ICH) are generally separated into those lying on the surface of the brain (extraaxial) that may exert compressive effects and those within the substance of the brain below the arachnoid layer (intra-axial or subarachnoid). Pneumocephalus (air within the brain) is an important finding as it often indicates the presence of an associated fracture either of the calvarium or sinuses. Identification of fractures is also important as this may predict the appearance of ICH on follow-up scans that were initially normal.

Subarachnoid hemorrhage (SAH) refers to any bleeding below the arachnoid layer and may be diffuse or focal. In cases where blood is diffuse, it appears as slightly brighter than the brain tissue and often layers over the convolutions of the sulci and gyri. Blood may also layer out on the reflections of the dura such as the tentorium. In the presence of large amounts of SAH, a concern may be raised for a "medical" (as opposed to traumatic) cause of bleeding such as a leaking cerebral aneurysm or arteriovenous malformation. Angiography (whether CTA, MRA, or conventional catheter based) can be used to resolve this question.

Small areas of SAH that are coalesced are sometimes referred to as "punctate hemorrhage"; these may be multiple and on follow-up scans may appear as discrete cerebral contusions. Contusions or intracerebral hematomas tend to be bright white in contrast to surrounding brain and may by unilateral or bilateral. Some contusions demonstrate an associated rim of darker gray brain that represents pericontusional vasogenic edema. It is common for contusions to increase in size on follow-up scans 24 to 48 h after injury particularly in patients taking anticoagulants or antiplatelet agents. For this reason, follow-up scans are often recommended by many neurosurgeons on a routine basis even if the neurological examination is unchanged.

Extraaxial collections of blood are generally classified into those that occupy the subdural space or the epidural space. Subdural hematomas (SDH) have an irregular contour as they conform directly to the brain surface, while epidural hematomas (EDH) separate the dural layer from the skull and have a smooth or "lenslike" contour. EDH is always acute. SDH may be acute or chronic and often demonstrate blood clot of different density depending upon the patient's age. These extraaxial blood collections are the most frequent neurosurgical emergencies after trauma, often requiring rapid surgical decompression for optimal patient outcomes.

The most important feature of any TBI with or without ICH is the presence or absence of mass effect. Mass effect indicates pressure exerted by blood or edema on the brain with the potential to produce herniation. Findings on CT scan that indicate the presence of increased intracranial pressure (ICP) and mass effect are the midline shift, collapse or effacement of the lateral ventricles on one side, and collapse or obliteration of the basilar cistern (most ominous sign). Obliteration of the fourth ventricle and basilar cistern suggests the presence of temporal herniation.

Diffuse axonal injury (DAI) refers to shearing and rotational forces that disrupt axons and may become manifest radiographically as a loss of the gray-white interface or a "homogeneous" appearance of the brain. When present early after trauma, it is indicative of a severe injury. Severe DAI may be present and should be on the differential diagnosis of any patient with an abnormal neurologic exam, even if the CT appears relatively unremarkable.

The decision to place an ICP monitor should be driven by clinical presentation and CT scan findings. Guidelines published by the Brain Trauma Foundation suggest ICP monitoring in any salvageable patient with a GCS 3–8 and with any abnormal finding (defined as hematoma, contusion, swelling, herniation, or compressed basilar cisterns) on CT scan of the brain. The guidelines also suggest ICP monitoring for patient with GCS 3–8 and a normal head CT if two of the following three criteria are met: age >40 years, unilateral or bilateral motor posturing, and systolic blood pressure <90 mm Hg. Some neurosurgeons and traumatologists selectively apply these criteria by incorporating the motor components of the GCS and specific appearance of the CT scan. Therefore, the ability to accurately interpret the initial CT scan is essential to the early management of TBI.

SUGGESTED READINGS

Brain Trauma Foundation. Guidelines for the management of severe traumatic brain injury. *J Neurotrauma*. 2007;24(1S):1–vi. Available at: http://www.braintrauma.org/

Quisling RG. Neuroradiologic imaging. In: Layton AJ, Gabrielli A, Friedman W, eds. *Textbook of Neurointensive Care*. Philadelphia, PA: Saunders; 2004:47.

Valadka A. Injury to the cranium. In: Moore E, Feliciano D, Mattox K, eds. *Trauma*. New York, NY: McGraw-Hill; 2004:385.

331

ALWAYS PERFORM A COMPLETE NEUROLOGIC ASSESSMENT OF THE TRAUMA PATIENT

MICHAEL D. GROSSMAN, MD, FACS AND MARC E. PORTNER, MD

Accurate neurologic assessment of the trauma patient is one of the most important components of the initial trauma evaluation. It provides valuable information for appropriate selection of diagnostic tests, emergency therapeutic modalities, and prognosis. Inaccurate assessments delay treatment and can lead to poor outcomes.

A rapid, brief neurologic assessment is a critical part of the primary survey, but this does NOT complete the neurologic assessment. Pupillary assessment and Glasgow coma scale (GCS) are components of the primary survey. It is essential to document pupillary asymmetry; even in the presence of periorbital swelling, every effort should be made to visualize the pupil. Asymmetry is present if there is a 1-mm difference between pupils; approximately 10% of the population have asymmetry due to physiologic anisocoria, but this is a diagnosis of exclusion in the trauma patient. Pupillary dilatation is defined as a diameter >4 mm; fixation is defined as absent response to light. In some cases of orbital trauma, the pupil may be nonreactive to light on the affected side but will react via a consensual response to light shined in the contralateral eye. Bilateral fixed dilated pupils may be produced by hypoxemia or severe brain trauma and should NOT be presumed to be secondary to medications.

GCS is both prognostic and guides immediate therapy. Mild head injury is defined by GCS as 13 to 15, moderate 9 to 12, and severe 8 or below. The score is weighted toward sensitivity in detecting severe injury as any patient who is "not speaking with eyes closed" is defined as having a severe injury irrespective of the motor score. The motor score is the most important component of the GCS and distinction between posturing and localization is essential, particularly in patients with relatively normal CT scans. Extensor posturing includes weak abduction and internal rotation. Flexor posturing may resemble withdrawal but abduction is minimal and does not approach midline. Posturing may be associated with tremor often confused with convulsion, while true withdrawal is not. Remember that patients may show brisk, unilateral localization or withdrawal in the presence of an expanding mass lesion.

The secondary survey should include a detailed assessment of neurological function. However, this key step is often inappropriately truncated or overlooked due to other injuries or a perceived need to "rush" patients to the radiology department for important diagnostic studies.

Head-to-toe assessment includes the inspection of the skull, scalp, and tympanic membranes; hemotympanum provides strong indirect evidence of head injury. Motor, reflex, and sensory testing are essential. Record any observations of movement prior to chemical paralysis and intubation; such observations are essential and easily forgotten. For example, a spinal cord injury diagnosis is commonly delayed in a patient with a gunshot to the abdomen who goes for immediate surgery before anyone notices he has not moved his legs. While evaluation may be obscured by medications and it is tempting to forego complete examination, thorough evaluation should always be carried out.

Motor and sensory evaluation begins with the presence or absence of voluntary movement and sensation. A *complete* spinal cord injury is diagnosed by complete paralysis and loss of sensation below a specific level. All other clinical findings are consistent with *incomplete* lesions. In the presence of spinal shock, these lesions may NOT be differentiated. Spinal shock does not necessarily imply neurogenic shock. The former is defined by loss of intraspinal reflex arcs; the latter by hypotension and bradycardia that *may* be associated with loss of sympathetic outflow in higher (cervical, upper thoracic) lesions. Examples include anal wink and bulbocavernosus reflex that are lost during spinal shock and return following resolution.

In the absence of spinal shock, neurological injury may be classified as upper or lower motor neuron based upon physical exam findings. Upper motor neuron implies loss of regulation of motor neurons originating in the spinal cord due to the injury of the cerebral cortex or cortical spinal tract above the level tested. This produces spastic paralysis with high motor tone, increased reflexes, and positive Babinski sign. Lower motor neuron implies direct injury to the motor neurons in the cord and flaccid paralysis and absent reflexes at that level.

The sensory exam is essential in distinguishing *complete* versus *incomplete* spinal cord lesions. Intact sensation of the toe/ankle indicates sparing of the S1 nerve, sensation in the perineum, and the S4–5 nerves. These findings indicate sacral sparing and are associated with injuries of the lower thoracic and/or upper lumbar spine. Prognosis is significantly better in the presence of sacral sparing. Cauda equina syndrome is also associated with lumbar spine injury; the lower extremities present lower motor neuron findings, with varying levels of sacral sparing and bowel or bladder function.

Central cord syndrome is one of the most common incomplete spinal cord lesions, particularly in older patients with underlying spinal canal stenosis. Contusion, edema, or ischemia of the central cord produces profound upper extremity deficits, often with greater preservation of the lower extremity function. For this reason, complete motor examination of all four limbs is mandatory.

Unilateral (lateralized) neurologic findings from spinal cord injury are rare because nerve fibers mediating pain and temperature cross immediately in the spinal cord so that injury to one "side" of the cord will produce bilateral findings (Brown–Sequard syndrome). In general, profound unilateral motor/sensory deficits derive from cortical lesions in the brain (stroke, mass lesion), blunt cerebrovascular injury (BCVI), or peripheral nerve injury. Examples of peripheral injuries include brachial plexus injury that is characterized by loss of function in the upper extremity. Complete loss of function indicates injury proximal to the clavicle and affected roots or trunks; an associated Horner syndrome (cervical sympathetic ganglion) or winged scapula (long thoracic nerve) may also be seen in proximal lesions. At or beyond the clavicle, specific nerves are affected and upper extremity movement/sensation is partially preserved.

SUGGESTED READINGS

Gluck EH, Samuel J, Sarrigiannidis A, et al. Altered mental status. In: Layton AJ, Gabrielli A, Friedman W, eds. *Textbook of Neurointensive Care.* Philadelphia, PA: Saunders; 2004:747.

Lindsey RW, Zbignew G, Pneumaticos SG. Injury to the vertebrae and spinal cord. In: Moore E, Feliciano D, Mattox K, eds. *Trauma.* New York, NY: McGraw-Hill; 2004:459.

332

KNOW WHEN A CHEST TUBE
IS TRULY NEEDED

CLINTON D. KEMP, MD AND ELLIOTT R. HAUT, MD, FACS

In the standard guidelines for the resuscitation of trauma patients as outlined in the Advanced Trauma Life Support developed by the American College of Surgeons' Committee on Trauma, there is an early emphasis on ensuring an adequate airway and breathing in the initial management of the injured patient. The rationale for the rapid evaluation of these systems is that potentially life-threatening injuries can rapidly become lethal if not immediately recognized and treated.

Injuries to the thoracic cavity which cause cardiopulmonary compromise necessitate the placement of a chest tube, many times on the basis of the primary survey and initial set of vital signs in the trauma bay. Tube thoracostomy, while easily completed by practitioners of various levels of experience, however, is not an entirely benign procedure as it can be associated with significant morbidity and even mortality. Complications such as bleeding and infection are relatively common, while damage to vital structures (i.e., heart, lungs, great vessels, spleen, liver, etc.) is more rare. It also can cause major anxiety and discomfort in the critically injured trauma patient. Tube thoracostomy should not be done if not indicated; however, this simple intervention can be lifesaving if properly performed on the correct patient population.

Commonly accepted absolute indications for the placement of a tube thoracostomy in the trauma patient include known or suspected hemothorax and/or pneumothorax causing hemodynamic compromise or respiratory distress and traumatic cardiac arrest. Relative indications include chest wall deformities, mild hypoxia and hypotension with physical evidence of thoracic trauma that localizes to one hemithorax, and occult hemo/pneumothorax that is asymptomatic and diagnosed on the basis of radiography alone. Knowledge of these common indications for chest tube placement as well as those which mimic them will ensure that those patients who need tube thoracostomies will receive them, whereas the placement of unnecessary chest tubes can be avoided.

Pneumothorax is the collection of air in the potential space outside the lung between the visceral and the parietal pleura of the thoracic cavity. A tension pneumothorax results when there is an injury to the pulmonary parenchyma or tracheobronchial tree, whereby air collects in the pleural space without an avenue for decompression. This results in an increased intrathoracic pressure on one side of the mediastinum, which can lead to collapse of the ipsilateral (and eventually contralateral) lung leading to hypoxia, and compression of the heart or vena cava, thereby decreasing preload and leading to tachycardia, hypotension, shock, and death. This will result in physical exam findings such as dyspnea, decreased breath sounds and unequal chest rise on the ipsilateral side, and/or tracheal deviation away from the tension pneumothorax toward the contralateral side. Tension pneumothorax should be a clinical (as opposed to radiographic) diagnosis and rapidly treated with needle decompression followed by tube thoracostomy. If this is a patient's only injury, he or she will improve rapidly.

Hemothorax, the intrathoracic collection of blood in the pleural space from an injury to the chest wall or structures within the thoracic cavity, can also be life threatening. The chest cavity is one of the major anatomic sites for significant blood loss in the trauma patient. This scenario commonly presents with hypotension and tachycardia due to hypovolemia and hypoxia due to pulmonary collapse. These patients may similarly exhibit dyspnea, decreased breath sounds, and unequal chest rise. The placement of a chest tube in this scenario is both diagnostic and therapeutic. Massive hemothorax (often defined as >1,000 mL blood return upon entry into the thoracic cavity or >200 mL drainage per h for >4 h) should prompt a thoracotomy for operative exploration to identify and treat the source of injury.

It is important to be aware of several groups of patients among whom a preintervention chest x-ray may save them from having a chest tube unnecessarily placed. For those patients who are hemodynamically stable with no signs of respiratory distress in the face of a potential thoracic injury necessitating an intervention, radiologic data as well as additional provider examination can further aid in making the correct diagnosis. We are not implying that every trauma patient with a clinically obvious tension pneumothorax needs a chest x-ray for confirmation of this diagnosis prior to a lifesaving tube thoracostomy; however, in select patients, the short delay associated with waiting for a chest x-ray will avoid the placement of an unnecessary chest tube.

Patients with subjective signs of decreased breath sounds or unilateral chest rise are among patients with injuries to the ipsilateral side. During the initial evaluation of a critically injured patient, the trauma bay can be full of distractions. During the primary survey, the primary surveyor should observe spontaneous breathing, look for chest rise, and listen for air movement with auscultation of bilateral chest cavities. It is tempting to diagnose a hemo/pneumothorax from the subjective determination of decreased breath sounds on the same side as an injury (often a penetrating stab or gunshot wound). In this case, the examiner "finds" the injury that one might expect given the mechanism of injury. In the hemodynamically stable patient without signs of respiratory distress (i.e., normal oxygen saturation and respiratory rate), it can be helpful to obtain a rapid chest x-ray to confirm (or refute) the findings before an urgent, but not emergent, chest tube placement begins. Should the patient become hemodynamically unstable or develop respiratory distress, tube thoracostomy can be performed rapidly without radiography.

Another group of patients at risk for "unnecessary" chest tube placement are those with a right main-stem intubation. This complication can occur when the endotracheal tube is advanced too far or migrates from its proper position above the carina into the right main-stem bronchus due to its shallow angle of takeoff from the trachea. These patients will have some confirmatory signs of correct endotracheal tube placement such as the direct visualization of the endotracheal tube passing through the vocal cords and positive carbon dioxide color change. A careful physical examination of this patient with a right main-stem intubation may include unilateral right-sided chest rise, absence of sounds over the left hemithorax, a tube in farther than would be expected, and possibly desaturation on the pulse oximetry monitor. It is easy to see how the examiner may assume that the patient has a left-sided hemo/pneumothorax. However, simply withdrawing the endotracheal tube several centimeters and/ or obtaining a rapid chest x-ray will lead to the true diagnosis, thus avoiding an unnecessary chest tube placement.

In conclusion, indications for immediate tube thoracostomy in the trauma bay are cardiopulmonary instability or arrest following trauma to the thoracic cavity, with the hemodynamic compromise often due to tension pneumothorax or life-threatening hemothorax. For those patients who are hemodynamically stable with no signs of respiratory distress, a rapid chest x-ray will ensure the correct diagnosis, potentially saving some patients from an unnecessary chest tube placement.

SUGGESTED READINGS

Brock MV, Mason DP, Yang SC. Trauma. In: Sellke F, Swanson S, del Nido P, eds. *Sabiston & Spencer Surgery of the Chest*. 7th ed. Philadelphia, PA: Saunders; 2004:79–103.

Gal TJ. Airway management. In: Miller RD, ed. *Miller's Anesthesia*. 6th ed. Philadelphia, PA: Elsevier; 2005:1617–1651.

Haut ER. Evaluation and acute resuscitation of the trauma patient. In: Evans SRT, ed. *Surgical Pitfalls: Prevention and Management*. Philadelphia, PA: Saunders; 2009:757–771.

Livingston DH, Hauser CJ. Chest wall and lung. In: Feliciano DV, Mattox KL, Moore EE, eds. *Trauma*. 6th ed. New York, NY: McGraw Hill; 2008.

Wisbach GG, Sise MJ, Sack DI, et al. What is the role of chest X-ray in the initial assessment of stable trauma patients? *J Trauma*. 2007;62(1):74–78.

333

STRONGLY CONSIDER ARTERIOGRAPHY IN PATIENTS WITH KNEE DISLOCATIONS

FAHAD KHAN, MD

A knee dislocation is a true orthopedic emergency. It is a relatively rare injury but an important one to recognize because a coexistent vascular injury, if missed, often leads to limb loss. In addition, the detection of a knee dislocation may be difficult because it often presents in the context of multisystem trauma or spontaneous reduction.

Knee dislocations are classified based on the position of the tibial displacement in relation to the femur. There are five main types of dislocations: anterior, posterior, medial, lateral, and rotary. The anterior dislocation is the most common and has the highest frequency of association with popliteal artery injury.

Knee dislocations require a significant force and usually occur in the context of a motor vehicle collision, auto-pedestrian collision, falls, or sporting accidents. These mechanisms result in tremendous ligamentous disruption due to forces applied to specific aspects of the knee joint. The knee consists of several stabilizers including the medial collateral, lateral collateral, anterior cruciate and posterior cruciate ligaments, the joint capsule itself, and the surrounding musculature. If a patient presents with a grossly unstable knee following trauma, with instability in at least three major ligaments, then a knee dislocation with spontaneous reduction should be suspected. In 50% of cases, the knee will be in the reduced position at presentation. Performing a thorough secondary survey and verifying that all extremities have full range of motion, specifically in the altered or unconscious patient, will help avoid missing a spontaneously reduced knee dislocation, as more overt injuries may be distracting.

If the knee is dislocated at presentation, then immediate reduction should be preformed in the ED with steady, sustained, longitudinal traction under moderate sedation, if necessary. Neurovascular exam should be checked before and after the reduction and the leg should then be immobilized in a posterior splint in 15-degrees flexion, as full extension of the knee applies tension on a potentially already injured popliteal artery.

Popliteal artery injury occurs in 10% to 40% of all knee dislocations. Controversy still remains between routinely obtaining arteriography in all knee dislocations versus observing patients with serial vascular exams and using the physical exam to determine the need for further imaging and/or surgical intervention. The physical exam alone cannot be relied upon as patients can have strong popliteal, dorsalis pedis, and posterior tibial pulses even in the context of popliteal arterial injury (e.g., intimal flap tears which can progress to full occlusion of the artery over the next several hours). Time is of the essence as revascularization of the lower limb becomes extremely difficult after 6 to 8 h from injury.

An ankle-brachial index (ABI) of <0.9 has had a sensitivity of 87% and a specificity of 97% for the diagnosis of arterial disruption when compared with the results of arteriography. The ABI compares the Doppler pressure of an arm to a leg to screen for lower limb ischemia. This straightforward measurement is performed by recording the highest Doppler sound of the brachial pulse and comparing it to the highest Doppler sound of the posterior tibial or dorsalis pedis artery. The ankle Doppler pressure is then divided by the brachial Doppler pressure to calculate the index. An index <0.9 indicates an abnormal result. Alternatively, CT angiography or a standard arteriogram should be obtained in a patient with an abnormal vascular exam or if the physician has a high clinical suspicion.

If immediate surgical intervention is indicated, then arteriography should be obtained in the operating room (OR), so that vascular repair may begin immediately, as arteriography obtained prior to going to the OR is associated with delays of 1 to 2 h. If vascular injuries are not detected and corrected in a timely fashion, salvage of the injured limb is much less likely and up to 86% of patients will require amputation of the lower limb.

TAKE HOME POINTS

- Knee dislocations require significant force, and a physician must have a high degree of suspicion for possible dislocation and spontaneous reduction of this dislocation and associated vascular injuries in the multisystem trauma patient.
- Even with a normal neurovascular exam distal to a dislocated knee, ABI and serial vascular exams should be performed to detect a possible vascular injury.
- CT angiography is a useful adjunct in patients requiring further investigation.
- Prompt surgical repair of vascular injuries is required within 6 to 8 h from time of injury to avoid lower limb amputation.

SUGGESTED READINGS

Hollis JD, Daley BJ. 10-year review of knee dislocations: Is arteriography always necessary? *J Trauma*. 2005;59(3):672–675; discussion 675–676.

Klineberg EO, Crites BM, Flinn WR, et al. The role of arteriography in assessing popliteal artery injury in knee dislocations. *J Trauma*. 2004;56(4):786–790.

Laing AJ, Tansey C, Hussey AJ, et al. Occult knee dislocation: The importance of secondary survey. *Emerg Med J*. 2004;21(5):635–636.

Mills WJ, Barei DP, McNair P. The value of the ankle-brachial index for diagnosing arterial injury after knee dislocation: A prospective study. *J Trauma*. 2004;56(6):1261–1265.

Patterson BM, Agel J, Swiontkowski MF, et al. LEAP Study Group. Knee dislocations with
    vascular injury: Outcomes in the Lower Extremity Assessment Project (LEAP) Study.
    J Trauma. 2007;63(4):855–858.
Stannard JP, Sheils TM, Lopez-Ben RR, et al. Vascular injuries in knee dislocations: The
    role of physical examination in determining the need for arteriography. *J Bone Joint Surg*.
    2004;86-A(5):910–915.
Wascher D. High-velocity knee dislocation with vascular injury. *Clin Sports Med*. 2000;
    19(3):457–477.

334

INTRAVENOUS ACCESS IN TRAUMA: CAREFULLY DECIDE WHERE TO PLACE IT AND WHICH CATHETER TO USE

ALICIA N. KIENINGER, MD AND ELLIOTT R. HAUT, MD, FACS

In addressing the circulation in the "ABCs" of trauma resuscitation, careful attention should be paid to the type and location of intravenous (IV) access placed. IV access represents the patient's lifeline in the case of an exsanguinating hemorrhage. The inability to effectively replace the patient's circulating blood volume renders other efforts at resuscitation futile. Effective IV access involves having an appropriately sized catheter to allow rapid administration of IV fluids and blood products placed in a location that ensures repletion of the patient's intravascular volume.

Do not place IV access smaller than 16 gauge or central lines other than introducer sheaths. IV access must allow the rapid administration of fluids and blood products. Rapid infusion is facilitated by large-bore access (14 or 16 gauge) placed in large peripheral or central veins. Resistance to flow through a catheter is directly proportional to the length of the conduit and inversely proportional to the fourth power of the radius, based on the equation:

$$R = \text{constant} \times (\text{length}/\text{cross-sectional area})^4$$

Doubling the diameter of a conduit actually quadruples its cross-sectional diameter, with a huge proportional decrease in resistance. On the other hand, increasing the length of the catheter results in a proportional increase in resistance. Based on this equation, a typical 16-gauge single- or double-lumen central venous catheter is a poor choice for trauma resuscitation. The length and smaller diameter of the catheter contribute to increased resistance that precludes rapid fluid administration. Peripherally placed

14- or 16-gauge IVs offer the best of both worlds: large bore and short in length, making them an ideal choice for trauma resuscitation. If central access is required, a large-bore introducer sheath of 7.5 to 8 French should be utilized. While these catheters are longer in length than a peripheral IV, their large diameter still accommodates rapid infusion of fluids and blood products.

Do not place IVs in anatomic locations that will result in ineffectual resuscitation or will interfere with further treatment of the patient's injuries. The second important consideration in vascular access for trauma patients is anatomic location. The goal of resuscitation of hemorrhagic shock is to maintain adequate filling of the heart in order to ensure cardiac output. While there is no published data regarding this topic, traditionally this is achieved via two large-bore IVs in the upper extremities, ideally in the antecubital veins. The patient's mechanism of trauma and suspected injuries must be carefully considered. For example, if a patient arrives with a penetrating injury to the abdomen and is at risk for a major intra-abdominal venous injury, upper extremity access is essential. In a patient with an injury to the inferior vena cava or an iliac vein, femoral access may be completely ineffectual. A femoral central line will result in resuscitative fluid delivery directly into the abdomen or pelvis, rather than into the venous circulation where it is intended.

While upper extremity access is preferred, certain injury patterns may eliminate one or both upper extremities as potential sites for IV access. Patients with penetrating wounds to the neck and potential internal jugular injuries are not good candidates for peripheral or subclavian access on the side of the injury, as this will result in poor delivery of fluids to the right atrium. Additionally, patients with fractures or other injuries to the upper extremities should not have lines placed in those extremities. IVs in these areas may interfere with further treatment of extremity injuries or result in extravasation of fluids into the extremity, exacerbating the existing injury. In these situations, femoral IV access may be the best option.

Do not continue with unsuccessful attempts at vascular access when other options are available. Think outside of the box. Occasionally, attempts at both percutaneous peripheral and central venous access fail. Venous cut-down, while not often used, remains a viable option in cases when other types of IV access have failed. The saphenous vein is frequently chosen as a site for venous cut-down and can be found at the level of the ankle approximately 2 cm superior and anterior to the medial malleolus. It is important to obtain circumferential control of the vessel, ligate the distal end, and place a peripheral IV catheter directly in the vein. Do not forget to suture this IV in place!

Another option for access is the use of intraosseous (IO) needles, which has played a long-standing role in pediatric resuscitation and is now being used more frequently in adults. Current ACLS algorithms have abandoned the use of endotracheal resuscitative drug administration in favor of IO access in patients without IV access. Military experience has led the way with the use of sternal IO needles for the initial field resuscitation of military trauma. They can be successfully placed in most patients and allow rapid fluid administration. Tibial IO access, more commonly used in children, is also an option for adults. While IO access represents a promising alternative, care must be taken with these lines to avoid complications such as infection at the insertion site or fluid extravasation. As IO access for adult resuscitation gains more popularity, increasing numbers of civilian trauma centers may stock these devices for use in trauma resuscitation.

SUGGESTED READINGS

American College of Surgeons Committee on Trauma. *ATLS Student Course Manual.* Chicago, IL: American College of Surgeons; 1997.
American Heart Association. *Advanced Cardiovascular Life Support Provider Manual.* Dallas, TX: American Heart Association; 2007.
Haut ER. Evaluation and acute resuscitation of the trauma patient. In: Evans SRT, ed. *Surgical Pitfalls: Prevention and Management.* Philadelphia, PA: Saunders; 2009:757–771.
Schwartz D, Amir L, Dichter R, et al. The use of a powered device for intraosseous drug and fluid administration in a national EMS: A 4-year experience. *J Trauma.* 2008;64(3):650–655.

335

ADMIT PATIENTS WITH DISPLACED SUPRACONDYLAR FRACTURES FOR FREQUENT NEUROVASCULAR CHECKS

JONATHAN KIRSCHNER, MD

Supracondylar humerus fractures are common in children and account for the majority of elbow fractures in this population. The incidence of distal humeral fractures in the elderly, while less common, is also rising. A supracondylar fracture is a transverse fracture of the distal humerus above the elbow joint capsule where the diaphysis dissociates from the condyles. Displacement occurs in >75% of these fractures. Supracondylar fractures can be divided based on the location of the distal fracture segment. In the extension-type fracture, accounting for 97% of supracondylar fractures, the condylar complex shifts posteriorly after a fall on the outstretched arm. Flexion-type fractures only constitute 2%

to 3% of supracondylar fractures and the condylar complex shifts anteriorly. In children, the strong anterior capsule and collateral ligaments of the elbow direct forces to the distal humerus leading to a fracture.

Neurovascular injury is more common in supracondylar fractures than in any other elbow fracture, with 12% to 20% of displaced fractures having associated nerve injury. The nerves and vessels of the arm are particularly vulnerable in extension-type fractures with posteromedial or posterolateral displacement of the distal fragment. Median nerve injury, anterior interosseous nerve injury, and radial nerve injury have each been reported as the most common type of nerve injury caused by the fracture.

Brachial artery injury is reported in 10% to 19% of displaced fractures, with 80% of these regaining pulses after closed reduction. In a pulseless extremity following displaced supracondylar fracture, the extremity should be splinted in 20 to 30 degrees of flexion while awaiting emergent reduction.

Further risk of injury to the nerves and vessels occurs during reduction and manipulation of the fracture. Multiple attempts at closed reduction are discouraged given the vulnerable position of the neurovascular structures.

Compartment syndrome is a rare but limb-threatening complication, estimated to be present in 0.1% to 0.3% of supracondylar fractures, though more common with concomitant forearm fractures. The clinical diagnosis of compartment syndrome in the setting of a possible nerve or artery injury is quite difficult. For example, median nerve injury may blunt the pain response of a volar forearm compartment syndrome. Pain is one of the earliest and most reliable indicators of increased compartment pressures. Ecchymosis and significant edema to the forearm despite a normal pulse and good capillary refill may indicate an early compartment syndrome. Splinting the elbow in >90 degrees of flexion, often required for appropriate fracture segment positioning, decreases perfusion to the distal extremity and should be avoided.

All displaced fractures require emergent consultation and admission for frequent neurovascular exams. Only nondisplaced fractures with minimal swelling can be safely discharged. Complications of displaced supracondylar fractures either present immediately or may be delayed (*Table 335.1*). Brachial artery injuries, such as an intimal tear, arterial wall contusion, or laceration of the artery, may be present despite palpable pulses. Furthermore, the initial clinical exam has a poor sensitivity for detecting compartment syndrome, and a reliable exam is difficult to obtain in the pediatric population.

A thorough physical exam is paramount in the initial ED evaluation of supracondylar humerus fractures. Despite a normal neurovascular exam, the risk of complications associated with supracondylar fractures is high, and all patients with displaced fractures should be admitted for frequent monitoring.

TABLE 335.1	COMPLICATIONS OF SUPRACONDYLAR FRACTURES
Median nerve injury	
Anterior interosseous nerve injury	
Radial nerve injury	
Brachial artery injury	
Compartment syndrome	

SUGGESTED READINGS

Battaglia TC, Armstrong DG, Schwend RM. Factors affecting forearm compartment pressures in children with supracondylar fractures of the humerus. *J Pediatr Orthop*. 2002;22(4):431–439.

Gosens T, Bongers KJ. Neurovascular complications and functional outcome in displaced supracondylar fractures of the humerus in children. *Injury*. 2003;34(4):267–273.

Kinik H, Atalar H, Mergen E. Management of distal humerus fractures in adults. *Arch Orthop Trauma Surg*. 1999;119(7–8):467–469.

Omid R, Choi PD, Skaggs DL. Supracondylar humeral fractures in children. *J Bone Joint Surg Am*. 2008;90(5):1121–1132.

Simon RR, Sherman SC, Konegsknecht SJ. *Emergency Orthopedics: The Extremities*. New York, NY: McGraw-Hill; 2001.

Strauss EJ, Alaia M, Egol KA. Management of distal humeral fractures in the elderly. *Injury*. 2007:38(S3):S10–S16.

336

KNOW THE RADIOGRAPHIC SIGNS OF A SCAPHOLUNATE DISLOCATION

SARAH J. LANNUM, MD

Scapholunate dislocation is the most common and most significant ligamentous injury of the wrist. The injury is usually caused by a forced hyperextension of the wrist or FOOSH—"fall on outstretched hand"—injury. The dislocation is caused by a tear in the scapholunate interosseous ligament, which may lead to a rotation of the scaphoid with the proximal pole displacing posteriorly and the distal pole displacing anteriorly. There are characteristic features on a radiograph that will assist in making the diagnosis and avoiding long-term complications such as joint instability, chronic pain, and degenerative arthritis (*Table 336.1*).

TABLE 336.1	SIGNS OF SCAPHOLUNATE DISLOCATION ON PLAIN FILM OF WRIST

>4 mm between the scaphoid and the lunate on PA view

Signet ring sign: scaphoid appears circular as opposed to oblong on PA view

>60 degree angle between the scaphoid and the lunate axis on lateral view

On a PA view of the wrist, the intercarpal spaces should be no more than 2 mm. A distance of >4 mm between the scaphoid and the lunate is specific for an injury to the scapholunate ligament and is called the Terry Thomas sign, named after a British comedian with a wide gap between his front teeth. If clinically suspicious, obtaining a clenched fist AP view with ulnar deviation will have better visualization of the scapholunate intercarpal space.

The cortical ring sign, or signet ring, is also seen on the posterior-anterior (PA) view of the wrist. Rotation of the scaphoid during a dislocation causes the image to project down the cylindrical shape of the scaphoid, making it appear as circular instead of its typical oblong shape.

On a lateral view of the wrist, the scapholunate angle should be evaluated. It is formed by an intersection of lines drawn down the longitudinal axes of the scaphoid and lunate. The angle should be between 30 and 60 degrees. When dislocated, the rotation of the scaphoid will increase this angle to >60 degrees.

Once identified, patients should be placed in either a radial gutter or a volar posterior mold splint. A hand surgery consult should be called as these injuries commonly require closed reduction with percutaneous pinning or open reduction.

SUGGESTED READINGS

Frankel VH. The Terry-Thomas sign. *Clin Orthop Relat Res.* 1978;135:311–312.

Meldon SW, Hargarten SW. Ligamentous injuries of the wrist. *J Emerg Med.* 1995;13(2): 217–225.

Perron AD, Brady WJ, Keats TE, et al. Orthopedic pitfalls in the ED: Lunate and perilunate injuries. *Am J Emerg Med.* 2001;19(2):157–162.

337

KNOW THE DIFFERENCE BETWEEN A JONES FRACTURE AND A PSEUDO-JONES FRACTURE

JARONE LEE, MD, MPH

Fifth metatarsal fractures of the foot are common injuries that present to the emergency department. Among children, 61% of foot fractures are in the metatarsal, with 41% of these fractures found in the fifth metatarsal specifically. The fifth metatarsal is particularly prone to injury because it has the widest range of motion of all the tarsal bones and the base of the fifth metatarsal has only loose ligamentous connections with the fourth. Two important fractures occur at the proximal fifth metatarsal: (1) fracture of the tuberosity (Pseudo–Jones fracture) and (2) fracture of the metaphyseal-diaphyseal junction (Jones fracture). It is important to distinguish between these fractures because they require very specific and significantly different treatments.

CLINICAL HISTORY/PATHOPHYSIOLOGY

Pseudo-Jones Factures. Acute fractures of the tuberosity of the fifth metatarsal are also known as Pseudo-Jones fractures. The typical mechanism is an inversion injury associated with a sprained ankle. These fractures are also called "dancer's fracture" or "tennis fracture" because the mechanism is usually related to dancing, sports, or physical exertion. The proposed mechanism for the injury is twofold. Both the peroneus brevis tendon and the plantar aponeurosis attach at the tip of the tuberosity and as a result, during rapid inversion of the ankle, the aponeurosis and tendon exact opposing forces that cause the avulsion of the tuberosity. Typically, radiographs show an avulsion fracture of the tuberosity of the fifth metatarsal (*Fig. 337.1, arrow B*).

Jones Fracture. Acute fractures of the metaphyseal-diaphyseal junction of the fifth metatarsal were first described by Sir Robert Jones in 1902 in a case report of four patients. Unlike the Pseudo–Jones fracture, patients present after a pivot injury, where they rapidly changed directions with their heel off the ground. This puts a rotational torque force on this weaker area of the metatarsal, thus causing a fracture. Fractures in this location are clinically important because there is a high incidence of poor healing, including delayed unions and nonunions. This is because of two reasons: (1) the metaphyseal-diaphyseal area of the fifth metatarsal is a watershed area with decreased blood supply and (2) the increased range of motion of the fifth metatarsal during weight bearing causes poor approximation of the fracture. Radiographs show a transverse fracture through the metaphyseal-diaphyseal junction of the fifth metatarsal (*Fig. 337.1, arrow A*).

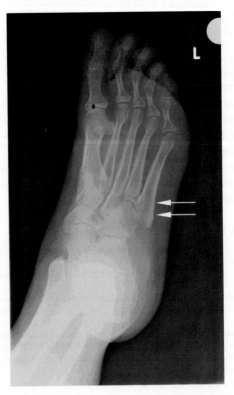

FIGURE 337.1. Location of Jones fracture (*A*) and Pseudo-Jones fracture (*B*).

TREATMENT

Pseudo-Jones Fractures. Nondisplaced Pseudo-Jones fractures are treated with a bulky dressing that is also known, confusingly, as a "Jones dressing." As a result, it is very important to understand that a Jones dressing is not the treatment for a Jones fracture. A hard shoe can also be used for comfort. Otherwise, treatment is weight bearing as tolerated, and most of these fractures heal in 3 to 6 weeks, with radiographic evidence of union by 8 weeks. Displacement of >1 to 2 mm from the cuboid requires referral to a foot specialist or an orthopedic surgeon.

Jones Fractures. Unlike the Pseudo-Jones fractures, Jones fractures require more aggressive management. Because of reasons described previously, these fractures have a higher incidence of delayed union and nonunion, with nonunion rates reported to be up to 44%. As a result, all of these should be referred urgently to a foot or orthopedic specialist, as the treatment should be individualized to the patient's level of activity. For example, athletes typically need early surgical reduction and fixation. Treatment for a Jones fracture typically is either early surgical fixation or non–weight-bearing cast for 6 to 8 weeks. A few studies have found that conservative treatment with casting only has similar healing rates.

TAKE HOME POINTS

- Distinguishing between tuberosity (Pseudo-Jones) and distal tuberosity fractures (Jones) is critical for proper healing and union of bones.
- Pseudo-Jones fractures are treated with conservative treatment (i.e., bulky "Jones dressing" with hard-sole shoe).
- Jones dressings are for Pseudo-Jones fractures and not Jones fractures.
- Urgent orthopedic referral or consultation is needed for Jones fractures but not Pseudo-Jones fractures.

SUGGESTED READINGS

Dameron TB Jr. Fractures of the proximal fifth metatarsal: Selecting the best treatment option. *J Am Acad Orthop Surg*. 1995;3(2):110–114.

Jones R. Fracture of the base of the fifth metatarsal bone by indirect violence. *Ann Surg*. 1902;35(6):697–700.

Konkel KF, Menger AG, Retzlaff SA. Nonoperative treatment of fifth metatarsal fractures in an orthopaedic suburban private multispeciality practice. *Foot Ankle Int*. 2005;26(9): 704–707.

Mologne TS, Lundeen JM, Clapper MF, et al. Early screw fixation versus casting in the treatment of acute Jones fractures. *Am J Sports Med*. 2005;33(7):970–975.

Zogby RG, Baker BE. A review of nonoperative treatment of Jones' fracture. *Am J Sports Med*. 1987;15(4):304–307.

338

CONSIDER OTHER CAUSES OF SHOCK (NEUROGENIC, CARDIOGENIC, OBSTRUCTIVE, ANAPHYLACTIC) IN THE NONBLEEDING TRAUMA PATIENT

BONNIE E. LONZE, MD, PHD AND KENT STEVENS, MD, MPH

Shock is defined as a pathophysiologic state in which there is inadequate oxygen delivery to end-organ tissues. In the setting of trauma, hemorrhage is the most common cause of shock and should be the primary consideration in the differential diagnosis. However, if shock persists and bleeding has been excluded, other causes—hemorrhagic, neurogenic, cardiogenic, obstructive, and anaphylactic—need to be considered. Causes of shock may be multifactorial, and alternative origins must be considered.

NEUROGENIC SHOCK

Injuries to the cervical or upper thoracic spinal cord interrupt sympathetic output to the peripheral vascular beds and the heart. Denervation of the peripheral vasculature causes vasodilation and decreased preload, resulting in hypotension. Additionally, myocardial denervation results in reduced myocardial contractility, leading to the inability to mount a proper cardiac response. A loss of motor and sensory functions below a "spinal level" is a finding suggestive of spinal cord transection and, in a hypotensive patient, must raise suspicion for neurogenic shock. A neurologic exam may be either unattainable or unreliable in trauma patients who are obtunded, in extremis, or intoxicated. A physical exam of the vertebral column should be done to evaluate for step-offs or deformities. Classic clinical findings include decreased blood pressure and bradycardia due to a disruption of the sympathetic chain. Other findings include warm extremities and loss of motor and sensory deficits. The mechanism of injury can also help to gauge the level of suspicion for an injury. Early cervical spine plain films may be helpful, and computed tomography (CT) or magnetic resonance imaging (MRI) can identify vertebral injuries and spinal canal compromise. The management of neurogenic shock begins with fluid resuscitation, with the goal of restoring euvolemia. While primary traumatic neurologic injuries are typically irreversible, prompt correction of hypotension can help ensure that secondary injuries related to CNS ischemia are minimized. If hypotension persists in spite of adequate volume resuscitation, vasopressor support with adrenergic agonists, such as phenylephrine, should be initiated. Dopamine may also be used in this situation, especially in patients with concomitant bradycardia.

CARDIOGENIC SHOCK

Arrhythmias, ischemia, or direct cardiac injury can result in decreased heart function and the development of cardiogenic shock. Patients with a history of heart disease who are injured in trauma have an increased risk for myocardial ischemia and infarction, as the combination of hypovolemia, anemia, and tachycardia results in inadequate myocardial perfusion. Blunt cardiac injuries involving rapid deceleration or blunt force can cause myocardial contusions, papillary muscle ruptures, or valvular injuries, resulting in myocardial dysfunction, arrhythmias, or both. Acute cardiac insufficiency can lead to pulmonary edema and hypoxemia. Clinical suspicion should be raised by mechanism, complaints of sternal or chest wall pain, chest wall injuries, or jugular venous distension. An electrocardiogram should be obtained on patients with thoracic trauma and when suspicion for blunt cardiac injury is high. This includes patients with chest pain, rib fractures, sternal fractures, and pulmonary injuries. Echocardiography and more invasive cardiac function studies can further elucidate cardiac injuries. Treatment should include judicious fluid management and correction of anemia. Patients with profound myocardial dysfunction may require inotropic, or rarely mechanical, cardiac support.

OBSTRUCTIVE SHOCK

In obstructive shock, hypoperfusion results from an anatomic process that impedes forward circulatory flow—the two most common causes in trauma are tension pneumothorax and pericardial tamponade. The presence of a tension pneumothorax is diagnosed clinically, with diminished breath sounds, hyperresonance, jugular venous distension, and mediastinal shift away from the affected side. The classic signs of Beck triad—hypotension, jugular venous distension, and muffled heart sounds—may be present. Clinical suspicion can be verified rapidly in the trauma bay using ultrasound and the FAST (Focused Assessment with Sonography for Trauma) exam. All clinical signs may be difficult to appreciate in the setting of a noisy trauma bay. Pleural decompression can be accomplished by a large-bore needle, typically in the 2nd intercostal space at the midclavicular line. Tube thoracostomy provides definitive treatment. In the absence of overt arrest, a suspicion for pericardial tamponade should prompt a percutaneous pericardiocentesis or subxiphoid pericardial window for definitive diagnosis. Tamponade that leads to cardiac arrest is managed with emergent thoracotomy.

ANAPHYLACTIC SHOCK

The causes of anaphylaxis are many and, in the trauma setting, include intravenous contrast, antibiotic administration, neuromuscular blocking agents, latex, and general anesthesia. Although shock due to anaphylaxis in the trauma setting may be rare, it should be considered if other more likely causes are not found.

SUGGESTED READINGS

Elie MC. Blunt cardiac injury. *Mt Sinai J Med.* 2006;73(2):542–552.

Haut ER. Evaluation and acute resuscitation of the trauma patient. In: Evans SRT, ed. *Surgical Pitfalls: Prevention and Management.* Philadelphia, PA: Saunders; 2009:757–771.

Moore EE, Feliciano DV, Mattox KL, eds. *Trauma.* 5th ed. New York, NY: McGraw-Hill; 2004:221–226.

339

KNOW WHICH TRAUMA PATIENTS NEED SCREENING FOR BLUNT CEREBRAL VASCULAR INJURY

YING WEI LUM, MD AND ELLIOTT R. HAUT, MD, FACS

Blunt cerebral vascular injury (BCVI) was first described over 30 years ago. It is a rare injury and has an incidence of <1%. Nevertheless, it is a devastating injury with stroke rates of up to 25% to 50% and mortality rates of 5% to 43%. The main mechanisms of injury include hyperextension injuries with contralateral rotation of the head (most common), direct blows to the neck, basilar skull fractures (involving the sphenoid or petrous bones), and intraoral trauma.

Diagnosis is difficult especially since the majority of patients with BCVI will initially have a normal neurologic exam. Patients who eventually develop focal neurologic deficits often do so only hours after their admission. Hence, identifying patients at high risk for BCVI is paramount in the initial evaluation of the trauma patient. Besides identifying patients from injury mechanisms, patients with severe soft tissue injuries to the cervical region (contusion, hematoma, or bruit) and polytrauma patients with combined head, neck, and chest injuries also appear to be at higher risk for BCVI (*Table 339.1*).

Catheter based four-vessel angiography remains the gold standard recommendation for patients suspected to have BCVI. However, there is now evidence that helical computer tomographic angiography (CTA) can be used as an effective screening tool without the embolic risk associated with invasive selective angiography of the cerebral vessels. Many trauma centers have adopted protocols and/or guidelines to screen high-risk patients based upon their history, physical exam, or radiographic findings.

Management of BCVI depends on the type (dissection, thrombosis, pseudoaneurysm) and location of the injury. Generally, systemic anticoagulation should be initiated early to prevent progression of the injury unless there are contraindications such as severe closed head injury, solid organ injury, or bleeding pelvic fractures. If such contraindications are present, open operative repair or endovascular techniques should be considered.

TABLE 339.1	PROPOSED REASONS FOR SCREENING FOR BCVI

- History
  - Injury mechanism consists of severe neck hyperextension, rotation, or hyperflexion
  - Hanging
  - Amaurosis fugax
- Physical exam
  - Arterial hemorrhage from the head or face and from the mouth, nose, ears, or wounds
  - Massive epistaxis
  - Expanding cervical hematoma
  - Bruit in the neck of a young patient (<50)
  - Complex facial or mandible fractures
  - Severe closed head injury
  - Seat belt sign across the neck
  - Anisocoria
  - Unexplained mono- or hemiparesis
  - Neurologic examination unexplained by head CT scan
  - Glasgow coma scale score ≤8 (in the field or in the emergency department)
  - Lateralizing neurologic signs
  - Cerebrovascular accident (CVA)
  - Transient ischemic attack (TIA)
  - Horner syndrome
- Radiographic findings
  - Complex facial or mandible fractures
  - Cervical spine fracture
  - Basilar skull fracture through or near the carotid canal
  - Fracture through the foramen transversarium
  - Cerebral infarction on CT scan

SUGGESTED READINGS

Bromberg WJ, Collier B, Diebel L, et al. *Blunt Cerebrovascular Injury Practice Management Guidelines. East Practice Management Guidelines.* Chicago, IL: The Eastern Association for the Surgery of Trauma; 2007. Available at: http://www.east.org/tpg/BluntCVInjury.pdf

Eastman AL, Chason DP, Perez CL, et al. Computed tomographic angiography for the diagnosis of blunt cervical vascular injury: Is it ready for primetime? *J Trauma.* 2006;60(5):925–929.

Fabian TC, Patton JH, Croce MA, et al. Blunt carotid injury: Importance of early diagnosis and anticoagulant therapy. *Ann Surg.* 1996;223:513–525.

Haut ER. Evaluation and acute resuscitation of the trauma patient. In: Evans SRT, ed. *Surgical Pitfalls: Prevention and Management.* Philadelphia, PA: Saunders; 2009:757–771.

340

ALWAYS SEARCH FOR OTHER INJURIES IN PATIENTS WITH SCAPULAR FRACTURE

CHRISTINA MANNINO, DO

Scapular fractures are rare, accounting for <1% of all fractures. The most common cause is blunt trauma in motor vehicle accidents as the leading mechanism, followed by falls, bicycle accidents, and assaults. Scapular fractures are most common in males at an average age of 25.

Scapular injuries alone do not cause significant morbidity or mortality. However, because they do require a significant amount of force, 80% to 96% of these fractures have other associated injuries and rarely occur in isolation. The most common of these injuries across multiple studies of blunt trauma patients is rib fracture. This is followed by pulmonary injuries (including pneumothorax, hemopneumothorax, and pulmonary contusion), clavicle fractures, head and neck injuries, brachial plexus and vascular injuries, intra-abdominal injuries, and other miscellaneous injuries. Although it has been classically taught that scapular fractures are associated with thoracic aortic injury, this association may have been overestimated. In a 10-year retrospective review of blunt trauma admissions to two level-one trauma centers in two different geographic locations (Washington Hospital Center and LA County Medical Center), only 1% of blunt trauma patients with scapular fractures were found to have concomitant thoracic aortic injury.

Fractures of the scapula most often occur in the body, followed by the neck, glenoid, and acromion. A patient with an isolated fracture may present with localized tenderness over the scapula and the ipsilateral shoulder.

Since most patients with scapular fractures are blunt trauma patients, the initial evaluation of these patients will be the same as for any other trauma patients, beginning with the ABCs. Often a fracture of the scapula will not be the injury first recognized. However, once a fracture has been recognized, it is imperative the clinician has a high index of suspicion for accompanying injury to the chest wall, lung, head and neck, or other parts of the body.

Plain radiographic evaluation of the scapula may include the chest x-ray as well as anteroposterior and apical oblique views of the shoulder. CT scanning with three-dimensional reconstructions is the most useful imaging modality to detect and define the extent of scapular injury.

The management of the majority of scapular fractures is nonoperative, consisting of a sling with early range of motion. Most scapular fractures will heal in 6 weeks. Operative management with internal fixation is reserved for unstable fractures. These consist of displaced fractures of the glenoid rim or fossa; intra-articular glenoid fractures with subluxation of the humeral head; extra-articular neck fractures with concomitant fracture of the acromion, clavicle, and coracoid or with angulation; and depressed acromion fractures that interfere with rotator cuff function.

Scapular fractures alone do not typically result in long-term disability; however, recognize the potential for other serious injuries.

SUGGESTED READINGS

Brown CV, Velmahos G, Wang D, et al. Association of scapular fractures and blunt thoracic aortic injury: Fact or fiction? *Am Surg.* 2005;71(1):54–57.
Stephens NG, Morgan AS, Corvo P, et al. Significance of scapular fracture in the blunt-trauma patient. *Ann Emerg Med.* 1995;26(4):439–442.
Tadros AM, Lunsjo K, Czechowski J, et al. Usefulness of different imaging modalities in the assessment of scapular fractures caused by blunt trauma. *Acta Radiol.* 2007;48(1):71–75.

341

USE ADJUNCTS INSTEAD OF PACKED RED BLOOD CELLS ALONE FOR TRAUMA PATIENTS WITH MASSIVE HEMORRHAGE

KAZUHIDE MATSUSHIMA, MD AND HEIDI L. FRANKEL, MD, FACS, FCCM

Despite advances in trauma care, uncontrolled hemorrhage remains a major cause of death in trauma patients. The incidence of injury in civilian trauma centers requiring massive transfusion, defined as 10 or more units of red blood cells (RBCs) in a 24-h period, ranges between 1% and 3%. Mortality rate for these massive transfusion patients may be as high as 50%.

Coagulopathy is one of the serious complications in the setting of massive transfusion. The mechanisms of this coagulopathy are multifactorial and include hypothermia and metabolic acidosis, the dilutional effect of massive resuscitation, impaired function of platelets and coagulation factors, and fibrinolysis activated by tissue trauma and endothelial damage. Although it has been believed that the coagulopathy develops over time, recent data have demonstrated that severe trauma patients are already suffering from coagulopathy before the resuscitation is initiated at the emergency room. Moreover, the results of coagulation profiles often take >30 min to obtain and do not necessarily represent the current coagulation status in rapidly bleeding trauma patients. Under such circumstances, administration of hemostatic blood products, including fresh frozen plasma (FFP), platelets, and other coagulating factor concentrates, should be instituted in a timely manner.

Recent studies have shown that early and intensive administration of FFP and platelets have improved the patient outcome. Most bleeding trauma patients require FFP and platelets before losing one blood volume. Some recommendations regarding the appropriate ratio of each type of blood product (plasma:packed red blood cells [PRBCs]:platelet) is 1:1:1 in patients at a high risk of requiring a massive transfusion.

Recombinant activated factor VIIa (rFVIIa) is a prohemostatic agent that is FDA approved in the United States for control of bleeding in patients with hemophilia with inhibitors to factor VIII concentrate. rFVIIa is active only in the presence of exposed tissue factor and has a rapid onset and a short half-time. rFVIIa has been used as an adjunct therapy to correct the coagulopathy in massively bleeding trauma patients in multiple trauma centers. One study of combat-related casualties has demonstrated decreased mortality with rFVIIa for patients who received massive transfusion without increased risk of thrombotic adverse effect. When used for this indication, a dose of 120 μg/kg is recommended after 4 to 6 U of PRBCs are transfused.

As the result of wide-ranging indications for anticoagulation therapy, it is common for trauma victims on preinjury warfarin to suffer a life-threatening hemorrhage. Prothrombin complex concentrate (PCC) can be used as a rapid method for warfarin reversal in the trauma patient with fatal bleeding, especially closed head injury. Although FFP is often administered to reverse the anticoagulation effect of warfarin, more rapid and complete replacement of vitamin K–dependent clotting factors can be achieved with lower volume of PCC. The optimal dose of PCC should be individualized based on the international normalized ratio of prothrombin time and body weight. The risk of thrombotic event may increase with higher dose of PCC. Factor VIIa has also been recommended for the reversal of the effect of warfarin in this patient population, although at a lower suggested dose.

A massive transfusion protocol including PRBCs, thawed plasma, cryoprecipitate, platelets, and recombinant factor VIIa is designed to guide the administration of a large volume of blood products given quickly and in appropriate ratios to optimize trauma patient outcomes. The most important factor guiding the success of a massive transfusion protocol is the early recognition of patients in whom it should be deployed. Once the massive transfusion protocol is activated, serial shipments with fixed blood components are sent at the request of trauma

	PRBCs	TP	PLATELET		RFVIIA
SHIPMENT	(U)	(U)	DOSE	CRYOPRECIPITATE	(MG)
1[a]	5 O–Negative	2 AB	NA	NA	NA
1[b]	5	2	NA	NA	NA
2	5	2	1	NA	NA
3	5	2	NA	10	4.8
4	5	2	1	NA	NA
5	5	2	NA	NA	NA
6	5	2	1	10	2.4
7	5	2	NA	NA	NA
8	5	2	1	NA	NA
9	5	2	NA	10	NA
10	5	2	1	NA	NA

TABLE 341.1 MASSIVE TRANSFUSION PROTOCOL

[a]If blood type is unknown, the first shipment consists of 5 U of blood group O Rh-negative PRBCs and 2 U of blood group AB TP.

[b]If blood type is known, shipment consists of type-specific PRBCs and TP.

NA, not applicable; PRBCs, packed red blood cells; rFVIIa, recombinant factor VIIa; TP, thawed plasma.

Reproduced with permission from O'Keeffe T, Refaai M, Tchorz, et al. A massive transfusion protocol to decrease blood component use and costs. *Arch Surg.* 2008;143(7):686–690; discussion 690–691.

team. *Table 341.1* illustrates the massive transfusion protocol utilized at Parkland Memorial Hospital, a high volume Level I trauma center in Dallas, Texas. Implementation of this massive transfusion protocol resulted in a reduction in the use of blood components with improved turnaround times and significant cost savings.

SUGGESTED READINGS

Ketchum L, Hess JR, Hiippala S. Indications for early fresh frozen plasma, cryoprecipitate, and platelet transfusion in trauma. *J Trauma.* 2006;60(6 Suppl):S51–S56; discussion S56–S58.

Leissinger CA, Blatt PM, Ewenstein B. Role of prothrombin complex concentrates in reversing warfarin anticoagulation: A review of the literature. *Am J Hematol.* 2008;83(2):137–143.

Malone DL, Hess JR, Fingerhut A. Massive transfusion practices around the globe and a suggestion for a common massive transfusion protocol. *J Trauma.* 2006;60(6 Suppl):S91–S96.

O'Keeffe T, Refaai M, Tchorz K, et al. A massive transfusion protocol to decrease blood component use and costs. *Arch Surg.* 2008;143(7):686–690; discussion 690–691.

Spinella PC, Perkins JG, McLaughlin DF, et al. The effect of recombinant activated factor VII on mortality in combat-related casualties with severe trauma and massive transfusion. *J Trauma.* 2008;64(2):286–293; discussion 293–294.

342

KNOW WHEN AND HOW TO DO AN ANKLE-BRACHIAL INDEX

KAMAL MEDLEJ, MD

The ankle-brachial index (ABI) is a cheap, fast, simple, and noninvasive procedure for assessing arterial blood flow in the lower extremities. It is primarily used in chronic arterial occlusive disease to assess for the extent of peripheral vascular disease (PVD) and to help predict the risk of mortality and cardiovascular disease. However, it has also been used successfully to screen for acute occult arterial injury of the lower extremities in the setting of blunt or penetrating trauma (dislocations, fractures, or penetrating injuries). ABI for suspected arterial injury is clinically useful, with a sensitivity and specificity of approximately 95% and 97%, respectively.

WHEN TO PERFORM THE TEST

The ABI is best used to screen for occult lower extremity arterial compromise. Any injury with obvious disruption to the arterial bed (significant bleeding, pulsatile bleeding, distal ischemia, shotgun wounds) should be investigated with contrast arteriography. Any suspected injury to the arterial vasculature of the leg in the absence of clinical signs should be screened with an ABI in the emergency department (see algorithm below). An ABI with a value of <0.9 is abnormal and should be followed by contrast arteriography to assess for the location and extent of the injury. Injuries with a normal ABI (>0.9) need not be followed by an arteriogram but can be observed with serial exams or follow-up for a repeat ABI (*Fig. 342.1*).

HOW TO PERFORM THE TEST

To perform the ABI, check the systolic brachial pressure in both arms as you would normally check a blood pressure (BP). Then, check the systolic pressure in the involved lower extremity. This can be done with a sphygmomanometer placed distal to the area of suspected injury and a Doppler over either the dorsalis pedis or posterior tibial ateries (i.e., ankle pressure).

The ABI is then calculated by dividing the systolic ankle pressure by the higher systolic brachial pressure:

$$ABI = P_{Leg}/P_{Arm}$$

P_{Leg} being the systolic pressure of the posterior tibial or dorsalis pedis artery.
P_{Arm} being the highest systolic pressure of the right and left brachial arteries.

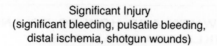

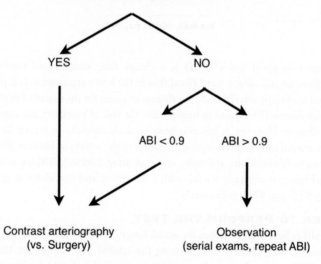

FIGURE 342.1. When to perform the ABI.

HOW TO INTERPRET THE RESULTS

In the event of trauma, a score of <0.9 serves as an indication to perform an arteriogram to locate the point of injury (*Table 342.1*).

The ABI has been a successful and accurate way of demonstrating an impaired arterial blood flow with a high specificity of 97% and a sensitivity of 87% for major arterial injury when compared to arteriography. However, the sensitivity improves to 95% when compared to significant clinical outcomes that require intervention (when eliminating findings such as pseudoaneurysms and arteriovenous fistulas that are clinically irrelevant in this setting).

LIMITATIONS

There are some limitations to the use of the ABI for the detection of vascular injury.

In certain circumstances, it is not possible to perform an ABI. These include situations where placing a BP cuff is not possible or when the BP is too low, such as in states of shock, to yield reliable distal pulses. Also, venous injuries or injuries to deep arteries such as the profunda femoris are not detected on the ABI, and it is not reliable for the screening of central injuries to the iliac artery.

TABLE 342.1	INTERPRETING THE ABI
ABI	**ARTERIAL DISEASE/ COMPROMISE**
>1.3	Abnormal (repeat)
1.0–1.3	Normal range
0.9–1.0	Indeterminate
0.8–0.9	Mild
0.5–0.8	Moderate
<0.5	Severe

TAKE HOME POINTS

- ABI is a cheap, quick, noninvasive bedside test to assess for lower extremity vascular injury that should be used in the appropriate trauma setting.
- An ABI <0.9 is abnormal and >0.9 is normal.
- An abnormal ABI should be followed by arteriography or CT angiography to determine the extent and location of the injury.
- A normal ABI (>0.9) can be observed with serial exams or follow-up for a repeat ABI.

SUGGESTED READINGS

Johansen K, Lynch K, Paun M, et al. Non-invasive vascular tests reliably exclude occult arterial trauma in injured extremities. *J Trauma*. 1991;31(4):515–519; discussion 519–522.

Mills WJ, Barei DP, McNair P. The value of the ankle-brachial index for diagnosing arterial injury after knee dislocation: A prospective study. *J Trauma*. 2004;56(6):1261–1265.

Nassoura ZE, Ivatury RR, Simon RJ, et al. A reassessment of Doppler pressure indices in the detection of arterial lesions in proximity penetrating injuries of extremities: A prospective study. *Am J Emerg Med*. 1996;14(2):151–156.

343

IN PATIENTS WITH A RADIAL HEAD FRACTURE, KNOW THE SIGNS OF AN ASSOCIATED ESSEX-LOPRESTI LESION

CHRISTIAN MENARD, PHD, MD

An Essex-Lopresti injury (ELI) involves radial head fracture, interosseous membrane (IOM) rupture, and distal radioulnar joint (DRUJ) dissociation. Some authors argue that triangular fibrocartilage complex (TFCC) disruption represents a fourth component. Curr and Coe described the injury in 1946, but Essex-Lopresti identified the defining elements of the injury mechanism, diagnosis, and repair in 1951. Discrimination of an ELI from an isolated radial head fracture can prevent a patient from experiencing chronic pain and dysfunction. Success rates approach 80% when the injury is diagnosed and treated acutely, whereas failure rates approach 80% when the injury is diagnosed and treated late.

When a patient presents with an ELI, the radial head fracture typically presents as the clinically and radiographically obvious injury. It is estimated that between 0.3% and 5.0% of radial head fractures co-occur with IOM disruption. DRUJ dissociation can occur acutely or gradually as the radius migrates proximally, inadequately restrained by the ruptured IOM.

Emergency department evaluation begins with a history of elbow pain secondary to forceful axial forearm loading, such as fall from height or at speed on an outstretched hand. An ELI is more likely when the forearm is pronated at the time of impact because the radial head and capitellum make maximal contact during pronation. As a result, the radial head bears the brunt of an impact and is likely to comminute. Unsupported by the radial head, the radius shifts proximally, tearing the IOM. Physical exam will likely reveal elbow pain and swelling but typically will not reveal wrist or forearm pain and swelling.

Radiography can reasonably begin with elbow imaging. If a radial head fracture is present, additional imaging above and below the fracture will reveal the diagnosis. Specifically, obtain true posteroanterior and lateral radiographs of the elbow and wrist, as well as grip views of both wrists with forearms pronated. Radiograph reading should focus on ulnar variance. Relative to the contralateral DRUJ, displacement >2 mm indicates DRUJ dislocation and variance >7 mm indicates IOM and TFCC injury. MR or ultrasound (US) can also be obtained to evaluate the integrity of the IOM.

To repair an acute injury, the orthopedist repairs the radial head by open reduction and internal fixation or by arthroplasty using a metal implant and secures the DRUJ in supination for 4 to 8 weeks by casting, K-wires, or screws with the hope that the IOM will heal. It remains unknown whether the collagenous IOM can truly heal. Alternatively, the IOM might be repaired. No repair method has yet proven comparable to an intact IOM, but several methods have been tried with mixed results.

TAKE HOME POINTS

- ELI involves radial head fracture, DRUJ dislocation, and IOM rupture.
- High-energy elbow injury warrants radiographic imaging of the wrist and follow-up US or MR if the ELI is suspected.
- Accurate diagnosis of acute injuries typically leads to successful surgical repair.
- Failure to initially diagnose an ELI results in significant long-term pain and functional impairment that currently cannot be fully corrected surgically.

SUGGESTED READINGS

Dodds SD, Yeh PC, Slade JF. Essex-Lopresti injuries. *Hand Clin*. 2008;24(1):125–137.

Edwards GS Jr, JupiterJB. Radial head fractures with acute distal radioulnar dislocation. Essex-Lopresti revisited. *Clin Orthop Relat Res*. 1988;234:61–69.

Fester EW, Murray PM, Sanders TG, et al. The efficacy of magnetic resonance imaging and ultrasound in detecting disruptions of the forearm interosseous membrane: A cadaver study. *J Hand Surg Am*. 2002;27(3):418–424.

Jaakola JI, Riggans DH, Lourie GM, et al. Ultrasonography for the evaluation of forearm interosseous membrane disruption in a cadaver model. *J Hand Surg Am*. 2001;26(6):1053–1057.

Jungbluth P, Frangen TM, Arens S, et al. The undiagnosed Essex-Lopresti injury. *J Bone Joint Surg Br*. 2006;88(12):1629–1633.

Jungbluth P, Frangen TM, Muhr G, et al. A primarily overlooked and incorrectly treated Essex-Lopresti injury: What can this lead to? *Arch Ortho Trauma Surg*. 2008;128(1):89–95.

Marcotte AL, Osterman AL. Longitudinal radioulnar dissociation: Identification and treatment of acute and chronic injuries. *Hand Clinics*. 2008;23(2):195–208.

344

RECOGNIZE AND CORRECT ROTATIONAL DEFORMITY OF BOXER'S/METACARPAL FRACTURES

KOUSTAV MUKHERJEE, MD

Injuries to the hand, such as boxer's fractures, are one of the most common traumatic conditions that an emergency physician will have to manage. Fractures of the metacarpals and phalanges represent 41% of all upper extremity fractures and account for approximately 10% of all fractures in the human body. The estimated cost (in terms of work days lost) from these injuries approaches 10 billion dollars. Though boxer's fractures of the hand are rarely life threatening, there can be significant morbidity associated with improper care. Timely reduction and immobilization in a functional position are the cornerstones of initial management. Moreover, identifying which cases will require referral to a hand surgeon for further reduction or open reduction and fixation is crucial in preventing further morbidity. Improper healing of fractures can result in significant pain, malunion, scissoring, cosmetic deformity, and ultimate loss of function. Most of this can be prevented by initially performing a thorough physical exam. A critical, sometimes overlooked, portion of the physical exam is assessing for rotational deformity, which is malalignment of the phalanges with respect to a fixed anatomic mark or as compared to the other fingers within the hand. This is usually a clinical judgment as traditional three-view x-rays do not show the presence of a rotational deformity.

In the normal hand, the presence of rotation can be assessed by examining the patient's fist or flexed fingers (*Fig. 344.1*). Lines drawn through the fingers should intersect at the scaphoid. Alternatively, the fingers can be flexed at the MCP joint and the fingertips examined. The presence of divergence, overlap, or scissoring suggests rotation. In a fractured extremity, however, these techniques are usually limited by pain or swelling. To correct this, some authors have suggested end-on examination of the fingernails held in flexion, examination of the nail plate in relation to the horizontal plane with the fingers held in full extension, or comparison to the uninjured hand. Recent studies, however, have shown that there is considerable variation in the horizontal lie of fingertips within and between hands when the fingers are held in full extension. Furthermore, there is some degree of overlap between fingertips held in flexion in the normal population. And these changes are often asymmetrical between both hands. To complicate matters, using modern photographic techniques, most people do not have convergence at the scaphoid and that simple swelling of the

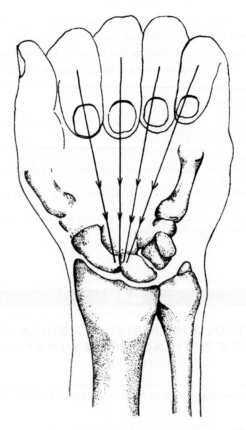

FIGURE 344.1. Normal anatomic position of the phalanges with respect to the scaphoid.

soft tissue can produce the appearance of rotation—so called "pseudorotation." Thus, it seems that the best way to assess for rotation is to ensure that there is no overlapping or scissoring with the fingers held in flexion at the MCP.

The presence of rotation can be seen with any metacarpal or phalangeal fracture, but it is more commonly found with spiral fractures. Even small degrees of overlap in the phalanges (up to 5%) can result in >0.5-cm overlap of the fingertips. In the metacarpals, one degree of overlap can result in up to five degrees of rotation at the fingertips. For this reason, some authors suggest that the presence of any rotational deformity after attempted reduction of a metacarpal fracture is an indication for operative reduction. Other studies, however, have shown that up to a 10% rotation is well tolerated in metacarpal fractures. If left untreated, though, rotational deformities can result in malunion of the fracture or disfiguring scissoring of the fingers. These crippling disabilities can decrease grip strength or render the hand functionally useless. A fresh fracture with a rotational deformity that is not reducible can be easily repaired with operative fixation. Once the fracture has begun to heal with rotation, much more invasive corrective osteotomies are needed to repair the defect.

SUGGESTED READINGS

Bansal R, Craigen MA. Rotational alignment of the finger nails in the normal population. *J Hand Surg Euro*. 2007;32(1):80–84.

Chin SH, Vedder NB. MOC-PSSM CME article: Metacarpal fractures. *Plast Reconstr Surg*. 2008;121(1 Suppl):1–13.

Freeland AE, Lindley SG. Malunions of the finger metacarpals and phalanges. *Hand Clin*. 2006;22(3):341–355.

Smith NC, Moncrieff NJ, Hartnell N, et al. Pseudorotation of the little finger metacarpal. *J Hand Surg*. 2003;28(5):395–398.

Tan V, Kinchelow T, Berediiklian PK. Variation in digital rotation and alignment in normal subjects. *J Hand Surg Am*. 2008;33(6):873–878.

345

BE METICULOUS IN GIVING MEDICATIONS TO PATIENTS WITH ACUTE TRAUMATIC BRAIN INJURY

DEBRAJ MUKHERJEE, MD, MPH AND ADIL HAIDER, MD, MPH

In patients with traumatic brain injury (TBI), little can be done to reverse the initial traumatic insult (primary brain injury). However, the secondary brain injury caused by decreased perfusion of the brain tissue can be prevented and is therefore the most important aspect in TBI management. Secondary injury is commonly a consequence of hypotension and/or hypoxia. In a study of the Trauma Coma Databank, mortality rates rose from 25% (in patients with neither factor) to 75% in patients with both factors. Medications that lead to hypoxia, hypotension, and/or decreased cerebral perfusion may also worsen secondary brain injury and must be avoided. Management of patients with acute TBI includes the avoidance of high-dose steroids and the judicious use of mannitol, anticonvulsants, sedatives, analgesics, barbiturates, antihypertensives, and anticoagulants for venous thromboembolic (VTE) prophylaxis.

Although regularly used to treat acute TBI patients through the 1960s and 1970s, several recent prospective studies and meta-analyses have shown that the use of steroids does not improve outcomes for patients with acute TBI. In fact, a recent prospective randomized clinical trial demonstrated that acute TBI patients receiving steroids had a higher mortality than their non–steroid-treated counterparts. The Brain Trauma Foundation (BTF) and the American Association for Neurological Surgery (AANS) currently recommend against the use of steroids after head injury.

Mannitol, an osmotic diuretic, demonstrates short-term efficacy in controlling intracranial pressure (ICP) in acute TBI patients. Mannitol works by decreasing blood viscosity and the diameter of peripheral blood vessels that helps maintain cerebral blood flow. It also shifts water from the intracellular to intravascular compartments preventing cellular edema. Mannitol is effective at acutely lowering ICP; however, no strong evidence exists supporting its repeated use to control ICP longer term. Furthermore, persistent use of mannitol may lead to hypovolemia and have the adverse effect of reducing cerebral blood flow. The use of mannitol should be avoided in acutely injured, hypotensive, (systolic blood pressure <90 mm Hg) polytrauma patients who may be in hypovolemic shock, as this will worsen perfusion to brain along with the entire body.

TBI patients with Glasgow coma scale (GCS) score <10, cortical contusions, depressed skull fractures, subdural/epidural/intracerebral hematomas, and/or penetrating head wounds are at elevated risk of developing early post-traumatic seizures (PTS). The prophylactic use of antiseizure medications such as valproic acid or phenytoin has been associated with a reduction in the early PTS occurring within the first 7 days of injury. However, prophylactic use of these anticonvulsants has not been associated with any reduction in the incidence of late PTS, occurring at any time >1 week after injury. With the myriad of adverse effects, including hematological abnormalities and neurobehavioral side effects, anticonvulsants should be judiciously used for the prevention of late PTS. If used, they should not be routinely continued past 7 days of injury.

Systemic hypertension is a natural response after TBI as the body attempts to autoregulate and augment cerebral blood flow. Do not attempt to correct these TBI patients to a "normal" blood pressure as this can be counterproductive to the body's attempt to improve cerebral perfusion. Sedation and analgesia are frequently better options than antihypertensives. Short-acting IV β-blockers (i.e., esmolol) or calcium channel blockers (i.e., nicardipine) are ideal agents in TBI patients needing control of severe hypertension.

Multiple studies support the use of both pharmacological and mechanical interventions to prevent the development of VTE (defined as both deep vein thrombosis and pulmonary embolism) in TBI patients. Mechanical interventions, such as intermittent pneumatic compression devices and/or graduated compression stockings, are recommended in all patients free of lower extremity injuries that would preclude their use. Among pharmacological interventions, there is clinical evidence favoring low molecular weight heparin (e.g., enoxaparin) versus unfractionated heparin for VTE prophylaxis in trauma patients. Some caution should be taken prior to initiating pharmacological therapy given that any anticoagulation may increase the risk of exacerbating an already existing intracranial hemorrhage. There is ongoing debate as to when pharmacologic DVT prophylaxis can be initiated in a patient with significant intracranial hemorrhage. Some authors wait for 7 days after a stable head CT scan, while others favor the earlier (48 h) start of prophylaxis.

SUGGESTED READINGS

Bratton SL, Chestnut RM, Ghajar J, et al. Guidelines for the management of severe traumatic brain injury. *J Neurotrauma*. 2007;24(Suppl 1):7–106.

Edwards P, Arango M, Balica L, et al. Final results of MRC CRASH, a randomised placebo-controlled trial of intravenous corticosteroid in adults with head injury-outcomes at 6 months. *Lancet*. 2005;365(9475):1957–1959.

346

USE A BEDSHEET TO STABILIZE OPEN-BOOK PELVIC FRACTURES WHEN MORE DEFINITIVE MEASURES ARE NOT IMMEDIATELY AVAILABLE

MÁRIA NÉMETHY, MD

Pelvic fractures account for 3% to 8% of skeletal fractures in the United States. The majority of pelvic fractures result from minimal or moderate trauma, such as a fall from standing height (particularly common among the elderly). However, injury resulting from considerable force—such as from a serious motor vehicle accident—can result in major pelvic trauma with significant associated morbidity and mortality. Pelvic fractures can involve the acetabulum, single bones, or complex fractures involving a break in the pelvic ring. In this latter group, the most dangerous are open-book fractures, which result from severe anterior-posterior compression forces. Open-book fractures are characterized by complete SI (sacroiliac) joint disruption with lateral displacement and opening of the pubic symphysis due to extensive ligamentous damage.

Pelvic ring disruptions are often highly unstable and are associated with a mortality rate as high as 20% to 50%. Early mortality is most commonly due to hemorrhage and subsequent coagulopathy; causes of delayed mortality include associated injuries and sepsis. With significant pelvic injury, hemorrhage can occur from fractured bone surfaces, direct arterial injury, and damage to the region's extensive venous plexus. An unstable pelvic ring also hinders clot formation, contributing to ongoing bleeding and risk of a hemorrhagic shock.

Pelvic fracture should be suspected based on the mechanism of injury as well as certain characteristic physical findings. These include

- Groin and/or suprapubic swelling or ecchymosis
- Tenderness of the symphysis pubis
- Palpable defect at the symphysis
- Hemipelvic mobility upon gentle compression at iliac crests
- Peripheral neuropathy

Severe open-book pelvic fractures are generally easily visualized on initial pelvic radiograph, most notably in the widening of the pubic symphysis and/ or SI joint(s).

In the case of suspected unstable pelvic ring fracture, primary resuscitative efforts should be directed at correcting hemodynamic instability and stabilizing the pelvis prior to definitive surgical treatment. Reduction of the pelvis facilitates physiologic tamponade by realigning fracture surfaces as well as by reducing the pelvic volume into which hemorrhage can occur. Increased pelvic stability also promotes clot formation. To this end, the advanced trauma life support course now recommends early use of circumferential compression of the unstable pelvis.

In the emergency department, circumferential compression can rapidly and effectively be achieved by binding the pelvis with a sheet.

- The patient's legs are gently lifted and a rolled-up pillow or sheet is placed behind the patient's knees.
- The lower thighs, as well as the ankles, are bound together (with appropriate padding). The internal rotation effected by this binding decreases the displacing force on the fractured pelvis. When binding the lower thighs, care should be taken not to bind at the level of the knees, so as not to risk injury to the common peroneal nerve.
- A bedsheet, folded longitudinally, is eased under the pelvis to the level of the greater trochanters. It is then applied circumferentially with gradual tightening and may be twisted once about itself to achieve secure compression. The sheet is then fastened with clamps.
- It is important to avoid any wrinkling of the sheet during placement, as this can increase risk of pressure ulcers.
- Obtain follow-up radiograph or CT scan to confirm reduction.
- Continue standard trauma fluid resuscitation measures, as patients are likely to require extensive ongoing resuscitation, even with an initial improvement in vital signs.

The use of a sheet to compress and stabilize the pelvis is advantageous for its ease and swiftness of application, safety, and effectiveness. The materials needed are inexpensive and can easily be obtained in the emergency department, and no specialized training is required. The binding sheet can be applied to conscious patients and may be used in the setting of acetabular fracture or other lower limb fractures. Furthermore, the binding sheet does not impede access to the abdomen or perineum during definitive treatment.

TAKE HOME POINTS

- Open-book pelvic fractures are associated with a high rate of mortality and require immediate, aggressive resuscitation and hemorrhage control.
- Initial resuscitation should focus on restoring hemodynamic stability with administration of intravenous crystalloid fluid and whole blood, as well as pelvic, stabilization.
- Circumferential compression using a sheet is an easy, safe, and effective way of stabilizing the pelvis and reducing hemorrhage and can be rapidly performed in the prehospital setting or in the emergency department.
- Avoid wrinkling the sheet to minimize risk of soft tissue pressure injuries.
- Always obtain follow-up imaging to confirm reduction.
- Continue aggressive fluid resuscitation after binding, even if vital signs are improved.

SUGGESTED READINGS

Bottlang M, Simpson T, Sigg J, et al. Noninvasive reduction of open-book pelvic fractures by circumferential compression. *J Orthop Trauma*. 2002;16(6):367–373.

Nunn T, Cosker TD, Bose D, et al. Immediate application of improvised pelvic binder as first step in extended resuscitation from life-threatening hypovolaemic shock in conscious patients with unstable pelvic injuries. *Injury*. 2007;38(1):125–128.

Routt ML Jr, Falicov A, Woodhouse E, et al. Circumferential pelvic antishock sheeting: A temporary resuscitation aid. *J Orthop Trauma*. 2002;16(1):45–48.

Simpson T, Krieg JC, Heuer F, et al. Stabilization of pelvic ring disruptions with a circumferential sheet. *J Trauma*. 2002;52(1):158–161.

Vermeulen B, Peter R, Hoffmeyer P, et al. Prehospital stabilization of pelvic dislocations: A new strap belt to provide temporary hemodynamic stabilization. *Swiss Surg*. 1999;5(2):43–46.

347

AVOID CONVERTING A METASTABLE AIRWAY TO AN UNSTABLE AIRWAY IN TRAUMA PATIENTS... BUT ALSO KNOW HOW TO DO A SURGICAL CRICOTHYROIDOTOMY

KELLY OLINO, MD AND ELLIOTT R. HAUT, MD, FACS

Guidelines for immediate intubation of critically injured trauma patients include Glasgow coma scale (GCS) score <9, acute airway obstruction, hypoventilation, persistent hypoxemia despite supplemental oxygen delivery, cardiac arrest, and/or massive hemorrhage. However, in certain scenarios, patients may fall into a gray area where decisions regarding the timing and necessity of intubation must be considered. The initial providers must always consider the risk/benefit ratio of intubation in every patient on a case-by-case basis. For example, in patients with a known or suspected "difficult airway," watchful waiting may be preferable to immediately beginning a rapid-sequence intubation which may ultimately fail.

Airway management in trauma patients introduces special concerns especially in patients with craniofacial injuries who are at risk for airway compromise. These injuries are often associated with brain injury, spinal cord injury, significant intraoral and/or facial bleeding, soft tissue damage to the face, and neck hematomas. The presence of intraoral foreign bodies or hyoid bone fractures or retropharyngeal injuries associated with cervical spine injury can all also cause delayed airway obstruction. Trauma or burn patients can present with concomitant inhalation injuries secondary to chemicals or burns with subsequent laryngeal swelling heralded by the presence of hoarseness, stridor, or difficulty in controlling secretions. Caution must always be given in this patient group as the degree of swelling often increases with IV fluid resuscitation. Trauma patients who are intoxicated from either alcohol or drugs have airways that are complicated by vomiting and aspiration.

In the cases described above, one may encounter patients who are agitated and attempt to sit up. In this scenario, the important question is: What is the cause of the patient's desire to sit up? Hypoxemia, brain injury, the need to vomit, and partial airway obstruction are common and should be considered before attempting to sedate the patient. In some cases with a severe mechanism of injury associated with evidence of spinal or pelvic fractures, the patient must remain supine to prevent axial loads or displacement of fractures. However, when this is less likely (i.e., isolated assault or gunshot to the face), patients may be allowed to sit up under supervision with the head supported. Often having the patient lean

TABLE 347.1	HOW TO PERFORM A CRICOTHYROIDOTOMY

1. Perform the procedure under universal precautions and quickly prep the area of the neck prior to incision.

2. The cricothyroid membrane lies between the thyroid cartilage (above) and cricoid cartilage (below). In men, the thyroid cartilage is the "Adam's apple" and is the most prominent cartilage palpated on the neck, with the membrane found inferior. In women, when running your finger up the neck, the cricoid cartilage is often more prominent with the membrane lying superior.

3. Place the nondominant hand over the thyroid cartilage to stabilize the area and do not remove your hand from this location during the procedure.

4. Make a vertical incision with a scapel. This is to avoid injury to the anterior jugular veins or venous tributaries as hemorrhage will obscure your view. The scapel is used to incise the pretracheal tissue until the membrane is reached.

5. A transverse incision is made through the cricothyroid membrane.

6. A hemostat, dilator, or a finger can be used to dilate the opening.

7. The tracheostomy tube is inserted into the opening. If a tracheostomy tube is not immediately available, an endotracheal tube can be used instead; however, it will have a long portion outside the neck and be harder to secure.

8. The tube placement should be confirmed with end-tidal carbon dioxide (CO_2) detector as well as bilateral breath sounds.

9. The tube should be safely secured.

forward will allow easier clearance of blood and secretions, relieve some partial airway obstruction, and may alleviate agitation. This is especially true of a patient who is able to speak. In the case of complex or bilateral mandibular fractures, lying flat may occlude the airway as the jaw and tongue retract. This patient may do better sitting up. In this case, mask ventilation while supine can be challenging; however, endotracheal intubation can usually be performed. Zygomatic fractures or fractures along the temporomandibular joint (TMJ) can cause trismus, which must be relieved with paralytics during rapid sequence intubation.

Maxillofacial trauma usually presents more challenges as both bag-mask ventilation and visualization during intubation may be difficult due to bleeding. Control of bleeding can be achieved by the reduction of facial fractures or reapproximation of soft tissue defects with the patient awake. Exploration of the oral cavity can also be quickly performed in the upright position to identify sources of bleeding.

If definitive airway management is necessary, decisions regarding the ideal location, personnel, and plan for intubation must be carefully considered. The above measures can temporarily maintain the metastable airway while all the appropriate equipment and personnel are gathered. If time allows, the combined expertise brought by emergency medicine, anesthesiology, trauma surgery, critical care medicine, and ENT surgery will allow for the safest route of intubation in the most controlled setting. At least one (if not more) backup plan should be discussed before it is needed. These may include videolaryngoscopy, light wand intubation, laryngeal mask airway, and/or fiberoptic intubation. The goal is to avoid the scenario where paralytics and/or sedatives are administered, leading to a loss of airway in a patient who cannot be intubated. At that point, if other routes are unsuccessful, emergency cricothyroidotomy (*Table 347.1*) will be the ultimate backup plan in all cases (except in children) and should be in the armamentarium of all health care practitioners who provide airway care.

SUGGESTED READINGS

Feliciano DV, Mattox KL, Moore EE. *Trauma*. 6th ed. New York, NY: McGraw-Hill; 2000: ch 12.

Haut ER. Evaluation and acute resuscitation of the trauma patient. In: Evans SRT, ed. *Surgical Pitfalls: Prevention and Management*. Philadelphia, PA: Saunders; 2009:757–771.

Hsiao J, Pacheco-Fowler V. Videos in clinical medicine: Cricothyroidotomy. *N Engl J Med*. 2008;358(22):e25.

Miller R, ed. *Miller's Anesthesia*. 6th ed. New York, NY: Churchill Livingstone; 2004:ch 63. 2006.

Perry M, Morris C. Advanced trauma life support (ATLS) and facial trauma: Can one size fit all? Part 2: ATLS, maxillofacial injuries and airway management dilemmas. *Int J Oral Maxillofac Surg*. 2008;37:309–320.

348

WHEN PATIENTS HAVE RIB FRACTURES, ALWAYS ASSUME ASSOCIATED SOLID ORGAN INJURIES AND TREAT PAIN AGGRESSIVELY

EMMANOUIL PAPPOU, MD AND KENT STEVENS, MD, MPH

Rib fractures are the most common injury in blunt trauma patients—occurring in 10% of patients. They also occur in penetrating trauma and nonaccidental trauma such as child abuse. Pneumothorax, pulmonary contusion, pneumonia, liver, and splenic injury are associated injuries that occur in association with rib fractures and can lead to serious morbidity and mortality.

The clinical presentation of patients, as well as the mechanism of injury and location of rib fractures, should guide management. Pain associated with rib fractures is felt on deep inspiration and point tenderness on palpation. Ribs 4 to 10 are the most commonly fractured. Physical examination should include careful inspection of the entire skin surface for chest wall asymmetry, paradoxical motion, lacerations, contusions, and deformities, as well as palpation of the rib cage for the presence of crepitus or point tenderness. Decreased or absent breath sounds on auscultation may reflect splinting from pain but can also be associated with a pneumothorax or hemothorax. Chest radiographs miss up to 50% of rib fractures and can therefore be used to confirm rib abnormalities but cannot rule them out. A pneumothorax or hemothorax can be seen on chest radiograph even when rib fractures are not evident.

Patients involved in severe trauma often have multiple rib fractures due to high energy transfer and are at increased incidence of associated intrathoracic or intra-abdominal injuries. Computed tomography can be used for the evaluation of intrathoracic or intra-abdominal injuries and should be utilized often in the trauma setting if there is a high clinical suspicion of internal injury. The location of rib fractures can give important clues to possible concomitant internal injuries. Fractures of the upper ribs (1 to 3), clavicle, or scapula are associated with injury to the aorta, brachial plexus, and subclavian vessels in 3% to 15% of cases. Up to 75% of patients with thoracic injury have significant injuries of the chest, abdomen, or extremities. Fractures of the lower ribs (9 to 12) are associated with underlying abdominal injuries. Patients with low right-sided rib fractures have a 20% to 50% probability of liver injury, whereas those who have low left-sided fractures have a 20% to 30% probability of splenic injury. Fracture of ribs 11 to 12 can be associated with renal injuries. Intrathoracic injuries such as pneumothorax, hemothorax, and pulmonary contusions can occur with rib fractures at any level.

Patients with only one or two isolated rib fractures can often be treated on an outpatient basis. They are instructed to take nonsteroidal anti-inflammatory drugs with additional prescription of narcotic pain medications if needed. They should avoid contact sports for 4 weeks and seek immediate medical care if they develop difficulty breathing or severe pain; otherwise, they should have a follow-up physical exam 4 to 8 weeks after the injury. Follow-up chest x-rays are not routinely indicated.

Injury to three or more ribs often requires hospital admission for analgesia and monitoring of respiratory status. Inadequate pain relief can lead to splinting, atelectasis, retained secretions, and pneumonia. Treatment is largely supportive and consists of early pain relief and respiratory care (incentive spirometry, chest physiotherapy). Pain control options include oral analgesia, intravenous opioids, patient-controlled analgesia (PCA), intercostals nerve blocks, local analgesia delivery systems, and epidural analgesia. Studies suggest that epidural analgesia for rib fractures is associated with a decreased rate of pneumonia and a shorter duration of mechanical ventilation.

The management of rib fractures in the pediatric and the elderly population merits special attention. Rib fractures in infancy require a great amount of force, and physical abuse should be considered. Radiographic findings will reveal multiple rib fractures in various stages of healing. The implications of such injuries must be recognized to ensure appropriate, safe, and consistent child protection outcomes. A skeletal survey should be obtained in cases where abuse is suspected. In the elderly, morbidity and mortality of rib fractures are twice that of younger populations. Studies have shown that for each additional rib fracture in patients over 65 years of age, mortality increases by 19%. Elderly patients with six or more fractured ribs should be admitted to the intensive care unit due to the increased incidence of morbidity and mortality.

SUGGESTED READINGS

Bulger EM, Edwards T, Klotz P, et al. Epidural analgesia improves outcome after multiple rib fractures. *Surgery*. 2004;136(2):426–430.

Easter A. Management of patients with multiple rib fractures. *Am J Crit Care*. 2001;10(5): 320–327; quiz 328–329.

Sharma OP, Oswanski MF, Jolly S, et al. Perils of rib fractures. *Am Surg*. 2008;74(4):310–314.

Shweiki E, Klena J, Wood GC, et al. Assessing the true risk of abdominal solid organ injury in hospitalized rib fracture patients. *J Trauma*. 2001;50(4):684–688.

349

DO NOT "POP THE CLOT": THE ROLE OF HYPOTENSIVE RESUSCITATION IN TRAUMA CARE

CATHERINE E. PESCE, MD AND ELLIOTT R. HAUT, MD, FACS

The traditional approach to the hypotensive trauma patient has been aggressive fluid resuscitation in order to preserve tissue perfusion and organ function. Universal implementation of this approach, however, is debated. Concern arises when hemorrhage is from an uncontrollable source such as the liver or spleen or other internal bleeding vessels. Overaggressive fluid resuscitation can disrupt the formed thrombus (pop the clot), further contributing to ongoing bleeding, and ultimately impact survival.

Deliberate hypotensive resuscitation during active hemorrhagic shock has been demonstrated to improve survival in a large number of animal trials. The first large, prospective, randomized trial in penetrating trauma patients was conducted in Houston, Texas, in 1994. Patients eligible for the study were >16 years of age with gunshot or stab wounds to the torso who had a systolic blood pressure (SBP) <90 mm Hg, including patients with no measurable blood pressure at the time of the initial on-scene assessment by paramedics. Patients were assigned to one of two groups: the immediate-resuscitation group, in which intravascular fluid resuscitation was given before surgical intervention in both the prehospital and trauma-center settings, or the delayed-resuscitation group, in which intravenous fluid resuscitation was delayed until operative intervention. Overall survival was significantly higher in the delayed-resuscitation group compared to the immediate-resuscitation group (70% vs. 62%, $p = 0.04$). Patients in the immediate-resuscitation group also had significantly longer hospital stays.

Other specific clinical findings in this study went along with the overall picture of worsening hemorrhage. The initial mean SBP was significantly higher in the immediate-resuscitation group. Also, despite the relatively small amount of crystalloid infused in the prehospital setting, the mean hemoglobin concentration at the emergency center was lower in the immediate-resuscitation group, suggesting accentuated bleeding and not just an associated effect of hemodilution. Similarly, the prothrombin and partial thromboplastin times were more prolonged in this group, suggesting that the fluid administration may worsen trauma-associated coagulopathy.

Current military medical teaching often promotes the hypotensive resuscitation strategy. According to the guidelines of the Israeli Defense Forces (IDF), hemorrhagic shock is defined as either *controlled* when the source of bleeding has been occluded or *uncontrolled* when bleeding has temporarily stopped because of hypotension, vasoconstriction, and/or clot formation. Fluid resuscitation of controlled hemorrhagic shock is aimed toward normalization of hemodynamic parameters, whereas in uncontrolled hemorrhagic shock, all principles are aimed at getting the patient to definitive care (i.e., surgery). Treatment is started in this group only when one of three parameters is documented: altered sensorium, radial pulse cannot be palpated, or SBP drops below 80 mm Hg. Massive fluid resuscitation is withheld until the time of surgical intervention.

Practice patterns and opinions regarding this management strategy vary among practicing trauma surgeons as demonstrated in a survey-based study of 345 trauma practitioners to determine opinions regarding prehospital interventions for critically injured patients. The majority of those surveyed recommended that prehospital personnel administer an initial 1- to 2-L bolus of crystalloid fluid. However, approximately two thirds of those surveyed suggested intravenous fluid replacement aimed at relative hypotension (SBP 70 to 80 mm Hg), while only one third of respondents suggested maintaining normotension (SBP 100 to 120 mm Hg).

A more recent randomized study did not show any benefit for patients treated with the hypotensive resuscitation approach. Titration of initial fluid therapy to a lower-than-normal SBP during active hemorrhage did not affect mortality. The authors cited many reasons for the decreased overall mortality and the lack of differentiation between groups, including the imprecision of SBP as a marker for tissue oxygen delivery. They also attributed their primary end point, in-hospital mortality, as too broad an end point to discriminate subtle difference in outcome between groups. Future studies hoped to focus on specific patient population most likely to benefit from deliberate hypotensive resuscitation and on the development of better markers for assessing tissue perfusion and ischemic risk.

The debate is not one of the overall value of fluid resuscitation but rather the optimal volume, timing, and extent of that resuscitation for certain patients. Further research in this area will help optimize the initial care for these patients.

SUGGESTED READINGS

Bickell WH, Wall MJ Jr, Pepe PE, et al. Immediate versus delayed fluid resuscitation for hypotensive patients with penetration torso injuries. *N Eng J Med.* 1994;331(17): 1105–1109.

Dutton RP, Mackenzie CF, Scalea TM. Hypotensive resuscitation during active hemorrhage: Impact on in-hospital mortality. *J Trauma.* 2002;52(6):1141–1146.

Krausa MM. Initial resuscitation of hemorrhagic shock. *World J Emerg Surg.* 2006;1:14.

Salomone JP, Ustin JS, McSwain NE Jr, et al. Opinions of trauma practitioners regarding prehospital interventions for critically injured patients. *J Trauma.* 2005;58(3):509–515; discussion 515–517.

350

ALWAYS PALPATE THE PROXIMAL FIBULA IN ANKLE INJURIES

JEFFREY S. RABRICH, DO

Ankle injuries are one of the most common orthopedic injuries seen in the emergency department (ED). Of all the patients presenting to the ED with ankle injuries, only approximately 15% of them will have fractures. The incidence of ankle fracture has been increasing over the last 20 years and is approximately 187 in 100,000 person-years. Even less common is the Maisonneuve fracture, which if missed can lead to long-term disability and delayed healing.

Jules German Francois Maisonneuve was a French surgeon who first described the fracture pattern bearing his name in 1840. The fracture is caused by an adduction or abduction with external rotation force on the ankle. The injury pattern consists of (1) a fracture of the medial malleolus or rupture of the deltoid ligament without fracture, (2) disruption of the interosseous ligament, and (3) a high (proximal third) fibula fracture. The fracture would be considered a Type C fracture on the commonly used Danis-Weber Classification of distal fibula fractures. The Maisonneuve fracture is estimated to occur in approximately 5% of ankle fractures.

There are several case reports of this injury being missed in the ED setting. Patients often only complain of ankle pain and physicians do not consider evaluation of the proximal fibula. When this injury is missed, it is almost always due to failure to simply palpate the proximal fibula, as radiographically the ankle injury may appear minimal. This examination is easily accomplished by gently squeezing the leg just inferior to the knee. If proximal fibula pain is present, radiographs of the tibia and fibula should be obtained, as well as the ankle.

The treatment of a Maisonneuve fracture depends on the stability of the ankle joint. Most often, the joint will not be stable, and operative repair followed by casting will be required. Therefore, early orthopedic consultation and referral are necessary. The patient's lower leg should be splinted, and it should be maintained nonweight bearing until orthopedic evaluation is obtained.

TAKE HOME POINTS

- Always palpate the proximal fibula with all ankle injuries. As a general rule, the joints above and below all injuries should be evaluated.
- If there is suspicion for this injury, but the mortise appears normal, stress views should be considered.
- Early orthopedic consultation is required for this injury.

Suggested Readings

del Castillo J, Geiderman JM. The Frenchman's fibular fracture. *JACEP*. 1979;8(10): 404–406.

Duchesneau S, Fallat L. The Maisonneuve fracture. *J Foot Ankle Surg*. 1995;34(5):422–428.

Pankovich AM. Maisonnueve fracture of the fibula. *J Bone Joint Surg Am*. 1976:58(3): 337–342.

351

Always consider domestic violence in women, elderly, and pediatric victims of trauma

Christina L. Roland, MD and Heidi L. Frankel, MD, FACS, FCCM

Violence or abuse directed at intimate partners, children, and elders is a major public health issue in the United States. It is vital that health care providers not miss signs of abuse in their treatment of pertinent patients.

Domestic violence or intimate partner violence (IPV) is the most common cause of nonfatal injury to women in the United States. As with all types of abuse, injuries in various stages of evolution or healing suggest IPV. Further, the given history often does not correlate with the physical findings, both in location and severity, and there may be a delay in seeking treatment. Head and neck injuries, usually caused by a punch to the face with a fist, are the most prevalent type of injuries after IPV, although musculoskeletal injuries including sprains and fractures or dislocations are also common with abuse. The diagnosis of IPV can be challenging, and many protocols or predictive models have been developed to assist in the diagnosis. Any women with facial or head and neck injuries and an inconsistent history should be confronted about the possibility of IPV.

Child abuse remains a significant problem in the United States with 872,000 cases of child abuse substantiated by state and local Child Protective Services (CPS) agencies in 2004. Children under the age of four are at greatest risk of severe injury and account for 79% of child maltreatment fatalities, with infants under 1 year accounting for 44% of deaths. The most common perpetrators of child abuse are, in the descending order of frequency, fathers, mothers' boyfriends, female babysitters, and mothers. Child abuse is suggested by the combination of historical inconsistencies, suspicious findings on physical examination, and social risk factors including poverty (although all groups are at risk). Signs of physical abuse include bruises and abrasions followed by lacerations, scratches, soft tissue edemas, strap marks, hematomas, burns, and bites. Bruising in an uncommon location (buttocks, back, trunk, genitalia, inner thighs, cheeks, earlobes, or neck), bruises in a child <9 months of age who is not independently mobile, bruising away from bony prominences, and bruises in a defined pattern or those that carry the imprint of an implement should alert the practitioner of potential abuse. Childhood burns are frequently due to abuse. Immersion burns have a clear delineation between burned and healthy skin, have a uniform depth, and may have a stocking-glove distribution. Oftentimes, splash marks are absent. Symmetrical burns and those involving the buttocks and perineum are especially suspicious. Burns may take on the shape of the object used, including such items as curling irons, radiators, and cigarettes. Finally, external signs of child abuse may not be outwardly visible, especially in the case of shaken baby syndrome, typified by shear hemorrhages of the brain and retinal damage. Clear documentation is paramount for the safety of the child. Physicians are under ethical and legal obligation to report cases suspicious for child abuse; however, procedures vary between hospitals and jurisdictions.

Elder abuse is a term that covers a broad spectrum of intentional or neglectful acts that cause harm or the potential for harm in an elderly adult. Abuse can be physical, sexual, psychological, financial exploitation, or neglect. Worrisome traumatic injuries include those to areas not commonly impacted during daily activities or even secondary to accidental trauma. The trauma may also leave a pattern such as from a shoe or a belt or abrasions from ligatures. Head trauma is especially prominent in severe cases of physical abuse and has high morbidity and mortality rates, with subdural hemorrhage being the most common cause of death in elder abuse. As with pediatric victims, inflicted contact burns and scalds can occur with elders. Patterned burns such as a cigarette burn or immersion lines with glove and stocking distribution can be identified. Like child abuse, elder abuse is a reportable offense.

Domestic violence and elder or child abuse are major health problems in the United States. Although abuse can be difficult to differentiate from nonintentional injuries, identifying injury patterns and inconsistencies in the history can help providers identify patients at risk. A suspicion for domestic, elder, or child abuse should prompt reporting to the proper authorities for the safety and protection of the patient. Clear documentation of the provider's findings is key to differentiating abuse from a nonintentional injury.

SUGGESTED READINGS

Akaza K, Bunai Y, Tsujinaka M, et al. Elder abuse and neglect: Social problems revealed from 15 autopsy cases. *Leg Med (Tokyo)*. 2003;5(1):7–14.

Bhandari M, Dosanjh S, Tornetta PR, et al. Musculoskeletal manifestations and physical abuse after intimate partner violence. *J Trauma*. 2006;61(6):1473–1479.

Collins KA. Elder maltreatment: A review. *Arch Pathol Lab Med*. 2006;130(9):1290–1296.

Dubowitz H, Bennett S. Physical abuse and neglect of children. *Lancet*. 2007;369(9576): 1891–1899.

Halpern LR, Perciaccante VJ, Hayes C, et al. A protocol to diagnose intimate partner violence in the emergency department. *J Traum*. 2006;60(5):1101–1105.

Halpern LR, Susarla SM, Dodson TB. Injury location and screening questionnaires as markers for intimate partner violence. *J Oral Maxillofac Surg*. 2005;63(9):1255–1261.

Rinker AG Jr. Recognition and perception of elder abuse by prehospital and hospital-based care providers. *Arch Gerontol Geriatr*. 2009;48(1):110–115.

Sheridan DJ, Nash KR. Acute injury patterns of intimate partner violence victims. *Trauma Violence Abuse*. 2007;8(3):281–289.

Swerdlin A, Berkowitz C, Craft N. Cutaneous signs of child abuse. *J Am Acad Dermatol*. 2007;57(3):371–392.

352

REDUCE HIP DISLOCATIONS IN A TIMELY MANNER

MICHAEL ROSSELLI, MD, MPH

Dislocation of the hip is a rare but serious orthopedic problem seen in the emergency department. Most often, this condition is secondary to direct trauma, such as a motor vehicle accident or a fall. Hip dislocations may also occur as the result of a congenital condition, such as developmental dysplasia of the hip. A hip dislocation requires immediate pain management and reduction of the dislocation within 6 to 12 h. The incidence of subsequent avascular necrosis of the femoral head is a time-dependent phenomenon, one most likely to occur if relocation is delayed beyond 6 h.

The hip is a very stable ball-and-socket joint. The head of the femur is deeply situated in the acetabulum, intensely supported by ligamentous and muscular structures. As a result, it takes a tremendous amount of force to dislocate a native hip.

Hip dislocations can be classified as anterior, posterior, and central. Posterior hip dislocations are the most common and account for approximately 90% of all hip dislocations. The mechanism of action is direct trauma to the flexed knee. On clinical examination, the extremity is found to be shortened, internally rotated and adducted. The remaining 10% of hip dislocations are either anterior or central hip dislocations. In anterior dislocations, the femoral head rests anterior to the coronal plane of the acetabulum. Anterior dislocations can be either superior or inferior depending on the degree of flexion at the time of injury. If the hip is abducted, externally rotated and flexed, inferior dislocation occurs. If the hip is abducted, externally rotated and extended, superior dislocation occurs. The mechanism of action is forced abduction that causes the femoral head to violate the anterior capsule. Comparatively, a central hip dislocation occurs with direct impact to the lateral aspect of the hip through the acetabulum and into the pelvis. This is a fracture dislocation of the hip.

The treatment of choice for all types of hip dislocations is closed reduction under conscious sedation or general anesthesia within 6 to 12 h. In these patients, time is of the essence. It is thought that with early reduction, the frequency of potential complications will decrease. Documented complications associated with posterior hip dislocations include avascular necrosis and sciatic nerve injury, whereas complications associated with anterior hip dislocation include femoral artery, nerve, and/or vein injury. It is recommended that there be no more than three attempts at closed reduction as the incidence of avascular necrosis increases with multiple attempts.

Although sciatic nerve injury is seen in 10% to 15% of patients with posterior hip dislocations, it is avascular necrosis of the femoral head that is most feared. Avascular necrosis is one of the most disabling complications of hip dislocation. It occurs because the artery of the round ligament of the femur head arises from the acetabulum. Therefore, when contact of the two articular surfaces is violated, blood to the proximal femur head is compromised. Even with immediate reduction, this complication, as well as the other complications mentioned above, may occur. Therefore, reduce hip dislocations as quickly as you can.

TAKE HOME POINTS

- Posterior dislocation of the hip is most common.
- Sciatic nerve injury and avascular necrosis of the hip are the most feared complications of a hip dislocation.
- Reduction of the hip should be performed within 6 to 12 h.

SUGGESTED READINGS

DeLee JC. Fractures and dislocations of the hip. In: Rockwood CA, Green DP, Bucholz RW, et al., eds. *Rockwood and Green's Fractures in Adults*. 4th ed. Philadelphia, PA: Lippincott-Raven; 1996:1659.
Dreinhöfer KE, Schwarzkopf SR, Haas NP, et al. Isolated traumatic dislocation of the hip: Long term results in 50 patients. *J Bone Joint Surg Br*. 1994;76(1):6–12.
Ufberg J, McNamara R. Management of common dislocations. In: Roberts JR, Hedges JR, eds. *Roberts and Hedges Clinical Procedures in Emergency Medicine*. 4th ed. Philadelphia, PA: Saunders; 2004:975–979.
Yang R, Tsuang Y, Hang Y, et al. Traumatic dislocation of the hip. *Clin Orthop Relat Res*. 1991;265:218–227.

353

PATIENTS WITH SNUFFBOX TENDERNESS AND NORMAL SCAPHOID X-RAYS SHOULD HAVE A SPLINT AND ORTHOPEDIC FOLLOW-UP

MICHAEL ROSSELLI, MD, MPH

The scaphoid is the most frequently fractured carpal bone, accounting for approximately 71% of all carpal bone fractures. A fracture of the scaphoid most commonly occurs in young and middle-aged adults. About 5% to 12% of these fractures are associated with other wrist fractures. The mechanism of action is classically a fall on an outstretched dorsiflexed hand or by an axial load directed along the thumb's metacarpal. The scaphoid itself articulates with the radius, lunate, capitate, trapezoid, and trapezium. Consequently, during a fall, it transmits compression forces from the hand to the forearm, leaving it susceptible to an injury.

Scaphoid injuries are concerning because of its unique blood supply. The dorsal and volar branches of the radial artery provide blood supply to the scaphoid. The prime blood supply comes from the dorsal branch of the radial artery that divides into multiple branches before entering the waist of the scaphoid, along the dorsal ridge. The branches course volarly and proximally within the bone, supplying 70% to 85% of the scaphoid. The volar scaphoid branch also supplies the distal 20% to 30% of the bone. Considering the distal to proximal vascular blood supply pattern, a scaphoid fracture may result in avascular necrosis, delayed union, malunion, and nonunion, leading to disabling osteoarthritis. As a result, one must have a high index of suspicion when evaluating these patients.

Even with an initial negative x-ray, it is recommended that all patients with anatomical snuffbox tenderness be treated with a short-arm thumb spica splint. Unfortunately, the incidence of nonunion of scaphoid fractures is about 10%, regardless of the type of immobilization employed in the emergency department.

Immobilization of such patients who have a negative x-ray is imperative because plain films fail to identify up to 25% of fractures. As a result, orthopedic follow-up is recommended in 10 to 14 days for reimaging and reevaluation. At this time, the orthopedic surgeon will repeat the x-ray. If the x-ray identifies a scaphoid fracture, the patient will be cast for another 4 weeks. If the x-ray still fails to identify a fracture, and the patient has anatomical snuffbox tenderness, the orthopedist will proceed to second-line imaging in the form of a CT or MRI. At that time, conservative versus surgical interventions are addressed.

TAKE HOME POINTS

- The scaphoid is the most frequently fractured carpal bone.
- An injury to the scaphoid presents unique challenges because of its tenuous vascular supply.
- Apply a short-arm thumb spica to all patients who present with anatomical snuffbox tenderness and a negative x-ray.
- Arrange orthopedic follow-up for these patients within 10 to 14 days.
- Delays in diagnosis and inadequate treatment may lead to avascular necrosis, nonunion, malunion, or delayed union, resulting in degenerative wrist arthritis.

SUGGESTED READINGS

Chudnofsky C, Byers S. Splinting techniques. In: Rockwood CA, Green DP, Bucholz RW, et al., eds. *Rockwood and Green's Fractures in Adults*. 4th ed. Philadelphia, PA: Lippincott-Raven; 1996:997–998.

Jenkins P, Slade K, Huntley J, et al. A comparative analysis of the accuracy, diagnostic uncertainty and cost of imaging modalities in suspected scaphoid fractures. *Injury*. 2008;39(7):768–774.

Kawamura K, Chung KC. Treatment of scaphoid fractures and nonunions. *J Hand Surg*. 2008;33(6):988–997.

Uehara D, Wolanyk D, Escarza R. Wrist injuries. In: Tintinalli JE, Kelen GD, Stapczynski JS, et al., eds. *Emergency Medicine: A Comprehensive Study Guide*. 6th ed. New York, NY: McGraw-Hill; 2003:1679.

354

USE COMPUTED TOMOGRAPHY SCANNING LIBERALLY FOR THE IDENTIFICATION OF SPINE FRACTURES

MIREN A. SCHINCO, MD, FACS AND
ANDREW J. KERWIN, MD

The identification of fractures in the cervical and/or thoracolumbar spine is of paramount importance for those providing care to trauma victims. The incidence of fractures of the cervical spine is 2% to 6% while that of thoracolumbar fractures may approach 20%. A prompt evaluation to identify injuries is required in order to prevent the development or progression of neurologic deficits. While debated by many, there is ample evidence to support physical examination alone for evaluating for spinal column injuries in patients who are awake and alert and have no spinal tenderness or neurologic deficits as long as there are no distracting injuries producing significant pain. The literature does not define what constitutes a distracting injury, so good clinical judgment from an experienced physician is important in making this determination. When these conditions cannot be met, anterior-posterior (A-P) and lateral films have typically been the historical gold standard for evaluating for spinal column injuries. Open mouth views must be incorporated to evaluate for odontoid fractures.

The advent of multidetector helical computed tomography (CT) scanners has given clinicians a new tool in the evaluation of the spinal column. With these CT scanners has come a much more liberal approach to using CT scan for the evaluation of the spine. While there are no prospective, randomized studies comparing CT to traditional x-rays, there is a growing body of literature demonstrating a higher sensitivity and negative predictive value for CT scan compared to traditional x-rays. CT scans identify clinically significant injuries missed by traditional x-rays and allow greater confidence that there are no missed fractures when the scan is negative. This assumes that there is an experienced radiologist reading the CT scan. These recent studies are prospective comparisons or retrospective reviews (Class II and Class III data) and have advocated replacing x-ray with CT scan. The additional injuries identified by CT scan typically require bracing but occasionally have required operative stabilization.

There are two ways to accomplish CT evaluation of the spine. Patients can either have images of the entire spine reformatted from the data obtained during CT scanning of the chest, abdomen, and pelvis or they can have a dedicated CT scan of their cervical, thoracic, and lumbar spine. There are benefits to each method. Several studies have shown that the use of a CT scan to evaluate the spinal column can exclude an injury in just 1 or 2 h as compared to lengthy delays of even up to 2 days in patients with life-threatening injuries. The decrease in evaluation time comes from the fact that the images for the thoracic and lumbar spine can be reformatted from data obtained during a CT scan of the chest, abdomen, and pelvis. This by no means should be interpreted to mean that every trauma patient should undergo a routine CT scan of the chest, abdomen, and pelvis, but rather, when a CT scan of the torso is indicated, the images of the thoracic and lumbar spine can be reconstructed to evaluate for a spinal column injury.

While the new generation of CT scanners has the ability to obtain this data quickly, reformatting of the data can take significant postprocessing time before the images become available for interpretation. Depending on the software and resources available for this processing, it may actually be faster to obtain dedicated CT images. In addition, some of the fine detail seen in dedicated scans which is needed for appropriate surgical planning may be lost with the reformatting techniques. This decision will have to be made after a discussion with the radiologist at your institution.

Benefits of the liberal CT approach in the evaluation of the spinal column include higher sensitivity, higher negative predictive value, shorter time to exclude a spinal column injury, and potentially less radiation. This will also decrease the need for multiple x-rays of the thoracic and lumbar spines as is commonplace, especially in obese patients. Although the radiation exposure from a CT is greater than that for a single x-ray, the need to repeat x-rays multiple times may actually *increase* the radiation exposure from x-rays. Considering all of the recent data combined with the above reasons, liberal use of CT scan for the evaluation of spinal column fractures is warranted.

SUGGESTED READINGS

Berry GE, Adams S, Harris MB, et al. Are plain radiographs of the spine necessary during evaluation after blunt trauma? Accuracy of screening torso computed tomography in thoracic/lumbar spine fracture diagnosis. *J Trauma*. 2005;59:1410–1413.

Diaz JJ, Cullinane DC, Altman DT, et al. Practice management guidelines for the screening of thoracolumbar spine fracture. *J Trauma*. 2007;63:709–718.

Griffen MM, Frykberg ER, Kerwin AJ, et al. Radiographic evaluation of blunt cervical spine injury: Plain radiograph or computed tomography scan? *J Trauma*. 2003;55:222–227.

Hauser CJ, Visvikis G, Hinrichs C, et al. Prospective evaluation of computed tomographic screening of the thoracolumbar spine in trauma. *J Trauma*. 2003;55:228–235.

355

REMEMBER TO X-RAY THE SPINE IN CASES OF CALCANEAL FRACTURES AFTER A FALL FROM HEIGHT

SONYA C. SECCURRO, MD, MS

Calcaneal fractures are usually sustained after a fall or jump from a significant height, usually at least 8 ft with the first impact on the feet. Alternatively, motor vehicle collision (MVC) can result in a fracture of the calcaneus from impact of the floor or toe pan. Calcaneal fractures are the most commonly injured tarsal bone and account for 60% of all tarsal fractures and 2% of fractures overall. The most common location for calcaneal fractures is intra-articular (75%), or through the body of the calcaneus. Intra-articular fractures occur commonly from direct impact of the foot from a fall or jump. Extra-articular fractures account for 25% of calcaneal fractures and usually result from a twisting mechanism or overuse.

Evaluating the mechanism of injury is critically important; a discussion with EMS providers about the scene of the accident can add additional information for the evaluation of the patient. Orientation of the body at impact strongly influences the pattern of an injury. "Jumpers" (as opposed to "fallers") tend to land on their feet; the force of impact is transmitted superiorly through the axial skeleton resulting in a calcaneal fracture (lover's fracture) that is then associated with a high incidence of pelvic and spinal injuries. Burst fracture of the spine associated with a calcaneal fracture is also called a "Don Juan" fracture. In feet-first landings, flexion forces cause an injury to the junctions of the fixed and mobile segments of the spine, specifically the lower cervical spine and the thoracolumbar junction.

On physical examination, the patient may present with pain, swelling, and ecchymosis on the sole of the foot as well as flattening of the heel. Fracture blisters can develop 1 to 2 days after the injury and may be blood or fluid filled. An initial radiographic evaluation should be with plain film, AP, lateral, and axial (Harris) views. In the lateral view, the calculation of Bohler angle (<30 degrees is abnormal) is helpful to identify subtle fractures and measure the degree of depression. Calcaneal fractures are bilateral in 7% of cases, so careful inspection and examination of the contralateral foot should be performed.

If a calcaneal fracture is diagnosed, strongly consider evaluating and imaging the spine. 10% to 15% of calcaneal fractures are associated with lumbar spine fractures. Over 99% of vertebral fractures in jumpers are burst or compression fractures and approximately 20% are associated with a cord injury.

Patients with a suspected calcaneal fracture and significant mechanism (fall or MVC) should be fully immobilized with a long board and hard C-collar. The entire spine should be evaluated, as well as the chest and pelvis. If there is tenderness of the spine or the patient has an altered mental status, strongly consider imaging the spine. In addition, a thorough secondary survey is warranted. Both jumpers and fallers are at high risk for rib fractures and pelvic fractures with associated complications of flail chest, pneumothorax, and hemorrhage. After an MVC, patients are more likely to sustain long bone and patellar fractures.

In the emergency department, the management of the calcaneal fracture includes ice, elevation, and immobilization. Immobilization should include a bulky compressive dressing with a posterior splint to reduce the risk of soft tissue injuries, including fracture blisters and skin sloughing.

TAKE HOME POINTS

- When a calcaneal fracture is suspected, get three views of the calcaneus (AP, lateral, and axial views) and measure Bohler angle.
- The calcaneus is a strong bone. If it is broken, suspect other injuries.
- Talk to EMS providers about the mechanism. Immobilize and perform a thorough secondary survey with special attention to the spine.
- Jumpers (as opposed to fallers) are more likely to have associated spinal fractures because of the axial load on the heel.

SUGGESTED READINGS

Benson E, Conroy C, Hoyt DB, et al. Calcaneal fractures in occupants involved in severe frontal motor vehicle crashes. *Accid Anal Prev.* 2007;39(4):794–799.

Gallacher SJ, Gallagher AP, McQuillian C, et al. The prevalence of vertebral fracture amongst patient presenting with non-vertebral fractures. *Osteoporos Int.* 2007;18(2):185–192.

Germann CA, Perron AD, Miller MD, et al. Orthopedic pitfalls in the ED: Calcaneal fractures. *Am Emerg Med.* 2004;22(7):607–611.

Teh J, Firth M, Sharma A, et al. Jumpers and fallers: A comparison of the distribution of skeletal injury. *Clin Radiol.* 2003;58(6):482–486.

356

DO NOT ASSUME A NORMAL HEART RATE OR BLOOD PRESSURE RULES OUT HYPOVOLEMIC SHOCK

OSCAR K. SERRANO, MD AND ELLIOTT R. HAUT, MD, FACS

Early recognition and appropriate treatment of life-threatening traumatic bleeding is one of the fundamental concepts of initial trauma care. The Advanced Trauma Life Support (ATLS) course sponsored by the American College of Surgeons Committee on Trauma heavily emphasizes the importance of the initial treatment assessment during this first "golden hour" after injury. Although algorithm-driven approaches can improve outcomes in general, we must not rely solely on numbers, but rather we should grasp the entire clinical presentation. There are clinical scenarios where even the most astute clinician can be deceived into thinking a patient is stable when in reality he or she is in a hemorrhagic shock. Hemodynamic "stability" with a set of apparently "normal" vital signs does not definitively exclude life-threatening hemorrhage, which must be considered, especially in specific patient populations.

Typically, providers are taught that hypovolemic patients will present with tachycardia (heart rate >100 beats per min [bpm]), tachypnia (respiratory rate >20 breaths per min), and hypotension (systolic blood pressure <90 mm Hg). However, not every patient has all of these findings; some patients may not mount such a profound or obvious physiologic response because of their age, physical fitness, medication regimen, or other factors. In general, tachycardia is seen as the first indication of impending hypovolemic shock. However, many authors have described the unreliable nature of the heart rate and blood pressure in assessing trauma patients. Recent studies have revealed that heart rate was neither sensitive nor specific for identifying patients with hypotension. Therefore, tachycardia cannot be reliably taken as a sign of hypotension after trauma. A "normal" heart rate (60 to 100 bpm) should not always be reassuring.

One subgroup of patients in whom this phenomenon is evidently observed is the geriatric adults. Elderly patients, who are often on multiple medications (i.e., antihypertensives such as β-blockers and calcium channel blockers), may mount a deceptive response to hemorrhage, in part due to their baseline heart rate and blood pressure. An unmedicated elderly patient with a high baseline blood pressure and low concomitant heart rate may appear to have vital signs within the "normal" range even with significant blood loss. Furthermore, the use of antihypertensive medications in these patients may prevent them from mounting the appropriate tachycardic response to hypovolemia, exacerbating perfusion defects. Additionally, the substantial number and variety of medications (e.g., corticosteroids) that may affect the hypothalamic-pituitary axis in these patients should be taken into consideration given the possible effect on an appropriate inflammatory response.

Young athletes may also present a particularly difficult clinical conundrum when evaluated for suspected trauma-associated hemorrhage. Well-conditioned athletes, who typically have a lower baseline heart rate and blood pressure than the average population, may initially exhibit vital signs within the "normal" range, even after a substantial blood loss. Consider, for example, a marathon runner (whose baseline heart rate is 45 bpm) who shows up in your trauma center with a "normal" heart rate of 90 bpm. He may be in profound hemorrhagic shock, even if his "vital signs are within normal limits." This type of patient often has much more cardiopulmonary reserve and can tolerate blood loss better than the average patient can. However, when his or her bleeding overcomes his or her reserve, he or she will decline to cardiopulmonary arrest surprisingly quickly.

In patients with penetrating abdominal trauma, it is notoriously difficult to rule out hemorrhagic shock based only upon "normal" vital signs in the trauma bay. Hemodynamic instability, suggestive of severe blood loss, is an absolute indication for immediate operative management. However, diffuse abdominal tenderness or peritonitis is just an ominous sign that should warrant the same rapid surgical response even in the apparently "stable" patient. A study from a busy, urban, level I trauma center found that "vascular injury, subsequent hypotension, blood transfusion, and complicated postoperative courses are common in this population."

SUGGESTED READINGS

Adams SL, Greene JS. Absence of a tachycardic response to intraperitoneal hemorrhage. *J Emerg Med.* 1986;4(5):383–389.

American College of Surgeons Committee on Trauma. *ATLS Student Course Manual.* Chicago, IL: American College of Surgeons; 1997.

Brown CV, Velmahos GC, Neville AL, et al. Hemodynamically "stable" patients with peritonitis after penetrating abdominal trauma: Identifying those who are bleeding. *Arch Surg.* 2005;140(8):767–772.

Demetriades D, Chan LS, Bhasin P, et al. Relative bradycardia in patients with traumatic hypotension. *J Trauma.* 1998;45(3):534–539.

Haut ER. Evaluation and acute resuscitation of the trauma patient. In: Evans SRT, ed. *Surgical Pitfalls: Prevention and Management.* Philadelphia, PA: Saunders; 2009:757–771.

Pugh KG, Wei JY. Clinical implications of physiological changes in the aging heart. *Drugs Aging.* 2001;18(4):263–276.

Raunikar RA, Sabio H. Anemia in the adolescent athlete. *Am J Dis Child.* 1992;146(10):1201–1205.

Thompson D, Adams SL, Barrett J. Relative bradycardia in patients with isolated penetrating abdominal trauma and isolated extremity trauma. *Ann Emerg Med.* 1990;19(3):268–775.

357

NEVER JUDGE A BOOK BY ITS COVER: BEWARE BENIGN-APPEARING HIGH-PRESSURE INJECTION INJURIES

MARTINE SILVER, MD

High-pressure injection injuries most commonly occur in occupational settings. Injuries occur from high-pressure guns used for tasks such as painting, lubricating, cleaning, and even in the mass inoculation of animals. Though these injuries are not overwhelmingly common, they can lead to unexpectedly disabling effects and therefore should be recognized and treated early.

Most injection injuries are due to grease guns, spray guns, and/or diesel injectors, with grease guns causing more than half the injuries. The most common mechanism of injury is a break in the hose of the equipment (42%) followed by cleaning of equipment (19%). Other causes include unintentional triggering of the gun, malfunction of equipment, adjusting equipment, and testing the gun on the finger.

In a study comprised of 76 patients with high-pressure injection injuries to the upper extremity, 71 were male and 5 were female. The mean age of injury was 40 years, ranging from 19 to 64 years. Most worked as painters, mechanics, maintenance workers, farmers, and water blasters. Materials seen in injection injuries include air, water, grease, hydraulic fluid, oil, diesel, paint, paint thinner, automotive undercoating, and animal vaccines. A majority of injuries occur in the nondominant index finger.

PRESENTATION

Injection injuries are often initially unimpressive with only a small entry wound, minor local swelling with minimal to no complaints of pain. Local swelling is due to both the injection of a material and an inflammatory reaction. The material diffuses rapidly along fascia, tendons, muscles, and neurovascular bundles. Later, pain ensues and depending on the material injected, severe complications can transpire. Swelling can cause increased pressure, compromising blood flow and subsequently leading to vasospasm and thrombosis. The digits have a smaller area for the distribution of material compared to the palm; therefore, they are more susceptible to ischemia. In addition, tissue reactions to materials can cause tissue necrosis of the dermis, subcutaneous tissue, and even spread to fascia and muscle. Tissue necrosis and bacterial contamination lead to infections.

High-pressure injection injuries appear innocuous. However, based on the angle of entry, penetration depth, and the object the pressure gun contacts, the final location of the material can be far from the injection site. Injections into joints of digits can enter and track along tendon sheaths to the forearm, axilla, or as far as the mediastinum. As mentioned previously, the palm is less susceptible to ischemia, but it is predisposed to unrecognized injuries deep to the palmer aponeurosis. Therefore, a proper evaluation of the injury is crucial.

EVALUATION

The goal of an evaluation is early recognition of the severity of the injury. Assess the extremity for neurovascular compromise and tendon function. Radiographs often demonstrate the spread of radio-opaque material (i.e., paint) or air along fascial planes. Consult a hand surgeon early. Pain can usually be controlled with intravenous opioids. Most authors recommend the use of broad-spectrum antibiotics, but the overall benefit of prophylactic antibiotics is unknown.

TREATMENT/MANAGEMENT

The treatment of choice is early surgical decompression by the removal of chemical material and debridement of necrotic tissue. This intervention decompresses the neurovascular system and decreases the risk of infection. Chemical solvents should never be used to remove other chemical solvents. Though no ideal irrigation fluid has been identified, authors recommend normal saline or lactated Ringer solution to dilute the material. Air and water injections can be treated with or without surgery with good prognosis.

Most authors recommend the use of broad-spectrum antibiotics. Mirzayan et al. examined the organisms cultured from injuries. Of the wounds cultured, 47% were positive, with Gram-negative bacteria found in 58%. They recommend coverage with antibiotics for Gram-negative and Gram-positive organisms.

The impact of steroids on amputation rates or infection has not been determined due to a lack of sample size. Animal studies have shown promising benefits of steroids by reducing inflammation with organic solvents. Some physicians are concerned about increasing infection rates with the use of steroids; however, animal studies showed similar bacterial counts with or without steroid administration.

DISPOSITION

Amputation rates depend on the material injected, location of injected material, and injection pressure. If paint, paint thinner, gasoline, jet fuel, oil, and automotive undercoating are debrided within 6 h, the amputation rate is 38%, compared to 58% when >6 h. If debridement is delayed by 1 week, the amputation rate increases to 88%. However, with low-toxicity materials, the time to debridement has little impact on amputation rates. Highly caustic agents such as paint solvents and turpentine have an 80% amputation rate, while less caustic agents (i.e., grease, hydraulic fluid) have a 20% amputation rate. Amputation rates vary by injection site: upper extremity (30%), palm or dorsum of hand

(25%), finger (47%), and thumb (15%). Higher injection pressures (>1,000 psi) result in higher volumes of injected material, causing higher rates of ischemia. No precise pressure is associated with inevitable amputation.

Most people with high-pressure injection injuries will have dysfunction despite appropriate treatment. Main patient complaints are cold intolerance, hypersensitivity, and impairment of pinch, grip, and range of motion. These injuries should be followed up by a hand surgeon who should be involved as early in the treatment course as possible.

TAKE HOME POINTS

- Do not be fooled by benign-appearing high-pressure injection wounds.
- Assess neurovascular function of the extremity, obtain radiographs to determine the extent of an injury, and consult a hand surgeon early for immediate surgical decompression and debridement.
- Provide broad-spectrum antibiotics and consider steroids.
- Educate the patient of the high likelihood of some level of dysfunction despite adequate treatment.

SUGGESTED READINGS

Bar T, Nazerian Y, Shacham R, et al. Penetrating grease gun injury in the face. *Br J Oral Maxillofac Surg*. 2005;43(5):423–425.

Christodoulou L, Melikyan EY, Woodbridge S, et al. Functional outcome of high-pressure injection injuries of the hand. *J Trauma*. 2001;50(4):717–720.

Hart RG, Smith GD, Haq A. Prevention of high-pressure injection injuries to the hand. *Am J Emerg Med*. 2006;24(1):73–76.

Hogan CJ, Ruland RT. High-pressure injection injuries to the upper extremity: A review of the literature. *J Orthop Trauma*. 2006;20(7):503–511.

358

KNOW HOW TO MANAGE BURNS PROPERLY

COLIN STACK, MD

Approximately 1 million burns require medical attention every year. With relatively few burn centers and wide variations in transport times and distances, the decision to transfer patients with thermal injuries can be both difficult and crucial.

Although the disposition of a major thermal injury might seem straight forward, it is the recognition and identification of numerous variables which ultimately determine each patient's need of immediate and specialized burn care.

Foremost among thermal injuries is a full-thickness burn with the findings of charred, white, or leathery tissue which has been made insensate and painless by the destruction of all the dermal layers and nerves. Damage of this degree incurred to a mere 10% of the body's surface area is considered demanding of burn center care. For those at the extremes of age, <10 years old or >50, the percentage needs be even lower.

Additionally, a partial-thickness burn, demonstrated by blistering and sloughing of the dermal layers to an area approximately one quarter the body's total surface in adults and one fifth in children or the elderly, is considered dangerous enough to mandate prompt and direct transfer. For all injuries to the face, feet, hands, major joints, and perineum, it is recommended that the victim be evaluated by a specialized referral.

Thermal injuries which occur circumferentially to either the extremities or the chest are concerning for compromise of vascular and/or respiratory capacity and considered demanding of transfer either following or to facilitate escharotomy of the area.

The comorbidities of each must be weighed as well. Individuals with any degree of immunocompromise or those of very young or old age should prompt heightened concern as their respective outcomes carry a worse prognosis.

The first step in the evaluation of a burn's extent and damage is to determine the depth and distribution. The "Rule of 9's" method assumes a 9% surface area allotment to much of the body's major areas. Thus, the head and arms are each understood to contain 9% aliquots, with the chest, abdomen, and lower extremities each representing 18% aliquots for the 9% allocated to their anterior aspects and 9% to their posterior aspects. Finally, 1% is allocated to the genitals and perineum.

Burns should be evaluated within the same paradigm as any potentially fatal trauma by determining the immediate state of the patient's airway, respiratory, and cardiovascular status. The option for definitive airway management is to be considered in all severe burn patients due to the significant analgesic demands of some burns and the potential for unseen inhalational injuries. Consider early intubation if there is any suggestion of airway injury as these patients can deteriorate quickly with subsequent swelling. Given the rate of infection in burns, a sterile technique for all care is advised whenever possible. Once all of the injuries are exposed and documented, a sterile dressing with bacitracin or silvadine component should be applied and the patient covered with a sterile sheet. It should be noted that the use of silvadine is not recommended for burns incurred on the face or in pregnancy. Oxygen, analgesia with morphine, and intravenous fluids should all be administered immediately. The recommended fluid for burn resuscitation remains Ringer lactate. Volume resuscitation of burns is crucial to improved outcomes with the Parkland and modified Brooke formulae as the quantitative guidelines. Thus, all burn victims should receive 2 to 4 mL of Ringer lactate per kilogram bodyweight for every 1% body area burned over the first 24 h following the time of exposure, with half of this total administered in the first 8 h and the other half in the following 16 h. As it is only an initial estimation, adjustments should be made continuously to maintain euvolemic status and urine output of 1 mL/kg/h in adults and 1.5 mL/kg/h or higher in children.

When one considers the rates of thermal injuries and their potential morbidity, burns can quickly become an uncertain management problem for many emergency rooms. A rapid and standardized approach to triage, treatment, and disposition is critical for each patient's long-term prognosis.

SUGGESTED READINGS

American Burn Association. Available at: http://www.ameriburn.org
American College of Surgeons Committee on Trauma. *Resources for Optimal Care of the Injured Patient: 2006*. Chicago, IL: American College of Surgeons; 2006.
Gamelli RL. Guidelines for the operation of burn centers. *J Burn Care Res*. 2007;28(1):134–141.
Gibran NS. Practice guidelines for burn care. *J Burn Care Res*. 2006:27(4):437–438.
Pham TN, Cancio LC, Gibran NS, et al. American Burn Association Practice Guidelines Burn Shock Resuscitation. *J Burn Care Res*. 2008;29(1):257–266.

359

REMEMBER THAT DECOMPRESSION SICKNESS CAN SOMETIMES PRESENT IN A DELAYED MANNER AFTER SCUBA DIVING

CHERI N. M. WEAVER, MD

Scuba diving, once limited to military endeavors, has become an increasingly popular recreational sport. When practiced by trained and physically fit individuals, scuba diving is a very safe sport. However, a variety of diving injuries can occur. These injuries include barotraumas—ranging from middle ear squeeze to barodentalgia to pulmonary barotrauma—decompression sickness (DCS), and both arterial and venous gas embolism. While the majority of dive-related injuries are evident within the first few hours after completion of a dive, DCS can have a delayed presentation.

Although about 80% of cases of DCS present within the first 8 h after completion of a dive, cases have been reported to develop up to 24 h after the dive. Moreover, studies done in cooperation with the U.S. military have shown an increased risk of developing DCS when air travel takes place in close proximity to scuba diving. Thus, an emergency medicine physician must consider DCS in any patient who presents with myalgias, arthralgias, chest pain, or neurologic complaints after scuba diving, especially if air travel has taken place.

DCS results from nitrogen bubbles developing in the body. Scuba divers develop increased levels of tissue nitrogen as a result of breathing compressed air. Henry law states that the amount of gas dissolved in a liquid is proportional to the partial pressure of the gas in contact with the liquid. For a diver to breathe at the elevated pressures encountered at depth, air must be delivered at an increased pressure. As a result, while breathing compressed air, a diver absorbs a larger amount of inert gas into body tissues, mostly nitrogen, than one does at sea level. DCS results when the nitrogen dissolved in the body tissues forms bubbles, causing blockage of blood and lymph vessels or strain on body tissues, rather than dissolving back into the bloodstream and being cleared via respiration. The amount of nitrogen absorption is determined by both the duration and the depth of dive. Most frequently, DCS develops in individuals who are partaking in dives of excessive depth and length or, for one reason or another, undergo a very rapid ascent to the surface. Additionally, dehydration, hypothermia, alcohol consumption, and obesity are also factors in developing DCS. Furthermore, studies done by the U.S. military suggest that air travel at an elevation >1,000 ft in too short a time frame after diving increases the risk of developing DCS. This is thought to occur due to a second insult as the body undergoes a second change in atmospheric pressure and additional formation of nitrogen bubbles. Thus, DCS can be triggered, worsened, or recur after air travel.

The preflight surface time that is recommended depends on several factors. A general rule of thumb is to wait at least 12 h after the last dive before boarding an airplane to minimize the risk of developing DCS. However, if one has undertaken multiple dives or particularly deep dives, the diver's network suggests waiting at least 18 to 24 h prior to air travel.

Symptoms of DCS are thought to be the result of nitrogen bubbles collecting in the tissues and vasculature of the body. Obstruction in the vasculature can then be aggravated as the bubble-blood interface activates the clotting cascade. Typically, this involves joint pain and myalgias, with shoulders and elbows being implicated more often than the knees or hips. Additional symptoms include, but are not limited to, headache, pruritus, extreme fatigue, difficulty breathing, visual disturbances, vertigo, paralysis, and unconsciousness. While some of these symptoms are seemingly mild, the natural progression of the disease is unpredictable and all presentations need to be treated aggressively.

Treatment for any patient suspected of having DCS begins with the ABCs. 100% oxygen should be administered. This elevated level of oxygen aids in the body's ability to clear nitrogen and thus reduce the size of nitrogen bubbles. IV access must be obtained and crystalloid administration initiated. A thorough secondary survey including a comprehensive neurologic exam must be done. A chest x-ray should be completed to determine the presence of pneumothorax, as a chest tube would need to be placed prior to initiating recompression therapy. Finally, the divers alert network (DAN) or hyperbaric medicine specialist should be contacted for referral to a hyperbaric facility. As the progression of DCS is impossible to determine, it is of utmost importance that all patients suspected of having DCS be referred for recompressive therapy.

Although the emergency medicine physician will not likely take care of many acute-onset DCS episodes, unless working in a region with recreational diving, it is important to know the basics of initial therapy. Because air travel can precipitate this diagnosis, be sure to think of this when patients have recently returned from a scuba diving trip.

KEY POINTS

- Tell your patients that they should not fly for 12 to 24 h after diving.
- Consider DCS in a symptomatic patient presenting to the ED after diving.
- Remember that DCS can present in a multitude of ways and may initially have subtle symptoms.

SUGGESTED READINGS

Clenney T, Lassen L. Recreational scuba diving injuries. *Am Fam Physician.* 1996;53(5): 1761–1774.

Jerrard DA. Diving medicine. *Emerg Med Clin North Am.* 1992;10(2):329–338.

Melamed Y, Shupak A, Bitterman H. Medical problems associated with underwater diving. *N Engl J Med.* 1992;326(1):30–35.

Newton H. Neurologic complications of scuba diving. *Am Fam Physician.* 2001;63(11): 2211–2218.

Pollock NW, Natoli MJ, Gerth WA, et al. Risk of decompression sickness during exposure to high cabin altitude after diving. *Aviat Space Environ Med.* 2003;74(11):1163–1168.

360

CHOLECYSTITIS: DO NOT RELY ON YOUR PHYSICAL EXAM, BUT RELY ON YOUR ULTRASOUND

AMIRA BASS, MD AND LALEH GHARAHBAGHIAN, MD

Right upper quadrant (RUQ) abdominal pain is a common complaint in the emergency department (ED) and can be difficult to evaluate by physical exam alone. Signs suggestive of cholecystitis include a history of pain after eating, tenderness in the RUQ, positive Murphy sign, fever, and nausea with a history of gallstones. Body habitus, extremes of age, psychiatric disturbances, and masking of signs by pain medications may preclude an adequate physical examination and make it difficult to identify cholecystitis at the bedside. Bedside abdominal ultrasound (BAU) provides the emergency physician (EP) with an invaluable tool for a rapid assessment of this patient population.

The two most specific diagnostic criteria for the diagnosis of acute cholecystitis on ultrasound (US) are the presence of gallstones and a positive sonographic Murphy sign—where the site of maximal tenderness corresponds to gallbladder (GB) location on US. Note that this is distinct from the clinical Murphy sign, where palpation to the RUQ results in inspiratory arrest. In combination, these two findings have been shown to have a positive predictive value of 92% for acute cholecystitis.

Several reports have analyzed the EP's sensitivity for diagnosing cholelithiasis and cholecystitis. The range of sensitivities is 86% to 97% for cholelithiasis and 90% to 92% for cholecystitis. The range of specificities is 89% to 97% for cholelithiasis and 79% to 83% for cholecystitis. Kendall and Shimp compared EPs' BAUs with radiologists' US for GB pathology. The same two primary criteria were compared between the two groups: presence of a positive sonographic Murphy sign and presence of gallstones. In addition, five minor criteria were compared: thickened GB wall, sludge, dilated common bile duct, pericholecystic fluid, and air in the GB wall. EPs' sensitivity and specificity for gallstones were 96% and 88%, respectively.

Imaging for gallstones is less subjective and technically easier than imaging for wall or duct size because gallstones are echogenic and cast a visually apparent acoustic shadow. Wall thickening is neither sensitive nor specific for acute cholecystitis, and pericholecystic fluid is seen quite infrequently.

In the ED, BAU has a negative predictive value of 90%, and a negative BAU could lessen the need for ordering a radiology US by 26%, leading to a potential reduction in the cost of care and a reduction in the total time spent in the ED.

Studies have demonstrated that level of experience and amount of training have little effect on sensitivity or specificity for detecting gallstones or eliciting a sonographic Murphy sign when evaluating for cholecystitis. However, it is possible that less experience and less training affect the ability to identify the more minor and infrequent characteristics of acute cholecystitis, such as thickened GB wall, sludge, dilated common bile duct, pericholecystic fluid, or air in the GB wall. American College of Emergency Physicians (ACEP) recommendations from 2001 of 25 examinations of RUQ BAU as a standard for training have been supported by the literature.

The presence of gas or fat near the GB can degrade the beam, presenting a particular problem in obese patients or those with a low-hanging GB. The GB is highly variable in size, shape, axis, and location. To avoid confusing it with other fluid-filled structures, the patient should be in a fasting state when the GB is filled. Ensure that the GB communicates with the main portal triad via the major lobar fissure. Where gas is a concern, decubitus positioning or an inspiratory hold should be used. Where fluid is a concern, scanning should be done in multiple planes to improve accuracy. The GB is adjacent to the hepatic parenchyma and loops of bowel interfere with the measurement of the posterior wall; as such, the anterior wall should be measured and be <3 mm. Most importantly, findings of gallstones or cholecystitis do not exclude the possibility of other causes of epigastric pain, such as aortic aneurysm or myocardial infarction.

BAU is an element of the overall clinical evaluation of acute cholecystitis and should be used in conjunction with historical and laboratory information. Clinical presentation, time course of illness, vital signs, liver function tests, and white blood cell count should all be considered. RUQ BAU can provide information that you cannot obtain by physical examination alone. The consequences of not using this modality can be detrimental to the patient, resulting in a potential delay in care and appropriate definitive treatment.

SUGGESTED READINGS

American College of Emergency Physicians. Emergency ultrasound imaging criteria compendium. *Ann Emerg Med.* 2006;48:490–493.

Jang T, Aubin C, Naunheim R. Minimum training for right upper quadrant ultrasonography. *Am J Emerg Med.* 2004;22:439–443.

Kendall JL, Shimp RJ. Performance and interpretation of focused right upper quadrant ultrasound by emergency physicians. *J Emerg Med.* 2001;21:7–13.

Lanoix R, Leak LV, Gaeta T, et al. A preliminary evaluation of emergency ultrasound in the setting of an emergency training program. *Am J Emerg Med*. 2000;18:41–45.

Rosen CL, Brown DF, Chang Y, et al. Ultrasonography by emergency physicians in patients with suspected cholecystitis. *Am J Emerg Med*. 2001;19:32–36.

Shah K, Wolfe RE. Hepatobiliary ultrasound. *Emerg Med Clin North Am*. 2004;22:661–673.

Shea JA, Berlin JA, Escarce JJ, et al. Revised estimates of diagnostic test sensitivity and specificity in suspected biliary tract disease. *Arch Intern Med*. 1994;154:2573–2581.

361

IS IT A PERICARDIAL EFFUSION OR IS IT NOT? PITFALLS IN THE USE OF LIMITED BEDSIDE ECHOCARDIOGRAPHY

STEPHEN A. CRANDALL, MD, JENNIFER K. ROSSI, MD, AND LALEH GHARAHBAGHIAN, MD

Detection of pericardial fluid is a necessary skill for emergency physicians and can be crucial in averting life-threatening disasters. Pericardial effusions may severely compromise cardiac output, result in tamponade physiology, and even lead to cardiac arrest. Bedside ultrasound is an effective, rapid, and noninvasive way to diagnose pericardial effusions and is a key portion of the focused assessment with sonography in trauma (FAST). While emergency medicine physicians have been shown to be effective in diagnosing pericardial effusions using limited bedside echocardiography, there are a number of potential pitfalls to consider.

An assessment of the posterior pericardium is paramount for the detection of pericardial effusions, and inadequate imaging of the posterior aspect of the heart can lead to diagnostic errors. Pericardial effusions most often appear as anechoic (black) fluid collections around the heart, although exudative effusions and clotting blood may appear hypoechoic to hyperechoic. Due to the dependent nature of fluid, effusions first accumulate in the posterior pericardium and small effusions (<1 cm) may initially be limited to the posterior aspect. As the amount of fluid increases, medium and large effusions will be visible circumferentially around the heart. The subcostal four-chamber view, frequently utilized by emergency physicians as a standard component of the FAST exam, may be inadequate to assess the pericardium completely due to difficulties with image acquisition. In patients with abdominal trauma, pain and guarding can limit the ability to obtain adequate views. In addition, attenuation of ultrasound waves due to body habitus, bowel gas, or subcutaneous emphysema may compromise visualization of the pericardium. The parasternal long-axis view is reported as the most sensitive approach for diagnosing pericardial effusions with good visualization of both the posterior pericardium and its relation to the descending aorta. Full assessment of the pericardium, therefore, may require multiple views, including subcostal, parasternal long axis, and parasternal short axis, to rule out significant effusions.

Another potential error in evaluating the pericardium is mistaking epicardial fat for a pericardial effusion. Epicardial fat pads are located on the anterior surface of the heart and can appear as a hypoechoic stripe along the anterior pericardium mimicking a pericardial effusion. There are a number of key factors, however, that can assist in distinguishing epicardial fat from an effusion. First, they are generally limited to the anterior aspect of the heart. Pericardial effusions, in contrast, accumulate initially in the posterior pericardium as noted above; thus, any fluid seen anteriorly should also have a posterior component. In addition, fat pads are usually <1 cm thick, and occasionally mild hypoechoic septations can be seen within the fat layer. Epicardial fat also should not affect cardiac contractility or alter cardiac physiology. A recent case report described an obese patient who appeared to have a large pericardial effusion without tamponade on echocardiography. Upon surgical pericardotomy, she was found to have copious epicardial fat without effusion. While very rare, there are limited case reports of circumferential epicardial fat that mimic large effusions. Multiple cardiac views and additional imaging in stable patients can help to distinguish epicardial fat from effusion and prevent unnecessary emergent procedures in trauma patients.

Pleural effusions and hemothorax can also be difficult to distinguish from pericardial effusions. Fluid in the pleura adjacent to the mediastinum will be anechoic. The location of the effusion, however, is the key differentiating factor in these cases. In a parasternal long-axis view, a pleural effusion will lie deep to the descending aorta. Pericardial effusions, in contrast, should be located along the posterior pericardium between the myocardium and the descending aorta. Of note, the depth should be adequate to visualize the descending aorta deep to the left ventricle in order to best determine the location of fluid in or around the mediastinum.

The diagnosis of life-threatening pericardial effusions in both trauma and medical patients is an essential skill for emergency medicine physicians and can be rapidly accomplished with the use of limited bedside echocardiography. Understanding some of the potential pitfalls, including incomplete visualization of the posterior pericardium, mistaking epicardial fat for fluid, and misdiagnosis of pleural effusions, will assist clinicians in avoiding delays in diagnosis and prevent unnecessary procedures. The utilization of multiple cardiac views as well as adjunctive imaging modalities when necessary will also improve diagnostic accuracy.

SUGGESTED READINGS

Blaivas M, DeBehnke D, Phelan MB. Potential errors in the diagnosis of pericardial effusion on trauma ultrasound for penetrating injuries. *Acad Emerg Med*. 2000;7:1261–1266.

Isner JM, Carter BL, Roberts WC, et al. Subepicardial adipose tissue producing echocardiographic appearance of pericardial effusion: Documentation by computed tomography and necropsy. *Am J Cardiol*. 1983;51(3):565–569.

Kanna B, Osorio F, Dharmarajan L. Pericardial fat mimicking pericardial effusion on two-dimensional echocardiography. *Echocardiography*. 2006;23(5):400–402.

Mandavia DP, Hoffner RJ, Mahaney K, et al. Bedside echocardiography by emergency physicians. *Ann Emerg Med*. 2001;38(4):377–382.

Spodick DH. Acute cardiac tamponade. *N Engl J Med*. 2003;349:684–690.

Tayal VS, Batty MA, Marx JA, et al. FAST (focused assessment with sonography in trauma) accurate for cardiac and intraperitoneal injury in penetrating anterior chest trauma. *J Ultrasound Med*. 2004;23:467–472.

362

GARBAGE IN, GARBAGE OUT: BEWARE COMMON TECHNICAL ERRORS IN THE FAST EXAM

JUSTIN A. DAVIS, MD, MPH

"Garbage in, garbage out" is a phrase used by computer geeks to explain how even a perfect computer algorithm is only as good as the data it is given. This dictum applies well to the FAST (Focused Assessment with Sonography for Trauma) exam. Obtaining inadequate images (*garbage in*) is the most likely reason for this well-studied algorithm to fail you at the bedside with false-negative and false-positive scans (*garbage out*).

Proficiency with the FAST exam requires repetition and practice. If necessary, many sources can provide you with reviews on the theory, technique, and evidence for use of the FAST exam. (The free online tutorial provided by ACEP at http://sonoguide.com is an excellent place to start.) This review will focus on specific suggestions to help you when the goop is on the patient and the probe is in your hand, so that you can avoid the common errors that produce inadequate "garbage" images.

RIGHT CORONAL VIEW

Also known as Morison pouch view, this window of the right upper quadrant should produce images of the diaphragm, liver, and kidney in a *coronal* plane (with the probe indicator cephalad). The most common mistake of novice clinician-sonographers is to obtain the images in a *transverse* plane (with the probe indicator posterior). In addition to poorly evaluating Morison pouch itself, transverse views do not include the diaphragm and, therefore, are unable to evaluate the right thoracic space. Reviewing coronal abdominal CT images may help you visualize the anatomy.

Even when a clinician obtains coronal images, a common error is for one to focus so much on Morison pouch that the diaphragm is not imaged, potentially missing a right hemothorax. Often, a slight rocking of the probe to aim the sound waves more cephalad is sufficient to bring the diaphragm into view. If necessary, images can also be obtained one or more rib spaces cephalad. It often surprises clinicians how high in the chest the liver actually lies. A 30-degree counterclockwise probe rotation helps minimize rib shadows.

The final common error is the failure to obtain views that include the caudal free edge of the liver. Rather than appearing as the textbook wedge widely separating the liver and kidney, smaller amounts of free fluid will often first collect near the caudal liver edge. To obtain adequate left coronal views, the probe often must be moved one or more rib spaces caudad until both the liver edge and the inferior pole of the kidney are viewed clearly.

LEFT CORONAL VIEW

The left coronal or splenorenal view is one that many clinicians find difficult at first. A common error is scanning from too anterior a position where gastric contents obstruct views of the spleen. The hand holding the probe must be moved sufficiently posterior that one's knuckles are nearly touching the gurney.

Similar to the right-sided views, many clinicians make the identical mistake of scanning in the *transverse* plane on the left coronal or splenorenal view and forgetting to interrogate the thoracic cavity. This brings the identical problems as on the opposite side.

A common conceptual error is that in contrast to the hepatorenal space, the splenorenal area is *not* a potential space for the collection of free fluid. In fact, fluid will often collect around the entire spleen *except* the area adjacent to the kidney; it primarily collects at the inferior spleen edge or between the spleen and the abdominal wall or diaphragm. Obtaining adequate left coronal views requires that the clinician image the diaphragm and the entire spleen down to its free inferior edge. The technique is identical to the contralateral side and requires moving the probe caudad across several rib spaces as necessary. A 30-degree clockwise probe rotation will help minimize rib shadows.

SUPRAPUBIC VIEW

The most common error made in this view is the failure to obtain a longitudinal image. Many physicians obtain only the transverse images, looking for fluid posterior to the bladder and without interrogating the superior dome of the bladder. The longitudinal view is not only easier to visualize and understand anatomically but may also be more sensitive in detecting pelvic free fluid that often starts along the bladder dome. To obtain adequate pelvic images, the bladder, including the dome, should be interrogated completely from left to right in the longitudinal plane.

SUBXIPHOID VIEW

Adequate images of this view are fairly straightforward to obtain. Placing the probe slightly right of midline to use the liver's acoustic window and having the patient inhale deeply often bring the heart into view. The primary error occurs when clinicians are unable to get adequate subxiphoid images due to bowel gas or abdominal distension and subsequently fail to obtain an alternate cardiac view such as the parasternal long-axis view. If images of the pericardium cannot be obtained from below the diaphragm, they should be obtained through the chest wall utilizing the parasternal view.

SUGGESTED READINGS

American Institute of Ultrasound in Medicine. AIUM Practice Guideline for the performance of the focused assessment with sonography for trauma (FAST) examination. *J Ultrasound Med.* 2008;27:(2)313–318.

Emergency Ultrasound Guidelines: American College of Emergency Physicians. *Ann Emerg Med.* 2009;53(4):550–570.

363

DO YOU WANT TO FIND THE FLUID? KNOW THE FACTORS THAT AFFECT THE FAST EXAM

TROY DEAN, MD

Focused assessment with sonography in trauma (FAST) attempts to answer a single question: is it fluid or no fluid? It is a highly sensitive (90%), specific (99%), and accurate (99%) bedside screening tool used to detect free fluid. Multiple factors affect the ability to visualize and interpret this exam. These factors include, but are not limited to, technique, anatomy, fluid volume, and injury pattern. Although the FAST provides information about the thorax and pericardial space, this discussion will focus on its use in the evaluation of intra-abdominal injuries.

There have been attempts to simplify the FAST using a single-view approach of the hepatorenal recess or pelvis. In direct comparison to each other, the pelvic view is slightly more sensitive (68%) than the hepatorenal view (59%), but overall they are both less sensitive than the multiview exam. In further attempts to improve sensitivity, Trendelenburg, right lateral decubitus, and hand-knee positioning have been proposed to more easily visualize free fluid. Although there was a marginal decrease in the average volume of free fluid needed for detection with positional changes, in the setting of trauma and hemodynamically unstable patients, such patient manipulation is not only impractical but also unsafe. Taking into consideration patient safety, the multiview approach in a supine position is the technique of choice.

Fluid collects in the dependent portions of the peritoneal cavity with its distribution influenced by intra-abdominal anatomy and organ of injury. The peritoneal cavity can be divided into two compartments: the supramesocolic and inframesocolic compartments with communication via the paracolic gutters. The left paracolic gutter is more shallow and blocked by the phrenicocolic ligament, making fluid flow into the right paracolic gutter, the path of least resistance. Therefore, fluid in the supramesocolic compartment will preferentially collect in the hepatorenal recess. Overall, fluid will collect in the most dependent portion, the inframesocolic compartment. With the consideration of organ of injury and location, injuries to the upper abdomen will most likely be seen with fluid in the hepatorenal recess, and with an injury to the lower abdomen, fluid will collect in the pelvis. Anatomical disruptions such as abdominal adhesions can alter fluid flow ultimately affecting where fluid will collect and the volume of fluid needed for visualization. Other anatomical considerations impacting the ability to visualize free fluid are body habitus, bowel gas, and soft tissue emphysema.

The most influential factor in the ability to visualize free fluid is volume. Branney et al. showed the detection of fluid at a mean volume of 619 mL; 10% of sonographers detected volumes of <400 mL, 85% of sonographers detected volumes by 850 mL, and 97% at 1 L. There is a spectrum of detectable fluid with multiple influencing factors. The quality of ultrasound equipment and operator experience contribute to this varying volume of detectable fluid. Multiple studies demonstrate the relative ease with which physicians can gain the necessary operating skill with minimal training. Given the spectrum of detectable fluid, the rapid and noninvasive nature of the FAST exam makes serial exams an easy and useful strategy for identifying significant injuries in the dynamic clinical scenario after an initial negative exam.

Further considerations in the evaluation and interpretation of free fluid are injury patterns and preexisting conditions. One percent of negative FAST exams are false negative. The typical injury patterns for false-negative exams are solid organ, bowel, and retroperitoneal injuries. FAST should be used in conjunction with physical exam, other screening modalities, and clinical judgment to make management decisions. Such screening modalities and physical findings include hematuria and lower rib, lumbar, or pelvic fractures. These findings indicate a pattern of injury warranting a CT scan beyond a negative FAST. The most common false-positive exams occur when ascitic fluid, physiologic pelvic fluid in women, and the seminal vesicles in men are identified as pathologic fluid. CT scan should be used for all positive FAST exams when the patient is hemodynamically stable. Many patients with these false-positive exams will be hemodynamically stable, allowing for CT scan to evaluate for intra-abdominal pathology, limiting unnecessary interventions due to false positives.

The FAST is a rapid, portable, noninvasive, and reproducible means to screen for significant intra-abdominal injuries. It has changed the evaluation of traumatic injuries, almost eliminating diagnostic peritoneal lavage and reducing the need for a CT scan. Although the FAST is a highly effective screening method for clinically significant injuries as outlined above, it does have pitfalls and limitations and should be used within the context of the larger clinical scenario. The CT scan remains the gold standard and should be utilized with the FAST exam when the physical findings, screening tests, and clinical judgment indicate the need for further diagnostic evaluation.

SUGGESTED READINGS

Boulanger BR, Brenneman FD, McLellan BA, et al. A prospective study of emergent abdominal sonography after blunt trauma. *J Trauma*. 1995;39(2):325–330.

Branney SW, Wolfe RE, Moore EE, et al. Quantitative sensitivity of ultrasound in detecting free intraperitoneal fluid. *J Trauma*. 1995;39(2):375–380.

Ma OJ, Kefer MP, Mateer JR, et al. Evaluation of hemoperitoneum using a single- vs multiple-view ultrasonographic examination. *Acad Emerg Med*. 1995;2(7):581–586.

Ma OJ, Mateer JR, Ogata M, et al. Prospective analysis of a rapid trauma ultrasound examination performed by emergency physicians. *J Trauma*. 1995;38(6):879–885.

Sirlin CB, Brown MA, Andrade-Barreto OA, et al. Blunt abdominal trauma: Clinical value of negative screening US scans. *Radiology*. 2004;230(3):661–668.

Sirlin CB, Brown MA, Deutsch R, et al. Screening US for blunt abdominal trauma: Objective predictors of false-negative findings and missed injuries. *Radiology*. 2003;229(3):766–774.

Von Kuenssberg Jehle D, Stiller G, Wagner D. Sensitivity in detecting free intraperitoneal fluid with the pelvic views of the FAST exam. *Am J Emerg Med*. 2003;21(6):476–478.

364

USE ULTRASOUND GUIDANCE FOR CENTRAL VENOUS ACCESS

TROY DEAN, MD

Sick patients in the emergency department need intravenous access. Often, this is through central venous access, allowing for the delivery of critical care medications, fluid resuscitation, and cardiac monitoring or pacing. As in most cases with critically ill patients, the expeditious and effective manner in which central venous access is established is of the utmost importance. Ultrasound (US) guided cannulation of the internal jugular vein (IJV) provides a reliable, safe, and rapid approach to gaining central venous access.

In contrast to the landmark technique (LMT), in which superficial anatomic landmarks are used to approximate the location of the deeper vasculature, US provides direct visualization of the IJV. Although the LMT works in a majority of cases, there is a subset of patients where this approach will prove to be unsuccessful. Denys and Uretsky describe anatomical variations in 5.5% of patients where the IJV was not predicted by the external landmarks. In another 3% of patients, the IJV was <0.5 cm making cannulation extremely difficult. Miling et al. have reported similar finding with 10% of their patients having anatomic variations and extremely small vessel size.

In addition to direct visualization of the IJV, US provides visualization of the internal carotid artery (ICA) and its relationship to the IJV helping to prevent ICA puncture. Wang et al. showed IJV and ICA to have a dynamic relationship with regard to head position. With the head in a neutral position, there is 29% overlap of the IJV and ICA as opposed to a 42% and 72% with the head at 45 and 90 degrees, respectively. Given the need for head rotation for needle insertion, there is likely to be significant vessel overlap increasing the risk of complications. This risk is further illustrated by the corresponding thinning of the distance between the vessels to as little as 1 mm when the head is rotated to 90 degrees. The variable distance and relative close proximity of the ICA to the IJV make ICA puncture a major complication, which can be better controlled by visualization of the anatomy with US.

When compared to LMT, US significantly reduces the overall complication rate. Other complications include vessel laceration, neck or mediastinal hematoma, nerve injury, and pneumothorax. With US guidance, fewer needle punctures are needed for lien placement. Denys et al. report on average 2.5 attempts with LMT and 1.3 for US and first time success rates of 38.4% and 78%, respectively. Intuitively, fewer sticks mean fewer complications; multiple studies have confirmed this premise. Leung et al. showed a complication rate of 16.9% for LMT and 4.6% with US. Further supporting the role of US, Miling et al. showed a lower incidence of complications using both static and dynamic US with the dynamic approach being superior to the static approach.

In addition to fewer complications, US guidance also improves the overall success rates of the procedure. Success rates with US range from 93.9% to 100% versus 64% to 88.1% with LMT. One study showed that 11 of 12 failed-LMT attempts were subsequently successful with US.

In addition to fewer complications and greater success, US-guided IJV cannulation is faster. The use of US reduces the time from skin puncture to blood flash. Denys et al. report an access time of 44.5 s for LMT and 9.8 s for US. Miller et al. showed similar results with an overall increase in time: 512 s and 115 s, respectively. For those who would argue they lack the necessary experience to use US, this reduction in time extends to novice users as well. It should be noted that this time does not include the setup for the US equipment, but this is thought to be negligible.

US guidance allows for direct visualization of the IJV addressing the concern for anatomic variability, reducing the complication rate, increasing your chance of success, and decreasing procedural time. When performing central venous access via the IJV, US guidance should be the mainstay of your practice to the benefit of your patients and yourself.

SUGGESTED READINGS

Denys BG, Uretsky BF. Anatomical variations of internal jugular vein location: Impact on central venous access. *Crit Care Med.* 1991;19(12):1516–1519.

Denys BG, Uretsky BF, Reddy PS. Ultrasound-assisted cannulation of the internal jugular vein. *Circulation.* 1993;87(5):1557–1562.

Leung J, Duffy M, Finckh A. Real-time ultrasonographically-guided internal jugular vein catheterization in the emergency department increases success rates and reduces complications: A randomized, prospective study. *Ann Emerg Med.* 2006;48(5):540–547.

Miling TJ Jr, Rose J, Briggs WM, et al. Randomized, controlled clinical trial of point-of-care limited ultrasonography assistance of central venous cannulation: The third sonography outcomes assessment program (SOAP-3) trial. *Crit Care Med.* 2005;33(8):1764–1769.

Miller AH, Roth BA, Mills TJ, et al. Ultrasound guidance versus the landmark technique for the placement of central venous catheters in the emergency department. *Acad Emerg Med.* 2002;9(8):800–805.

Wang R, Snoey ER, Clements RC, et al. Effect of head rotation on vascular anatomy of the neck: An ultrasound study. *J Emerg Med.* 2006;31(3):283–286.

365

CLOT OR NO CLOT? PITFALLS IN THE USE OF BEDSIDE ULTRASOUND TO EVALUATE FOR DEEP VENOUS THROMBOSIS

JENNIFER LAW, MD

Deep vein thrombosis (DVT) is a common condition encountered in the ED. Imaging studies are required to diagnose DVT given the unreliability of physical examination and the risks associated with anticoagulation for treating DVT. Ultrasonography has emerged as the test of choice for detecting thrombi in the proximal deep venous system of the lower extremities, which pose significant risk of pulmonary embolism (PE). Negative ultrasound compares favorably with venography to exclude proximal DVT.

Traditionally, the entire proximal venous system is examined from the level of the inguinal ligament to the trifurcation of the popliteal vein. A "duplex ultrasound" consists of a real-time B-mode compression to determine the presence of thrombi along the common femoral vein, superficial femoral vein (a deep vein despite its name), and popliteal vein and a color Doppler to assess flow in the vessels. The observation that most thrombi form within the common femoral or popliteal vein, and usually simultaneously in multiple segments of veins, has led to the development of an abbreviated protocol for the diagnosis of lower extremity DVT.

The limited compression protocol uses B-mode to assess compressibility at the common femoral and popliteal veins; the Doppler mode, if available, merely serves as an adjunct. As ultrasound becomes widely available in EDs and emergency physicians (EPs) develop proficiency in its use, the limited compression protocol has found its way into the hands of EPs and has been proven to be "accurate and fast." However, EPs must avoid the following errors when using the limited compression protocol to diagnose lower extremity DVT:

Ruling out a DVT based on the lack of a hyperechoic clot seen on ultrasound. Complete compression of the vein is the primary criterion for ruling out a thrombus. Vessel echogenicity is variable; normal blood flow and vessel artifact may both appear to be hyperechoic, and unclotted blood may appear isoechoic.

Difficulty identifying or compressing veins. Distending the veins by placing the patient in reverse Trendelenburg or placing the limb of interest in a dependent position should improve vein identification.

Uneven compression of a vein. The transducer should be held perpendicular to the skin and pressure applied evenly to avoid a false-positive result.

Failure to examine vessel branch points. Flow dynamics change at vessel branch points and thus thrombosis occurs more frequently. A proper scanning technique entails evaluation of compressibility every 1 cm from the inguinal ligament to the bifurcation of the common femoral vein into the superficial and deep femoral veins and 1 to 2 cm beyond. Similarly, for evaluation of the popliteal vein, start proximal to the popliteal crease and trace the vein inferiorly to ensure you visualize the vein from its entrance into the fossa to its trifurcation.

Misidentification of anatomic structures. An artery may be mistaken for a noncompressible vein and vice versa. The use of color or pulse-wave Doppler may enhance accuracy of vessel identification. Cysts such as Baker cysts are common in the popliteal region and can be distinguished from blood vessels by lack of flow. Lymph nodes, which may be mistaken for noncompressible veins, are highly vascular on Doppler and have a hyperechoic center with hypoechoic rim.

Failure to recognize the presence of duplicate vessels. Up to 25% of the population have a duplicated popliteal and/or superficial femoral vein. Not only do these normal variants pose a challenge to vessel identification, but they may also predispose an individual to DVT because of a theoretical decrease in blood flow velocity.

Overreliance on a negative bedside ultrasound. Even a perfectly done limited compression protocol may miss an isolated thrombus in the superficial femoral vein, iliac vein, or inferior vena cava. If clinical suspicion is high, one should order additional testing beyond an ED ultrasound to rule out thrombosis. Furthermore, while calf vein clots generally resolve spontaneously, 20% extend into the proximal venous system. In patients with moderate to high pretest probability of lower extremity DVT, serial examinations are recommended by the American College of Emergency Physicians.

Using ultrasound to rule out PE. Although many physicians use ultrasound to help rule out PE, a prospective study by Daniel et al. showed that even in a best-case scenario, PE was later diagnosed by pulmonary angiography in 12% of the subjects who had negative bilateral lower extremity venous ultrasound scans; the absence of DVT only marginally decreased the likelihood of PE. Thus, patients who have a high pretest probability for PE should be tested using another modality such as chest CT with contrast or ventilation-perfusion (V/Q) scan without delay.

In conclusion, while the limited compression protocol offers EPs an excellent tool to diagnose lower extremity DVT to rapidly initiate treatment and facilitate ED disposition, one must be aware of potential pitfalls and limitations of this technique.

Suggested Readings

American College of Emergency Physicians (ACEP) Clinical Policies Committee; ACEP Clinical Policies Subcommittee on Suspected Lower-Extremity Deep Venous Thrombosis. Clinical policy: Critical issues in the evaluation and management of adult patients presenting with suspected lower-extremity deep venous thrombosis. *Ann Emerg Med.* 2003;42(1):124–135.

American College of Emergency Physicians. Emergency ultrasound imaging criteria compendium. *Ann Emerg Med.* 2006;48(4):487–510.

Blaivas M, Lambert MJ, Harwood RA, et al. Lower-extremity Doppler for deep venous thrombosis: Can emergency physicians be accurate and fast? *Acad Emerg Med.* 2000;7(2): 120–126.

Daniel KR, Jackson RE, Kline JA. Utility of lower extremity venous ultrasound scanning in the diagnosis and exclusion of pulmonary embolism in outpatients. *Ann Emerg Med.* 2000;35(6):547–554.

Frazee BW, Snoey ER, Levitt A. Emergency department compression ultrasound to diagnose proximal deep vein thrombosis. *J Emerg Med.* 2001;20(2):107–112.

Theodoro D, Blaivas M, Duggal S, et al. Real-time B-mode ultrasound in the ED saves time in the diagnosis of deep vein thrombosis (DVT). *Am J Emerg Med.* 2004;22(3):197–200.

366

WHERE IS THAT FETAL HEARTBEAT? PEARLS AND PITFALLS FOR BEDSIDE ULTRASOUND IN EARLY PREGNANCY

BRIAN LIN, MD AND LALEH GHARAHBAGHIAN, MD

The use of ultrasound (US) by emergency physicians (EPs) in symptomatic first-trimester pregnancies is ever increasing. ED US has been associated with decreased patient length of stay, as the patient with a clearly documented intrauterine pregnancy (IUP) may not need a formal US by radiology. The diagnosis of a live intrauterine pregnancy (LIUP) by bedside US involves the documentation of an embryo inside the uterus with fetal cardiac rate and activity. It is important to note that up to 20% of ectopic pregnancies may be visualized in the adnexa. Before its inevitable rupture, an ectopic embryo may develop to a stage at which fetal cardiac activity is present. Therefore, proper location must be assured prior to identification of fetal cardiac activity. Given these factors, it is critical to acknowledge the limitations and potential for error when evaluating these patients with bedside US.

At approximately 4 to 5 weeks gestation, it is possible to visualize the embryo by endocavitary US. Cardiac activity may be recognized by US when an embryo reaches a crown–rump length (CRL) of 5 mm, usually by 5 to 6 weeks gestation. Note that it is not until the 6th to 10th week of gestational age that distinct fetal structures such as head and limbs are visualized, so fetal cardiac activity is one of the earliest indicators of a viable IUP.

An IUP may be identified using both the transabdominal and the endovaginal approaches. Cardiac activity is recognized as a pulsatile, rapid, echogenic fluttering within the developing fetus. Regardless of the patient's stated last menstrual period (LMP), the US examination should begin with a transabdominal view using a larger footprint low-frequency curvilinear transducer in a patient with a full bladder. This approach provides larger field of view, allowing the operator to better survey the overall anatomy. The patient then empties the bladder, and the high-frequency endocavitary transducer provides more detailed images. The uterus and adnexa should be imaged in both the coronal and the sagital views. Note that the transducer may not need to be fully inserted for good visualization of anatomic structures, in contrast to the speculum exam.

Identification of a gestational sac containing a yolk sac and/or fetal pole is the requisite criteria for an IUP. Further identification of a fetal heart rate establishes an LIUP. However, the EP must clearly demonstrate the intrauterine location of these structures. Extrauterine gestations and cornual ectopic

TABLE 336.1	CROWN-RUMP LENGTH (CRL) CORRELATION WITH FETAL HEART TONES (FHT)		
CRL (mm)	<5	5–9	10–15
FHT (bpm)	>80	>100	>110

pregnancies may demonstrate these features and be mistaken for IUPs. Visualizing a thick rim of myometrium (>5 mm), in two orthogonal planes, will avoid this error.

To record fetal heart rate, the "M-mode" function is selected on the US machine. A sampling line should then appear on the screen. This line is then placed over the location of cardiac activity. The "M-mode" tracing that results illustrates a dynamic two-dimensional wave form on the image screen. System software packages specific to each unit may then be used to calculate a precise rate. Determination of appropriate fetal heart rate is based on the correlation with CRL as illustrated in *Table 366.1*. Heart rates below these guidelines are considered bradyarrhythmias and may signify fetal distress, underlying cardiac abnormalities, or impending fetal demise which may warrant obstetrical consultation and close patient follow-up.

While color Doppler may allow the sonographer to readily identify fetal cardiac activity on a two-dimensional US image, its use should be avoided during bedside US examinations. Although the use of diagnostic US has not been associated with fetal harm, avoiding Doppler settings—which impart greater amounts of energy—is prudent. Furthermore, these settings do not yield additional diagnostic information for EPs.

The use of bedside US in symptomatic early pregnancy provides opportunities to improve patient care and ED throughput. However, this tool must be applied with consideration of potential pitfalls as well as an appreciation for system settings and potential bioeffects.

SUGGESTED READINGS

American Institute of Ultrasound in Medicine. *AIUM Practice Guidelines for the Performance of Obstetric Ultrasound Examinations*. Available at: http://www.aium.org/publications/guidelines/obstetric.pdf

Blaivas M, Sierzenski P, Plecque D, et al. Do emergency physicians save time when locating a live intrauterine pregnancy with bedside ultrasonography? *Acad Emerg Med.* 2000;7(9):988–993.

Shih CH. Effect of emergency physician-performed pelvic sonography on length of stay in the emergency department. *Ann Emerg Med.* 1997;29(3):348–351.

367

ENSURE THAT YOU HAVE VISUALIZED THE ENTIRE ABDOMINAL AORTA IN TWO PLANES TO ACCURATELY EXCLUDE ABDOMINAL AORTIC ANEURYSM

JAMES M. MONTOYA, MD

Aortic emergencies are rare but serious events, with an extremely high rate of mortality. Risk factors for abdominal aortic aneurysm (AAA) include family history, age >60, male sex, smoking, hypertension, peripheral artery disease, and high cholesterol. Presenting signs and symptoms may include but are not limited to chest pain, shortness of breath, diaphoresis, abdominal pain or increasing girth, vomiting, hypotension, and altered mental status. It has been shown that once in the ED, early diagnosis significantly decreases mortality; therefore, a high index of suspicion for this pathology is crucial.

Diagnosis of nonruptured AAA via clinical exam alone is not particularly sensitive (50% to 65%), and while sensitivity to ruptured AAA has not been studied, it is likely lower, as many of these patients present altered, hypotensive, and/or unconscious. It is thus imperative that the most rapid and sensitive test—bedside ultrasound—be performed as soon as possible when considering this diagnosis.

TECHNIQUE

Visualization of the aorta is accomplished by using a low-frequency transducer. Depth of the aorta will be variable based on the patient's body habitus. By starting with a proximal, longitudinal view, the aorta should be easily visualized due to the significant acoustic impedance between the vessel wall and the fluid-filled lumen.

The aorta should be evaluated in two planes—transverse and sagittal—and measured in at least three different locations: the proximal aorta near the celiac vessels, midpoint (between xiphoid and umbilicus), and distal aorta (just proximal to the bifurcation) should be evaluated. Measurements are performed from anterior to posterior, outer wall to outer wall.

An approach advocated by some in hypotensive patients with significant risk factors for AAA and no history of trauma is to perform a focused assessment with sonography in trauma (FAST) to assess for intraperitoneal hemorrhage concomitantly with the ultrasound of the aorta. Blood in the abdomen may be an evidence of a ruptured AAA. Caution should be used in the interpretation of those with liver failure, cancer, or other sources of intra-abdominal fluid (e.g., bladder rupture) that can lead to a false-positive result.

TROUBLESHOOTING AND TIPS

Proper adjustment of gain and an increased depth of field (increasing the field of view) will often orient the operator initially and allow the identification of the aorta. The most common reason for inability to visualize the aorta is interference from bowel gas. Often, gentle, steady pressure over the region of interest will displace the artifact. Alternatively, the aorta may be evaluated from the right side, with the patient in the left lateral decubitus position, scanning through the liver during sustained deep inspiration. Finally, if longitudinal scanning proves difficult, coronal view from the left will provide a provisional second view.

SOURCES OF ERROR

There are four primary sources of error when undertaking an abdominal aortic scan for AAA. The first involves improper identification of the aorta itself. Other fluid-filled structures exist in the region of interest, including the inferior vena cava (IVC), splenic vein, superior mesenteric artery, and left renal vein. Identification of regional landmarks (most prominently the vertebral body) in close association with the vessel of interest is critical. The aorta is round and has a thick echogenic wall. The IVC is generally almond shaped and compressible and should also have a respiratory variation in size; it may, however, be pulsatile so caution is warranted in using this as the only criteria for identification. If available, evaluation of the structure with color-flow Doppler will confirm the structure as the aorta.

The second source of error is improper measurement of the aorta. If there is a clot within the lumen, it may lead to false identification of the edge of the thrombus as the aortic wall and a false-negative test, with disastrous consequences. Color-flow Doppler may falsely reassure the examiner that flow is good through a normal-sized aorta, when in fact the area is leaking and clotted within the larger aneurysm, leading to a "normal-appearing" aortic diameter. Careful identification of the true aortic wall by evaluating in two planes is crucial. The presence of a double lumen suggests thrombus or significant plaque that mandates further evaluation.

The final two sources of error are failure to evaluate the entire length of the aorta and failure to evaluate the aorta in two planes. Each of these errors can lead to false-negative results. Saccular aneurysms would be most likely missed on longitudinal scans, although the rate of this type of error is unknown. A tortuous aorta can confound attempts to visualize the aorta throughout its length in the transverse plane.

TAKE HOME POINTS

- Image the full length of the abdominal aorta, in two planes; failure to do so results in an indeterminate test. Measure proximal, midpoint, and distal aorta in two planes from outside wall to outside wall.
- Color-flow Doppler, if available, will assist in identifying the aorta and its branches and is helpful in the diagnosis of aortic dissection.

- While perhaps useful for incidental diagnosis of aortic dissection, it cannot be used to exclude a dissection. CT scan and transesophageal echocardiogram remain the tests of choice for diagnosis and characterization.

- Supine positioning and gentle pressure on the transducer often will eliminate gas/bowel artifact; however, in some cases, patients may have to be repositioned to a side-lying position to encourage bowel gas to fall away from the field.

- Patients with a presumed diagnosis of ruptured AAA need a FAST to assess for blood in the peritoneal cavity, immediate resuscitation, and surgical consult. Do NOT delay resuscitation or consultation while performing the aortic ultrasound examinations.

SUGGESTED READINGS

Tayal VS, Graf CD, Gibbs MA. Prospective study of accuracy and outcome of emergency ultrasound for abdominal aortic aneurysm over two years. *Acad Emerg Med*. 2003;10:867–871.

Kuhn M, Bonnin RLL, Davey MJ, et al. Emergency department ultrasound scanning for abdominal aortic aneurysm: Accessible, accurate, and advantageous. *Ann Emerg Med*. 2000;36:219–223.

368

USE BEDSIDE ULTRASOUND INSTEAD OF NEEDLE ASPIRATION IN THE ASSESSMENT OF SOFT TISSUE INFECTIONS

MASARU RUSTY OSHITA, MD AND WARREN WIECHMANN, MD

Your next patient has a red, warm, tender skin infection that you are sure is an abscess. After gathering your supplies, cleaning the skin, providing local anesthesia of the area, and 12 min of an unsuccessful aspiration, your patient states he or she just wants to leave—dissatisfied. The use of the bedside ultrasound (US) as an extension of your physical exam can allow for an appropriate clinical decision, increase patient throughput, and improve patient satisfaction.

The use of US for the interpretation of soft tissue redness, swelling, and pain can be a rapid and accurate diagnostic tool to differentiate cellulitis from a suspected abscess. The use of US may dictate the management of a patient, as the initial treatment and subsequent follow-up (e.g., wound care, etc.) of a patient with an abscess may be profoundly different than that of a patient with cellulitis. Studies have demonstrated that US is more accurate than clinical exam in diagnosing abscesses and documented changes in management based on sonographic findings.

There are typical sonographic findings, which represent cellulitis and abscess. In order to understand some potential pitfalls, it is important to first recognize the common findings, which will be obtained with the high-frequency linear probe in most cases. For the evaluation of cellulitis, an appearance of "cobblestones"—anechoic edema tracking among hyperechoic fat and subcutaneous tissue—is characteristic of this diagnosis (*Fig. 368.1*). Conversely, a hypoechoic, fluid-filled collection—often with identifiable debris of mixed echogenicities—is consistent with an abscess (*Fig. 368.2*). In some cases, posterior acoustic enhancement may also be present.

One common pitfall in using US to differentiate between cellulitis and abscess is the overexuberance of stating inflammatory changes as those consistent with an abscess. While the inflammatory changes of cellulitis may be similar to some features of an abscess (i.e., hyperemia of the tissues when using color Doppler), there will be absence of a "swirl" of purulent material or definitive confined space. Exerting gentle pressure with the transducer to create movement or "swirling" has been studied as a useful adjunct for differentiating the two entities.

The use of ultrasonography in the diagnosis of a peritonsillar abscess (*Fig. 368.3*) is a facile procedure, which again has profound treatment implications. "Diagnostic" needle aspirations may be avoided, due to the accuracy of US in differentiating peritonsillar cellulitis versus abscess. US in this clinical scenario may also be used for procedural guidance. Caution, however, needs to be applied as the presence of a lymph node may appear as a dark, fluid-filled, well-circumscribed structure. The application of power flow to the suspected structure revealing flow would be consistent with a lymph node.

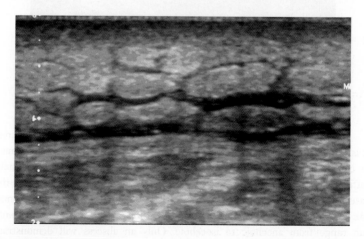

FIGURE 368.1. Cobblestones.

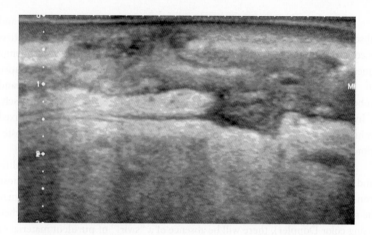

FIGURE 368.2. Abscess.

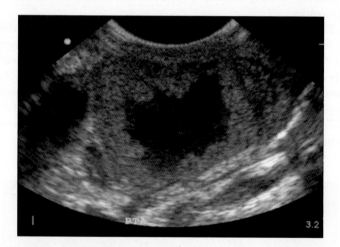

FIGURE 368.3. Peritonsillar abscess.

Finally, in an effort to avoid misdiagnosis and unwarranted procedures, it is important to recall that hematoma and seroma are two entities that may be confused for an abscess. In most cases, the clinical scenario alone can help differentiate the three; however, in the postoperative patient, this may not be the case. Typically, a seroma is homoechoic with well-defined margins. Hematomas can be homoechoic or heteroechoic and, depending on the age of the hematoma, can range from anechoic to isoechoic. Only an abscess will demonstrate "swirling" with gentle pressure by the transducer.

SUGGESTED READINGS

Araujo Filho BC, Sakae FA, Sennes LU, et al. Intraoral and transcutaneous cervical ultrasound in the differential diagnosis of peritonsillar cellulitis and abscesses. *Braz J Otorhinolaryngol.* 2006;72(3):377–381.

Arslan H, Sakarya ME, Bozkurt M, et al. The role of power Doppler sonography in the evaluation of superficial soft tissue abscesses. *Eur J Ultrasound.* 1998;8(2):101–106.

Blankenship RB, Baker T. Imaging modalities in wounds and superficial skin infections. *Emerg Med Clin North Am.* 2007;25(1):223–234.

Loyer EM, Kaur H, David CL, et al. Importance of dynamic assessment of the soft tissues in the sonographic diagnosis of echogenic superficial abscesses. *J Ultrasound Med.* 1995;14(9):669–671.

Robben SG. Ultrasonography of musculoskeletal infections in children. *Eur Radiol.* 2004;14(Suppl 4):L65–L77.

Squire BT, Fox JC, Anderson C. ABSCESS: Applied bedside sonography for convenient evaluation of superficial soft tissue infections. *Acad Emerg Med.* 2005;12(7):601–606.

Taval VS, Hasan N, Norton HJ, et al. The effect of soft-tissue ultrasound on the management of cellulitis in the emergency department. *Acad Emerg Med.* 2006;13(4):384–388.

369

UnStable Patient = UltraSound: Use Ultrasound to Evaluate Hemodynamically Unstable Patients

JAMES PENG, MD

A patient with undifferentiated hypotension presents a particular challenge for the emergency physician (EP). In such patients, many diagnoses are considered: trauma, myocardial infarction, cardiac tamponade, abdominal aortic aneurysm (AAA), aortic dissection, massive pulmonary embolism (PE), tension pneumothorax, septic shock, hypovolemia, etc. To initiate proper treatment, it is critical for the EP to have an approach that can quickly identify reversible causes of unstable and undifferentiated hypotension. Bedside ultrasound is a cornerstone of this approach.

The FAST (Focused Assessment with Sonography in Trauma) examination is such an application in the trauma patient, allowing rapid identification of free fluid in the peritoneal, pericardial, and pleural spaces, and has revolutionized the ED evaluation of these patients. Additional emergency bedside ultrasound applications are now available that are equally important in the undifferentiated hypotensive patient (UHP). Emergency bedside ultrasound is used to rapidly and systematically visualize the heart, the inferior vena cava (IVC), and abdominal aorta facilitating rapid diagnosis. A simple assessment of the heart's global contractility, chamber sizes, and surrounding pericardium is a high yield in the UHP, allowing a rapid narrowing of the differential diagnosis. For example, the absence of a pericardial effusion effectively excludes cardiac tamponade as the cause of a patient's unstable hypotension. Detection of a large circumferential pericardial effusion, right ventricular diastolic collapse, and hyperdynamic contractility may necessitate emergent pericardiocentesis in the same patient. Similarly, findings of massive right ventricular dilatation (or right-heart strain), poor right ventricular contractility, small and hyperdynamic left ventricle, plethoric IVC, and "paradoxical septal motion" (interventricular septum moves toward the left ventricle during diastole) in an UHP may substantiate clinical suspicious of massive PE, which would necessitate early thrombolytic therapy or even embolectomy. Absence of such findings in an UHP refutes massive PE as the etiology.

Studies have demonstrated EPs with focused training can accurately measure left ventricular ejection fraction (LVEF) based on simple visual estimation, allowing identification of systolic pump failure and cardiogenic shock as a contributing etiology. This type of assessment requires only visualization of the anterior mitral leaflet during systole or two-plane views of change in LV size between the diastole and the systole and does not require quantitative measurements. Thus, a rough assessment of LVEF may allow EPs to identify cardiogenic shock using bedside ultrasound and appropriately cater management decisions.

Moving away from the heart, a rapid, noninvasive method of estimating fluid status is invaluable in the UHP. With emergency bedside ultrasound, the proximal IVC may be quickly evaluated to assess right atrial filling pressure and provide a rough estimation of CVP, confirming or refuting hypovolemia. Viewing the IVC as it passes the diaphragm through the liver, a very large IVC (>2.5 cm) correlates an elevated CVP and a small, flat IVC reflects a low CVP. In addition, because of changes in intrathoracic and intraluminal pressures, there is respiratory variation in the size of the IVC. EPs can take advantage of this variation by performing the "sniff test" while viewing the IVC. Ask the patient to "sniff" quickly as the IVC is viewed. If there is >50% collapse of the IVC, the CVP is estimated as low; if there is <50% collapse of the IVC, the CVP is estimated as normal. A plethoric IVC with no respiratory variation is consistent with an elevated CVP. In the patient who cannot follow the sniff command, various studies have shown the use of IVC diameter and change with respiration to estimate right atrial pressure. Such measurements can also be taken during the course of fluid resuscitation, introducing a measure of objectivity in the guidance of volume replacement.

In the older patient presenting with hypotension, the additional findings of abdominal pain and/or altered mental status would mandate an evaluation for a ruptured AAA. As most symptomatic AAAs do not present with the classic triad of abdominal or back pain, hypotension, and a palpable abdominal mass, the EP must have a low threshold for the use of emergency bedside ultrasound to evaluate the aorta in this patient population. This can be accomplished rapidly at the bedside by visualizing the continuity of the aorta from the epigastrium to the bifurcation of the aorta into the common iliac arteries.

In summary, emergency bedside ultrasound allows the EP to quickly narrow the differential in an otherwise undifferentiated, unstable, hypotensive patient. Evaluation of cardiac contractility, chamber size, ejection fraction, and the pericardial space quickly suggest the cause of the hypotension to be due to tamponade, PE, or other causes of cardiogenic shock. Visualization of the IVC yields valuable information regarding the patient's fluid status, confirming or refuting hypovolemia as the cause of hypotension. Analyses of the abdominal aorta further confirms or denies ruptured AAA as the catastrophic cause of a patient's unstable hemodynamic status. Failure to employ this safe, rapid, portable diagnostic tool may delay diagnoses and definitive, targeted therapy.

SUGGESTED READINGS

Bessen H. Abdominal aortic aneurysm. In: Marx JA, Hockberger RS, Walls RM, eds. *Rosen's Emergency Medicine: Concepts and Clinical Practice.* 6th ed. St. Louis, MO: Mosby; 2006: 1330–1341.

Moore CL, Rose GA, Taval VS, et al. Determination of left ventricular function by emergency physician echocardiography of hypotensive patients. *Acad Emerg Med.* 2002;9(3):186–193.

Randazzo MR, Snoey ER, Levitt MA, et al. Accuracy of emergency physician assessment of left ventricular ejection fraction and central venous pressure using echocardiography. *Acad Emerg Med.* 2003;10(9):973–977.

370

IT IS NOT THE MACHINE'S FAULT! USE BASIC SYSTEM CONTROLS TO IMPROVE YOUR ULTRASOUND IMAGES

JENNIE K. ROBIN, MD AND STEPHEN A. CRANDALL, MD

The use of ultrasound by the emergency physician is now considered a standard part of the algorithm in evaluating patients with both traumatic and medical emergencies. For novice users of bedside ultrasound, it is difficult at times to acquire and interpret ultrasound images. There is a steep learning curve not only with using the transducer but also with familiarizing oneself with the basic system controls (knobology) on the ultrasound machine. All systems do not have the same interface, but many of the basic controls such as gain and depth are uniform across models. A basic understanding of these features is essential to both obtain and correctly interpret images.

One of the most common errors is the inadequate use of the gain control. The gain control can lighten or darken the viewing screen as it amplifies or dampens the returning sound waves. All machines will have either a knob or buttons that can adjust the overall gain. In addition, most machines allow for independent adjustment gain at varied segments of the image, by the use of time gain compensation.

Novice users will often increase the gain to attempt to improve the detail and "visibility" of the images. An inappropriate gain level, however, may reduce contrast between structures and obscure subtle findings such as free fluid. Normally, black, anechoic areas may appear more echogenic as the overall image becomes brighter. This can be potentially catastrophic if the intra-abdominal free fluid is unrecognized, especially when assessing a trauma patient or a patient with an ectopic pregnancy. Additionally, posterior shadowing from gallstones, foreign bodies, or other hyperechoic structures may be significantly reduced with inappropriately elevated gain settings. Comet-tail artifacts and lung rockets, which can be essential in evaluating pulmonary pathology such as pneumothoraces or pulmonary edema, can also be minimized or obliterated. While overgaining images is more common, insufficient gain can also result in poor image acquisition and interpretation. *Figure 370.1* provides examples of images that are under-, over-, and appropriately gained. Note that the top image may fail to identify a small collection of fluid in Morison pouch. Conversely, the bottom image does not use sufficient gain to display the normal finding of a mirror-image artifact superior to the diaphragm. The ability to appropriately adjust gain settings is essential to maximize diagnostic sensitivity and avoid potential errors.

Another common error during image acquisition is an inappropriate depth setting for the object in question. The depth helps to define both the surrounding anatomy as well as the perceived size and clarity of the images. Ultrasound displays provide a scale along the side of the screen and a number that denotes the depth of the entire viewing field. A knob or button will increase/decrease the depth of the overall viewing field from the probe. Too much displayed depth may actually decrease the size of structures on the screen and obscure subtle findings, such as a small layer of free fluid or a mural thrombus. Too little displayed depth may distort or hide surrounding anatomy or may exclude additional significant areas of interest, such as the posterior pericardium in a cardiac view or the rectouterine pouch when assessing the pelvis. *Figure 370.2* provides an example, with the middle image demonstrating appropriate depth for imaging this aortic dissection in the transverse plane. The top image has too little depth displayed, failing to identify the posterior extent of the aorta and the bony landmark of the vertebral body. In contrast, the

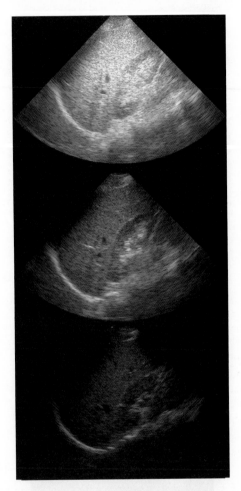

FIGURE 370.1. Images that are undergained, overgained, and appropriately gained. **Top:** May fail to identify a small collection of fluid in Morison pouch; **bottom:** does not use sufficient gain to display the normal finding of a mirror-image artifact superior to the diaphragm.

bottom image displays too much depth, wasting nearly a third of the screen on posterior acoustic shadowing deep to the spine. Familiarity with the concept of scale, and how to interpret this on individual ultrasound machines, is important when performing procedures, as well as to assess the location of a foreign body, vascular structures, and absecesses.

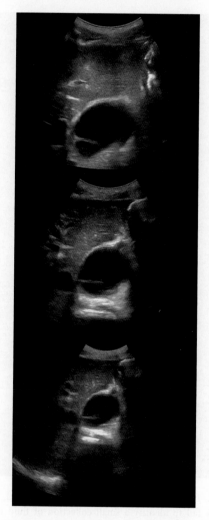

FIGURE 370.2. Top: too little depth displayed; **middle:** appropriate depth for imaging this aortic dissection in the transverse plane; **bottom:** displays too much depth.

A basic understanding of the depth, gain, and other fundamental system controls enables the emergency physician to more accurately interpret findings, perform ultrasound-guided procedures, avoid diagnostic errors, and better direct patient care.

SUGGESTED READINGS

Beck-Razi N, Gaitini D. Focused assessment with sonography for trauma. *Ultrasound Clin.* 2008;3(1):23–31.

Cosby KS, Kendall JL. *Practical Guide to Emergency Ultrasound.* Philadelphia, PA: Lippincott Williams & Wilkins; 2006.

Gaspari RJ, Fox JC, Sierzenski PR. *Emergency Ultrasound: Principles and Practice.* Philadelphia, PA: Mosby; 2006.

Ma OJ, Mateer JR, Blaivas M. *Emergency Ultrasound.* New York, NY: McGraw Hill; 2008.

371

TREAT PATIENTS WITH EPIDIDYMITIS AND THEIR PARTNERS FOR SEXUALLY TRANSMITTED DISEASES

MARY SADEGHI, MD AND
JORGE A. FERNANDEZ, MD, FAAEM, FACEP

Despite established guidelines in place for the treatment of epididymitis, epidemiologic studies of practice patterns have shown that for patients between the ages of 18 and 35, fewer than one third receive the appropriate diagnostic evaluation and fewer than half receive appropriate treatment.

Epididymitis is the fifth most common urological diagnosis in men, ages 18 to 50. Acute epididymitis is characterized by pain, swelling, and inflammation of the epididymis and can present as lower abdominal, inguinal canal, scrotal, or testicular pain. In patients younger than 35 years, epididymitis is generally caused by sexually transmitted diseases (STDs), most frequently *Chlamydia trachomatis* and/or *Neisseria gonorrhoeae*.

The ultimate goals for treatment of acute epididymitis caused by *C. trachomatis* and *N. gonorrhoeae* are cure of infection, improvement of signs and symptoms, prevention of transmission to others, and a decrease in potential complications. The Center for Disease Control and Prevention (CDC) recommends initiating empiric therapy for treatment of acute epididymitis before laboratory results are available. The recommended regimen is ceftriaxone 250 mg IM in a single dose AND doxycycline 100 mg orally twice a day for 10 days. Patients who are allergic to cephalosporins or tetracyclines and with negative gonococcal culture may be given ofloxacin 300 mg orally twice a day for 10 days OR levofloxacin 500 mg orally once daily for 10 days. As of April 2007, the CDC no longer recommends the use of fluoroquinolones to treat *N. gonorrhea* because of the high rate of resistance. The best available treatment for *N. gonorrhea* in patients with cephalosporin allergy is desensitization. Unfortunately, there is no standard approach to desensitization to cephalosporins, and many documented cases have taken hours to days, which may prove to be impractical in the emergency department. In one study, the shortest time that patients underwent intravenous cephalosporin desensitization safely was 2.25 h. Patients were given an initiating dose of 0.1 mg. Each subsequent dose was then increased by half-log$_{10}$ at 15-min intervals. An alternative to desensitization is azithromycin 2 g orally. The guidelines also recommend that the patient be told to refer any recent sexual partners (within 60 days) for evaluation and treatment. Patients should also be instructed to avoid sexual intercourse until they (and all sexual partners) have completed treatment and are symptom free.

Acute epididymitis, if not treated adequately, may result in serious complications including epididymo-orchitis, scrotal abscess formation, sepsis, and infertility. Unfortunately, patients with epididymitis secondary to *C. trachomatis* are often asymptomatic, and scarring may lead to infertility. The female partners of men with epididymitis caused by *C. trachomatis* may also be asymptomatic, and they are also at risk of serious complications such as pelvic inflammatory disease and infertility. In a prospective study in the United Kingdom, 80% of female partners of men under age 35 with epididymitis tested positive for chlamydia, regardless of the results of the patient's chlamydial test. Unfortunately, patients may be unreliable in referring their sexual partners for treatment. One comparative study of males with nongonococcal urethritis demonstrated that provider referral was three times more successful at identifying partners with chlamydia infection than self-referral.

An emerging alternative to partner referral is expedited partner therapy (EPT). EPT is a practice of treating the sexual partners of patients with STDs and involves the delivery of medications or prescriptions by the patients for their partners without the clinical assessment of the partners. Studies show that the rate of reinfection of patients with *C. trachomatis* and/or *N. gonorrhoeae* who underwent patient-delivered partner therapy was significantly less than those with standard partner referral. EPT has its risks and limitations and is not legal in all states. Partners who undergo EPT are at risk for drug toxicity and allergic reactions and may not benefit from prevention counseling by a clinician.

SUGGESTED READINGS

Centers for Disease Control and Prevention. *Expedited Partner Therapy in the Management of Sexually Transmitted Diseases.* Atlanta, GA: US Department of Health and Human Services; 2006.

Collins MM, Stafford RS, O'Leary MP, et al. How common is prostatitis? A national survey of physician visits. *J Urol.* 1998;159:1224–1228.

Drury NE, Dyer JP, Breitenfeldt N, et al. Management of acute epididymitis: Are European guidelines being followed? *Eur Urol.* 2004;46:522–525.

Geisler WM, Krieger JN. Epididymitis and the acute scrotum syndrome. In: *Current Diagnosis and Treatment of Sexually Transmitted Diseases.* New York, NY: McGraw-Hill; 2007.

Luzzi GA, O'Brien TS. Acute epididymitis. *BJU Int.* 2001;87(8):747–755.

Macke BA, Maher JE. Partner notification in the United States. *Am J Prev Med.* 1999;17: 230–242.

National Guideline Clearinghouse. Epididymitis. Sexually transmitted diseases guidelines 2006. Center for Disease Control and Prevention; August 4, 2006.

Robinson AJ, Grant JB, Spencer RC, et al. Acute epididymitis: Why patient and consort must be investigated. *Br J Urol.* 1990;66(6):642–645.

Win PH, Brown H, Zankar A, et al. Rapid intravenous cephalosporin desensitization. *J Allergy Clin Immunol.* 2005;116(1):225–228.

372

DO NOT FAIL TO CONSIDER TORSION IN PATIENTS WITH INTERMITTENT SCROTAL PAIN

SAI-HUNG JOSHUA HUI, MD AND
JORGE A. FERNANDEZ, MD, FAAEM, FACEP

The modern word *torsion* has several origins: from the French *torsion* meaning "wringing pain in the bowels," from the Latin *tortionem* or *tortio* meaning "torture or torment," and from the late Latin *tortus*, past participle of *torquēre*, meaning "to twist." Given its significant medicolegal risks to the emergency physician, all of these origins ring true for the diagnosis of testicular torsion. Although it is not fatal, the infertility that may result when diagnosis is delayed continues to yield huge payouts in malpractice suits.

How promptly must one make the diagnosis and treatment? Immediately, as emergent surgical detorsion is necessary if manual detorsion is unsuccessful. Irreversible damage from ischemia of the testicle starts after 6 h, and the odds of infertility increases as the duration of ischemia goes on. Salvage rates of 80% to 100% are possible if intervention happens within 6 h. Currently, the imaging study of choice is testicular color Doppler ultrasound, which detects decreased blood flow to the affected testis in the case of active torsion and identifies other potential causes of acute scrotal pain such as acute epididymo-orchitis, hydroceles, varicoceles, or trauma. Based on the timing of the patient's presentation, the sensitivity of ultrasound in the diagnosis of active testicular torsion is estimated to be between 86% and 100% with a specificity near 100%.

However, there is an important urological syndrome that emergency physicians must be aware of: intermittent testicular torsion (ITT). By definition, patients with ITT have prior episodes of acute scrotal pain followed by spontaneous resolution. ITT is considered to predispose patients toward acute testicular torsion because 55% to 100% of ITT patients have an underlying bell clapper deformity. In fact, multiple reports show that about 50% of males diagnosed with acute testicular torsion have had previous episodes of similar testicular pain, suggesting that they may have had ITT.

Instead of decreased blood flow to the affected testis as in active torsion, patients with ITT usually will have increased blood flow as a reaction to spontaneous detorsion, if ultrasound is performed shortly after the scrotal pain resolves. Doppler ultrasound has been found to be less effective in differentiating ITT from acute epididymo-orchitis in patients with acute scrotal pain, as both may demonstrate increased blood flow. In a study by Eaton et al., the finding of horizontal lie of the affected testis and a previous history of similar pain are highly suggestive of ITT.

Discharging a patient with acute scrotal pain simply based on the presence of increased blood flow with a diagnosis of acute epididymo-orchitis is therefore a significant and dangerous pitfall because the patient may very well have ITT.

The risk of missing ITT is minimized if there is no past history of scrotal pain, the testicular lie is vertical, and signs of infection suggestive of epididymo-orchitis on physical examination are present and documented. On the other hand, if ITT is suspected based on history, urologists should be consulted emergently, because patients with ITT have a high risk of complete torsion and subsequent infertility.

SUGGESTED READINGS

Boopathy Vijayaraghavan S. Sonographic differential diagnosis of acute scrotum: Real time whirlpool sign, a key of torsion. *J Ultrasound Med.* 2006;25:563–574.

Eaton SH, Cendron MA, Estrada CR, et al. Intermittent testicular torsion: Diagnostic features and management outcomes. *J Urol.* 2005;174:1532–1535.

Kahler J, Harwood-Nuss AL. Selected urologic problems. In: *Rosen's Emergency Medicine Concepts and Clinical Practice.* 6th ed. Philadelphia, PA: Mosby Elsevier; 2006.

Kim ED. Segmental ischemia of testis secondary to intermittent testicular torsion. *Urology.* 2006;68:670–671.

Swartz D. The acute scrotal mass. In: Harwood-Nuss AL, Linden CH, Luten RC, et al., eds. *The Clinical Practice of Emergency Medicine.* 2nd ed. Philadelphia, PA: JB Lippincott; 1996.

373

CONSULT A UROLOGIST IMMEDIATELY FOR SUSPECTED TESTICULAR TORSION

MARY LOUISE MARTIN, MD

AND JORGE A. FERNANDEZ, MD, FAAEM, FACEP

Testicular torsion is a devastating etiology of acute scrotal pain. While not life threatening, it is a leading cause of male infertility. Affected patients may also develop delayed torsion or autoantibody-mediated destruction of the uninvolved testicle. The medicolegal implications of delayed or missed diagnosis of testicular torsion are obvious. Therefore, the emergency physician should consider testicular torsion in all presentations of acute scrotal pain.

The most important and necessary step in the evaluation and management of testicular torsion is early urologic consultation. Testicular salvage rates approach 100% if vascular supply is returned to the affected testicle within 4 to 6 h. This rate drops to <70% after 6 h; after 12 h, the salvage rate is a dismal 20%.

Unfortunately, the diagnosis of testicular torsion is often not straightforward. Diagnostic findings that suggest the diagnosis of torsion include acute onset of symptoms (<12 h), absent cremasteric reflex, elevation, and abnormal lie of the testicle into a horizontal, rather than vertical, plane. A critical pitfall, however, is to rule out the diagnosis based on the absence of any one or more of these findings.

Historically, all acute scrotal presentations were diagnosed by surgical exploration. Since the advent of nuclear medicine scintigraphy and Doppler ultrasound as diagnostic tools in evaluating the acute scrotum, not all presentations require exploration. However, imaging is indicated only in those cases in which the clinical diagnosis is uncertain or when torsion appears unlikely. In these cases, surgery may be prevented with documented evidence of normal or increased blood flow seen to the testicle, suggesting a diagnosis of epididymitis or torsion of an epididymal appendix. In cases where imaging results are equivocal and in those that give a history suspicious for torsion-detorsion, surgical exploration is indicated. It should be noted that there is as high as an 8% false-negative rate with nuclear medicine studies; Doppler ultrasound has been shown to have sensitivity as low as 82% to 86% in some studies.

The urologist should be present to evaluate the results of imaging tests and, if necessary, initiate surgical repair or exploration immediately. When a consultant is not immediately available, the emergency physician should attempt manual detorsion after adequate analgesia to restore blood flow to the affected testicle. However, consultation and surgical intervention should not be delayed in an attempt to obtain imaging or perform manual detorsion. If a urologist requests an imaging study and to be recontacted with results, the emergency physician should hold firm about the need for immediate evaluation. In cases with classic symptoms of torsion, the urologist should require no further testing, and surgical exploration should be immediately performed without a confirmed diagnosis. In these cases, a high rate of negative surgical exploration (up to 30% in some series) may be acceptable in exchange for missed or delayed diagnosis.

Although urologists are the most frequently litigated specialty in cases of malpractice involving testicular torsion, emergency physicians are second. When named in malpractice suits, emergency physicians are most frequently cited for delayed referral to the surgical consultant. This stresses the need to involve the consultant early in all cases where there is any reasonable suspicion for torsion. The emergency physician should never allow for "castration by procrastination."

SUGGESTED READINGS

Corbett HJ, Simpson ED. Management of the acute scrotum in children. *ANZ J Surg.* 2002;72(3):226–228.

Lindsey D, Stanisic TK. Diagnosis and management of testicular torsion: Pitfalls and perils. *Am J Emerg Med.* 1988;6(1):42–46.

Marcozzi D, Suner S. The nontraumatic, acute scrotum. *Emerg Med Clin North Am.* 2001;19:547–568.

Marx J, Hockberger R, Walls R, eds. *Rosen's Emergency Medicine: Concepts and Clinical Practice.* 6th ed. Philadelphia, PA: Mosby Elsevier; 2006.

Matteson JR, Stock JA, Hanna MD, et al. Medicolegal aspects of testicular torsion. *Urology.* 2001;57:783–787.

McCollough M, Sharieff GQ. Abdominal surgical emergencies in infants and young children. *Emerg Med Clin North Am.* 2003;21:909–935.

Ringdahl E, Teague L. Testicular torsion. *Am Fam Physician.* 2006;7410:1739–1743.

374

DO NOT EXCLUDE THE DIAGNOSIS OF RENAL COLIC PURELY BASED ON THE URINALYSIS

SAI-HUNG JOSHUA HUI, MD
AND JORGE A. FERNANDEZ, MD, FAAEM, FACEP

More than 1 million emergency room visits annually are due to renal colic with an estimated cost at $1.83 billion. Although renal colic may strike at any age, the peak incidence is age 35 to 45. Male sex, Caucasian race, high socioeconomic status, and a positive family history are all associated with a higher incidence of the disease. The majority of cases are secondary to calcium oxalate crystal formation. Less common causes include struvite stones, associated with urea-splitting bacteria such as *Proteus*, *Klebsiella*, and *Pseudomonas*; uric acid stones; and congenital cysteine stones. When a patient presents with acute flank pain or pain radiating toward the genitalia, the emergency physician should consider renal colic in the differential diagnosis. A common pitfall, however, is to rely solely on urinalysis (UA; both dipstick and microscopic) to rule out renal colic.

UA is the initial diagnostic modality of choice in patients with suspected renal colic. It may reveal useful information regarding the underlying cause of urolithiasis as well as potential emergency complications. Highly acidic urine pH (<6.0) suggests uric acid stones; highly alkaline pH (>8.0) suggests struvite stones. Furthermore, crystals may be seen in the urine, and the underlying composition of these crystals is highly predictive of the underlying cause. UA is necessary in all patients with renal colic in order to rule out associated urinary tract infection. In the presence of urinary obstruction, a urinary tract infection becomes a urologic emergency.

The sensitivity of urine dipstick and UA in diagnosing renal colic ranges from 70% to 90% at best. Urine dipstick is a fast, low-cost, and first-line diagnostic test. Multiple studies have shown that urine dipstick actually carries a slightly higher sensitivity than formal laboratory microscopy. This may be because centrifugation during urine sample preparation causes RBC hemolysis and the resulting absence of RBCs in the supernatant. The sensitivity of UA also depends on the timing of the presentation. In a retrospective study of 537 patients with suspected renal colic by Kobayashi et al., it was found that sensitivity was highest in patients who presented on the first day of pain compared to those patients who presented several days later.

Symptomatic nephrolithiasis may result in significant morbidity such as hydronephrosis, pyelonephritis, ruptured renal capsule with uroma, and acute renal failure. Emergency physicians should be particularly vigilant in pursuing the diagnosis of renal colic in those patients at highest risk for complications. These include patients with diabetes mellitus, preexisting renal insufficiency, solitary or transplanted kidneys, polycystic kidney disease, and functional urological disorders such as spinal cord injuries. Bedside renal ultrasonography is a useful initial imaging modality for screening for renal anomalies and ruling out alternative life-threatening diagnoses such as abdominal aortic aneurysm. Furthermore, some studies have demonstrated an excellent negative predictive value of the combination of negative renal ultrasonography and flat plate radiography of the abdomen (KUB). However, ultrasound is most often unable to visualize the calculus itself, and in many cases, it is necessary to proceed with CT. Noncontrast CT is superior to ultrasound for both the delineation of renal anatomy as well as the detection and characterization of calculi. The downsides of routinely performing CT are increased cost and exposure to ionizing radiation. This becomes an increasingly important concern when repeat or serial CT imaging is being considered.

In summary, UA should routinely be performed in all patients suspected of renal colic. UA may reveal potential causes of nephrolithiasis, such as cysteine crystalluria, as well as potentially emergent complications, such as infection. However, the diagnosis of renal colic cannot be ruled out with a normal UA alone.

SUGGESTED READINGS

Bove P, Kaplan D, Dalymple N, et al. Reexamining the value of hematuria testing in patients with acute flank pain. *J Urol.* 1999;162(3 pt 1):685–687.

Clark JY, Thompson IM, Optenberg SA. Economic impact of urolithiasis in the United States. *J Urol.* 1995;154:2020–2024.

Kobayashi T, Nishizawa K, Mitsumori K, et al. Impact of date of onset on the absence of hematuria in patients with acute renal colic. *J Urol.* 2003;170(4 pt 1):1093–1096.

Li J, Kennedy D, Levine M, et al. Absent hematuria and expensive computerized tomography: Case characteristics of emergency urolithiasis. *J Urol.* 2001;165(3):782–784.

Luchs JS, Katz DS, Lane MJ, et al. Utility of hematuria testing in patients with suspected renal colic: Correlation with unenhanced helical CT results. *Urology.* 2003;59(6):839–842.

Press SM, Smith AD. Incidence of negative hematuria in patients with acute urinary lithiasis presenting to the emergency room with flank pain. *Urology.* 1995;45(5):753–757.

375

Provide Adequate Treatment and Appropriate Disposition for Patients with Renal Colic

Jennifer Taitz Soifer, MD and
Jorge A. Fernandez, MD, FAAEM, FACEP

Urinary tract stones are one of the most common urologic diseases, occurring in approximately 10% of the population. They have a recurrence rate of 50%. Patients may present with stones anywhere along the urinary tract. In general, ureteral stones cause the worst pain, secondary to hydroureter and hydronephrosis. The rate of spontaneous stone passage and the time required for passage are both related to the size of the stone. Small stones, those ≤5 in size, have spontaneous passage rates >60% to 70%. Stones between 5 and 10 mm are less likely to pass, with rates <50%, and will often take much longer to pass. Stones larger than 10 mm are unlikely to pass spontaneously. Struvite stones, formed by urease-producing bacteria, often fill the entire collecting system (so-called staghorn calculi); these will never pass spontaneously into the bladder.

The identification of stone composition is important for therapy; uric acid stones are nearly 100% preventable with allopurinol and dietary modification. Notably, there has been successful litigation against physicians who failed to identify uric acid stones in patients with recurrent renal colic. Therefore, all emergency physicians should instruct patients to strain their urine and to take the stone to their primary physician.

Medical expulsive therapy refers to the use of medications to dilate the smooth muscle in the ureter, prostate, and urethra. It has been demonstrated to achieve clinically significant improvements in the rate of stone passage. Agents that have shown to facilitate stone passage include calcium channel blockers, α-adrenergic blockers, corticosteroids, and NSAIDs. The most commonly prescribed calcium channel blocker for urolithiasis is nifedipine; however, α-adrenergic blockers, such as terazosin, and α_1 selective blockers, such as tamsulosin, have each been shown to be superior to nifedipine. Corticosteroids provide a marginal benefit when added to these agents; therefore, the adjunctive use of corticosteroids is controversial. NSAIDs play a similar role as corticosteroids; both induce smooth muscle relaxation and arteriolar vasoconstriction, thereby reducing inflammation and edema. A 10-day course of medical expulsive therapy is generally prescribed. Patients who fail to improve require urologic follow-up for possible surgical intervention. Unfortunately, there are no studies that explore the use of medical expulsive therapy for stones larger than 10 mm. In patients with stones smaller than 10 mm, medical expulsive therapy has become standard. Therefore, all emergency physicians should become familiar with this treatment modality.

In general, urologic consultation is indicated for all patients with (1) stones >10 mm, (2) stones smaller than 10 mm that fail medical expulsive therapy, (3) struvite stones, and (4) stones associated with acute urinary tract infection, acute renal failure, or solitary kidneys, including transplant recipients. Surgical interventions in these situations include percutaneous nephrostomy tube or ureteral stent placement. The use of extracorporeal shock wave therapy is controversial and at the discretion of the treating urologist.

The combination of urinary tract obstruction and infection represents a true urologic emergency. These patients may rapidly develop septic shock and multisystem organ failure. Furthermore, urinary obstruction impairs glomerular filtration, so antibiotics cannot be effectively delivered to the collecting system. Therefore, all cases require emergent decompression of the collecting system by a urologist. Failure to identify urinary tract infections associated with obstruction is a devastating pitfall. Similarly, failure to identify urinary obstruction in a septic patient is also potentially lethal.

Finally, do not forget that renal colic is an extremely painful condition! Pain should be treated aggressively, and diagnostic certainty is not necessary to initiate analgesia. A combination of intravenous morphine and ketorolac has been documented to be more effective than either given alone; therefore, this should be the initial analgesic treatment modality in most situations, unless contraindications exist. Ketorolac is contraindicated in patients with impaired renal function or when there is a good reason to suspect renal insufficiency (e.g., a patient with a history of multiple, bilateral, or congenital stones). Lastly, because ketorolac takes longer to have effect, narcotics should not be withheld in patients with acute colic.

SUGGESTED READINGS

Preminger GM, Tselius HG, Assimos DG, et al. 2007 Guideline for the management of ureteral calculi. *Urology.* 2007;178(6):2418–2434.

Safdar B, Degutis LC, Landry K, et al. Intravenous morphine plus ketorolac is superior to either drug alone for treatment of acute renal colic. *Ann Emerg Med.* 2006;48:173–181.

Singh A, Alter HJ, Littlepage A. A systematic review of medical therapy to facilitate passage of ureteral calculi. *Ann Emerg Med.* 2007;50(5):552–563.

Teichman JMH. Acute renal colic from ureteral calculus. *N Engl J Med.* 2004;350:684–693.

Yoshimura K, Utsunomiya N, Ichioka K, et al. Emergency drainage for urosepsis associated with upper urinary tract calculi. *J Urol.* 2005;173(2):458–462.

376

DO NOT DELAY SUPRAPUBIC
CATHETERIZATION WHEN NEEDED

DIEGO ABDELNUR, MD
AND JORGE A. FERNANDEZ, MD, FAAEM, FACEP

Most cases of acute urinary retention can be successfully treated in the emergency department with Foley catheter placement. Familiarity with the placement of a suprapubic catheter, however, is a necessity for any physician working in the emergency department where urologic specialists may not be readily available. The placement of a suprapubic catheter can provide immediate relief to a patient with a full bladder and may avert postobstructive renal failure in these situations. Although the procedure may seem daunting, in practice, suprapubic catheterization is simple, fast, and has few adverse side effects.

There are a number of indications for the placement of a suprapubic urinary catheter. These include urinary retention from prostatic hypertrophy, prostatic or gynecological malignancy, spinal cord injury, urethral stricture, urethral trauma, and phimosis. The majority of cases of urinary retention involve men over the age of 50 suffering from either benign prostatic hypertrophy (BPH) or prostatic malignancy. In fact, it is estimated that 50% of men have histologic evidence of BPH by the age of 50, with almost half of these cases being clinically significant. Urethral strictures are either of congenital origin or due to infections such as gonorrhea and chlamydia. Phimosis often affects patients with sickle cell anemia but increasingly affects patients taking prescription medication for erectile dysfunction. In all these cases, suprapubic catheterization should be initiated if attempts at Foley catheterization are unsuccessful or contraindicated, such as in cases of urethral trauma. A delay in the placement of a suprapubic catheter, in addition to prolonging extreme patient discomfort, can lead to acute and often permanent renal failure.

The placement of a suprapubic catheter can be accomplished in several easy steps. Perhaps the most important advance has been the advent of bedside ultrasonography. The location of the bladder is simple with ultrasonography, and real-time monitoring of catheter placement is possible. Recent studies using ultrasound guidance have shown a 100% success rate and no complications. If no ultrasound machine is available, a general landmark for needle insertion is 2 cm above the pubic symphysis, in the midline of the lower abdomen. A 22-gauge needle may be used to aspirate the urine; commercial cystotomy kits may be used to achieve permanent drainage. Similar to the Seldinger technique of central line placement, after the needle (18 or 20 gauge) is inserted into the bladder, a guide wire is threaded through the needle. The needle is removed, a small cut is made in the skin, and an introducer is threaded over the guide wire. The guide wire is then removed, a 10F Foley catheter is threaded through the introducer, the balloon is inflated with 10 mL of normal saline, and the introducer sheath is peeled away.

Complications of suprapubic catheter placement include peritoneal perforation, bowel perforation, infection, and hematuria. Perforation of the peritoneum does not necessarily indicate bowel perforation, and perforation of the bowel oftentimes does not cause clinically significant complications if the introducer has not yet been placed. Patients with known bladder tumors or a history of lower abdominal scars have a higher incidence of adherent bowel to either the bladder or the abdominal wall, so suprapubic catheter placement should be avoided; simple aspiration may still be necessary. The second major complication, infection, can be minimized by using a strict aseptic technique. In fact, studies have shown a *decreased* rate of infection with suprapubic catheters when compared with Foley catheters (5% vs. 12.5%). And, one recent study of 219 patients showed that 89% of the patients actually *preferred* suprapubic catheter insertion over traditional Foley insertion.

In summary, the insertion of a suprapubic catheter is a simple and safe endeavor. Emergency physicians should not hesitate to perform suprapubic catheter placement in situations where urologic consultation will be delayed.

SUGGESTED READINGS

Aguilera PA, Choi T, Durham BA. Ultrasound-guided suprapubic cystostomy catheter placement in the emergency department. *J Emerg Med.* 2004;26(3):319–321.

Ahluwalia RS, Johal N, Kouriefs C, et al. The surgical risk of suprapubic catheter insertion and long-term sequelae. *Ann R Coll Surg Engl.* 2006;88(2):210–213.

Johnson CD. Suprapubic catheterization at laparotomy. *Dig Surg.* 2006;23(5–6):281–282.

Tintinalli JE, Kelen GD, Stapczynski JS, eds. *Emergency Medicine: A Comprehensive Study Guide.* 6th ed. New York, NY: McGraw-Hill Companies; 2004:618–619.

377

Do not confuse simple with complicated urinary tract infections

Samuel N. Melton, MD
and Jorge A. Fernandez, MD, FAAEM, FACEP

Recognizing and properly managing a urinary tract infection (UTI) in the emergency department are important to prevent the potential morbidity associated with disease progression. Delayed diagnosis and treatment may lead to treatment failure, renal abscess, bacteremia, sepsis, emphysematous pyelonephritis, or recurrent UTI. Longer term sequelae of untreated UTIs include papillary necrosis, renal scarring, and renal failure.

Acute, uncomplicated UTIs are generally limited to young, immunocompetent, adult, nonpregnant women with normal anatomy. The term "honeymoon cystitis" has been used to describe acute, uncomplicated UTIs that occur presumably due to the introduction of perineal flora into the urethra during sexual activity. In young, well-appearing, nonpregnant women with classic UTI symptoms (and absence of vaginal symptoms), a 3-day course of appropriate oral antibiotics is sufficient treatment. Any UTI that occurs outside this population of young, healthy, nonpregnant women is, by definition, a complicated UTI and must be managed more conservatively.

Complicated UTIs are defined as urinary infections occurring in a patient with structural or functional abnormalities that may predispose to treatment failure. Structural abnormalities may include indwelling catheters, prostatic enlargement, calculi, vesicoureteral reflux, a history of genitourinary surgery, obstructing mass, malignancy, or other abnormalities that may impede the normal flow of urine. Functional abnormalities include advanced age, chronic illness, HIV, diabetes, drug or alcohol abuse, immunosuppressant medications, neurologic abnormality, renal impairment, sickle cell anemia, recent antibiotic use, and atypical organisms. UTIs in males, pregnant women, and neonates are also considered complicated. Although more evidence is needed to support this strategy, it is currently recommended that all patients with complicated UTIs have urinalysis and urine cultures obtained. Whereas *Escherichia coli* is the pathogen in uncomplicated UTIs, a multitude of organisms across the full spectrum of bacteria and fungi may be responsible for complicated UTIs. Moreover, complicated UTIs should be treated with much longer courses of antibiotics (7 to 14 days), using broad-spectrum agents until culture results are available. Indications for admission are generally based on clinical judgment, and there is evidence to support outpatient management of complicated UTIs, provided the patient is well appearing, has normal vitals signs, can tolerate oral medication, and has good access to outpatient follow-up. Otherwise, the patient should be admitted for IV antibiotics and inpatient management.

All UTIs in neonates, infants, and young children are presumed to be due to structural abnormalities, such as vesicoureteral reflux, until proven otherwise. Neonates and infants may present with atypical symptoms, such as fever without apparent source, failure to thrive, irritability, jaundice, constipation, or diarrhea, making the diagnosis more difficult. Catheterized urinalysis and urine cultures should be sent for all presumed UTIs in infants and young children. Although follow-up imaging is controversial, currently, renal ultrasound plus either voiding cystourethrogram (VCUG) or radionuclide cystography (RNC) are recommended following the first UTI in children aged 2 months to 2 years of age. For older children, recommendations are less clear, although all males should be referred for further urologic consultation regardless of age. Most authors suggest that females over 4 years old should be referred for evaluation upon the diagnosis of their second episode of acute, uncomplicated UTI.

Occasionally, complicated UTIs may present with unusual physical exam and laboratory findings. Atypical organisms such as fungal or mycoplasma species should be suspected in patients with repeated diagnosis of UTI and nondiagnostic urine cultures. Also, urinalysis may be falsely negative for urine infection in upper UTIs with obstruction. CT imaging should be performed in ill-appearing patients with upper UTI symptoms to rule out surgical complications such as emphysematous pyelonephritis or perinephric abscess. These patients need emergency surgical consultation for drainage.

In summary, physicians should be cautious when diagnosing acute, uncomplicated UTIs, and the diagnosis should only be made in healthy, nonpregnant, young adult females. Male patients or patients with UTI and underlying structural and functional abnormalities should be diagnosed with complicated UTI, a urine culture should be sent, and appropriate 7- to 14-day courses of antibiotics given with appropriate consultation and follow-up.

SUGGESTED READINGS

Alper BS, Curry SH. Urinary tract infection in children. *Am Fam Physician*. 2005;75(12): 2483–2488.

Bergman DA, Baltz RD, Cooley, et al. Practice parameters: The diagnosis, treatment, and evaluation of the initial urinary tract infection in febrile infants and young children. *Pediatrics*. 1999;103:834–853.

Marx JA, ed. *Rosen's Emergency Medicine: Concepts and Clinical Practice*. 6th ed. Philadelphia, PA: Mosby; 2006:1573–1586.

Neal DE Jr. Complicated urinary tract infections. *Urol Clin North Am*. 2008;35(1):13–22.

Orenstein R, Wong ES. Urinary tract infections in adults. *Am Fam Physician*. 1999;59(5): 1225–1234, 1237.

378

Treat pyelonephritis in the pregnant patient aggressively

Jennifer Taitz Soifer, MD
and Jorge A. Fernandez, MD, FAAEM, FACEP

Acute pyelonephritis occurs in approximately 1% to 2% of pregnant women and is associated with significant risk for both the mother and the fetus. Pregnant women are at increased risk of developing pyelonephritis due to the physiologic and anatomic changes caused by pregnancy. Bacterial growth is facilitated by changes in urine chemistry, such as elevated urine pH and glucose levels, as well as due to urinary stasis, caused by ureteral dilatation and increased renal perfusion. As in nonpregnant patients, the majority of cases are caused by an ascending bacterial infection in the urethra and urinary bladder. In rare cases, usually in immunocompromised patients, pyelonephritis may occur secondary to hematogenous spread.

Complications of pyelonephritis in the pregnant patient are reportedly common. Bacteremia may be seen in up to 20% of patients; serious cases may become complicated by endotoxin-mediated hemolysis, disseminated intravascular coagulopathy, acute respiratory distress syndrome, acute renal failure, and/or septic shock. Renal insufficiency, lasting days to weeks, may occur even in the absence of bacteremia. Uterine contractions are common and may result in spontaneous abortion or preterm labor.

The diagnosis of pyelonephritis may be difficult because symptoms of cystitis, such as dysuria, urinary frequency, urgency, and suprapubic tenderness, may not be present in pregnant patients. A prudent recommendation is that emergency physicians should routinely order urinalysis and urine culture in any febrile or vomiting pregnant patient. Urinalysis findings suggestive of pyelonephritis include positive nitrites, leukocyte esterase, or white blood cell casts. While a urine culture of >10,000 colony-forming units establishes the diagnosis, counts of 1,000 to 9,999 may be seen in partially treated or early infections.

Historically, the recommended treatment of acute pyelonephritis in the pregnant patient was hospital admission for intravenous hydration and parenteral antibiotics. Patients were transitioned to oral therapy when afebrile for 48 h. A recent, small randomized study demonstrated comparable risk to the mother and fetus with inpatient versus outpatient treatment in carefully selected patients at >24 weeks gestation. Although no poor outcomes occurred in the study patients, a 30% rate of treatment failure was observed in the outpatient group, requiring prolonged subsequent hospitalization. Notably, all patients were initially treated with intramuscular ceftriaxone and observed in the hospital for 24 h. Furthermore, patients with serious medical comorbidities, obstetric complications, or penicillin allergy were excluded from this study. As there is still much controversy regarding the optimal disposition of pregnant patients with pyelonephritis, these decisions should be made by an obstetrician.

Prior to the initiation of antibiotics, it is important to obtain a catheter urine specimen. By definition, a urinary tract infection (UTI) in pregnancy is complicated. A specific bacteriologic pathogen should be sought in a complicated UTI because the risks of serious sequelae and treatment failure are greater. Regardless of patient disposition, the initial antibiotic therapy should be empiric and broad spectrum, covering typical urinary pathogens.

Ceftriaxone is an effective and safe first-line agent in pregnancy. Importantly, fluoroquinolones and trimethoprim-sulfamethoxazole are contraindicated in pregnancy due to risks of teratogenicity. After treatment is completed, prophylaxis with nitrofurantoin is recommended until 4 to 6 weeks postpartum in order to minimize the risk of recurrent episodes.

All toxic-appearing patients and those with evidence of renal failure should be imaged to rule out obstruction or perinephric abscess. Ultrasonography or magnetic resonance imaging is preferred in pregnancy; computed tomography should be avoided, if possible, to minimize excessive fetal radiation exposure.

SUGGESTED READINGS

DeCherney AH, Nathan L, eds. *Current Obstetric and Gynecologic Diagnosis and Treatment.* 9th ed. New York, NY: Lange/McGraw Hill; 2003.

Ramakrishnan K, Scheid DC. Diagnosis and management of acute pyelonephritis in adults. *Am Fam Physician.* 2005;71:933–942.

Wing DA. Pyelonephritis. *Clin Obstet Gynecol.* 1998;41:515–526.

Wing DA, Hendershott CM, Debuque L, et al. Outpatient treatment of acute pyelonephritis in pregnancy after 24 weeks. *Obstet Gynecol.* 1999;94(5 pt 1):683–688.

379

DOSE RENALLY EXCRETED MEDICATIONS BASED ON RENAL FUNCTION

JENNIFER TAITZ SOIFER, MD
AND JORGE A. FERNANDEZ, MD, FAAEM, FACEP

Emergency physicians are required to have a working knowledge of a wide variety of medications. Usually, a single dose is memorized for the most commonly used medications. Unfortunately, many medications commonly prescribed by emergency physicians can potentially harm patients with renal insufficiency due to adverse side effects and medication toxicity.

Failure to recognize renal insufficiency is an important pitfall to avoid. Physicians should remember that serum creatinine levels alone are inadequate in determining renal function. Furthermore, approximately 60% of renal function may be lost prior to the elevation of the serum creatinine level about normal limits. Renal function may be reliably estimated using the Cockcroft-Gault formula: Estimated creatinine clearance = ([140 − Age] × Ideal body weight [kg] × 0.85 [if female])/(72 × Serum creatinine [mg/dL]). The Cockcroft-Gault formula demonstrates why creatinine clearance may be overestimated in thin, elderly, or female patients, if the serum creatinine level alone is used to determine renal function. Estimated creatinine clearance levels <60 mL/min/m^2 indicate renal insufficiency; as a result, medication dosages may need to be adjusted.

Analgesics are some of the most commonly prescribed medications in the emergency department. The majority of narcotic analgesics are metabolized by the liver; however, meperidine is renally metabolized. In patients with renal insufficiency, some experts say that repeated doses of meperidine should be avoided in order to avoid a reduction in the seizure threshold. Nonsteroidal anti-inflammatory drugs (NSAIDs) are a particular problem and should be either avoided or used with extreme caution. NSAIDs may precipitate nephrotic syndrome, interstitial nephritis, hyperkalemia, and sodium retention. In patients with renal insufficiency, chronic therapy with oral NSAIDs such as ibuprofen and aspirin should be avoided. If ketorolac is used, doses should be decreased in these patients in order to avoid both gastrointestinal and renal toxicities. There have been numerous reports of acute renal failure directly attributable to ketorolac, particularly when intravenous doses exceed 30 mg in patients with underlying renal insufficiency.

Antihypertensives are available in many different drug classes, each with varied mechanisms of action and metabolism. In patients with renal insufficiency, hyperkalemia is a potential complication of numerous antihypertensive agents, including potassium-sparing diuretics, angiotensin-converting enzyme inhibitors, angiotensin II receptor antagonists, and β-blockers. Potassium levels must be closely monitored in all cases, and potassium-sparing diuretics should be avoided altogether in patients with a creatinine clearance <30 mL/min/m². Notably, calcium channel blockers and nitroglycerin require no dosing adjustments, and loop diuretics frequently require *higher* dosages to achieve therapeutic effects in patients with renal insufficiency.

Many diabetic medications also require dosing adjustments in renal insufficiency. The dosage of insulin should be lowered in most patients because insulin metabolism is significantly reduced in the setting of renal dysfunction. Furthermore, when administering insulin in conjunction with D50 to treat hyperkalemia, half the usual insulin dosage should be given to avoid hypoglycemia. Metformin is contraindicated in renal insufficiency, and the dosage of glipizide should be reduced in these patients as well in order to avoid life-threatening hypoglycemia. Notably, glucophage is metabolized by the liver, and it requires no dosage adjustments in renal insufficiency.

In general, most antimicrobial agents require reductions in both frequency of administration and dose in renal insufficiency. Two notable exceptions include ceftriaxone and metronidazole. Aminoglycoside and vancomycin, however, require special attention. With both, levels must be frequently monitored in order to avoid nephrotoxicity. Nitrofurantoin and many antifungals generally should be avoided in cases of renal insufficiency.

The dose of many sedative-hypnotics should be adjusted in the setting of renal insufficiency. Both benzodiazepines and haloperidol can cause deep and prolonged sedation in renal failure patients. Additionally, benzodiazepines can cause encephalopathy, and haloperidol may lead to hypotension. Most drugs used for rapid sequence intubation do not need dosing adjustments; however, succinylcholine should be avoided in patients entirely in the emergency setting, as it may cause significant hyperkalemia in these patients.

In summary, emergency physicians should recognize that serum creatinine levels alone are inadequate in calculating renal function. Furthermore, in the setting of renal insufficiency, emergency physicians should remember to think about dosage adjustments; failure to do so could result in serious or even fatal complications. In general, a drug reference should be used or a pharmacist consulted in cases of suspected or confirmed renal insufficiency, in order to ensure the proper dosage of medications and to avoid toxicity.

SUGGESTED READINGS

Aronoff GR, Bennett WM, Berns JS, et al., eds. *Drug Prescribing in Renal Failure: Dosing Guidelines for Adults.* 5th ed. Philadelphia, PA: American College of Physicians; 2007.

Marx JA, Hockberger RS, Walls RM, eds. *Rosen's Emergency Medicine: Concepts and Clinical Practice.* 6th ed. Philadelphia, PA: Mosby; 2006.

380

KNOW THE INDICATIONS FOR EMERGENT HEMODIALYSIS

JENNIFER TAITZ SOIFER, MD

Failure to perform hemodialysis when it is emergently indicated could be a fatal error. A useful mnemonic is AEIOU: acidosis, electrolyte derangement, intoxication, (volume) overload, and uremic encephalopathy. Each of these entities may present across the spectrum of disease, but when severe and refractory to medical therapy, each is an indication for dialysis. Moreover, the clinical manifestations of each should drive the decision, not necessarily absolute laboratory values.

During hemodialysis, blood is pumped through an extracorporeal unit where it makes contact with a semipermeable membrane. On the other side of this membrane is a physiologically balanced dialysate solution. Water and solutes move across the membrane according to concentration and osmotic gradients. Dialysis can correct electrolyte abnormalities, remove toxins from the blood, and adjust fluid imbalances. In order for a substance to be removed by traditional dialysis, it must be water soluble, have a molecular weight <500 daltons, have low protein binding, and have a small volume of distribution. Newer high-flux dialysis units utilize higher flow rates and are able to push the limits of what can be dialyzed.

Most commonly, renal failure patients present to the emergency department with volume overload due to their decreased ability to handle fluid and salt loads. This may manifest as pulmonary edema and/or severe hypertension. Although dialysis is the most effective method to reduce intravascular volume, temporary treatment with preload and afterload reduction should occur as in the patient without renal failure. This includes preload reduction with nitroglycerin, bilevel or continuous positive airway pressure, and diuretics in patients with enough preserved renal function to make urine. Prolonged use of nitroprusside to reduce afterload in patients with severe hypertension will produce cyanide toxicity due to an accumulation of its metabolite, thiocyanate, but this is also dialyzable. A newer agent, fenoldopam, may be preferable in these cases. It is equally titratable and, unlike nitroprusside, may improve renal blood flow. While hypertension is common in renal failure patients, emergent dialysis is only necessary in cases of acute end-organ damage, such as hypertensive encephalopathy and cardiovascular decompensation.

Uremia is a syndrome caused by the accumulation of metabolic waste products normally excreted in the urine. It is characterized by derangements of homeostasis and metabolism. This eventually leads to the kidney's inability to regulate sodium and water balance. Acid-base balance is also deranged, leading to nonanion gap metabolic acidosis. Uremic encephalopathy may result, which is a clear indication for hemodialysis. Pericarditis, with or without effusion, is another potentially serious side effect of uremia and is also an indication for emergent dialysis. It occurs in 12% to 20% of patients on hemodialysis and may be a sign of worsening uremia. Cardiac tamponade may require emergent pericardiocentesis before dialysis can be undertaken.

Dialysis can be lifesaving in the treatment of most serious electrolyte or acid-base disturbances. Hyperkalemia is a frequent problem in patients who miss a treatment or are noncompliant with their diets. It may also occur in the setting of hemolysis or rhabdomyolysis. Emergent dialysis is indicated in patients with hyperkalemia that is refractory to medical treatment. Whereas emergency medical therapy with calcium, bicarbonate, insulin/glucose, and albuterol is aimed at stabilizing the myocardium and shifting potassium into cells and out of the plasma, total body elimination of potassium is only achieved through fecal and urinary excretion or blood filtration (e.g., using kayexalate resin, loop diuretics, and hemodialysis). Caution should be exercised when using sodium bicarbonate if there is any question of volume overload. Dialysis is also used to treat hypernatremia and hypermagnesemia but is only a temporizing treatment for hypercalcemia.

Several intoxications require treatment with hemodialysis, in both patients with normal and compromised renal function. These include poisonings with lithium, theophylline, metformin, salicylates, valproic acid, and toxic alcohols. In each case, in addition to emergent consultation with a nephrologist, there are stabilizing measures that should occur while awaiting dialysis.

SUGGESTED READINGS

De Pont A. Extracorporeal treatment of intoxication. *Curr Opin Crit Care.* 2007;13:668–673.
Marx JA, Hockberger RS, Walls RM, eds. *Rosen's Emergency Medicine: Concepts and Clinical Practice.* 6th ed. Philadelphia, PA: Mosby; 2006.
Wolfson AB, Singer I. Hemodialysis-related emergencies—part I. *J Emerg Med.* 1987;5: 533–543.
Wolfson AB, Singer I. Hemodialysis-related emergencies—part II. *J Emerg Med.* 1988; 6:61–70.

381

DEEP SUTURES: WHEN, WHY, AND WHY NOT?

JENNIFER M. BAHR, MD

Goals of placement of deep sutures include improving cosmetic outcome and eliminating dead space within the wound to minimize hematoma or seroma formation and the associated increased risk of infection. If superficial sutures are placed in a gaping wound, the wound will dehisce to some extent and may result in a scar as wide as the initial gape. This occurs because the early healing process has low tensile strength. The fibroblasts and collagen cannot hold the skin tension, so the edges drift apart, widening the scar tissue defect. Using deep sutures to bring the edges of dermis together allows the epidermis to be approximated without tension, thereby significantly reducing the risk of large depressions in the skin surface and wide scars.

Deep sutures should be placed at the junction of the subcutaneous tissue and dermis with absorbable suture material. The needle is passed from deep to shallow, then from shallow to deep again. When the knot is then tied, it will be "buried" in the subcutaneous tissue so that it does not interfere with skin surface closure. The suture ends should be cut short, about 2 mm, for the same reason. For a more detailed description of the technique, including diagrams, refer to the suggested readings.

Deep sutures are not always appropriate, however. In surfaces such as hands and feet, there is little subcutaneous tissue to reapproximate and the resulting knot may form a sensitive nodule that bothers the patient. Also, in heavily contaminated wounds, the placement of large amounts of absorbable suture material into the wound can cause increased inflammation and infection. Caution should also be used when considering the placement of deep sutures in areas of poor vascularity due to slightly increased risk of infection to these areas. This would include areas such as lower extremities in vasculopathic patients and areas of prior scar formation, such as burned areas.

Scalp wounds are frequently seen in the emergency department. If the laceration extends through the galea aponeurotica, this requires special attention. The galea is a functional part of the frontalis and occipitalis muscles, so repair of this layer is necessary. This can be performed either with a deep suture closing the galea and staples at the skin surface or with a large trilayer "bite" closing the wound in one step.

Deep sutures can greatly enhance wound closure and cosmesis by apposing the skin surfaces, thus preparing the skin surface for precise vertical alignment of the epidermis. However, care should be taken if considering the placement of deep sutures in certain locations of the body, in wounds with poor vascularity, and in contaminated wounds to prevent poor outcomes.

KEY POINTS

When?

- Gaping wounds
- Deep wounds
- Scalp wounds through the galea

Why?

- Improved cosmetic outcome of gaping wounds
- Decreased risk of infection in deep wounds

Why not?

- Heavily contaminated wounds
- Skin with little or no subcutaneous tissue
- Caution should be used in regions of poor vascularity

SUGGESTED READINGS

Capellan O. Management of lacerations in the emergency department. *Emerg Med Clin North Am.* 2003;21:205–231.
Moreira ME, Markovchick VJ. Wound management. *Emerg Med Clin North Am.* 2007;25: 873–899.

382

BE CERTAIN TO PERFORM A NEUROLOGIC EXAMINATION OF THE HAND PRIOR TO ANESTHETIZING A LACERATION

CHARLES A. BRUEN, MD

Proper wound evaluation and closure are enhanced by good anesthesia; however, it is imperative that a detailed neurologic examination be performed before anesthetizing and repairing a hand laceration. The application of anesthesia, while providing substantial patient comfort, can often mask the clinical findings of acute nerve injuries.

SENSORY TESTING

The two distinct sensory nerve fiber functions that should be evaluated by the emergency physician after an acute injury are light touch/localization and static two-point discrimination. Light touch is conveyed by sensory fibers that travel in the anterolateral spinal tract. These fibers are only able to crudely localize pressure sensation. Separate sensory fibers located in the dorsal columns rely on final cortical interpretation to provide accurately localized spatial discrimination. Two-point discrimination testing provides a mechanism of testing isolated digital nerve injuries in a highly sensitive manner.

Light touch/localization testing is performed by lightly stroking the patient's skin with a blunt point while the patient looks away. The patient should then be asked to localize and characterize the sensation. Care should also be taken in phrasing during this test. It is preferable to ask, "Does this feel normal?" to account for the patient's baseline function. A reported change in sensation or ability to localize light touch implies an injury to the nerve being tested. The unique areas of nerve innervation in the hand that should be specifically tested are the dorsal web space between the thumb and the index finger (radial nerve), the tip of the index finger (median nerve), and the tip of the small finger (ulnar nerve).

Two-point discrimination is the ability of peripheral sensory nerves to distinguish the sensation between one and two points of contact on the skin. Two-point discrimination is commonly performed with a paper clip bent to yield to blunt ends. The two points must make contact simultaneously, be in the finger's axial line, and not cross the digit's midline. This technique avoids inadvertently testing the distribution of different digital nerves and ensures separate assessment of each digital nerve at the finger tip. The points are initially 1 cm apart and are then moved progressively closer. Two-point discrimination is the point at which the patient can no longer differentiate one from two points.

A normal finding is 5 mm or less at the volar finger tips, but normal variation and age may affect the patient's ability to discriminate; thus, it is advisable to compare findings with results from the contralateral side.

MOTOR FUNCTION

Motor nerves are best examined by having the patient contract a muscle that is reliably innervated by the nerve being tested. The specific muscle belly should be palpated as it is contracting against resistance to prevent the examiner from being misled by anatomical variations in innervation and overlapping functions of different muscle groups.

Motor function of the median nerve is tested by placing the patient's dorsal hand on a flat surface, and have the patient palmar abduct the thumb against resistance while the examiner palpates the radial border of the thenar eminence for the belly of the abductor pollicis brevis. Testing of the radial nerve is best accomplished by placing the volar surface of the patient's forearm on a table and having the patient extend the wrist, thumb, and fingers against resistance. Finally, for the ulnar nerve evaluation, place the patient's ulnar forearm on a table and have the patient elevate the index finger (abduct) against resistance. The belly of the first dorsal interosseous muscle can be palpated in the web space of the radial side of the index finger.

TENDON FUNCTION

A tendon injury may also be suspected when weakness is noted during full examination of the motor function of the hand. Patient discomfort may contribute to weakness noted during strength examination; therefore, it is important to repeat the exam after the application of anesthesia. Regardless of the motor exam, the tendon should be directly visualized during wound inspection. The tendon must be visualized through a full range of motion in order to safely rule out an injury that may have occurred in a position different from the resting position most patients assume during examination. Direct visualization of the tendon may also be the only way to rule out partial lacerations, since a tendon can maintain normal function with up to a 90% laceration.

Once nerve function has been fully evaluated, then proceed with the application of anesthesia to make the patient more comfortable for the repair.

KEY POINTS

- Perform a thorough neurologic exam prior to anesthetizing hand wounds.
- Motor abnormalities may be secondary to nerve or tendon injury or discomfort; provide anesthesia, repeat the exam, and directly visualize the wound through full range of motion to differentiate.
- Carefully document all findings.

SUGGESTED READINGS

DeBoard RH, Rondeau DF, Kang CS, et al. Principles of basic wound evaluation and management in the emergency department. *Emerg Med Clin North Am.* 2007;25:23–29.

Moreira ME, Markovchick VJ. Wound management. *Emerg Med Clin North Am.* 2007;25: 873–899.

Overton DT, Uehara DT. Evaluation of the injured hand. *Emerg Med Clin North Am.* 1993;11:585–600.

Singer AJ, Hollander JE, Quinn JV. Evaluation and management of traumatic lacerations. *NEJM.* 1997;337(16):1142–1148.

Sloan EP. Nerve injuries in the hand. *Emerg Med Clin North Am.* 1993;11(3):651–670.

383

KEEP IT CLEAN: PITFALLS IN TRAUMATIC WOUND IRRIGATION

RICHARD J. CHANG, MD

Traumatic wounds are one of the most common presenting complaints encountered by emergency physicians, accounting for approximately eight million ED visits in the United States annually. Proper wound cleaning is essential to prevent infection and ensure wound healing. Wounds can vary greatly in size, depth, shape, location on the body, and degree of contamination. It is difficult to produce a single set of recommendations for irrigation to effectively clean all wounds; however, research shows that there are several common errors in wound cleaning and irrigation that are easily avoidable.

What type of irrigation solution should be used to clean the wound? Antiseptic solutions such as hydrogen peroxide or concentrated Betadine are poor choices due to tissue toxicity which can impair wound healing. Furthermore, the practice of soaking contaminated wounds in 1% Betadine has been shown to be ineffective in reducing wound bacterial counts. In many settings, the standard of care is irrigation with sterile saline. There is a theoretical advantage to using a sterile solution to avoid further introduction of bacteria into an open wound. However, standard tap water is an acceptable alternative that can achieve the same results. Several randomized controlled trials comparing sterile solutions to tap water have shown equivalence in infection rates.

One study randomized 715 adult patients at two large urban trauma centers either to irrigation with running tap water from the ED sink or to normal saline via a sterile syringe. Bite wounds, grossly contaminated wounds, and wounds in immunocompromised patients were excluded. Follow-up wound checks at 5 to 14 days showed essentially identical infection rates of 4% and 3.3% for the tap water and sterile saline groups, respectively. Tap water irrigation has additional advantages in that it is inexpensive, widely available in large volumes, and requires few additional hospital resources and little clinician time. Sink irrigation is particularly convenient for upper extremity wounds. However, for other wound sites, clear plastic tubing attached to the faucet may be required.

Does the irrigation pressure matter? Many sources recommend an irrigation pressure of at least 8 psi (pounds per square inch) for the effective removal of surface bacteria. In vivo studies have compared conventional gravity flow and bulb syringe techniques to high-pressure jet irrigation. The high-pressure group had lower wound bacterial counts and lower incidence of infections. One method of achieving up to 8 psi is to utilize a 19-gauge needle on a 60-mL syringe. Of note, standard tap water faucet pressures are more than adequate, measuring up to 45 psi in some studies. Inadequate pressures have been demonstrated with both intravenous bags (4 psi) and bulb syringes (0.5 psi).

The volume of irrigation solution needed to sufficiently decontaminate a wound should also be considered. The volume depends on both the location and the level of wound contamination. For example, bite wounds on the foot, an area particularly prone to infections, will most likely require at least 500 mL of pressurized irrigation. On the other hand, a clean laceration to a well-vascularized region such as the scalp may not require any irrigation at all. One cross-sectional study investigated 1,923 patients with noncontaminated facial and scalp lacerations who received primary closure either with or without wound irrigation. No significant differences in infection rates or cosmetic appearance ratings were observed between the two treatment groups.

KEY POINTS

- Effective wound irrigation depends more on adequate pressure than on the type of solution used; tap water is a safe and convenient option.
- Avoid antiseptic solutions such as Betadine or hydrogen peroxide in open wounds as they can slow wound healing.
- The volume of irrigation required to prevent infection depends on both the location on the body and the degree of contamination.

SUGGESTED READINGS

Brown LL, Shelton HT, Bornside GH, et al. Evaluation of wound irrigation by pulsatile jet and conventional methods. *Ann Surg*. 1978;187(2):170–173.

Hall Angeras M, Brandberg A, Falk A, et al. Comparison between sterile saline and tap water for the cleaning of acute traumatic soft tissue wounds. *Euro J Surg*. 1992;158(6–7):347–350.

Hollander JE, Richman PB, Weblud M, et al. Irrigation in facial and scalp laceration: Does it alter outcome? *Ann Emerg Med*. 1998;31(1):73–77.

Morse JW, Babson T, Camasso C, et al. Wound infection rate and irrigation pressure of two potential new irrigation devices: The port and the cap. *Am J Emerg Med.* 1998;16(1):37–42.

Moscati RM, Reardon RF, Lerner EB, et al. Wound irrigation with tap water. *Acad Emerg Med.* 1998;5(11):1076–1080.

384

DO NOT BELIEVE THE OLD ADAGE THAT EPINEPHRINE CANNOT BE USED IN DIGITAL BLOCKS

PRAKASH RAMSINGHANI, MD

In 1905, Braun first described the synergistic effect of using epinephrine with procaine, an anesthetic developed the year previously. Many texts recommend against the use of epinephrine with an anesthetic when performing a digital block due to the theoretical risk of gangrene in the "fingers, nose, toes, and penis." With respect to the fingers and toes, this is a myth. The use of epinephrine with lidocaine in standard concentrations for digital blocks is not harmful and is likely beneficial to the physician and the patient.

In 1998, Wilhelmi et al. enrolled 23 patients with finger injuries in a study with no control group where all received digital blocks with lidocaine with epinephrine. There were no complications. The study was repeated in 2001 using a control group where 29 patients did not receive epinephrine during the digital block and 31 patients received lidocaine with epinephrine. Of those receiving epinephrine, only 29% required a tourniquet for additional hemostasis compared to 69% of those who did not receive epinephrine. In addition, 5 of the 29 who did not receive epinephrine required an additional block compared to 1 of the 31 who received epinephrine. This study showed that epinephrine prolongs the effect of lidocaine fourfold, decreases the amount of local anesthetic needed through vasoconstriction, and, of course, decreases the amount of bleeding. One additional small prospective randomized trial has been published with similar results.

Lindblad et al. studied the risk of ischemia from vasoconstriction through Doppler assessment of iontophoretically applied norepinephrine to the third digit. The control group, which received saline, did not have any change in blood flow. In the group receiving norepinephrine, there was a noticeable decrease in blood flow by 37% in the treated group. Blanching of the skin usually wore off after 30 min. There were no ischemic outcomes noted.

There are a few comprehensive literature reviews of epinephrine use with lidocaine that all fail to report any cases of digital necrosis. The reports of necrosis and gangrene following digit blocks are believed to occur from factors other than epinephrine. Those factors include inappropriate use of a tourniquet, administration of excessive volume, burns from hot soaks, nonstandardized epinephrine concentrations, and poor surgical technique.

Digital blocks using epinephrine as an adjunct to lidocaine result in decreased bleeding into the field, prolongation of anesthetic effect, and prevention of additional need for anesthetic and, most importantly, do not result in permanent ischemia to tissue. Epinephrine provides rapid, temporary vasoconstriction while still allowing blood flow through the patent lumen of the artery and thus can be safely used in digit blocks.

SUGGESTED READINGS

Lindblad EL, Ekenvall L, Ancker K, et al. Laser doppler flow-meter assessment of iontophoretically applied norepinephrine on human finger skin circulation. *J Invest Dermatol*. 1986;87:634–636.

Sylaidis P, Logan A. Digital blocks with adrenaline: An old dogma refuted. *J Hand Surg Br*. 1998;23(1):17–19.

Waterbrook A, Germann C, Southall J. Is epinephrine harmful when used with anesthetics for digital nerve blocks? *Ann Emerg Med*. 2007;50:472–475.

Wilhelmi BJ, Blackwell ST, Miller J, et al. Epinephrine in digital blocks: Revisited. *Ann Plast Surg*. 1998;41:410–414.

Wilhelmi BJ, Blackwell ST, Miller J, et al. Do not use epinephrine in digital blocks: Myth or truth? *Plast Reconstr Surg*. 2001;107(2):393–297.

385

PROPHYLACTIC ANTIBIOTIC USE FOR SIMPLE, NONBITE WOUNDS IS NOT NECESSARY

STEPHEN J. DUNLOP, MD

Over the past 50 years, there has been much debate in the literature attempting to pin down exactly when the use of prophylactic antibiotics is indicated in traumatic wounds presenting to the emergency department (ED). One study found that if the decision was left to the discretion of the physician, there was an associated fourfold increase in wound infections. The majority of the debate can be settled by using the host's health, the environment in which the wound occurred, and the characteristics of the wound itself to risk stratify the situation.

"High-risk" wound situations have been defined by emergency medicine and infectious disease specialists providing a guideline for the use of prophylactic antibiotics in less than ideal circumstances. Patients with significant immunocompromise from any cause (e.g., AIDS, chronic steroid use, poorly controlled diabetes, chemotherapy, extremes of age, chronic renal failure, peripheral vascular disease, and obesity) have been associated with increased wound infection rates. Likewise, wounds that are created in unsanitary environments are also more prone to infections. Common examples of this include bites (dog, cat, human, or otherwise), through and through intraoral wounds, and wounds grossly contaminated with a foreign material. Lastly, the characteristics of the wound itself play a significant role in the decision to use prophylactic antibiotics. Puncture wounds (which drive bacteria and foreign material deep under the skin surface), crush wounds (which have devitalized and necrotic tissues that inhibit healing and foster bacterial growth), and wounds involving cartilage, tendon, ligaments, and joint spaces (all relatively avascular structures) are at high risk for infection and subsequent morbidity.

Many wounds presenting to the ED are simple, nonbite traumatic wounds. The most cited article that addresses prophylactic antibiotics in these wounds is a meta-analysis published in 1995 by Cummings et al. In this article, literature from 1966 to 1993 was reviewed including studies that had randomly assigned patients with uninfected nonbite wounds to an antibiotic treatment group or control group. After the analysis, they found that not only were prophylactic antibiotics not helpful, but they were also associated with a slightly greater incidence of infection compared with untreated controls generating an odds ratio of 1:16.

It is of note that irrigation using normal saline 50 to 100 mL/cm wound and removal of devitalized tissue are likely to be more effective at infection prevention than prophylactic antibiotics. However, if you decide to use prophylactic antibiotics, the choice should be made based on the likely etiology of the infection. Superficial skin wounds are likely to be colonized with predominantly staphylococcal and streptococcal species which can be covered with simple first-generation cephalosporins, antistaphylococcal penicillins, or a macrolide. Bite wounds, however, are more likely to be polymicrobial with *Pasteurella multocida* contributing to a large percentage of infections and are appropriately covered with amoxicillin or clavulanate. Finally, wounds which involve bone fractures, tendons, ligaments, or joints can be covered with first-generation cephalosporins if the wound is <2 cm, relatively noncontaminated, and treated in <6 h. If there is extensive soft tissue damage, a grossly contaminated wound, or a delay in treatment, then therapy should be directed at both Gram-positive and Gram-negative organisms.

Although 40% of all cases of tetanus in the United States occur in patients who either do not recall an injury or have relatively minor wounds, the most recent CDC guidelines are based on wound severity and perceived contamination. It is a good idea to look at the recommendations from the CDC, but in short, for people who have completed a primary vaccination series, you should give a tetanus booster at 5 years for large contaminated wounds and at 10 years for clean minor wounds. If no primary vaccination series has been completed, you should consider giving a tetanus booster and tetanus immune globulin.

In short, prophylactic antibiotics are not necessary unless the wound is

- On an immunocompromised patient
- A bite wound
- A through and through intraoral wound
- A puncture or crush wound
- An open fracture or involving avascular structures such as tendon, cartilage, or joint space
- A grossly contaminated wound
- At risk for communicable disease transmission

SUGGESTED READINGS

Baker MD. The management and outcome of lacerations in urban children. *Ann Emerg Med.* 1990;19:1001–1005.

Centers for Disease Control and Prevention. Preventing tetanus, diphtheria, and pertussis among adults: Use of tetanus toxoid, reduced diphtheria toxoid and acellular pertussis vaccine. *MMWR Recomm Rep.* 2006;55(RR-17):1–37.

Cruse PJ, Foord R. A five year prospective study of 23,649 surgical wounds. *Arch Surg.* 1973;107(2):206–210.

Cummings P. Antibiotics to prevent infection of simple wounds: A meta-analysis of randomized studies. *Am J Emerg Med.* 1995;13:396–400.

Hollander J, Singer AJ. Laceration management. *Ann Emerg Med.* 1999;34:356–367.

Moran GJ, Talan DA, Abrahamian FM. Antimicrobial prophylaxis for wounds and procedures in the emergency department. *Infect Dis Clin North Am.* 2008;22(1):117–143.

Simon B, Hern G. Wound management principles. In: Marx J, Hockberger R, Walls, eds. *Rosen's Emergency Medicine: Concepts and Clinical Practice.* 6th ed. St. Louis, MO: Mosby Elsevier; 2006:842–858.

386

EXPLORE AND IMAGE: DO NOT MISS A FOREIGN BODY IN A WOUND

SALAH BAYDOUN, MD

Prioper wound management is an integral part of emergency medicine as traumatic open wounds account for approximately 4% of all annual emergency department (ED) visits. Current standards of care necessitate that the health care provider have a high index of suspicion for wound-related foreign bodies and actively search for their presence through exploration and the judicious use of radiography. In fact, the most common error in the treatment of retained foreign debris is the failure to identify it due to omission of an active search. A practitioner may incorrectly assume that a wound is too small or superficial to harbor a foreign body.

Retained foreign bodies delay healing through localized inflammation and granuloma formation, infection, and toxic and allergic reactions. Foreign bodies are a clear risk factor for localized soft tissue infections and may develop into serious complications such as cellulitis, abscess formation, lymphangitis, bursitis, synovitis, arthritis, and osteomyelitis. Such infections are typically resistant to antibiotics until removal of the foreign body occurs. Local inflammation is common and results from the body's attempt to eliminate or isolate the foreign body through an immune response involving granulocytes, fibroblasts, and macrophages. The severity of the inflammatory process is highly dependent on the composition and size of the foreign body.

Adequate local wound exploration is essential to detect imbedded foreign bodies. While history and mechanism of injury should raise the practitioner's level of suspicion for a retained body, it is important to recognize that the presenting history may be misleading and is not a reliable means of ruling out foreign objects. In addition, superficial examination of a laceration is an insensitive means of retained foreign body detection and should not be confused with careful full-depth wound exploration.

Exploration must be gentle but thorough. The wound should be adequately anesthetized via a local injection or a regional nerve block prior to any exploration. Achieving hemostasis prior to visualization is vital and can be facilitated through the use of a tourniquet or by an injection of a local vasoconstricting agent when appropriate. Direct careful visualization of the field can be performed once hemostasis is achieved. In addition, the wound may be gently probed with a sterile instrument such as a metal clamp as a way of both feeling and listing for an imbedded foreign body. It is important to recognize that some wounds such as those found in the neck or on the anterior chest should never be explored due to the risk of damage to fragile or vital surrounding structures. Once adequate exploration is complete, the wound can be irrigated as a means of sterilization.

Radiography is the second step for the detection of wound-related foreign bodies. The ability to detect a foreign object with plain films depends on size, orientation, and relative density as compared to the surroundings. Fortunately, most foreign bodies are denser than the local soft tissue and hence tend to project well on x-ray. A practitioner may choose to place surface markers such as paper clips over the wound as a method of easing localization of the foreign object.

Examples of highly radio-opaque substances that are easily recognizable on plain films include glass, gravel, and metal. Early studies using plain films of tissue embedded with foreign objects have demonstrated that glass and metal could be identified in 96% and 100% of cases, respectively. In fact, recent trials utilizing animal and cadaver subjects have demonstrated an 83% to 99% sensitivity of two-view plain radiographs in the detection of all glass particles. Of note, organic plant matter such as wood has been shown to be highly radio-lucent and be poorly visualized on x-ray.

Finally, when compared to radiographs, ultrasound detection of imbedded foreign bodies has yielded significantly lower sensitivity and specificity even when conducted by skilled operators. This is particularly true in regions of varying tissue interfaces such as the hand and feet where bone, tendon, muscle, and fat may distort the acoustic window. Ultrasound is an option in the patient with suspected wood or other objects not seen on plain radiographs.

SUGGESTED READINGS

Anderson MA, Newmeyer WL, Kilgore ES. Diagnosis and treatment of retained foreign bodies in the hand. *Am J Surg*. 1982;144:63–67.

Arbona N, Jedrzynski M, Frankfather R, et al. Is glass visible on plain radiographs? A cadaver study. *J Foot Ankle Surg*. 1999;38:264–270.

Courter BJ. Radiographic screening for glass foreign bodies-what does a "negative" foreign body series really mean? *Ann Emerg Med*. 1990;19:997–1000.

Manthey DE, Storrow AB, Milbourn JM, et al. Ultrasound versus radiography in the Zdetection of soft-tissue foreign bodies. *Ann Emerg Med*. 1996;28:7–9.

Weinberger LN, Chen EH, Mills MA. Is screening radiography necessary to detect retained foreign bodies in adequately explored superficial glass-caused wounds? *Ann Emerg Med*. 2008;51:666–667.

387

EXPLORE WOUNDS PROPERLY PRIOR TO REPAIR

LISA M. HAYDEN, MD

Before closure of any wound in the emergency department, full exploration of the entire wound is of utmost importance. By visualizing the full depth of a wound, injuries to tendons and neurovasculature structures can be identified, foreign bodies may be found, and involvement of bones and joints may be recognized. Important components of wound exploration include recognizing regional anatomy, obtaining hemostasis and anesthesia, removing foreign bodies whenever possible, and identifying common mechanisms of injury and associated complications. By making these simple and often overlooked steps routine to emergency wound care, many common mistakes can be avoided. This will result in a lower incidence of infection, earlier consultation with specialists when important anatomical structures are involved, and increased patient satisfaction.

Adequate visualization is the first step of wound exploration. This requires obtaining hemostasis so that the whole wound may be probed and visualized. Usually direct pressure is adequate, though occasionally additional measures such as elevation are necessary. If bleeding persists, a tourniquet can and should be used, a blood pressure cuff proximal to the wound may be placed and inflated, or a Penrose drain can be tied proximal to the wound. If using a blood pressure cuff, inflate it to slightly higher than the patient's systolic blood pressure. The accepted time of tourniquet inflation varies, though many sources suggest that it is unlikely to cause injury when left in place for <2 h.

Full wound exploration can begin once adequate hemostasis is established and the wound is anesthetized. (Refer to the chapter on performing a neurologic exam prior to anesthetizing wounds.) A thorough sensory and motor examination distal to the wound can help identify possible neurovascular or tendon injuries. A careful functional examination generally reveals full tendon lacerations, but wound exploration may be necessary to reveal partial tendon lacerations. Keep in mind that injuries sustained while a body part was in a specific position may necessitate moving joints in a full range of motion while exploring the wound to reveal the injury. Identifying and characterizing the degree of injury are important to management and referral after emergency care. Any injury to major vessels requires early surgical consultation for operative repair to prevent or reduce tissue ischemia and irreversible damage.

Identification, visualization, and removal of foreign bodies are necessary prior to laceration repair. Though useful, adjuncts such as ultrasound or x-ray may not reveal glass, metal objects, or organic materials such as wood or dirt. Exploration of foreign bodies, especially organic materials, is important as they are associated with a high incidence of wound infection if left behind. Irrigation and gentle probing throughout the base of the wound help identify and extract many foreign bodies. Extensively contaminated wounds should be left open and dressed properly to heal by secondary intention.

The mechanism of injury is an important consideration. A knife cut wound while chopping vegetables, for example, often has a simple path with an easily identifiable wound base. A knife stab wound in an assault, however, can penetrate deeply and in any direction. If the mechanism involves shear stress, for example, from a limb being dragged on the ground, extensive damage to deeper tissues is not easily recognized. If the base of the wound cannot be visualized, consider extending the wound with an incision along the longitudinal axis of the limb until exploration is adequate.

Thorough wound exploration will help identify joint, tendon, or bony involvement as well as foreign bodies. In general, consultation with an orthopedic surgeon is necessary in the case of open fracture, joint exposure, retained foreign bodies, or certain tendon injuries such as digital flexor tendons. Appropriate antibiotic prophylaxis can also be determined by identifying these types of injuries.

KEY POINTS

- Obtain hemostasis before wound exploration.
- Perform a complete functional exam.
- Visualize the base of the wound to identify foreign bodies, neurovascular injury, and bone, tendon, or joint involvement.
- Consult an orthopedic surgeon early in the event of open fracture, joint or tendon involvement, and retained foreign bodies.

SUGGESTED READINGS

Capellan O, Hollander JE. Management of lacerations in the emergency department. *Emerg Med Clin North Am*. 2003;21:205–231.

Moreira ME, Markovchick VJ. Wound management. *Emerg Med Clin North Am*. 2007;25: 873–899.

388

DO NOT NEGLECT PROPER WOUND CARE FOR PATIENTS WITH MAMMALIAN BITES

LINDSAY ROBERTS, MD

Mammalian bite wounds raise concern for infection given that the mouth contains multiple organisms that are introduced into the broken skin during a bite. Infection rates vary widely in the literature and are reported to be as high as 50%. Based on the high reported rates of infection, some physicians choose to provide antibiotic prophylaxis for all mammalian bites. However, given that animal bites account for approximately 1% of all emergency department (ED) visits, the impact of a "treat all" policy is significant in terms of both the financial burden and the implications of antibiotic overuse. The available evidence supports treating only high-risk category mammalian bites with antibiotics. However, all bites require extensive wound care, which is the most important component of infection prophylaxis, especially in low-risk bites.

High-pressure irrigation of wounds is the standard of care for cleansing and infection prophylaxis for lacerations in the ED: "Dilution is the solution to pollution." Wound cleansing practices for mammalian bites at EDs varied dramatically and often consisted of merely wiping the bite wound with saline gauze or gentle washing.

The standard of care for cleansing mammalian bites, like other wounds, is high-pressure irrigation for wound cleansing. The solution of choice is normal saline, sterile water or perhaps, as supported by several studies, even tap water. Iodine or other tissue destructive agents should be avoided. It is the mechanical force generated by the high pressure that helps to clear the tissue of any debris or bacteria, as opposed to the properties of the solution used. High-pressure irrigation requires a 30 mL or larger syringe and an approximately 20-gauge catheter or other attachment (splash guard attachment). The volume of irrigation performed should be based on the size and depth of the wound, approximately 100 to 150 mL/cm.

Once the wound is adequately irrigated and explored for deeper damage, the question left is whether to send the patient home with antibiotics? Although the evidence is limited, the consensus is that all bites are not equal: only high-risk bites require antibiotics. Higher-risk bites include bites on the hand, human bites, cat bites, and puncture-type bites, bites that damage underlying structures, and bites in high-risk individuals (patients with diabetes, peripheral vascular disease, or end-stage renal disease).

Hand bites are of special concern given the potentially disastrous consequences of infection in the closed spaces of the hand. Prophylactic treatment with antibiotics has been proven to be of benefit. Of particular importance for hand bites is to irrigate and explore the bite in the position that the hand was bitten: If the hand was bitten while in a clenched fist, irrigation and exploration must occur in this position or serious injuries will be missed.

Puncture bites, such as those typically inflicted by cats, do not create a cosmetically disruptive wound, and patients often present after an infection has already developed. Those that do present prior to infection should be given prophylactic antibiotics. Puncture wounds that cats inflict are difficult to properly irrigate and thus create a setup for infection. However, antibiotics do not replace the need for irrigation. These bites must be irrigated as best as is possible.

Bites deeper than the dermis are concerning for damage to tendons and other deep structures. These bites deserve extensive exploration, consultation as appropriate, as well as prophylactic antibiotics.

Mammalian bites are polymicrobial with an average of five different bacteria per bite. An assortment of aerobes and anaerobes are common, with specific consideration given to pasteurella as the most common pathogen in dog and cat bites and eikenella for human bites. Because of the bacteriology, ampicillin-sulbactam and amoxicillin-clavulanate as first-line parenteral and oral treatment, respectively. For the penicillin-allergic patient, doxycycline, bactrim, or a fluoroquinolone plus clindamycin is appropriate.

Lastly, "Don't Forgets" for mammalian bites:

- To think about rabies vaccine status in the offending animal and evaluate the necessity for rabies vaccine in the patient
- To update tetanus status: last Td in >5 years needs to be updated
- To have the patient follow up in 1 to 2 days for a wound evaluation

SUGGESTED READINGS

Cummings P. Antibiotics to prevent infection in patients with dog bite wounds: A meta-analysis of randomized trials. *Ann Emerg Med.* 1994;23(3):535–340.
Dire DJ. Cat bite wounds: Risk factors for infection. *Ann Emerg Med.* 1991;20(9):973–979.
Dire DJ, Hogan DE, Walker JS. Prophylactic oral antibiotics for low-risk dog bite wounds. *Pediatr Emerg Care.* 1992;8(4):194–199.
Turner T. Do mammalian bites require antibiotic prophylaxis? *Ann Emerg Med.* 2004;44: 274–276.

389

BE AWARE OF THE HIGH RISK ASSOCIATED WITH "FIGHT BITES"

CHAD E. ROLINE, MD AND SEAN WANG, MD

A "fight bite" refers to a clenched fist laceration injury sustained by striking another individual in the mouth. This causes a tooth to penetrate the dorsum of the patient's hand, most often over a metacarpophalangeal joint. The visible laceration can be very small. In addition to the often unimpressive physical exam findings immediately after the injury, it may be difficult for the treating emergency physician to elicit an accurate history of how the wound occurred due to the patient's reluctance to admit to acts of physical violence or alcohol intoxication at the time of the injury. However, despite the initial innocuous appearance of a fight bite, these wounds can have serious complications due to their potential for the development of devastating infections if not treated early and correctly. Therefore, in order to prevent possibly serious patient morbidity, it is critical for emergency physicians to consider a fight bite in the evaluation of any hand injury.

The incidence of fight bites is hard to determine as many people may not seek immediate medical attention or may not seek help at all. The rate of infection in these injuries is estimated to be approximately 10%. One study from New York City states that the incidence of fight bites may be 11.8/100,000 in a population per year. Most of these injuries occur in males with a male-to-female ratio of 4:1. Most injuries occur among individuals between 10 and 34 years of age and mostly during the summer months. Aside from injuries as a result of physical altercations, clenched fist injuries may also occur during sports or sexual activities.

The potential for serious infections due to these injuries is attributable to both mechanical and microbiological factors. Mechanically, the skin overlying the metacarpophalangeal joints is relatively thin. This allows even for small lacerations to not only damage the underlying soft tissue but also possibly violate the extensor tendon or even the joint space. This leads to the potential for the development of septic arthritis and the resulting sequelae of chronic problems with joint stiffness, mobility, and pain. In addition, as the fingers are extended following the injury, the extensor tendon and soft tissues are retracted proximally, thereby pulling bacteria deep into the wound. Finally, the extensor tendons and metacarpophalangeal joints are relatively avascular structures, making it difficult for these areas to combat infection. From a microbiological standpoint, the human mouth and saliva contain a high concentration of a number of organisms. Because of this, infections associated with fight bite wounds are typically polymicrobial in nature. The most common organisms isolated from fight bite infections include the Gram-positive organisms *Streptococcus* sp., *Staphylococcus aureus*, and *Corynebacterium* sp. and the Gram-negative organism *Eikenella corrodens*.

A patient presenting late to the emergency department (ED) with an obvious infection following a fight bite suffered several days prior does not present a diagnostic or treatment challenge. In this case, the patient clearly requires admission to the hospital for prompt operative intervention by a hand surgeon and IV antibiotics. Ideal management of a patient with an acute, often asymptomatic, injury is more difficult. Some researchers have concluded that all patients with fight bite injuries should be admitted to the hospital for surgical debridement regardless of their appearance at presentation due to the potential for mismanagement of these injuries. However, a more conservative approach is considered acceptable by most clinicians if several key components are carefully followed (*Table 389.1*).

First, the wound must be adequately explored. This includes ensuring that the injury is thoroughly examined through the joint's entire range of motion with adequate lighting and hemostasis. Any signs of damage to the tendon or joint space should lead the emergency physician to carefully consider consultation with a hand surgeon and possible admission for debridement. Second, plain film radiographs should be obtained to evaluate the patient for fractures as well as to investigate for retained tooth fragments. Third, the wound must be copiously irrigated and then left open to heal slowly via secondary intention. Under no circumstances should a suspected fight bite be repaired with sutures as doing so acts to trap organisms within the wound. Fourth, the affected hand should

TABLE 389.1	MANAGEMENT OF "FIGHT BITES"[a]

- Plain film
- Anesthetize the wound
- Explore the wound
- Irrigate copiously
- Allow to heal by secondary intention
- Tetanus prophylaxis
- Antibiotic prophylaxis
- Close follow-up for wound check

[a]if already infected or open fracture, give IV antibiotics and consult orthopedics or hand surgery.

be splinted in a position of function and tetanus status evaluated and updated as needed. Fifth, prophylactic antibiotics should be given. The evidence for this is admittedly limited. However, one small prospective randomized study performed in 1991 divided patients with acute human bite injuries of the hand into groups to receive a placebo, oral antibiotics, or IV antibiotics. Of the 15 patients receiving the placebo, 7 (46.7%) developed an infection. None of the 16 patients treated with oral antibiotics or 17 patients treated with IV antibiotics developed subsequent infections. According to the 2005 Infectious Diseases Society of America guidelines, options for effective IV antibiotics for the treatment of a fight bite include ampicillin-sulbactam, cefoxitin, or ertapenem. Amoxicillin-clavulanate is the preferred oral medication, although in patients with a history of anaphylaxis to penicillins, clindamycin plus a fluoroquinolone in adults or clindamycin plus trimethoprim-sulfamethoxazole in children is an appropriate alternative regimen. Finally, and probably most importantly, close follow-up must be ensured. If the patient cannot be referred to be evaluated by a hand surgeon in the next 24 to 48 h, a return visit to the ED is needed for a wound check. Strong consideration for admission is recommended in unreliable patients in whom follow-up or outpatient antibiotic treatment regimen adherence is questionable.

SUGGESTED READINGS

Goon PK, Mahmoud M, Rajaratnam V. Hand trauma pitfalls: A retrospective study of fight bites. *Europ J Trauma Emerg Surg*. 2008;34(2):135–140.

Perron AD, Miller MD, Brady WJ. Orthopedic pitfalls in the ED: Fight bite. *Am J Emerg Med*. 2002;20(2):114–117.

Stevens DL, Bisno AL, Chambers HF, et al. Practice guidelines for the diagnosis and management of skin and soft tissue infections. *Clin Infect Dis*. 2005;41:1378–1406.

Talan DA, Abrahamian FM, Moran GS, et al. Clinical presentation and bacteriologic analysis of infected human bites presenting to emergency departments. *Clin Infect Dis*. 2003;37:1481–1489.

390

CONSIDER THE DIAGNOSIS OF SPIDER ENVENOMATION AND MAINTAIN A BROAD DIFFERENTIAL DIAGNOSIS IN PATIENTS WITH UNEXPLAINED LOCAL OR SYSTEMIC ILLNESS

KEVIN GREER, MD

Spider envenomation can be a challenging clinical entity to diagnose in the emergency department (ED). Patients will frequently present with a complaint of "spider bite" to explain a cutaneous lesion of unknown origin. It has been suggested that to avoid over attribution of clinical presentations to spider bites, the diagnosis be reserved for patients who have a witnessed bite, have recovered the spider, and have undergone a full workup to rule out other possible etiologies. However, spider envenomation rarely meets all of these criteria and may result in a local or systemic disease that requires therapy. The two most common venomous spiders in the United States are the brown recluse spider and the black widow spider.

The brown recluse spider (or *Loxosceles reclusa*) is also known as the fiddleback or violin spider due to a dark violin–like pattern on the body. The reclusa spider typically lives in human dwellings hiding during the day in baseboards, woodpiles, or undisturbed clothing. Brown recluse venom contains hyaluronidase and loxosotoxin, which cause hemolysis. *L reclusa* are located in the Midwest and south central region of the United States. Recent data suggest that skin lesions may not be attributed to brown recluse bites in regions that do not have endemic loxosceles spiders. Inappropriate presumption of a brown recluse bite may lead to missed diagnosis of other clinical entities such as neoplasm, vasculitis, or other infectious etiologies including cutaneous anthrax. Brown recluse bites result in a local reaction of tingling or swelling with blistering that may progress to induration, necrosis, and eschar within hours to weeks. This phenomenon, often referred to as necrotic arachnidism, may result in ulcerative skin lesions that heal slowly. Some common presenting symptoms of brown recluse bites are pain, puritis, malaise, chills, sweats, and rash. Most cases of a brown recluse bite do well with local wound care, tetanus prophylaxis, and pain control. Other treatments including dapsone, electric shock, hyperbaric oxygen, and excision have not proven to be more effective than a "benign neglect" approach for local tissue necrosis. Wounds should be reevaluated for progression of necrosis in 24- to 48-h intervals for 3 to 5 days. Systemic effects of brown recluse bites (or loxoscelism) are presumed the result of toxin-mediated hemolysis resulting in fever, hemolytic anemia and hematuria, and rarely anuria. Pregnant women, young children, and debilitated victims are at greater risk to develop loxoscelism, but death is extremely rare. Hemolysis should be treated with corticosteroids and component therapy as needed. In the ED, patients with presumed brown recluse bite should have a baseline CBC and urinalysis as well as further hemolytic workup as warranted.

The black widow (or *Latrodectus* species) spider is found throughout the United States. These spiders are black with a red or yellow hourglass marking over the abdomen. They reside in solitary environments such as wood piles, under rocks, or low-level benches. Female black widows are the only gender of the species large enough to be toxic to humans. The venom of the *Latrodectus* species contains α-atrotoxin, a potent neurotoxin that causes presynaptic neurotransmitter release. Typical bites display local erythema with fang marks and central clearing producing a "target lesion" as well as local piloerection and perspiration. Hematogenous spread of neurotoxin leads to Latrodectism which typically occurs in three phases. The first phase occurs in 2 to 24 h and includes muscle spasms presenting with generalized abdominal, back, or leg pain. Other symptoms that commonly occur include diaphoresis, chest pain, hypertension, tachycardia, headache, nausea/vomiting, and dyspena. Children may present with agitation, anxiety, diaphoresis, jerky movements, abdominal rigidity, and altered mental status. The second phase of latrodectism occurs 1 to 3 days after the bite with the decline of symptoms, and the third phase is characterized by persistence of muscle spasms, tingling, and weakness for weeks to months. Historically, the mortality rate was reported as high as 10% before the development of antivenom, but death is now considered a rare complication of latrodectism. The treatment of black widow spider envenomations focuses on symptom control and prevention of complications. Minimal treatment is needed for patients with pure local envenomation site pain. For systemic effects, treatment focuses on opioid and benzodiazepine treatment of symptoms. Patients with uncontrolled hypertension may benefit from a short-acting antihypertensive such as nitroprusside. Calcium gluconate has long been a first-line treatment, but recent data find it ineffective. Antivenom results in a rapid resolution of symptoms within 30 to 120 min. Antivenom should be reserved for patients with systemic symptoms and no contraindications because a risk of anaphylaxis and death exists. Subcutaneous antivenom skin testing is often recommended prior to IV administration. Abnormal presentations have included priapism, myocardial ischemia, myocarditis, paralysis, and cardiac dysrhythmias. Reported cases exist of presentations mistaken for an acute abdomen and taken to surgery as well as presumed cholecystitis. Pregnant patients with abdominal pain and hypertension may be mistaken for preeclampsia or onset of labor.

SUGGESTED READINGS

Bulunt E, Ibrahim T, Aytac B, et al. Uncommon cardiovascular complications after a latrodectus bite. *Am J Emerg Med.* 2007;25(2):232–235.

Clark RF, Western-Kestner S, Vance MV, et al. Clinical presentation and treatment of black widow spider envenomation: A review of 163 cases. *Ann Emerg Med.* 1992;21(7):782–787.

Kemp ED. Bites and stings of the arthropod kind: Treating reactions that can range from annoying to menancing. *Postgrad Med.* 1998;103(6):88–90, 93–96.

Pneumatikos I, Galiatsou E, Goe D, et al. Acute fatal toxic myocarditis after black widow spider envenomation. *Ann Emerg Med.* 2003;41:158.

Sherman R, Groll J, Gonzales D, et al. Black widow spider (*Latrodectus mactans*) envenomation in a term pregnancy. *Curr Surg.* 2000;57(4):346–348.

Swanson DL, Vetter RS. Bites of brown recluse spiders and suspected necrotic arachnidism. *N Engl J Med.* 2005;352:700–707.

Williams ST, Khare VK, Johnston GA, et al. Severe intravascular hemolysis associated with brown recluse spider envenomation: A report of two cases and review of the literature. *Am J Clin Pathol.* 1995;104(4):463–467.

391

LOCAL ANESTHETICS FOR ABSCESS INCISION AND DRAINAGE ARE USUALLY INADEQUATE

EDWARD S. BESSMAN, MD, MBA

Local anesthetics are the mainstay for pain control during brief, painful procedures in the ED. They are suitable for a wide variety of situations, but they are not, as it turns out, ideal for incision and drainage (I&D) of cutaneous abscesses. To understand why requires a brief refresher in biochemistry.

Local anesthetics are weak bases that, in aqueous solution, exist in ionized (protonated) and nonionized (unprotonated) equilibriums. The nonionized form is relatively water insoluble. Lowering the pH of the solution shifts the equilibrium to the ionized form, which makes the molecules easier to dissolve in water. Most local anesthetics are therefore formulated as hydrochloride salt.

Local anesthetics exert their effect by diffusing across the bilipid layer of nerve cell membranes and blocking sodium channels. This interrupts the transmission of nerve impulses. However, it is the nonionized form of the molecule that will more readily enter the lipid environment of the cell membrane. Thus, anesthetics that exist in greater proportion as nonionized molecules at tissue pH will in general penetrate into nerves faster and result in faster onset of action. Hence, at lower pH, local anesthetics are more soluble in body fluids but less able to diffuse into nerves, and at higher pH, the reverse is true.

In the presence of inflammation, tissue pH is lowered. One would expect, therefore, that local anesthetics would be less effective in the presence of inflammation and this is the case. The resulting shift to a more acidic environment means that more of the local anesthetic molecules exist in the ionized form and thus are less able to diffuse across nerve cell membranes. This is seldom an important consideration in the repair of fresh wounds, where inflammation is minimal, but presents a problem in the case of abscess I&D. Normal tissue pH is roughly 7.35, but the pH of an abscess cavity can range from 5.5 to 7.2. Given the logarithmic nature of the pH scale, this implies a many thousandfold decrease in the proportion of nonionized molecules of local anesthetics that are present. Practically speaking, this means that local anesthesia simply may not work well, if at all, for a highly inflamed abscess.

There are some strategies to help overcome this problem. One potential approach is to raise the pH of the tissue environment by the addition of sodium bicarbonate to the local anesthetic injection. This increases the proportion of nonionized molecules and improves the performance of the agent. For a typical lidocaine solution, the addition of 1 mL of a standard 1-mEq/mL sodium bicarbonate preparation to 9 mL of lidocaine can be beneficial. Too much alkalinization must be avoided or else the anesthetic may precipitate; certain agents such as bupivacaine are very sensitive in this regard. A second strategy involves avoiding injection into the cavity itself and instead injecting circumferentially around the abscess or else superficially across it. This may provide some anesthesia for the incision but likely will prove insufficient for pain relief while breaking up loculations or during packing.

Alternatives or adjuncts to local anesthetic injection include topical freezing agents, regional nerve blocks where anatomically feasible, inhalational agents such as nitrous oxide, or else some form of intravenous sedation and analgesia. The take-home message, however, is that in the presence of extreme inflammation, such as in an abscess, reliance upon local anesthesia for analgesia is often insufficient.

SUGGESTED READINGS

Gmyrek R, Dahdah M. Local anesthesia and regional nerve block anesthesia. eMedicine.com. Available at: http://emedicine.medscape.com/article/1127490-media. Accessed February 28, 2009.

Wagner C, Sauermann R, Joukhadar C. Principles of antibiotic penetration into abscess fluid. *Pharmacology*. 2006;78(1):1–10.

392

Eyelid lacerations: Use a three-step approach to repair

Esther I. Chang, MD

Eyelid lacerations are frequently seen in the emergency department in the setting of trauma and should be approached with care. First, all eyelid lacerations should wait until the orbit and globe have been examined for injury and treated as necessary. A delay of 36 to 48 h in repairing eyelid lacerations is acceptable and has not been shown to affect outcomes. Often while waiting for repair, a dressing of xeroform gauze followed by an eye patch is sufficient to keep the tissues moist. Ice as tolerated, or gauze soaked in iced saline, can help with decreasing swelling until repair occurs.

A basic understanding of eyelid anatomy is crucial to determining when to refer a laceration to an ophthalmology or plastics specialist and when it is safe to repair yourself. The innermost aspect of both upper and lower eyelids is lined with a layer of conjunctiva that is continuous with the conjunctiva that covers the whites of the eyes. Just anterior to the conjunctiva is the tarsus, a dense plate of connective tissue that extends for the entire width of the eyelids horizontally and extends vertically 10 to 12 mm from the margin in the upper lids and 4 mm from the margin in the lower lids. Anterior to the tarsus lies the orbicularis muscle and skin. It is particularly important to be aware of the tarsus when evaluating eyelid lacerations.

Where the tarsus ends, the septum begins. This layer of connective tissue separates the preseptal structures, including the orbicularis muscle and skin, from the postseptal structures, including the levator aponeurosis and levator muscle in the upper lid and the capsulopalpebral fascia and inferior tarsal muscle in the lower lid. The orbital fat pads lie posterior to the septum.

The horizontal edge of the eyelid margin contains, from posterior to anterior, the meibomian gland orifices, the gray line where the orbicularis muscle ends, and the lash line where the eyelashes exit the skin.

When managing an eyelid laceration, there are three important questions to ask. Firstly, how deep is the laceration? If the laceration is superficial or only involving the skin and orbicularis, simple primary closure is sufficient. If the laceration is full-thickness, the tarsus is involved and must be closed as a separate layer in addition to skin closure, a procedure that should be referred to a specialist. If orbital fat is exposed, the septum has been breached with possible damage to the underlying levator muscle, and the patient should be referred for possible orbital exploration in addition to repair.

Second, does the laceration involve the lid margins? Closely inspect to examine whether or not there is extension to the edge of the eyelid or whether the edge itself is involved separately. The latter results in a notch or irregularity of the margin that can be quite subtle. Lacerations involving the margin should be referred to a specialist as they require anatomical closure along the meibomian line and the lash line. Missing margin-involving lacerations, or hastily closing them without referral, often results in notching or improper realignment of the margins that can cause chronic tearing, irritation of the conjunctiva or cornea, or turning in or out of the lid margin.

Third, does the laceration involve the tear duct system? The upper and lower lids each have a puncta located just adjacent to the inner canthus, each of which connect to an upper and lower canaliculus that extends horizontally 8 to 10 mm before joining to form the lacrimal sac just inferomedial to the inner canthus. Any laceration that extends medial to the inner canthus or along the inferomedial area where the lacrimal sac is located should be referred to a specialist for examination. Probing and instillation of fluorescein dye can be used to determine whether the canalicular system is intact, but often simple examination under a slit lamp will suffice. Repair of canalicular-involving lacerations involves placing a stent to reapproximate the severed canaliculus.

When repairing a superficial, nonmargin-involving, noncanalicular-involving laceration, simple approximation using the general principles of laceration repair is sufficient. 8-0 nylon is usually used, with removal of sutures in 7 to 10 days, though absorbable sutures can be considered in patients for whom follow-up is a concern. Care must be taken not to exert undue vertical tension in reapproximation, as this can distort the fragile and thin lid surface and lead to scarring that results in abnormal lid function. Any suture ends approaching the lid margin must be trimmed closely to avoid irritative contact with the eye surface. Steroid and/or antibiotic ointment, such as prednisolone-gentamicin or ophthalmic erythromycin, can be applied after repair for 1 week.

In summary, when presented with an eyelid laceration, ask three questions: How deep does the laceration extend? Does it involve the margin? Does it involve the canalicular system? Careful irrigation of the area, followed by close and probing examination, will help to determine if referral is appropriate and will allow you to repair simple lacerations with confidence.

SUGGESTED READINGS

Brown DJ, Jaffe JE, Henson JK. Advanced laceration management. *Emerg Med Clin North Am.* 2007;25(1):83–99.

Chang EL, Rubin PA. Management of complex eyelid lacerations. *Int Ophthalmol Clin.* 2002;42(3):187–201.

Mehta JK. Primary repair of eyelid lacerations. *Trans Ophthalmol Soc UK.* 1978;98(1):75–80.

393

KNOW THE ALTERNATIVES TO THE SIMPLE INTERRUPTED SUTURE METHOD

JAMES E. CORWIN, MD

Emergency physicians should have expertise in the management of traumatic wounds. It is clear that not all wounds need to be closed, but those that are at low risk for infection or other complication should be closed with the method that will expedite healing and minimize scar formation. Several types of closure are available to the emergency physician including the use of tissue adhesives, tapes, and various types of suture methods and materials. Each wound is different and should be evaluated individually to decide which material and method would provide the optimal outcome. Ultimately, the timely closure of wounds, with an aesthetically pleasing scar, should be the goal.

It is helpful to consider the "reconstructive ladder" that has been described as beginning with simple linear closure and advancing to grafts and flaps for more complex wounds. This chapter will focus on simple linear closures.

Linear closures may be performed using a number of different suturing techniques, including simple interrupted percutaneous sutures (which are commonly used), (partially buried) running continuous sutures, vertical or horizontal mattress sutures, half-buried horizontal or vertical mattress sutures, or (totally buried) dermal or subcutaneous running sutures. This is only a partial listing of suturing variations, and each has its own indications, advantages, and disadvantages. Mastering these (and others) gives the plastic surgeon-wannabe a potent armamentarium for dealing with the myriad wounds presenting to the ED.

In the ideal linear closure, there will be no "dog ears" (redundant mounds of skin at the wound ends) and skin edges are coapted under minimal tension. A linear closure may be done in layers, in which like tissue is approximated to like tissue (such as periosteum, perichondrium, muscular fascia, dermis, and epidermis). While disruption of some of these deeper layers should be repaired by a surgical specialist, simple two-layered closure of dermal and subdermal layers is well within the scope of an emergency physician.

Dermal approximation, using totally or partially buried sutures, permits the dermis to bear practically all of the tension so the epidermis can be finely aligned for ideal scar formation. With good dermal closure, the skin will appear almost completely closed, with edges aligned and slightly everted along the length of the wound. When this has been accomplished, the skin can be closed

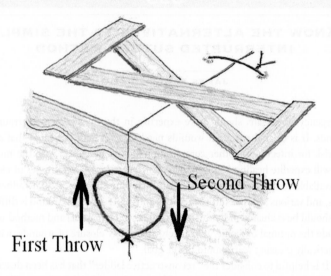

Second Throw

First Throw

FIGURE 393.1. Buried-inverted vertical suture (note the knot at the bottom); skin closed with a combination of simple percutaneous suture and Steri-Strips (note crisscross pattern with ends secured).

with interrupted (simple) or running subcuticular sutures, or even skin tapes (*Fig. 393.1*) or wound adhesive (Dermabond or Indermil).

Buried sutures can be used primarily to reduce tension at the wound edges. At one time, it was thought that buried sutures should be used primarily to obliterate dead space, but this has been disproven. Dead space has been defined as "gaps in the soft tissues that can result in hematoma or seroma formation, serve as a locus for infection, and produce soft tissue contractures." While dead space definitely has been associated with higher rates of infection, aggressive use of buried sutures in an attempt to completely obliterate dead space can also lead to higher rates of infection, particularly in lacerations repaired in an ED setting.

Good alternatives to totally buried sutures are those that are partially buried, such as vertical or horizontal mattress (included the half-buried varieties), the figure-eight and the near-far-far-near suture method. The vertical mattress (far-far-near-near) is an old standby that reduces tension, closes dead space, and everts skin edges. In areas where the skin is under tension yet is also thin (e.g., eyelids), the near-far-far-near method makes an excellent choice (*Fig. 393.2*). It has all the strength of a vertical mattress but allows for more meticulous alignment of skin edges.

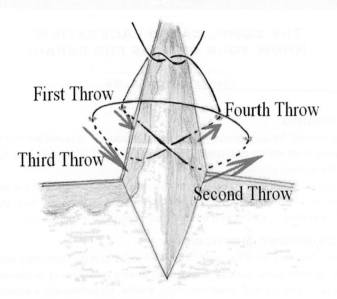

FIGURE 393.2. Near-far-far-near suture.

SUMMARY

Not all wounds should be closed, but if a wound is appropriate for primary closure, several options exist. Simple interrupted sutures are commonly used. Two-layered closures can be considered to reduce tension at the wound edges. Buried sutures can also be an option when trying to reduce wound tension. Vertical and horizontal sutures can help evert skin edges, and the near-far-far-near suture in combination with a few simple interrupted sutures and/or Steri-Strips is a worthwhile consideration for a wound that is under tension but needs meticulous closure and good skin eversion.

SUGGESTED READINGS

Bodiwala GG, George TK. Surgical gloves during wound repair in the accident-and-emergency department. *Lancet.* 1982;2(8289):91–92.

Georgiade G, Georgaide N, Riefkohl R, et al., eds. *Textbook of Plastic, Maxillofacial, and Reconstructive Surgery.* 2nd ed. Baltimore, MD: Williams & Wilkins; 1992:ch 15.

Thirlby RC, Blair AJ III, Thal ER. The value of prophylactic antibiotics for simple lacerations. *Surg Gynecol Obstet.* 1983;156(2):212–216.

Townsend CM Jr, Beauchamp RD, Evers BM, et al., eds. *Sabiston Textbook of Surgery.* 18th ed. Philadelphia, PA: Saunders; 2008:ch 73.

394

THE COMPLICATED LACERATION:
KNOW YOUR OPTIONS FOR REPAIR

JAMES E. CORWIN, MD

SCENARIO

A 32-year-old female presents with "wound infection." A laceration had been repaired in an urgent care center several days ago, but it "doesn't look right" and she wants it checked.

On exam, the patient has a 3-cm chevron-shaped laceration in the preauricular area with a necrotic tip (*Fig. 394.1*). The old chart notes a "deep arrowhead laceration ... closed with 6 simple interrupted 5-0 nylon sutures."

BACKGROUND METHODS

Wound closure is one of the most common procedures in the emergency department. In most cases, standard interrupted sutures are sufficient to adequately close an uncomplicated linear traumatic wound. Unfortunately, a significant number of lacerations will pose some difficulty highlighting the need to consider alternate suture strategies.

This chapter reviews several common interrupted nonburied and partially buried techniques that every ED physician should master.

Before proceeding, I would like to highlight one of Halsted's basic tenets of surgical technique that is often overlooked in a busy ED: careful handling of

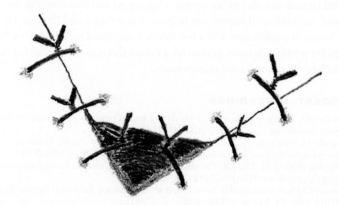

FIGURE 394.1. A wound showing ischemia-induced tip necrosis caused by poor choice of suturing technique.

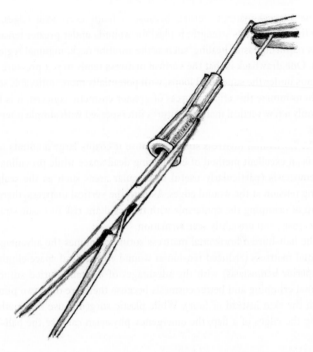

FIGURE 394.2. A needle driver and/or hemostat to make a skin hook out of a 19-gauge needle.

tissues. Its interesting to note that a typical ED "lac tray" contains—in addition to instruments such as a needle driver, hemostat, and scissors—the Adson tissue forceps, usually with teeth. It is hard to imagine a pair of forceps more traumatizing to epidermis than forceps with teeth. An excellent alternative is the skin hook, which is usually more difficult to find in an ED than a hospital administrator. Nothing beats a skin hook for gentle, nontraumatic handling of skin during a laceration repair. A skin hook can be fashioned using a hemostat to bend two right angles at the end of a 19- or 20-gauge needle (*Fig. 394.2*).

APPROPRIATE USE

In deciding which suturing technique to use, one must keep in mind the geometry of tissue movements affected by methods and factors such as likelihood of complications (e.g., infection), long-term cosmesis, patient acceptability, ease of placement, and ease of post-op management.

Simple interrupted percutaneous sutures may be used in wounds extending only as deep as the dermal-subdermal junction, when there is little tension on the wound edges and no significant dead space or tissue loss.

The vertical mattress suture, because it helps evert skin edges, closes deeper tissue, and adds strength, is ideal for wounds under greater tension and in areas requiring faster healing, such as the anterior neck, inguinal region, and eyelids. One drawback is that the vertical mattress tends to put pressure on the epidermis under the superficial loops, with potentially more noticeable scars. In order to minimize this effect in areas of greater cosmetic concern, it is helpful to use only a few vertical mattress sutures interspersed with simple interrupted sutures.

The horizontal mattress suture, because it coapts large amounts of deep tissue, is an excellent method of eliminating dead space while providing excellent hemostasis (particularly useful in vascular areas such as the scalp) and reducing tension at the wound edges. As with the vertical mattress, there is the problem of crimping the epidermis with the resultant risk of tissue strangulation, necrosis, and unsightly scar formation.

The half-buried horizontal mattress suture combines the advantages of a horizontal mattress (reduced tension at wound edges, dead space elimination, and superior hemostasis) with the advantages of a totally buried suture (less epidermal crimping and better cosmesis because there are only two punctures through the skin instead of four). While plastic surgeons use this method for securing the edges of a flap, the emergency physician can use the half-buried

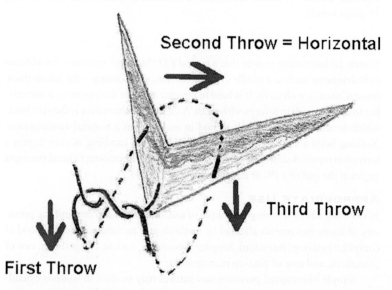

FIGURE 394.3. Half-buried horizontal mattress suture to safely secure the tip in chevron-shaped wound.

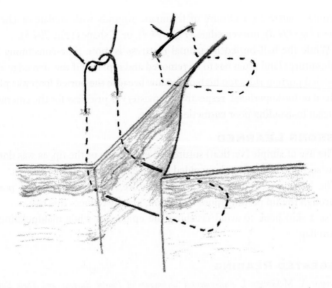

FIGURE 394.4. Half-buried horizontal sutures used to level uneven edges.

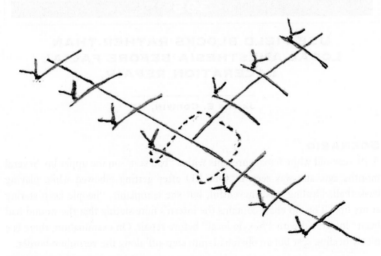

FIGURE 394.5. Half-buried horizontal mattress to close four-point wound.

horizontal mattress for closure of traumatic wounds with stellate or chevron shapes (*Fig. 394.3*), uneven edges (*Fig. 394.4*), or T shapes (*Fig. 394.5*).

While the half-buried horizontal mattress is more time-consuming than simple sutures (and often has to be removed and replaced if the skin edge above the buried portion rides too high or too low because the buried loop was placed too deep or too superficial, respectively), mastery is priceless for the emergency physician in avoiding poor cosmetic outcome.

LESSONS LEARNED

1) The use of simple (vertical) sutures on either side of the tip, as was done in the scenario above, is to be avoided because of the risk of tip necrosis.
2) The half-buried horizontal mattress suture, because the buried portion through the tip permits more blood flow, greatly reduces this risk.
3) Use a skin hook to avoid crushing the epidermis while manipulating the skin flap.

SUGGESTED READING

McGregor A, McGregor I. *Fundamental Techniques of Plastic Surgery and Their Surgical Applications*. 10th ed. Edinburgh, UK: Churchill Livingstone; 2000.

395

USE FIELD BLOCKS RATHER THAN LOCAL ANESTHESIA BEFORE FACIAL LACERATION REPAIR

JAMES E. CORWIN, MD

SCENARIO

A 19-year-old white female presents with a "bad scar" on the upper lip. Several months ago, she was seen in your ED after getting elbowed while playing basketball. Healing was uneventful, but she complains, "people keep staring at my lip." The old chart contains the intern's note stating that the wound had been "infiltrated with 1% xylo local" before repair. On examination, there is a nicely healing scar but an obvious 1-mm step-off along the vermilion border.

BACKGROUND

Most surgical procedures require anesthesia to reduce pain; because of the absence of cardiovascular and respiratory disturbance, ease of administration, rapid onset and effectiveness, and low cost, local anesthesia is usually preferable to general.

There are several options to use with local anesthesia, each has its advantages and should be considered when deciding to close a traumatic wound.

Western physicians began using cocaine (an ester similar to the synthetic procaine or tetracaine) as a local anesthetic in the 1880s, with the newer amides like lidocaine and bupivacaine coming into play since the 1940s. Because of a higher risk of toxicity and allergic reactions, esters are limited to topical use and amides are preferred for infiltration.

Infiltrative anesthesia techniques include local infiltration, field (or ring) blocks, and nerve (or regional) blocks. Using no anesthesia should be considered when placing a very limited number of staples (usually <4, depending on patient tolerance), because the fleeting pain associated with the rapid stapling process is often less than the more prolonged pain of anesthetic infiltration.

Local infiltration is the simplest technique and, in a traumatic laceration, is generally introduced through the cut surface of the open wound, parallel to the dermis into the subcutaneous tissue. To lessen the burning pain of the anesthetic, use the smallest diameter needle available and inject slowly and steadily. Because infiltration will distort tissues, it is helpful to mark important landmarks (e.g., vermilion border or eyebrow) *before* the injection to guide alignment during suturing.

Field blocks are performed by injecting anesthetic through intact skin encircling the laceration. They work by blocking all of the nerves supplying that particular area and have the advantage of avoiding distortion of tissues to be repaired, causing less pain by injecting into more distensible tissue (e.g., skin *around* nose or ear instead of directly into those structures) and often requiring less anesthetic than local infiltration.

Nerve blocks are performed by injecting anesthetic through intact skin at a precise anatomic location (trunk of a peripheral nerve supplying the region containing the laceration). This is the most challenging of the three techniques. It requires knowledge of the relevant neuroanatomy and depends on injection near the membrane of the nerve trunk (not *into* it). Adequate concentration of the anesthetic, the length of nerve anesthetized, and the amount of time allowed for diffusion of the anesthetic, the nerve block has all the pluses of a field block with the added advantages of fewer injections, larger area of anesthesia, and ability to anesthetize highly sensitive areas by directly injecting into them.

Finally, the central part of the face (eyes, nose, and mouth) is the most visible and notable portion of the human façade. The naked eye of the beholder can discern uneven borders of these structures (eyebrows, eyelids, nares, and lips) with incredible precision. The closure of wounds involving these structures is essential to prevent an unsightly outcome. Local infiltration of anesthesia can distort these structures and make proper alignment impossible.

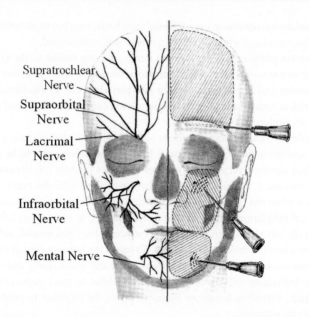

FIGURE 395.1. Peripheral nerves of the face and injection sites for nerve blocks.

APPROPRIATE USE

Which technique to use depends on factors such as location and size of the wound, distensibility and distortability of skin, and the number of injections and amount of anesthetic required.

A reasonable goal is to use the lowest possible dose of anesthetic by using the smallest volume of the lowest concentration to effect the greatest amount of anesthesia. Because local infiltration uses the most anesthetic, it should be used for the smallest wounds. A field block should be considered for medium-sized wounds, and a nerve block should be considered for the largest wounds. The latter requires fewer injections and a smaller volume of anesthetic than the former, while both use less than the local infiltration.

Much of the face (*Fig. 395.1*) can be anesthetized using nerve blocks, as can the digits, hands, and plantar surface of the foot, by blocking digital nerves, the ulnar and/or median nerves at the wrist, and the sural nerve, respectively.

As mentioned earlier, both field and nerve blocks are useful in any location for avoiding tissue distortion. The field block is excellent for less distensible areas (with little subcutaneous fat) such as the nail folds, ear, nose, or penis. Use of the nerve block obviates the need to inject directly into sensitive areas such as the lips, anterior cheek, lateral nose, ears, and lower eyelids. Complete anesthetization of the external nose often requires a combination of nerve and field blocks.

LESSONS LEARNED

1) Local infiltration distorts the skin architecture.
2) Meticulous alignment of structures such as the vermilion border is critical for successful cosmetic outcome.
3) Infraorbital nerve block would have been a much better choice for anesthesia of the upper lip than local infiltration.

SUGGESTED READING

Bennett RG, ed. *Fundamentals of Cutaneous Surgery*. St. Louis, MO: C.V. Mosby; 1988:ch 6.

396

KNOW WHICH WOUNDS TO CLOSE... AND WHICH ONES CAN BE LEFT OPEN

JAMES E. CORWIN, MD

SCENARIO

A 58-year-old diabetic smoker presents to the ED with "leg pain." She had been jogging a few days ago when an immunized dog bit her leg. Several hours later she went to her local hospital ED, where the wound was cleansed; received a Td booster; and was told such a gaping wound would need to be closed. The old chart contains a note stating, "wound closed with excellent approximation using a series of vertical nylon mattress sutures." On examination, there are mounds of skin at the ends of the wound (dog-ear deformity), the edges have separated, and there is frank pus draining. The surrounding 5 to 6 cm of skin is cellulitic.

BACKGROUND

In order to consider the best approach to wound closure, one needs to understand the classification of wounds, different mechanisms of wound healing, types of wound repair, and factors affecting healing.

Superficial wounds have lost epidermis and occasionally superficial (or papillary layer) dermis. These wounds are usually wide (e.g., abrasion), spare the deeper structures of the dermis (e.g., sebaceous and sweat glands), and heal by epithelialization.

Deep wounds extend into, and usually through, the dermis. They can be narrow, as is found in the typical traumatic laceration, but may be wide with significant tissue loss. A deep and narrow wound heals by epidermization, with little granulation and contraction. A deep and wide wound heals primarily by granulation with resultant contraction and subsequent epidermization.

The difference between epithelialization and epidermization is subtle, but the result can be quite noticeable. In the former, the epidermis resurfaces from both the wound edges *and* the dermal structures (e.g., hair follicle) below the wound; in the latter, the epidermis migrates across a granulated base from the wound edges only. With epithelialization, the result is almost a normal skin in form and function; with epidermization, the result is a skin with form but little function (e.g., no hair or sweat glands).

Proper wound management also requires consideration of the available types of wound repair. Primary closure (or primary intention) consists of apposing fresh skin edges on the day of the wound's creation. Healing by secondary intention is the process of natural healing without surgical intervention. Delayed primary closure (or tertiary intention) is a surgical repair performed anytime after the day of the wound's creation, typically in a wound that has begun to granulate.

Whether a wound will become infected depends on factors such as level of bacterial contamination and degree of pathogenicity, local wound defenses, and systemic host resistance. Based on the degree of contamination, all wounds can be classified as clean, clean-contaminated, contaminated, or dirty. By definition, all fresh, traumatic wounds (such as those seen in the ED) are considered contaminated. Wounds with large areas of devitalized tissue, foreign bodies, and possibly hematomas are more likely to get infected. All animal bites present risk for infection; those that produce punctures (cats, rodents) are at a higher risk than dogs. Because of variations in vascular supply, wounds of the head, face, and neck are less likely to get infected than those of the trunk and upper extremities, which in turn are less likely to get infected than those of the lower extremities.

APPROPRIATE USE

Superficial wounds, after thorough cleansing, can readily be left to heal by secondary intention or simple primary closure using skin tapes and/or wound adhesive. Because they heal by epithelialization, and risk of complication is rare with proper wound care, there is every expectation of restoration of form and function.

Deep and wide wounds with significant loss of tissue may require immediate plastic surgery consultation or appropriately cleansed and dressed with plastics referral in 1 to 2 days to evaluate for possible delayed closure.

Deciding on the type of repair for the typical deep and narrow traumatic laceration requires consideration of timing, contamination, location, and cosmesis. With adequate blood supply and absent bacterial invasion, these wounds can be closed at any time (in contrast to the outmoded "golden period" rule that proscribed primary closure beyond 6 to 8 h). In fact, delaying closure for up to 3 to 6 days can *reduce* the risk of infection. This is because the advancing sheet of proliferating vascular tissue seen during granulation forms an excellent barrier to bacterial invasion. Contaminated wounds of the trunk and extremities are suitable for delayed closure after completely granulating, as long as there is no gross infection.

Contaminated wounds of the richly vascular head and neck, without foreign material or tissue devitalization, may be considered for immediate primary closure after vigorous cleansing. Finally, areas that contract easily, with minimal distortion of surrounding areas (preauricular and postauricular, nasolabial fold, neck), are suitable for healing by secondary intention because the resultant scar is often more cosmetically acceptable than that seen in surgical closure. Wounds under tension (e.g., arm), where suture closure can result in dog ears, often heal better with secondary intention (because dog ears cannot occur with natural healing).

LESSONS LEARNED

1) A dog bite is always contaminated and consideration needs to be given to risk of infection (especially one in a less vascular area such as the leg).
2) Host factors such as macro- and microvascular compromise (as is likely in this diabetic smoker) also increase the risk of infection.
3) Even a deep and wide ("gaping") wound does not need to be closed primarily.
4) Allowing a contaminated wound to granulate reduces bacterial invasion and forms a suitable base upon which to perform a delayed closure.
5) Healing by secondary intention would have been a reasonable option, especially in a wound at moderate-to-high risk of infection and dog-ear deformity if closed primarily.

SUGGESTED READINGS

Richard L. Lammers. Principles of wound management. In: Roberts, Hedges, Custalow, Chanmugam, eds., *Clinical Procedures in Emergency Medicine.* 5th edn. Saunders, Elsevier Philadelphia, 2010:563–633.

Dire DJ. Emergency Management of dog and cat bite wounds. *Emerg Med Clin North Am.* 1992;10(4):719–736.

397

THE KEYS TO GOOD STAPLING

JAMES E. CORWIN, MD

SCENARIO

A 19-year old presents with "chest pain" to the ED. On further questioning, you understand the pain is very superficial and is related to a stab wound that was repaired in your ED several days ago. On examination, there is a 2.5-cm laceration on the upper abdomen with 19 staples, many jammed together and overlapping and/or deeply imbedded with marked crimping of the epidermis

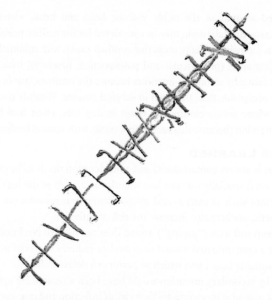

FIGURE 397.1. Wound at presentation.

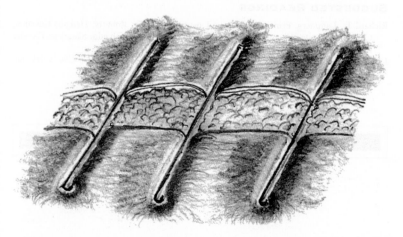

FIGURE 397.2. Close-up showing crimping and dehiscence.

with areas of dehiscence and uneven wound edges (*Figs. 397.1* and *397.2*). The patient tells you that, after the CT was done and the trauma team left the room, the repair was done by a student after the resident physician told him that the student could "easily handle this by himself."

BACKGROUND

The advance of modern surgery dates back to the end of the nineteenth century when William H. Welsh invited William Halsted to head a department of surgery at the nascent Johns Hopkins Hospital. Halsted had already established himself as a free thinker and immediately began to challenge the reigning dogma of his time. Out of his work grew his well-known basic tenets of surgical technique: asepsis, hemostasis, obliteration of dead space, preservation of blood supply, gentleness, and reduction of tension at the suture line.

Because of his meticulous technique, Halsted was notoriously slow, leading a contemporary of his to quip that Halsted was the only surgeon he knew who was still suturing the bottom of a wound when the top had already healed. In the intervening years, numerous developments have sought to maintain Halsted's basic tenets while reducing surgery time.

In the modern ED, few advances stand out like the skin stapler, which came into use for cutaneous surgery in 1980. Years of experience have established stapling's supremacy as a time saver, with numerous studies showing that one can staple a wound in 25% to 35% of the time it takes with conventional suturing technique.

Staples work by creating an *incomplete* rectangle which, besides the time-saving factor, is the other big advantage of stapling wounds. Because the tips bend inward but do not advance as far as the wound cavity, this incomplete rectangle does not form a tract from the skin surface into the wound (*Fig. 397.3*), thus eliminating further wound contamination and reducing the likelihood of infection.

Because staples are made of a strong, nonreactive material, and they gather a significant amount of tissue (depending on the leg length and size of

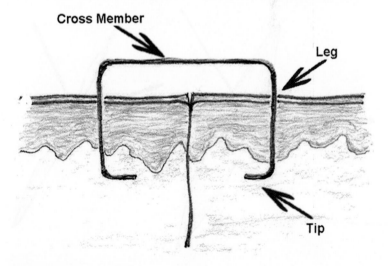

FIGURE 397.3. Cross section of a staple.

cross member), they are ideal for closing wounds under tension. This makes them particularly suitable for wounds on the scalp and torso.

The biggest challenges with skin stapling are achieving decent wound edge alignment and avoiding uneven skin edge height, overriding staples, and bunching of skin between the legs on either side of the wound. Also, staples can be uncomfortable in some areas (intertriginous areas such as the axilla and inguinal regions), leading to inflammation and patient dissatisfaction.

APPROPRIATE USE

Skin staples are ideally suited for linear closure of traumatic wounds under tension (scalp, torso, proximal extremities) when time is of the essence. However, because the wire diameter of skin staples is larger than the typical suture material (approximately five times as thick as 5-0 nylon), their use is often avoided in highly visible areas (such as the face). On the other hand, because they remove more tension from wounds than sutures, they can be removed sooner and are thus less likely to leave epithelial tracts into the punctures. With meticulous technique and close postoperative follow-up, excellent cosmetic results can be achieved.

Wound edges need to be completely apposed before stapling. This would seem to be self-evident, but many a novice assumes that when the stapler bends in the tips of the legs, it pulls the tissue together. This is simply not true and is evident in the scenario above with significant separation of the wound edges. Typical methods of skin apposition include using the thumb and index finger of the nonstapling hand to appose and slightly evert skin edges, using one or more buried dermal sutures, or placing a temporary silk suture (*Fig. 397.4*).

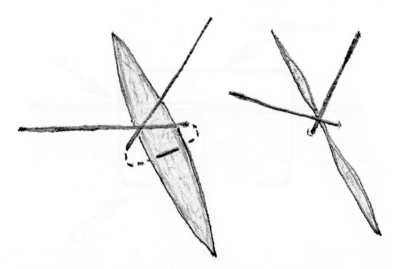

FIGURE 397.4. Use of temporary silk suture to appose skin edges.

Because it requires no additional time, thus taking full advantage of the time-saving benefit of stapling over suturing, many prefer "two person stapling method" for ideal skin apposition (*Fig 397.5*). In this method, the experienced physician stands opposite the assistant and, using skin hooks or Adson forceps (these have the disadvantage of traumatizing tissue more than skin hooks), the physician apposes and slightly everts the skin edges while the assistant places the staple at the point of maximal apposition. The physician uses his or her knowledge of tissue dynamics to determine the order and location of staples while keeping a watchful eye on the angle and depth of the entry of staples. This simple technique eliminates problems with unapposed and uneven edges, flat or inverted edges, improper spacing and depth, and bunching of skin under the cross member.

Regardless of the method used to appose skin edges, the stapler should only be held very lightly against (or even hovering above) the surface of the skin,

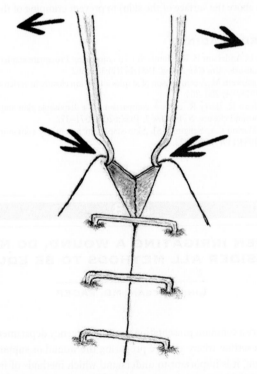

FIGURE 397.5. Two person stapling technique using skin hooks to align and appose skin edges. *Arrows* show direction of force used by surgeon in a "scissoring" fashion to pull skin edges together.

as close to perpendicular as possible so the staple enters the skin squarely. In a properly placed staple, the cross member should be left "riding high" above the skin surface, with 1 to 2 mm of each leg visible on either side of the wound. This prevents the cross member from crimping the epidermis with resultant cross-hatching. If the staple is not riding high, it should be removed and replaced.

LESSONS LEARNED

1) Use the two person stapling technique to avoid much of the bad outcome in this case.

2) If an assistant is not available, use a well-placed buried dermal suture or two, apposition and eversion of skin edges using the nonstapling hand, or placement of a temporary silk suture.

3) Staples should be spaced more appropriately (placed just enough to appose the skin edges closer together in areas of greater tension and further apart where there is lesser tension).

4) Care should be taken to ensure the staples are "riding high" (cross member 1 to 2 mm above the surface of the skin) to prevent crimping of the epidermis.

SUGGESTED READINGS

Eldrup J, Wied U, Anderson B. Randomized trial comparing Proximate stapler with conventional skin closure. *Acta Chir Scand*. 1981;147(7):501–502.

Lennihan R, Mackereth M. A comparison of staples and nylon closure in varicose vein surgery. *Vasc Surg*. 1975;9(4):200–204.

Meiring L, Cilliers K, Barry R, et al. A comparison of a disposable skin stapler and nylon sutures for wound closure. *S Afr Med J*. 1982;62(11):371–372.

Stillman RM, Marino CA, Seligman SJ. Skin staples in potentially contaminated wounds. *Arch Surg*. 1984;119(7):821–822.

398

WHEN IRRIGATING A WOUND, DO NOT CONSIDER ALL METHODS TO BE EQUAL

LINDA REGAN, MD, FACEP

Lacerations are a common presentation to any emergency department. Whether you work in a setting where you are preparing the wound or support staff prepares it for you, it is important to understand which methods of irrigation are considered acceptable for maintaining low infection rates and producing good cosmetic outcomes. Given the chaotic and busy environment within which we work, shortcuts or creative solutions often become "tricks of the trade." While such tricks are often handy, one must be cautious not to resort to choosing a suboptimal technique that may lead to poor wound healing or infection.

What are the optional methods to reduce contamination in wounds and thereby reduce infection? First, one must answer the question of why wounds become infected. In order to maintain low levels of infection, it is important to know which intrinsic wound characteristics place them at high risk. Certainly, there are patient characteristics that can contribute to their risk; patients with poor circulation, diabetes, or other forms of immunocompromise are at higher risk for infection. There is consensus that wounds with devitalized tissue, such as crush wounds and bites, have an increased risk of infection. This is likely because devitalized wounds require a lower quantity of bacteria to become infected than wounds with healthy tissue. The numbers are in the range of 10^6 bacteria/g of tissue in normal wounds versus 10^4 bacteria/g of tissue in wounds with devitalized tissue. Again, consensus agrees that the number one way to reduce the bacterial contamination in a wound is to irrigate it.

The ultimate questions here are what is the optimal solution and pressure to use for wound irrigation? The sentinel study citing the use of goal pressures between 5 and 8 psi comes from the 1970s but presents good data regarding how much pressure you need to lower the quantity of bacteria to 10^2/g of tissue. This is clearly below the 10^4 bacteria/g of tissue in wounds in which a wound with devitalized tissue may become infected. Options currently in use are shown in *Table 398.1*. Note that some common "easy" methods do not generate adequate pressures at the tissue surface (which has been calculated to be about 40% of the peak pressures measured at the device). Thus, the only acceptable equipment setup (that you can make yourself!) that generates adequate pressures is the needle and syringe combinations. Alternatively, tap water irrigation usually

TABLE 398.1 IRRIGATION OPTIONS CURRENTLY IN USE (PSI)	
METHODS OF IRRIGATION	**MEDIAN PEAK PRESSURE**
NS bag pierced by 19-G needle	4
NS bottle pierced by 19-G needle	2.3
NS bag using tubing, 16-G needle and pressure cuff (400 mm Hg)	4–6
NS bag using tubing, 19-G needle and pressure cuff (400 mm Hg)	6–10
19-G needle and 35-mL syringe	35
19-G needle and 65-mL syringe	27.5
Tap water faucet	50–60

generates adequate pressure, and when high-quality tap water is available, studies note that the infection rates are similar. Lastly, some commercial irrigation systems report adequate pressures can be generated when they are used. Just remember to check whether or not they are reporting the median peak pressure of the device or at the tissue surface. Remember, what gets to the tissue is only 40% of what comes out of the device!

In terms of the appropriate solution, hydrogen peroxide is clearly hemolytic and lifts off any newly formed epithelium. The three main options discussed are normal saline (NS), 1% povidone iodine, and tap water. All three options have been studied to varying degrees.

NS is the standard by which all other solutions are measured. Povidone iodine, when diluted to <1%, maintains low-infection rates that are similar to NS. At concentrations >1%, povidone iodine is toxic to wound defenses by decreasing neutrophil migration into the area. Tap water has been studied in both children and adults, and multiple studies have shown that infection rates are not increased when tap water is used. However, it is important to note that in most, if not all, of these studies, patients who are at high risk for infection (diabetics, HIV, vascular disease, on steroids, highly contaminated wounds, or devitalized tissue present) are always excluded.

So, what is the answer? Simply put, not all methods of irrigation are the same. So, why risk it? Stick with what we know. Use a 19-gauge needle and a 35- or 65-mL syringe and a bottle of sterile saline or 1% povidone iodine. If your institution stocks a commercially available irrigation system, feel free to use it; just investigate the pressure that can be generated. Alternatively, if your patients are at low risk for infection, just stick them under the tap!

SUGGESTED READINGS

Dire DJ, Welsh AP. A comparison of wound irrigation solutions used in the emergency department. *Ann Emerg Med.* 1990;19:704–708.

Edlich RF, Rodeheaver GT, Thacker JG, et al. Management of soft tissue injury. *Clin Plast Surg.* 1977;4:191–198.

Fernandez R, Griffiths R. Water for wound cleansing. *Cochrane Database Syst Rev.* 2008;(1):CD003861 [Review].

Hollander JE, Singer AJ, Valentine S, et al. Wound registry: Development and validation. *Ann Emerg Med.* 1995;25:675–685.

Moscati RM, Mayrose J, Reardon RF, et al. A multicenter comparison of tap water versus sterile saline for wound irrigation. *Acad Emerg Med.* 2007;14:404–409.

Singer AJ, Hollander JE, Fincher L, et al. Pressure dynamics of various irrigation techniques commonly used in the ED. *Ann Emerg Med.* 1994;24:36–40.

Valente JH, Forti RJ, Freundlich LF, et al. Wound irrigation in children: Saline solution or tap water? *Ann Emerg Med.* 2003;41:606–609.

INDEX

Note: Page numbers in *italics* denote figures; those followed by a "t" denote tables.

A

Abdominal aortic aneurysm (AAA)
 back pain, 413
 error sources, 855
 low-frequency transducer, 854
 ruptured, 39, 63–64
Abdominal compartment syndrome, paracentesis, 591
Abdominal/gastrointestinal pain
 acute appendicitis, atypical presentations of, 29–31
 analgesics
  morphine, 37
  opiates, 37
  sphincter of Oddi spasm, 37, 38
 cholangitis, 20–22, 21t
 CT scans, acute pancreatitis, 17–19, 18t, 19t
 dislodged feeding tube management, 56–58
 diverticulitis, 60–62
 elderly patients, intraabdominal condition in
  computed tomography (CT), 39
  laboratory studies, 39
  myocardial infarction (MI), 40
  vascular catastrophes, 39–40
 focused assessment with sonography for trauma (FAST), 48–50
 geriatrics, 259–260
 hernias, 58–60
 imaging modalities
  acute abdomen, 1–2
  acute cholecystitis, 2–3, 3t
  radiograph, 1
 inflammatory bowel disease (IBD), 34–36
 liver failure, medications administration
  initial PO dose, 12t, 13
  risks, 11–12
 mesenteric ischemia (MI), 54–56
 painless jaundice, 9–10
 postcholecystectomy pain, 27–28
 post-ERCP complications
  bleeding, 26
  pancreatitis, 25
  perforation, 25–26
 pregnant patients, radiography in, 32–33
 rectal bleeding, 46–48
 right upper quadrant (RUQ), 22–24
 sigmoid volvulus (SV), 4–6, *5*
 small bowel obstruction (SBO)
  intravenous fluid resuscitation, 6–8
  US *vs.* CT in, 2, 2t
 spontaneous bacterial peritonitis (SBP), 14–16
 transplant patients, 52–53

upper gastrointestinal bleeding (UGIB), 41–43, 42t, 43t
 variceal bleeding, 44–45
Aberrant conduction (AC), 115
Abscess, *858*
Acetaminophen, 9–10
Acetyl salicylic acid (ASA)
 acid–base disturbances, 741
 management, 741–742
 medicinal properties, 740
Acid–base (*see* Anion gap acidosis)
Acidosis, 369–370
ACS (*see* Acute coronary syndrome)
Acute abdomen, 1–2
Acute appendicitis, 29–31
Acute asthma exacerbations, steroids administration, 646–647
Acute bronchitis, 677–679
Acute chest syndrome, pediatric patient, 282–283
Acute coronary syndrome (ACS)
 chest pain
  mortality rates, 120
  myocardial ischemia, 119
 geriatrics, 257–258
 negative angiogram
  lesions, 133–134
  stenoses, 133
 stress test
  cardiac catheterization, 136
  nuclear cardiac imaging, 135–136, 136t
 troponin, 129–130, 129t
Acute mountain sickness (AMS), 250–251
Acute myocardial infarction (AMI), pacemakers, 149–151, *150*
Acute otitis media (AOM), 520–522
Acute pancreatitis, computed tomography scans, 17–19, 18t, 19t
Acute psychosis, 633–634
Acute salt-wasting syndrome, 512
Acutely decompensated heart failure (ADHF), nitroglycerin (NTG) dosing, 151–152
Adamantanes, 319
Advanced life support (ALS), 180–181
Adverse drug reactions (ADRs), 81–82
AF (*see* Atrial fibrillation)
β_2-Agonist therapy, asthma, 665
Airways assessment, pediatrics
 equipment size selection, 494–495
 gentle handling, 495
 positioning method, 494
 preoxygenation, 495
 respiratory reserve limit, 494

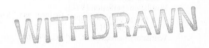